What Radiology Residents Need to Know

Series Editor
Ronald L. Eisenberg, Harvard University
Boston, MA, USA

The books in the *What Radiology Residents Need to Know* series act as an introduction to radiology, specifically designed for the needs of residents on their first rotation in a specific subspecialty. Radiology residents are asked to learn significant amounts of information at a fast and unrelenting space. The current available literature for residents, though, is dense and includes more information than they can easily digest, while the number, variety, and quality of images is often limited. This forces residents to turn to quick searches on the internet to seek out information that often is not at their exact level of knowledge and leaves gaps in their learning. *What Radiology Residents Need to Know* answers resident needs for each radiology rotation, presenting the material in bullet fashion and dividing it into convenient sub-units, such as introductory clinical information followed by "imaging findings" and, when appropriate, "management." In most cases, an individual pathological condition is presented in one page or less, allowing residents to quickly review the essential information on a specific pattern or disease. Books in the *What Radiology Residents Need to Know* series contain a large number of high-quality images, as well as a downloadable set of additional images that give readers a comprehensive library of illustrations. With both readable text and a broad spectrum of images, the books in the *What Radiology Residents Need to Know* series serve as an ideal guide for radiology residents.

Behroze A. Vachha • Gul Moonis
Max Wintermark • Tarik F. Massoud
Editors

What Radiology Residents Need to Know: Neuroradiology

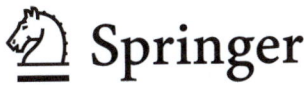

Editors
Behroze A. Vachha
Department of Radiology, UMass Chan Medical School
Chief of Neuroradiology, Associate Professor
Worcester, MA, USA

Max Wintermark
Neuroradiology
The University of Texas MD Anderson Canc
Houston, TX, USA

Gul Moonis
Professor, Department of Radiology
NYU Langone Medical Center
New York, NY, USA

Tarik F. Massoud
Department of Radiology
School of Medicine
Stanford University
Stanford, CA, USA

ISSN 2662-9569 ISSN 2662-9577 (electronic)
What Radiology Residents Need to Know
ISBN 978-3-031-55123-9 ISBN 978-3-031-55124-6 (eBook)
https://doi.org/10.1007/978-3-031-55124-6

© The Editor(s) (if applicable) and The Author(s), under exclusive license to Springer Nature Switzerland AG 2024, corrected publication 2025

This work is subject to copyright. All rights are solely and exclusively licensed by the Publisher, whether the whole or part of the material is concerned, specifically the rights of translation, reprinting, reuse of illustrations, recitation, broadcasting, reproduction on microfilms or in any other physical way, and transmission or information storage and retrieval, electronic adaptation, computer software, or by similar or dissimilar methodology now known or hereafter developed.

The use of general descriptive names, registered names, trademarks, service marks, etc. in this publication does not imply, even in the absence of a specific statement, that such names are exempt from the relevant protective laws and regulations and therefore free for general use.

The publisher, the authors, and the editors are safe to assume that the advice and information in this book are believed to be true and accurate at the date of publication. Neither the publisher nor the authors or the editors give a warranty, expressed or implied, with respect to the material contained herein or for any errors or omissions that may have been made. The publisher remains neutral with regard to jurisdictional claims in published maps and institutional affiliations.

This Springer imprint is published by the registered company Springer Nature Switzerland AG
The registered company address is: Gewerbestrasse 11, 6330 Cham, Switzerland

If disposing of this product, please recycle the paper.

Preface

Neuroradiology is a complex and ever-evolving field, integral to the diagnosis and management of numerous neurological, spinal, and head and neck conditions. For radiology residents navigating this intricate specialty, the need for a concise and accessible resource is paramount. This book was designed with that purpose in mind: to provide a clear, straightforward guide that distils essential information into a format that is both practical and easy to reference.

The content is divided into three main sections—Brain, Spine, and Head and Neck—each covering high-yield topics that are crucial for understanding the core principles of Neuroradiology. These sections address the most commonly encountered pathologies, imaging findings, and diagnostic challenges faced during residency. We have adopted a streamlined, bullet-point format that allows for quick review without sacrificing depth, making this book an ideal companion during clinical rotations, exam preparation, and on-call shifts.

Recognizing that imaging is central to Neuroradiology, we have included valuable tips for interpreting CT and MRI studies. These practical insights aim to build confidence and enhance diagnostic accuracy when reviewing complex imaging cases. Our goal is to bridge the gap between theoretical knowledge and its practical application in a busy clinical environment.

In addition to the printed text, this book is supported by an accompanying e-platform, which provides an expanded collection of high-quality images. These supplementary visuals are intended to further illustrate key concepts and reinforce learning. We believe this integrated approach—combining concise written content with comprehensive visual aids—will enhance the learning experience and make the material more engaging and accessible.

It is our hope that this book will serve as a reliable and effective tool throughout your residency, helping you navigate the challenges of Neuroradiology with confidence. Thank you for choosing to embark on this journey with us, and we hope you find this resource as useful and rewarding as we intended it to be.

Worcester, MA, USA Behroze A. Vachha
New York, NY, USA Gul Moonis
Houston, TX, USA Max Wintermark
Stanford, CA, USA Tarik F. Massoud

The original version of this book was inadvertently published without a Preface, editor's biography text and the list of contributors. The above listed front matter elements have been included in the revised publication.

The original version of the book has been revised. A correction to this book can be found at https://doi.org/10.1007/978-3-031-55124-6_46

Contents

1. **Basic Imaging Techniques** 1
   Kevin Yuqi Wang and Raag Airan

2. **Neuroimaging Structural Anatomy** 11
   D. Kenneth Jamison and Tarik F. Massoud

3. **Neuroimaging Functional Anatomy** 43
   Behroze A. Vachha and Erik H. Middlebrooks

4. **Congenital and Developmental Brain Malformations** 53
   Edward Yang

5. **Stroke** 69
   Yuh-Shin Chang and Pamela W. Schaefer

6. **Intracranial Hemorrhage** 97
   Eric K. van Staalduinen and Tarik F. Massoud

7. **Intracranial Aneurysms and Vascular Malformations: Imaging Findings and Clinical Considerations** 109
   Justin E. Vranic and Javier M. Romero

8. **Head Trauma** 127
   Sara G. Tedla, Tarik F. Massoud, and Elizabeth Tong

9. **Post-operative Appearances** 137
   Francis Scott, Tarik F. Massoud, and Tomasz Matys

10. **Congenital and Neonatal Infections** 149
    Pamela Nguyen

11. **Brain Infections** 159
    Rosaura Suazo Aguero and Rafael Rojas

12. **Noninfectious Inflammatory Processes** 177
    Derek Hsu and Ranliang Hu

13. **Inherited Metabolic Disorders** 187
    Sara Fardin and Neel Madan

14. **Demyelinating Diseases** 197
    Komal Manzoor, Behroze A. Vachha, and Susie Y. Huang

15. **Tumors and Tumor-Like Lesions** 207
    Susie Yi Huang, Raymond Y. Huang, and Behroze A. Vachha

16. **Toxic and Metabolic Diseases of the CNS** 231
    Harry Subramanian and Amit Mahajan

17	**Neurodegenerative Disorders**..245	
	Johannes H. Decker, Max Wintermark, and Michael Zeineh	
18	**Hydrocephalus and CSF Disorders**..255	
	Afshin Ameri and Neel Madan	
19	**Intracranial Cysts**..263	
	Angela L. Kanna, Salar Hakham, and Neel Madan	
20	**Normal Spine Anatomy and Imaging**..273	
	Peter Liaw, Charissa Kim, Mike Bao, Elisa Flower, and Yu-Ming Chang	
21	**Congenital and Developmental Malformations of the Spine**.................289	
	Anna Y. Li, Tarik F. Massoud, and Hisham Dahmoush	
22	**Spine Trauma**...307	
	Alexander M. Khalaf, Tarik F. Massoud, and Syed S. Hashmi	
23	**Degenerative Disease of the Spine and Spinal Arthritides**...................319	
	Brian Rigney, Shivam Kaushik, and Amish Doshi	
24	**Tumors and Tumor-Like Lesions of the Spine and Spinal Cord**.............333	
	Kimberly Seifert, Tarik F. Massoud, and Austin Trinh	
25	**Spine Infection**...349	
	Nicole Levy and Michael J. Hoch	
26	**Spinal Cord Inflammation and Demyelination**..................................361	
	Jason R. Lauer and William A. Mehan Jr.	
27	**Spine: Vascular Pathologies**..369	
	Victor Lam Shin Cheung and Sachin Kishore Pandey	
28	**Imaging Anatomy of the Orbit, Sinus, and Mucosal Surfaces of the Neck**..377	
	Nahil Matari and Akinrinola Famuyide	
29	**Imaging of the Orbit (Infection, Inflammation, Benign, and Malignant Lesions)**..385	
	Michael T. Starc and Azita Khorsandi	
30	**Imaging of Sinonasal Disease (Infection, Tumors)**.............................399	
	Nathan Gruenhagen and Mohit Agarwal	
31	**Temporal Bone Imaging**...413	
	Daniel Thomas Ginat	
32	**Anterior Skull Base**...423	
	Gopi Nayak, Jesi Kim, and Mari Hagiwara	
33	**Central Skull Base**..433	
	Nikdokht Farid, Soudabeh Fazeli, Paul Manning, and Michael Shroads	
34	**Posterior Skull Base**..445	
	Yuh-Shin Chang and Gul Moonis	
35	**Embryology and Anatomy of the Sella and Parasellar Region**.............465	
	Anil Vasireddi and Katie Suzanne Traylor	
36	**Facial and Skull Base Fractures**..481	
	Suehyb G. Alkhatib, Francis Deng, Dan Cohen-Addad, and Suyash Mohan	

Contents

37 Neck Infections 489
Emma Lindsey, Parth Vaghasia, and Evan G. Stein

38 Imaging of Neck Spaces 499
Shehanaz K. Ellika, Anthony Portanova, Devanshi Mistry,
and Edward Lin

39 Imaging of the Nasopharynx 519
Harry Griffin and Amy Juliano

40 Imaging of the Oral Cavity and Oropharynx 531
Jennifer M. Watchmaker, Laura B. Eisenmenger, and Jacqueline C. Junn

41 Imaging of the Larynx and Hypopharynx 541
Kevin Byunghoon Oh and Xin Cynthia Wu

42 Vascular Lesions of the Head and Neck 553
Yang M. Jiang and Alok A. Bhatt

43 Cystic Neck Masses 561
Kathryn E. Dean and Oren Jaspan

44 Noninterpretive Skills Including Quality and Safety 575
Syed S. Hashmi and Tarik F. Massoud

45 Advanced Imaging Techniques 589
Brian Dang, Max Wintermark, Behroze A. Vachha, and Michael Iv

Correction to: What Radiology Residents Need to Know: Neuroradiology C1
Behroze A. Vachha, Gul Moonis, Max Wintermark, and Tarik F. Massoud

Index 611

Editors and Contributors

About the Editors

Behroze A. Vachha is Chief of Neuroradiology and Associate Professor of Radiology at UMass Chan Medical School. Prior to her current role, she was a neuroradiologist at Memorial Sloan Kettering Cancer Center and served on the faculty of Weill Cornell Medical College in New York. Dr. Vachha received her clinical training in Diagnostic Radiology at the Beth Israel Deaconess Medical Center, Harvard University followed by a Neuroradiology fellowship at the Massachusetts General Hospital, Harvard University. She also has a PhD in Human Development and Communication Sciences. Dr. Vachha is the Neuroradiology co-Section Editor of *Cancer Imaging* and the Chair of the Research Committee of the American Society of Functional Neuroradiology. Her academic and research interests include using advanced imaging tools to link pathophysiology, neurocognition, and clinical medicine to improve care for people with various neurological disorders. She is actively involved in teaching and supervising radiology residents, neuroradiology fellows, and medical students in the clinical aspects of neuroradiology as well as mentoring them in neuroimaging research.

Gul Moonis is a Professor of Radiology at NYU Langone Medical Center in New York. Her academic responsibilities also include teaching and supervising radiology residents, neuroradiology fellows and medical students. Dr. Moonis is a member of the Radiological Society of North America and the American Society of Neuroradiology and a senior member of the Eastern Neurological Society and the American Society of Head and Neck Radiology. In addition to all aspects of general neuroradiology, Dr. Moonis has clinical expertise in radiology of the head and neck. Dr. Moonis' research currently focuses on imaging of the temporal bone which has resulted in publications, book chapters, and review articles. She is particularly dedicated to mentoring residents and fellows in clinical research projects. A gifted educator, Dr. Moonis has won numerous teaching awards and has been an invited speaker at various national and international meetings in the field of head and neck radiology.

Max Wintermark is a neuroradiologist with a specific interest and expertise in imaging brain, neck and spine tumors, stroke, traumatic brain injury, and psychiatric disorders. He received his training in Diagnostic Radiology at the University of Lausanne in Switzerland followed by a fellowship in Diagnostic Neuroradiology at the University of California, San Francisco. He has a degree in biomedical engineering from the Swiss Federal Institute of Technology and a master's in clinical research from the University of San Francisco. He worked as a faculty at the University of California, San Francisco, at the University of Virginia, at Stanford, and he is currently a Professor and Chair of Neuroradiology at the University of Texas MD Anderson Center, Dr. Wintermark is the Editor-in-Chief of the American Journal of Neuroradiology (AJNR) and the President of the American Society of Neuroradiology (ASNR).

Tarik Massoud is a physician-scientist and Professor of Neuroradiology at Stanford University School of Medicine. He trained in Radiology and Neuroradiology in Oxford, UCLA, and Michigan, and held academic positions at UCLA, Cambridge, and Stanford. His academic interests include molecular and translational imaging of the brain especially in neuro-oncology and cerebrovascular diseases, experimental aspects of neuroimaging, clinical neuroradiology, neuroradiological anatomy, and research training of radiologists and scientists.

Contributors

Mohit Agarwal Medical College of Wisconsin, Milwaukee, WI, USA

Rosaura Suazo Aguero Tufts Medical Center, Boston, MA, USA

Raag Airan Division of Neuroimaging and Neurointervention, Department of Radiology, Stanford University, Stanford, CA, USA

Materials Science and Engineering and Psychiatry and Behavioral Sciences (by courtesy), Palo Alto, CA, USA

Suehyb G. Alkhatib Division of Neuroradiology, Department of Radiology, Perelman School of Medicine at the University of Pennsylvania, Philadelphia, PA, USA

Afshin Ameri Tufts University School of Medicine, Boston, MA, USA

Mike Bao Radiology Department, Beth Israel Deaconess Medical Center, Boston, MA, USA

Alok A. Bhatt Mayo Clinic, Jacksonville, FL, USA

Yuh-Shin Chang Division of Neuroradiology, Department of Radiology, Massachusetts General Hospital, Boston, MA, USA

Department of Radiology, Massachusetts Eye and Ear, Boston, MA, USA

Yu-Ming Chang Radiology Department, Beth Israel Deaconess Medical Center, Boston, MA, USA

Victor Lam Shin Cheung Department of Medical Imaging, Western University, Schulich School of Medicine and Dentistry, London, ON, Canada

Dan Cohen-Addad Division of Neuroradiology, Department of Radiology, Perelman School of Medicine at the University of Pennsylvania, Philadelphia, PA, USA

Hisham Dahmoush Department of Radiology, Lucile Packard Children's Hospital at Stanford, Palo Alto, CA, USA

Brian Dang Radiology Resident, Stanford University, Stanford, CA, USA

Kathryn E. Dean Weill Cornell Medical College, New York, NY, USA

Johannes H. Decker Division of Neuroimaging and Neurointervention, Stanford University School of Medicine, Stanford, CA, USA

Francis Deng The Russell H. Morgan Department of Radiology and Radiological Science, Johns Hopkins University, Baltimore, MD, USA

Amish Doshi Icahn School of Medicine at Mount Sinai, New York, NY, USA

Laura B. Eisenmenger Department of Radiology, University of Wisconsin School of Medicine and Public Health, Madison, WI, USA

Shehanaz K. Ellika Department of Imaging Sciences, University of Rochester Medical Center, Rochester, NY, USA

Akinrinola Famuyide Columbia University Irving Medical Center, New York, NY, USA

Department of Radiology, CUMC, New York, NY, USA

NewYork-Presbyterian, New York, NY, USA

Sara Fardin Massachusetts General Hospital, Boston, MA, USA

Nikdokht Farid University of California, San Diego, La Jolla, CA, USA

Soudabeh Fazeli University of California, San Diego, La Jolla, CA, USA

Elisa Flower Radiology Department, Beth Israel Deaconess Medical Center, Boston, MA, USA

Daniel Thomas Ginat Department of Radiology, University of Chicago, Chicago, IL, USA

Harry Griffin Department of Radiology, Massachusetts General Hospital, Boston, MA, USA

Harvard Medical School, Boston, MA, USA

Nathan Gruenhagen Medical College of Wisconsin, Milwaukee, WI, USA

Mari Hagiwara Department of Radiology, NYU Langone Medical Center, New York, NY, USA

Salar Hakham Beverly Hospital, Montebello, CA, USA

Syed S. Hashmi Division of Neuroimaging and Neurointervention, Stanford University School of Medicine, Stanford, CA, USA

Michael J. Hoch Department of Radiology, Hospital of the University of Pennsylvania, Philadelphia, PA, USA

Derek Hsu Department of Radiology and Imaging Sciences, Emory University School of Medicine, Atlanta, GA, USA

Raymond Y. Huang Department of Radiology, Division of Neuroradiology, Brigham and Womens Hospital, Boston, MA, USA

Susie Yi Huang Department of Radiology, Division of Neuroradiology, Massachusetts General Hospital, Boston, MA, USA

Ranliang Hu Department of Radiology and Imaging Sciences, Emory University School of Medicine, Atlanta, GA, USA

Michael Iv Department of Radiology (Neuroradiology), Stanford University, Center for Academic Medicine, Palo Alto, CA, USA

D. Kenneth Jamison Division of Neuroimaging and Neurointervention, Stanford University School of Medicine, Stanford, CA, USA

Oren Jaspan NewYork-Presbyterian Weill Cornell, New York, NY, USA

Yang M. Jiang Mayo Clinic, Jacksonville, FL, USA

Amy Juliano Harvard Medical School, Boston, MA, USA

Jacqueline C. Junn Department of Radiology and Imaging Sciences, Emory School of Medicine, Atlanta, GA, USA

Angela L. Kanna Tufts University School of Medicine, Boston, MA, USA

Shivam Kaushik Rowan School of Osteopathic Medicine, Stratford, NJ, USA

Alexander M. Khalaf Division of Neuroimaging and Neurointervention, Stanford University School of Medicine, Stanford, CA, USA

Azita Khorsandi Department of Radiology, New York Eye and Ear Infirmary of Mount Sinai, New York, NY, USA

Charissa Kim Radiology Department, Beth Israel Deaconess Medical Center, Boston, MA, USA

Jesi Kim Department of Radiology, NYU Langone Medical Center, New York, NY, USA

Jason R. Lauer Department of Neuroradiology, Massachusetts General Hospital, Boston, MA, USA

Nicole Levy Department of Radiology, Hospital of the University of Pennsylvania, Philadelphia, PA, USA

Anna Y. Li Department of Radiology, Stanford University School of Medicine, Palo Alto, CA, USA

Peter Liaw Radiology Department, Beth Israel Deaconess Medical Center, Boston, MA, USA

Emma Lindsey NYU Grossman School Medicine, New York, NY, USA

Edward Lin Department of Imaging Sciences, University of Rochester Medical Center, Rochester, NY, USA

Neel Madan Tufts University School of Medicine, Boston, MA, USA

Amit Mahajan Yale University School of Medicine, New Haven, CT, USA

Paul Manning University of California, San Diego, La Jolla, CA, USA

VA Health System, San Diego, La Jolla, CA, USA

Komal Manzoor Department of Radiology, Massachusetts General Hospital, Boston, MA, USA

Tarik F. Massoud Department of Radiology, School of Medicine, Stanford University, Stanford, CA, USA

Nahil Matari Diagnostic Radiology and Internal Medicine, Yale New Haven Health Greenwich Hospital, Greenwich, CT, USA

Columbia University Irving Medical Center, New York, NY, USA

Tomasz Matys Department of Radiology, Cambridge University Hospitals NHS Foundation Trust, Addenbrooke's Hospital, Cambridge, UK

Department of Radiology, University of Cambridge, Cambridge, UK

William A. Mehan Jr Harvard Medical School, Boston, MA, USA

Department of Radiology, Massachusetts General Hospital, Boston, MA, USA

Erik H. Middlebrooks Department of Radiology, Mayo Clinic, College of Medicine and Science, Jacksonville, FL, USA

Department of Neurosurgery, Mayo Clinic, College of Medicine and Science, Jacksonville, FL, USA

Devanshi Mistry University of Pennsylvania, Philadelphia, PA, USA

Suyash Mohan Division of Neuroradiology, Department of Radiology, Perelman School of Medicine at the University of Pennsylvania, Philadelphia, PA, USA

Gul Moonis Department of Radiology, NYU Langone Medical Center, New York, NY, USA

Gopi Nayak Department of Radiology, NYU Langone Medical Center, New York, NY, USA

Pamela Nguyen Columbia University Irving Medical Center, New York, NY, USA

Kevin Byunghoon Oh Department of Radiology and Imaging Sciences, Emory University School of Medicine, Atlanta, GA, USA

Sachin Kishore Pandey Department of Medical Imaging, Western University, Schulich School of Medicine and Dentistry, London, ON, Canada

Anthony Portanova Department of Imaging Sciences, University of Rochester Medical Center, Rochester, NY, USA

Brian Rigney Icahn School of Medicine at Mount Sinai, New York, NY, USA

Rafael Rojas Neuroradiology Section, Radiology Department, Harvard Medical School, Beth Israel Deaconess Medical Center, Boston, MA, USA

Javier M. Romero Division of Neuroradiology, Department of Radiology, Massachusetts General Hospital, Boston, MA, USA

Pamela W. Schaefer Division of Neuroradiology, Department of Radiology, Massachusetts General Hospital, Boston, MA, USA

Francis Scott Department of Radiology, Cambridge University Hospitals NHS Foundation Trust, Addenbrooke's Hospital, Cambridge, UK

Kimberly Seifert Division of Neuroimaging and Neurointervention, Stanford University School of Medicine, Stanford, CA, USA

Michael Shroads Clinical Radiology & Imaging Sciences, Indiana University, Indianapolis, IN, USA

Michael T. Starc Department of Radiology, Memorial Sloan Kettering Cancer Center, New York, NY, USA

Evan G. Stein NYU Grossman School Medicine, New York, NY, USA

Harry Subramanian Department of Radiology and Biomedical Imaging, New Haven, CT, USA

Sara G. Tedla Division of Neuroimaging and Neurointervention, Stanford University School of Medicine, Stanford, CA, USA

Elizabeth Tong Division of Neuroimaging and Neurointervention, Stanford University School of Medicine, Stanford, CA, USA

Katie Suzanne Traylor Neuroradiology Division, University of Pittsburgh School of Medicine, Pittsburgh, PA, USA

Austin Trinh Division of Neuroimaging and Neurointervention, Stanford University School of Medicine, Stanford, CA, USA

Behroze A. Vachha Department of Radiology, Division of Neuroradiology, UMass Chan Medical School, UMass Memorial Medical Center, Worcester, MA, USA

Parth Vaghasia Maimonides Medical Center, Brooklyn, NY, USA

Eric K. van Staalduinen Division of Neuroimaging and Neurointervention, Stanford University School of Medicine, Stanford, CA, USA

Anil Vasireddi Neuroradiology Division, University of Pittsburgh School of Medicine, Pittsburgh, PA, USA

Justin E. Vranic Division of Neuroradiology, Department of Radiology, Massachusetts General Hospital, Boston, MA, USA

Department of Neurosurgery, Massachusetts General Hospital, Boston, MA, USA

Kevin Yuqi Wang Moran, Rowen and Dorsey, Inc., Orange, CA, USA

Jennifer M. Watchmaker Department of Diagnostic, Molecular and Interventional Radiology, Icahn School of Medicine at Mount Sinai, New York, NY, USA

Max Wintermark Division of Neuroimaging and Neurointervention, Stanford University School of Medicine, Stanford, CA, USA

MD Anderson Cancer Center, Houston, TX, USA

Xin Cynthia Wu Neuroradiology Division, Department of Radiology and Biomedical Imaging, University of California San Francisco, San Francisco, CA, USA

Edward Yang Department of Radiology, Boston Children's Hospital, Boston, MA, USA

Michael Zeineh Division of Neuroimaging and Neurointervention, Stanford University School of Medicine, Stanford, CA, USA

Basic Imaging Techniques

Kevin Yuqi Wang and Raag Airan

COMPUTED TOMOGRAPHY

Basic Principles

- In **Computed Tomography** (CT), an X-ray beam is projected through the patient at multiple angles and read on a detector. A computer then uses the detected photon intensities to calculate the attenuation induced by each chunk of tissue, which is plotted as an image where each voxel is assigned a grayscale value according to the calculated X-ray attenuation.
- Hounsfield units (HU)—A quantitative scale of X-ray attenuation as displayed in CT images. Named after one of the Nobel laureates who helped to invent CT [1].
   - The attenuation of air is defined as −1000, water as 0, and everything else scaled from there.
   - Typical values: Gray matter: 40, White matter: 25, Fat: −100, cortical bone: 1000.
   - Note: the measured HU can change with certain parameters, especially kVp.
- CT image quality is determined by acquisition parameters and reconstruction parameters:
   - Acquisition parameters—set by protocol, cannot be adjusted post hoc:
     - kVp—peak energy of the X-ray beam. Lower energy (e.g., 80 kVp) helps for soft tissue differentiation; higher energy (e.g., 150 kVp) helps for bone, metal, and contrast agent (iodine) differentiation. Most routine single energy CT uses a middle of the road energy (100 or 120 kVp).
     - mAs—Number of photons shot through subject. Tradeoff of dose vs. image quality; higher mAs is more dose but lower image noise. Usually scanners modulate this depending on degree of attenuation seen on scout, but modulated around a setpoint set by the protocol.
     - Pitch—for a helical acquisition, how fast the table moves with respect to the beam. Higher pitch means less projections and dose per volume of tissue and potentially poorer quality; lower pitch means more projections and dose per volume of tissue and better quality.
   - Reconstruction parameters—can be adjusted post hoc (so long as the primary data is saved!):
     - Algorithm/kernel—in making the image the computer makes certain assumptions about the type of tissue being imaged. A "sharp" algorithm assumes there are sharp edges of, e.g., bone against air, and is more likely to assign disparate numbers to neighboring voxels. A "smooth" algorithm assumes less variation of neighboring voxels and is used for soft tissue imaging. A sharper image has higher edge detail but looks grainier; a smoother image is less grainy but has blurred edges at bone, metal, or contrast opacified vessel interfaces [2].
     - Iterative reconstruction and other computer vision (AI) algorithms—recently more sophisticated algorithms have been developed to reduce streak and other artifacts in the image. The degree to which this is applied and how it is applied can be set depending on what the vendor software allows. There is a tradeoff of potentially better image quality and the degree to which these algorithms permit their own artifacts to enter the image, when their assumptions about the image break down.

K. Y. Wang
Moran, Rowen and Dorsey, Inc., Orange, CA, USA
e-mail: yuqi.wang@ucla.edu

R. Airan (✉)
Division of Neuroimaging and Neurointervention, Department of Radiology, Stanford University, Stanford, CA, USA

Materials Science and Engineering and Psychiatry and Behavioral Sciences (by courtesy), Palo Alto, CA, USA
e-mail: rairan@stanford.edu

- Scanner types:
  - Most modern scanners are helical, multi-row scanners with the X-ray source and detector on a gantry that rotates around the table. The table can move with respect to the gantry so the X-ray beam projects in a spiral pattern with respect to the patient. The computer then uses all that information in its back calculation (Fig. 1.1).
    - These scanners can have multiple sources/detector pairs so one half-rotation yields the same information as a full rotation of single headed scanner, yielding faster acquisition that is less motion sensitive.
  - Another type is cone-beam CT in which a cone-shaped beam with a wide flat detector rotates with no table movement. Single gantry rotation acquires whole volume. High spatial resolution (typical: 0.3–0.4 mm) of fixed, limited volume with minimal dose. Used in dentistry and ENT given high detail of high contrast (bone, metal) structures.

Dual Energy

- Dual energy protocols use two X-ray beams at two different energy levels, e.g., 80 kVp and 150 kVp. The traditional CT images can be reconstructed from the average of the two scans at a radiation dose similar to marginally higher than a single energy scan.

- Different materials attenuate X-rays to different degrees at different energy levels due to different atomic structures of the material. With a model of how each material (gray vs. white matter; iron in blood vs. iodine in contrast) attenuated each energy level, one can estimate the material composition of a given voxel by comparing the attenuation level of the low vs. high energy beams.
- Used clinically to help differentiate if hyperdensity is from blood or prior contrast administration, by comparing a calculated "iodine only" or the converse "virtual non-contrast" (or other names depending on the scanner vendor) images to the usual image.
- More advanced techniques are coming out now routinely in the literature—e.g., giving a probability of fracture or marrow infiltration in bone.

Radiation Dose

- CT-specific dose parameters include CT Dose Index (CTDI) and Dose-Length Product (DLP).
  - CTDI estimates absorbed dose for a given field of view, measured in mGy, and is commonly written as something like $CTDI_{100}$ given the phantom used to measure CTDI is typically 100 mm long (and 160 or 320 mm in diameter). $CTDI_{100}$ is the estimated absorbed dose delivered to a single slice as indicated by a 100 mm long phantom.

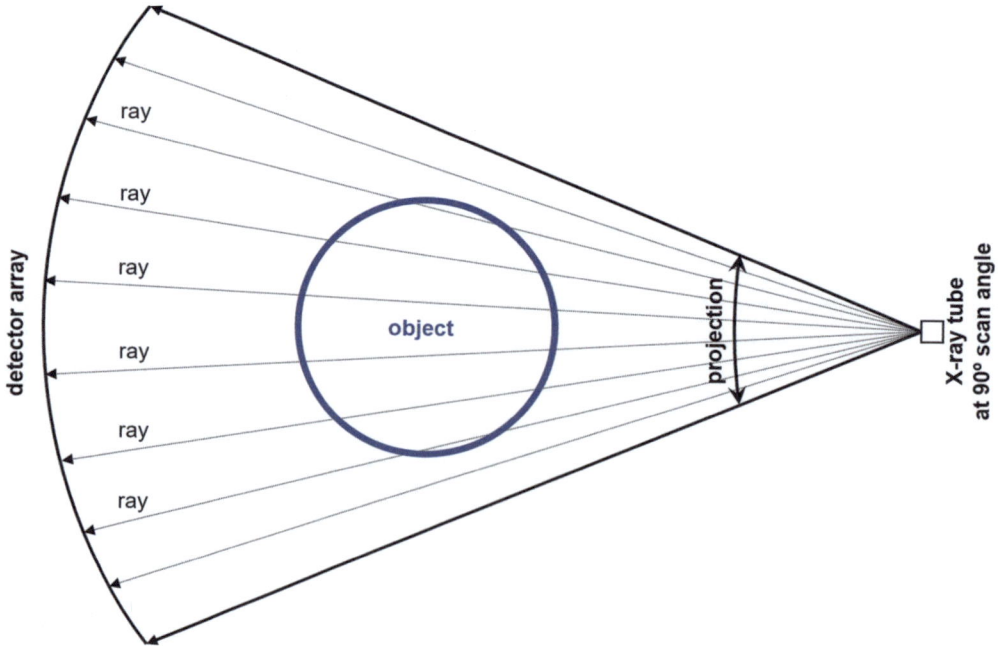

Fig. 1.1 In this example, we see the gantry at a scan angle of 90° and the collection of rays originating from the X-ray tube on the right and striking the detector elements on the left. Hence, a fan beam shot at one particular scan angle is synonymous to one projection

- Governing bodies like the American College of Radiology use $CTDI_{vol}$ as a quality-control parameter with set "reference levels," for instance, adult head, adult abdomen, and pediatric abdomen $CTDI_{vol}$ indicated at 75 mGy, 25 mGy, and 20 mGy, respectively, at the 75th percentile of doses in a registry.
- DLP measures total absorbed dose across the scan volume, measured in mGy-cm: $DLP = CTDI_{vol} \times$ scan length (in cm).
- DLP can be converted to an effective dose (in mSv-cm) for an average 70 kg patient using a conversion factor constant derived from simulations or phantoms.
- *These values are only estimates based on phantoms*, and do not account for the patient's actual anatomy. There is no practical way to measure exactly the dose delivered to a given patient in CT. We can only report these estimates.
- Dose adjustment is set by the protocol, which is determined by the radiologist, usually in consultation with a medical physicist or the scanner vendor, to optimize between the tradeoffs of image quality and radiation dose to the patient.

MAGNETIC RESONANCE IMAGING (MRI)

MRI Safety

- Most critical: *The magnet is always ON.* There is strict control over access to the scanner room with screening of people and things based on how magnetic they are, with space divided into zones.
  - Zone 1: Freely accessible to public.
  - Zone 2: The patient screening area (e.g., waiting room).
  - Zone 3: Screened patients and staff (e.g., the scanner control room).
  - Zone 4: Scanner room itself; only people and things (including their clothes and jewelry!) that are confirmed as OK to go in.
- Devices/hardware classified as MRI Safe, Conditional, or Unsafe by a trained physicist.
  - Can look up status of known devices on mrisafety.com "The List."
  - Must assume something is MRI Unsafe unless there is specific documentation.
  - Some MRI Safe/Conditional items can become unsafe; e.g., coiled loops of wires, like EKG leads, can act as a coil dissipating the energy and leading to burns.
- SAR = specific absorption rate. MRI sequences use radiofrequency electrical radiation and this energy can deposit in the body causing heating not unlike how a cell phone with poor signal heats up.
  - Governed by the FDA and other regulatory bodies and limited to certain ranges; cannot violate these limits without an IRB. Generally limited so there is <1 °C temperature rise in tissue.
  - SAR varies with each MRI sequence and there are two limits: one for the overall protocol and one for each sequence. The vendor hardware should indicate the SAR per sequence and protocol, to help guide the technician and radiologist.
  - Since devices can lead to differential RF absorption, there are specific considerations for patients with implants (AICD, DBS leads; spinal hardware).
- Contrast: MRI contrast agents generally contain Gd^{3+}, which can cause two related potential consequences of indeterminate current significance if the ion dissociates from its chelate and deposits in tissue, making MR contrast administration a potential relative contraindication in patients with renal impairment or who are pregnant (particularly in first trimester). Refer to your institutional policy.
  - Nephrogenic systemic fibrosis (NSF)—a scleroderma-like reaction to unchelated Gd^{3+}, which is mainly associated with older forms of Gd^{3+}-based agents. Considered "nephrogenic" since it mainly arises in those with renal impairment who cannot renally excrete the contrast agent, so there is prolonged circulation time and higher chances for Gd^{3+} to dissociate. There is limited evidence of its association with newer contrast agents, to the point that some institutions have stopped prospective checking of renal function prior to administration.
  - Gd^{3+} deposition—on MRI, T1 shortening (brightness on T1w) is seen in certain structures in patients with prior Gd^{3+}-based contrast administration, indicating possible deposition of Gd^{3+} in these tissues. No definite clinical syndrome has been described as a result of this deposition although there are informal reports online and elsewhere of potential interactions. This remains an area of active inquiry.
- Other considerations:
  - MRIs can be loud. Give hearing protection!
  - MRI sequences involve rapidly shifting magnetic fields, which can lead to peripheral nerve stimulation via electromagnetic induction, which can be painful or at least unnerving (pun intended). Generally, if within SAR limits then there is limited risk of this, but it could happen in particularly excitable patients.
  - Varying magnetic fields can induce forces on tubes of electrolytes—like the IVC and the semicircular canals. This can induce nausea if the patient moves their head or body too fast in or around the scanner. More a potential issue at 3 T than 1.5 T.

- MRI can be claustrophobic. Screen for claustrophobia and make patients comfortable; it will lead to better images!

How MRI Images Are Made

- When placed in the magnetic field of an MRI scanner, each chunk of tissue will act as a tiny bar magnet, with a **net magnetization** aligned with the **main magnetic field**, with a strength of magnetization that depends on the tissue's magnetic **susceptibility**.
- If radiofrequency (**RF**) energy is applied by a **transmit coil** at a particular frequency called the **Larmor frequency**, the magnetization tips away from its initial state so that at the end of this **excitation**, the tissue magnetization forms an angle with the main magnetic field called the **flip angle** [3].
  - The Larmor frequency depends on the atom in the tissue that is being excited and the strength of the local magnetic field. In usual clinical MRI we excite and use the signal of hydrogen atoms, whose nuclei are protons.
  - The flip angle depends on the RF strength and duration and can be any amount: 5°, 45°, 90°, 180°, 270°, 360°, 405°….
- After excitation, the tissue magnetization **precesses** around the direction of the main magnetic field, akin to a top precessing in the Earth's gravitational field (Fig. 1.2). Over time the tissue magnetization aligns back toward the main magnetic field; this process is called **relaxation**. During relaxation the excitation energy is emitted back and can be picked up as an electrical signal in our **receiver coil**; this signal's frequency will be the Larmor frequency. This is the signal we use to eventually generate an MRI image.
- The tissue magnetization can be split into a **longitudinal** component that is always aligned with the main magnetic field, and a **transverse** component perpendicular to the main magnetic field. The relaxation process of the longitudinal component is called **T1 relaxation**; relaxation of the transverse component is called **T2 relaxation**.
- So that the signal in MRI contains spatial information, and we can use it to make an image, we use **gradients**. Gradients are variations of the main magnetic field so that the magnetic field is slightly stronger on one end (e.g., the left side, or the head) and weaker on the other end (the right side, or the toes). The gradient field is aligned with the main magnetic field; the gradient field just varies along a particular direction.
  - Since the rate of precession of magnetization depends on the local magnetic field strength, after a set of gradients turns on and then off, the individual magnetizations of each chunk of tissue are then labeled with a phase added to their precession, with the amount of this phase now dependent on the position in space of that tissue. This phase label comes through in the signal emitted during relaxation.
  - There are usually three gradient coils in the bore of the MRI oriented along the head-toe, left-right, or front-back directions. By combining gradients, the imaging plane can be oriented along any direction intrinsically—no post hoc reformats needed!
- To make an MRI image, after placement in the bore of a scanner with a high-strength magnetic field, RF excitation excites the tissue's magnetization to tip it by a particular flip angle. Then gradients turn on and off to impart spatial patterning so that the signal that is produced during relaxation has some spatial information in it.
  - The signal produced in MRI corresponds to what a particular spatial frequency is doing in the image. After one round of excitation/gradient application and signal recording, we need to iterate and vary the gradients to see what each spatial frequency is doing in the image. After all that data is collected, we computationally process it to produce the final image.

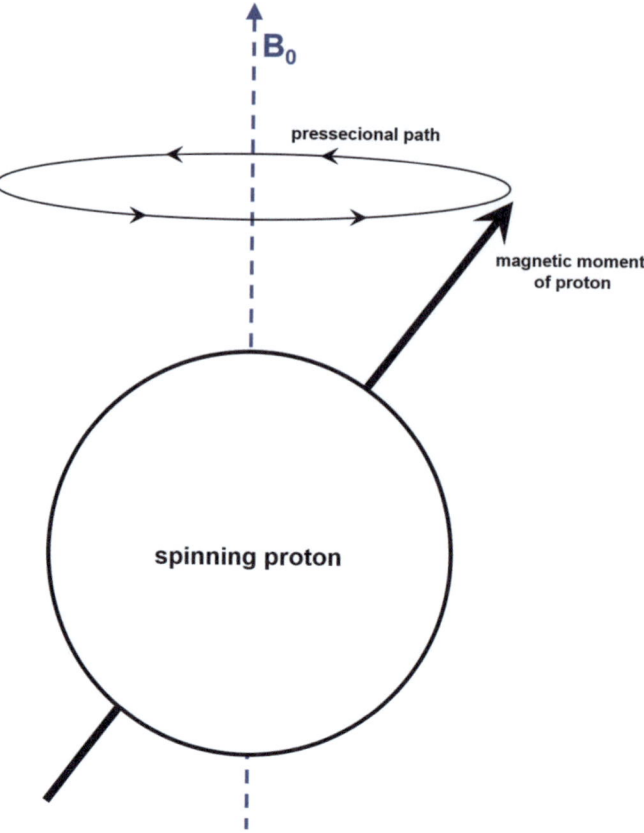

Fig. 1.2 When induced by the B_0 external magnetic field, the proton not only spins with respect to the axis of its magnetic moment but also precesses about a second axis. This is similar to that of a spinning top toy. The axis of the precession is aligned either parallel (seen here) or antiparallel with respect to the external magnetic field

- o This is definitely not as intuitive as X-ray or CT imaging. An analogy would be reconstructing a piece of music (image) by finding out the strength and timing of each note (spatial frequency) and then combining that information together [4].
- o By playing with the RF and gradient strength and timing, we can weight the image toward different contrasts (T1, T2, T2*, diffusion, flow, etc.).
- o The signal in MRI is also called the **echo**, because we are shouting a Larmor frequency "sound" into the tissue and listening for the return of a Larmor frequency signal. The time from excitation to signal emission is called the **TE** (time of echo).
- o The time between successive RF excitations is **TR** or time of repetition. Without any advanced processing, making a 256 × 256 pixel MRI image will take 256*TR time to acquire.

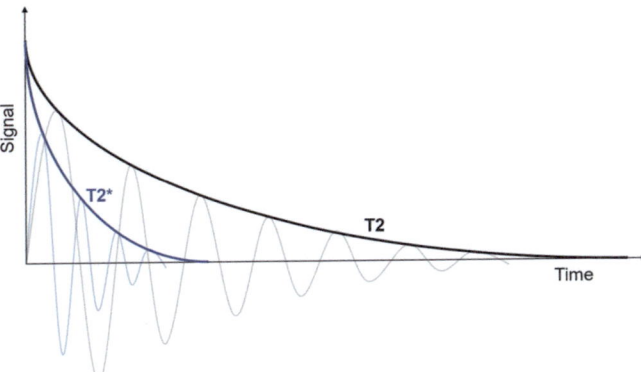

Fig. 1.3 While T2 relaxation occurs due to spin–spin interactions (local field inhomogeneity), in reality, a much faster relaxation occurs when accounting for additional field inhomogeneities (including B_0 magnetic field inhomogeneity, magnetic field gradients, and magnetic susceptibility), known as T2* relaxation. This is depicted in the free induction decay curve governed by T2* in which the amplitude of the sinusoidal wave decreases to zero much more rapidly than by T2

Spin Echoes

- MRI signal is made by the action of the transverse component of the magnetization, which decays quickly after RF excitation. This decay happens because the magnetization of the tissue is due to the summed effect of what the magnetization of each hydrogen nucleus in the voxel is doing and after excitation they are all in phase, with strong transverse magnetization, but then because of differences in the environment each atom and nucleus sees, they quickly become out of phase and that transverse magnetization goes away.
- If we apply a 180° pulse soon after RF excitation, then that flips the direction of precession and those individual nuclei that precessed differentially faster or slower to yield signal decay before the 180° flip will then turn around and actually refocus to regain coherence as quickly as they initially decayed.
  - o As an analogy, if a set of racers, some slower and some faster, agreed to run out until they heard a siren and then run back at the same speed, they would all return to the starting position at the same time, regardless of their individual speed. Before the siren the runners' phases (distances from start) disperse; after the siren their phases recohere or refocus.
- So, if we apply a 180° refocusing pulse at TE/2, we would recohere or refocus the phases so they are realigned at TE, yielding a maximal signal or a refocused echo at TE. This type of signal or echo is termed a **"spin echo."**
- The rate of decay of the signal after RF excitation is termed **T2*** (Fig. 1.3). If we continually applied 180° refocusing pulses following RF excitation, we would see an echo generated for each refocusing pulse. The amplitudes of successive echoes would decay at a slower rate than T2*. This slower rate of echo decay is **T2**.
  - o T2* decay results from the dephasing effects of all sources of heterogeneity of the local magnetic field in the chemical environment of the tissue. T2 decay results from decay due to sources that are nonconstant before and after the 180° refocusing pulse; static sources of dephasing like field inhomogeneities are negated by the refocusing. Typical values for T2 are ~100 ms, while for T2* are ~10 ms or less.
- In clinical MRI, we do not routinely measure T1 or T2 times, but instead make images weighted toward differences in the tissue T1 or T2 times, or other parameters such as proton density, diffusivity, susceptibility, flow, etc.
- T1-weighted (T1w) spin echo imaging.
  - o T1 decay results from excitation energy from RF dissipating into the medium, allowing the magnetization to fall back toward the main magnetic field. This dissipation happens most efficiently when molecules in the environment are tumbling at a rate close to the Larmor frequency. For clinical MRI strengths (1.5 or 3 T) this corresponds to medium sized molecules like fat or proteins.
  - o Materials with medium sized molecules such as protein or fat, or with paramagnetic ions such as Gd^{3+} or Fe^{3+} (methemoglobin), will have a short T1 time, and show as brighter on T1w images. Long T1 materials are devoid of T1 shortening agents, such as simple fluids (e.g., CSF), and are darker on T1w MRI.
  - o For spin echo T1w imaging, we use excitation to flip the longitudinal magnetization to the transverse plane and then look at the signal generated to indicate the rate of recovery of longitudinal magnetization. This means that a **short TR** (<750 ms) is used to discern differences in the rate of longitudinal recovery; and a **short TE** (<40 ms) is used to minimize the effects of T2 decay of the signal (Fig. 1.4).

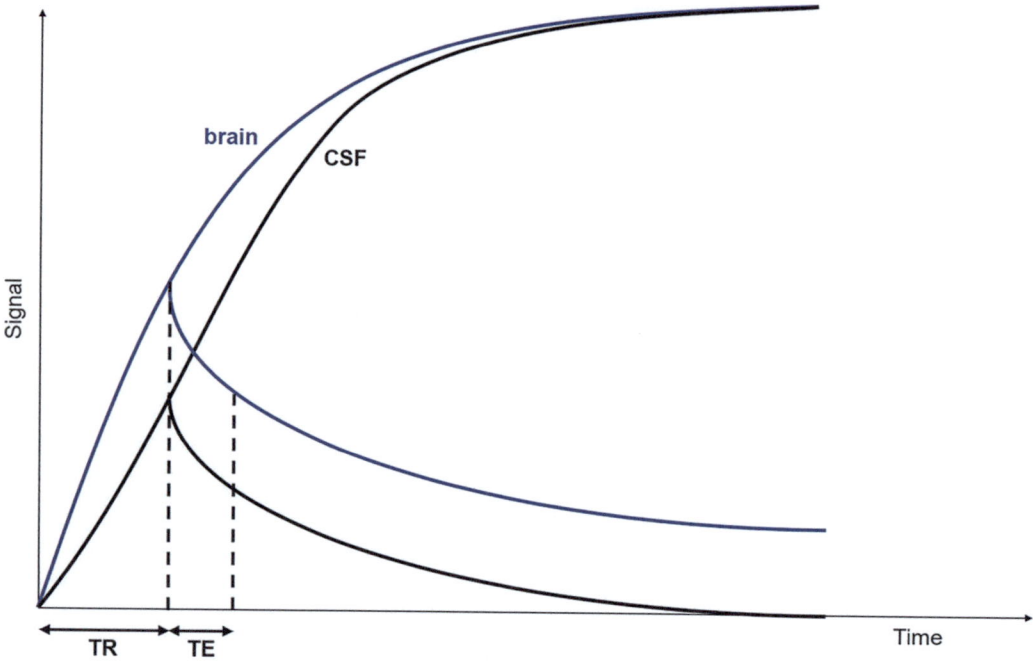

Fig. 1.4 Imaging early in T1 relaxation provides the best T1 tissue contrast as the difference in the level of longitudinal magnetization recovered between two tissues is greatest sooner after the RF pulse. Therefore, for T1-weighting imaging, a short TR and a short TE is desired to maximize T1 tissue contrast and minimize T2 tissue contrast

- T2-weighted (T2w) spin echo imaging.
  - For T2w imaging, materials with inhomogeneity and anisotropy such as axons (white matter) or hypercellular tumors (with inhomogeneous distribution of intracellular vs. extracellular fluid) will have an environment that accelerates dephasing of the individual atomic nuclei and therefore have a shorter T2 time and so less signal overall; these are darker on T2w images. Conversely, long T2 material is brighter since it has more long-lived transverse magnetization that yields more signal and includes homogenous isotropic materials such as simple fluid (e.g., CSF).
  - A long TE would differentiate the longer vs. shorter-lived echoes and therefore impart T2 weighting in the image. So, for a spin echo T2-weighted image, a **long TE** (>75 ms) is used, combined with a **long TR** (>1.5 s), to weight against T1 time differences (Fig. 1.5).
- Proton density weighting (PDw) spin echo imaging.
  - Proton density refers to the concentration of hydrogen nuclei, which mainly indicates the concentration of water. With T1 and T2, PD is the main other determinant of MRI signal intensity.
  - In spin echo imaging, by shortening TE (<40 ms) and increasing TR (>1.5 s), one can mitigate both T1 and T2 effects, weighting toward PD differences. Of the three weightings, proton density has the highest SNR as there is a relative lack of T1 and T2 relaxation effects, which tend to reduce signal strength. With the advent of FLAIR (discussed below) PD has been largely displaced in neuroimaging.
- Mnemonic: TE/TR: short/short (T1w), long/long (T2w), short/long (PDw).

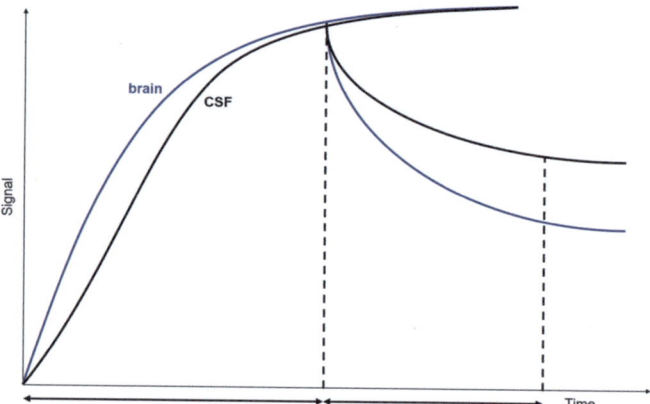

Fig. 1.5 Imaging later in T2 relaxation provides the best T2 tissue contrast as the difference in the level of dephasing between two tissues is greatest later in the T2 relaxation curve. Therefore, for T2-weighting imaging, increasing the TR in a T2-weighted sequence will minimize T1 effects and T1 tissue contrast

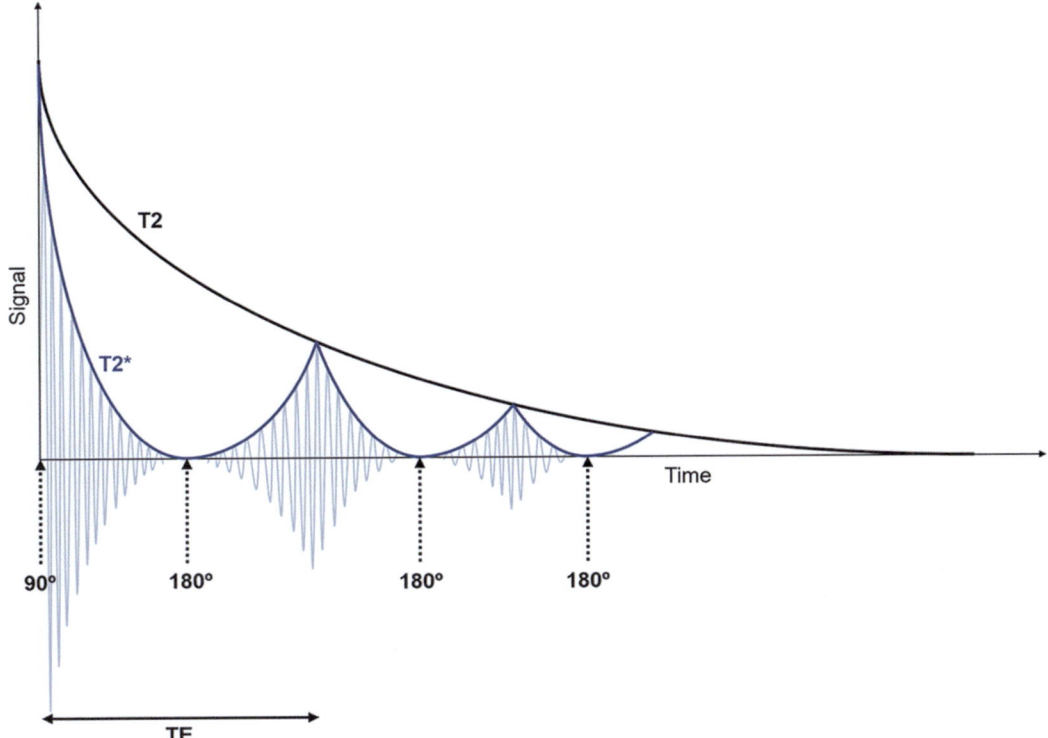

Fig. 1.6 Because T2* relaxation occurs so quickly, the decaying signal is partly recovered using a 180-degree RF pulse (refocusing pulse) and in essence eliminates the effects of T2*. Dephasing of spins due to local field inhomogeneity cannot be corrected by the refocusing pulse and therefore signal decay continues at the time constant T2. Therefore, the signal recovered is weaker than the initial FID due to the continued T2 relaxation

Fast Spin Echo, Ultrafast Spin Echo, and Inversion Recovery

- Most modern MR scanners use Fast Spin Echo (FSE) or turbo SE, to reduce scan time.
  - Instead of one inversion pulse to yield one spin echo per TR, multiple inversion pulses are applied to generate multiple spin echoes per TR, accelerating the image acquisition (Fig. 1.6).
  - The "echo train length" (ETL), or "turbo factor," is how many echoes are generated per TR. Acquisition time is divided by the ETL. A conventional spin echo 256 × 256 image takes 256*TR acquisition time; if four echoes are generated per TR with fast spin echo, the same image would take 256*TR/4 = 64*TR acquisition time. Tradeoff is the echo signal decreases with T2 decay across the train, making for a practical ETL limit. Due to factors beyond the scope of this chapter, multiple refocusing pulses in FSE reduce "J coupling" among fat protons, making fat appear brighter on T2w FSE compared to conventional spin echo.
- Ultrafast spin echo and Half-Fourier acquisitions.
  - As a reminder, in MRI acquisitions, each echo corresponds to the amplitude and phase of one spatial frequency in the image. We have to acquire as many spatial frequencies (i.e., echoes) as there are rows of pixels in the image. If you have enough signal to acquire as many echoes as there are pixel rows using one excitation, that is a **"single shot"** or **"ultrafast"** spin echo technique.
  - Further, there are mathematical similarities between the different spatial frequencies we can take advantage of so that, in the right conditions, we can only acquire half or even one quarter of the spatial frequencies and computationally fill in the rest of the information for the image, reducing acquisition time accordingly and making it easier to use a single shot or ultrafast technique.
  - Common names of such sequences are "half Fourier acquisition single shot turbo spin echo" (HASTE; Siemens), "single-shot fast spin echo" (SSFSE; GE), or "single-shot half turbo spin echo" (SSH-TSE; Philips).
  - While spatial resolution is maintained with this technique, the drawback is lower edge detection due to more limited SNR for echoes for the higher spatial frequencies. And, because of long effective TE, single-shot sequences are often T2 weighted.

- These sequences are used commonly as localizers, in fetal imaging, MR angiography (MRA), and non-breath-hold abdominal imaging.
- Inversion recovery can be used to suppress the signal of specific tissues.
  - A 180° RF pulse is first transmitted to flip the magnetization to point in the opposite direction. As the longitudinal magnetization recovers for a particular tissue, it passes through zero as it goes from the opposite/negative orientation to the original. At that point, it has net zero magnetization. If an MRI sequence is initiated at that time, that tissue will not contribute signal and will be suppressed in the image.
  - The time between the inversion pulse and the RF excitation is called the "inversion time" and is a characteristic for each tissue based on its particular T1 time.
  - Examples are "short tau inversion recovery" (**STIR**), in which fat is suppressed, and "fluid attenuated inversion recovery" (**FLAIR**), in which CSF is suppressed, prior to initiating a T2w sequence in either case.

Gradient-Recalled Echo and Susceptibility-Weighted Imaging

- Gradient-recalled echo (GRE).
  - As an alternative to spin echoes, one can make an echo using gradient pulses alone.
  - A basic GRE sequence starts with an RF pulse with flip angle usually <90°. Then, a gradient pulse is applied, which induces some phase dispersion as the inhomogeneous gradient field has differential effects on the nuclei across the voxel. Then, an oppositely oriented gradient is applied, which cancels some of the dephasing induced by the first pulse. When the amplitude of the two opposite gradients net cancel there is net rephasing, yielding an echo.
  - Gradient echoes can be generated much faster than spin echoes yielding much shorter TEs and TRs, yielding greatly reduced scan time vs. spin echo (Fig. 1.7).
  - GRE TRs may be so short that there is residual transverse magnetization that has not fully decayed at the end of each TR, and the next RF pulse will inadvertently produce its own *spin* echo, similar to the effect of the 180° refocusing pulse of spin echoes.
    - This residual transverse magnetization can be taken advantage of for advanced gradient echo sequences including SSFP, CISS, FIESTA, VIBE, and so on. These are beyond the scope of this chapter. See Chavhan et al. for further details [5].
    - Alternatively, a "spoiling" gradient may be used at the end of each TR to dephase or "spoil" and eliminate the residual transverse magnetization.

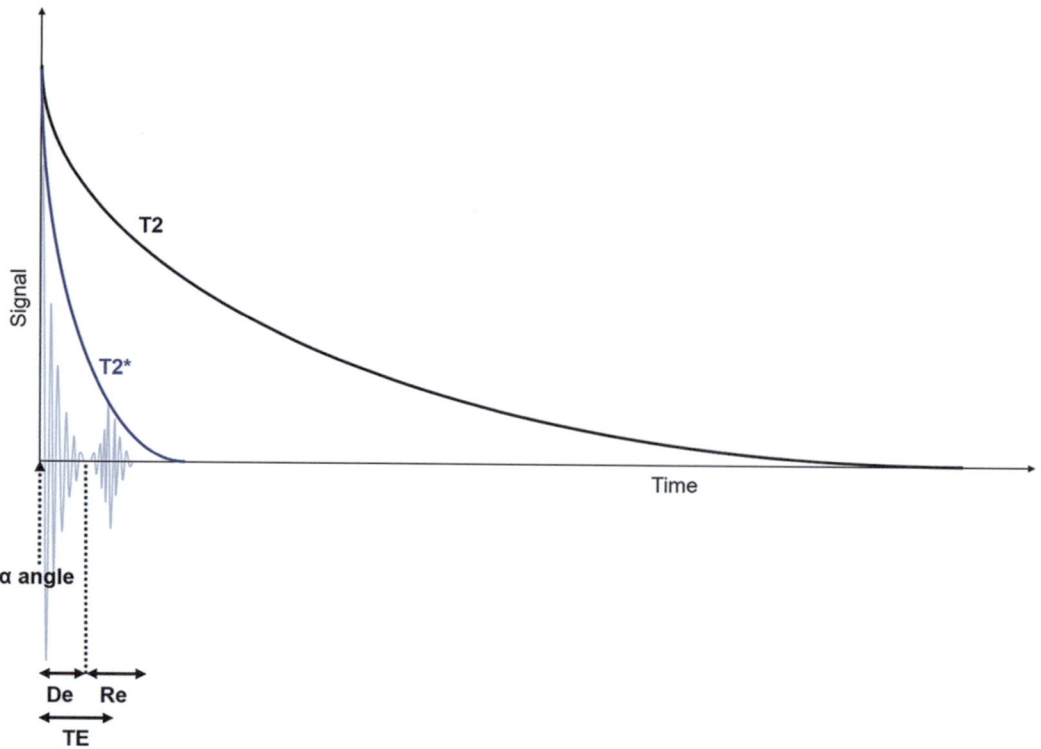

Fig. 1.7 To form an echo in GRE, the frequency encoding gradient is turned on to purposely dephase the protons and destroy the transverse magnetization even more quickly than that governed by T2* (De). The gradient is then turned on at the same strength but in reverse polarity to rephase to protons and recover the transverse magnetization (Re) to generate the echo

- o Because of the role of dephasing as the mechanism of GRE, these sequences are sensitive to field inhomogeneities and susceptibility interfaces (e.g., at bone and around hemosiderin and calcification), which compound the effects of dephasing. This can be taken advantage to detect such substances.
- o A drawback is that the signal-to-noise ratio of gradient echo sequences are typically lower compared to spin echo, and with conventional gradient echo can only generate T2*w not T2w images.
- o Typical scan parameters used in gradient echo sequences are:
  - T1w: "large" flip angle (70–110°), "short" TE (5–10 ms).
  - T2*w: "small" flip angle (5–20°), "long" TE (15–25 ms).
  - PDw: "small" flip angle (5–20°), "short" TE (5–10 ms).
  - Note a "long" TE for GRE is "short" for spin echo!
- Susceptibility-weighted imaging (SWI).
  - o Susceptibility defines the degree to which a material becomes magnetized when placed in an external magnetic field and either aligns with (paramagnetic or ferromagnetic) or is opposite (diamagnetic) to the external field.
  - o In SWI typically a 3D GRE sequence is acquired and its signal is split into magnitude and phase components; phase and magnitude images can be acquired for any sequence but are specifically utilized in SWI. T2*-related changes can occur in both the phase and magnitude images. The magnitude image is essentially the same as any T2*-weighted GRE image.
  - o The phase data is filtered to scale each voxel by how much its phase is deflected due to T2* effects; this makes a "filtered phase image."
  - o The changes on the magnitude image are then amplified by the degree of phase difference seen in the filtered phase image to produce the final SWI image.
  - o The net result is an image with heightened sensitivity to changes in susceptibility, like a super T2*-weighted GRE with higher contrast resolution and generally higher spatial resolution.
  - o In addition, the filtered phase image adds clinical information as paramagnetic and diamagnetic substances yield opposite effects on the phase images. For example, hemosiderin (which is paramagnetic) on the filtered phase images exhibit a signal intensity opposite to that of calcification (which is diamagnetic). With this you can tell if the hyperdense lesion on CT represents a hemorrhagic or calcified lesion, shifting the differential diagnosis and perhaps avoiding a biopsy!

Echo-Planar Imaging

- Warning: This is abstract. In MRI, we acquire signals corresponding to spatial frequencies. This spatial frequency information is plotted in a chart where instead of having a spatial domain along each axis, we have a frequency domain along each axis with higher spatial frequencies corresponding to edge detail of the image (borders between materials of different intensity) and lower frequencies corresponding to the contrast information.
- The conventional readout for MRI fills the spatial frequency chart one row at a time. An accelerated filling is provided by echo planar imaging (EPI) and can be used following either GRE, spin echo, or any MRI contrast generating initial sequence module.
- Following RF excitation and gradient phase encoding, during readout in EPI, instead of collecting one row only, the gradients oscillate rapidly back and forth generating a train of gradient echoes (and scanner noise!) that collectively rapidly fill the rows of the frequency chart in a "zig-zag" pattern (Fig. 1.8).
- Because of the long train of gradient echoes, EPI imaging is sensitive to susceptibility artifacts (e.g., near the mastoid air cells or near blood products) and to motion artifacts.

Diffusion-Weighted Imaging (DWI)

- In many pathologies, the free diffusion of water is altered, for instance, when the proportion of extracellular vs. intracellular water shifts during states of cytotoxic edema (ischemia, trauma, inflammation) or hypercellularity (tumor).
- To image diffusion, a variant of both spin and gradient echoes is used. In a spin echo, an inversion pulse flips the trajectory of phase dispersion to refocus the nuclear magnetizations at the echo time. Now, if gradient pulses of the same amplitude and timing are applied before and after the inversion pulse, they will accentuate this dephasing and rephasing process, similar to how gradient echoes are gen-

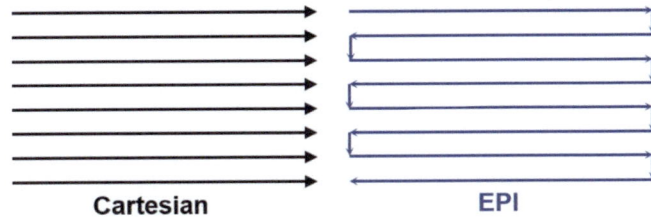

Fig. 1.8 The filling of k-space is conventionally performed "line-by-line" in the same left-to-right direction. In EPI, the filling occurs line-by-line but in a zig-zag fashion much akin to a "Pacman" pattern

erated. However, this only applies to stationary molecules—if a molecule moves between these gradient pulses, it will not experience the exact same effects of the second gradient as the first and will have a net dephasing compared to the stationary molecules. This means that stationary (or "diffusion-restricted") hydrogen nuclei will generate a brighter signal than moving, freely diffusing ones. In this manner, diffusion weighting is encoded into the signal.
- The timing and amplitude of the gradient pulses defines a "**b-value**" that is essentially the motion sensitivity of the sequence—higher b-value images are more sensitive to subtler motion differences.
- Because gradients are direction selective, in practice, the diffusion motion-encoding gradients are successively applied along different directions in separate acquisitions. For usual **diffusion-weighted imaging (DWI)**, the acquisitions (usually six directions, two along each of the three cardinal axes) are averaged on a voxel-by-voxel basis to form the DWI image of the typical diffusivity of each voxel, without regard to directionality. If instead direction sensitivity is desired, more directions (~35–50) are acquired and the set of data is analyzed to determine the typical direction of motion in each voxel for **diffusion tensor imaging (DTI)**.
- Given the number of directions that need to be acquired, to make DWI scan times more reasonable, EPI readout is usually used to accelerate the process.
- Note, a b = 0 image in which the motion-encoding gradients are off, is a standard spin echo image with a T2 weighting given the long TE. This indicates that any diffusion-weighted image will have an element of T2 weighting. To account for this, a "b0" image with the motion-encoding gradients off is acquired in addition to images with the different gradient directions on. This b0 image is used to computationally take the T2-weighting out of the DWI image to produce an **"apparent diffusion coefficient" (ADC)** map, which is a voxel-by-voxel map of the measured diffusion constant across the image. True diffusion restriction will be low intensity on the ADC map; diffusion facilitation will be bright.

Flow-Related Phenomenon

- Flow-related enhancement, bright blood, black blood.
  - In a GRE acquisition, recall that the TR is usually quite short, especially for T1-weighted images (TR <50 ms).
  - Successive application of excitations with short TRs will constantly flip the recovered longitudinal magnetization to the transverse plane, yielding net limited magnetization available to contribute to signal in the aggregate. This state is known as "partial saturation," since the net signal generatable is less than the initial.
  - However, fresh protons that move into/through the slice will not have such saturation. So inflowing protons will look brighter on a short TR (T1-weighted) GRE study. This is known as "flow related enhancement" of the inflowing protons vs. the partially saturated stationary background tissue. This makes such GRE sequences a "bright blood" technique.
    - Similar flow-related enhancement makes for flow artifacts in FLAIR where the in-flowing CSF is not completely suppressed.
  - In contrast, for spin echo images, protons need to see both the RF excitation and the inversion refocusing pulse to then generate an echo. So flowing protons, as with through plane arterial blood, would not yield signal if they move through the slice too fast. This makes spin echo images generally a "black blood" technique.
    - Similar effects result in CSF flow voids on T2w images, particularly 3D T2w images.
- Time of flight MR angiography.
  - Flow-related enhancement can be taken advantage of to permit noncontrast MR angiography. Indeed, most noncontrast MR angiography is completed with a spoiled T1-weighted short TE gradient echo sequence, with other tricks to accentuate the signal from the inflowing blood.
  - To isolate arterial flow in these images, a saturation pulse is usually performed more superior to the slice of interest, to prevent imaging venous flow moving downward into the slice.
  - Importantly, turbulent flow or blood flow parallel to the slice plane will not exhibit optimal flow-related enhancement, artifactually limiting the opacification of blood vessels with non-laminar flow or flow within the slice of interest.
  - In addition, as the base sequence is T1-weighted, stationary tissues with intrinsically short T1 relaxation (e.g., mural hematoma) will be suppressed poorly and shine through. Make sure to double check the raw images!

References

1. Bushberg JT, Seibert JA, Leidholdt EM, et al. The essential physics of medical imaging. 3rd ed. Philadelphia: Lippincott Williams and Wilkins; 2011.
2. Brink JA, Heiken JP, Wang G, et al. Helical CT: principles and technical considerations. Radiographics. 1994;14(4):887–93.
3. Hashemi RH, Bradley WG, Lisanti CJ. MRI: the basics. Philadelphia: Lippincott Williams and Wilkins; 2010.
4. Mezrich R. A perspective on K-space. Radiology. 1995;195(2):297–315.
5. Chavhan GB, Babyn PS, Jankharia BG, et al. Steady-state MR imaging sequences: physics, classification, and clinical applications. Radiographics. 2008;28(4):1147–60.

Neuroimaging Structural Anatomy

D. Kenneth Jamison and Tarik F. Massoud

Abbreviations

aka	Also known as
3T/7T	3 Tesla/7 Tesla
ACA	Anterior cerebral artery
ACOM	Anterior communicating artery
AICA	Anterior inferior cerebellar artery
AX	Axial
BRAVO	Brain volume imaging (GE Healthcare)
BVoR	Basal vein of Rosenthal
COR	Coronal
CSF	Cerebrospinal fluid
CT	Computed tomography
CTA	CT angiography
DTI	Diffusion tensor imaging
EAC	External auditory canal
ECA	External carotid artery
FIESTA	Fast Imaging Employing Steady-state Acquisition (GE Healthcare)
FSE	Fast spin echo
IAC	Internal auditory canal
ICA	Internal carotid artery
ICV	Internal cerebral vein
MCA	Middle cerebral artery
MIP	Maximum intensity projection
MPR	Multiplanar reconstruction
MPRAGE	Magnetization Prepared Rapid Gradient Echo (Siemens)
MR	Magnetic resonance
MRA	MR angiography
PCA	Posterior cerebral artery
PCOM	Posterior communicating artery
PICA	Posterior inferior cerebellar artery
SAG	Sagittal
SCA	Superior cerebellar artery
T1	Longitudinal relaxation time
T2	Transverse relaxation time
TSV	Thalamostriate vein
VoG	Vein of Galen

Introduction

Learning neuroanatomy can be a challenging undertaking. The goal of this chapter is to give a cohesive account of the neuroanatomy of the brain and surrounding structures sufficient to approach the disease processes encountered when on clinical service and during board examinations, while valuing brevity. This prioritization means that issues such as variant anatomy are omitted or given a cursory review.

Anatomical symmetry is most often regarded as implicit; however, many normal subtle asymmetries of the brain exist [1]. Additionally, there is often variability or disagreement in the literature regarding the names, boundaries, or typical relationships of structures. Thus, we provide the most common anatomical understanding or interpretation while striving to remain accurate and consistent. For a more comprehensive review of neuroimaging anatomy of the brain and skull, see Massoud [2]. The skull base, face, neck, and spine are reviewed in separate chapters.

The reversed right/left radiologic convention of image display is maintained throughout. When appropriate, images are displayed with the AC-PC line as the reference axial plane (see further description in the White Matter section). Also, recall that owing to the curved neuroaxis of the brain, ventral/dorsal mean inferior/superior in anatomy positioned toward the face (or rostrally), and ventral/dorsal mean anterior/posterior in anatomy positioned toward the brainstem

D. K. Jamison
Division of Neuroimaging and Neurointervention, Stanford University School of Medicine, Stanford, CA, USA
e-mail: d.kenneth.jamison@stanford.edu

T. F. Massoud (✉)
Department of Radiology, School of Medicine, Stanford University, Stanford, CA, USA
e-mail: tmassoud@stanford.edu

and spine (or caudally). Most anatomical terms are provided in English, rather than Latin, and eponyms are avoided, except when the Latin or eponymous terms are far more commonly used in practice than their counterparts. We describe the anatomy from the exterior to the interior, beginning with the skull, meninges, and extra-axial spaces, moving inward to the cortical brain, deep brain, white matter, and ventricles, and finally the brainstem, cerebellum, cisterns, cranial nerves, and vasculature.

The international standard for terms that describe the intricate anatomy of the brain and skull can be found in the *Terminologia Anatomica* or *Neuroanatomica*. We recommend that the anatomical terms we have placed in italics at first mention or where explained under their own headings be, at a minimum, the ones that residents should understand, be familiar with, and adopt in clinical practice.

SKULL

- The *skull* is composed of two parts: the viscerocranium (aka: facial bones) and the neurocranium—the bones that encase the brain, which will be the focus of this review.
- Neurocranium: composed of the calvarium and skull base.
- *Calvarium* (aka: cranial vault, calvaria): an assortment of bones that form a dome that surround and protect the brain.
   - Composed of the squamous part of the frontal bone, parietal bones, squamous parts of the temporal bones, and squamous part of the occipital bone (Fig. 2.1).
- *Skull base*: floors of the neurocranium that support the brain and allow passage of nerves and blood vessels through many foramina (aka: holes) and fissures (narrow openings).
   - Divided into *anterior, middle, and posterior cranial fossae* (surfaces).
   - See Chaps. 32–34 for further description of the skull base.

Bones of the Calvarium

Frontal bone: Forms the forehead, superior orbits, and most of the anterior cranial fossa.
Frontal bone parts:

- *Squamous part*: outward convex component that forms the forehead.
   - Frontal crest: attachment for the anterior falx cerebri (divides the two brain hemispheres) on the midline inner surface of the squamous part.
- *Nasal part*: between the orbits.
   - Glabella: prominence between the superior orbits.
- *Orbital plate*: roughly flat plate that forms the roofs of the orbits and majority of the anterior cranial fossa.

Frontal bone variant:

- *Hyperostosis frontalis interna*: in a minority of patients, the inner cortex (aka: inner table/plate) of the squamous part may demonstrate irregular benign overgrowth, often in elderly women [3].

Parietal bones: paired bones that form the sides and posterior roof of the calvarium.
Occipital bone: forms the lower posterior skull.
Occipital bone parts:

- Squamous part: interparietal portion that forms the posterior calvarium.
   - *Opisthion*: the posterior-most aspect of the foramen magnum.
- Lateral parts: form the base of the bone and sides of the foramen magnum.
   - *Occipital condyles*: project inferiorly at both sides of the foramen magnum and rest upon the atlas (first cervical vertebra).
   - *Jugular tubercles*: bony eminences on the inner surfaces beitween the *hypoglossal canals* and *petrous apices* (see below).
- Basilar part (aka: *basiocciput*): forms the caudal aspect of the clivus. "Caudal" is Latin for "tail" and means toward the tail.
   - *Basion*: the anterior-most aspect of the foramen magnum.

Occipital bone foramina and contents:

- *Hypoglossal canals*: found between the occipital condyles and jugular tubercles and contain the hypoglossal nerves (CNs XII).
- *Foramen magnum*: medulla, spinal accessory nerves (CNs XI), vertebral arteries, anterior/posterior spinal arteries, and meninges.
- *Condylar canals*: posterior to the occipital condyles, they contain emissary veins and small branches of the ECA.

Temporal bones: paired bones that form the sides of the skull and contain the middle and inner ear elements.
Temporal bone parts:

- *Squamous part*: forms a side of the skull and a majority of a middle cranial fossa.
- *Petrous part* (aka: pyramid): triangular elevation rising from the skull base, it contains middle and inner ear elements.
   - *Petrous apex*: the apex of the "pyramid" forms part of the posterior wall of the carotid canal. Asymmetric pneumatization can be mistaken for pathology.

Fig. 2.1 Bones, sutures, and foramina of the skull. MPRs of the skull: (**a**) from a superior view with anterior upward, (**b**) from a left posterolateral view, and (**c**) a superior view with the calvarium cut away to reveal the skull base

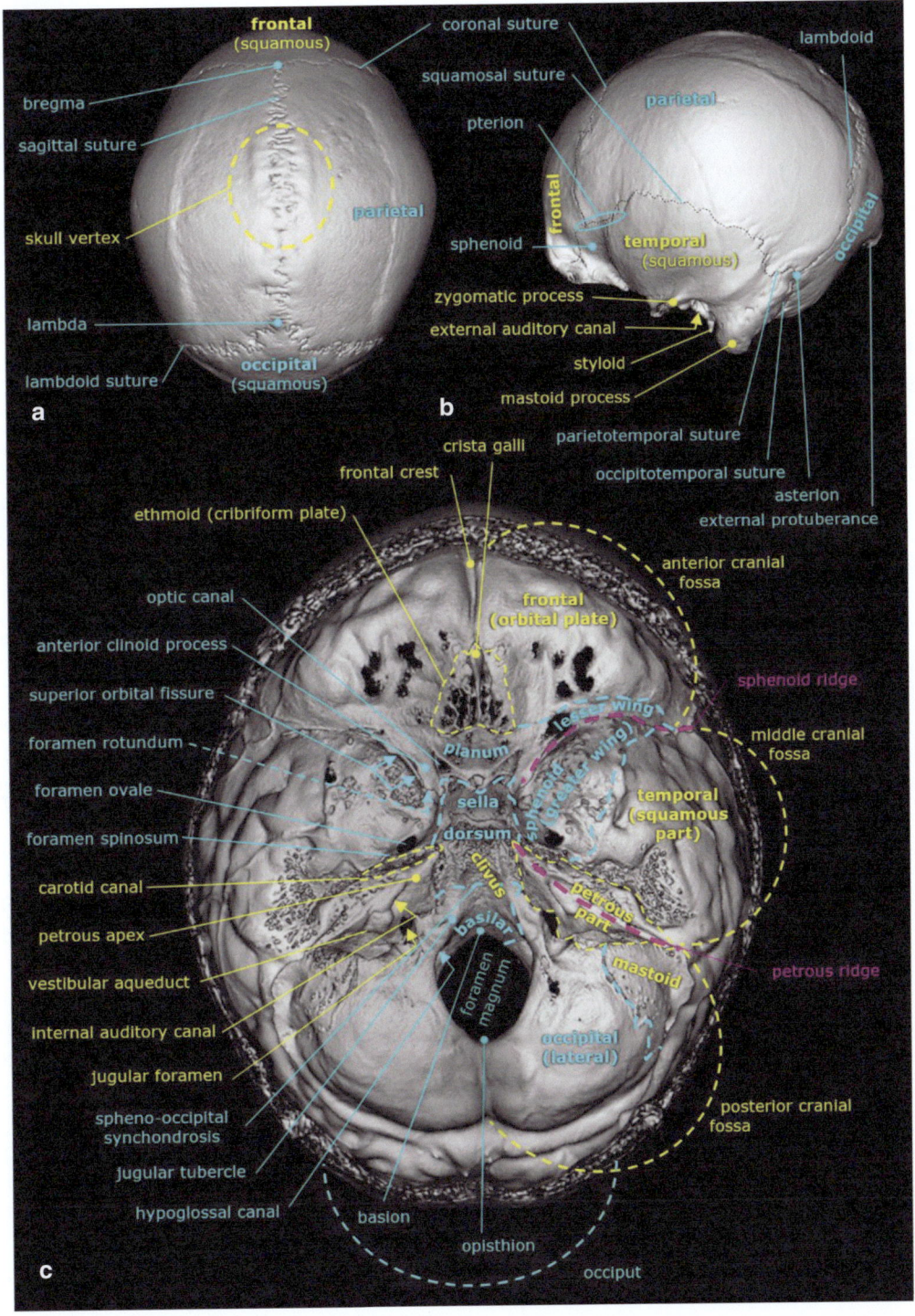

- *Petrous ridge*: the most superior edge of the "pyramid" that forms a portion of the boundary between the middle and posterior cranial fossae.
- *Mastoid part*: pneumatized by mastoid air cells.
  - *Mastoid process* (aka: mastoid tip): caudal projection behind the auricle (aka: pinna).
- *Tympanic part*: contains the external auditory canal.
- *Styloid process*: long cone-shaped projection extending caudally below the EAC.
- *Zygomatic process*: articulates with the zygoma of the face.
  o *Mandibular fossa*: the mandible articulates at this surface.

Temporal bone foramina, canals, and contents:

- *Stylomastoid foramen*: between the styloid and mastoid processes, it contains a facial nerve (CN VII) and stylomastoid artery (ECA).
- *Carotid canal*: in the petrous part, it contains a segment of an ICA.
- *Internal auditory (aka: acoustic) canal (meatus* is the entrance to this): facial nerve (CN VII), vestibulocochlear nerve (CN VIII), labyrinthine artery (most often a branch of AICA that supplies the inner ear).
- *Vestibular aqueduct*: endolymphatic duct posterior to IAC.
- *External auditory canal and meatus*.

Sphenoid bone: complex midline bone near the center of the skull base, possibly named for its wasp-like shape [4].
Sphenoid bone parts:

- *Greater wings*: forms a minority of the middle cranial fossae and contains *foramina rotundum*, *ovale*, and *spinosum*.
- *Lesser wings*: contain the *optic canals*.
  - *Sphenoid ridge*: posterior margin of the lesser wings that forms most of the border between the anterior and middle cranial fossae.
  - *Anterior clinoid process*: common landmark for the ICA and aneurysms.
- *Body*: midline portion pneumatized by the sphenoid sinuses in adolescents and adults.
  - *Planum sphenoidale*: flat area between lesser wings.
    - A common site for meningiomas.
  - *Sella turcica* ("Turkish saddle," aka: sella): saddle-shaped depression that houses the pituitary gland.
    - *Tuberculum sellae*: transverse ridge that forms the anterior sella.
    - *Pituitary fossa* (aka: hypophyseal fossa): floor of the sella.
    - *Dorsum sellae*: transverse ridge forms the posterior sella.

Sphenoid bone foramina, fissures, and contents:

- *Optic canal*: optic nerve (CN II), ophthalmic artery.
- *Foramen rotundum*: maxillary nerve (CN V_2).
- *Foramen ovale*: mandibular nerve (CN V_3), accessory meningeal artery (often from middle meningeal artery), emissary veins connecting cavernous sinus to pterygoid plexus.
- *Foramen spinosum*: middle meningeal artery/vein, meningeal branch of mandibular nerve (CN V_3).
  - The appearance of ovale and spinosum in an axial plane is often likened to the footprint made by a high-heeled shoe and is a useful landmark.
- *Superior orbital fissure*: between greater and lesser wings, it contains: an oculomotor nerve (CN III), trochlear nerve (CN IV), ophthalmic nerve (CN V_1), abducens nerve (CN VI), and superior ophthalmic vein.

Ethmoid bone: midline bone that separates the intracranial space from the underlying nasal cavities.
Ethmoid bone parts:

- *Cribriform plate*: perforated to transmit olfactory nerve filaments. The intracranial surface of the cribriform plate forms the *olfactory fossa* (where the olfactory bulb is positioned) and the *olfactory groove* at its base.
- *Crista galli* ("rooster's crest"): serves as an attachment site for the falx cerebri.

Ethmoid bone foramen and contents:

- Olfactory foramina of the cribriform plate: olfactory neurons.

Other Calvarial Fissures, Foramina, and Their Contents

- *Inferior orbital fissure*: between sphenoid greater wing and orbital surface of the maxilla contains: branches of maxillary nerve CN V_2, inferior ophthalmic veins, infraorbital artery/vein.
- *Foramen lacerum*: predominantly formed by the sphenoid greater wing anteriorly and petrous part of the temporal bone posteriorly, with slight contribution from the occipital bone medially, it contains: Vidian artery/nerve, branch of the ECA.
- *Jugular foramen*: anterolateral margin formed by the temporal petrous bone, posteromedial margin formed by the occipital bone, divided into two parts by a fibrous septum and the bony jugular spine:
  - *Pars nervosa*: anterior aspect of jugular foramen, it contains: glossopharyngeal nerve (CN IX), Jacobson's nerve (tympanic branch of the glossopharyngeal nerve).
  - *Pars vascularis*: posterior aspect of jugular foramen, contains: vagus nerve (CN X), Arnold's nerve (auricular branch of vagus), spinal accessory nerve (CN XI), and junction of internal jugular vein, sigmoid sinus, and inferior petrosal sinus.

Other Skull Terminology

- *Skull vertex*: the most superior region of the midline skull.
- *Anterior cranial fossa*: roughly axial plane that supports the inferior frontal lobes of the brain, it is composed of the frontal bone orbital plate, ethmoid cribriform plate, sphenoid lesser wings, and planum sphenoidale.

- *Middle cranial fossa*: plane that supports the inferior temporal lobes and the pituitary gland, composed of the sphenoid greater wings, temporal squamous parts, and the sella turcica.
- *Posterior cranial fossa*: surfaces of the skull base bounded by the foramen magnum inferiorly and tentorium superiorly (see Meninges), which contain the cerebellum and brainstem.
- *Occiput*: the posterior skull; it does not correspond exactly to the occipital bone.
  - *External occipital protuberance*: on the midline posterior outer surface (its tip is referred to as the inion).

Sutures and Synchondroses

Sutures: Sutures are irregularly sinuous lines where cranial bones meet, and fuse when bone growth is complete. A suture is a slightly mobile fibrous joint versus a synchondrosis, which is a relatively immobile hyaline cartilaginous joint. With a few notable exceptions, sutures and synchondroses are named for the two bones they join (Fig. 2.1).

- *Coronal suture*: between the frontal bone and parietal bones in a coronal plane.
- *Sagittal suture*: between the parietal bones in a sagittal plane.
  - *Bregma*: point where the sagittal suture bisects the coronal suture and the location of the anterior fontanelle in infancy.
- *Lambdoid sutures*: form inverted "V" shape between the parietal bones and occipital bone.
  - *Lambda*: point where the sagittal suture and bilateral lambdoid sutures meet.
    - The location of the posterior fontanelle in infancy.
- *Squamosal sutures* (aka: squamous sutures): have a semicircular shape between parietal and squamous temporal bones on the sides of the skull.
- Sphenosquamosal sutures: between the sphenoid greater wings and squamous temporal bones.
- Sphenofrontal suture: between the frontal bone orbital plate and sphenoid lesser wings and planum sphenoidale.
- *Pterion*: where the frontal, parietal, temporal, and sphenoid bones come together on the side of the skull near the "temples."
- *Occipitotemporal sutures (aka: occipitomastoid sutures)*: lateral continuation of the lambdoid suture between the occipital bone and a temporal mastoid.
- Parietotemporal sutures (aka: parietomastoid sutures): posterior continuation of the squamous sutures between a parietal bone and a temporal mastoid.
- *Asterion*: point where the parietal, temporal, and occipital bones meet behind the auricle.

Synchondrosis

- *Spheno-occipital synchondrosis* (aka: basiocciput synchondrosis): joins the posterior sphenoid body (*basisphenoid*) and basilar occipital bone (*basiocciput*) to form the *clivus*.

MENINGES

(Singular: meninx): three membranes that surround and protect the brain and spinal cord, namely, the dura mater, arachnoid mater, and pia mater (Fig. 2.2). Cerebrospinal fluid (CSF) is present in the subarachnoid space between the arachnoid and pia mater. "Meninx" is derived from a Greek word meaning "membrane" [4].

Pachymeninx

(Plural: *pachymeninges*): the dura mater. "Pachy-" is derived from a Greek word meaning "thick."

1. **Dura mater**: outermost fibrous double-layer membrane immediately underlying the skull and spinal canal. "Dura" is from a Latin word meaning "hard" and "mater" meaning "mother." An early description of this structure was in Arabic, which often uses familial terms to describe relationships between things [4].
   - Outer layer: periosteal (aka: endosteal), inner layer: meningeal.
   - Often referred to as the "thecal/dural sac" in the spine.
- *Dural venous sinuses* (aka: dural sinuses): valveless channels between periosteal and meningeal layers that receive venous blood from cerebral and cerebellar veins and CSF from arachnoid granulations (see below) and drain predominantly to the internal jugular veins.
- Dural partitions (aka: dural reflections/folds): two meningeal layers come together to form septa that partition the brain.
  - *Falx cerebri* (aka: cerebral falx, falx): C-shaped partition between the left and right cerebral hemispheres in a midline sagittal plane.
    - Attaches to the frontal crest and crista galli anteriorly.
  - *Tentorium cerebelli* (aka: cerebellar tentorium): C-shaped partition between the cerebrum (specifically the posterior temporal and occipital lobes) and cerebellum in a roughly axial plane.
    - Attaches anteriorly to the anterior clinoid processes and petrous ridges.
    - *Tentorial leaflet*: left or right half of the tentorium.

Fig. 2.2 The meninges and extra-axial spaces. (a) MPR of the brain from a left superolateral view with the dura mater partially retained posteriorly and a magenta line designating the plane of (b) a coronal T1 BRAVO post-contrast cross section

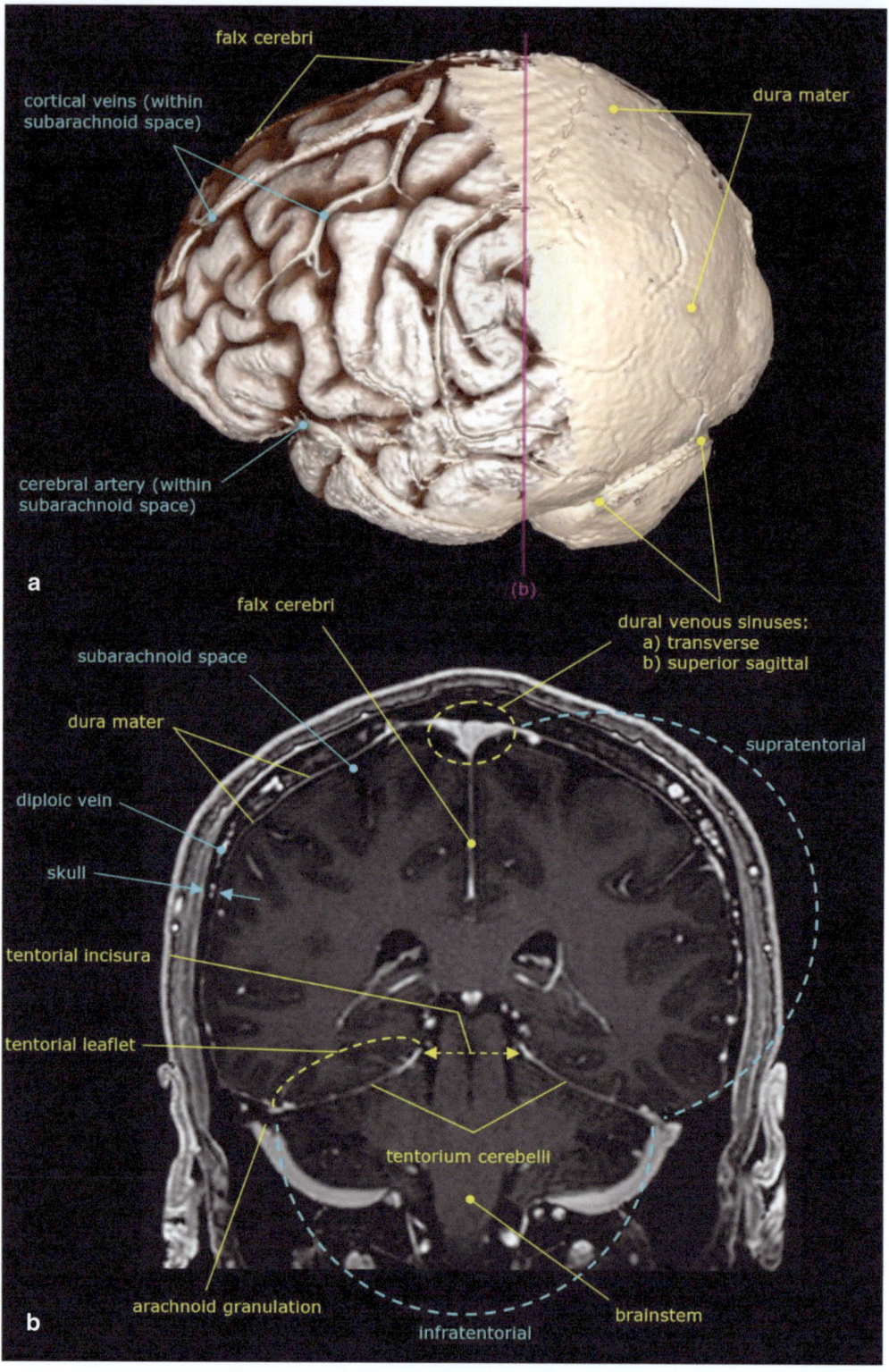

- *Tentorial incisura* (aka: tentorial incisure/notch/hiatus): plane between the U-shaped anterior edge of the tentorium and the clivus where the brainstem meets the cerebrum.
  - Tentorial apex: the posterior-most and highest edge of the incisura.
- *Supratentorial*: above the tentorium, roughly synonymous with cerebrum.
- *Infratentorial*: below the tentorium, roughly synonymous with cerebellum and brainstem, or posterior fossa.

- *Diaphragma sellae* (aka: sellar diaphragm): roof of the sella.
- Dural recess/pouch: CSF-filled space between periosteal and meningeal dural layers.
  - *Meckel's caves* (aka: trigeminal caves): contain the trigeminal ganglions (groups of nerve cell bodies) between the prepontine cistern and cavernous sinuses (see Fig. 2.9d).
- Dural sleeve: channel formed by a dural double layer.
  - *Dorello's canals*: transmit CNs VI from the prepontine cistern to the cavernous sinuses. The inferior petrosal sinuses merge with the cavernous sinuses at the apices (deep/anterior aspect) of the canals (see Fig. 2.9e).

Leptomeninges

Composed of the *arachnoid mater* and *pia mater*. "Lepto-" is derived from a Greek word meaning "thin" [4].

2. **Arachnoid mater**: middle meningeal layer with spiderweb-like fibrous trabeculae/filaments crossing the subarachnoid space to the pia mater.
   - *Arachnoid granulations* (aka: arachnoid villi): globular projections of arachnoid mater that cross the dura mater inner meningeal layer into dural venous sinuses and allow CSF to enter the venous blood stream.
     - Most often found in the superior sagittal sinus and transverse sinuses where they can be mistaken for thrombus.
3. **Pia mater**: the innermost meningeal layer is adherent to brain parenchyma and therefore enters sulci, which is a differentiating characteristic relative to other meningeal layers. "Pia" is from a Latin word meaning "soft" [4].

EXTRA-AXIAL SPACES

"*Intra-axial*" is a term synonymous with the brain tissues or brain parenchyma. "*Parenchyma*" is derived from a Greek word meaning "to pour in," as organs were considered by some in antiquity to be formed from congealed blood [4]. "*Extra-axial*" means outside the brain parenchyma. Understanding of the extra-axial spaces is most frequently useful in the context of intracranial hemorrhage or precise localization of a mass to aid differential diagnosis.

- *Epidural* space (aka: extradural space): the potential space between the skull or vertebral spinal canal and the outer periosteal layer of the dura mater.
- *Subdural* space: the potential space between the dura mater inner meningeal layer and the arachnoid mater.
- *Subarachnoid* space: the space between the arachnoid mater and pia mater filled with CSF as well as cerebral arteries and veins.

CEREBRUM

- The brain is composed of the *cerebrum*, *cerebellum*, and *brainstem*.
- The cerebrum is divided into left and right *cerebral hemispheres* each composed of *cerebral cortex*, underlying *cerebral white matter*, and *subcortical (deep) brain structures*.
- The cerebral cortex is generally divided into four paired *lobes: frontal, temporal, parietal, and occipital* (Figs. 2.3 and 2.4). Sometimes a fifth insular lobe is included and occasionally a sixth limbic lobe is described.

Fissures, Lines, and the Central Sulcus

Fissures and *sulci* (singular: sulcus) both describe grooves in the surfaces of the brain. "Sulcus" is Latin for "furrow." Fissures are generally thought of as deeper and separating lobes, while sulci are shallower and separating gyri (singular: gyrus) or folds within a lobe; however, these conventions are not always followed. "*Gyrus*" is derived from a Greek word meaning "curved." A "line" in this context is a conceptual division between lobes where no anatomical fissure or sulcus exists.

- *Interhemispheric fissure* (aka: medial longitudinal cerebral fissure): separates the left and right cerebral hemispheres and contains the falx cerebri (Fig. 2.4).
- *Sylvian fissures* (aka: lateral fissures): separate portions of the frontal and parietal lobes superiorly from the temporal lobes inferiorly, on the lateral surfaces of the brain.
- *Central sulcus* (aka: *central sulcus of Rolando*, Rolandic fissure): separates frontal and parietal lobes and more specifically a precentral gyrus (primary motor cortex) from a postcentral gyrus (primary somatosensory cortex) (Fig. 2.3a).
- *Parieto-occipital fissures*: separate the parietal and occipital lobes on the medial surfaces of each cerebral hemisphere and more specifically separate the precunei from the cunei.
- Basal temporo-occipital lines (aka: basal parietotemporal lines): straight lines between the preoccipital notches on the lateral surfaces of the brain and the posterior ends of

Fig. 2.3 The lateral and medial surfaces of the brain. MPRs of (**a**) the left lateral brain surface and (**b**) right medial brain surface

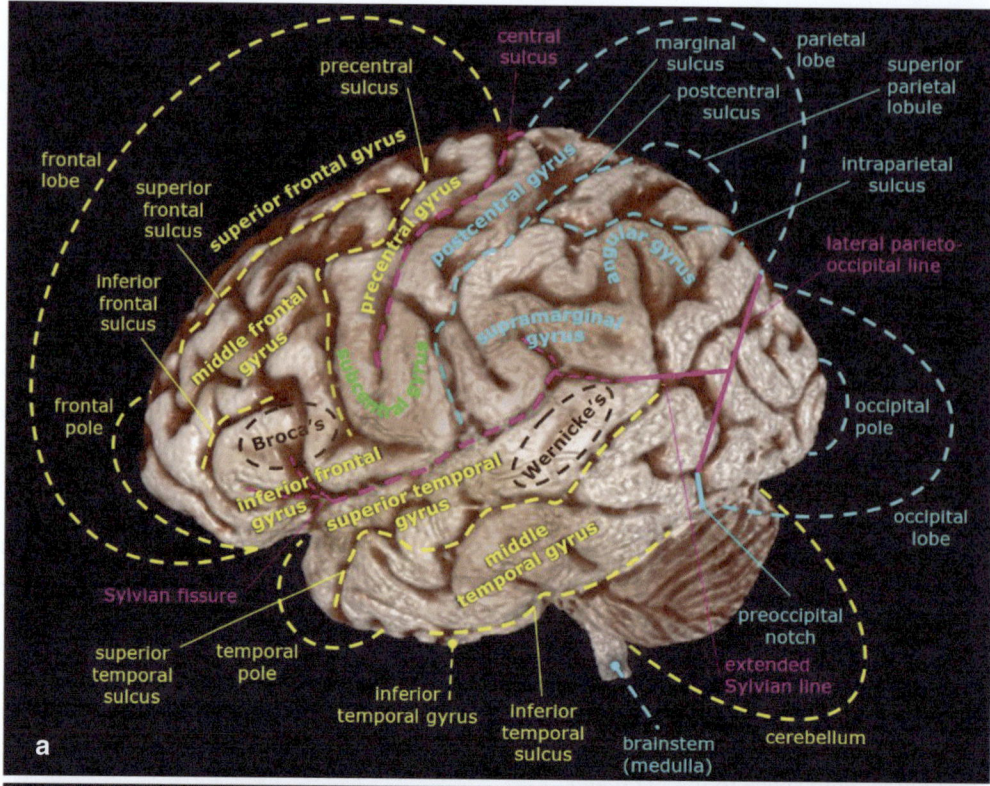

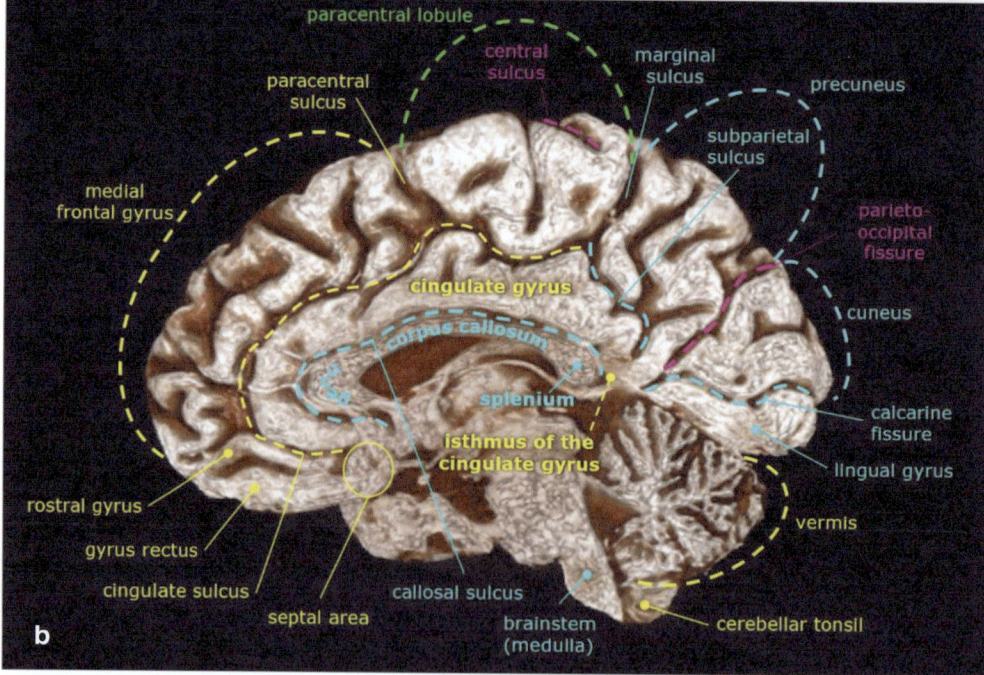

the calcarine fissures on the medial surfaces; they separate the temporal and occipital lobes at the basal surfaces of the brain (Fig. 2.4d).

- Lateral parieto-occipital lines (aka: lateral parietotemporal lines): straight lines between the preoccipital notches laterally and the superior ends of the parieto-occipital fissures medially; they separate the parietal and temporal lobes from the occipital lobes on the lateral surfaces of the brain (Fig. 2.3a).

- Extended Sylvian lines (aka: temporo-occipital lines): straight lines from the posterior descending rami of the Sylvian fissures to the mid-points of the lateral parieto-occipital lines; they separate the parietal and temporal lobes on the lateral surfaces of the brain.

Fig. 2.4 Four orthogonal views of the left brain. MPRs of (**a**) the left hemibrain superior view, (**b**) anterior view, (**c**) posterior view, and (**d**) basal view with the cerebellum removed

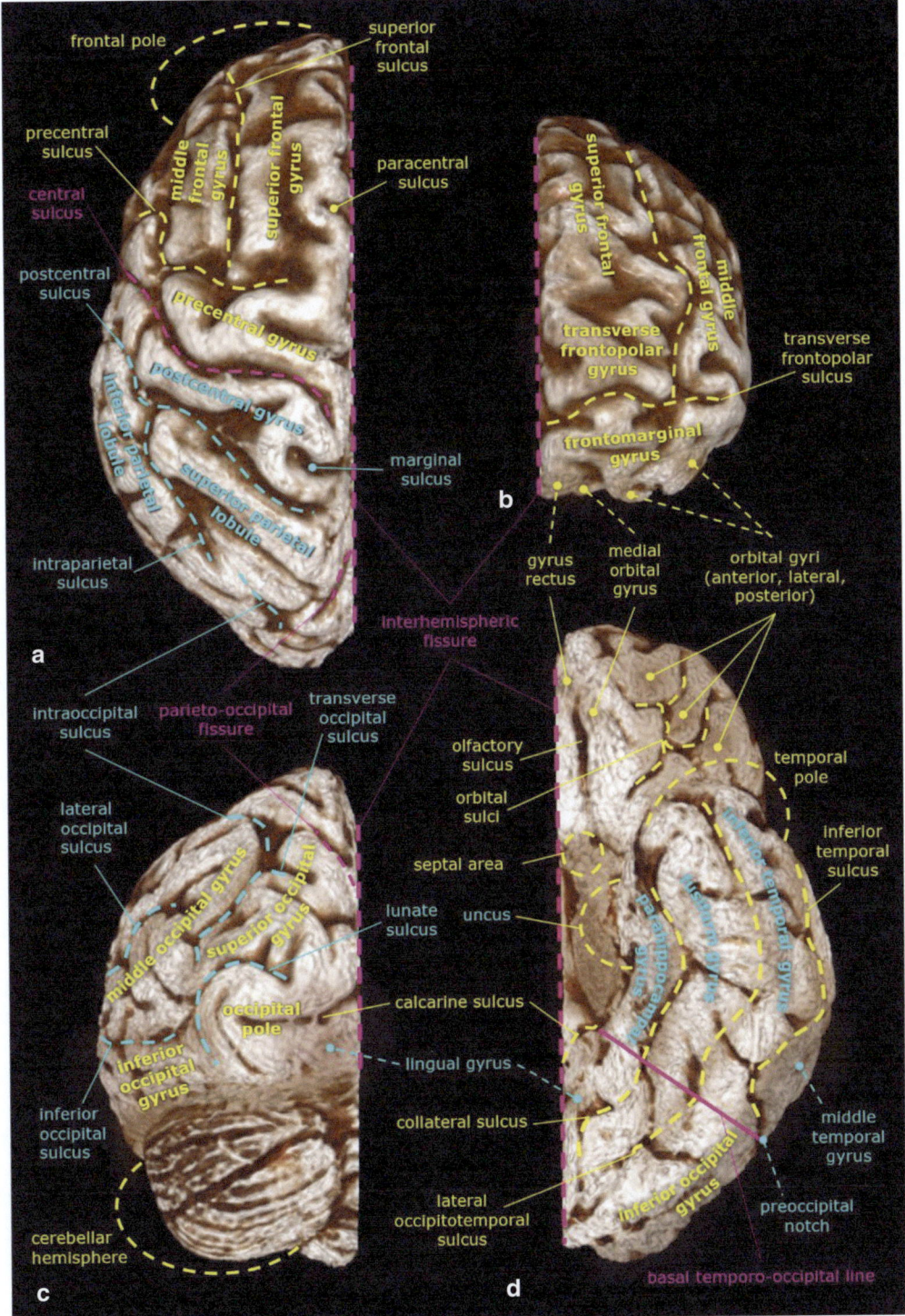

Lobes

Anatomic divisions of the cerebral cortex. Cortical gyri and their dividing sulci have many variations, and the following description provides an internally consistent approach to describe the surface anatomy.

Frontal lobes: the largest and most anterior lobes of the cerebrum.

Frontal lobe surfaces, gyri, and divisions:

- Lateral frontal surfaces (aka: frontal convexity, Fig. 2.3a): "*convexity*" is a term that may be used to describe a lateral surface of the brain, the adjacent meninges, or nearby extra-axial spaces.

- ○ *Precentral gyrus* (aka: primary motor cortex): anterior to the central sulcus. Recall the organization of the motor homunculus, which depicts the regions of the precentral gyrus dedicated to processing motor information for different body parts. The hips sit on the superior margin of the gyrus and the lower extremities fall into the interhemispheric fissure along the medial surface. The trunk, arms, and hands lie superior to superolateral, with a disproportionately large region dedicated to the hands. On the lateral surface the face, eyes, lips, and tongue are also disproportionately represented, and turning inward along the inferior surface within a Sylvian fissure (Fig. 2.5a), pharyngeal and secretomotor functions are represented.
  - ○ *Superior frontal gyrus*: the most superior sagittally oriented gyrus on the lateral surface.
  - ○ *Middle frontal gyrus*: lateral to the superior frontal gyrus.
  - ○ *Inferior frontal gyrus*: lateral to the middle frontal gyrus. Composed of three parts:
    - Pars orbitalis: the anterior portion.
    - Pars triangularis: the middle portion with a characteristic triangular shape.
    - Pars opercularis: the posterior portion.
- Basal frontal surface (Fig. 2.4b and d):
  - ○ *Gyrus rectus* (aka: *straight gyrus*): the most medial gyrus on the inferior surface.
  - ○ Medial *orbital gyrus*: parallels the gyrus rectus laterally.
  - ○ There are also anterior, posterior, and lateral orbital gyri.
- Medial frontal surface (Fig. 2.3b):
  - ○ Rostral gyrus: lies superior to the gyrus rectus. "Rostrum" is Latin for the "beak" of a bird and directionally refers to something toward the face.
  - ○ Medial frontal gyrus: the medial surface of a frontal lobe between a rostral gyrus and paracentral lobule.
  - ○ Paracentral lobule (a majority portion): defined by the paracentral sulcus anteriorly, cingulate sulcus inferiorly and marginal sulcus posteriorly. The thin posterior portion between central and marginal sulci is part of the parietal lobe.
- *Frontal pole* (aka: frontopolar cortex): corresponds to anteroinferior portions of a lateral surface, and anterior portions of a gyrus rectus and orbital gyri.

Frontal lobe sulci:

- *Precentral sulcus*: parallel to a central sulcus and anterior to a precentral gyrus.
- Paracentral sulcus: an ascending branch of the cingulate sulcus on a medial surface that forms the anterior margin of a paracentral lobule.
- *Superior frontal sulcus*: divides superior and middle frontal gyri.
- *Inferior frontal sulcus*: divides middle and inferior frontal gyri.
- Olfactory sulcus: divides a gyrus rectus and medial orbital gyrus.

Other frontal lobe divisions:

- Supplementary motor cortex: often corresponds to portions of the superior frontal gyrus and medial frontal gyrus immediately anterior to the primary motor cortex.
- Premotor cortex: often immediately anterior to the primary motor cortex and lateral to the supplementary motor cortex.
- Prefrontal cortex: portions of the frontal lobe anterior to motor, premotor, and supplementary motor cortices.
- Orbitofrontal cortex: comprises the straight gyri and orbital gyri.
- *Frontal operculum*: the portions of the inferior frontal gyrus and precentral gyrus that appose the temporal lobe forming the anterior Sylvian fissure (Fig. 2.5a). "Operculum" is a Latin word meaning "lid" or "cover" [4]. The frontal, parietal, and temporal opercula cover the insular cortex.
- *Broca's area*: important for speech production, comprises the pars triangularis and pars opercularis, generally on the left (Fig. 2.3a).

Temporal lobes: the second largest cerebral lobes composed of five gyri, the hippocampal formations, and the amygdalae.

Temporal gyri, hippocampal formations, and amygdalae: listed from superolateral to inferior to medial.

- Lateral temporal surfaces (aka: temporal convexities, Fig. 2.3a):
  1. *Superior temporal gyrus* (STG): between the Sylvian fissure and superior temporal sulcus.
     - ○ *Temporal operculum*: portion of the STG that apposes the frontal and parietal lobes to form the Sylvian fissure.
     - ○ Heschl's gyrus (aka: transverse temporal gyrus): transverse fold on the superior surface of the STG that serves as the primary auditory cortex. It lies opposite to the postcentral gyrus across the Sylvian fissure.
     - ○ Wernicke's area: important for speech recognition, generally considered to be in the posterior aspect of the STG, most often on the left.
  2. *Middle temporal gyrus*: bounded by superior and inferior temporal sulci.
  3. *Inferior temporal gyrus*: between inferior temporal and lateral occipitotemporal sulci.

Fig. 2.5 The hippocampus and insular lobe. (a) Oblique T2 coronal oriented perpendicular to the long axes of the hippocampi through the level of the insula, and (b) T1 MPRAGE oblique sagittal through the right insular lobe. A solid magenta line crossing each image designates the imaging plane of the other image

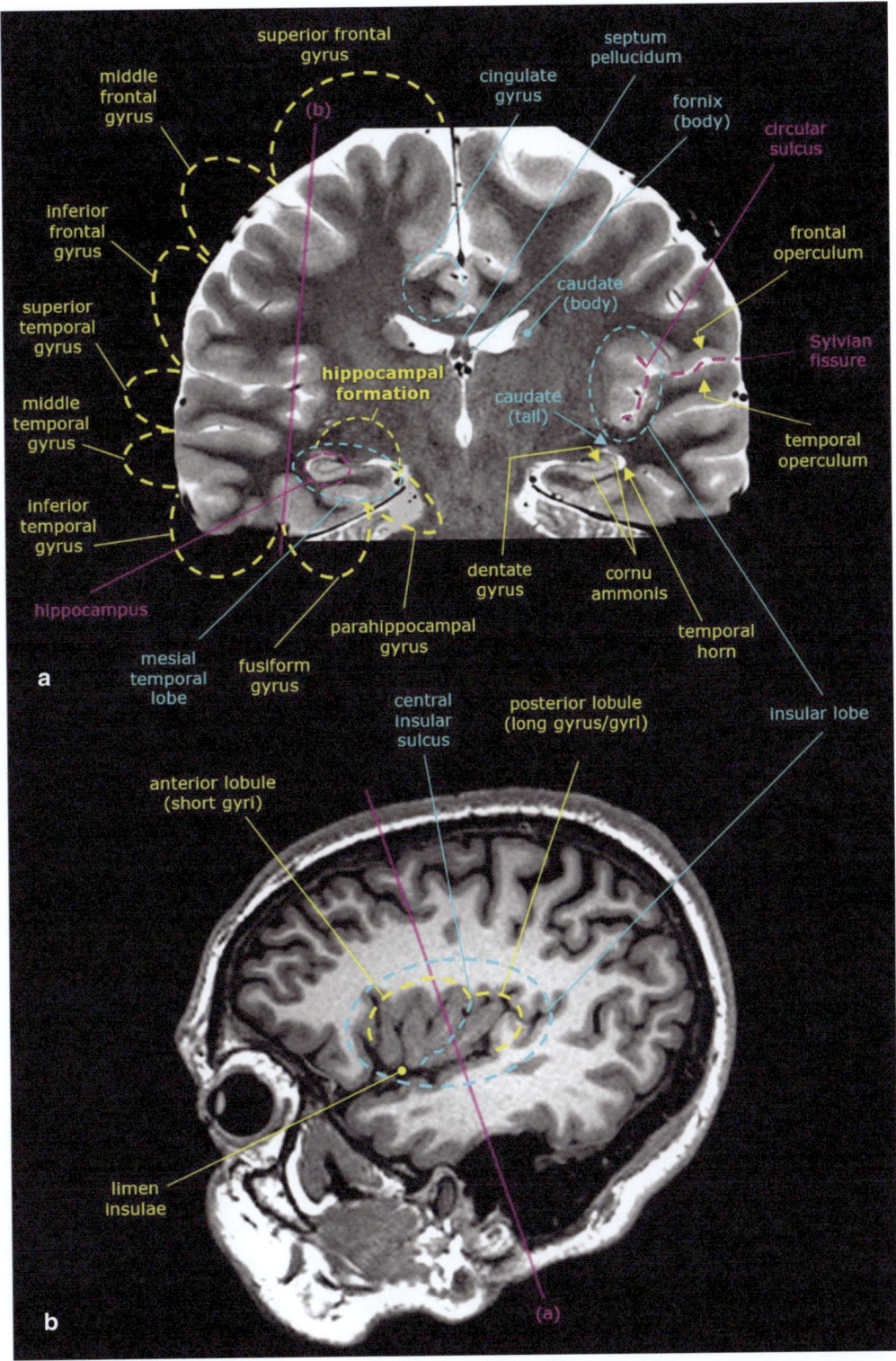

- Basal temporal surfaces (Fig. 2.4d):
  4. Fusiform gyrus (aka: lateral occipitotemporal gyrus): between the lateral occipitotemporal sulcus and collateral sulcus.
- *Mesial temporal lobes* (aka: medial temporal lobes): composed of the hippocampal formations, amygdalae, and parahippocampal gyri (Fig. 2.5a).

5. *Parahippocampal gyrus* (PHG, aka: medial occipitotemporal gyrus when combined with the lingual gyrus of the occipital lobe): between the collateral sulcus and hippocampal formation.
   o *Uncus* (aka: uncinate gyrus): medial-most part of the anterior temporal lobe and anterior portion of the PHG. It is a major component of the olfactory

cortex. "Uncus" is Latin for "hook," describing its morphology.
  - Entorhinal cortex: loosely corresponds to the medial surface of an anterior PHG that connects to the subiculum.
  - Subiculum (aka: subicular complex): loosely corresponds to the superior surface of an anterior PHG that connects to the cornu ammonis (see below).
 6. *Hippocampal formation* (aka: postcommissural hippocampus): the exact components are not agreed upon, but it is variably considered to include the following:
    - Entorhinal cortex: (see above)
    - Subicular complex: (see above)
    - *Hippocampus*: Composed of two interlocking gray matter structures: the cornu ammonis and dentate gyrus, which are in a mesial temporal lobe medial to a temporal horn (see Ventricles). "Hippocampus" is Greek for "seahorse," reflecting its distinctive shape composed of an anterior expanded "head," tapering "body," and curved "tail" posteriorly.
      - Cornu ammonis (aka: Ammon's Horn, hippocampus proper): gray matter of a hippocampus with a spiral appearance when viewed in a coronal cross section. Amun is an ancient Egyptian god with ram-shaped horns.
      - Dentate gyrus: gray matter of a hippocampus seen within the central spiral when viewed in a coronal cross section.
      - Fimbria: hippocampal white matter outputs that collect on the superomedial surface of a hippocampus, ultimately forming the fornix (see White Matter).
      - Pes hippocampi: anterior head of the hippocampus. "Pes" is Latin for "foot"; a hippocampal head has digitations that give it a gross paw-like appearance.
 7. *Amygdala* (aka: amygdaloid body): collection of gray matter nuclei anterosuperior to a pes hippocampi. "Amygdala" is derived from a Greek word meaning "almond," reflecting its shape.
- *Temporal pole* (aka: temporopolar cortex): anterior-most portion of a temporal lobe where temporal gyri merge.

Temporal lobe sulci (Figs. 2.3a and 2.4d):

- *Superior temporal sulcus*: parallel to the Sylvian fissure on the lateral brain surface separating the superior and middle temporal gyri.
- *Inferior temporal sulcus*: parallel to the Sylvian fissure on the inferolateral brain surface separating the middle and inferior temporal gyri.
- Lateral occipitotemporal sulcus (aka: occipitotemporal sulcus): courses anteroposteriorly on the basal brain surface separating the inferior temporal gyrus laterally from the fusiform gyrus medially.
- Collateral sulcus (aka: medial occipitotemporal sulcus): parallels the lateral occipitotemporal sulcus on the basal brain surface. In the temporal lobe, it separates the fusiform gyrus laterally from the parahippocampal gyrus medially. In the occipital lobe it separates the fusiform gyrus laterally from the lingual gyrus medially.
- Hippocampal sulcus: between a dentate gyrus and subiculum.
- *Choroidal fissure*: dorsal to hippocampal fimbria, medial to a temporal horn (see Fig. 2.8b).

Parietal lobes: the third largest cerebral lobe.
Parietal lobe divisions:

- Lateral parietal surfaces (aka: parietal convexities, Fig. 2.3a): composed of three divisions.
  1. *Postcentral gyrus* (aka: primary somatosensory cortex, ascending parietal gyrus): posterior to the central sulcus. Recall the organization of the sensory homunculus, which depicts the regions of the postcentral gyrus dedicated to processing sensory information for different body parts. The hips sit on the superior margin of the gyrus and the lower extremities fall into the interhemispheric fissure along the medial surface, with the genitalia at the most inferior region. The trunk, arms, and hands lie superior to superolateral, with a disproportionately large region dedicated to the hands. On the lateral surface the face, eyes, lips, and tongue are also disproportionately represented, and turning inward into the parietal operculum, sensation of the abdominal organs is represented.
  2. Superior parietal lobule: superior to the intraparietal sulcus and posterior to the postcentral sulcus.
  3. Inferior parietal lobule: inferior to the intraparietal sulcus, posterior to the postcentral sulcus, and superior to the Sylvian fissure.
     - Supramarginal gyrus: rostral portion of the inferior parietal lobule; it arches over the posterior ascending ramus of the Sylvian fissure.
     - Angular gyrus: caudal portion of the inferior parietal lobule; it arches over the posterior end of the superior temporal sulcus.
- Medial parietal surfaces (Fig. 2.3b):
  – *Precuneus*: bounded by the marginal sulcus anteriorly, subparietal sulcus inferiorly, and parieto-occipital fissure posteriorly. It is anterior to the cuneus of the occipital lobe, which has a triangular shape (see below). "Cuneus" is Latin for "wedge."
  – Paracentral lobule (a minority portion): the portion between the central, cingulate, and marginal sulci is

the posterior portion of the paracentral lobule (see frontal lobe above).

Parietal lobe sulci:

- *Postcentral sulcus*: parallel to the central sulcus and posterior to the postcentral gyrus.
- Marginal sulcus (aka: pars marginalis, ramus marginalis): the superoposterior extension of the cingulate sulcus that separates the paracentral lobule from the precuneus on the medial surface of the brain.
- Subparietal sulcus: has the appearance of a posterior extension of the cingulate sulcus on the medial surface of the brain; it separates the precuneus from the posterior cingulate gyrus.
- *Intraparietal sulcus*: separates the superior and inferior parietal lobules on the lateral surface of the brain. Anteriorly terminates at the postcentral sulcus and posteriorly terminates at the transverse occipital sulcus.

Other parietal lobe divisions:

- Parietal operculum: the portions of the parietal lobe that appose the temporal operculum forming the posterior Sylvian fissure.
- Secondary somatosensory cortex (aka: somatosensory association cortex): roughly corresponds to the supramarginal gyrus and the parietal operculum.

Occipital lobes: the most posterior lobes of the cerebrum. "Occiput" is Latin for the back part of the head [4].
Occipital gyri:

- Medial occipital surfaces (Fig. 2.3b):
  o *Cuneus*: triangular-shaped surface bounded by parieto-occipital and posterior calcarine fissures.
  o *Lingual gyrus* (aka: lingula): bounded superiorly by the calcarine fissure and inferiorly by the collateral sulcus. Also comprises the medial aspect of the basal surface.
- Lateral occipital surface (aka: occipital convexity, Fig. 2.4c): has highly variable morphology, but some structures are frequently preserved as below [5].
  o Superior occipital gyrus: forms the superolateral edge of the lobe.
  o Middle occipital gyrus: bounded by the intraparietal sulcus superiorly and divided by or bounded by a lateral occipital sulcus inferiorly.
  o Inferior occipital gyrus: forms the inferolateral edge of the lobe.
- *Occipital pole*: posterior-most portion of an occipital lobe where superior, middle, inferior, and lingual gyri merge.
- Basal occipital surface (Fig. 2.4d): the medial edge is formed by the lingual gyrus and the lateral edge by the inferior occipital gyrus.
  o Fusiform gyrus (posterior portion): lies entirely on the basal surface.

Occipital lobe fissures and sulci:

- *Calcarine fissure*: separates the cuneus and lingual gyrus.
- Preoccipital notch (aka: temporo-occipital incisure): a short sulcus at the anterior margin of an occipital lobe where the lateral and basal surfaces meet.
- Intraoccipital sulcus (aka: superior occipital sulcus): often a posterior continuation of an intraparietal sulcus; it separates the superior and middle occipital gyri.
- Lateral occipital sulcus: often a posterior continuation of the superior temporal sulcus or arises independently near the angular gyrus. It may merge posteriorly with the transverse occipital sulcus or lunate sulcus. It separates middle and inferior occipital gyri or divides a middle occipital gyrus.
- Inferior occipital sulcus: sometimes a continuation of the inferior temporal sulcus.

Other occipital lobe divisions:

- Primary visual cortex (aka: calcarine cortex, striate cortex): gyri bordering the calcarine fissures on the medial surfaces of the occipital lobes.
- Secondary visual cortex (aka: visual association cortex): roughly corresponds to the remainder of the occipital lobe.

Insular lobes: (aka: *insula*, insular cortex, island of Reil): sometimes described as a "fifth" cerebral lobe, it lies deep to the frontal, parietal, and temporal opercula (Fig. 2.5).
Insular lobe divisions and gyri:

- Anterior lobule:
  o Short gyri: often three, but sometimes four short gyri.
    - May include anterior, middle, and posterior short gyri.
    - Limen insulae: "apex" of an insula where the short gyri meet at its anteroinferior margin.
- Posterior lobule:
  o Long gyri: there may be one or two long gyri.
    - These may include anterior and posterior long gyri.

Insular lobe sulci:

- Central insular sulcus: separates anterior and posterior lobules.
- Circular sulcus (aka: peri-insular sulcus): separates an insula from overlying opercula.

Limbic lobes: occasionally described as a sixth cerebral lobe or alternatively as the *limbic "system"* with variation of included structures, some of which overlap with temporal lobe components.

- Its name is derived from the Latin word for "border" [4], as it is composed of a collection of structures on the medial margins of the frontal, parietal, occipital, and temporal lobes that have a somewhat C-shaped orientation that roughly parallels the caudate nuclei (see Deep Brain).
- Components include a cingulate gyrus, septal area, indusium griseum, fasciolar gyrus, hippocampus, parahippocampal gyrus, and piriform cortex.

Limbic gyri and cortical areas (Figs. 2.3b and 2.5a):

- *Cingulate gyrus*: C-shaped gyrus that lies dorsal to the corpus callosum on a medial surface of the brain.
  - Isthmus of the cingulate gyrus: thin strip of cortex that connects a cingulate gyrus to a parahippocampal gyrus inferior to the splenium.
- Septal area: variably described depending on the source, it is composed of two vertical gyri on the medial surface of a hemisphere, inferior to the rostrum of the corpus callosum [6].
  - Parolfactory area (aka: subcallosal area): gyrus anterior to a vertically oriented middle subcallosal sulcus.
  - Paraterminal gyrus (aka: subcallosal gyrus, precommissural hippocampus, subgenual area, geniculate gyrus, peduncle of the corpus callosum): gyrus posterior to a middle subcallosal sulcus and continuous with the supracallosal gyrus superiorly.

Limbic lobe sulci:

- *Callosal sulcus*: runs along the dorsal margin of the corpus callosum separating it from a cingulate gyrus.
- *Cingulate sulcus*: runs along the dorsal margin of a cingulate gyrus separating it from a frontal lobe.

Other Cerebral Terminology

- Perisylvian cortex: encompasses the frontal, parietal, and temporal opercula.
- Perirolandic cortex: comprises the precentral, postcentral, and subcentral gyri, as well as a portion of the paracentral lobule.
- Secondary auditory cortex: surrounds the primary auditory cortex largely within the superior temporal gyri.

DEEP BRAIN

Basal ganglia: (aka: basal nuclei) large clusters of neurons in the central deep brain generally described in four parts: striatum, pallidum, substantia nigra, and subthalamic nuclei.

1. *Striatum*: named for its characteristic striated appearance owing to alternating bands of gray and white matter between the caudate and putamen (Fig. 2.6a).
   - Ventral striatum: located inferomedial to the dorsal striatum.
     - Nucleus accumbens: interposed between a fundus striatum (where a caudate head and putamen meet ventromedially at their rostral ends) and a parolfactory area [7].
     - Olfactory tubercle: an anterior portion of an anterior perforated substance on the basal surface of the brain posterior to olfactory striae and ventral to a fundus.
   - *Dorsal striatum* (aka: neostriatum): composed of the *caudate nucleus and putamen.*
     - *Caudate nucleus*: C-shaped nucleus composed of a "head" and a tapering "body" inferolateral to a lateral ventricle body, and a slender "tail" overlying the temporal horns of the lateral ventricles (Fig. 2.5a).
     - *Putamen*: separated from a caudate nucleus by the anterior limb of an internal capsule (see White Matter).
2. Pallidum: divided into the ventral pallidum and dorsal pallidum with the boundary between the two partially defined by the anterior commissure [8] (see White Matter).
   - Ventral pallidum: inferior to the anterior commissure.
   - Dorsal pallidum (aka: globus pallidus, paleostriatum): "*Globus pallidus*" is Latin for "pale globe."
     - Globus pallidus internus (aka: medial segment).
     - Globus pallidus externus (aka: lateral segment).
3. *Substantia nigra*: in the ventral midbrain dorsal to the cerebral peduncles (see Brainstem, Fig. 2.9b).
4. *Subthalamic nuclei*: the major constituents of the subthalami.

Other basal ganglia terminology:

- *Corpus striatum*: a name that comprises a caudate nucleus, putamen, and globus pallidus.
- Lenticular nuclei (aka: *lentiform nuclei*): comprises the putamen and globus pallidus, which are collectively somewhat lens-shaped when viewed in an axial or coronal cross section.

- Basal forebrain: roughly comprises the ventral striatum and ventral pallidum.
- Anterior perforated substance: posterior to olfactory trigones, lateral to the optic chiasm, anterior to optic tracts, and medial to lateral olfactory striae (see Cranial Nerves). The "perforations" are where the tissue is pierced by lenticulostriate arteries to supply the basal ganglia. The anterior aspect is the olfactory tubercle.

Claustrum: thin strip of gray matter lying between an insular lobe and lentiform nucleus (Fig. 2.6a).

Capsules: white matter that divide deep brain gray matter nuclei.

- *Internal capsule*: white matter fibers that divide a caudate head and thalamus from lenticular nuclei (see White Matter for further details).
- *External capsule*: separates a putamen from a claustrum and contains the uncinate fasciculus and inferior fronto-occipital fasciculus anteriorly (see White Matter—Association Fibers).
- *Extreme capsule*: separates a claustrum from an insular lobe.

Thalamus: large ovoid groups of nuclei that sit atop the midbrain (see Brainstem) posteromedial to a lenticular nucleus. "Thalamus" is derived from a Greek word meaning "chamber" [4].

- In an axial cross section, there is a "Y-shaped" internal medullary lamina made of white matter fibers that separates a thalamus into three major groups: anterior, medial, and lateral nuclei.
- *Massa intermedia* (aka: interthalamic adhesion, intermediate mass): connects the medial nuclei of the thalami across midline, sometimes erroneously referred to as the "middle commissure."
- *Pulvinar*: posterior group of nuclei that are physically located with the lateral nuclei, but functionally distinct.

Metathalamus: ovoid nuclei on the posterior margin of a pulvinar (Fig 2.6a).

- Medial geniculate nucleus (aka: *medial geniculate body*): part of the auditory pathway.
- Lateral geniculate nucleus (aka: *lateral geniculate body*): part of the visual pathway.

Epithalamus: collection of structures between and posterior to the thalami that form the posterior wall of the third ventricle (Fig 2.6b).

- *Pineal gland* (aka: epiphysis, pineal body): midline ovoid endocrine gland that sits between the tectum and splenium; its name is derived from the Latin word for "pine cone" reflecting its shape. It often calcifies, a normal variant.
  - Pineal stalk: connects the pineal gland to the habenular and posterior commissures.
- *Habenula*: group of nuclei anterolateral to the pineal gland.
- *Posterior commissure*: fiber bundle that crosses midline situated between the cerebral aqueduct and the pineal gland.

Subthalamus (aka: prethalamus): nuclei below the thalamus.

Hypothalamus: several small, paired nuclei situated along the walls of the anteroinferior third ventricle.

  o *Tuber cinereum*: an inferior portion of the hypothalamus.
  - Median eminence: inferior conical projection of the tuber cinereum that connects to the pituitary stalk.
  o *Mammillary bodies*: paired mounds posterior to the tuber cinereum at the basal surface of the brain separated by the mammillary sulcus.

Pituitary gland (aka: hypophysis): endocrine gland extending inferiorly from the hypothalamus that sits on the pituitary fossa within the sella turcica of the sphenoid body at midline.

- *Anterior pituitary* (aka: anterior lobe, adenohypophysis): larger than the posterior pituitary, it is composed of the pars distalis, pars tuberalis, and pars intermedia.
- *Posterior pituitary* (aka: posterior lobe, neurohypophysis): an extension of the hypothalamus composed of the pars nervosa and infundibular stem.
- *Pituitary stalk* (aka: *infundibulum*): combination of the pars tuberalis of the anterior pituitary and infundibular stem of the posterior pituitary.

WHITE MATTER

Myelinated axons of the brain are generally categorized into three groups: projection fibers, commissures, and association fibers [10] (Fig. 2.7).

Projection fibers: connect deep brain structures, brainstem, or cerebellum to cortex.

- *Internal capsule*: a collection of projection fibers conceptually divided into five parts (Fig. 2.6a).

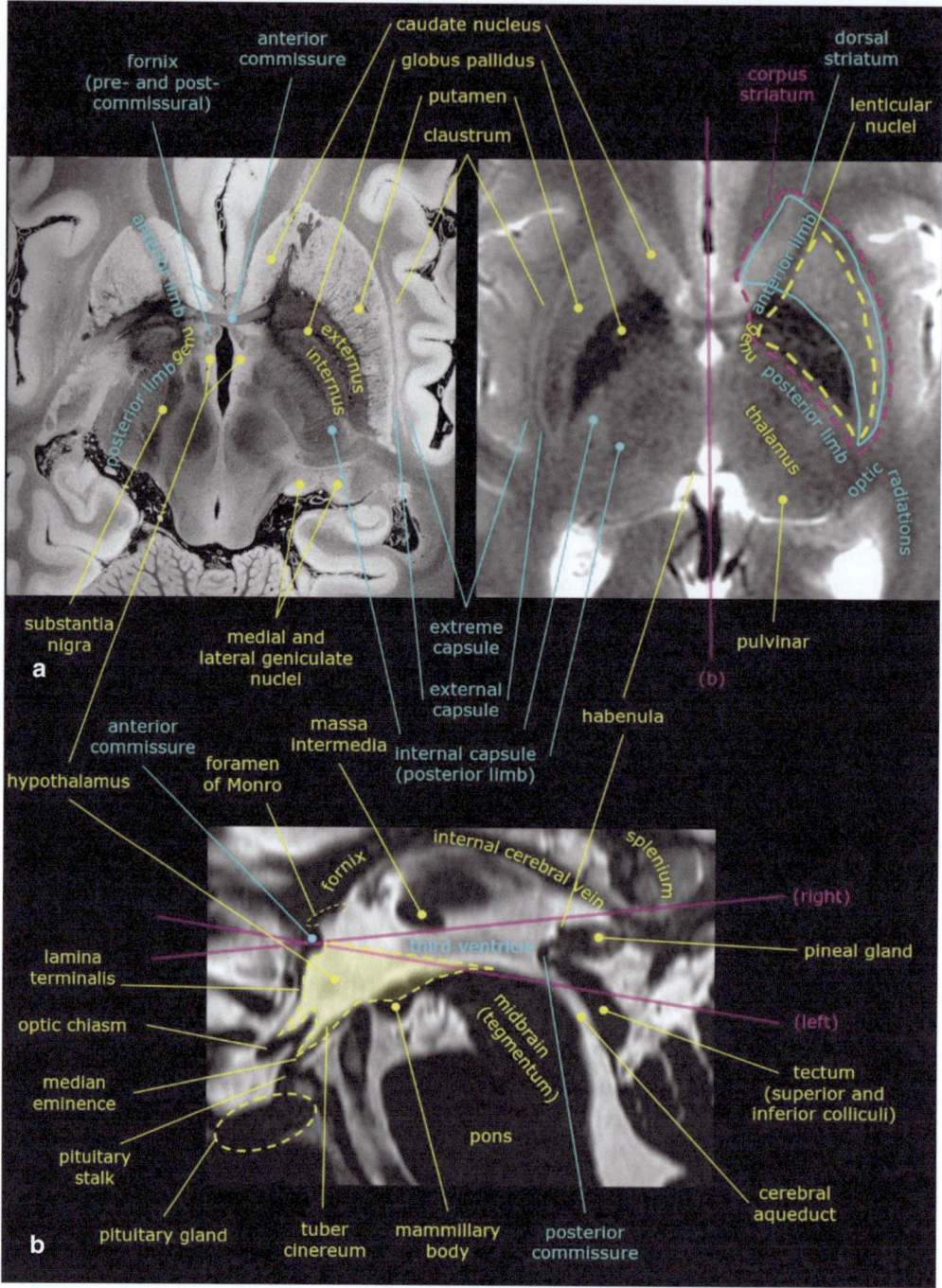

Fig. 2.6 The deep brain. (a) Paired T2 axial images through the basal ganglia at slightly different obliquities as designated by the solid magenta lines in image "**b**." The left image is an ex vivo specimen scanned at 7T providing 100-micron resolution [9] allowing for better visualization of deep brain structures. The right image is a typical T2 FSE acquired at 3T for comparison to clinical imaging. (**b**) A midline sagittal highly T2-weighted FIESTA demonstrates the deep brain structures between the basal ganglia situated around the third ventricle. The shaded yellow region represents the approximate location of paired hypothalamic nuclei in parasagittal planes

1. *Anterior limb* (aka: anterior crus, frontal part): separates a caudate head and lenticular nucleus.
2. *Genu*: in an axial cross section it appears as a bend between anterior and posterior limbs. "Genu" is Latin for "knee."
    - *Corticonuclear tract*: (aka: corticobulbar tract): motor fibers of the head and neck.
3. *Posterior limb* (aka: posterior crus, occipital part): separates a thalamus and globus pallidus.
    - *Corticospinal tract*: motor fibers of the trunk and extremities in the anterior aspect of the posterior limb.
    - Superior *thalamic radiations* (aka: thalamoparietal fibers): somatosensory fibers from dorsal thalami to parietal lobes.
4. *Retrolenticular part* (aka: retrolentiform part).
    - *Optic radiations* (aka: geniculocalcarine tract): connect lateral geniculate nuclei (LGN) to visual

Fig. 2.7 White Matter. Two axial and two coronal DTI color maps demonstrate major white matter tracts. Red areas represent tracts in a transverse orientation, green reflects fibers in an anterior-posterior alignment, and blue areas denote tracts in a superior-inferior direction. Each dashed magenta line indicates the imaging plane of the adjacent image

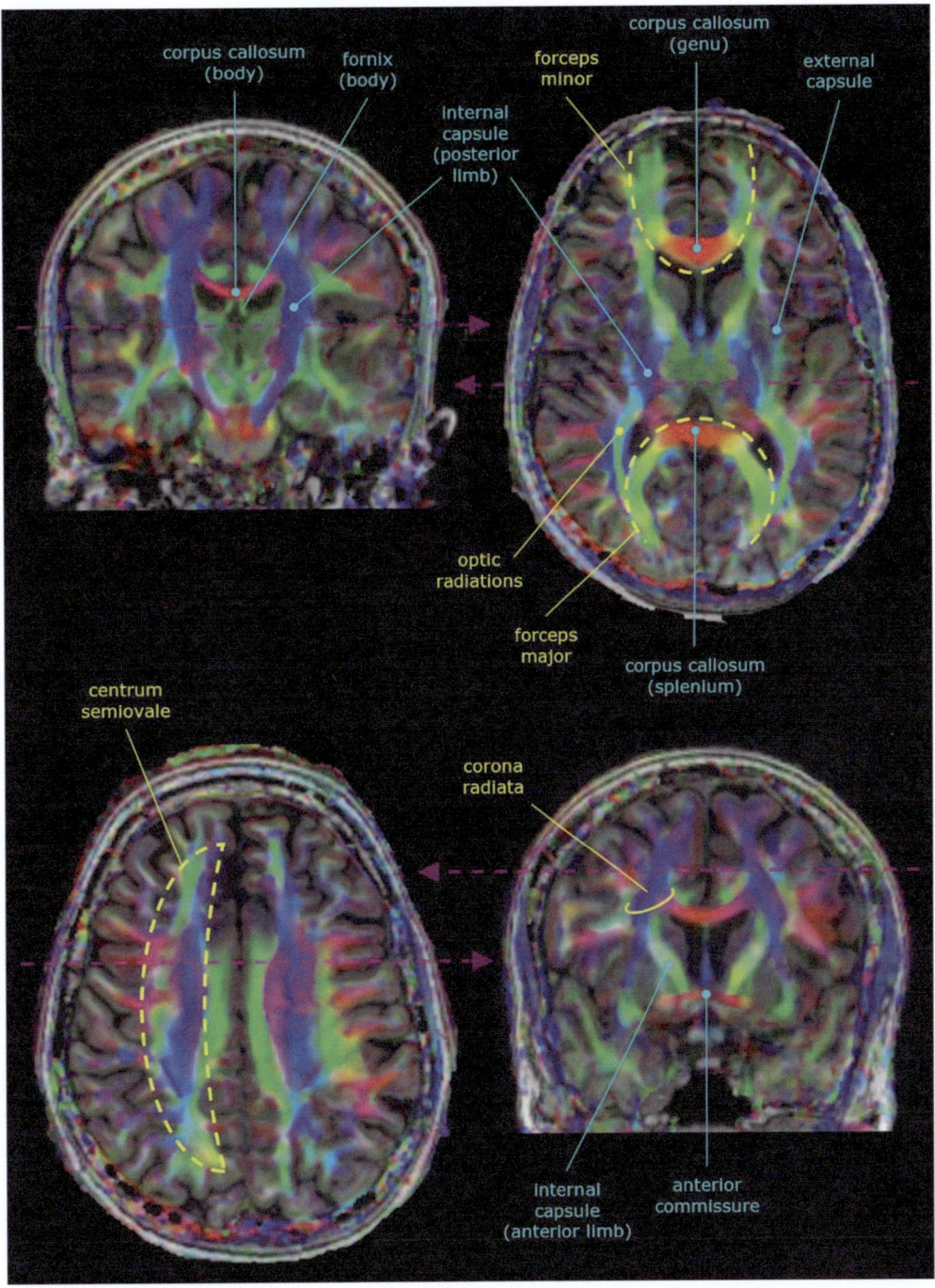

cortex in three horizontal bundles (Meyer's loops, central, and dorsal bundles) [11].
- Meyer's loops (aka: anterior bundle): the inferior-most bundle exit anterolaterally from the LGN passing over the temporal horns and meeting anterior commissure fibers before coursing posteriorly along the lateral margins of the temporal horns and occipital horns.
5. *Sublenticular part* (aka: sublentiform part).

  o *Auditory radiations* (aka: acoustic radiations): connect the medial geniculate nuclei to the transverse temporal gyri.
- *Fornix* (plural: fornices): a paired C-shaped fiber bundle (open-side down) that connects a hippocampus to a septal area, nucleus accumbens, hypothalamus, and thalamus (Figs. 2.5a, 2.6b, 2.7, 2.9a). Grossly, it has the appearance of terminating at a mammillary body of the hypothalamus. "Fornix" is Latin for "arch."

- *Crus* (aka: posterior column, posterior pillar): the white matter of a hippocampus (alveus) bundles medially to form the fimbria of a hippocampus, which becomes the vertical crus of a fornix as it leaves a hippocampal tail posteriorly. "Crus" is Latin for "leg."
- *Body*: the crura join superiorly to form the bodies of the fornices. The inferior margin of the septum pellucidum attaches to the superior aspect of the bodies (Fig. 2.5a).
- *Anterior columns* (aka: *anterior pillars*): the bodies then diverge as they turn downward forming the anterior columns, which further split into precommissural and postcommissural fibers on either side of the anterior commissure (Fig. 2.6a).

Commissures: fibers that traverse midline connecting brain regions in one hemisphere to their counterparts in the other hemisphere.

- *Corpus callosum*: the largest commissure is composed of five parts in a C-shaped configuration when viewed in a mid-sagittal cross section (Fig. 2.3b):
    - *Rostrum*: anteroinferior portion connects inferior frontal lobes.
    - *Genu*: anterior bend that connects the frontal lobes.
        - *Forceps minor* (aka: anterior forceps): U-shaped fibers, when viewed in an axial plane, which connect the frontal lobes through the genu (Fig. 2.7).
    - *Body* (aka: trunk): connects large portions of the cerebral cortex.
    - *Isthmus*: a slightly thinned mid-portion, it is often omitted and considered part of the body.
    - *Splenium*: thick posterior bend that connects the occipital lobes (Figs. 2.3b, 2.6b, 2.7, 2.9a).
        - *Forceps major* (aka: posterior forceps): U-shaped fibers, when viewed in an axial plane, which connect the occipital lobes through the splenium (Fig. 2.7).
- *Anterior commissure*: thin fiber bundle in the anterior wall of the third ventricle that passes through the globi pallidi connecting olfactory cortex and temporal lobes (Figs. 2.6 and 2.7).
- *Posterior commissure*: thin fiber bundle between the pineal stalk and cerebral aqueduct (see Ventricles) that connects nuclei of the thalami, habenulae, and tectum (see Brainstem).
- Commissure of the fornix (aka: hippocampal commissure, psalterium): as the crura of the fornices rise from the posterior hippocampi and approach each other, fibers cross midline forming a commissure connecting hippocampi.
- *Habenular commissure*: connects the habenulae, amygdalae, and hippocampi across midline [12]; may calcify as a normal variant.

Association fibers: connect brain regions within a hemisphere.

- Long-range:
    - Arcuate fasciculus: C-shaped fiber bundle that connects Broca's (inferior frontal gyrus), Geschwind's (inferior parietal lobule) and Wernicke's (superior temporal gyrus) speech areas.
    - Uncinate fasciculus: hook-shaped fiber bundle that connects an inferior frontal lobe to a mesial temporal lobe and temporal pole as part of the limbic system.
    - External capsule: inferiorly contains uncinate and inferior longitudinal fasciculi, superiorly connects the claustrum with frontal and parietal cortices.
    - Extreme capsule: connects an insula primarily to a parietal lobe [10].
- Short-range.
    - U-fibers (aka: arcuate fibers): connect adjacent gyri immediately below cortical gray matter.

Other White Matter Terminology

- *Corona radiata*: a crown-like structure formed by projection fibers of the internal capsules extending above the basal ganglia, intermixing with commissural fibers of the corpus callosum, and dispersing toward cortical destinations (Fig. 2.7).
- *Centrum semiovale*: the central masses of white matter seen in an axial cross section superior to the corpus callosum, which have shapes reminiscent of a parenthesis in each hemisphere. It is formed by fibers of the corona radiata extending to frontal, parietal, and/or occipital cortices depending on the angle of the chosen axial plane.
- *Anterior commissure-posterior commissure line* (aka: AC-PC line, bicommissural line): the imaginary line that crosses through the anterior and posterior commissures in a mid-sagittal plane is regarded as the standard axial plane for CT and MR neuroimaging.

VENTRICLES

Four CSF-filled cavities that are lined with ependymal cells and contain choroid plexus (Fig. 2.8).

- *Choroid plexus*: specialized ependymal cells that produce CSF.
- Tela choroidea: double layer of pia mater adherent to ependyma from which choroid plexus arises. It is present in the lateral ventricle bodies, in the atria, temporal horns, roof of the third ventricle, lower roof of the fourth ventricle, and the foramina of Luschka. "Tela" is Latin for "web."

Lateral ventricles: the two largest ventricles extend into all four of the major cerebral lobes.

- *Frontal horn* (aka: anterior horn): extends toward a frontal lobe medial to a caudate head (Fig. 2.5a).
- *Body*: courses over a thalamus in a paramedian plane within frontal and parietal lobes.
  - *Septum pellucidum*: double-layer membrane that separates the bodies of the lateral ventricles in the midsagittal plane. It attaches to the rostrum, genu, and body of the corpus callosum superiorly and the fornical bodies inferiorly.
- *Temporal horn* (aka: inferior horn): courses within a temporal lobe superolateral to a hippocampus (Fig. 2.8).
  - Uncal recess: a medial outpouching of the temporal horn at its anterior end that separates a hippocampal head and amygdala.
  - *Choroidal fissure* (aka: choroid fissure): C-shaped fissure is the site of tela choroidea attachment along the medial margin of a temporal horn (between a hippocampal fimbria and a stria terminalis), and between a fornix and thalamus on the floor of a lateral ventricle.
- *Occipital horn* (aka: posterior horn): courses within the occipital lobe deep to its calcarine fissure.
- *Atrium* (aka: *trigone*): where the lateral ventricle body, temporal horn, and occipital horn meet. "Trigone" is Greek for "triangle."
- *Foramen of Monro* (aka: interventricular foramen): paired channels that connect the lateral ventricle frontal horns/bodies to the superior third ventricle behind the anterior commissure (Figs. 2.6b and 2.8).

Third ventricle: thin midline ventricle between the thalami, hypothalamus, midbrain, and fornical bodies (Figs. 2.6b and 2.8).

- Anterior wall: anterior fornical columns, anterior commissure, and lamina terminalis.
  - *Lamina terminalis*: thin membrane between the anterior commissure and optic chiasm (see Cranial Nerves).
- Floor: tuber cinereum, mammillary bodies, posterior perforated substance, and tegmentum (of the midbrain).
  - Posterior perforated substance: thin triangular strip of gray matter posterior to the mammillary bodies that forms the roof of the interpeduncular cistern (see Cisterns). It is perforated by small branches of the posterior cerebral arteries that supply the thalami.
- Posterior wall: epithalamus (see Deep Brain).
- Roof:
  - Velum interpositum: tela choroidea encasing the internal cerebral veins (see Veins).
- Lateral walls: the thalami and hypothalamus.
  - Hypothalamic sulcus: horizontal groove in the lateral walls of the third ventricle that marks the dorsal margin of the hypothalamus.
- Recesses: small hollow ventricular protrusions.
  - Supraoptic recess (aka: optic recess, preoptic recess, chiasmatic recess): a spade-shaped recess pointing anteroinferior toward the optic chiasm.
  - *Infundibular recess*: conical recess pointing anteroinferior toward the pituitary stalk.
  - Pineal recess: tiny triangular recess between the posterior and habenular commissures that points toward the pineal gland.
  - Suprapineal recess: above the habenula and pineal gland.
- *Cerebral aqueduct* (aka: *aqueduct of Sylvius*): slender tunnel that passes through the dorsal midbrain connecting the third and fourth ventricles.

Fourth ventricle: a midline ventricle between the brainstem and cerebellum.

- *Foramen of Magendie* (aka: median aperture): tapering midline channel opens inferiorly to the cisterna magna (see Cisterns).
- *Foramina of Luschka* (aka: lateral apertures): tapering channels directed ventrolaterally that open to the cerebellopontine cisterns.
- Roof: the dorsal walls of the ventricle.
  - Superior medullary velum (aka: anterior medullary velum): a white matter membrane lined by pia mater dorsally and ependyma ventrally suspended between the superior cerebellar peduncles that forms the upper half of the roof.
  - Inferior medullary velum (aka: posterior medullary velum): a white matter membrane lined by tela choroidea that forms the lower half of the roof in combination with the teniae.
  - Fastigium: most dorsal point of the midline roof. "Fastigium" is Latin for "summit" (Fig. 2.9a).
- Floor: the ventral wall of the ventricle, formed by the dorsal pons and medulla.
  - *Obex*: inferior-most point that empties into the central canal of spinal cord.
- Lateral walls: superior, middle, and inferior cerebellar peduncles (see Cerebellum).

BRAINSTEM

Composed of the midbrain, pons, and medulla oblongata, the brainstem connects the cerebrum, cerebellum, and spinal cord, and is the site of many white matter tracts and nuclei

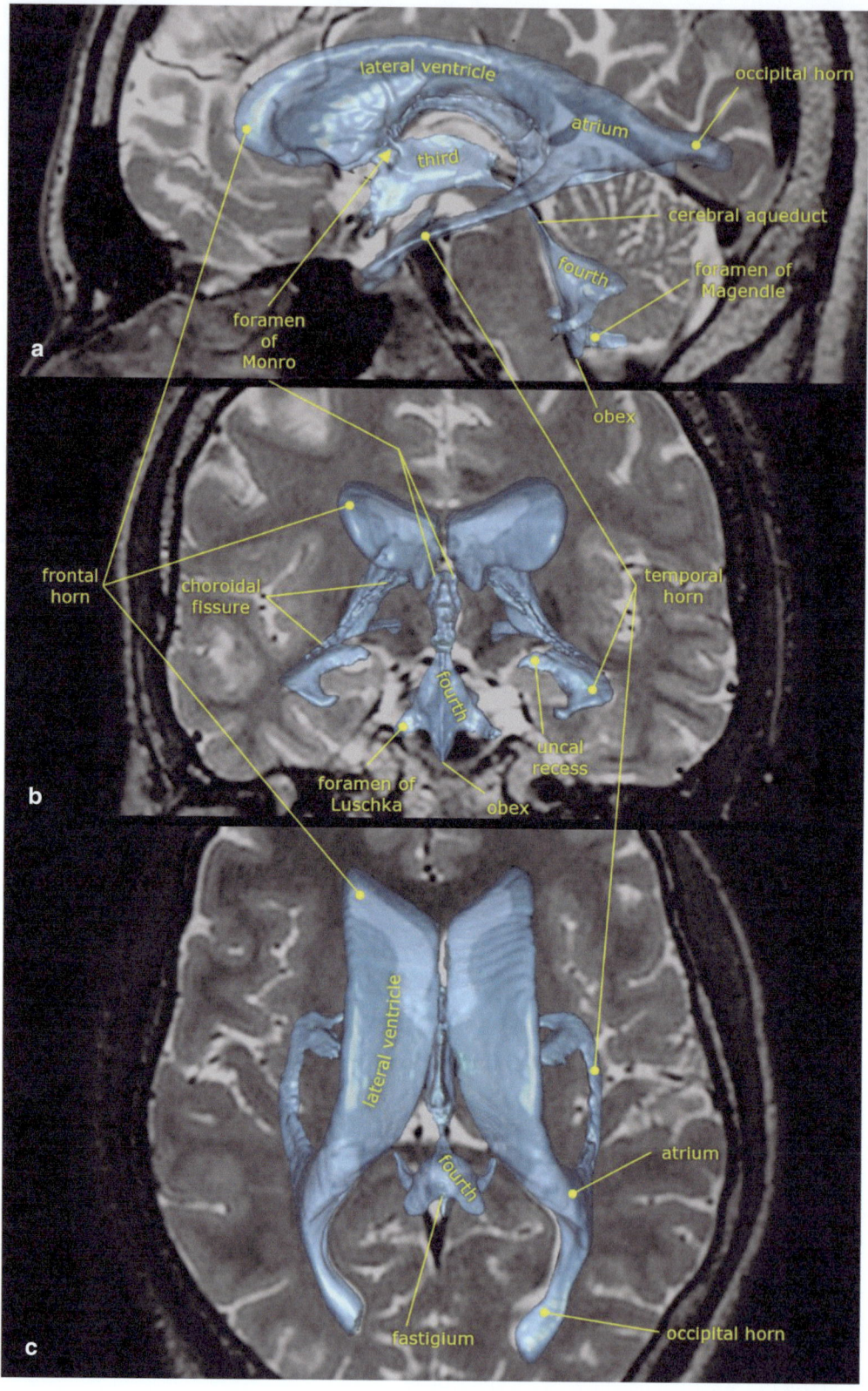

Fig. 2.8 Cerebral ventricles. (**a**) Left lateral, (**b**) anterior, and (**c**) superior orthogonal views of a 3D rendering of the ventricular system overlaid on sagittal, coronal, and axial T2 cross-sectional images, respectively. The left-right convention of image "**c**" is reversed to show a superior view

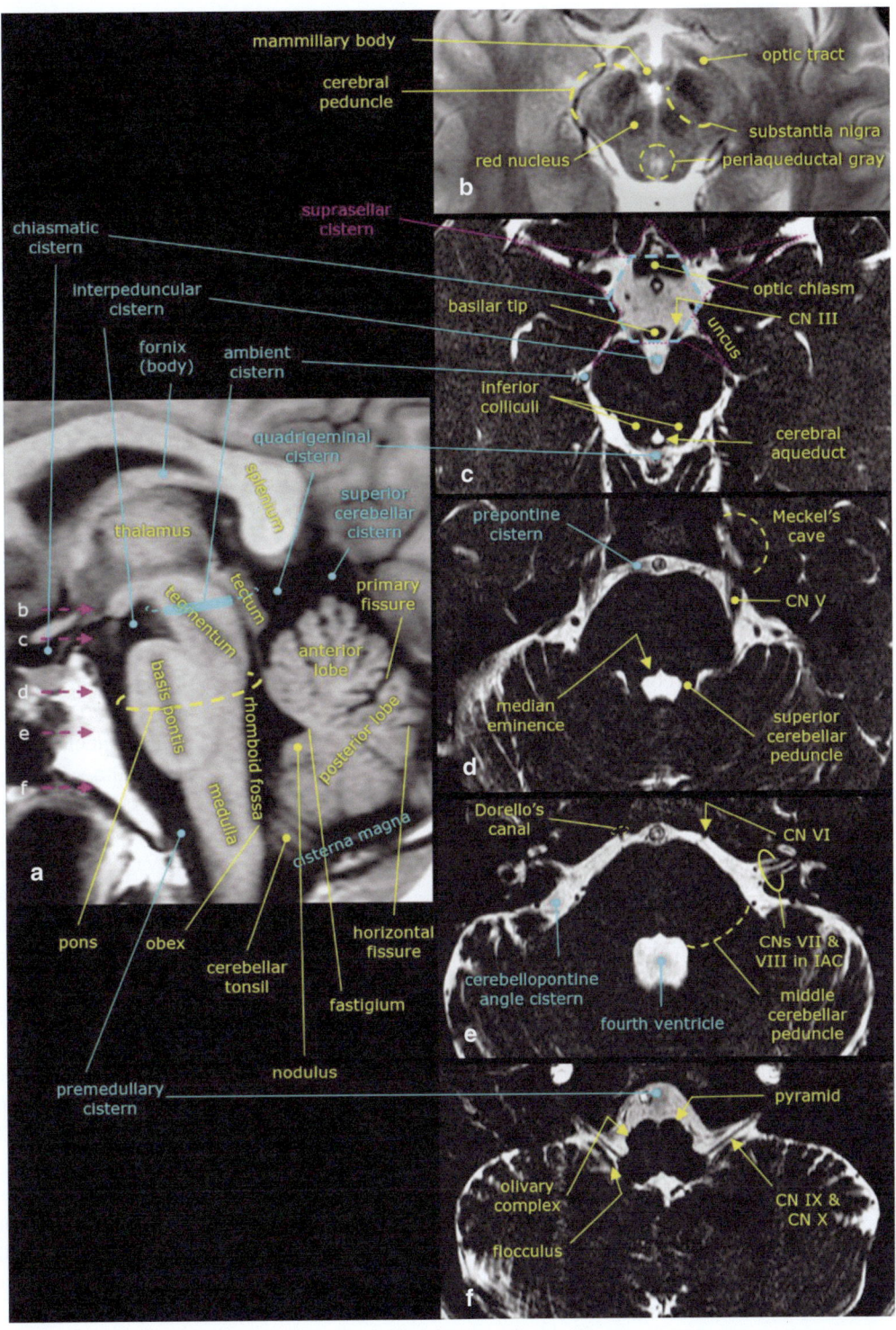

Fig. 2.9 The brainstem, cerebellum, cisterns, and cranial nerves. (**a**) T1 FSE midline sagittal image of the brainstem and cerebellum with dashed magenta lines indicating the levels of five T2-weighted FIESTA axial images (**b–f**)

(Fig. 2.9), including the nuclei for 9 of the 12 paired cranial nerves (CNs).

Midbrain: the most superior part of the brainstem, it contains nuclei for CNs III-V.

- *Cerebral peduncles* (aka: *crus cerebri*, pes pedunculi): large paired vertical fiber bundles form the ventral surfaces of the midbrain; they are the inferior continuation of the corticospinal and corticonuclear tracts (in the middle 3/5ths of the peduncles), as well as corticopontine tracts of the internal capsule.
- Midbrain *tegmentum*: portion between the cerebral peduncles ventrally and cerebral aqueduct dorsally.
  - *Substantia nigra*: largest midbrain nucleus, each composed of two parts.

- Pars reticulata: reddish iron-containing ventrolateral strip.
- Pars compacta: dark neuromelanin-containing dorsomedial strip.
  - *Red nucleus*: large round nucleus is an important part of the extrapyramidal (involuntary motor) system.
  - *Periaqueductal gray matter* (aka: central gray matter): roughly cylindrical column of gray matter surrounding the cerebral aqueduct.
  - Oculomotor and Edinger-Westphal nuclei (CN III): ventral to the periaqueductal gray in the upper midbrain.
  - Trochlear nuclei (CN IV): inferior to oculomotor nuclei.
  - Mesencephalic nuclei of the trigeminal nerves (CN V): one of three CN V sensory nuclei, lateral to the periaqueductal gray, extends to upper pons.
  - Decussation of the superior cerebellar peduncles: dorsomedial to the substantiae nigrae at midline in the lower midbrain and upper pons.
- *Tectum* (aka: *quadrigeminal plate*): portion of the midbrain dorsal to the cerebral aqueduct composed of four colliculi (singular: colliculus). "Tectum" is Latin for "to cover."
  - *Superior colliculi*: paired mounds are part of the vision pathway.
  - *Inferior colliculi*: paired mounds are part of the auditory pathway.
- Basis pedunculi: comprises the cerebral peduncles and substantiae nigrae.
- *Superior cerebellar peduncles* (aka: brachium conjunctivum): white matter bundles that connect the cerebellum and midbrain.
- *Interpeduncular fossa*: the surfaces of the basal brain bound by the optic tracts and chiasm anteriorly and cerebral peduncles and basis pontis posteriorly.
- Pontomesencephalic junction: describes where the midbrain and pons meet; CN IV leaves the brainstem at this level.

Pons: the middle section of the brainstem; it contains nuclei for CNs V-VIII. "Pons" is Latin for "bridge."

- *Basis pontis* (aka: *basilar pons*): the rotund ventral pons, it contains descending tracts from the cerebral peduncles as well as transverse fibers of the middle cerebellar peduncles.
- Pontine tegmentum: the portions of the pons dorsal to the basis pontis.
  - Motor trigeminal nuclei (CN V): ventral to the superior cerebellar peduncles at the level of the mid-pons.
  - Main/chief/principal/pontine sensory trigeminal nuclei (CN V): lateral to the motor trigeminal nuclei.
  - Rhomboid fossa: a depressed roughly diamond-shaped surface of the dorsal pons and medulla that forms the floor (ventral surface) of the fourth ventricle.
    - Median sulcus: vertically bisects the rhomboid fossa.
    - Median eminences: vertical ridges to each side of the upper median sulcus. Distinct from the median eminence of the tuber cinereum (see Hypothalamus).
    - Facial colliculi: mounds at the caudal ends of the median eminences with underlying abducent nuclei (CNs VI) and, more ventrally, facial nuclei (CNs VII).
    - Vestibular areas (aka: area acustica): triangular surfaces lateral and inferolateral to the facial colliculi with underlying vestibular nuclei (CN VIII) and more ventral spinal trigeminal nuclei (CN V, sensory), both of which extend caudally into the medulla.
    - Hypoglossal trigones: thin triangular ridges on each side of the lower median sulcus with underlying hypoglossal nuclei (CN XII).
    - Vagal trigones: thin triangular ridges lateral to the hypoglossal trigones with underlying dorsal vagal nuclei (CN X) and much more ventral nucleus ambiguus (CNs IX and X).
    - Solitary nuclei (CNs VII, IX, X): immediately lateral to the vagal trigones, with functions related to taste, chemoreceptors, and mechanoreceptors.
    - Cochlear nuclear complexes (CN VIII): lateral to the vagal trigones and solitary nuclei at the level of the foramina of Luschka.
- *Middle cerebellar peduncles* (aka: *brachium pontis*): thick white matter bundles that connect the pons to the cerebellum.
- Pontomedullary junction: describes where the pons and medulla meet.

Medulla oblongata: the most inferior part of the brainstem, it contains nuclei for CNs VII-X, and XII).

- *Medullary pyramids*: contain the descending corticospinal and corticonuclear tracts on the ventromedial surface.
- Anterior median fissure (aka: ventral median fissure): vertically bisects the pyramids on the ventral surface.
- Anterolateral sulcus (aka: ventrolateral sulcus, pre-olivary sulcus): separates a pyramid from a more lateral olivary complex; CNs XII exit the brainstem here.
- Olivary complexes (aka: olivary bodies, *olives*): ovoid bulges on the ventrolateral surface of the upper medulla with underlying olivary nuclei.
- Post-olivary sulcus: demarcates the lateral margin of an olive; CNs IX and X exit here.
- Medullary tegmentum: the medulla dorsal to the pyramidal tracts and olivary complexes.

- Posterior median sulcus (aka: dorsal median sulcus): bisects the dorsal surface of the medulla.
- Gracile fasciculus: tract that communicates sensation from the lower body.
  - Gracile tubercles: the gracile nuclei underlie these bulges at the upper extent of the gracile fasciculi.
- Posterolateral sulci: form the lateral margin of the gracile fasciculi.
- Cuneate fasciculus: tract that communicates sensation from the upper body.
  - Cuneate tubercles: the cuneate nuclei underlie these bulges at the upper extent of the cuneate fasciculi.
- Pyramidal decussation (aka: motor decussation): descending corticospinal tracts decussate at the caudal ventral medulla.
- Inferior cerebellar peduncles: white matter bundles that connect the cerebellum and medulla.
- Cervicomedullary junction: the border between the medulla and spinal cord, generally thought of as below the pyramidal decussation or at the level of the foramen magnum.

Key Brainstem Tracts

- Pyramidal tracts: comprise the corticospinal and corticonuclear motor tracts. Cerebral peduncles → basis pontis → medullary pyramids.
- Dorsal column-medial lemniscus pathway: communicate fine touch, vibration, and proprioception. Fibers ascending from the gracile and cuneate nuclei in the dorsal medulla decussate and ascend dorsal to the pyramidal tracts in the ventral medulla. In the pons, they ascend dorsally and move dorsolateral in the midbrain until reaching the thalami.
- Spinothalamic tracts: communicate pain, temperature, pressure, and coarse touch sensations. In the medulla these tracts ascend in the ventrolateral cord, lateral to the pyramidal tracts and olives. In the pons, they ascend dorsally joining the medical lemnisci, and move dorsolateral in the midbrain until reaching the thalami.

CEREBELLUM

- Cerebellum is Latin for "little brain."
- It is located within the posterior fossa, separated from the temporal and occipital lobes by the overlying tentorium, and posterior to the brainstem centered at the level of the pons (Fig. 2.9).
- Its most established role is to coordinate motor activity.
- The cerebellum can be thought of as a large cellular sheet regularly folded in a fashion comparable to the bellows of an accordion, but far more extensively, and opened 360° in a mid-sagittal plane.
- Vermis: the midline region of the cerebellum that bridges the left and right cerebellar hemispheres (Fig. 2.3b).

Vermis and hemispheres: divided by eight named fissures into three lobes (anterior, posterior, and flocculonodular) and several named lobules.

- Flocculonodular lobe: the medial component is the nodulus (aka: nodule, Fig. 2.9a) and the lateral component is the flocculus (Fig. 2.9f).
- Primary fissure (aka: tentorial fissure): separates the anterior and posterior lobes.
- Horizontal fissure (aka: petrous fissure, intercrural fissure): nearly encircles the cerebellum like an equator.
- Posterolateral fissure (aka: dorsolateral fissure, uvulonodular fissure): separates the posterior and flocculonodular lobes.
- Folium (plural: folia): each lobule is composed of many thin folia; the cerebellar analog of cerebral gyri.
- Arbor vitae: the bulk of white matter underlying the cerebellar cortex, named for its tree-like branching appearance when seen in a coronal cross section (Fig. 2.2b, unlabeled).

Nuclei: there are four pairs of cerebellar nuclei encompassed by cerebellar white matter located slightly dorsal to the fastigium, listed from paramedian to lateral: fastigial, globose, emboliform, dentate.

- Dentate nuclei: the largest and most lateral of the cerebellar nuclei have a crescent shape when viewed in an axial cross section and are generally the only visible cerebellar nuclei on MR.

Other Cerebellar Terminology

- Cerebellopontine angle: the horizontal fissure nearly encircles the cerebellum like an equator. As it wraps around the ventral surface it encounters the middle cerebellar peduncles and splits above and below them forming the superior and inferior limbs of the V-shaped cerebellopontine fissures, which define the cerebellopontine angles.
- Paravermis (aka: intermediate hemisphere): paramedian regions lateral to the vermis.

CISTERNS

The cisterns are dilated CSF-filled subarachnoid spaces (Fig. 2.9).

- Paramesencephalic cisterns: spaces surrounding the midbrain.
  - *Interpeduncular cistern* (aka: basal cistern): between the cerebral peduncles (*interpeduncular fossa*), below the floor of the third ventricle, and above the basis pontis. The term "basal cistern" refers to its relationship to the basis peduculi and basis pontis (see Brainstem).
  - *Ambient cisterns* (aka: circummesencephalic cistern): lateral to the cerebral peduncles and midbrain tegmentum.
    - *Crural cisterns*: this term may be used to refer to the spaces between the cerebral peduncles and opposing mesial temporal lobes, in which case the term "ambient cisterns" refers to the CSF spaces lateral to the midbrain tegmentum.
  - *Quadrigeminal cistern*: dorsal to the quadrigeminal plate and extending over the cerebellum.
    - Cerebellomesencephalic cistern: tiny cistern between the midbrain and cerebellum, more specifically between superior cerebellar peduncles and the central lobule of the vermis.
- *Superior cerebellar cistern* (aka: superior cistern): between the cerebellum and tentorium, posterior to the tentorial apex.
- *Suprasellar cistern* (aka pentagonal cistern, Fig. 2.9c): shaped like a 5-pointed star in an axial plane, it is composed of the chiasmatic cistern centrally with the Sylvian cisterns, ambient cisterns, and interhemispheric fissure forming the 5 points.
  - *Chiasmatic cistern*: above the sella turcica and below the floor of the third ventricle, when viewed in an axial plane it forms a hexagonal shape bounded by the tuberculum sellae anteriorly, interpeduncular cistern posteriorly, unci posterolaterally, and carotid cisterns anterolaterally.
  - The *MCA cistern* leading to the *Sylvian cistern* or insular cistern): deep extensions of the Sylvian fissures containing the proximal middle cerebral arteries.
- Pontomedullary cistern: ventral to the pons and medulla.
  - *Prepontine cistern* (aka: pontine cistern): ventral to the pons.
  - *Premedullary cistern* (aka: medullary cistern): ventral to the medulla.
- *Cerebellopontine angle cisterns* (aka: cerebellopontine cistern): between the cerebellopontine angles and petrous bones.
- *Cisterna magna* (aka: posterior cerebellomedullary cistern, cerebellomedullary cistern): dorsal to the medulla and caudal to the cerebellum, above the foramen magnum.
- *Basal cisterns*: a somewhat ambiguous term, it is sometimes meant as a synonym for all cisterns, perhaps with the exceptions of the pericallosal, lamina terminalis, and velum interpositum cisterns. Clinically, the term is often used to communicate the presence or absence of mass effect or herniation at the tentorial incisura. In this context, the meaning resembles the definition of the paramesencephalic cisterns given above.
- Internal arachnoid membranes: thin sheets of connective tissue in the subarachnoid spaces that partially separate cisterns but allow for CSF flow between compartments. Typically, not visible expect on high-resolution T2 sequences.
  - Liliequist membrane: the most well-known of the arachnoid membranes, it separates the chiasmatic, interpeduncular, and prepontine cisterns. When viewed in a midline sagittal plane it is somewhat Y-shaped stretching between the dorsum sellae, mammillary bodies, and pontomesencephalic junctions [13].

CRANIAL NERVES

Twelve paired nerves that arise directly from the cerebrum or brainstem and pass through skull base foramina (Fig. 2.9). The descriptions below will focus on the anatomical path of these nerves to aid in imaging evaluation when symptoms are attributable to a cranial nerve.

CN I—*olfactory nerve*: sensory nerve for olfaction. Components:

- *Olfactory filaments*: first-order neurons reside in the nasal mucosa, their axons bundle into filaments and cross the cribriform plate to the olfactory bulb.
- *Olfactory bulb*: second-order neurons reside in the bulbous end of the olfactory tract.
- *Olfactory tract*: formed by second-order neuronal axons, which extend posteriorly between an olfactory groove (anterior cranial fossa) and olfactory sulcus (inferior frontal lobe).

Olfactory pathway: nasal mucosa → cribriform plate → olfactory bulb and tract → olfactory cortex (septal area, piriform cortex, entorhinal cortex, and parts of the amygdala).

CN II—*optic nerve*: sensory nerve for vision.

- *Optic nerve segments*: intraocular (optic nerve head), intraorbital, intracanalicular (within optic canal), intracranial.
- *Optic nerve sheath*: CSF-filled meninges surrounding the optic nerves.
- *Optic chiasm*: where the medial fibers in each optic nerve decussate (Figs. 2.6b and 2.9c).
- *Optic tracts*: continuation of optic nerve fibers posterior to the chiasm (Fig. 2.9b).

Vision pathway: retinal neurons → optic nerve (orbit, optic canal, and chiasmatic cistern) → optic chiasm → optic tracts (crural cisterns) → lateral geniculate nucleus → optic radiations (including Meyer's loops) along lateral occipital horns → primary visual cortex (posteromedial occipital lobes).

AND retina → CN II → superior colliculus → pulvinar → secondary visual cortex (much of the remainder of the occipital lobes).

CN III—*oculomotor nerve*: a motor nerve, it partially controls eye movement by innervating the superior/inferior/medial recti, levator palpebrae superioris, inferior oblique, ciliary and sphincter pupillae muscles (Fig. 2.9c).

Pathway: midbrain nuclei (paramedian and ventral to the periaqueductal gray) → exits brainstem at interpeduncular cistern → courses between PCA and SCA arteries (see Arteries) → cavernous sinus (superolateral wall) → superior orbital fissure → eye muscles.

CN IV—*trochlear nerve*: motor nerve, it partially controls eye movement by innervating the superior oblique muscle. "Trochlea" is Greek for "pulley" referring to the cartilaginous loops that the muscle passes through. Typically, it is not visible by MRI.

- It is the only cranial nerve to arise from the dorsal brainstem, and the only cranial nerve to cross midline.

Pathway: midbrain nucleus (caudal to CN III nuclei) → crosses midline and exits brainstem caudal to inferior colliculi → ambient and prepontine cisterns → cavernous sinus (lateral wall) → superior orbital fissure → superior oblique muscle.

CN V—*trigeminal nerve*: sensory and motor nerve, it provides facial sensation and innervates the muscles of mastication (Fig. 2.9d).

Common Sensory Pathway: *3 sensory divisions* (as below) → merge at trigeminal ganglion to form CN V sensory root (in Meckel's cave) → pre-pontine cistern → enter brainstem at lateral pons → several dorsal brainstem nuclei (from caudal midbrain through medulla).

Motor Pathway: nucleus in dorsal pons → exits brainstem at lateral pons → pre-pontine cistern → Meckel's cave (bypasses trigeminal ganglion) → foramen ovale → joins V$_3$ at infratemporal fossa → muscles of mastication.

Three sensory divisions of the trigeminal nerve:

- **CN V$_1$—*ophthalmic nerve***: sensation of upper face (frontal scalp, forehead, upper eyelids, eyes, midline nose), paranasal sinuses and nasal cavity mucosa.
  ○ Pathway: three branches from orbit (frontal, lacrimal, and nasociliary nerves) → superior orbital fissure → merge to CN V$_1$ → cavernous sinus (lateral wall) → trigeminal ganglion → (continue as above).

- **CN V$_2$—*maxillary nerve***: sensation of middle face (lower eyelids, cheeks, lateral nose, temples, upper lip, maxillary teeth).
  ○ Pathway: many branches from orbit, nasal cavity, and oral cavity (zygomatic, infraorbital, nasopalatine, pharyngeal, and greater/lesser palatine nerves) → pterygopalatine fossa → merge to CN V$_2$ → foramen rotundum → cavernous sinus (inferolateral wall) → trigeminal ganglion → (continue as above).

- **CN V$_3$—*mandibular nerve***: sensation of lower face (chin, jawline, pre-/supra-auricular skin, oral mucosa, mandibular teeth, tongue sensation, temporomandibular joint), and muscles of mastication plus a few additional muscles of the head and neck.
  ○ Pathway: many branches from infratemporal fossa → foramen ovale → trigeminal ganglion → (continue as above).

CN VI—*abducens nerve*: motor nerve, it partially controls eye movement by innervating the lateral rectus muscle (Fig. 2.9e).

Pathway: dorsal pons (nucleus underlies a facial colliculus in the rhomboid fossa) → exits at ventral pontomedullary junction → pre-pontine cistern → Dorello's canal → cavernous sinus (inferolateral to ICA) → superior orbital fissure → lateral rectus muscle.

CN VII—*facial nerve*: sensory and motor nerve, it is responsible for taste (anterior 2/3rds of the tongue), sensation (skin of ear canal, parts of the ear, and retro-auricular skin), and innervates the muscles of facial expression and additional head and neck muscles. It also has secretomotor function involving mucous membranes of palate, as well as lacrimal, submandibular, and sublingual glands.

- *Facial nerve segments*: cisternal (aka: pontine), canalicular (aka: meatal, in IAC), labyrinthine, first genu (geniculate ganglion), tympanic (aka: horizontal), second genu, mastoid (aka: vertical), extratemporal.

Motor Pathway: nuclei in dorsal pons → exit brainstem at ventrolateral pontomedullary junction → cerebellopontine angle cistern → IAC → geniculate ganglion → temporal bone (beneath lateral semicircular canal and through mastoid) → stylomastoid foramen → several branches into the face.

CN VIII—*vestibulocochlear nerve*: sensory nerve, responsible for hearing (cochlear nerve) and balance (vestibular nerve).

Vestibular Pathway: vestibular apparatus (vestibular nerve) → merges with cochlear nerve in IAC to CN VIII → cerebellopontine angle cistern → enter brainstem at ventrolateral pontomedullary junction (lateral to CN VII) → vestibular nuclei in caudal dorsal pons and rostral dorsal medulla → many connections to other regions of brainstem, spinal cord, and cerebellum.

Auditory Pathway: cochlea (cochlear nerve) → merges with vestibular nerve in IAC to CN VIII → cerebellopontine angle cistern → enter brainstem at ventrolateral pontomedullary junction → cochlear nuclei in dorsolateral rostral medulla → olive → inferior colliculus → medial geniculate → auditory cortex (superior temporal gyrus).

CN IX—*glossopharyngeal nerve*: sensory and motor nerve, responsible for taste (posterior 1/3rd of tongue), sensation (tongue and throat), and innervates pharyngeal muscles, as well as secretomotor function involving the parotid glands.

Sensory Pathway: several branches at skull base → merge to CN IX → jugular foramen (pars nervosa) → lateral cerebellomedullary cistern → enters brainstem at lateral medulla posterior to an olive → nuclei in central and dorsolateral rostral medulla.

CN X—*vagus nerve*: sensory and motor nerve, responsible for taste (tongue root and epiglottis), sensation (larynx, pharynx, thoracoabdominal organs), and innervates some muscles of the tongue, pharynx and larynx, and thoracoabdominal organs.

Pathway: nuclei in central and dorsal medulla → exits brainstem dorsal to olive → lateral cerebellomedullary cistern → jugular foramen (pars nervosa) → branches at skull base.

CN XI—*spinal accessory nerve*: a motor nerve, it innervates sternocleidomastoid and trapezius muscles.

Pathway: anterior horns of upper and mid-cervical spinal cord → exits lateral cervical spinal cord as multiple rootlets → ascends and merges to CN XI → foramen magnum → jugular foramen (pars nervosa) → branches into neck.

CN XII—*hypoglossal nerve*: motor nerve, it innervates the tongue muscles except the palatoglossus muscles.

Pathway: nucleus in the paramedian dorsal medulla beneath a vagal trigone → exits medulla between pyramids and olives as several rootlets → merge to CN XII in premedullary cistern → hypoglossal canal of occipital bone.

ARTERIES, VEINS, AND DURAL VENOUS SINUSES

- The arteries of the head are divided into extracranial vessels and intracranial vessels.
- There are many variations in the origins, branching patterns, course, and vascular territory of arterial branches. The descriptions below are typical.
- The intracranial arterial system is divided into anterior and posterior circulations (Fig. 2.10).
- The anterior circulation is composed of the internal cerebral arteries and their branches, together supplying most of the brain.

Arteries: *Anterior Circulation*

Internal cerebral artery (**ICA**): originates at the bifurcation of a common carotid artery near the angle of a hemimandible, it is typically described in seven segments (C1–C7), but with many variations in labeling schemes.

Segments and branches:

- Cervical (C1, aka: vertical): the only extracranial segment, it ascends to the skull base.
- Petrous (C2, aka: horizontal): within the carotid canal of the petrous part of a temporal bone, the intracranial ICA starts at this segment.
- Lacerum (C3): sometimes omitted from the ICA labeling scheme, it is above the foramen lacerum.
- Transitional (C3–C4): often omitted from the ICA labeling scheme.
- Cavernous (C4): within a cavernous sinus.
  ○ Meningohypophyseal trunk (aka: posterior trunk): branches posteromedially near the dorsum sellae, typically not visible on CTA/MRA.
    - Branches include the dorsal meningeal artery (aka: lateral tentorial artery), tentorial artery (aka: marginal/medial tentorial artery, artery of Bernasconi and Cassinari, Italian artery), and inferior hypophyseal artery, which supply the clival dura, tentorium, and CNs III, IV, and VI.
  ○ Inferolateral trunk: branches laterally supplying CN V_2.
- Clinoid (C5, aka: paraclinoid): near the anterior clinoid process of the lesser sphenoid wing.
- Ophthalmic (C6): the first intradural segment.
  ○ Ophthalmic artery: it extends anteriorly passing through an optic canal to supply an orbit including its globe. The origin is typically visible on CTA/MRA.
  ○ Superior hypophyseal artery: extends medially supplying the pituitary gland and stalk, median eminence, and optic nerve and chiasm.
- Terminal (C7, aka: communicating): begins at the posterior communicating artery and ends at the bifurcation of an ICA into anterior and middle cerebral arteries.
  ○ Posterior communicating artery (PCOM): extends posteriorly to anastomose with the posterior circulation as part of the circle of Willis (see below). It has many miniscule perforators that supply the optic chiasm and tract, posterior hypothalamus including mammillary bodies, anterior thalamus (anterior thalamoperforating arteries), and anterior optic radiations.

Fig. 2.10 The intracranial arteries. (**a**) Anteroinferior view, (**b**) left lateral view of an MRA MPR with the MCAs and C1–C3 segments of the ICA removed on the lateral view, and (**c**) a CTA MPR with the calvarium and brain removed for a superior view of the circle of Willis in situ

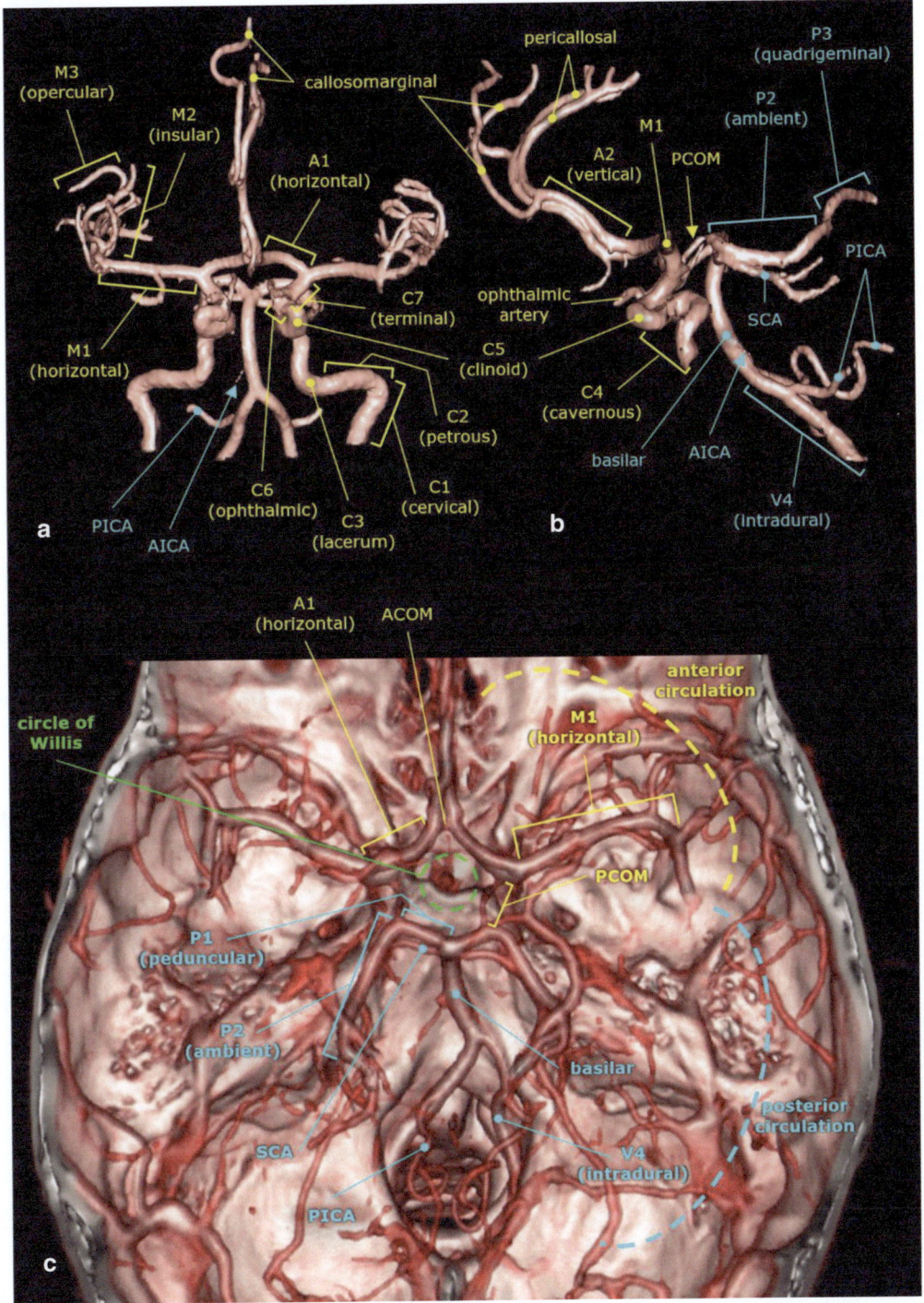

- Anterior choroidal artery: extends posteriorly to the choroidal fissure supplying many critical structures along the way such as the optic chiasm and tract, uncus, caudate tail, temporal horn choroid plexus, cerebral peduncle, internal capsule (genu, posterior limb, and retrolenticular parts), globus pallidus internus, thalamus, lateral geniculate nucleus, and anterior optic radiations.

Other arterial terminology:

- Perforating artery: a small end-artery (supplies a region without other sources of oxygenated blood) that supplies deep brain structures.
- Carotid siphon: loosely includes the cavernous through terminal ICA segments, often used to describe the location of atherosclerotic plaques.

- Supraclinoid ICA (aka: cisternal, cerebral part): variably considered synonymous with the ophthalmic segment, or the combined ophthalmic and terminal ICA segments.

Anterior cerebral artery (**ACA**): begins at the terminal ICA bifurcation directed anteromedially, its segmentation is typically described in three to five segments. The ACAs supply the medial frontal lobes, parts of the medial parietal lobes, the hypothalamus, and parts of the striatum and internal capsule.

Segments and branches:

- *A1* (horizontal, aka: pre-communicating): from the origin to the anterior communicating artery.
  - Medial *lenticulostriate arteries*: may supply the caudate head, anterior limb of the internal capsule, anterior lenticular nuclei, and optic tract.
  - *Anterior communicating artery* (ACOM): anastomosis between ACAs, perforators may supply the lamina terminalis, anterior commissure, hypothalamus, and nearby corpus callosum [14].
- *A2* (vertical, aka: post-communicating, subcallosal, infracallosal): courses beneath the rostrum of the corpus callosum and ends at the callosomarginal artery or anterior to the genu of the corpus callosum.
  - Recurrent artery of Heubner (aka: medial striate artery): variably arises near the A1/A2 junction and may supply the anterior caudate head and putamen, anterior limb of the internal capsule, ventral striatum, and hypothalamus [14].
  - Orbitofrontal artery (aka: frontobasal artery): extends anteriorly to supply the orbital gyri and gyrus rectus.
  - Frontopolar artery: extends anteriorly to supply the frontal pole.
- *A3* (precallosal, aka: pericallosal artery): rises anterior to the genu of the corpus callosum. The pericallosal artery comprises the A3-A5 segments beyond the callosomarginal artery and courses posteriorly within the callosal sulcus.
  - Callosomarginal artery: often courses superiorly then posteriorly within a cingulate sulcus and branches into medial frontal arteries (anterior, middle, posterior) that may supply a cingulate gyrus, medial frontal lobe, and prefrontal lobule.
- A4 (supracallosal): along the anterior body of the corpus callosum.
- A5 (postcallosal): along the posterior body of the corpus callosum.

Middle cerebral artery (**MCA**): begins at the terminal ICA bifurcation, it is larger and with a broader vascular distribution than the ACA and described in four segments. It supplies the lateral surfaces of the brain including large portions of the frontal, parietal, and temporal cortex, the temporal poles, as well as portions of the basal ganglia, internal capsules, and thalami.

Segments and branches:

- *M1* (horizontal, aka: sphenoidal): courses laterally within the Sylvian cistern and generally bifurcates near a limen insula into superior and inferior divisions, which supply large portions of the lateral surfaces of the frontal/parietal and temporal lobes, respectively.
  - Lateral lenticulostriate arteries: arise from the proximal to mid-M1, they supply the internal capsule (anterior limb, genu, and posterior limb), caudate head and body, and lenticular nuclei.
- *M2* (insular): course in a roughly sagittal plane over an insular lobe within a circular sulcus.
- *M3* (opercular): course laterally over frontal, parietal, or temporal opercula.
- M4 (cortical): disperse over frontal, parietal, or temporal lateral surfaces, and are generally described by the territory they supply (i.e., orbitofrontal, temporopolar, prefrontal, precentral, central, angular, anterior/posterior parietal, anterior/middle/posterior temporal, and temporo-occipital arteries) [15].

Arteries: *Posterior Circulation*

The posterior circulation (aka: vertebrobasilar system) is composed of two vertebral arteries, which merge to form the basilar artery, and their branches. Together these structures supply the brainstem, cerebellum, occipital lobes, medial/inferior temporal lobes, some of the medial parietal lobes, and thalami.

Vertebral arteries: paired arteries, generally described in four parts, they supply the lower brainstem and inferior cerebellum:

Segments and branches:

- *V1* (preforaminal, aka: extraosseous): most commonly arise from the subclavian arteries and ascend in the neck to the level of the C6 vertebral body transverse foramen.
- *V2* (foraminal): ascend through the transverse foramina of C6 through C2.
- *V3* (atlantal, extradural, extraspinal, suboccipital): exit the C2 transverse foramina laterally to reach the C1 transverse foramina, once through they sweep posteriorly past the C1 lateral bodies and medially over the posterior arches of C1 to enter the skull and pass through the dura at the foramen magnum.
- *V4* (intradural, aka: intracranial): once intracranial, the vertebral arteries merge near the level of the lower pons to become the basilar artery.

- *Posterior inferior cerebellar arteries* (PICA): one of the three primary paired arteries to supply the cerebellum; one of the vertebral arteries often terminate as a PICA instead of joining at the vertebrobasilar junction.
  - *Anterior spinal artery*: classically arises from the medial surfaces of both vertebral arteries; these two branches then merge to a single artery that courses caudally along the ventral medulla and spinal cord.

Basilar artery: formed near the lower pons at the confluence of the vertebral arteries; it supplies most of the brainstem and cerebellum.

- *Anterior inferior cerebellar arteries* (AICA): supply the anterior inferior cerebellum and pons.
  - Labyrinthine arteries (aka: internal auditory arteries): supply the inner ears (vestibular apparatuses and cochlea), CNs VII and VIII, and may alternatively arise directly from basilar artery.
- *Pontine arteries*: there are typically a few pairs arising from the mid-basilar artery that supply the pons and superior medulla [14].
- *Superior cerebellar arteries* (SCA): arise at the superior end of the basilar artery just before the basilar artery bifurcates (at the basilar apex or tip) wrapping posteriorly around the cerebral peduncles. In addition to the superior cerebellum, they typically supply the midbrain and superior/middle cerebellar peduncles.

Posterior cerebral arteries (PCAs): paired arteries that begin as the bifurcation of the basilar artery within the interpeduncular cistern and supply the occipital lobes, medial/inferior temporal lobes, and some of the medial parietal lobes.

- *Fetal origin of a PCA*: alternatively, one or both PCAs may be a continuation of a PCOM.

Segments and branches:

- *P1* (peduncular, aka: mesencephalic, pre-communicating): a short segment measuring typically less than 1 cm, it courses laterally from the basilar apex until reaching a PCOM.
  - Interpeduncular perforating arteries, posterior thalamoperforating arteries, and thalamogeniculate arteries pass through the posterior perforated substance to supply the medial midbrain, subthalamus, thalamus, medial geniculate nuclei, internal capsule posterior limbs, and optic tracts [14].
- *P2* (ambient, aka: post-communicating): courses posteriorly from a PCOM to the posterior margin of quadrigeminal plate.
  - Medial posterior choroidal artery: supplies a posteromedial pulvinar, posteromedial thalamus, pineal gland, tela choroidea, quadrigeminal plate, and cerebral peduncle [14].
  - Lateral posterior choroidal artery: supplies a lateral pulvinar, dorsal thalamus, posterior fornix, and lateral ventricle choroid plexus [14].
- *P3* (quadrigeminal): within the quadrigeminal cistern.
- *P4* (distal, aka: cortical): through and beyond tentorial incisura.
  - Calcarine artery: supplies the primary visual cortex.
  - Parietooccipital artery: supplies the precuneus and cuneus.

Circle of Willis (COW): anastomoses between the anterior and posterior circulations, it is composed of several arterial segments that encircle the pituitary stalk within the suprasellar and interpeduncular cisterns.

- Components of the COW listed clockwise when viewing the intracranial skull base (as in Fig. 2.10c), beginning rostrally: ACOM, right A1, right terminal ICA, right PCOM, right P1, basilar tip, left P1, left PCOM, left terminal ICA, left A1.
- The complete circle is typically not present, with frequent absence or hypoplasia of an A1 segment or absence of one or both PCOMs related to fetal origin of a PCA.

Arteries: Extracranial Circulation

Middle meningeal artery: a branch of the maxillary artery, which is a terminal artery of the external carotid artery originating at the carotid bifurcation.

- Branches off a maxillary artery in the infratemporal fossa and enters the skull via a foramen spinosum.
- Gives off small branches that supply a trigeminal ganglion and CN VII.
- Splits into an anterior division that crosses the middle cranial fossa laterally headed toward the pterion, and a posterior division that extends posterolaterally toward the posterior parietal region to supply large regions of the dura mater.
- When injured, it is frequently the cause of an epidural hematoma.

Cerebral Veins and Dural Venous Sinuses

- Dural venous sinuses: valveless venous channels between the meningeal and periosteal layers of the dura mater; they are generally triangular in cross section. In addition to draining veins, CSF drains into the sinuses via arachnoid granulations.
- Intracranial venous system: can be conceptually divided into superficial and deep venous systems.

Superficial venous system (aka: external/cortical venous system): numerous superficial medullary veins drain to *cortical veins* lying predominantly within cerebral sulci on the lateral surfaces of the brain and then, as bridging veins, empty into *dural venous sinuses* (Fig. 2.11).

Drainage pathway:

1. *Superior sagittal sinus*: at the superior aspect of the falx coursing below the sagittal suture, it drains posteriorly toward the venous sinus confluence.

    Tributaries:
    - *Superior cerebral veins* (aka: superficial/external cerebral veins): approximately ten *"bridging veins"* that drain the superior paramedian cerebral cortex by crossing the subarachnoid space and meningeal dural layer to empty into the superior sagittal sinus.
    - *Superior anastomotic vein of Trolard*: often the largest vein on the lateral surfaces of the frontal and parietal lobes and often found in the postcentral sulcus. It may anastomose with the superficial middle cerebral vein and *inferior anastomotic vein of Labbé* near the angular gyrus on the lateral brain surface.

2. *Venous sinus confluence* (aka: confluence, *torcula, torcular Herophili*): It is located at the midline occiput near the internal occipital protuberance. It drains the superior sagittal, straight, and occipital sinuses into the transverse sinuses. Herophilos was an anatomist in ancient Greece [4].

    Tributaries:
    - *Straight sinus*: drains posteriorly along the midline tentorium at its junction with the posterior falx.
      - *Vein of Galen* (VoG, aka: *great cerebral vein*): large caliber, short vein at the tentorial incisura.
        - Internal cerebral veins (ICVs): within the tela choroidea in the midline roof of the third ventricle (Fig. 2.6b), they converge posteriorly into the vein of Galen and receive deep venous drainage (see below).
        - Basal veins of Rosenthal (BVoR): begin as a convergence of the anterior cerebral and deep middle cerebral veins deep to the anterior perforated substance, they course posteriorly through the ambient cisterns draining the mesial temporal lobes and course along a similar path as the PCAs before emptying into the VoG.
        - Superior cerebellar vein: often a convergence within the quadrigeminal cistern of the precentral cerebellar vein in the cerebellomesencephalic cistern and the superior vermian vein in the superior cerebellar cistern that empties directly into the VoG.
    - *Inferior sagittal sinus*: within the inferior margin of the falx, it drains posteriorly into the straight sinus at a confluence with the vein of Galen.

3. *Transverse sinuses* (aka: lateral sinuses): receive blood from the confluence at their origins and course laterally along the posterior margins of the tentorium within a transverse groove in the occipital bone to drain at the sigmoid sinuses.

    Tributaries:
    - Cerebellar veins: superficial veins that drain the cerebellar hemispheres and inferior vermis directly into the transverse sinuses.
    - Inferior anastomotic vein of Labbé: often the largest vein on the lateral surface of a temporal lobe, it may anastomose with a vein of Trolard and/or a superficial middle cerebral vein on the lateral brain surface near the angular gyrus to drain into a transverse sinus.

4. *Sigmoid sinuses*: S-shaped sinuses are a continuation of the lateral transverse sinuses; they curve downward along the posteromedial walls of the mastoids toward the jugular foramina.

    Tributaries:
    - *Superior petrosal sinuses*: drain the cavernous sinuses anteromedial to Meckel's caves, run posteriorly along the petrous ridges and lateral margin of the tentorium to drain into the sigmoid sinuses near their origins.
    - *Inferior petrosal sinuses*: drain the cavernous sinuses and basilar venous plexus by coursing between the petrous bones and clivus toward the jugular foramen within the inferior petrosal sulcus.

5. *Internal jugular veins* (IJV): the sigmoid sinuses mildly dilate to become the *jugular bulb* as they pass through the pars vascularis of the jugular foramen, merge with the inferior petrosal sinuses, and caudally exit the skull as the internal jugular veins. The IJVs descend through the neck lateral to the internal carotid and then common carotid arteries draining into the subclavian veins.
    - *Cavernous sinuses*: on either side of the sella turcica, they contain the cavernous segments of the ICAs as well as segments of CNs III, IV, V_1, V_2, and VI, they primarily drain to the internal jugular veins via the inferior and superior petrosal sinuses and basilar venous plexus (aka: clival venous plexus), and they also drain to the external jugular veins via the *pterygoid venous plexus*.
    - Major tributaries:
      - *Superior ophthalmic veins*: drain the orbits by passing through the superior orbital fissures and emptying into the cavernous venous sinuses.
      - *Sphenoparietal sinuses*: run medially along the sphenoid ridges draining into the cavernous sinuses.

Fig. 2.11 The cerebral veins and dural venous sinuses. (a) Left lateral, (b) superior left posterolateral oblique, and (c) inferior views of an MPR of the cerebral venous system

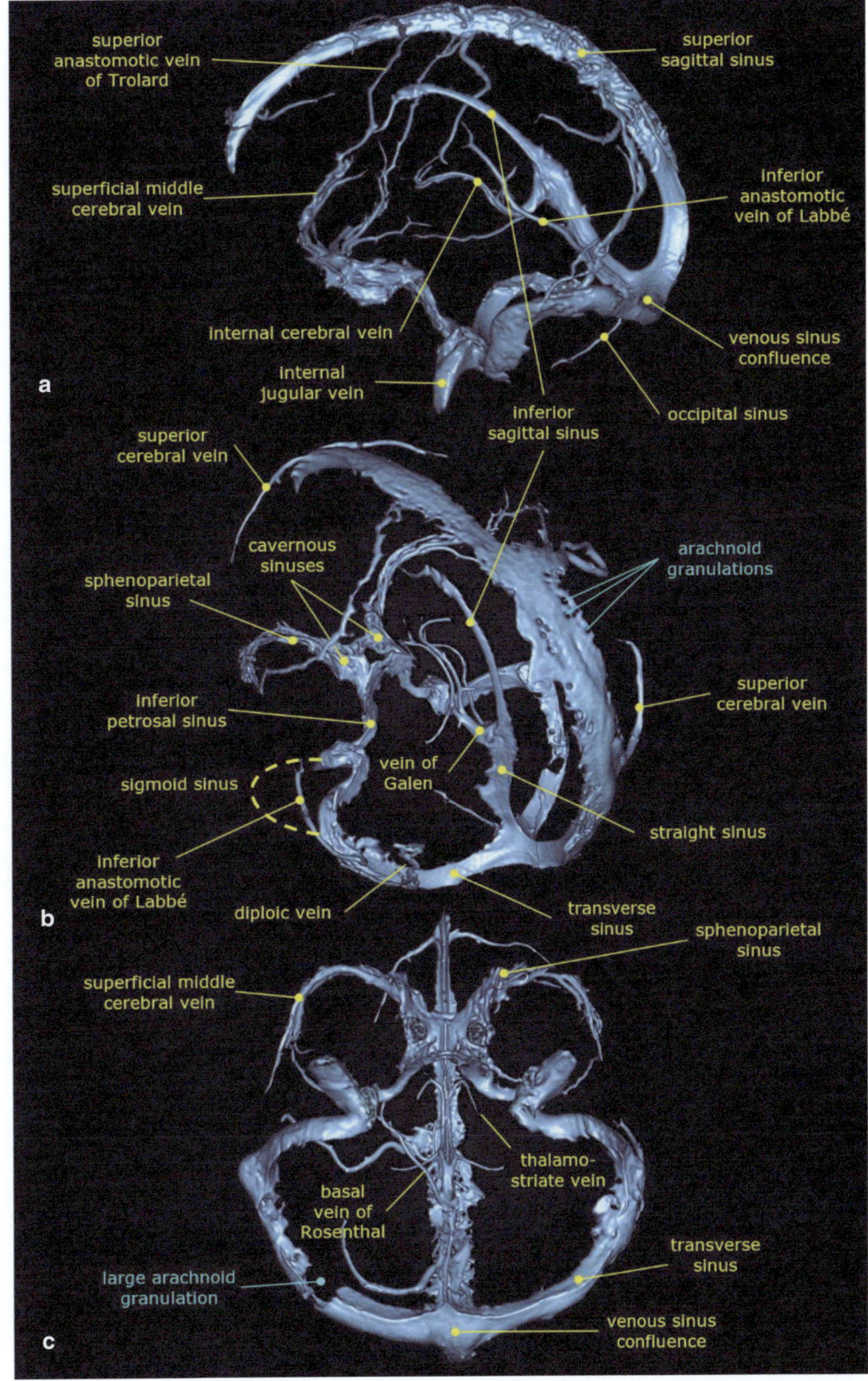

- Superficial middle cerebral veins (aka: superficial Sylvian veins): run superficially within the Sylvian fissures draining the superior temporal lobes to the cavernous or sphenoparietal sinuses. They may anastomose with the veins of Trolard and/or Labbé on the lateral brain surfaces near the angular gyri.
- Anterior and posterior intercavernous sinuses: small channels that connect the cavernous sinuses across midline.

Deep venous system (aka: internal/subependymal venous system): extensive *deep medullary veins* originate deep to cerebral cortex and pass through white matter bulk such as the centrum semiovale or corona radiata, or originate within the deep brain structures, to drain generally perpendicular to ventricular surfaces and empty into larger subependymal veins.

- Internal cerebral veins (ICVs): within the tela choroidea in the midline roof of the third ventricle, they converge posteriorly and drain into the vein of Galen to join the superficial venous drainage system via the straight sinus (see above).
  - Thalamostriate veins (TSVs, aka: superior thalamostriate veins): course anteriorly within the caudothalamic grooves, draining these structures, before turning posteriorly at the venous angles and merging with the septal veins and choroidal veins to become the ICVs. The venous angles: are a nearly 180° anterior to posterior bend in the TSVs at the anterodorsal margins of the thalami.
  - Septal veins: drain frontal lobe and corpus callosum medullary veins, they course posteriorly along the medial frontal horns and septum pellucidum to flow into the ICVs.

Extracranial Venous System

- *Emissary veins*: many small valveless veins cross the skull through foramina and bony channels, draining extracranial venous blood from the scalp into large intracranial cortical veins and dural venous sinuses. Collectively, they are a key pathway between the extracranial and intracranial venous systems. Emissary veins may also connect with *diploic veins* and venous lakes found in the bony medulla between the inner and outer cortices (tables) of the skull.

References

1. Kuo F, Massoud TF. Structural asymmetries in normal brain anatomy: a brief overview. Ann Anat. 2022;241:151894.
2. Massoud TF. Neuroimaging anatomy. Part 1: brain and skull. In: Neuroimaging clinics of North America. London: Elsevier; 2022. (in press).
3. Raikos A, Paraskevas G, Yusuf F, Kordali P, Meditskou S, Al-Haj A, Brand-Saberi B. Etiopathogenesis of hyperostosis frontalis interna: a mystery still. Ann Anat. 2011;193:453–8.
4. Skinner HA. The origin of medical terms. 2nd ed. Baltimore: Williams & Wilkins; 1961.
5. Koutsarnakis C, Komaitis S, Drosos E, Kalyvas A, Skandalakis G, Liakos F, Neromyliotis E, Lani E, Kalamatianos T, Stranjalis G. Mapping the superficial morphology of the occipital lobe: proposal of a universal nomenclature for clinical and anatomical use. Neurosurg Rev. 2019;44:335–50.
6. Spasojević G, Malobabić S, Šuščević D, Stijak L, Nikolić V, Gojković I. Morphological variability of the subcallosal area of man. Surg Radiol Anat. 2010;33:313–8.
7. DeArmond SJ, Fusco MM, Dewey MM. Structure of the human brain. 3rd ed. New York: Oxford University Press; 1989.
8. Mai JK, Voss T, Paxinos G. Atlas of the human brain. Amsterdam: Elsevier; 2008.
9. Edlow BL, Mareyam A, Horn A, Polimeni JR, Witzel T et al. Data from: 7 tesla MRI of the ex vivo human brain at 100 micron resolution. Dryad, Dataset. 2019. https://doi.org/10.5061/dryad.119f80q.
10. Yeh F, Panesar S, Fernandes D, Meola A, Yoshino M, Fernandez-Miranda J, Vettel J, Verstynen T. Population-averaged atlas of the macroscale human structural connectome and its network topology. Neuroimage. 2018;178:57–68.
11. Hofer S, Karaus A, Frahm J. Reconstruction and dissection of the entire human visual pathway using diffusion tensor MRI. Front Neuroanat. 2010;4:15.
12. Jinkins JR. Atlas of neuroradiologic embryology, anatomy, and variants. Philadelphia: Lippincott Williams & Wilkins; 2000.
13. Lu S, Brusic A, Gaillard F. Arachnoid membranes: crawling back into radiologic consciousness. Am J Neuroradiol. 2021;43:167–75.
14. Vogels V, Dammers R, van Bilsen M, Volovici V. Deep cerebral perforators: anatomical distribution and clinical symptoms. Stroke. 2021;52:e660–74.
15. Gibo H, Carver C, Rhoton A, Lenkey C, Mitchell R. Microsurgical anatomy of the middle cerebral artery. J Neurosurg. 1981;54:151–69.

Neuroimaging Functional Anatomy

Behroze A. Vachha and Erik H. Middlebrooks

INTRODUCTION

- A detailed understanding of neuroanatomy is essential for interpretation of neuroimaging.
- With the rise in advanced imaging techniques, such as functional magnetic resonance imaging (fMRI) and diffusion tractography, such understanding is more important than ever.
- Accurate and informative descriptions of pathology relative to functional anatomy not only provide greater insight into the potential clinical manifestations of disease, but also can help guide safe surgical interventions.

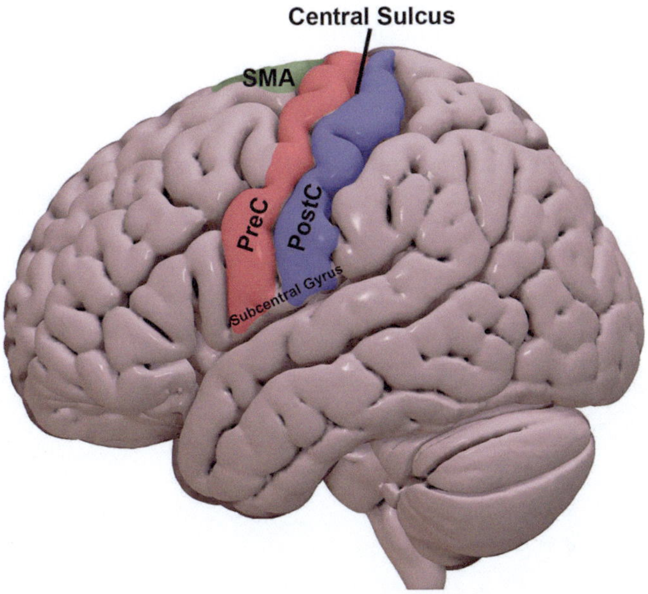

SENSORIMOTOR SYSTEM

Overview

- The primary sensorimotor cortex is centered in the pre- and postcentral gyri, which are separated by the central sulcus (Fig. 3.1) [1–3].
- At the superior termination of the central sulcus, the pre- and postcentral gyri connect to form the paracentral lobule [2].

B. A. Vachha (✉)
Department of Radiology, UMass Chan Medical School, UMass Memorial Medical, Worcester, MA, USA
e-mail: Behroze.Vachha@umassmemorial.org

E. H. Middlebrooks
Department of Radiology, Mayo Clinic, College of Medicine and Science, Jacksonville, FL, USA

Department of Neurosurgery, Mayo Clinic, College of Medicine and Science, Jacksonville, FL, USA
e-mail: middlebrooks.erik@mayo.edu

Fig. 3.1 Surface anatomy of the primary and supplementary sensorimotor regions including the primary motor cortex in the precentral gyrus (PreC), primary sensory cortex in the postcentral gyrus (PostC), and the supplementary motor area (SMA)

- Along the inferior central sulcus, the U-shaped subcentral gyrus is formed by the connection of the pre- and postcentral gyri [3, 4].
- Defining the central sulcus can be challenging and several landmarks or signs have been described to identify the sulcus and pre-/postcentral gyri.
  - The "inverted T sign" refers to the shape of the junction between the superior frontal sulcus and precentral sulcus, which is the anterior border of the precentral gyrus [5].
  - The "reverse omega" sign is also a commonly cited sign for identifying the hand motor cortex. On axial images, a focal bend in the precentral gyrus, forming an epsilon-shaped structure, approximates the hand motor region and is referred to as the "motor hand knob" [1, 3].

© The Author(s), under exclusive license to Springer Nature Switzerland AG 2024
B. A. Vachha et al. (eds.), *What Radiology Residents Need to Know: Neuroradiology*, What Radiology Residents Need to Know,
https://doi.org/10.1007/978-3-031-55124-6_3

- Another useful feature for separating the pre- and postcentral gyri is that the precentral gyrus is generally thicker in anterior-posterior dimension compared to than the postcentral gyrus [1, 2].

Primary Motor Cortex

- The primary motor cortex (PMC) encompasses the posterior precentral gyrus, anterior bank of the central sulcus, and anterior paracentral lobule [6].
- Within the PMC, there is discrete representation of body parts, or "homunculus" that can be used to estimate the body regions controlled by each part of the PMC.
  - Extending from superomedial to infero-lateral is the foot, legs, trunk, arm, hands, face, and tongue motor function (Fig. 3.2) [3, 7].
- The size of each region varies and is proportional primarily to the complexity of the motions within each body part (e.g., larger regions representing hands, fingers, face, and lips) [8].

Somatosensory Cortex

- The primary somatosensory cortex occupies the postcentral gyrus and mirrors the precentral gyrus in configuration (Fig. 3.1) [3, 9].
- As seen with the PMC, there is a somatotopic representation with similar distribution including larger representation for face, lips, fingers, hands, and genitals [10].

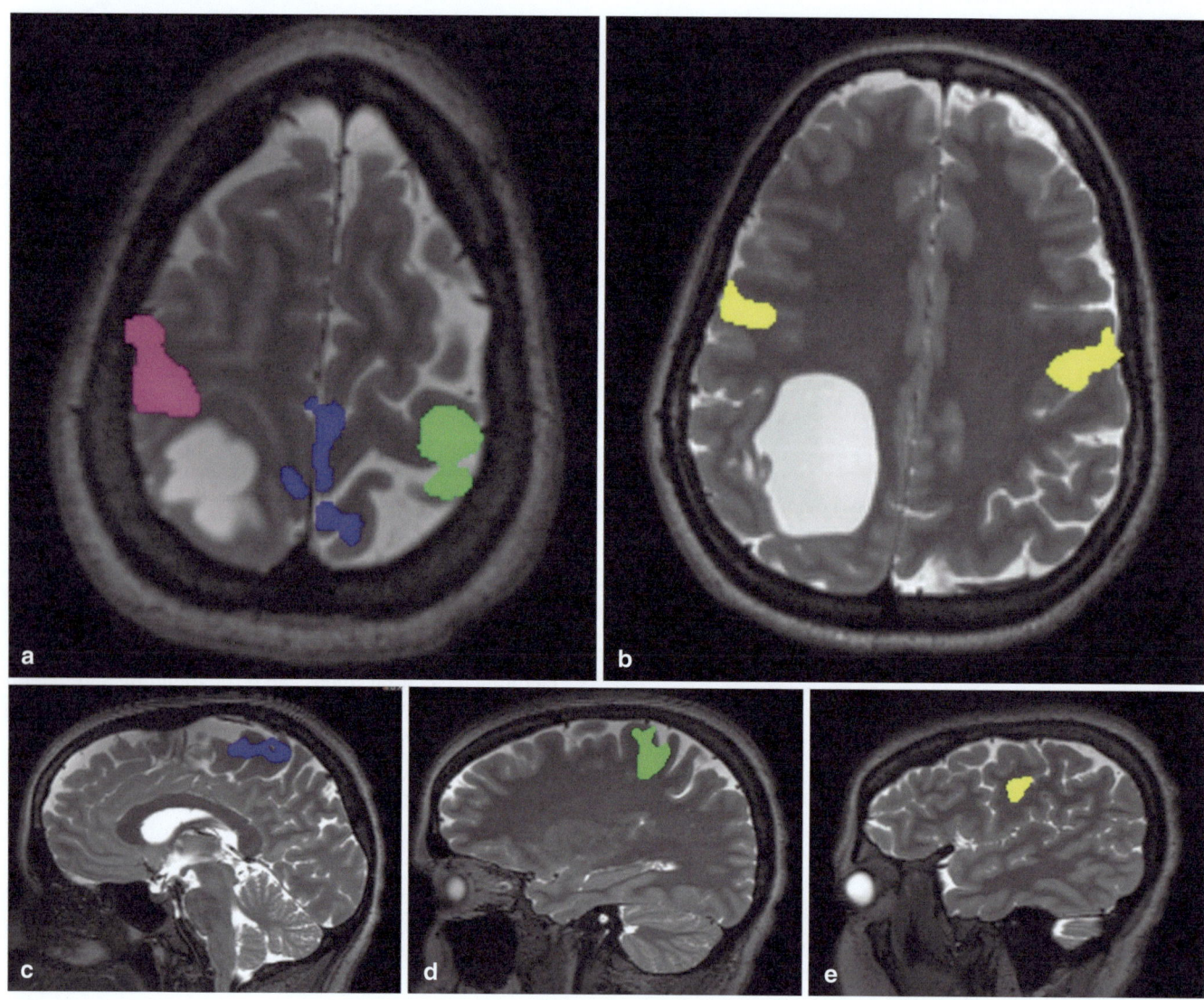

Fig. 3.2 (a, b) Axial functional MRI images of the primary sensorimotor cortex showing locations of right hand (green), left hand (pink), feet (blue), and tongue (yellow). Sagittal functional MRI images illustrating the medial-to-lateral locations of the feet (c), hand (d), and tongue (e)

Supplementary Motor Area

- The supplementary motor area (SMA) complex is found in the dorsomedial superior frontal gyrus, just anterior to the foot motor representation of the PMC (Fig. 3.1).
- The SMA complex is generally divided into the SMA proper (posterior portion; from here on referred to as SMA) and the pre-SMA (anterior portion) [3, 6].
- The boundaries of the SMA include the falx cerebri medially, cingulate sulcus and gyri inferiorly, premotor cortex laterally, foot motor area of PMC posteriorly, and pre-SMA anteriorly [2, 6].
  - The border between SMA proper and pre-SMA can be approximated by a vertical line through the anterior commissure that is perpendicular to a line joining the anterior and posterior commissures [3, 11].
- The SMA proper is involved in the planning, initiation, and execution of movements [12].
- The SMA proper also has a somatotopic organization reflecting parts of the body with the lower extremity posteriorly, followed by upper extremity, trunk, and head when moving anteriorly [2].
  - A helpful way of recalling this layout is to image a person standing on the PMC and falling face forward onto the medial superior frontal gyrus so that the head is the most anterior and feet most posterior.

Fiber Tracts of Sensorimotor System

Fiber Tracts of the Primary Motor Cortex

- The primary output of the PMC consists of the corticospinal tract (CST; Fig. 3.3) that synapse on neurons in the spinal cord and the more lateral corticobulbar tracts that synapse on neurons in the brainstem.
- The CST descends from the PMC into the centrum semiovale and through the posterior limb of the internal capsule, cerebral peduncle, and anterior pons.
  - Within the medulla, most CST fibers cross to the contralateral side through the pyramidal decussation and descend within the lateral corticospinal tract to synapse directly or indirectly on lower motor neurons in the spinal cord supplying distal muscles [13].
  - The non-decussating fibers continue ipsilaterally in the anterior corticospinal tract of the spinal cord and innervate proximal muscles and trunk [13]. The CST also transmits fibers from the SMA, somatosensory, and premotor cortices [6].
- The corticobulbar tract (Fig. 3.3) originates in the lateral portions of the PMC, primarily in regions of the face and neck regions, and descend alongside the corticospinal tract, but synapse with neurons in the brainstem motor cranial nerve nuclei [3].
  - The main exception is the lack of cortical synapse with the facial nucleus of the lower face. This fact explains why patients with complete facial paralysis can be localized to a lower motor neuron process due to the lack of upper motor neuron projection to the lower face portion of the nucleus.
  - The corticobulbar tracts are primarily involved in movements of the head, neck, and face [13].

Fiber Tracts of the Primary Sensory Cortex

- Input to the primary somatosensory area, including conscious recognition of fine touch, two-point discrimination, conscious proprioception, and vibration sensations from the body are via the dorsal column medial lemniscus pathway via the ventral posterolateral nucleus of the thalamus [3, 8, 14].

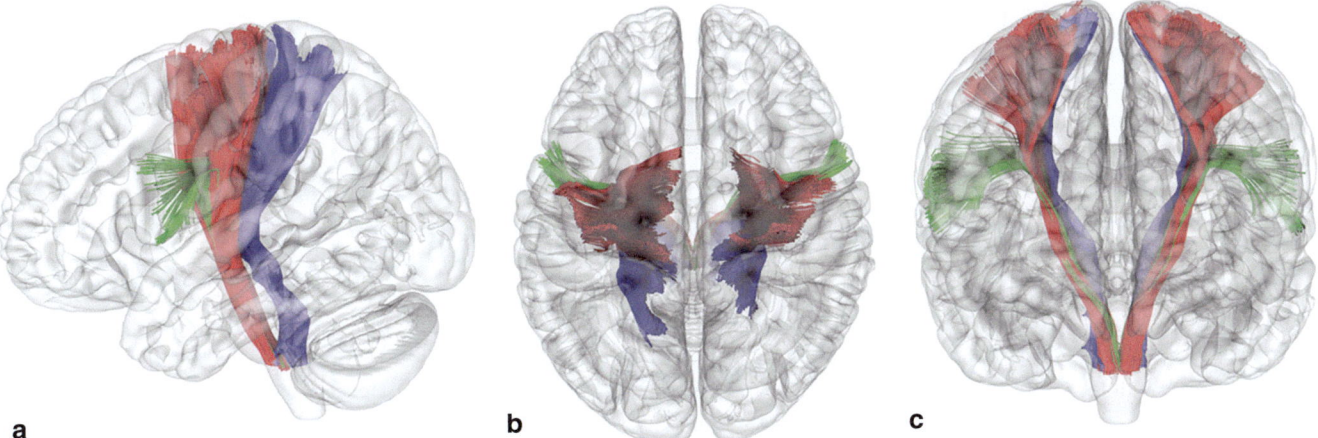

Fig. 3.3 (a) Sagittal, (b) axial, and (c) coronal views of the corticospinal tracts (red), corticobulbar tracts (green), and medial lemniscus (blue)

- Input regarding crude touch (via anterior spinothalamic tract) and temperature and pain (via lateral spinothalamic tract) project from the ventral posterolateral nucleus of the thalamus (Fig. 3.3) [8, 14].

Fiber Tracts of the Supplementary Motor Area

- The SMA is extensively connected to the motor, premotor, and cingulate cortex, as well as the contralateral SMA, insula, superior parietal lobule, basal ganglia, thalamus, and cerebellum [3, 6, 11].
- Projections from the SMA to the corticospinal tract arise only from the SMA proper, while the pre-SMA only consists of association tracts to other brain regions [12].
- Many of the connections of the SMA to adjacent motor and premotor areas are via short U-fibers [12].
- Connection to the contralateral SMA is via the corpus callosum fibers.
- The frontostriatal tract connects the SMA and pre-SMA to the caudate and putamen, which functions in aspects of motor and speech control [12].
- The SMA is also connected to the thalamus, in particular the ventralis oralis nucleus, which may play a role in various movement disorders, such as tremor related to multiple sclerosis [15] and dystonic tremor [16].
- The most medial portion of the superior longitudinal fasciculus (SLF I) connects the SMA to the precuneus and anterior cingulate cortex, functioning in initiation of motor activity and higher-order control of body-centered action [12].

SPEECH AND LANGUAGE SYSTEM

Overview

- While medical texts commonly reference the traditional "localizationist" models of language largely based on works by Paul Broca and Carl Wernicke, these models have largely been disproven in the century subsequent to their initial work [3].
- Currently, the most accurate model of human language is the "connectomic" model known as the "dual stream" model (Fig. 3.4) [3, 17].
  - Dual-stream model posits that language is a complex function widely distributed across numerous areas of the brain.
  - The core pathways in this dual-stream model include a dorsal "phonologic" stream (sounds of words) and a ventral "semantic" stream (meaning of words) [3, 18].
- Notable discrepancy with the traditional models includes the fact that no discrete areas of language comprehension or language production exist.

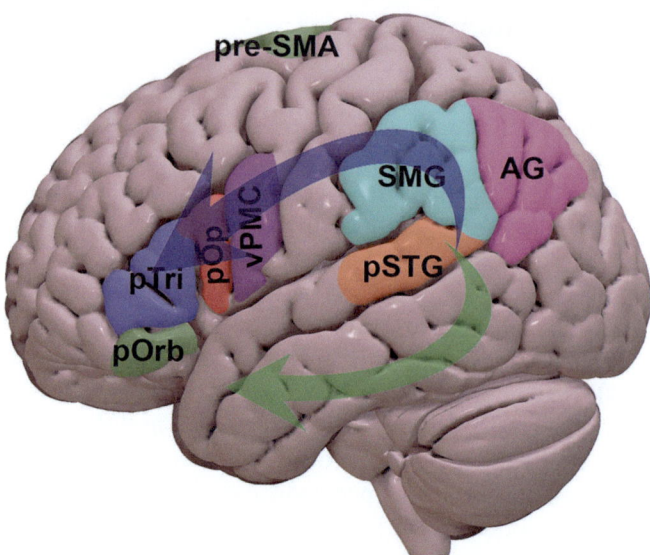

Fig. 3.4 Surface anatomy of the most eloquent cortical regions of language processing. The dorsal stream of language is highlighted by the blue arrow and the ventral stream by the green arrow. *AG* angular gyrus, *pOp* pars opercularis, *pOrb* pars orbitalis, *pSTG* posterior superior temporal gyrus, *pTri* pars triangularis, *pre-SMA* pre-supplementary motor area complex, *SMG* supramarginal gyrus, *vPMC* ventral premotor cortex

- In the following section, we will focus only on a small number of brain regions implicated in speech and language with a focus on those believed to be most critical for language function, but it is important to acknowledge that numerous additional areas play a role in language but have a low incidence of severe language dysfunction, presumably related to compensation by other pathways or by playing a less critical role in language function.

Dorsal Stream

Inferior Frontal Gyrus

- The inferior frontal gyrus (IFG) has long been known to play a role in language since the pioneering work of Paul Broca.
- The IFG constitutes the most inferior gyrus along the lateral frontal lobe making up the frontal opercular region [3].
  - It is bound by the inferior frontal sulcus superiorly and the Sylvian fissure inferiorly.
  - The IFG consists of three continuous parts, the pars orbitalis, pars triangularis, and pars opercularis (Fig. 3.4) [1, 3, 19].
  - The pars orbitalis, the most anterior portion, is separated from the middle pars triangularis by anterior ramus of the Sylvian fissure.

- o The pars triangularis is separated from the posterior pars opercularis by the ascending ramus of the Sylvian fissure (Fig. 3.4) [1].
- While there is some debate about the anatomic correlate of Broca's area [20], it is generally considered as part of the pars opercularis and pars triangularis [21].
- Traditionally, Broca's area is found in the language dominant hemisphere (most commonly the left hemisphere) and functions in speech production; however, this theory has been disproven despite its persistence in many medical texts and literature.
- More recently, the dominant pars opercularis has been shown to function in pre-articulatory planning and lexical retrieval. Importantly, activation in this area precedes the onset of speech motor function and is also elicited in the absence of overt speech [3, 17, 22].
  - o The function of the pars opercularis can be regarded as the gateway to releasing phonetic codes to be subsequently processed by the more important ventral premotor cortex prior to speech initiation.
- The nondominant hemisphere homolog functions in linguistic prosody and attention [21].
- Awake brain stimulation of the traditional Broca's area can produce transient speech disturbances (e.g., anomia); however, permanent speech deficits rarely occur after damage to this cortical area alone [23].
- Patients with more severe and long-term speech dysfunction from IFG damage likely result from concomitant damage to the more vital ventral premotor cortex (discussed below) or underlying white matter tracts.

Ventral Premotor Cortex

- The pars opercularis is separated posteriorly from the ventral premotor cortex (vPMC) by the inferior aspect of the precentral sulcus (Fig. 3.4) [3, 17].
- The inferior portion of the vPMC is critical in phonologic processing and the bridge to speech motor function.
- Awake brain mapping commonly reveals dysarthria or anarthria with stimulation of the vPMC and resection of this area is highly associated with permanent defects of speech given its limited plasticity.
- The superior half of the vPMC overlaps with motor cortex of speech functions, such as tongue movement.

Supplementary Motor Area

- As previously discussed, the SMA can be divided into two primary components.
- The pre-SMA is located directly anterior to the SMA proper in the dorsomedial superior frontal gyrus (Fig. 3.4) [2, 3, 12].
- The pre-SMA has a greater role in cognitive function, such as higher-order language production.
- Damage to the SMA and/or pre-SMA may result in a SMA syndrome (temporary global akinesia that is more pronounced contralaterally, and mutism if the lesion is in the dominant hemisphere).
  - o While symptoms may be disabling, they are commonly transient as there is a high plasticity associated with SMA complex injury, particularly with greater preservation of the underlying frontal aslant tract and frontostriatal tract.

Supramarginal Gyrus

- The supramarginal gyrus is an important node in the dorsal language stream.
- Anatomically, the supramarginal gyrus is within the inferior parietal lobule at the posterior termination of the Sylvian fissure (Fig. 3.4) [3].
- The supramarginal gyrus functions in phonologic working memory, and stimulation or damage to this region may result in an apraxia of speech or anomia [17].

Fiber Tracts of the Dorsal Stream

- The key association fibers that connect the aforementioned eloquent regions of the dorsal stream include the arcuate fasciculus, superior longitudinal fasciculus part III, and the frontal aslant tract [3].
- The arcuate fasciculus (Fig. 3.5a) originates in the posterior superior temporal gyrus, mid superior temporal gyrus, and mid middle temporal gyrus.
  - o Terminations include the pars opercularis and ventral premotor cortex. The arcuate fasciculus reaches the pars triangularis in 40% of subjects [17, 24].
  - o Most common deficits resulting from damage to the arcuate fasciculus include phonologic paraphasia and impaired repetition.
- The frontal aslant tract is a more recently described frontal lobe tract that primarily connects the pre-SMA and pars opercularis (Fig. 3.5b and c) [3, 12].
  - o The frontal aslant tract is a critical pathway for verbal fluency.
  - o Damage to the dominant frontal aslant tract is associated with impaired articulatory planning and speech initiation [12, 17].
- The superior longitudinal fasciculus is an associative tract that consists of three parts (Fig. 3.6): SLF I, SLF II, and SLF III [3].
- SLF III is the only component of the superior longitudinal fasciculus that functions primarily in language.

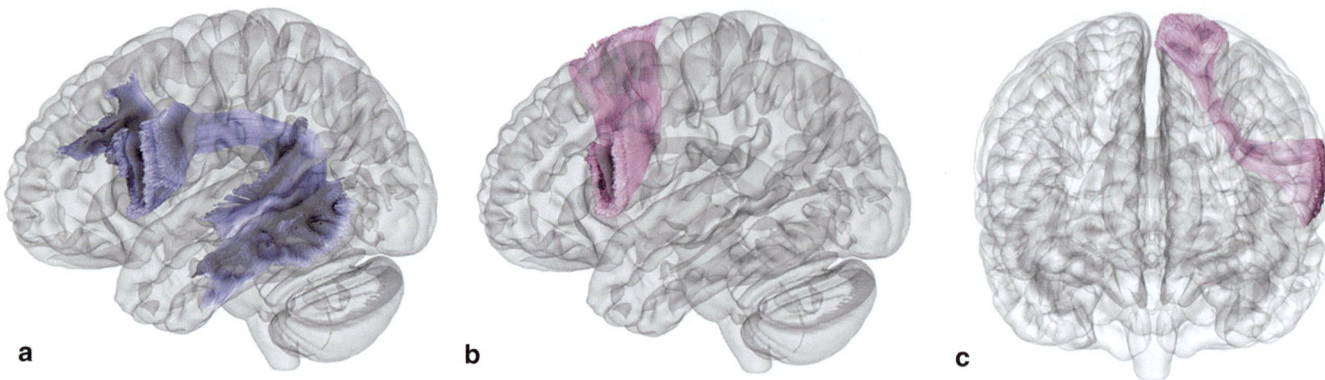

Fig. 3.5 (**a**) **Sagittal image of the course of the arcuate fasciculus**. (**b**) Sagittal and (**c**) coronal images of the frontal aslant tract

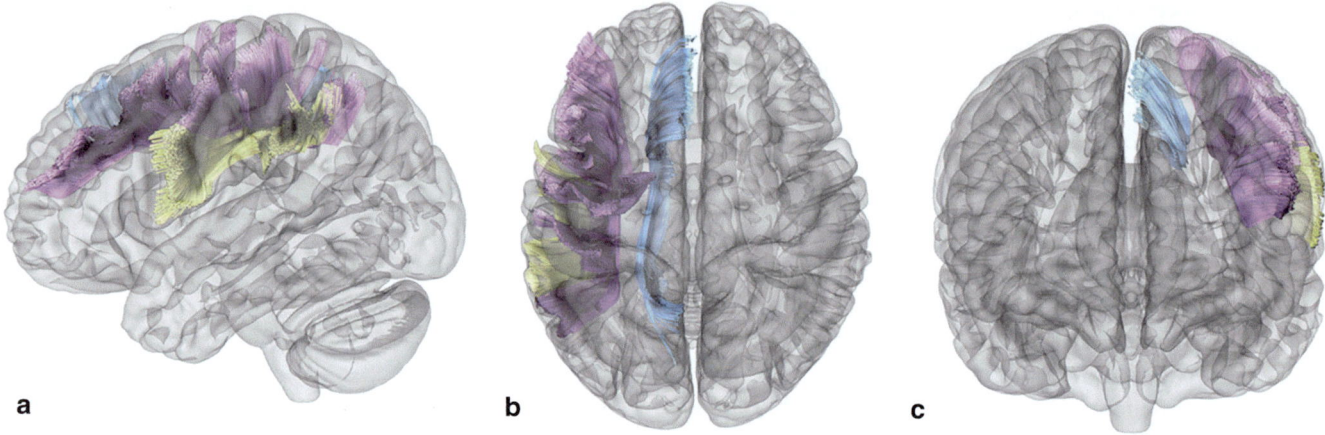

Fig. 3.6 (**a**) Sagittal, (**b**) axial, and (**c**) coronal views of the superior longitudinal fasciculus (SLF), which consists of the more medial and superior SLF I (cyan), slightly more lateral and inferior SLF II (purple), and the most lateral and inferior SLF III (yellow)

- o SLF III connects the supramarginal gyrus to the pars opercularis forming a phonologic working memory loop in the language-dominant hemisphere [17, 24]. The nondominant SLF III functions in visuospatial attention, prosody, and music processing. Damage to the dominant SLF III results in a high occurrence of anarthria/dysarthria and can produce a severe speech output disorder [17, 24].

Ventral Stream

Temporal Language Areas (Wernicke's Area)

- The ventral stream encompasses broad areas of the temporal lobe with a hypothesized "gradient" of increasing processing complexity moving from posterior temporal lobe to the temporal pole.
- The classic Wernicke area constitutes variable anatomic definitions that are primarily centered on the posterior temporal lobe, although there is no consensus on the anatomic structures [20].
  - o In most definitions, the dominant hemisphere posterior superior temporal gyrus is a key component (Fig. 3.4) [2].
  - o While commonly described as functioning in language comprehension, this theory has been repeatedly disproven with more recent language studies [3].
- The posterior superior temporal gyrus most likely functions in early processing of phonemes.
  - o Initially, phonologic information is perceived in the visual word form area (written) or middle superior temporal gyrus and superior temporal sulcus (audio) and then retrieved in the posterior superior temporal gyrus before passing into the dorsal and ventral streams [17].
  - o Posterior superior temporal gyrus injury in the dominant hemisphere can produce impairments in word retrieval, phonemic paraphasia, or anomia [17].

Angular Gyrus

- The angular gyrus is located in the inferior parietal lobule and surrounds the posterior termination of the superior temporal sulcus (Fig. 3.4) [17].

- The angular gyrus is a commonly activated region in semantic tasks, and evidence from awake mapping studies suggests that damage to the dominant angular gyrus may result in anomia, agraphia, speech arrest, and difficulty with reading tasks.
- Classically, lesions within the dominant angular gyrus are also associated with Gerstmann syndrome, a classic tetrad of left-right disorientation, finger agnosia, acalculia, and agraphia [17].

Visual Word Form Area

- Within the dominant ventral occipitotemporal cortex lies the visual word form area (vWFA).
- The vWFA has connectivity to multiple regions, including the superior temporal, inferior parietal, and lateral prefrontal areas.
- The vWFA is known to be a critical hub in decoding written words.
- Damage or stimulation of the vWFA can produce pure alexia [25].

Fiber Tracts of the Ventral Stream

- The major fiber tracts of the ventral stream can be envisioned as a "parallel circuit" connecting posterior parietal, occipital, and temporal regions with the anterior temporal lobe and frontal lobe.
- The first pathway (direct pathway) is the inferior fronto-occipital fasciculus (IFOF), and a paralleling (indirect) pathway made up by the inferior longitudinal fasciculus (ILF) and uncinate fasciculus (UF) [3].
- The IFOF is one of the longest associative pathways in the human brain.
  - IFOF connects the middle occipital gyrus, inferior occipital gyrus, and precuneus with the dorsolateral prefrontal cortex, pars orbitalis, and pars triangularis (Fig. 3.7a and b) [26].
  - As IFOF extends anteriorly in the temporal lobe, it narrows into a bowtie shape at the insula where it travels with the uncinate fasciculus through the ventral external capsule and into the frontal lobe.

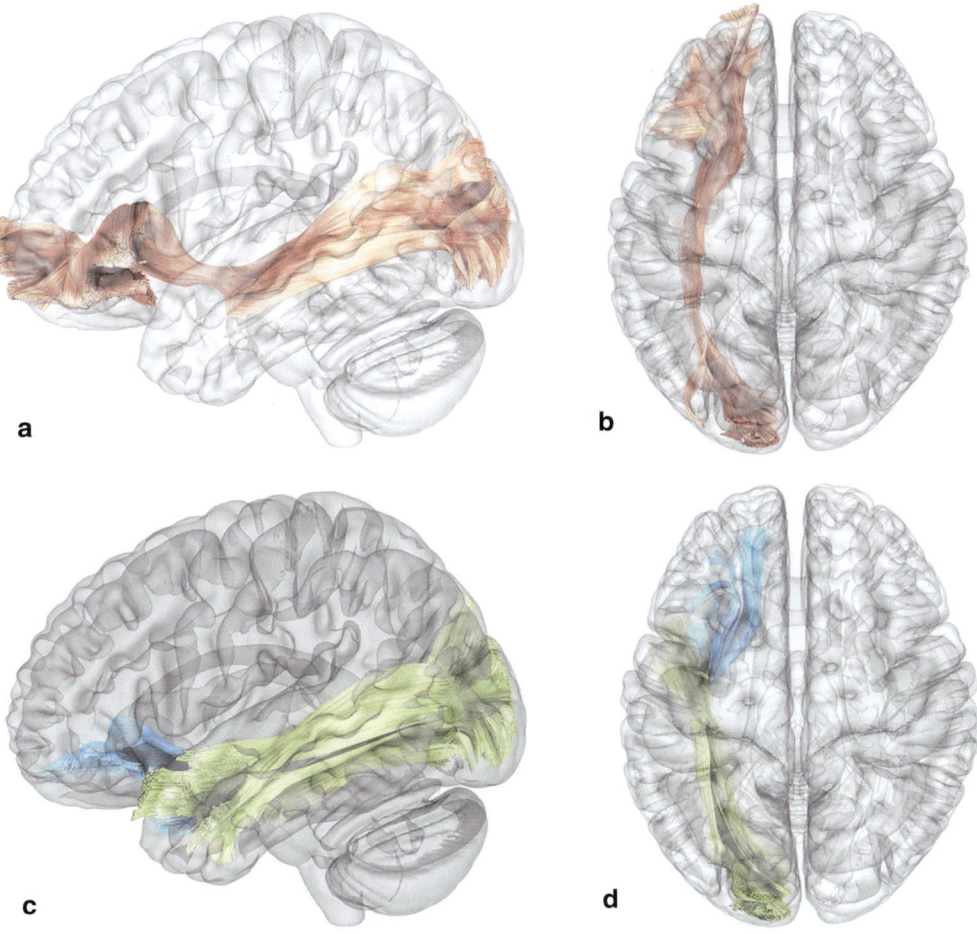

Fig. 3.7 (a) Sagittal and (b) axial images of the inferior fronto-occipital fasciculus. (c) Sagittal and (d) axial images of the uncinate fasciculus (cyan) and inferior longitudinal fasciculus (yellow)

- o The IFOF plays a critical role in semantic processing and assignment of meaning to language.
- o Damage to IFOF has a high association with semantic paraphasia and anomia [17].
- The ILF traverses from the dorsolateral occipital cortex to the temporal pole, paralleling the posterior portion of the IFOF (Fig. 3.7c and d).
  - o The cortical connections of ILF include extrastriate areas, middle and inferior temporal gyri, parahippocampal gyrus, hippocampus, amygdala, and temporal pole.
  - o ILF has been proposed to function in reading and visual orthographic processing.
  - o Damage to ILF may result in alexia and impaired reading [17].
- The second portion of this indirect pathway, the UF, traverses from the temporal pole to the frontal lobe after passing through the ventral external capsule paralleling the anterior portion of the IFOF (Fig. 3.7c and d) [26].
  - o The cortical connections of UF include the temporal pole, dorsolateral frontal lobe, amygdala, parahippocampal gyrus, medial orbitofrontal cortex, and nucleus accumbens.
  - o Damage to UF can lead to impairments in memory and semantic function, such as impaired famous face naming and object naming.

VISION AREAS

Overview

- The visual cortex can largely be divided into a primary visual cortex versus extrastriate and visual association cortices [3, 27, 28].
- The extrastriate and association regions are those visually responsive areas outside of the primary visual cortex, which have complex function and broad connectivity.
- This chapter will focus only on the primary visual cortex, as this is more commonly a source of significant visual impairments.

Primary Visual Cortex

- The primary visual cortex is located primarily around the calcarine fissure of the occipital lobe (Fig. 3.8a).
- The calcarine fissure can be identified by its nearly perpendicular intersection with the mid portion of the parieto-occipital fissure.
- The primary visual cortex receives the primary visual input via the retinogeniculocortical pathways, which are then transmitted to various extrastriate cortical areas for further integration into other higher-order functions [28].
- Visual fields have distinct representations within the primary visual cortex.
  - o The fovea, the central part of gaze, is represented at the occipital pole.
  - o The fovea represents the area of highest visual acuity, and as such, there is a larger cortical region representing the fovea versus the peripheral visual field [27].
  - o Peripheral visual fields project more anteriorly near the junction of the parieto-occipital fissure and calcarine sulcus [28].

Fiber Tracts of Primary Visual Pathway

- The primary tracts involved in primary visual processing are the optic nerve, optic tracts, and optic radiations (Fig. 3.8b and c) [3].

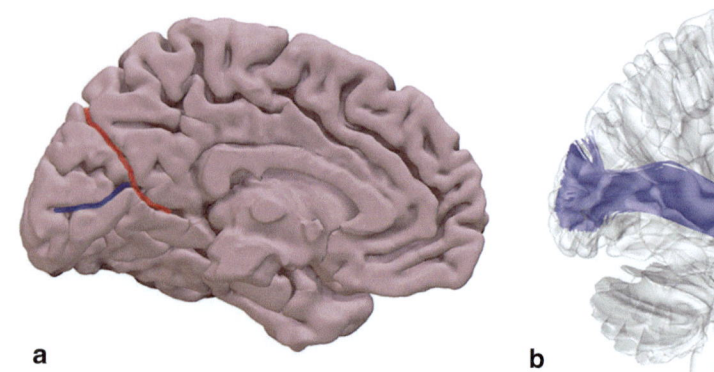
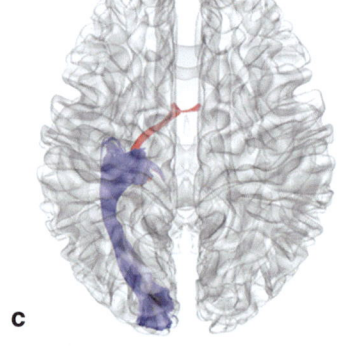
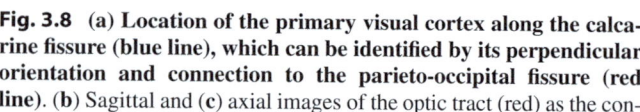

Fig. 3.8 (a) Location of the primary visual cortex along the calcarine fissure (blue line), which can be identified by its perpendicular orientation and connection to the parieto-occipital fissure (red line). (b) Sagittal and (c) axial images of the optic tract (red) as the connection from the optic chiasm to the lateral geniculate nucleus and the optic radiations (blue) connecting the lateral geniculate nucleus to the primary visual cortex

- The optic tracts represent the continuation of the optic nerve and connect the optic chiasm with the lateral geniculate nucleus.
- The optic radiations then project from the lateral geniculate nucleus of the thalamus to the primary visual cortex [28].
- The human visual cortex is organized into multiple retinotopic maps [27].
  - The inferior visual field (superior retina) is projected via the retrolenticular fibers of the optic radiation and terminate in the superior lip of the calcarine fissure [19].
  - The superior visual field (inferior retina) projects via sublenticular fibers of the optic radiation that extend anteriorly from the lateral geniculate nucleus around temporal horn of the lateral ventricle ("Meyer's loop") before terminating in the inferior lip of the calcarine fissure [19].

Disclosures B.A.V. has no disclosures. E.H.M. receives unrelated research support from Varian Medical Systems, Inc., Boston Scientific Corp., and Vigil Neuroscience, Inc. E.H.M. is a consultant for Boston Scientific Corp. and Varian Medical Systems, Inc.

References

1. Naidich T, Tang C, Ng J, Delman B. Surface anatomy of the cerebrum. In: Naidich T, Castillo M, Cha S, Smirniotopoulos J, editors. Imaging of the brain. Philadelphia: Elsevier; 2013.
2. Naidich T, Yousry T. Functional neuroanatomy. In: Stippich C, editor. Clinical functional MRI: presurgical functional neuroimaging. Berlin-Heidelberg: Springer-Verlag; 2007. p. 53–86.
3. Vachha BA, Middlebrooks EH. Brain functional imaging anatomy. Neuroimaging Clin N Am. 2022;32(3):491–505.
4. Wagner M, Jurcoane A, Hattingen E. The U sign: tenth landmark to the central region on brain surface reformatted MR imaging. AJNR Am J Neuroradiol. 2013;34(2):323–6.
5. Kido DK, LeMay M, Levinson AW, Benson WE. Computed tomographic localization of the precentral gyrus. Radiology. 1980;135(2):373–7.
6. Hill VB, Cankurtaran CZ, Liu BP, et al. A practical review of functional MRI anatomy of the language and motor systems. AJNR Am J Neuroradiol. 2019;40(7):1084–90.
7. Schellekens W, Petridou N, Ramsey NF. Detailed somatotopy in primary motor and somatosensory cortex revealed by Gaussian population receptive fields. Neuroimage. 2018;179:337–47.
8. Watson C, Kirkcaldie M, Paxinos G. The brain: an introduction to functional neuroanatomy. Amsterdam: Elsevier; 2010.
9. Ulmer S. Neuroanatomy and cortical landmarks. In: Ulmer S, Jansen O, editors. fMRI: basics and clinical applications. 3rd edition ed. Cham: Springer Nature; 2020. p. 5–13.
10. Roux FE, Djidjeli I, Durand JB. Functional architecture of the somatosensory homunculus detected by electrostimulation. J Physiol. 2018;596(5):941–56.
11. Potgieser AR, de Jong BM, Wagemakers M, Hoving EW, Groen RJ. Insights from the supplementary motor area syndrome in balancing movement initiation and inhibition. Front Hum Neurosci. 2014;8:960.
12. Bozkurt B, Yagmurlu K, Middlebrooks EH, et al. Microsurgical and tractographic anatomy of the supplementary motor area complex in humans. World Neurosurg. 2016;95:99–107.
13. Lemon RN. Descending pathways in motor control. Annu Rev Neurosci. 2008;31:195–218.
14. Vanderah T, Gould D. Nolte's the human brain an introduction to its functional anatomy. 8th ed. Philadelphia: Elsevier; 2021.
15. Foote KD, Seignourel P, Fernandez HH, et al. Dual electrode thalamic deep brain stimulation for the treatment of posttraumatic and multiple sclerosis tremor. Neurosurgery. 2006;58(4 Suppl 2):ONS-280–5; discussion ONS-285-286.
16. Tsuboi T, Wong JK, Eisinger RS, et al. Comparative connectivity correlates of dystonic and essential tremor deep brain stimulation. Brain. 2021;144(6):1774–86.
17. Middlebrooks EH, Yagmurlu K, Szaflarski JP, Rahman M, Bozkurt B. A contemporary framework of language processing in the human brain in the context of preoperative and intraoperative language mapping. Neuroradiology. 2017;59(1):69–87.
18. Hickok G, Poeppel D. Dorsal and ventral streams: a framework for understanding aspects of the functional anatomy of language. Cognition. 2004;92(1–2):67–99.
19. Boling W, Olivier A. Anatomy of important functioning cortex. In: Byrne R, editor. Functional mapping of the cerebral cortex. Cham: Springer International Publishing; 2016.
20. Tremblay P, Dick AS. Broca and Wernicke are dead, or moving past the classic model of language neurobiology. Brain Lang. 2016;162:60–71.
21. Sibilla L. Functional anatomy of the major lobes. In: Agarwal N, Port J, editors. Neuroimaging: anatomy meets function. Cham: Springer International Publishing; 2018. p. 81–99.
22. Flinker A, Korzeniewska A, Shestyuk AY, et al. Redefining the role of Broca's area in speech. Proc Natl Acad Sci U S A. 2015;112(9):2871–5.
23. Gajardo-Vidal A, Lorca-Puls DL, Team P, et al. Damage to Broca's area does not contribute to long-term speech production outcome after stroke. Brain. 2021;144(3):817–32.
24. Yagmurlu K, Middlebrooks EH, Tanriover N, Rhoton AL Jr. Fiber tracts of the dorsal language stream in the human brain. J Neurosurg. 2016;124(5):1396–405.
25. Sabsevitz DS, Middlebrooks EH, Tatum W, Grewal SS, Wharen R, Ritaccio AL. Examining the function of the visual word form area with stereo EEG electrical stimulation: a case report of pure alexia. Cortex. 2020;129:112–8.
26. Baydin S, Gungor A, Tanriover N, Baran O, Middlebrooks EH, Rhoton AL Jr. Fiber tracts of the medial and inferior surfaces of the cerebrum. World Neurosurg. 2017;98:34–49.
27. DeYoe EA, Raut RV. Visual mapping using blood oxygen level dependent functional magnetic resonance imaging. Neuroimaging Clin N Am. 2014;24(4):573–84.
28. Gill S, Ulmer J, DeYoe E. Vision and higher cortical function. In: Holodny A, editor. Functional neuroimaging a clinical approach. New York: Informa Health Care; 2008. p. 67–80.

Congenital and Developmental Brain Malformations

Edward Yang

Embryology in a Nutshell

- Understanding brain malformations requires at least a schematic understanding of brain embryology (Fig. e4.1. All electronic images (Figs. e4.1–e4.12) can be found in this chapter's website on SpringerLink: https://doi.org/10.1007/978-3-031-55124-6_4) [1].
- After induction of the neural plate, the nervous system folds dorsally into a neural tube at *4 weeks postconception*. Failure in this process underlies open rostral or caudal defects in the neuraxis as seen in anencephaly and myelomeningoceles, respectively.
- By *4–6 weeks postconception*, rudimentary vesicles bud off the rostral neural tube on each side, defining the nascent cerebral hemispheres.
- By *6 weeks postconception*, cerebellar tissue is defined and there is fenestration of a membrane separating the ventricular system from the subarachnoid space, the posterior membranous area or Blake's pouch.
- Between *6 and 16 weeks*, neuronal precursor cells proliferate in holding compartments in the lining of the lateral ventricles (the *ventricular zone* or *germinal matrix*) as well as an adjacent compartment in the periventricular white matter (*subventricular zone*).
- Between *8 and 24 weeks*, the neuronal precursors migrate radially outward investing the cortex in excitatory neurons.
- Between *11 and 20 weeks*, the nascent connections between the hemispheres form and then massively expand defining the major interhemispheric connection, the corpus callosum.
- From 16 weeks postconception until term, the brain undergoes massive growth and gyrification, which define the normal surface anatomy of the brain (i.e., sulci), a process tightly linked with neuronal precursor proliferation and neuronal migration.

Abnormalities of Hemispheric Cleavage

- *Holoprosencephaly* (HPE) refers to incomplete separation of the cerebral hemispheres, reflecting failed cleavage of the rudimentary hemispheric vesicles at 4–6 weeks postconception [1, 2].
- Etiologies include single gene disorders, aneuploidy, and environmental causes (e.g., teratogen exposure, maternal diabetes).
- Holoprosencephaly is classified according to severity of interhemispheric fusion with three classically recognized forms (in order of decreasing severity): *alobar, semilobar*, and *lobar* (Fig. 4.1).
- Although descriptions of holoprosencephaly focus on degree of hemispheric separation, it is important to note that other midline anomalies occur more frequently with severe holoprosencephaly (e.g., cyclopia, a nasal probiscus, hypotelorism, absent olfactory apparatus, and a single median maxillary central incisor are typically seen in alobar rather than lobar holoprosencephaly).

Alobar HPE

- *Alobar* holoprosencephaly is the most severe form of holoprosencephaly.
- The parenchyma consists of a single lobe, which encloses a single ventricle, frequently with decompression dorsally as a cyst.
- Basal ganglia (sometimes also thalami) are fused and the third ventricle is small.
- Septum pellucidum, corpus callosum, and falx cerebri are all absent.

Supplementary Information The online version contains supplementary material available at https://doi.org/10.1007/978-3-031-55124-6_4.

E. Yang (✉)
Department of Radiology, Boston Children's Hospital, Boston, MA, USA
e-mail: edward.yang@childrens.harvard.edu

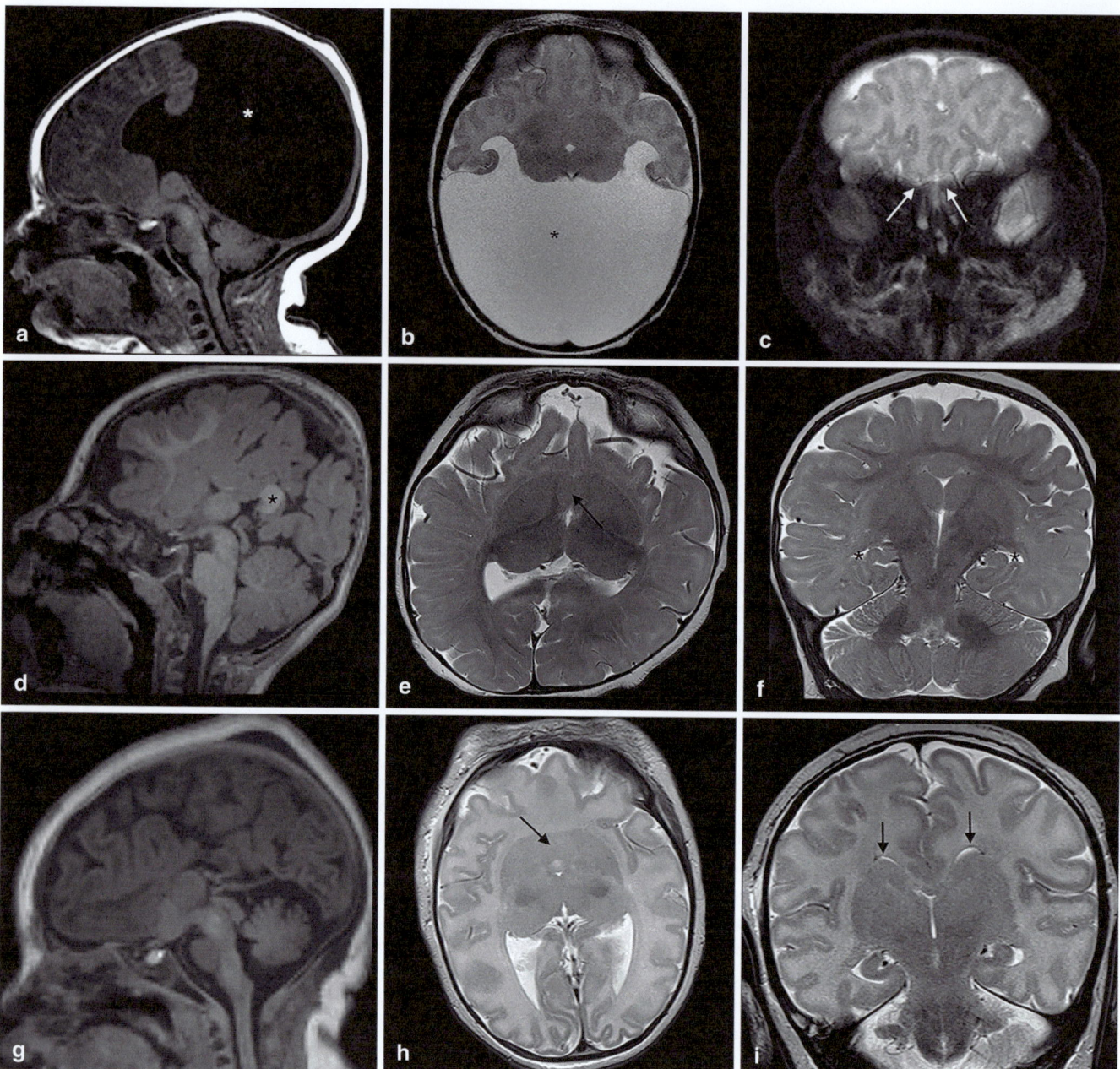

Fig. 4.1 Spectrum of classic holoprosencephaly. As disorders of ventral induction, the classic holoprosencephalies share failure of cleavage of the ventral forebrain but have varying degrees of cleavage of the dorsal/posterior forebrain. This concept is illustrated (in order of decreasing severity) by infants with alobar (**a–c**), semilobar (**d–f**), lobar (**g–i**) holoprosencephaly using sagittal T1 (**a, d, g**), axial T2 images through the deep gray matter (**b, e, h**), and coronal T2 images (**c, f, i**). In *alobar holoprosencephaly* (**a–c**), there is an undivided cerebrum enclosing a monoventricle frequently in communication with a dorsal cyst (asterisk, **a/b**). There is no falx/callosum/septum pellucidum, and the deep gray matter structures are fused (arrow, **b**). Often, the olfactory apparatus will be absent (arrows, **c**). In semilobar holoprosencephaly (**d–f**), there is rudimentary separation of the posterior hemispheres by a posterior falx and short posterior callosum (asterisk, **d**). The temporal horns (asterisk, **f**) may be formed but not the frontal horns. The frontal lobes and the basal ganglia remain fused (arrow, **e**). In lobar holoprosencephaly (**g–i**), this partitioning of the hemispheres is more complete with at least half the posterior corpus callosum being formed along with the frontal horns (arrows, **i**). However, the deep gray matter remains abnormally fused (arrow, **h**). (Adapted with permission from [1])

Lobar and Semilobar HPE

- These milder holoprosencephaly variants demonstrate at least partial cleavage of the hemispheres, which is most evident posteriorly.
- Septum pellucidum is still absent for these forms of holoprosencephaly.
- For *lobar holoprosencephaly*, the posterior cerebral hemispheres are separated to sufficient extent that the posterior falx and posterior corpus callosum are formed.
- Lobar holoprosencephaly also typically results in cleavage of the lateral ventricles sufficient to define the frontal/temporal horns as well as the hippocampi.
- *Semilobar holoprosencephaly* falls in between lobar and alobar holoprosencephaly with one arbitrary discriminator being that semilobar has less than half the posterior corpus callosum formed.

Less Common Holoprosencephalies

- In addition to classic HPE, it is important to be aware of attenuated forms of holoprosencephaly and disorders, which have been historically associated with holoprosencephaly (Fig. e4.2).
- *Middle interhemispheric variant of HPE* features a segmental fusion of the hemispheres midway along the anterior-posterior axis with cleavage anterior and posterior to the fusion (e.g., genu/splenium present but callosal body obscured by cerebral fusion).
  - This form of holoprosencephaly does not typically have basal ganglia fusion.
  - Endocrine abnormalities are less common with this holoprosencephaly variant.
  - Unlike other holoprosencephalies, cortical malformations such as polymicrogyria are reportedly frequent.
- *Septopreoptic HPE* is a form of very mild holoprosencephaly where the hemispheric fusion is confined to a small area of the inferomedial frontal lobes anterior to the fornix.
  - Unlike the other holoprosencephalies, some rudimentary septum pellucidum can be identified.
- *Septo-optic dysplasia* is a clinical syndrome defined by optic pathway hypoplasia and endocrine deficiencies, some but not all having an absent septum pellucidum.
  - Because HPEs were originally ascertained in research projects based on absence of the septum pellucidum, there is a lingering tendency to lump septo-optic dysplasia with holoprosencephaly though this does not appear entirely justified on the basis of the genetic understanding of these two disorders.
  - Radiographic findings include hypoplasia of the optic nerves, olfactory apparatus, and pituitary gland.
  - Patients with radiographically recognizable septo-optic dysplasia have associated schizencephaly and/or polymicrogyria in upward of 50% of cases.

Abnormalities of the Midline Commissures

- An understanding of normal and abnormal callosal anatomy is an important part of characterizing any brain malformation (Fig. 4.2) [2].
- The corpus callosum (CC) is the major midline white matter structure or commissure connecting the cerebral hemispheres and consists of five segments (*rostrum, genu, body, isthmus, and splenium*).
- The five segments become defined 11–20 weeks postconception after fusion of a nascent midline crossing of forebrain axons anteriorly (*lamina reuniens*) and crossing of fibers from the fornix posteriorly (the *hippocampal commissure*).
  - At one time, the CC was thought to elongate during embryogenesis by sequential formation of segments anterior to posterior (genu to splenium) culminating with formation of the rostrum.
  - However, the elongation of the CC is now understood to reflect relative density of crossing fibers, which is driven by the disproportionate growth of the frontal lobes rather than de novo fiber crossings.
- Callosal anomalies are frequently associated with other brain malformations and neurodevelopmental conditions, making their recognition an important sentinel sign of brain maldevelopment on midsagittal imaging.
  - *Callosal hypoplasia* refers to normal length and overall shape of the callosum with relative thinning.
  - *Callosal dysgenesis* refers to foreshortening of the corpus callosum and associated abnormalities in shape, including *agenesis* and *partial agenesis*.
- Morphologic abnormalities of the brain parenchyma and the ventricular system are a consequence of CC dysgenesis.
  - Incomplete formation or absence of the cingulate gyrus with radially oriented gyri extending from a high riding third ventricle.
  - Relative dilation of the atria of the lateral ventricles or so-called *colpocephaly*.
  - Parallel configuration of the lateral ventricles in the axial plane and "steer horn" appearance of the frontal horns in the coronal plane.
  - Under rotation of the hippocampi.
  - Absence of the normal septum pellucidum.
  - Redirection of white matter tracts along the medial surface of the lateral ventricles as *Probst bundles* rather than across the midline, resulting in an impression on the medial walls of the lateral ventricles.

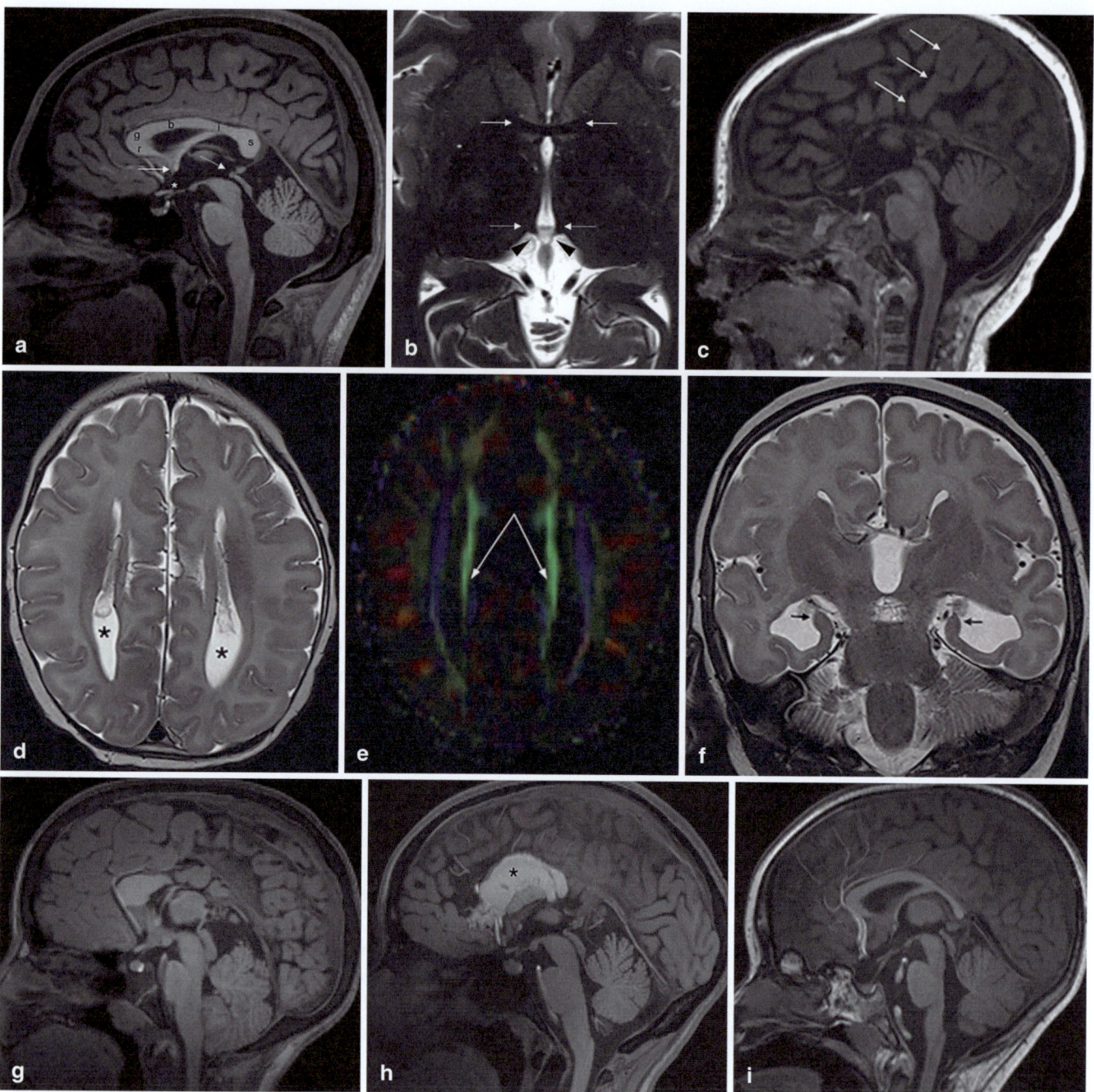

Fig. 4.2 Normal and abnormal midline commissures. Sagittal T1 (**a**) and axial T2 (**b**) images of a healthy child demonstrate the rostrum (r), genu (g), body (b), isthmus (i), and splenium (s) segments of a fully formed corpus callosum as well as the anterior commissure (arrow with solid stem) and posterior commissure (arrow with dashed stem). Sagittal T1-weighted (**c, g, h, i**), axial T2 (**d**), axial color fractional anisotropy map (**e**), and coronal T2 (**f**) images illustrate the range of callosal anomalies. In *complete agenesis of the corpus callosum* (**c, d, e, f**), the callosum and septum pellucidum are not identifiable, and there are typical morphological abnormalities that include: gyral folds radiating to a high-riding third ventricle on sagittal imaging (arrows, **c**: sagittal T1 weighted) due to absence of the cingulate gyrus; parallel configuration of the ventricles with dilation of the atria or colpocephaly (asterisks, **d**); steerhorn appearance of the frontal horns in the coronal plane (**f**); redirection of Probst bundles along the medial walls of the lateral ventricles on directionally coded fractional anisotropy maps (medial green fibers marked with arrows in **e**); and under-rotation of the hippocampi (arrows, **e**). Partial callosal agenesis can be associated with abnormalities of callosal thickness (**g**), interhemispheric cysts, and pericallosal lipomas (asterisk, **h**). Callosal hypoplasia refers to a normal anteroposterior length of the callosum but with relative thinning of one or more of the callosal segments (e.g., splenium in **i**). (Adapted with permission from [1])

4 Congenital and Developmental Brain Malformations

- o Associated interhemispheric cysts and pericallosal lipomas may be present.
- o While these abnormalities are obvious in callosal agenesis, mild forms of dysgenesis and hypoplasia can benefit from comparison to age-expected normative values [3].
- Additional commissures connect the hemispheres including the anterior commissure, which is embedded in the anterior wall of the third ventricle (*lamina terminalis*) and several fiber tracts connecting the thalamus (*massa intermedia, habenular commissure, posterior commissure*).

Malformations of Cortical Development (MCD)

- Malformations of cortical development (MCD) encompass abnormalities of neuronal precursor proliferation, neuronal migration, and cortical organization (Fig. e4.3) [1, 2, 4].
- Focal and diffuse abnormalities in these processes explain the major types of MCD though it should be acknowledged that sometimes multiple processes may be defective.

Gray Matter Heterotopia (GMH)

- Gray matter heterotopia (GMH) represent focal or multifocal failure of neuronal migration, resulting in unorganized neuronal tissue deposited midway between their origin in the germinal matrix and their normal destination, the cortex.
- The key imaging feature of GMH is that *they follow gray matter signal on all sequences including diffusion imaging* (Fig. 4.3).
- They are grouped by location: *periventricular/subependymal, subcortical, and transmantle* (i.e., spanning the entire cerebral mantle).

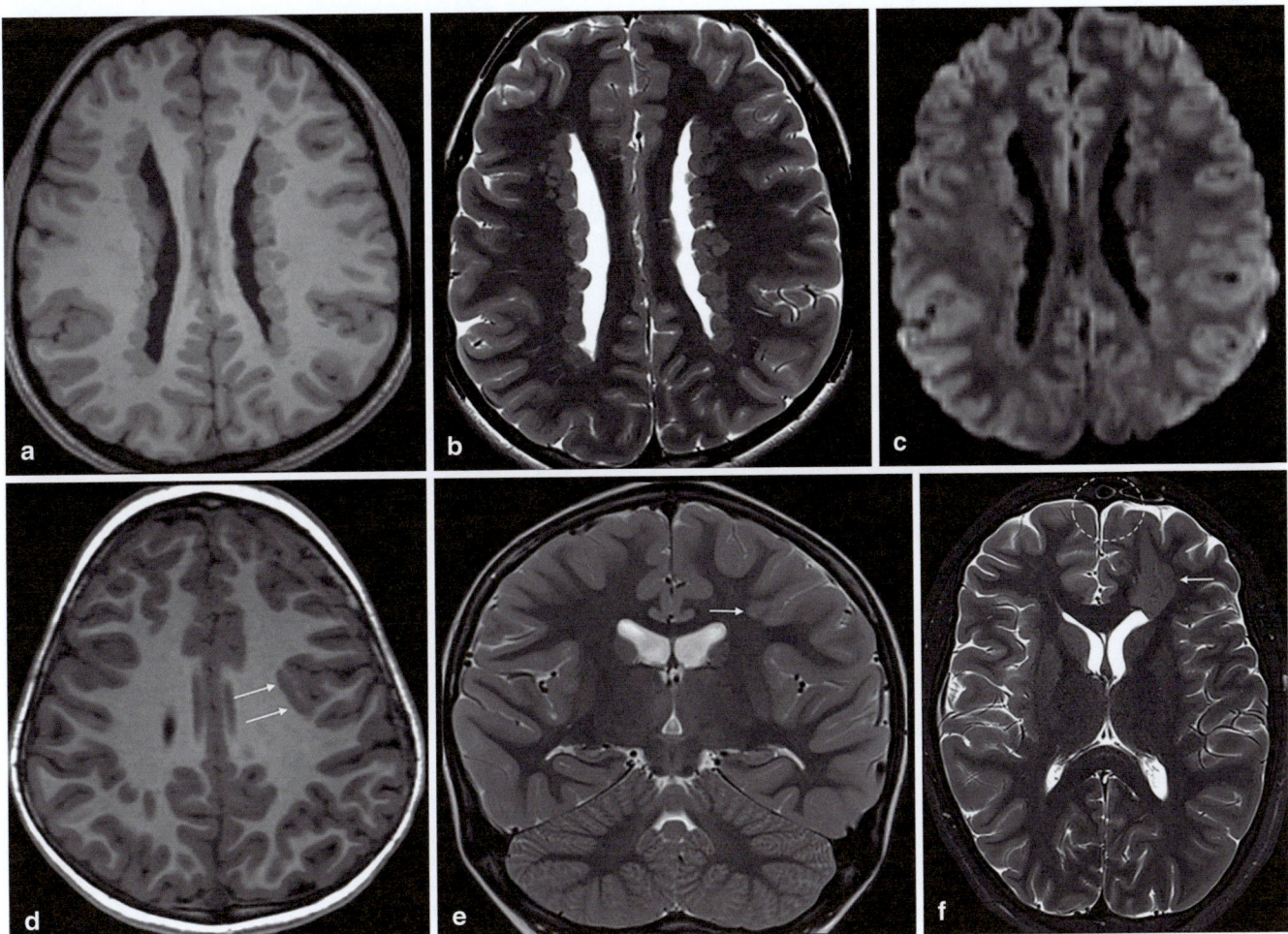

Fig. 4.3 Gray matter heterotopia. Gray matter heterotopia are islands of gray matter, which are classified according to location: periventricular/subependymal (**a**–**c**), subcortical (arrows in **d**, **e**), and transmantle (arrow, **f**). As illustrated by these examples, gray matter heterotopia will follow the signal characteristics of other gray matter structures on T1-weighted (**a, d**), T2-weighted (**b, e, f**), and diffusion-weighted (**c**) sequences. In the case of transmantle heterotopia, overlying cortical malformations such as polymicrogyria are common (circle **f**). (**d, e**, and **f** adapted with permission from [1])

- While historical case series suggested a high incidence of epilepsy in patients with GMH, small heterotopias can be encountered as an incidental finding with high quality imaging.
- Transmantle gray matter heterotopias frequently have overlying cortical abnormalities such as polymicrogyria.
- Syndromic causes of GMH may be suggested by additional clinical or radiographic findings. For example, mutations in filamin A (*FLNA*) cause extensive periventricular GMH and are associated with joint laxity and valvular heart disease.

Pachygyria

- In pachygyria, there is a global failure of neurons to migrate into a compact six-layer cortex.
- As a result, the cortical ribbon is markedly thickened and overlying sulcation is attenuated (Fig. 4.4).
- *Lissencephaly* or *agyria* refers to severe pachygyria where the brain has scarcely any recognizable sulci.
- In some instances, the thick cortex will have a *cell-sparse zone*, which lacks gray matter signal, reflecting an absent cortical layer.

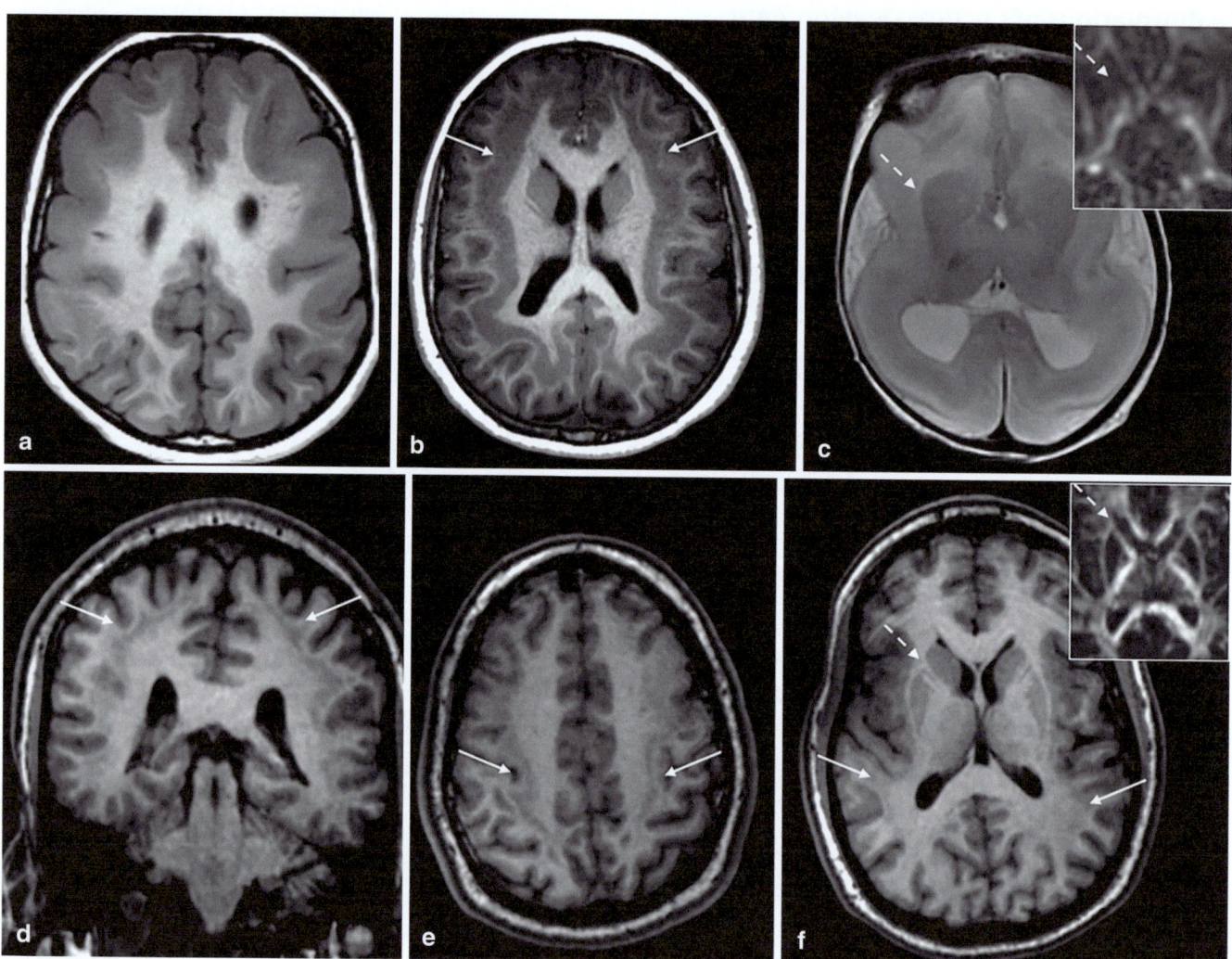

Fig. 4.4 Pachygyria and subcortical band heterotopia. Pachygyria features thick cerebral cortex with attenuated sulcation as demonstrated by these axial T1 (**a**) and axial T2 (**c**) images from two different patients. The most severe form of pachygyria is referred to as lissencephaly or agyria and features near total lack of sulcation (**c**). The gradient of severity (anterior versus posterior predominance) is determined by the underlying gene mutation. For example, mutations in the *DCX* gene cause anterior predominant pachygyria (**a**) whereas mutations in the *TUBA1A* gene cause posterior predominant pachygyria (**c**). When a pachygyria-associated gene mutation is present in mosaic form (i.e., not present in every cell of the brain), an attenuated phenotype known as subcortical band heterotopia (arrows in T1-weighted images **b**, **d**, **e**, **f**) results where a normal thickness cortex is accompanied by gray matter heterotopia parallel to the cortex. In subcortical band heterotopia, the anterior-posterior gradient is still generally preserved. For example, females who are obligate mosaics for *DCX* (located on the X-chromosome) have anterior predominant subcortical band heterotopia (**b**), and mosaic mutations in *TUBA1A* cause posterior predominant band heterotopia (**d**, **e**, **f**); the *TUBA1A* variants in **c** and **d/e/f** are p.R402C in both cases. Note that the basal ganglia are fused in the germline *TUBA1A* case with pachygyria (**c**) but not the mosaic *TUBA1A* case with an identical mutation (**f**), a difference which can be most easily appreciated by looking for the anterior limb of the internal capsule on the fractional anisotropy maps (arrows with dashed stems mark the absent anterior limb of the right internal capsule in **c** and its presence in **f**; fractional anisotropy maps shown as insets)

- With modern sequencing, upward of 80% of pachygyria patients will be found to have an underlying genetic cause, typically due to mutations in genes essential to neuronal migration (e.g., *DCX, LIS1, ACTB, ACTG1*, various tubulin genes).
- Features that distinguish the different genetic etiologies of pachygyria include:
  o Severity of cortical thickening.
  o Severity of attenuated sulcation.
  o Anterior to posterior gradient of severity.
  o Head size.
  o Basal ganglia fusion (seen in MCDs caused by tubulin mutations).
- Dilution of a pachygyria genetic variant attenuates the severity of the brain malformation and can produce *subcortical band heterotopia (SBH)*.
  o In SBH, there is a normal thickness six-layer cortex with minimally attenuated sulcation.
  o Gray matter signal deep to the cortex is not part of the cortex and is histologically similar to gray matter heterotopia.
  o SBH and mild pachygyria may be difficult to differentiate on imaging, but since the same genetic mutations can cause SBH or pachygyria depending on prevalence in tissue, this distinction will not influence appropriate genetic testing.

Focal Cortical Dysplasia (FCD)

- Focal cortical dysplasias (FCDs) are focal areas of abnormal neuronal tissue due to incomplete migration of neurons to the cortex and organization into normal cortical layers.
- FCDs are highly epileptogenic and represent the single most common malformation underlying refractory epilepsy.
- Resection of an FCD can render an epilepsy patient seizure-free, and therefore detection of an FCD can be life changing.
- Several types of FCD are generally recognized.
  o *Mild MCD* refers to microscopic neuronal heterotopia within the cortex or the subjacent white matter.
  o *FCD type I* refers to abnormal layering of the cortex.
  o *FCD type II* refers to abnormal cortical layering with dysmorphic neurons (e.g. balloon cells in FCD IIb).
  o *FCD type III* refers to abnormal cortical layering in conjunction with another lesion type such as mesial temporal sclerosis.
- The signature imaging finding of FCD is indistinctness of cortical gray-white matter differentiation on one or multiple tissue weightings, frequently with apparent cortical thickening or abnormal cortical folding (Fig. 4.5).
  o FCD I or mild MCD may be radiographically occult.
  o FCD II may be mildly expansile.
  o FCD IIb and less frequently FCD IIa may have a *transmantle sign*, which consists of a funnel or wedge-shaped signal abnormality that is narrow toward the ventricular margin and expands toward the cortex. The transmantle sign represents a fate-map of a mutated clone of neuronal precursor cells.
  o Upward of 50% of FCD II will have activating somatic mutations in the PI3 kinase—AKT—MTOR signaling pathway. Somatic mutations underlying FCD I are an active area of current research.
  o It is important to realize that although detection of a transmantle sign is specific for cortical dysplasia and specifically FCD II, regional signal abnormality, which obscures the cortex, has a differential that includes low-grade neoplasm and gliosis.

Hemimegalencephaly (HMEG)

- Dysplastic megalencephaly (DMEG) refers to regional brain overgrowth attributed to excessive neuronal precursor proliferation with disorganized cortex in one or multiple areas of the brain.
- HMEG is the most common subtype of DMEG wherein an entire hemisphere is affected.
- Imaging features of DMEG include (Fig. 4.5):
  o Increased volume of the affected brain parenchyma.
  o Abnormal cortex, which can have features of pachygyria, polymicrogyria, and cortical dysplasia.
  o Advanced myelination compared to the remaining brain.
  o Areas of heterotopic gray matter signal (variable).
  o HMEG/DMEG have been recently shown to be caused by activating somatic mutations in the PI3 kinase—AKT—MTOR signaling pathway, similar to FCD II.

Polymicrogyria (PMG)

- As the name suggests, PMG features an excessive number of small gyri.
- Histologically, this appearance reflects fusion of the most superficial layer of the cortex, which effectively clumps adjacent gyri to one another, but the migration of the neurons to the cortex is normal.
- In addition to a high incidence of seizure and developmental disability, PMG can be associated with abnormal tone and when found in the perisylvian region oromotor apraxia.

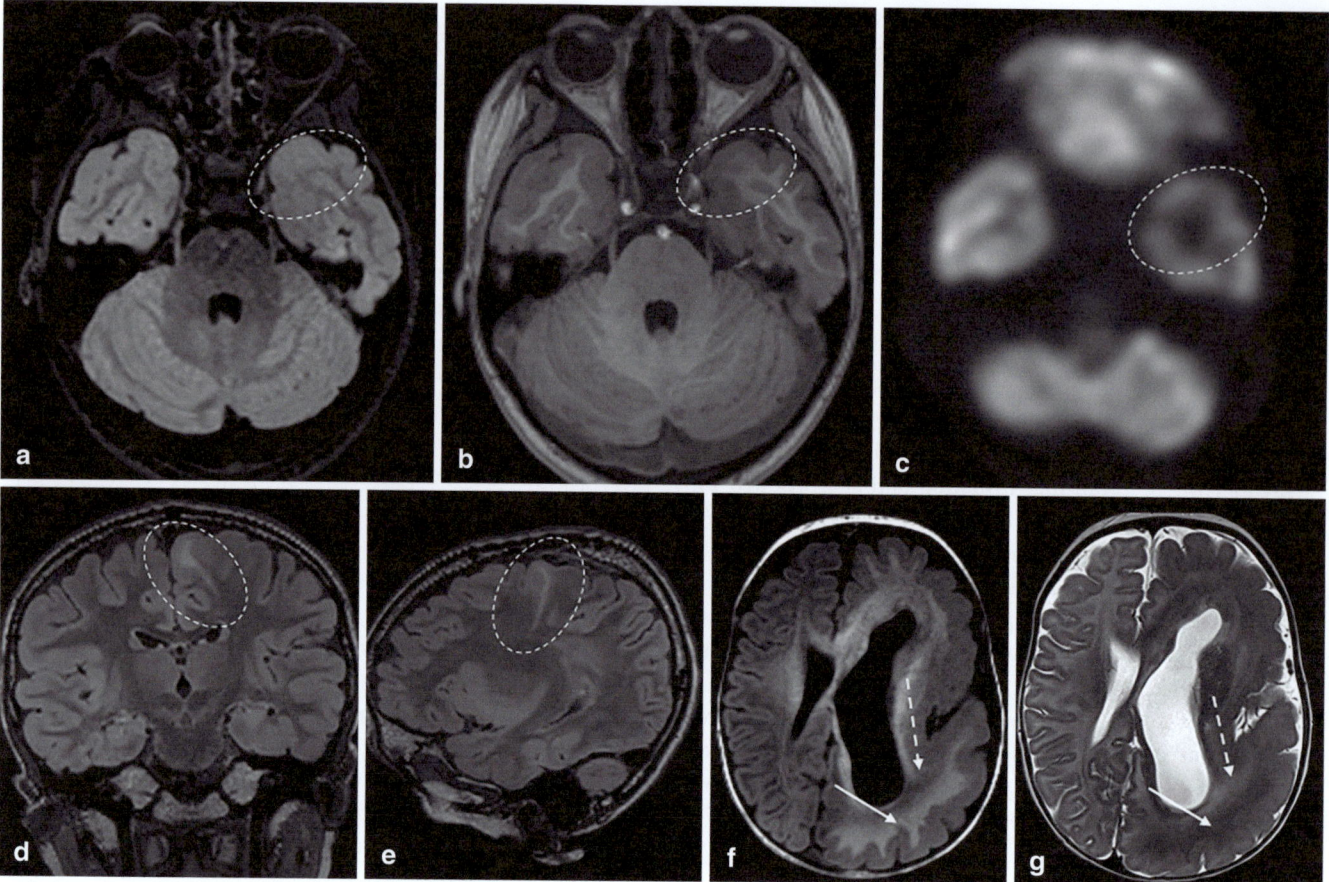

Fig. 4.5 Focal cortical dysplasia and hemimegalencephaly. Axial FLAIR (**a**), axial T1 (**b**), and axial FDG-PET (**c**) images of a child with left temporal FCD IA prior to resection demonstrate subtle loss of gray-white matter differentiation at the left temporal pole (circles, **a** and **b**) and hypometabolism over a wider area on FDG-PET (circle, **c**). The poor conspicuity of this finding on the T1 sequence (**b**) demonstrates the challenges of detecting FCD I, but the indistinctness of the peripheral white matter compared to the contralateral side on FLAIR drew attention to the left temporal pole (as did the PET data and correlative EEG data). By contrast, coronal (**d**) and sagittal oblique (**e**) 3D-FLAIR images of a patient who underwent resection of a left frontal FCD IIB demonstrates a conspicuous *transmantle sign* (circles, **d** and **e**), which fans out as it approaches cortex. Though FCD II shares genetic commonality with hemimegalencephaly, the imaging appearance is markedly different as illustrated by axial T1 (**f**) and axial T2 (**g**) images of a neonate with hemimegalencephaly who subsequently underwent functional hemispherectomy. In addition to enlargement of the affected left hemisphere, there are areas of thickened cortex reminiscent of pachygyria and areas of bumpy cortex reminiscent of polymicrogyria. There is also advanced myelination for age (arrows with solid stems, **f** and **g**) and patchy signal abnormality consistent with dysmyelination (arrows with dashed stems, **f** and **g**) in the left hemisphere

- On imaging, PMG has a number of unusual features not seen in other MCDs (Fig. 4.6).
    - Increased frequency of gyri within affected areas.
    - Obscuration or disruption of normal sulci.
    - Characteristic locations of involvement, most commonly the perisylvian region.
    - Fusion of the basal ganglia and cerebellar dysplasia may be present in cases of PMG due to tubulin mutations, making this feature alone insufficient to distinguish PMG from pachygyria.
    - However, a sharp gray-white matter interface and normal cortical thickness distinguish PMG from FCD and pachygyria, respectively (usually possible with modern MRI scanners in a patient with mature myelination).
- The causes of PMG are myriad but include megalencephaly syndromes (e.g., megalencephaly capillary malformation polymicrogyria syndrome) and environmental causes (e.g., congenital CMV infection) with extremes of head circumference and basal ganglia fusion being one of the few clues to a specific etiology.

Cobblestone Malformation

- Cobblestone malformations reflect excessive migration of neurons *past* the pial surface into the subarachnoid space.
- Cobblestone malformations are caused by mutations in structural proteins necessary for integrity of the basement membrane at the pial surface.

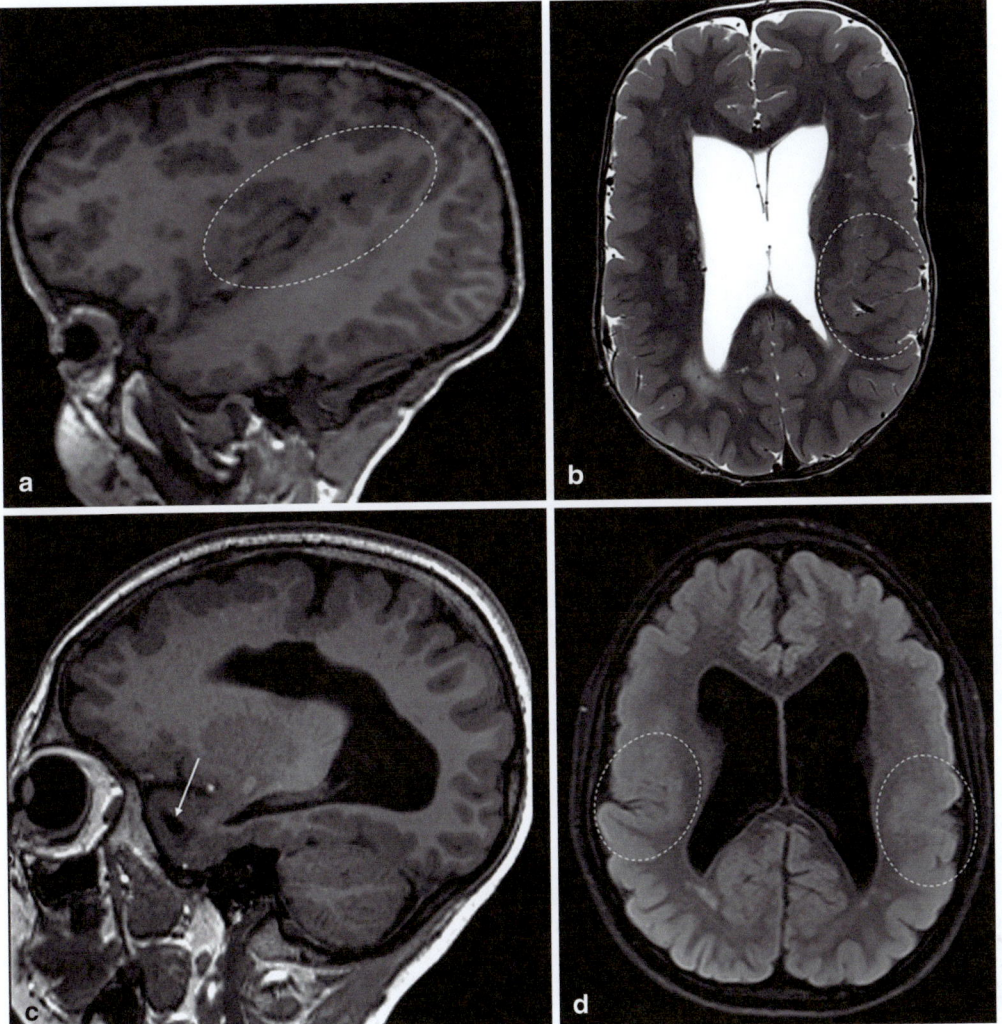

Fig. 4.6 Polymicrogyria. Sagittal T1 (**a**, **c**), axial T2 (**b**), and axial FLAIR (**d**) images of patients with megalencephaly capillary malformation polymicrogyria (MCAP) syndrome (**a**, **b**) and congenital CMV infection (**c**, **d**) demonstrate typical imaging features of polymicrogyria. In both cases, there is diffuse increase in gyral frequency, which leads to a bumpy appearance of the cortex and obscuration of the normal surface anatomy of the brain. As is often the case for polymicrogyria, these changes are most conspicuous in the perisylvian region in these two patients (circles in **a**, **b**, and **d**). Notice that the cortex is not actually thickened and the gray–white matter interface is sharp once individual gyri are resolved, allowing differentiation from pachygyria and cortical dysplasia, respectively. Polymicrogyria can be caused by many genetic mutations and environmental exposures. Head circumference can narrow the potential etiologies and is often reflected on imaging. As seen on the sagittal images, there is frontal bossing of the MCAP case indicative of macrocephaly (**a**) and posterior sloping of the forehead in the CMV case indicative of microcephaly (**c**). Additionally, CMV frequently has temporal horn cysts (arrow, **c**), calcification, and gliotic changes (not specific in isolation as demonstrated by periatrial gliosis in both **b** and **d**). The septum pellucidum is fenestrated in B from an endoscopic third ventriculostomy used to manage the patient's hydrocephalus, a complication of MCAP syndrome

- Because the same structural proteins are critical to muscle function and eye formation, cobblestone malformations can be associated with muscular dystrophy and congenital eye malformations.
- The surface of the brain in cobblestone malformations has superficial resemblance to polymicrogyria, namely, bumpiness from increased gyral frequency and obscuration of normal sulci (archaic term for cobblestone malformation was "type II lissencephaly").
- Some authorities actually conflate polymicrogyria and cobblestone malformation for this reason, and some genetic causes of cobblestone malformation are erroneously described as polymicrogyria even when there is contradictory histopathology (e.g., some of the tubulinopathies).
- However, cobblestone malformations have additional imaging features that assist with their recognition (Fig. 4.7).
  o Reduction of the subarachnoid spaces due to encroachment by neuronal migration.
  o Centrifugal islands of cortical gray matter at sites of pial basement membrane perforation.

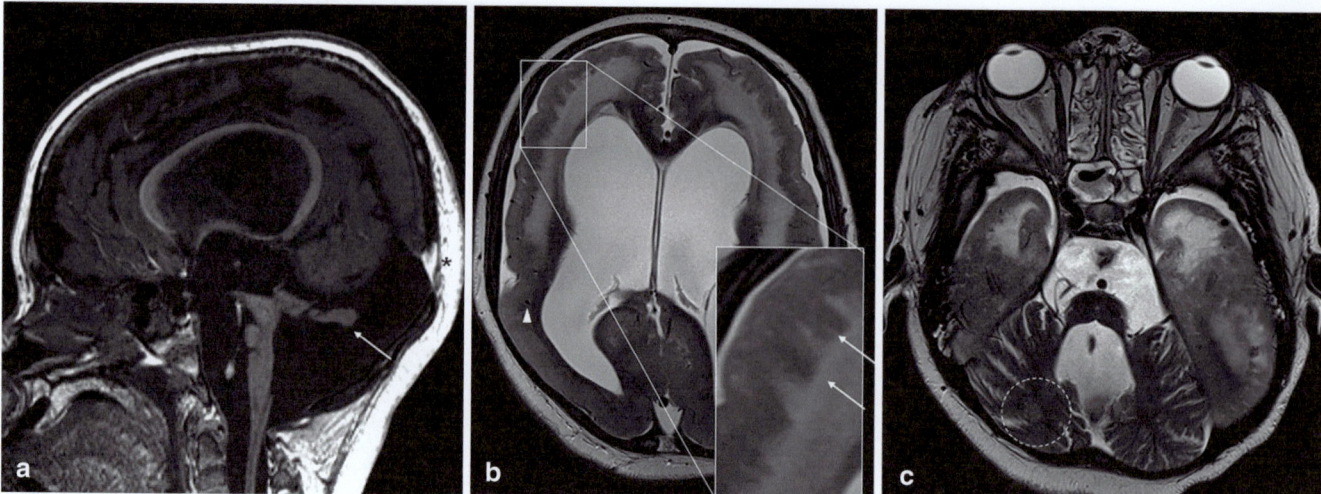

Fig. 4.7 Cobblestone malformation. Sagittal T1 (**a**) and axial T2 (**b**, **c**) images of a patient with Walker-Warburg syndrome demonstrate typical features of cobblestone malformation. The signature morphologic abnormality in cobblestone malformation is the absence of normal sulcation accompanied by apparent undulation of the cortical ribbon; with high quality imaging this cortical ribbon undulation can be demonstrated to represent centrifugal streaks of gray matter perforating the pial limiting membrane (arrows in **b** inset). Another manifestation of this spillage of gray matter into the subarachnoid space is the engulfment of major cerebral arteries by brain matter (e.g., the major right MCA opercular branch marked with an arrowhead in **b**). This case demonstrates additional features of a dystroglycanopathy, a common cause of cobblestone malformation: repaired cephalocele (asterisk in **a**), vermian/brainstem hypoplasia (arrow in **a**), high T2 signal of white matter from dysmyelination (**b**, **c**), and microcystic changes in the cerebellum (circle in **c**)

- Patchy areas of signal abnormality in the subcortical white matter due to abnormal myelination.
- Microcystic foci in the cerebellum.
- Unusual distribution of abnormal cortex compared to polymicrogyria in some subtypes of cobblestone malformation (e.g., frontal predominance of abnormal cortex in *GPR56* related cobblestone malformation).
- Association with hindbrain malformations (e.g., primitive, kinked configuration of the brainstem), and cephaloceles.

Non-MCD Pathologies

- While MCDs are common explanations for epilepsy, it is important to acknowledge other lesional causes of epilepsy (Fig. e4.4).
- *Mesial temporal sclerosis* (also called *hippocampal sclerosis*) is a common cause of temporal lobe epilepsy and results from an inciting event such as febrile seizure.
  - Histologically, there is neuronal loss in the hippocampus.
  - Radiographically, the hippocampus is reduced in volume, high in T2 signal intensity, and lacking normal gray-white matter differentiation ("internal architecture").
  - Presence of mesial temporal sclerosis does not preclude a genetic etiology or another structural cause of epilepsy.
- *Rasmussen encephalitis* is a progressive neurodegenerative process with underlying inflammatory changes and a poorly understood pathogenesis.
  - The most characteristic imaging finding is progressive volume loss, especially cortical volume loss.
  - Associated signal abnormality is variable but typically mild.
  - Findings are typically unilateral, which could prompt consideration of an FCD upon initial imaging.
  - Epilepsy can be severe and result in continuous focal epilepsy referrable to the affected region of the brain (*epilepsia partialis continuua*).
- Other forms of injury can incite seizure including arterial ischemic stroke, trauma, and hemorrhage.
- Cortically based neoplasms are a common acquired cause of epilepsy and low-grade gliomas in particular may be initially difficult to distinguish from an FCD without a transmantle sign.

Hindbrain Malformations

- Although the embryology of the hindbrain (cerebellum, pons, medulla) is not as well understood as for the forebrain/cerebrum, there are several reproducible patterns of malformation and normative data, which assist with recognition of subtle abnormalities (Fig. 4.8) [2, 5].

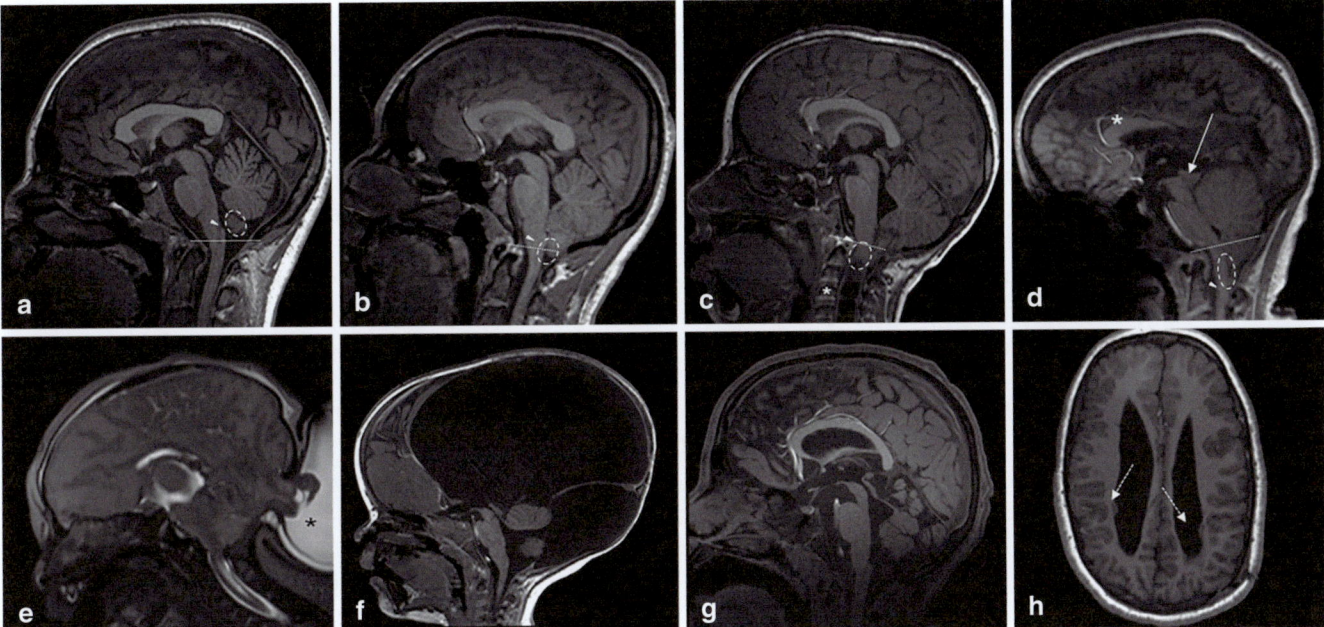

Fig. 4.8 Posterior fossa and cervicomedullary junction anomalies. Sagittal images provide a quick overview of abnormalities affecting the posterior fossa and cervicomedullary junction (**a–g**, all T1-weighted except for E, which is T2 weighted). Defining the foramen magnum as a line between the basion and opisthion (dashed line in **a–d**), the cerebellar tonsils (circle) and obex (arrowhead) are normally both above the foramen magnum (**a**). In tonsillar ectopia (**b**), the tonsils terminate below the foramen magnum, but there is a normal rounded configuration of the tonsils as well as preservation of the foramen magnum CSF space and normal position of the obex. In a Chiari I malformation (**c**), the cerebellar tonsils protrude into the upper cervical canal by more than 5 mm, resulting in pointed configuration of the tonsils and effacement of the foramen magnum CSF space. While the obex is still typically above the foramen magnum in a Chiari I malformation, it can become obstructed by soft tissue crowding, resulting in syringohydromyelia as seen in the shown case (asterisk, **c**). By comparison, the entire hindbrain herniates below the foramen magnum in a Chiari II malformation (**d** and axial T1 reformat **h**), a finding best appreciated by abnormal position of the obex below the foramen magnum. Additional common features of a Chiari II malformation include tectal beaking (arrow with solid stem, **d**), callosal dysgenesis (asterisk, **d**), and subependymal gray matter heterotopia (arrow with dashed stem, **h**). There is frequently stenogyria or increased gyral frequency in Chiari II patients. Stenogyria can be differentiated from polymicrogyria by lack of persistent increase of gyral frequency upon review of an area of concern in multiple planes and lack of cortical ribbon nodularity (compare **d** and **h**). A Chiari III malformation results from herniation of hindbrain into a cephalocele/myelocystocele involving the foramen magnum and upper cervical spine. This term is also sometimes applied to suboccipital cephaloceles, which share contraction of the posterior fossa CSF space and traction on the hindbrain toward the cephalocele (**e**, cephalocele sac marked with asterisk). A classic Dandy Walker malformation (**f**) and Joubert syndrome (**g**) are shown for comparison in midsagittal views but are further discussed separately

Chiari Malformations

- *Chiari I malformation* (C1M) refers to protrusion of the cerebellar tonsils below the foramen magnum with regional compression of soft tissue structures [2].
  - The foramen magnum is most easily defined by the *basion-opisthion line* on sagittal imaging.
  - Imaging criteria for C1M require descent of the tonsils by at least 5 mm AND tonsillar pointing due to crowding of the foramen magnum CSF space.
  - Resulting compression of the cervicomedullary junction in C1M can cause syringohydromyelia, presyrinx (edema, which is a precursor to syringohydromyelia), syringobulbia ("syrinx" in the brainstem), and (rarely) hydrocephalus from obstruction of the fourth ventricle outlet foramina.
  - Predisposing anatomic variation include shortening of the clivus, retroflexion of the odontoid, a hypoplastic posterior arch of C1, and basilar invagination.
  - Despite the term "malformation," C1M is an acquired rather than congenital abnormality, and some have therefore advocated the term *Chiari I deformation*.
  - C1M is distinguished from generic cerebellar tonsillar ectopia by the absence of tonsillar and cervicomedullary compression in ectopia.
  - C1Ms are associated with posterior headaches and symptoms referrable to the brainstem (e.g., gagging), but not all C1Ms will be symptomatic.
- *Chiari II malformation* (C2M) refers to protrusion of the hindbrain as a whole through the foramen magnum [2].
  - Although variable quantities of cerebellar tissue herniate below the foramen magnum in C2M, the key morphologic differentiator from C1M is the descent of the cervicomedullary junction.
  - The hindbrain herniation can be best identified by locating the *obex*, the opening to the central canal of the cord at the caudal extent of the medulla; in C2M the obex descends below the foramen magnum.

- The hindbrain herniation in C2M is a result of CSF egress from a myelomeningocele, but myelomeningoceles will occasionally lack a C2M due to limited CSF egress (i.e., a C2M may not develop if the myelomeningocele sac has skin overgrowth and a C2M can resolve after fetal repair).
- Unlike C1M, C2M is a true congenital malformation and can be seen on fetal MRI.
- Syringohydromyelia, presyrinx, syringobulbia, and hydrocephalus are commonly associated with C2M due to the severe compression of the cervicomedullary junction.
• *Chiari III malformation* (C3M) refers to hindbrain herniation in association with a low occipital cephalocele and/or high cervical myelocystocele. Due to the location, there is tenting of the cerebellum, brainstem, and upper cord, which are variably included within the cephalocele or myelocystocele sac.

Dandy-Walker Continuum

• *Dandy-Walker Continuum* (DWC) refers to a range of hindbrain malformations between the *classic Dandy-Walker malformation* (DWM) and milder dysmorphology, which some consider in the spectrum of normal variation (Fig. e4.5) [6, 7].
• *Classic Dandy-Walker Malformation* (DWM) refers to cystic expansion of the posterior fossa in association with a deficient cerebellar vermis.
  - Mechanistically, DWM is thought to arise from failure of the posterior membranous area to fenestrate.
  - As a result, there is ballooning of the posterior membranous area, which fills the posterior fossa as a cystic structure and classically elevates the torcula above the lambdoid suture (*torcular-lambdoid inversion*).
  - Hydrocephalus is usually present due to obstructed outflow from the fourth ventricle.
  - Due to coupling of posterior membranous area fenestration and cerebellar vermis embryogenesis, there is vermian hypoplasia, which is usually severe.
• Other entities in the DWC can be conceptualized as increasingly less severe vermian hypoplasia and failure of posterior membranous area fenestration.
  - *Inferior vermian hypoplasia* (IVH) with/without rotation is a morphologic descriptor of an abnormality in the DWC without expansion of the posterior fossa and typically without hydrocephalus either.
  - *Blake's pouch cyst* (BPC) refers to expansion of the foramen Magendie and rotation of a normally formed vermis with retrocerebellar CSF space enlargement (some authors also require hydrocephalus to be present for BPC).
  - *Mega cisterna magna* (MCM) refers to enlargement of the CSF space posterior to the cerebellum without vermian hypoplasia/rotation or mass effect.
  - Posterior fossa arachnoid cysts are differentiated from MCM by the presence of mass effect.
  - Due to differing definitions for entities short of DWM and circulation of confusing archaic terms such as "Dandy Walker variant," a morphologic description of findings in a DWC dictation is helpful for avoiding miscommunication.

Joubert Syndrome

• Joubert syndrome refers to a group of disorders with a *molar tooth malformation* (MTM) (Fig. e4.6) [2].
  - MTMs consist of thickened superior cerebellar peduncles, which have the appearance of molar tooth roots when viewed in the axial plane.
  - MTMs are associated with an absent superior cerebellar peduncle decussation on diffusion tensor imaging.
  - Vermian agenesis or severe hypoplasia are present.
  - In general, there is no distension of the posterior fossa CSF spaces so the vermian hypoplasia results in a midline cerebellar cleft.
• A large number of single gene disorders has been implicated in MTMs many of which are associated with cilia function.
• Recognition of a MTM is important as Joubert syndrome can be associated with renal and ophthalmologic abnormalities as well as supratentorial brain malformations.

Rhombencephalosynapsis

• *Rhombencephalosynapsis* (RES) refers to partial or absent cleavage of the cerebellar hemispheres (Fig. e4.6) [8].
  - The vermis is absent or partially absent.
  - But unlike IVH or MTM, the cerebellar parenchyma is in continuity across the midline.
  - Cerebellar fissures and the dentate nucleus can be followed from side to side.
  - The *fastigial point*, which defines the roof of the fourth ventricle, has a curved rather than sharply angled appearance.
  - Frequently, there are thalamic or midbrain fusion anomalies, which cause obstructive hydrocephalus.

Cephaloceles

• *Cephaloceles* refer to protrusion of intracranial contents (meninges, CSF, brain matter) through a defect in the dura and/or skull (Fig. e4.7) [2].

4 Congenital and Developmental Brain Malformations

- o *Meningoceles* contain CSF and meninges only.
- o *Encephaloceles* contain brain matter.
- Cephaloceles are classified by location.
  - o *Occipital cephaloceles* are the most common type in the Western hemisphere and can be associated with venous ischemic complications when they involve the dural sinuses.
  - o *Sincipital cephaloceles* involve the anterior skull base (e.g., frontonasal suture and foramen cecum) and can result in complex facial deformities due to encroachment on the sinonasal cavity as well as the orbits.
  - o *Skull base cephaloceles* are significant for their potential cause CSF leaks and meningitis.

Cysts

- Cysts are common incidental findings on brain imaging (Fig. e4.8) and are described in more detail in Chap. 19.
- *Rathke's cleft cysts* are benign cysts in the sella turcica or the pituitary gland itself.
  - o They can be differentiated from craniopharyngiomas by their lack of enhancing soft tissue and absence of chunky calcification.
  - o When large, they may have areas of T2 hypointensity from inspissated material.
- *Pars intermedia cysts* are located between the posterior pituitary bright spot and the adenohypophysis [9].
  - o Pars intermedia cysts can be found in over half of children with high quality imaging and do not require imaging follow-up.
  - o Some authors consider them a subtype of Rathke cleft cyst.
- *Pineal cysts* are intraglandular cysts of the pineal gland [10, 11].
  - o Have historically elicited concern because of potential overlap with cystic pineal neoplasms.
  - o However, published literature suggests that pineal cysts are found in up to a couple percent of patients, and they are encountered clinically substantially more frequently than that.
  - o Non-neoplastic pineal cysts lack nodularity or significant mass effect on adjacent structures.
  - o Cysts, which cause mass effect or have atypical features, are followed though there are no widely accepted criteria.
  - o FLAIR hyperintensity of pineal cysts is generally the rule, but hematocrit levels are a more specific sign of prior hemorrhage.
- *Arachnoid cysts* (ACs) are encysted areas of the arachnoid membrane, which cause local mass effect [12].
  - o ACs are common incidental findings, especially in the middle cranial fossa.
  - o AC growth is most commonly seen in the first 5 years of life and especially the perinatal time frame.
  - o Large cysts with mass effect warrant periodic follow-up in younger patients.
  - o Rarely, ACs can rupture into the subdural space or hemorrhage, triggering symptoms.
- *Neuroenteric cysts* are remnants of embryologic communications between the neuroectoderm and endoderm.
  - o Most commonly found in the spine where they can be associated with spinal formational anomalies.
  - o Intracranially, infratentorial location is more common than supratentorial.
  - o Most common location is ventral to the cord or brainstem.
- *Choroid plexus cysts* are benign cysts, typically in the glomus of the choroid plexus.
  - o Generally small and asymptomatic though they are considered a risk marker when detected in utero.
  - o Accumulation of lipid material results in a high proportion of diffusion signal abnormality in choroid plexus cysts.
- *Subependymal cysts* are cysts located along the ventricular system where they elevate the ependymal surface.
  - o Most common location is at the caudothalamic groove where they are termed *germinolytic cysts* due to their association with germinal matrix hemorrhage.
  - o Usually asymptomatic but can obstruct the ventricular system when large.

Phakomatoses

- *Phakomatosis* refers to multisystem disorders with congenital anomalies and/or neoplasms involving the skin, eye, and brain [13].
  - o With genetic characterization, the diseases in this group are now understood to have little mechanistic commonality.
  - o However, the syndromic associations do highlight the common embryogenesis of neuroectodermal structures.

Neurofibromatosis Type 1 (NF1)

- Autosomal dominant disorder due to loss of function mutations in *neurofibromin*, a tumor suppressor gene located on chromosome 17q11.2 [14].
- NF1 features tumors of the peripheral and central nervous system as well as tumors outside the nervous system (e.g., pheochromocytoma, rhabdomyosarcoma) and non-neoplastic abnormalities (Fig. e4.9).

- Low-grade gliomas present as expansile T2 hyperintensity infiltrating the optic pathway*, the brain parenchyma, and less commonly the spinal cord with variable enhancement (can be nonenhancing or avidly enhancing).
- Individual and plexiform neurofibromas* consisting of fusiform T2 hyperintense expansion of peripheral nerves, which classically have enhancement and central T2 hypointensity.
- *Buphophthalmos* refers to enlargement of the globe due to congenital glaucoma.
- Dysplastic bone* can be present at the greater sphenoid wing, tibia, and other locations adjacent to plexiform neurofibromas.
- Like dermatologic findings such as café-au-lait macules, many of the neuroimaging features are included in clinical criteria for diagnosis of NF1 (asterisked above).
• Areas of *myelin vacuolization* in NF1 (also called *spongiform change* or *focal areas of signal intensity*) produce ill-defined T2 hyperintensities in characteristic locations (basal ganglia, thalami, mesial temporal lobe, brainstem, cerebellar white matter).
- Myelin vacuolization tends to accumulate during the first decade of life and wane in the second decade of life.
- Differentiation of myelin vacuolization from low-grade gliomas can be challenging though the former do not have the circumscribed appearance, mass effect, and enhancement seen in low-grade gliomas.

Neurofibromatosis Type 2 (NF2)

• Autosomal dominant disorder due to loss of function mutations in *merlin*, a tumor suppressor gene unrelated to neurofibromin on chromosome 22q12.2 [15].
• NF2 is associated with multiple CNS tumors (Fig. e4.10).
- Spinal nerve, cranial nerve (e.g. vestibular), or extra-CNS schwannomas.
- Intracranial and spinal meningiomas.
- Spinal cord ependymomas (usually with indolent growth characteristics).
- Clinical criteria for NF2 are met in a patient with bilateral vestibular schwannomas or some combination of the above tumors, positive family history, and peripheral cataracts.
- Adult presentations commonly involve hearing loss but other focal neurologic deficits are more common in children with NF2 (e.g., facial palsy).

• Imaging of NF2 patients is directed at detecting extraaxial tumors so fat suppressed postcontrast imaging is essential.

Von Hippel Lindau (VHL)

• Autosomal dominant disorder due to loss of function mutations in *VHL*, a tumor suppressor gene located on chromosome 3p25.3, which regulates responses to hypoxia [16].
• VHL manifests as vascular CNS tumors as well as extra-CNS tumors (Fig. e4.11).
- Cerebellar and spinal hemangioblastomas present as superficial areas of nodular enhancement with surrounding edema and cysts/syrinx, the latter frequently posing the primary neurosurgical issue for VHL patients.
- Retinal hemangioblastomas also present as nodular enhancement with potential complication by retinal detachment.
- Endolymphatic sac tumors are malignant tumors, which destroy bone at the endolymphatic sac (vestibular aqueduct), uncommon even in VHL but not generally seen in other clinical settings.
- Pheochromocytomas and other neuroendocrine tumors.
- Renal cell carcinomas.

Tuberous Sclerosis Complex (TSC)

• Autosomal dominant disorder due to loss of function mutations in *hamartin* (TSC1) on chromosome 9q34.13 or *tuberin* (TSC2) on chromosome 16p13.3, both of which are negative regulators of the oncogenic PI3-kinase-AKT-MTOR signaling pathway [17].
• TSC manifests as hamartomatous overgrowths in multiple tissues of the central nervous system and torso (e.g., lymphangioleiomyomatosis, cardiac rhabdomyomas, renal angiomyolipomas).
• TSC can be clinically diagnosed in the presence of two major or 1 major plus 2 minor features where the neuroimaging findings are each considered major features (Fig. 4.9).
- Retinal hamartomas occur in as many as 25% of TSC patients though they may not always be readily visible on routine brain MRI.
- Subependymal nodules (SENs) are small hamartomas with mild T1/T2 shortening along the course of the caudates; as many as a quarter of these nodules will be calcified.

Fig. 4.9 Tuberous sclerosis complex. Axial T1 (**a**), T2 (**b**), and FLAIR (**c**) sequences demonstrate a dominant right foramen of Monro mass (arrows with solid stems, **a–c**), which grew over time in this TSC patient, consistent with a subependymal giant cell tumor. Smaller nodules elsewhere along the lateral ventricles (arrows with dashed stems, **a–c**) represent subependymal nodules of TSC, which differ from subependymal giant cell tumors in their long-term stability and smaller absolute size. Notice the slightly larger size of the right lateral ventricle, which highlights the potential for abnormal CSF dynamics secondary to subependymal giant cell tumors. The axial (**c**) and sagittal (**d**) FLAIR sequences from this patient also demonstrate numerous centrifugal streaks of signal abnormality denoting tubers (largest such foci are circled in **c, d**). These tubers are radiographically indistinguishable from the transmantle sign seen with sporadic FCDIIB (e.g., Fig. 4.8d and e)

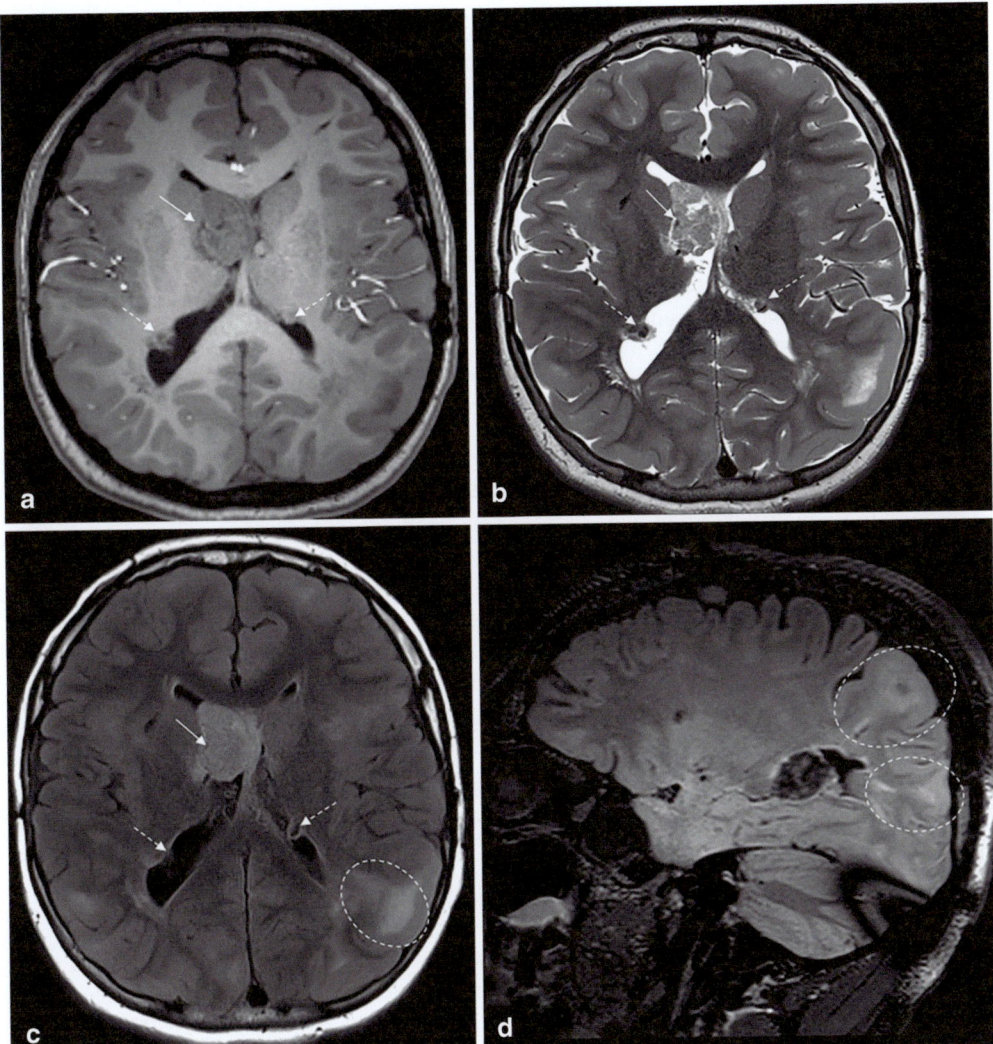

- Subependymal giant cell tumors (also called subependymal giant cell astrocytomas or SEGAs) are WHO grade I neoplasms, which are differentiated from SENs by their growth over time and may have less T1/T2 shortening (both SEGA and SEN may enhance). SEGAs at the foramina of Monro can cause obstructive hydrocephalus and are the major reason for periodic surveillance brain MRIs in TSC patients.
- Tubers are transmantle regions of signal abnormality, which progressively fan out as they extend centrifugally toward cortex; while T1 hyperintense and T2 hypointense relative to unmyelinated white matter, tubers demonstrate T2/FLAIR hyperintensity and magnetization transfer effect in a fully myelinated background.
- Tubers may demonstrate calcification, cystic change, and/or enhancement with enhancement particularly common in cerebellar tumors.
- Individual tubers are indistinguishable from FCD IIb, a resemblance explained by their common genetic etiology: tubers and FCD IIb are both thought to result from somatic activating PI3K-AKT-MTOR pathway mutations, but multiple lesions (tubers) develop in TSC due to the germline TSC1/2 mutations, which allow for lesions with a single additional hit (more likely than a double spontaneous mutation).

Sturge Weber Syndrome (SWS)

- SWS is caused by a recurrent activating somatic mutation in the GNAQ signaling molecule encoded on chromosome 9q21.2.
- Distribution of findings in SWS depends on precise timing of the somatic mutation event, but classic findings include ipsilateral involvement of the skin, eye, and brain (Fig. e4.12).
  - Capillary malformation (port wine stain) in the V1 and possibly the V2 distribution of the face.
  - Choroidal angioma (hyperenhancement) and glaucoma.

- Obliteration of the cortical veins and possibly the deep cerebral veins in the posterior quadrant.
- Early on, there is leptomeningeal enhancement, hyperperfusion, and the appearance of advanced myelination for age attributed to venous congestion.
- Chronically, the brain parenchyma undergoes atrophy, calcification, and decreased blood flow.
- Engorgement of the choroid plexus and deep venous collaterals may be present as secondary effects of the venous congestion present in SWS patients.

Brain Malformation Tips

- Detection and characterization of brain malformations require high quality imaging.
- For brain MRIs obtained for evaluation of epilepsy or developmental delay, the best possible magnet and head coils should be used (e.g., 3 T MRI, highest density multichannel head coil).
- Three-dimensional isotropic imaging should be obtained using T1 and FLAIR sequences to enable reformatting in multiple planes.
- High resolution axial and coronal T2 images are necessary for detailed characterization of the cortical ribbon and hippocampal architecture.
- Myelination can impact detection of brain malformations.
  - Immature brain myelination can obscure subtle abnormalities (e.g., in a 1 year old), and it is reasonable to offer follow-up imaging in this scenario if there is a high index of suspicion for an undetected abnormality.
  - With intermediate brain myelination, it is critical to review earlier imaging studies as cortical dysplasias can become transiently obscured as the brain myelinates.
  - Although brain myelination appears superficially complete by approximately 2 years of age, some degree of haziness of the frontal and temporal subcortical white matter is not uncommon in children less than 10 years old, and symmetry can be critical in differentiating pathology from incomplete myelination in this situation.
- When in doubt regarding subtle findings, review them in all imaging series as a "real" malformation will persist in multiple planes.
- Head circumference is often critical for suggesting a specific diagnosis.
- EEG data and seizure semiology can be used to direct attention to areas of the brain requiring added scrutiny.

References

1. Yang E, Chu WCW, Lee EY. A practical approach to supratentorial brain malformations: what radiologists should know. Radiol Clin North Am. 2017;55(4):609–27.
2. Barkovich AJ, Raybaud C. Congenital malformations of the brain and skull. In: Barkovich AJ, Raybaud C, editors. Pediatric neuroimaging. Philadelphia: Wolters Kluwer; 2019. p. 405–632.
3. Garel C, Cont I, Alberti C, Josserand E, Moutard ML, Ducou le Pointe H. Biometry of the corpus callosum in children: MR imaging reference data. AJNR Am J Neuroradiol. 2011;32(8):1436–43.
4. Severino M, Geraldo AF, Utz N, Tortora D, Pogledic I, Klonowski W, et al. Definitions and classification of malformations of cortical development: practical guidelines. Brain. 2020;143(10):2874–94.
5. Jandeaux C, Kuchcinski G, Ternynck C, Riquet A, Leclerc X, Pruvo JP, et al. Biometry of the cerebellar vermis and brain stem in children: MR imaging reference data from measurements in 718 children. AJNR Am J Neuroradiol. 2019;40(11):1835–41.
6. Whitehead MT, Barkovich MJ, Sidpra J, Alves CA, Mirsky DM, Oztekin O, et al. Refining the neuroimaging definition of the Dandy-Walker phenotype. AJNR Am J Neuroradiol. 2022;43(10):1488–93.
7. Whitehead MT, Vezina G, Schlatterer SD, Mulkey SB, du Plessis AJ. Taenia-Tela choroidea complex and choroid plexus location help distinguish Dandy-Walker malformation and Blake pouch cysts. Pediatr Radiol. 2021;51(8):1457–70.
8. Whitehead MT, Choudhri AF, Grimm J, Nelson MD. Rhombencephalosynapsis as a cause of aqueductal stenosis: an under-recognized association in hydrocephalic children. Pediatr Radiol. 2014;44(7):849–56.
9. Mahdi ES, Webb RL, Whitehead MT. Prevalence of pituitary cysts in children using modern magnetic resonance imaging techniques. Pediatr Radiol. 2019;49(13):1781–7.
10. Al-Holou WN, Maher CO, Muraszko KM, Garton HJ. The natural history of pineal cysts in children and young adults. J Neurosurg Pediatr. 2010;5(2):162–6.
11. Al-Holou WN, Terman SW, Kilburg C, Garton HJ, Muraszko KM, Chandler WF, et al. Prevalence and natural history of pineal cysts in adults. J Neurosurg. 2011;115(6):1106–14.
12. Al-Holou WN, Yew AY, Boomsaad ZE, Garton HJ, Muraszko KM, Maher CO. Prevalence and natural history of arachnoid cysts in children. J Neurosurg Pediatr. 2010;5(6):578–85.
13. Vezina G, Barkovich AJ. Neurocutaneous disorders. In: Barkovich AJ, Raybaud C, editors. Pediatric neuroimaging. Philadelphia: Wolters Kluwer; 2019. p. 633–702.
14. Friedman JM. Neurofibromatosis 1. In: Adam MP, Ardinger HH, Pagon RA, Wallace SE, Bean LJH, Gripp KW, et al. editors. GeneReviews((R)). Seattle; 1993.
15. Evans DG. Neurofibromatosis 2. In: Adam MP, Ardinger HH, Pagon RA, Wallace SE, Bean LJH, Gripp KW, et al. editors. GeneReviews((R)). Seattle; 1993.
16. van Leeuwaarde RS, Ahmad S, Links TP, Giles RH. Von Hippel-Lindau syndrome. In: Adam MP, Ardinger HH, Pagon RA, Wallace SE, Bean LJH, Gripp KW, et al. editors. GeneReviews((R)). Seattle; 1993.
17. Northrup H, Koenig MK, Pearson DA, Au KS. Tuberous sclerosis complex. In: Adam MP, Ardinger HH, Pagon RA, Wallace SE, Bean LJH, Gripp KW, et al. editors. GeneReviews((R)). Seattle; 1993.

Stroke

Yuh-Shin Chang and Pamela W. Schaefer

Introduction

Stroke is a leading cause of both disability and death worldwide [1], with approximately 795,000 individuals in the United States experiencing a new or recurrent stroke each year [2]. Recent acute stroke guidelines [3] emphasize that the early evaluation and treatment of eligible patients, by intravenous (IV) thrombolytic and/or endovascular therapy, lead to improved functional outcomes. Acute stroke patients should first be assessed by unenhanced head CT or brain MR imaging and CT or MR angiogram (CTA or MRA) to determine whether or not they are candidates for reperfusion therapies [4]. Subsequent radiological studies in stroke patients are also essential because they allow the early identification of stroke complications, and help predict clinical outcomes [5].

Definition

- A stroke is defined as a neurological deficit attributed to an acute focal injury of the central nervous system by a vascular cause, including cerebral infarction, intracerebral hemorrhage (ICH), and subarachnoid hemorrhage (SAH) [6].
- An ischemic stroke is defined as an episode of neurological dysfunction caused by focal cerebral, spinal, or retinal infarction. An ischemic stroke requires clinical symptoms, and evidence of infarction based mainly on clinical and neuroimaging data.
- The definition of ischemic stroke is limited to focal ischemia and does not include global ischemia resulting from decreased cerebral perfusion. A transient ischemic attack requires symptoms lasting <24 h, without clinical or imaging evidence of infarction.
- ICH and SAH correspond, respectively, to bleeding within the brain parenchyma or into the subarachnoid space that is not caused by trauma. ICH and SAH will be discussed in their respective chapters.

Pathophysiology

- In acute ischemic stroke (AIS), the severely hypoperfused area ("ischemic core"), will undergo infarction. A surrounding moderately hypoperfused area ("ischemic penumbra") is an area at risk of infarction unless perfusion is reestablished in a timely fashion.
- The lack of oxygen and glucose leads to neural injury through diverse mechanisms, including failure of cells to maintain ATP-dependent ionic gradients, excitotoxicity, mitochondrial alterations, free radical release, protein misfolding, and inflammatory changes [7].
- Irreversible ischemic injury triggers cell death through necrotic, apoptotic, or, less commonly, autophagocytic pathways.
- The temporal evolution of stroke includes four phases [8]:
  o Hyperacute stroke: 0–6 h.
  o Acute stroke: 6–24 h.
  o Subacute stroke: 24 h to approximately 2 weeks.
  o Chronic stroke: Greater than 2 weeks.
- Pathological changes in ischemic stroke [6]:
  o Hyperacute and acute ischemic stroke:
    - Cytotoxic edema related to ionic pump failure evolves within minutes to hours after the event, and declines within 1 day.

Supplementary Information The online version contains supplementary material available at https://doi.org/10.1007/978-3-031-55124-6_5.

Y.-S. Chang · P. W. Schaefer (✉)
Division of Neuroradiology, Department of Radiology,
Massachusetts General Hospital, Boston, MA, USA
e-mail: ychang3@partners.org; pschaefer@partners.org

© The Author(s), under exclusive license to Springer Nature Switzerland AG 2024
B. A. Vachha et al. (eds.), *What Radiology Residents Need to Know: Neuroradiology*, What Radiology Residents Need to Know,
https://doi.org/10.1007/978-3-031-55124-6_5

- Ionic edema, an extracellular edema caused by early endothelial dysfunction, appears shortly after cytotoxic edema [9].
- In areas of irreversible injury, histopathological changes appear after 6–10 h. Neuronal cell bodies are eosinophilic, and their nuclei become pyknotic.
  o Subacute ischemic stroke:
    - Vasogenic edema results from breakdown of the blood–brain barrier, and peaks approximately 24–48 h after acute ischemic injury.
    - Migration of polymorphonuclear neutrophils appear 1–2 days after stroke onset.
    - Neovascularization: 5–10 days after stroke onset.
    - Migration of macrophages and microglia into the infarcted area appears 5–6 days to 4–5 weeks after stroke onset.
  o Chronic ischemic stroke:
    - Development of cystic gliosis (cystic cavitation lined with rim of reactive astrocytes). The cavity is traversed by gliovascular bundles.

Anatomy

ARTERIAL ANATOMY

Extracranial Cerebral Arteries (Fig. 5.1)

- Carotid arteries (Fig. 5.1a, b).
  o In the classic configuration, the right common carotid artery (CCA) originates from the bifurcation of the brachiocephalic trunk, while the left CCA originates from the aortic arch.
  o The CCA branches into the internal (ICA) and external carotid arteries (ECA) at the carotid bifurcation at approximately the C3–C4 level. In 90% of cases, the ICA courses posterolateral to the ECA.
  o Cervical segment of the ICA:
    - Carotid bulb = focal dilatation of the ICA at its origin.
    - Courses superiorly in the carotid space of the neck, where it enters the carotid canal at the skull base.
    - No branches.
- Vertebral arteries (Fig. 5.1c).
  o Arise from the posterosuperior aspect of the proximal subclavian arteries:
    - In 6% of cases, the left vertebral artery (VA) originates from the aortic arch.
  o Common variations in size between sides:
    - A unilateral, atretic VA is found in 15% of individuals.
  o VA segments:
    - V1: Origin to the C6 transverse foramen.
    - V2: Passes through the transverse foramina of C6 to C2.
    - V3: From the C2 transverse foramen to the site where the VA pierces the dura mater at the level of the foramen magnum.
    - V4: Intracranial segment that joins the contralateral VA to form the basilar artery (BA).
      - Main branch of the V4 segment: Posterior inferior cerebellar artery (PICA).

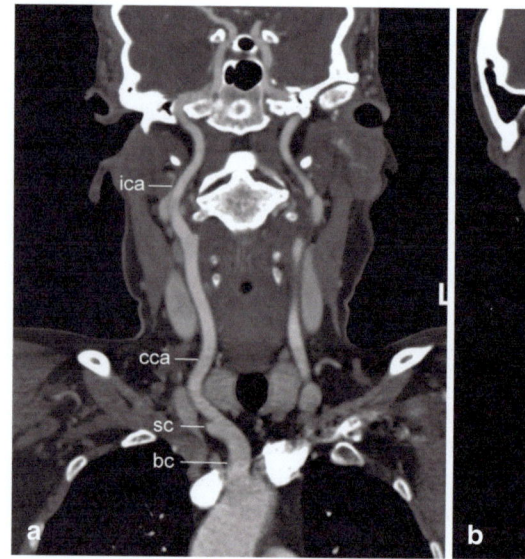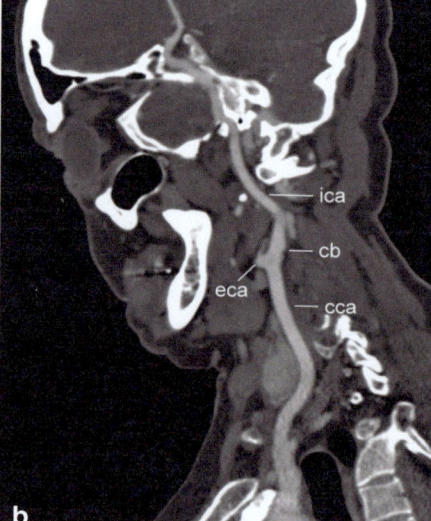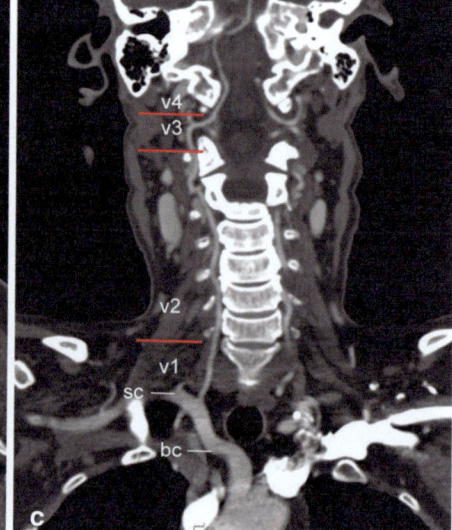

Fig. 5.1 **Extracranial cerebral arteries: Anatomy**. Overview of the extracranial cerebral arteries on CTA MIP images of the neck in coronal (**a**, **c**) and sagittal (**b**) views. (**a**, **b**) Extracranial carotid arteries. (**c**) Cervical vertebral arteries (VA). *bc* Brachiocephalic artery, *cb* carotid bulb, *cca* common carotid artery, *eca* external carotid artery, *ica* internal carotid artery, *sc* subclavian artery, *v1* V1 segment VA, *v2* V2 segment VA, *v3* V3 segment VA, *v4* V4 segment VA

Grading of ICA Stenosis (Fig. e5.1)

- Measurement methods that are derived from two major carotid endarterectomy trials, the North American Symptomatic Carotid Endarterectomy Trial (NASCET) and the European Carotid Surgery Trial (ECST) [10, 11] (Fig. e5.1a).
- (All electronic images (Figs. e5.1–e5.9) can be found on this chapter's website on SpringerLink: https://doi.org/10.1007/978-3-031-55124-6_5).
- The NASCET criteria compares the diameter of residual lumen to the diameter of the distal normal ICA lumen (beyond the post-stenotic dilatation).
  - The distal location is meant to avoid overestimation of stenosis when measured within the bulb or post-stenotic dilatation.
- The ECST criteria compares the diameter of the residual lumen with an estimate of the total arterial diameter at the level of the stenosis (usually the carotid bulb).
- The ECST criteria usually overestimate stenosis severity relative to NASCET criteria, which are more reliable.
- Caveats to stenosis grading:
  - Carotid near-occlusion (Fig. e5.1b): decreased contrast opacification and caliber of a collapsed ICA distal to a severe stenosis, which can result in underestimating the degree of stenosis using the NASCET grading criteria.
    - CT angiogram (CTA)-based criteria for carotid near-occlusion [12]:
      - Residual lumen diameter of ≤1.3 mm.
      - Presence of distal ICA caliber reduction:
        - Ipsilateral distal ICA diameter of ≤3.5 mm.
        - Ipsilateral distal ICA/contralateral distal ICA ratio of ≤0.87.
        - Ipsilateral distal ICA/ipsilateral ECA of ≤1.27.
  - Pseudo-Occlusion [13, 14] (Fig. 5.11b):
    - Apparent absent contrast opacification and caliber of the cervical ICA on CTA, but patency on digital subtraction angiography.
    - Seen in ~50% of patients with acute occlusion in the distal intracranial ICA, most commonly at the terminus ("T-occlusion").
    - Due to sluggish or absent contrast opacification in a stagnant column of unopacified blood proximal to the occlusion.
    - Imaging: flame-shaped tapering of the proximal cervical ICA, may mimic a long segment extracranial-intracranial ICA occlusion or dissection. Can be differentiated from true occlusion or dissection by opacification of the proximal ICA on the delayed CTA sequence.

Intracranial Cerebral Arteries [15] (Figs. 5.2 and e5.2)

- Internal carotid artery.
  - Various internal carotid artery (ICA) classification systems exist [16].
    - The most widely used system by Bouthillier et al. from 1996 divides the internal carotid artery into seven segments (Fig. e5.2):
      - C1: cervical segment (from the carotid bifurcation to the carotid canal).
      - C2: petrous segment (from the carotid canal to the posterior edge of the foramen lacerum).
      - C3: lacerum segment (from the posterior edge of the foramen lacerum to the superior margin of the petrolingual ligament).
      - C4: cavernous segment (from the superior margin of the petrolingual ligament to the proximal dural ring/anterior clinoid process).
      - C5: clinoid segment (between the proximal and distal dural rings of the cavernous sinus).
      - C6: ophthalmic (supraclinoid) segment (from the distal dural ring to just below the origin of the posterior communicating artery (PCoA)).
      - C7: communicating (terminal) segment (from below the PCoA to the bifurcation into the anterior cerebral artery (ACA) and middle cerebral artery (MCA).
- Middle cerebral artery.
  - Largest major branch of the ICA.
  - Arterial segments [17, 18]:
    - M1: Horizontal segment extending from the ICA to its bifurcation or trifurcation into M2 branches.
      - Bifurcates into superior and inferior M2 divisions in approximately 90% of cases.
      - Trifurcates into frontal, parietal, and temporal branches in approximately 10% of cases with many variations.
      - The lateral lenticulostriate arteries originate from the M1 segment.
    - M2: Ascending branches of the MCA overlying the insula, and ending in a sharp bend at the level of the circular sulcus of the insula.
    - M3: Branches originate within the opercular compartment, and end as the MCA exits the sylvian fissure.
    - M4: MCA branches extending along the brain convexity.
- Anterior cerebral artery.
  - A simplified classification of the ACA segments divides it into:

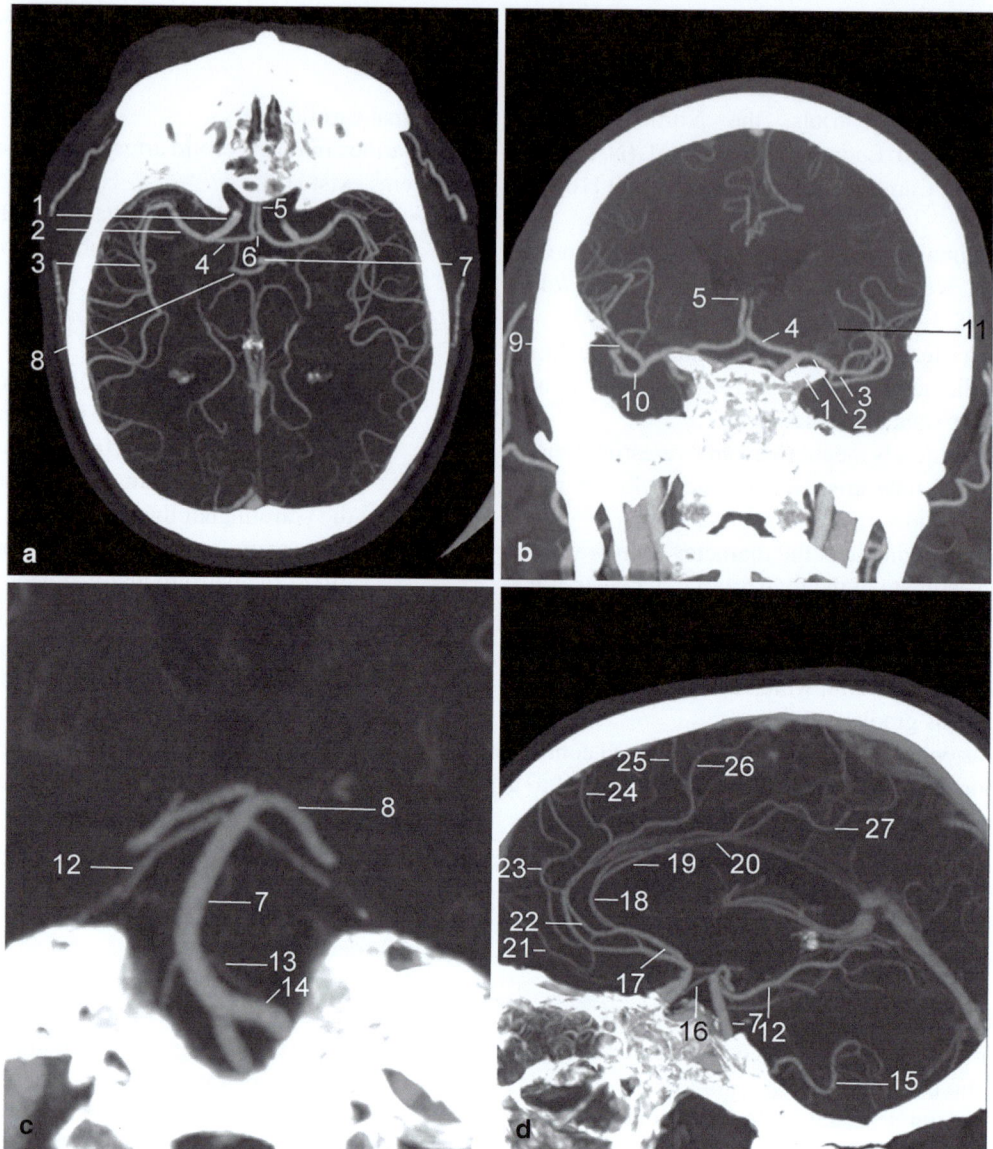

Fig. 5.2 Intracranial cerebral arteries: Anatomy. Intracranial cerebral arteries anatomy demonstrating major cerebral arteries and the circle of Willis. (**a**) Axial CTA MIP of the head. (1) Internal carotid artery (ICA), (2) middle cerebral artery (MCA, M1 segment), (3) MCA (M2 segment), (4) anterior cerebral artery (ACA, A1 segment), (5) ACA (A2 segment), (6) anterior communicating artery (ACoA), (7) basilar artery (BA), (8) posterior cerebral artery. (**b**) Coronal CTA MIP of the head at the level of the ICA terminus. (9) MCA (M2 segment, superior division), (10) MCA (M2 segment, inferior division), (11) lateral lenticulostriate arteries. (**c**) Coronal CTA MIP of the head at the level of the BA. (12) superior cerebellar artery (SCA), (13) anterior inferior cerebellar artery (AICA), (14) vertebral artery. (**d**) Sagittal CTA MIP of the head. (15) Posterior inferior cerebellar artery (PICA), (16) posterior communicating artery (PCoA), (17) ACA (A2 or postcommunicating/infracallosal segment), (18) ACA (A3 or precallosal segment), (19) ACA (A4 or supracallosal segment, pericallosal artery), (20) ACA (A5 or postcallosal segment), (21) frontopolar artery, (22) callosomarginal artery, (23) anterior internal frontal artery, (24) middle internal frontal artery, (25) posterior internal frontal artery, (26) paracentral artery, (27) parietal artery

- A proximal or A1 segment, located between the ICA and its junction with the anterior communicating artery (ACoA).
- An A2 segment—originating at the ACoA, extending anterior to the lamina terminalis and rostrum of the corpus callosum. The A2 typically branches into the callosal marginal artery lying in the cingulate sulcus and the pericallosal artery lying in the pericallosal cistern.
- More distal segments labeled A3 to A5.
  ○ Major ACA branches:
    - Proximal (A1) segment: Medial lenticulostriate arteries, ACoA.

- A2 segment: Recurrent artery of Heubner (originates less commonly from A1) and small basal perforating arteries.
    - A3–A5 segments—Cortical branches predominantly arising from the callosal marginal or pericallosal arteries: Orbitofrontal artery; frontopolar artery; anterior, middle and posterior frontal arteries; paracentral artery, superior parietal artery.
- Posterior cerebral artery.
  - The posterior cerebral artery (PCA) originates from the rostral BA, and is divided into four segments:
    - P1: From the BA to the PCoA.
    - P2: From the PCoA to the posterior aspect of the midbrain.
    - P3: From the pulvinar to the anterior limit of the calcarine fissure.
    - P4: Within the calcarine fissure.
  - PCA branches:
    - P1 and P2 branches: PCoA, tuberothalamic arteries, thalamoperforating arteries, thalamogeniculate and posterior thalamic arteries, posterolateral choroidal artery, posteromedial choroidal artery.
    - P3 and P4 branches: Splenial artery, anterior and posterior inferior temporal arteries, occipitotemporal artery, occipitoparietal artery, calcarine artery.
- Anterior choroidal artery (AChA) [19, 20].
  - Originates from the internal carotid artery, distal and posterolateral to the PCoA origin.
  - Divided into two segments:
    - Cisternal segment: from its origin to the choroidal fissure.
    - Intraventricular segment: enters the choroidal fissure at the plexal point.
  - Hyperplastic AChA [21]: anatomical variant, in which a prominent AChA supplies a part of the PCA territory.
- Basilar artery.
  - Originates at the pontomedullary junction from the joining of the two VAs.
  - Ends near the pontomesencephalic junction where it divides into the PCAs.
  - Branches:
    - Branches to the brainstem: Median arteries, short and long circumferential arteries.
    - Cerebellar arteries: Anterior inferior cerebellar artery (AICA), and superior cerebellar artery (SCA).
- Circle of Willis.
  - The ACoA and PCoA allow a redistribution of blood flow to the brain in case of a proximal vessel occlusion.
  - Anatomical variations are common [15], with a missing or hypoplastic PCoA found in more than 50% of subjects [22].

Arterial Vascular Territories [23, 24] (Fig. 5.3)

- MCA: Lateral aspects of cerebral hemispheres (frontal, temporal, and parietal lobes).
- Lateral lenticulostriate arteries: Lentiform nucleus, upper part of internal capsule [25].
- Medial lenticulostriate arteries and recurrent artery of Heubner: Head of caudate nucleus, inferior part of anterior limb of internal capsule.
- AChA: Hippocampus, inferior part of posterior limb of internal capsule, optic tract, cerebral peduncle, choroid plexus in the anterior temporal horn of the lateral ventricle.
- ACA: Medial parts of frontal and parietal lobes, anterior corpus callosum.
- PCA: Rostral midbrain, hippocampus, thalamus (P1 and P2 branches), inferomedial temporal lobe, occipital lobe, splenium of corpus callosum.
- SCA: Superior aspect of cerebellum.
- AICA: Anteroinferior aspect of cerebellum.
- PICA: Posteroinferior aspect of cerebellum.
- VA: Medulla.
- BA: Pons and caudal midbrain.

VENOUS ANATOMY [26]

Intracranial Venous System (Fig. 5.4)

- The cerebral venous system can be divided into cerebral veins and dural venous sinuses.
  - Cerebral veins can be further subdivided into superficial and deep veins:
    - Superficial cortical veins.
      - The major superficial cortical veins are:
        - Superficial middle cerebral vein.
        - Superior anastomotic vein (of Trolard).
        - Inferior anastomotic vein (of Labbé).
    - Deep veins.
      - The medullary veins drain into subependymal veins.
      - The subependymal veins merge into septal veins, thalamostriate veins, internal cerebral veins, and basal veins of Rosenthal.
      - The internal cerebral veins join the basal veins of Rosenthal to form the vein of Galen.
      - The vein of Galen joins the inferior sagittal sinus to form the straight sinus.
  - Dural venous sinuses.
    - Can be divided into superior and inferior dural sinuses.
    - Main dural venous sinuses:
      - Superior dural sinuses: Superior sagittal sinus, inferior sagittal sinus, straight sinus, and the transverse and sigmoid sinuses.

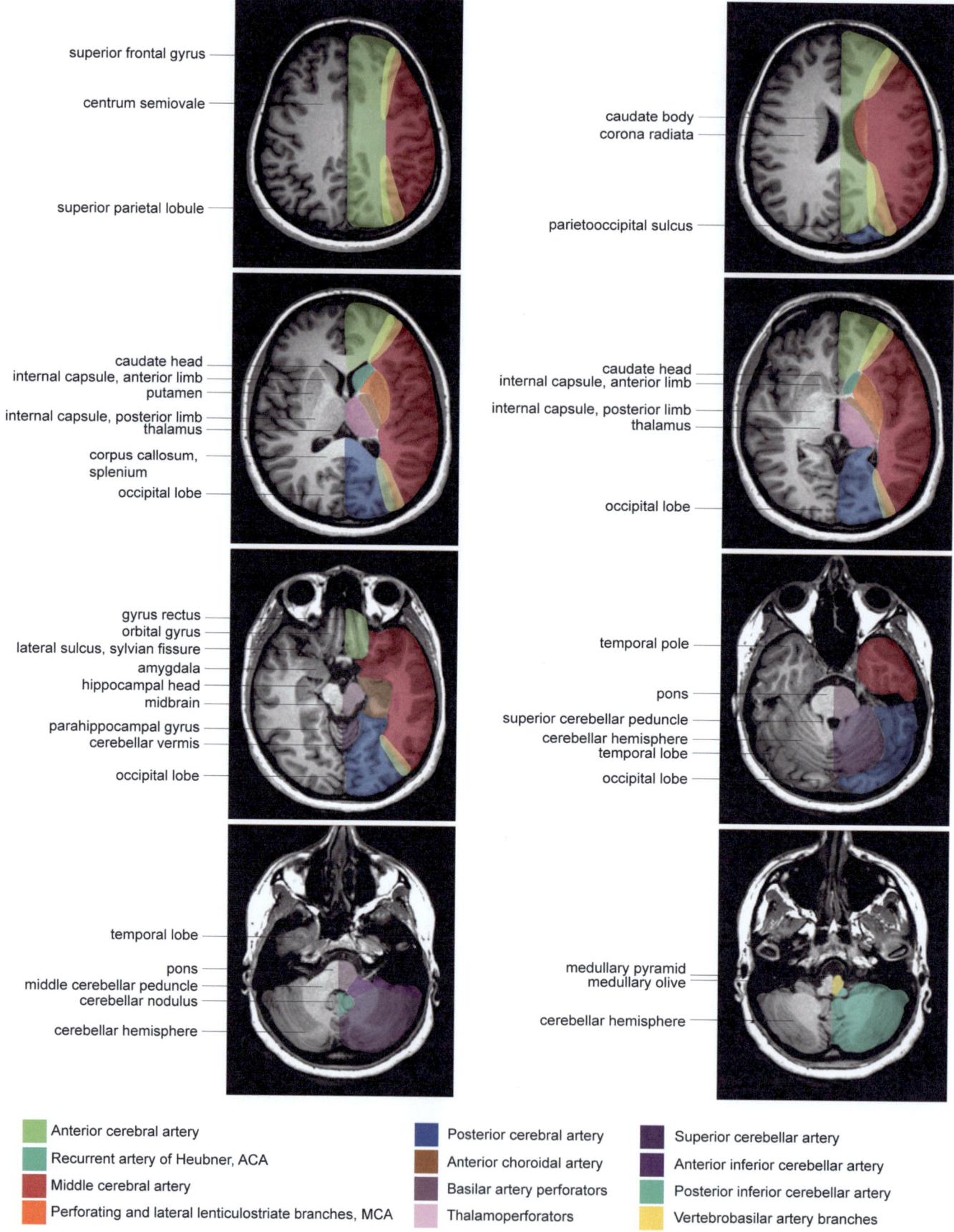

Fig. 5.3 Intracranial arterial vascular territories. Multilevel axial T1 MR images of the brain outlining the vascular territories on the left hemisphere and major anatomical structures on the right hemisphere

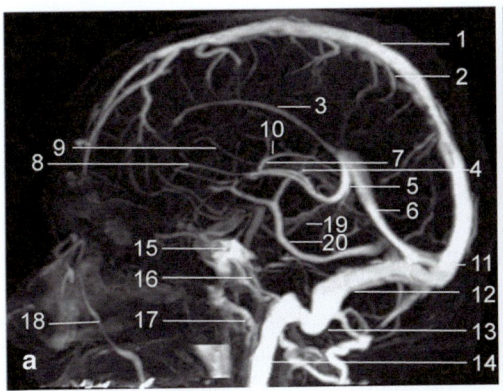

Fig. 5.4 Intracranial venous anatomy. Overview of the major superficial and deep cerebral veins. (**a**) Sagittal CTV Head MIP. (1) Superior sagittal sinus, (2) superficial cortical veins, (3) inferior sagittal sinus, (4) internal cerebral vein, (5) vein of Galen, (6) straight sinus, (7) thalamostriate vein, (8) septal vein, (9) anterior caudate vein, (10) terminal vein, (11) confluence of sinuses/torcula Herophili, (12) transverse sinus, (13) sigmoid sinus, (14) internal jugular vein, (15) cavernous sinus, (16) superior petrosal vein, (17) inferior petrosal vein, (18) common facial vein, (19) basal vein of Rosenthal, (20) inferior anastomotic vein of Labbé. (**b**) Coronal CTV Head MIP. There is a dominant left transverse sinus, an anatomical variant

- Inferior dural sinuses:
  - Cavernous sinuses and adjoining anterior and posterior intercavernous sinuses.
  - Superior and inferior petrosal sinuses.
  - Occipital sinus.
- Torcula herophili: Site of the confluence of superior sagittal sinus, straight sinus, occipital sinus, and transverse sinuses.

Venous Vascular Territories (Fig. e5.3)

- Superficial cortical veins: Drain the venous blood from the cerebral cortex and the subcortical white matter toward the dural sinuses.
- Deep veins: Drain the thalami, basal ganglia, upper brainstem, and cerebral deep white matter.
- Dural venous sinuses: Last point of confluence before the venous blood drains into the sigmoid sinuses and the internal jugular veins.

Stroke Treatment Options

TREATMENT OF ACUTE ISCHEMIC STROKE

Medical Treatment [3, 27]

- ≤4.5 h from symptom onset.
  - IV thrombolysis with alteplase for eligible patients with acute ischemic stroke presenting within 4.5 h of symptom onset.
  - In most patients, neuroimaging with noncontrast-enhanced CT (NCCT) provides information (e.g., lack of intracranial hemorrhage), which is sufficient to initiate IV thrombolysis [3, 28, 29].
- 4.5–9 h from symptom onset.
  - Patients with AIS that are seen 4.5–9 h from "time last seen well" can benefit from IV thrombolysis with alteplase [27] (WAKE-UP trial, EXTEND trial). These patients should have MRI DWI-FLAIR mismatch as defined in the WAKE-UP trial [30] or CT/MR evidence of core/perfusion mismatch as defined in the EXTEND trial [31], and not be candidates for endovascular treatment.

Endovascular Treatment [3]

- ≤6 h from symptom onset.
  - Mechanical thrombectomy with a stent retriever is indicated in patients with ischemic stroke and large vessel occlusion (LVO) in the anterior circulation, in which treatment can be initiated within 6 h of symptom onset.
  - LVO is defined as occlusion of the internal carotid artery or MCA M1 segment [3].
  - Other inclusion criteria for mechanical thrombectomy include:
    - ASPECTS of ≥6.
    - NIHSS score of ≥6.
    - Pre-stroke modified Rankin Score of 0–1.
    - Age ≥18 years.
  - Benefits of thrombectomy are less clear with occlusions involving M2 or M3 segments.
- 6–24 h from symptom onset.
  - The DAWN [32] and DEFUSE 3 [33] trials have shown that selected patients presenting with AIS within 6–24 h of "time last known seen well," and who have LVO in the anterior circulation, can benefit from mechanical thrombectomy.
- Thrombectomy is recommended in selected patients with occlusion of the ACA, VA, BA, or PCA when treatment can be initiated within 6 h of symptom onset [3, 23].

- Secondary stroke prevention [2].
  - Medical management of vascular risk factors (hypertension, diabetes, dyslipidemia), and lifestyle modifications for all patients.
  - Antithrombotic therapy, either with antiplatelet agents or anticoagulants, for most patients.
  - Long-term treatment with antiplatelet agents for patients with extracranial and intracranial vascular disease.
  - Anticoagulation for patients with stroke secondary to atrial fibrillation or other cardioembolic sources, and for patients with cerebral venous thrombosis (CVT).
  - Carotid endarterectomy or carotid artery stenting should be considered in patients with ipsilateral symptomatic severe (≥70%) carotid artery stenosis.
  - Percutaneous closure of a patent foramen ovale can be considered in patients with a non-lacunar ischemic stroke of undetermined cause, and a patent foramen ovale.
  - Treatment options for less common causes of stroke are described in [2].
- Secondary stroke work-up [2, 34].
  - Imaging studies recommended in the initial evaluation of acute stroke and TIAs: NCCT, MRI, and CTA or MRA.
  - Identification of atrial fibrillation either by Holter or by prolonged ECG recording.
  - The use of transthoracic echocardiography should be considered for patients with embolic stroke of unknown source [35].

Surgical Treatment [3, 9]

- Possible decompressive craniectomy for patients with mass effect, and ventriculostomy for patients with obstructive hydrocephalus.

Stroke Imaging

CT OF HEAD

Noncontrast Head CT (NCCT) Imaging in AIS (Fig. 5.5)

- NCCT of head should be obtained in all patients suspected of having an AIS to assess for the presence of a

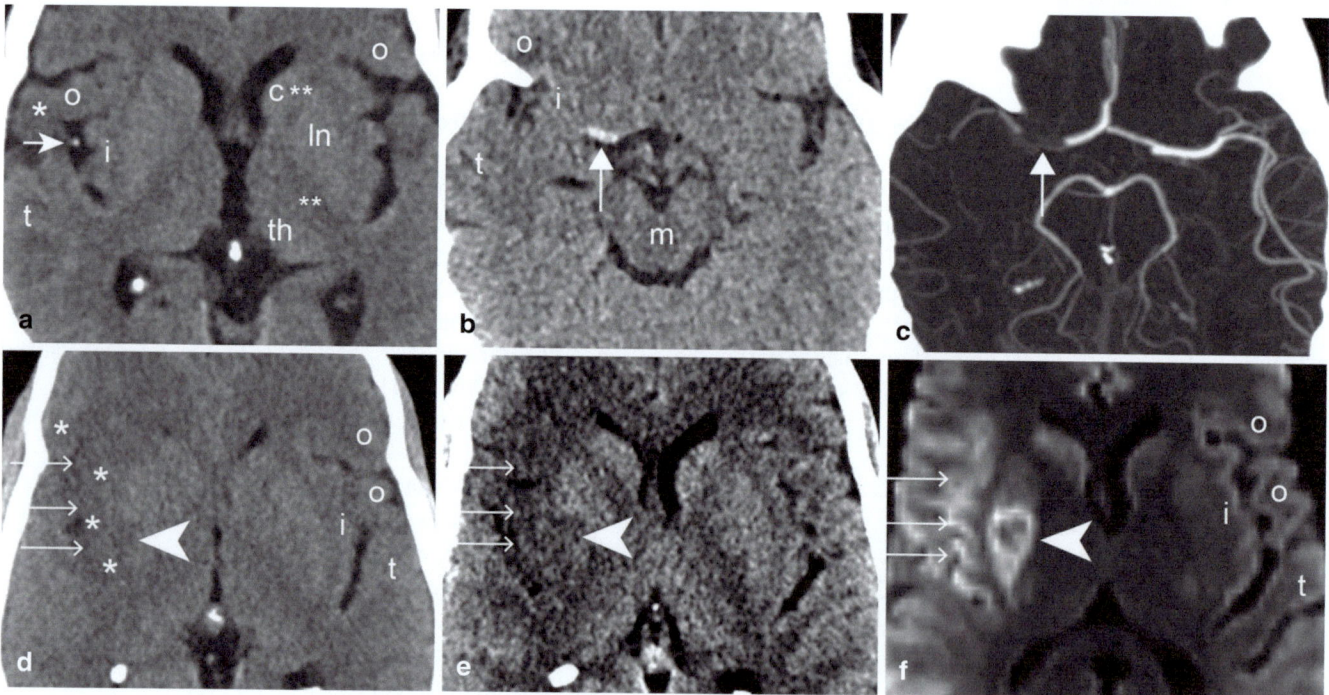

Fig. 5.5 NCCT findings in acute ischemic stroke. Findings in AIS on axial NCCT imaging. (**a**) MCA dot sign: punctate hyperdense thrombus (white arrow →) in a M2/M3 branch of the right MCA. There is subtle gray-white matter differentiation loss (*) in the right frontal operculum (o) compared to the normal contralateral side. (**b**) Hyperdense MCA sign: hyperattenuation in the proximal M1 branch of the right MCA at the site of a thrombus (white arrow →) seen on the concurrent CTA (**c**). (**d**) Insular ribbon sign: subtle loss of gray-white matter differentiation (*) in the right insular cortex (white arrow →) and in the posterior aspect of the right putamen (white arrowhead). There is also mild gyral swelling, resulting in effacement of the right sylvian sulcus. (**e**) Narrowing the CT window width setting to window width 8HU and window level 32 HU ("stroke window") markedly increases the sensitivity for detection of acute infarcts. (**f**) Axial DWI of the brain at the same level shows the extent of infarcted area. *c* Caudate head, *i* insula, *ln* lentiform nucleus, *m* midbrain, *t* temporal lobe, *th* thalamus, ** internal capsule

hemorrhage, extent of ischemic changes, or stroke mimic [3, 34].
- o NCCT is highly sensitive and specific (>95–98%) in detection of ICH [36].
- o Widespread availability, rapid image acquisition.
- o Variable sensitivity and specificity in detecting early ischemic changes [37].
  - Related to duration of stroke, infarct size, and location.
  - Within the first 3 h, detection rate ≤67%, increases to 82% at 6 h [37].
  - Higher sensitivity and specificity for the detection of acute anterior compared to posterior circulation infarcts.
  - Narrowing the CT window width settings increases the conspicuity of the infarct ("stroke window": window width, 8HU; window level, 32 HU) [34].
  - Addition of CT perfusion increases the sensitivity for detection of acute ischemic infarcts by 18.2% over NCCT alone.
- Early imaging findings of ischemic infarct [4, 8, 34] (Fig. 5.5).
  - o Appear within an hour of an AIS.
    - Subtle hypodensity in the lentiform nucleus.
    - Insular ribbon sign (loss of gray-white matter differentiation at the insula).
    - Cortical ribbon sign (loss of gray-white matter differentiation at the cortex).
  - o Imaging findings are secondary to reduced blood volume and edema.
- Other signs.
  - o Hyperdense artery sign.
    - Hyperdense MCA sign (M1 segment).
      - High specificity (~100%); low sensitivity (17–50%).
    - MCA dot sign: Hyperdense M2/M3 MCA branches.
    - Hyperdense basilar artery sign [38].
      - High specificity (98%); moderate sensitivity (71%).
  - o Eye deviation sign.
    - Gaze preference toward the side of infarct involving the corticospinal tract or frontal eye fields.

Alberta Stroke Program Early CT Score (ASPECTS) (Fig. e5.4) [5, 34]

- A 10-point scoring system based on early ischemic changes on NCCT scan.
  - o A score of 10 is normal. One point is deducted for each area in the MCA territory in which ischemic change is identified.
- Correlates with prognosis, clinical stroke severity, and presence and location of an intra-arterial occlusion.
- Insufficient evidence to suggest that there is a threshold that affects response to IV thrombolysis [3].
- Guidelines recommend that eligible patients with ASPECTS ≥6 should be treated with mechanical thrombectomy [3].
- A similar scoring system has been devised for posterior circulation ischemic strokes (pc-ASPECTS), but its use is still limited [23].

Evolution of Ischemic Infarct on CT and Complications (Fig. 5.6, Table 5.1) [8, 34]

- Hyperacute stage (0–6 h):
  - o Low sensitivity in detecting early ischemic changes.
    - Lower sensitivity for posterior circulation, small or deep infarcts.
  - o Early ischemic changes may not be present for up to 8 h.
- Acute stage (6–24 h):
  - o Wedge-shaped hypodensity, sulcal effacement, and gyral swelling without other mass effect.
- Subacute stage (24 h to approximately 2 weeks):
  - o Increased edema and mass effect [9], usually maximal at 48–72 h and decreasing after 7 days.
    - Mass effect may lead to cerebral herniation.
  - o Hypodensity becomes more apparent, then decreases.
  - o Fogging effect [39] (Fig. e5.5): Approximately 2 weeks after a stroke, the ischemic areas may regain near-normal density on NCCT due to inflammatory cell infiltration, capillary proliferation, and decreasing edema, causing an apparent disappearance of the infarct on imaging.
    - Occurs in up to 40% of medium to large-sized infarcts.
  - o Hemorrhagic transformation (HT), most commonly at 24–48 h after onset [40, 41].
    - Described in up to 50% of patients.
    - Petechiae or parenchymal hematoma.
    - ECASS classification [42]:
      - HI1: Small petechiae along the margins of the infarct.
      - HI2: Confluent petechiae within the infarcted area, without mass effect.
      - PH1: Hematoma ≤30% of the infarcted area, with mild mass effect.
      - PH2: Hematoma >30% of the infarct volume, with significant mass effect.
    - Multiple risk factors [40, 41].
      - Major risk factors: Atrial fibrillation, anticoagulant use, thrombolysis, mechanical thrombectomy, diabetes mellitus, poor collateral flow, large ischemic core, and high NIHSS.
      - Associated with poor clinical outcome.

- Increased risk following thrombolysis and thrombectomy [27].
  - Parenchymal hematoma reported in 5–6% of patients following thrombolysis and thrombectomy [28].
  - Symptomatic parenchymal hematoma in less than 2%.
  - >10 cerebral microbleeds on baseline MRI associated with increased bleeding risk (30–47%) following IV thrombolysis [3].
- HT should be differentiated from parenchymal contrast staining [41].
  - Contrast staining conforms to the boundaries of normal anatomic structures.
  - Contrast has a lower HU density than HT (<50 HU—100% specificity and 56% sensitivity for contrast staining) [43].
  - Contrast effect can last up to 48 h.
  - MRI T2*-weighed GRE or SWI sequences, or dual-energy CT imaging done after endovascular treatment can reliably distinguish contrast staining from HT.
- Chronic stage (Greater than 2 weeks):
  - Affected areas undergo volume loss, cavitation, and gliosis.

MRI OF HEAD (Fig. 5.7; Table 5.2)

MR Imaging Findings in Acute Ischemic Stroke

- MRI is more sensitive and specific at detecting early ischemic changes than NCCT [4].
  - DWI—88–100% sensitivity; 95–100% specificity [44].
  - DWI hyperintensity and ADC hypointensity appear within minutes of ischemic stroke onset.
  - DWI allows the most accurate quantification of ischemic core volume with low measurement error. A volume of 70 cc has been used in a number of trials as a cutoff for receiving intra-arterial thrombectomy.
  - DWI reflects alterations in water diffusion due to cytotoxic edema.
- MRI with SWI or T2* GRE is more sensitive and specific than NCCT at detecting ICH.
- Advantages are offset by lower availability, longer procedure time, and patient restrictions (incompatible metallic devices; claustrophobia) associated with MR imaging [4].
- The probability of positive findings on DWI increases in a time-dependent fashion after symptom onset [45].
  - Low false-negative rate on DWI scan performed >2 h from symptom onset.
- DWI-negative AIS [44]:
  - Patients with neurological deficits consistent with posterior circulation AIS have five times greater odds of having a negative DWI study.
  - Small AIS in the brainstem or hyperacute ischemia (≤6 h of symptom onset) may be underestimated or missed by DWI.
- Temporal evolution of ischemic stroke on MRI sequences (Fig. 5.7; Table 5.2) [4, 46, 47].
  - DWI: Hyperintensity for 10–14 days, then iso- or hypointense.
    - Persistence of high DWI signal in the late stages after an ischemic event reflects a T2 shine-through effect.
    - DWI signal can remain elevated due to marked T2 hyperintensity associated with vasogenic edema, tissue cavitation, and gliosis.
  - ADC: Signal intensity lowest at days 2–3, remains low up to approximately 1 week, then increases.
    - Pseudonormalization (when ADC values become similar to the surrounding brain) occurs 1–2 weeks after stroke onset.

Fig. 5.6 CT findings of evolving acute ischemic infarct. (**a**) Axial NCCT at <6 h after symptom onset shows very subtle gray-white matter differentiation loss in the right insula (white →) adjacent to two hyperdense thrombi in the occluded M2/M3 branches (small white →). This is better seen on stroke window (**b**). There is no significant mass effect. (**c**) One day later, the infarcted region corresponds to a wedge-shaped hypoattenuating area with gray-white matter differentiation loss and edema. The associated mass effect results in effacement of the sulci (black →) and partial effacement of the right frontal horn (*). (**d**) Early subacute infarct. On day 2, there is increased hypoattenuation and conspicuity of the now early subacute infarct with increased mass effect, resulting in further effacement of the right frontal horn and a subtle leftward midline shift. (**e**) Subacute infarct. On day 6, the edema and mass effect are maximal. There is near complete effacement of the right frontal horn (*), a mild midline shift and diffuse sulcal effacement. Early gyriform iso- to hyperattenuation in the cortices of the infarcted region (black →) could represent early cortical laminar necrosis or petechial hemorrhage. (**f**) Early chronic infarct. Increased hypoattenuation in the infarcted region corresponds to gliosis/developing encephalomalacia. The mass effect has decreased, resulting in reexpansion and asymmetric passive dilatation of the right frontal horn (*). (**g**) Late chronic infarct. In a different patient with a large PCA territory infarct involving the right hippocampal body and tail, medial temporal and occipital lobes, there is development of focal dystrophic calcification in the encephalomalacia (white ≫). Also note the asymmetric volume loss in the right cerebral peduncle, consistent with Wallerian degeneration

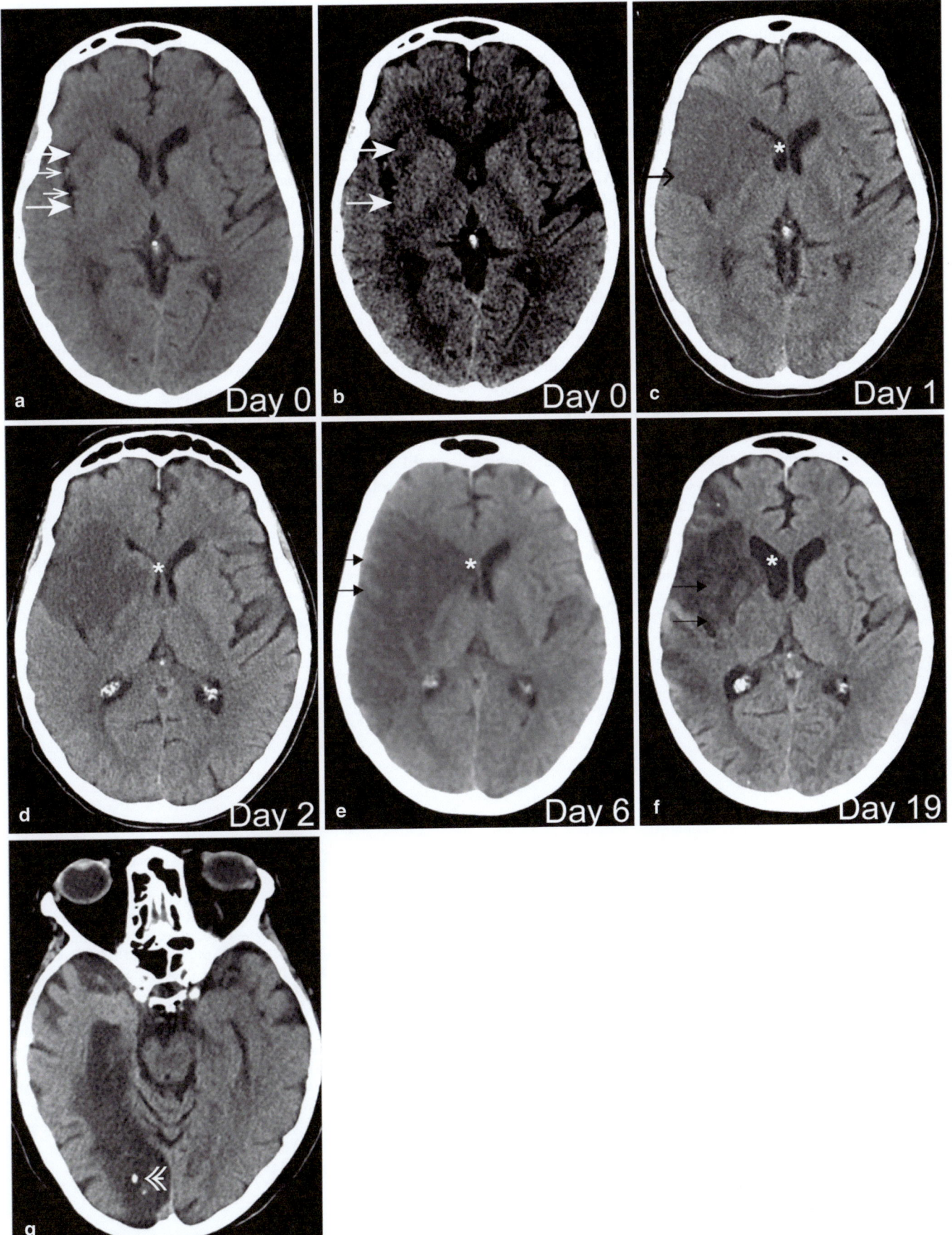

- Pseudonormalizaton reflects persistence of cytotoxic edema and development of vasogenic edema.
- The ADC continues to rise above normal tissue values as the development of gliosis and tissue cavitation occur.
o FLAIR: FLAIR hyperintensity, representing breakdown of the blood–brain barrier, appears approximately 6 h after the onset of an AIS. The signal intensity remains high during the subacute phase, then becomes low in the phase of cystic cavitation.
  - Early FLAIR hyperintensity is associated with increased extracellular water.
  - MRI DWI-FLAIR mismatch: defined as DWI hyperintense area of infarction with little to no associated hyperintensity on FLAIR. According to the WAKE-UP trial [30], AIS patients with unknown time of onset and DWI-FLAIR mismatch on MR imaging have better functional outcome after IV alteplase treatment.
o T1WI: Hypointense signal appears 16 h after stroke onset, and persists into the chronic phase.
o T2WI: Hyperintense T2 signal appears about 8 h after an AIS, and persists into the chronic phase.
  - In 50% of patients, there is fogging of the infarct on T2-weighed MR [39].
  - Most common during the second week after stroke.
  - The T2 signal becomes isointense due to decreasing vasogenic edema and the accumulation of inflammatory cells in the infarcted tissue.
o T2*-weighted GRE sequences and SWI: Highly sensitive in detecting hemorrhagic transformation, remote hemorrhages, and microbleeds.
o T1 C+: Collateral vessels with slow flow show enhancement in the acute phase. In the subacute and early chronic phases, there is gyriform enhancement from approximately 1 week to several months.
- Vascular signs on MR brain imaging.
o T2WI: Absent vascular flow void indicates arterial occlusion or slow flow.
o FLAIR: Vascular hyperintensities distal to an occluded vessel.

Table 5.1 Evolution of an AIS on NCCT. CT has a low sensitivity for the initial diagnosis of AIS. Factors such as size, duration, and location of infarct (anterior vs posterior circulation) will influence the depiction of early ischemic changes

Hyperacute 0–6 h	Acute 6–24 h	Subacute 24 h–2 weeks	Chronic >2 weeks
Obscuration of lentiform nucleus Insular ribbon sign Cortical ribbon sign Vascular signs: Hyperdense artery (hyperdense MCA sign, MCA dot sign, hyperdense basilar artery sign)	Wedge-shaped hypodensity Sulcal effacement Gyral swelling	↑ edema ↑ mass effect ↓ density then near-normal density—40% fogging at 2 weeks Hemorrhagic transformation ~50% at 24–48 h	Volume loss Cystic cavitation Gliosis

Fig. 5.7 MRI appearance of ischemic infarcts of various ages. First row: hyperacute infarct: axial MRI shows a DWI hyperintense, markedly ADC hypointense, FLAIR iso- to slightly hyperintense area in the frontal operculum, insula/subinsular region, and basal ganglia in the right MCA territory. Note that the DWI hyperintense region is larger than the FLAIR hyperintense region ("DWI-FLAIR mismatch") (arrowhead ▶), indicating a stroke onset ≤6 h. Second row: acute infarct: in a different patient, there is a large area of DWI hyperintense, ADC hypointense, FLAIR hyperintense diffusion restriction involving most of the left inferior cerebellar hemisphere, consistent with a large acute left PICA territory infarct. There is mild mass effect from the associated gyral edema, resulting in effacement of the foliae (white arrow →). On the axial postcontrast T1 images, there are engorged leptomeningeal vessels in the foliae (white arrow ⇒). Third row: Subacute infarct. In a different patient on day 3 after onset of symptoms, an infarct in the globus pallidus shows DWI hyperintensity, ADC hypointensity, and FLAIR hyperintensity without contrast enhancement. A likely older subacute infarct in the left posterior left putamen shows mild DWI hyperintensity, iso- to mildly hyperintense ADC ("pseudonormalization"), increased FLAIR hyperintensity and contrast enhancement (white open arrow →). Fourth row: chronic infarct. MR imaging in a different patient 2.5 years after a right PCA infarct shows a DWI hypointense, ADC hyperintense ("facilitated diffusion"), and FLAIR hyperintense (gliosis) and hypointense (cavitation) area of encephalomalacia involving the right occipital lobe (→). There is parenchymal volume loss, resulting in passive dilatation of the atrium of the right lateral ventricle. On SWI, tiny foci of susceptibility artifact within this region could represent petechial microhemorrhage or mineralization. In the right basal ganglia, there is focal cystic gliosis at the site of an old infarct (*). Fifth row: axial T1 image shows intrinsic T1 hyperintensity in the cerebral cortex of the right occipital lobe, consistent with cortical laminar necrosis

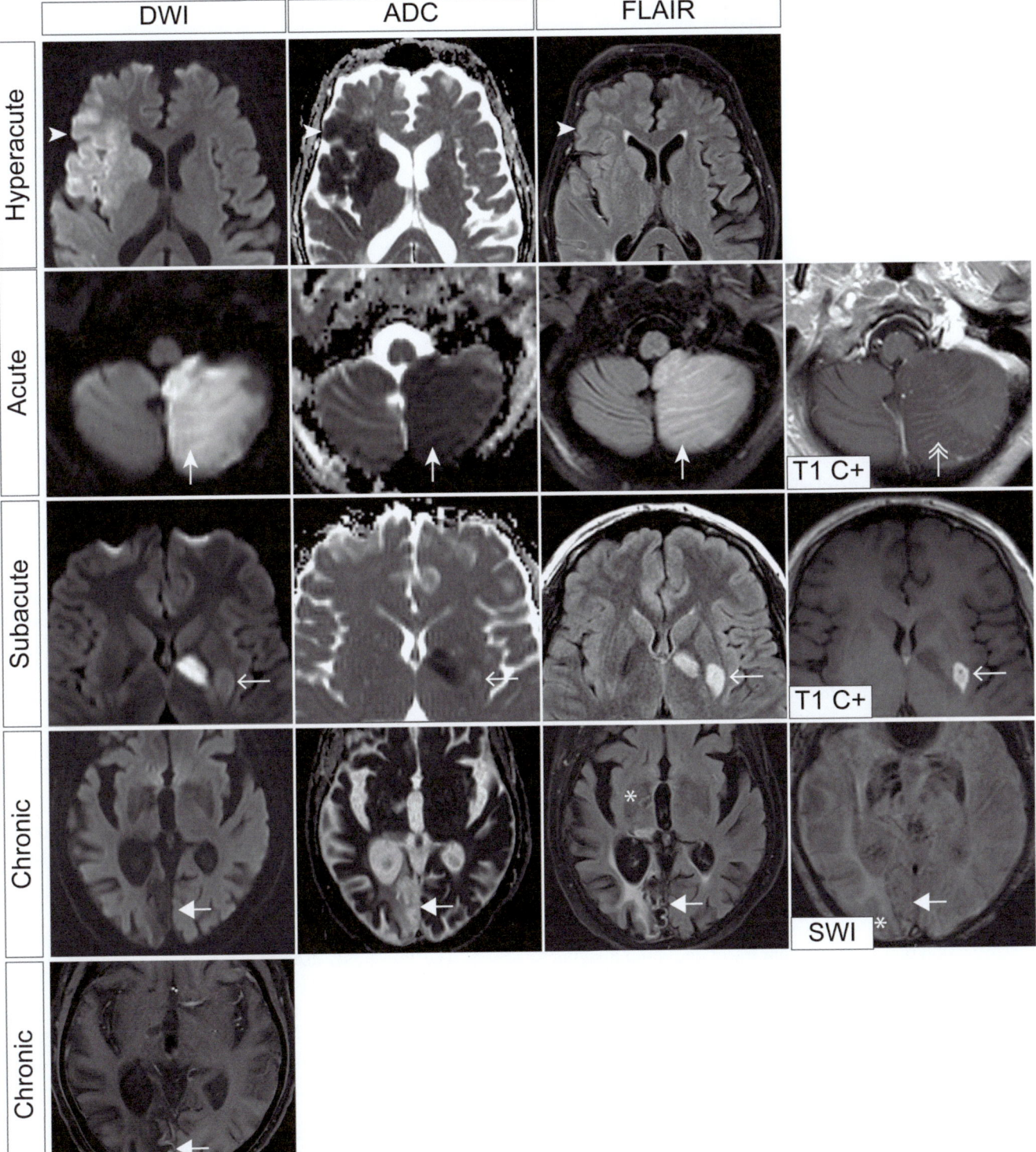

Table 5.2 Time course of MRI findings in AIS. Additional vascular signs seen on MRI sequences include an absence of arterial flow void on T2WI, T2*WI GRE/SWI blooming related to an intravascular thrombus, and FLAIR hyperintensity distal to an arterial occlusion

MRI sequence	Hyperacute 0–6 h	Acute 6–24 h	Subacute 24 h–2 weeks	Chronic >2 weeks
DWI	↑ within minutes	↑	↑ for 10–14 days	Iso or ↓; T2 shine-through if persistence of ↑
ADC	↓ within minutes	↓ Lowest at days 2–3	↓ Pseudonormalizes weeks 1–2	↑
FLAIR	iso	↑ at >~6 h	↑	↑ (↓ in cystic cavitation)
T1-WI	iso	↓	↓	↓
T2-WI	iso	↑ at ~8 h	↑ or iso: 50% fogging in second week	↑
T2*-WI GRE/SWI	–	–	Hemorrhagic transformation 24–48 h	–

- Indicate slow flow and good collateral retrograde flow.
- Favorable prognostic indicator.
  ○ T2*-weighted GRE and SWI:
  - Intraarterial blooming artifact is highly specific (99%) for detection of a large vessel thrombus (susceptibility vessel sign). SWI has superior sensitivity and better contrast resolution compared to T2* GRE and is more sensitive in the detection of distal M2 and M3 thrombi compared to Time-of-flight (TOF) MRA [48–50].
  - Prominent SWI hypointense medullary veins in the area of infarction indicate increased deoxygenation secondary to increased oxygen extraction ("misery perfusion") in that region [51, 52].
  - A discrepancy between a smaller area of infarct core and a larger area of misery perfusion on SWI (DWI-SWI mismatch) indicates the penumbra and predicts the risk for infarct expansion if left untreated [51].

PERFUSION IMAGING IN ACUTE ISCHEMIC STROKE (Figs. 5.8, e5.6, e5.7, e5.8, and e5.9; Table 5.3)

- Utilization of an intravascular tracer and serial imaging to measure blood flow in the brain parenchyma [53].
- Purposes: (1) improves the diagnostic accuracy, (2) assess the extent of infarcted, irreversibly damaged tissue ("ischemic core") and potentially salvageable ischemic tissue at risk of infarction ("ischemic penumbra"), (3) prognostication of functional outcome [53, 54].
- The two main perfusion imaging techniques are CT perfusion (CTP) [4, 55] and MR perfusion (MRP) [53, 56].
  ○ In CTP and dynamic susceptibility contrast MRP, the intravenous contrast agent is the tracer.
  ○ In Arterial spin labeling (ASL) [57], a more recent technique for MRP imaging, the protons of the arterial water molecules traveling to the brain are the tracer and no injected contrast agent is required (Fig. e5.6).
- Cerebral blood flow (CBF), cerebral blood volume (CBV), time to max (Tmax), and mean transit time (MTT) obtained through CTP or MRP are used to outline the extent of the ischemic core and penumbra. They are related through the following formula: CBF = CBV/MTT.
- Pathophysiology in AIS: Occlusion or significant stenosis → ↑MTT in the affected vascular territory → vasodilatation of the distal vessels → ↑CBV; CBF remains initially unchanged to slightly increased; once maximum vasodilatation is reached, further ↑MTT due to persistent stenosis/occlusion and decreased vascular supply cannot be further compensated and CBF then ↓.
- The core-penumbra mismatch [34, 55] allows for selection of patients with a high mismatch ratio, corresponding to a low hemorrhagic risk (small core) and a high likelihood of treatment benefit (large penumbra) [58] (Table 5.3) (Figs. 5.8 and e5.7).
  ○ The extent of the collateral circulation has a primary role in determining the mismatch between infarct core and penumbra and the rate of infarct growth.
  ○ Mismatch ratio: Ratio between the volumes of critically hypoperfused tissue and the ischemic core.
  ○ The thresholds used to define a core-penumbra mismatch are variable.
    - A mismatch ratio of ≥1.2 with a minimal penumbra volume of 10 mL are usually considered significant. A mismatch ratio of ≥1.8 has been used in a number of trials.

MR VESSEL WALL IMAGING (VWI) [59–61]

- Advanced MR imaging technique used to characterize vessel wall characteristics. When used in conjunction with conventional stroke imaging, it can help assess for the etiology of vascular stenosis in an ischemic stroke or TIA and help guide management.

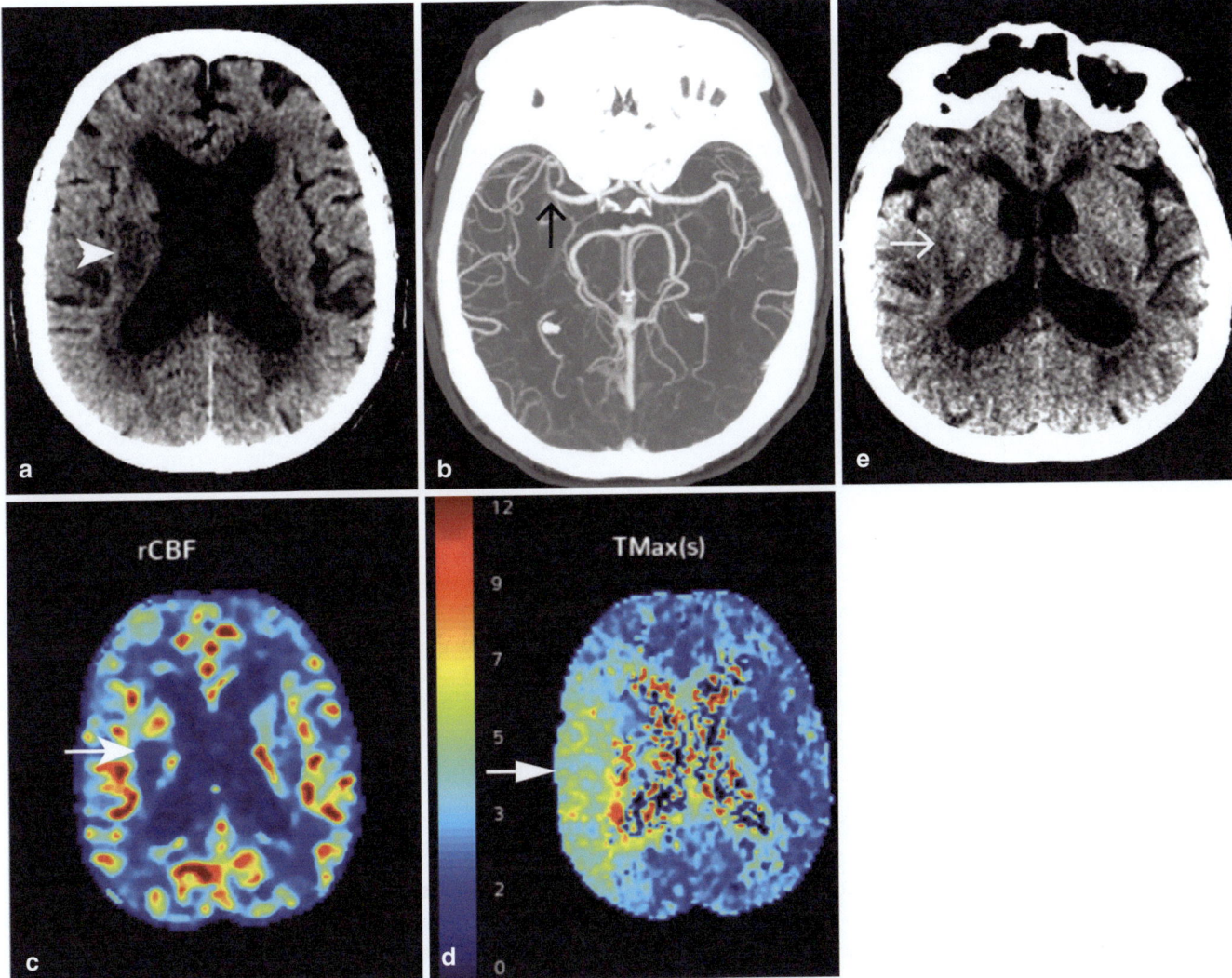

Fig. 5.8 CT perfusion of AIS with a large mismatch ratio. (**a**) Nonenhanced CT head shows a small hypodense area of gray white matter differentiation loss in the posterior superior right putamen (white arrowhead). (**b**) Axial CTA head MIP demonstrates an acute occlusion in the right M1 MCA segment (black arrow). (**c**) CT perfusion rCBF <30% sequence shows that the finding in (**a**) corresponds to a small volume acute ischemic infarct core (white arrow ➙). (**d**) Tmax CT perfusion map shows a large area of ischemic penumbra (Tmax >6 s) (white arrow ➙). This corresponds to a large mismatch ratio. The patient underwent thrombectomy. (**e**) Follow-up MRI/CT 2 days later demonstrates no enlargement of the ischemic core, but new hyperdensity from petechial microhemorrhage (white open arrow →)

Table 5.3 Perfusion imaging in AIS

Region	Definition	Threshold	Clinical significance
Ischemic core	• Irreversibly infarcted brain parenchyma • ↓↓CBF, ↓↓CBV, ↑MTT or Tmax	• Relative CBF (rCBF) ≤30% compared with the normal contralateral hemisphere most accurately estimates final infarct size after successful IA therapy/reperfusion • In very early time window (0–90 min) and after EVT, a rCBF of ≤20% may provide a more accurate estimate of the final infarct size and infarct core • Summarized in [53, 56]	• Non-salvageable brain tissue • Reperfusion therapy is associated with increased risk of hemorrhage • Using CBF alone may overestimate infarct core • CTP has lower signal to noise and higher core volume measurement error compared to DWI and can significantly underestimate or overestimate infarct core ("ghost infarct core"—tissue that has CBF ≤30% on CTP, but appears normal on follow-up imaging). Small subcortical, lacunar, and infratentorial infarcts are usually not detected with CTP

(continued)

Table 5.3 (continued)

Region	Definition	Threshold	Clinical significance
Ischemic penumbra	• Salvageable ischemic brain parenchyma at risk of infarction • ↓CBF, normal to ↑CBV, ↑MTT or Tmax	• Tmax >6 s is commonly used as a threshold for penumbra • Most accurately estimates final infarct size when no recanalization/reperfusion occurs	• Salvageable brain tissue if reperfusion is established in a timely fashion
Large core-penumbra mismatch ratio	Large area of ischemic penumbra, small area of ischemic core	• A mismatch ratio of ≥1.2 with a minimum penumbra volume of 10 mL (EXTEND-IA) or mismatch ratio ≥1.8 with mismatch volume ≥ 15 mL (DEFUSE3) is usually considered significant [55] • A mismatch ratio of >1.8 has also been used (SWIFT PRIME trial [5])	• Associated with high likelihood of treatment benefit • Summarized in [53]
None to small core penumbra mismatch ratio	Similar to slightly increased area of penumbra relative to area of ischemic core	• Mismatch ratio of <1.2	• Associated with high likelihood of reperfusion hemorrhage • No treatment advised as risk outweighs the benefit of reperfusion therapy.

- Conventional CTA, MRA, and DSA techniques assess the vascular lumen for the presence of occlusion, stenosis, dissection, but are limited in the assessment of the underlying etiology.
- In VWI, very high spatial and contrast resolution images are acquired before and after intravenous contrast with suppression of the blood ("black blood" signal) and CSF signals.
- The vessel walls are then assessed for the presence and pattern of vessel wall enhancement, lumen contour, and atherosclerotic plaque characteristics.
- VWI is useful to differentiate between atherosclerotic plaque (eccentric thickening, eccentric enhancement correlates with ischemic stroke), vasculitis (smooth concentric thickening and enhancement), reversible cerebral vasoconstriction syndrome (RCVS) (variable concentric thickening with no enhancement), intracranial dissection (detection of flap and vessel wall hematoma with variable enhancement), and Moyamoya vasculopathy (concentric thickening, enhancement correlates with infarction within 3 months), amongst others.

MODIFIED THROMBOLYSIS IN CEREBRAL INFARCTION (MTICI) GRADING [62]

- A recanalization grading scale that evaluates the degree of angiographic reperfusion following revascularization treatment.
- Ranges from 0 to 3, with grades of mTICI 2b or 3 indicating reperfusion of >50% of the affected territory.
- Current guidelines [3] recommend achieving grades of mTICI 2b or mTICI 3 following thrombectomy in order to maximize the probability of a good functional clinical outcome.
- Grading:
  - Grade 0: No perfusion.
  - Grade 1: Reperfusion past the occlusion, but limited or no distal reperfusion.
  - Grade 2a: Incomplete reperfusion. Reperfusion <50% of territory of occluded artery.
  - Grade 2b: Incomplete reperfusion. Reperfusion ≥50% of territory of previously occluded target artery.
  - Grade 3: Complete antegrade reperfusion of previously occluded target artery ischemic territory.
- A TICI 2c grading has been proposed to describe near-complete distal reperfusion, but has not met widespread use [63].

Ischemic Stroke Classification and Etiologies

ISCHEMIC STROKE SUBTYPE CLASSIFICATION SYSTEMS [64, 65]

- Trial of ORG 10172 in acute stroke treatment (TOAST) classification [66].
  - Most widely used etiologic classification of stroke subtypes.
  - Five ischemic stroke subtypes (Table 5.4):
    1. Large artery atherosclerosis.
    2. Cardioembolism.
    3. Small vessel occlusion (or lacunes).
    4. Stroke of other determined etiology.
    5. Stroke of undetermined etiology.
       - Meets one of the following criteria:
         a. Two or more causes.
         b. Indeterminate cause.
         c. Incomplete evaluation.

LARGE ARTERY ATHEROSCLEROSIS (Fig. 5.9, Table 5.4)

- Imaging findings: Cortical, cerebellar, brainstem, or subcortical infarcts >15 mm.

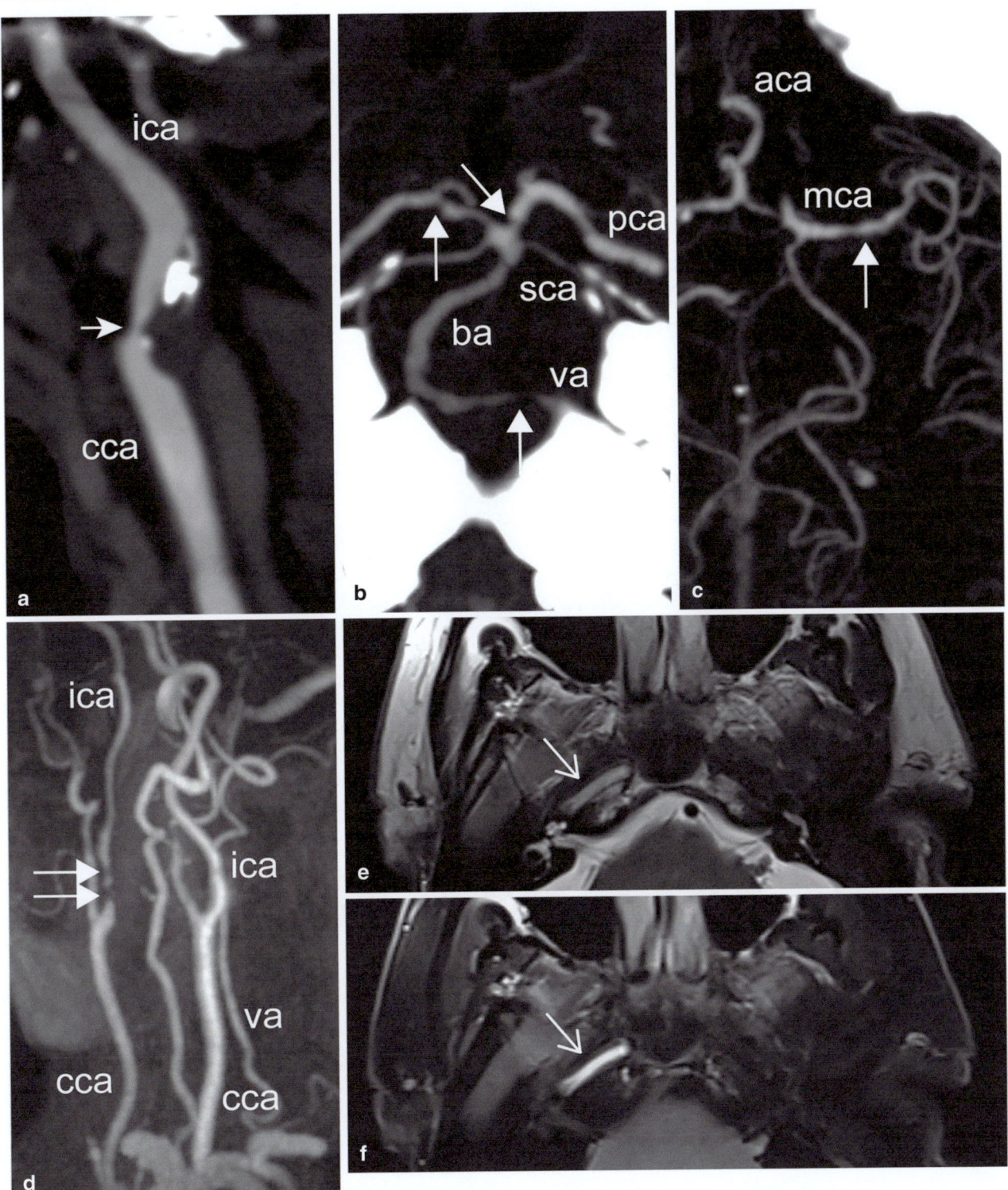

Fig. 5.9 Atherosclerotic disease. Extracranial and intracranial atherosclerotic disease. (**a**) CTA of the neck demonstrates atheromatous calcified and noncalcified plaques at the carotid bifurcation, resulting in severe stenosis of the proximal internal carotid artery (→). (**b** and **c**) CTA Head in the same patient shows severe intracranial atherosclerotic disease. (**b**) Luminal irregularities and multifocal stenoses in the intradural vertebral, basilar, left superior cerebellar and both posterior cerebral arteries. Note the severe stenoses in the intradural left vertebral and proximal left PCA (→). (**c**) In the same patient, luminal irregularities with multifocal mild stenoses are also present in the left MCA. (**d–f**) In a different patient, contrast-enhanced MRA of the neck demonstrate two foci of severe/critical stenosis in the proximal right ICA (→), resulting in decreased caliber distally compared to the contralateral left ICA and T2/FLAIR hyperintense slow flow in the ipsilateral right petrous ICA on axial T2 (**e**) and axial FLAIR (**f**) brain MRI. *Aca* anterior cerebral arteries, *ba* basilar artery, *cca* common carotid artery, *eca* external carotid artery, *ica* internal carotid artery, *mca* middle cerebral artery, *pca* posterior cerebral artery, *sca* superior cerebellar artery, *va* vertebral artery

Table 5.4 Overview of subtypes of ischemic strokes

Subtype	Pattern		Etiologies	Imaging appearance	Differential diagnosis
Extracranial vasculopathies			• Atherosclerosis • Dissection • Radiation-induced vasculopathy • Connective tissue disease (Ehlers Danlos) • Fibromuscular dysplasia (FMD) • Large vessel vasculitis (Takayasu's) • Giant cell arteritis	• Regional gray and white matter in one vascular territory • CTA, MRA: large vessel occlusion, stenosis or dissection	• Venous thrombosis • Seizures, postictal deficits • Migraine headache • Brain tumors • Hypoglycemia • Transient global amnesia • Herpes simplex encephalitis
Intracranial vasculopathies	Abnormal COW		• Atherosclerosis • Vasculitis (PACNS, others) • Moyamoya vasculopathy • Infection • Drug-related • Radiation-induced vasculopathy	• Wedge-shaped infarcts or lacunes: Punctate infarct ≤15 mm in the subcortical and deep white matter, internal capsule, thalamus, brainstem, cerebellar nuclei • CTA, MRA: abnormal vascular imaging	
	Normal COW		• Cerebral amyloid angiopathy • CADASIL • Susac syndrome • Arteriolosclerosis	• White matter infarcts	
Lacunar infarct, basal ganglia infarct			• Arteriolosclerosis • Infection (Tuberculosis)	Deep gray matter (basal ganglia, thalami)	• Hypoxic-ischemic encephalopathy • Carbon monoxide poisoning • Wernicke's encephalopathy • Extra pontine osmotic myelinolysis • Creutzfeldt-Jakob Disease • Vigabatrin toxicity • Nonketotic hyperglycemia • Venous thrombosis

5 Stroke

Borderzone infarct	Internal border zone infarct:	Punctate infarcts in internal border zones		• Cerebral hyperperfusion syndrome • Reversible cerebral vasoconstriction syndrome (RCVS) • Posterior reversible encephalopathy (PRES)
	External border zone infarct:	Punctate infarcts in external border zones		• Diffuse axonal injury • Active demyelination • Metastases
Central embolic infarct		Multifocal, multi-territorial infarcts	• Cardioembolic • Fat emboli • Air emboli • Calcific emboli • Septic emboli	

- Vascular imaging: Extracranial or intracranial atherosclerosis causing ≥50% luminal stenosis, or occlusion in the clinically relevant vessel.
- Evidence for accelerated atherosclerosis risk factors (hypertension, diabetes, dyslipidemia), or symptomatic atherosclerotic disease in other locations (coronary artery disease, aortic disease, and peripheral arterial disease).
- Stroke mechanisms.
  - Artery-to-artery embolism from atherosclerotic plaque, most commonly from the proximal internal carotid artery, just distal to the carotid bifurcation.
  - In situ thrombosis in intracranial atherosclerosis, more commonly in Asians.
  - Hemodynamic insufficiency due to progression of luminal stenosis.
- Border zone (or watershed) infarct [67].
  - Ischemic lesions that occur at the junction between two main arterial territories.
  - More often associated with extracranial than intracranial atherosclerotic disease.
  - Two main categories:
    - External or cortical border zone infarct.
      - At the junctions of the ACA, MCA, and PCA territories.
    - Internal or subcortical border zone infarct.
      - At the junction of penetrating vessels of the ACA, MCA, and PCA and deep perforating branches (mainly lenticulostriate arteries).
    - Cerebellar border zone infarcts also seen at the junctions of the PICA, AICA, and SCA territories.
  - Imaging findings:
    - External border zone infarct: Wedge-shaped cortical and subcortical infarct at the junction between vascular territories.
    - Internal border zone infarct: Series of bead-like ischemic lesions localized in the periventricular regions.
    - Can be unilateral or bilateral, depending on the location of the stenosis.
  - Mechanisms:
    - External border zone infarcts result more commonly from artery-to-artery embolism or cardiac microembolism but can also result from hypoperfusion.
    - Internal border zone infarcts are caused by hypoperfusion at the level of the distal penetrating arterial branches.

SMALL VESSEL OCCLUSION (OR LACUNES) (Table 5.4)

- Imaging findings: lacunar infarct (subcortical or brainstem infarct whose diameter is less than 15 mm [66]), leukoaraiosis (patchy or confluent CT hypodense lesion or T2/FLAIR hyperintense lesion in the subcortical or periventricular white matter), cerebral microbleeds or intracerebral hemorrhage in the subcortical white matter, deep gray nuclei or brainstem.
- Most common locations: Basal ganglia, internal capsule, thalamus, or brainstem, supplied by smaller caliber perforating arteries (e.g., pontine perforating arteries, lenticulostriate arteries, thalamoperforating arteries).
- History of hypertension or diabetes mellitus.
- Vascular imaging should not demonstrate findings consistent with large artery atherosclerosis.
- Stroke mechanisms [68]:
  - Hemodynamic insufficiency.
    - Narrowing of small penetrating arteries due to arteriolosclerosis.
    - Branch atheromatous disease with occlusion of the origin of penetrating arteries.
  - Embolism.
    - Uncommon cause of lacunar infarcts.

CARDIOEMBOLISM [69] (Table 5.4)

- Supportive imaging findings include acute ischemic lesions in multiple vascular territories.
- Vascular imaging shows abrupt occlusions of distal or branch arteries.
- Abnormal cardiac evaluation with the presence of a cardiac source for embolization.
- Causes: Atrial fibrillation, mechanical prosthetic valve, heart failure, recent myocardial infarction, atrial myxoma, infective endocarditis, patent foramen ovale.

STROKE OF OTHER DETERMINED ETIOLOGY (NON-ATHEROSCLEROTIC VASCULOPATHIES, PROTHROMBOTIC DISORDERS, AND OTHERS) (Figs. 5.10, 5.11, and 5.12; Table 5.4)

- Diagnostic studies (such as blood tests or arteriography) reveal the cause of stroke.
- 34% of ischemic strokes in individuals 18–45 years [70].
- 1% of ischemic strokes >45 years.

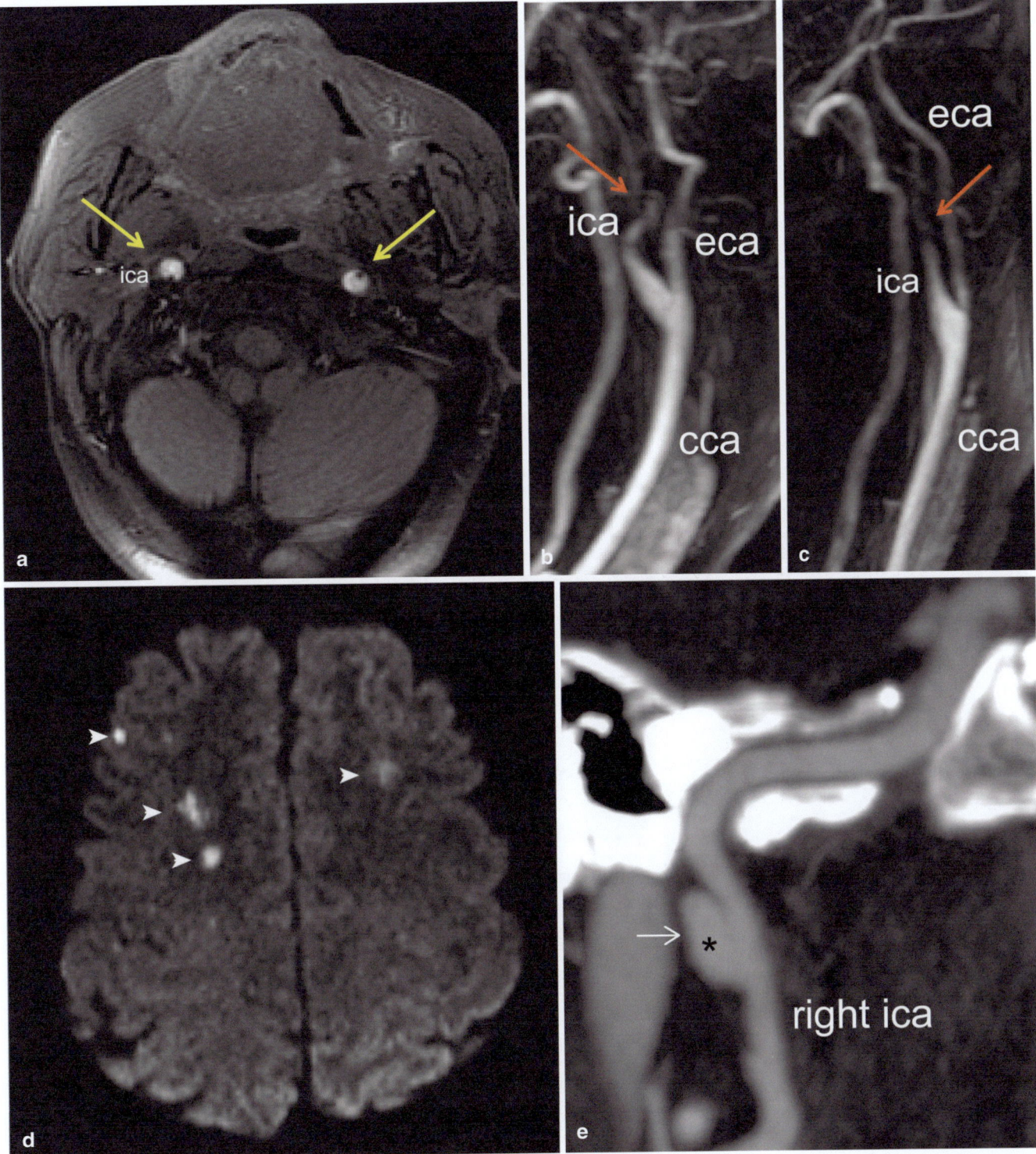

Fig. 5.10 Nonatherosclerotic extracranial vasculopathies— Carotid dissection. Forty-four-year-old female with acute symptoms following prolonged neck extension for dental extraction. (**a**) Axial T1 fat-saturated image shows a T1 hyperintense crescentic false lumen containing an intramural hematoma and a peripheral thin T1 hypointense true lumen with flow void in both distal cervical internal carotid arteries, consistent with acute dissections (yellow arrows). (**b**, **c**) Sagittal contrast-enhanced MRA neck images demonstrate flame-shaped tapering of the right (**b**) and left (**c**) ICA true lumens due to the intramural hematoma (orange arrows). (**d**) Axial DWI image shows multiple focal infarcts in the right frontal cortex and anterior centrum semiovale bilaterally (arrowhead). (**e**) In a different patient with history of posttraumatic carotid dissection, there is a dissecting traumatic pseudoaneurysm (open arrow, *)

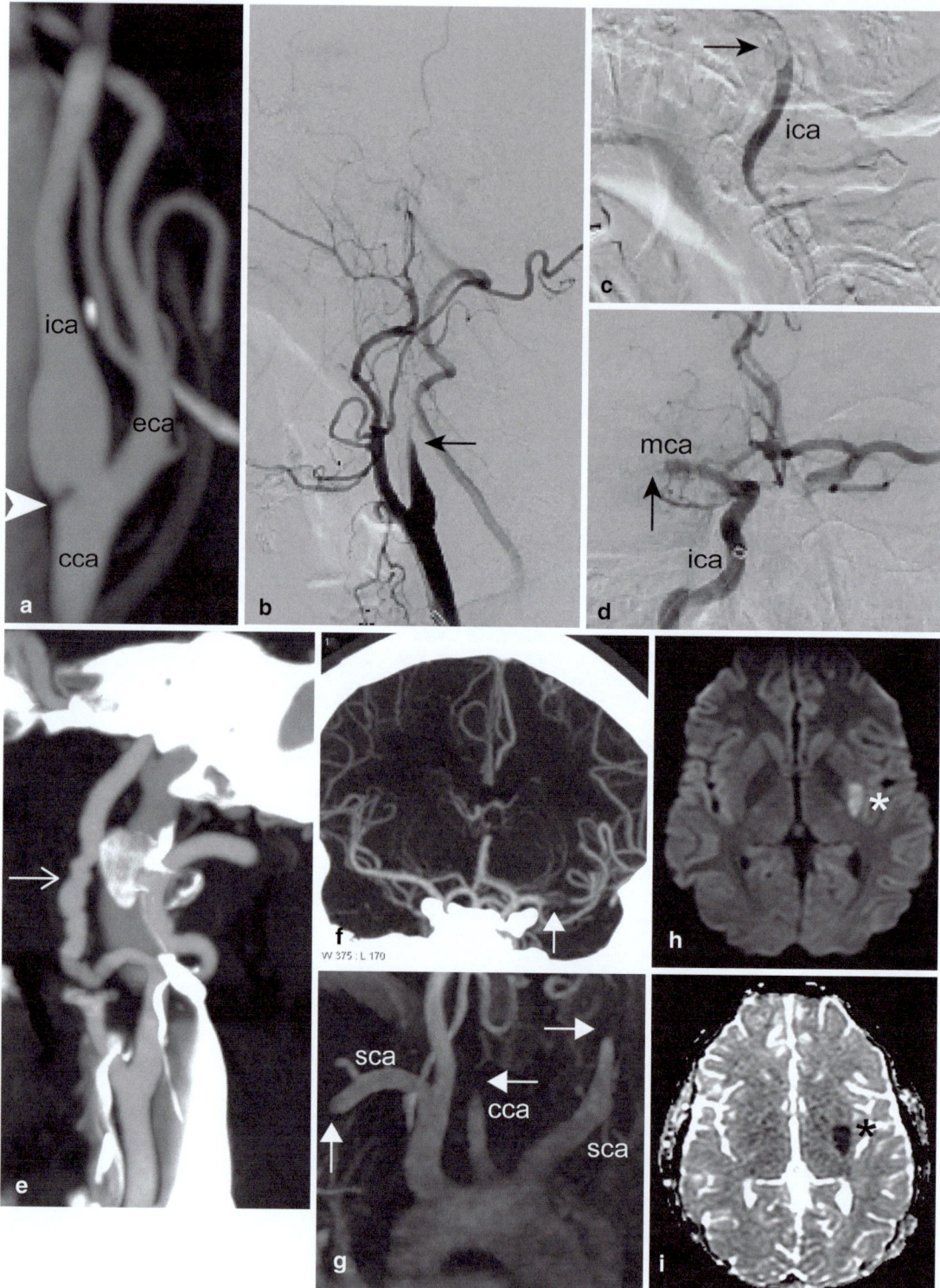

Fig. 5.11 Nonatherosclerotic extracranial vasculopathies. (a) Carotid web (intimal variant fibromuscular dysplasia). CTA neck shows a thin, linear, shelf-like filling defect extending from the posterior wall of the carotid bulb into the proximal ICA lumen (arrowhead). (b) Carotid pseudo-occlusion. Sagittal view digital subtraction angiography shows a flame-shaped tapering of the proximal ICA, mimicking an acute ICA dissection (black arrow →). On further advancement of the catheter, there is filling of the distal cervical ICA (c) up to a long segment filling defect in the ICA terminus, consistent with an occluding thrombus (white arrow →). (d) After thrombectomy, there is recanalization of the right ICA, but a second thrombus is located distally in the right M1 MCA segment (black arrow →). (e) Fibromuscular dysplasia. CTA neck demonstrates the "string and pearl" beaded appearance of the cervical ICA, consistent with fibromuscular dysplasia (white open arrow →). (f) Takayasu arteritis in a 19-year-old female with right facial droop and hemiplegia. Coronal CTA head shows a partially occluding thrombus in the left M1 MCA segment (closed arrow). (g) Coronal CTA of the arch and proximal vessels shows occlusion of the left common carotid and both subclavian arteries (white closed arrow →). (h) Axial DWI and ADC (i) images demonstrate a small acute infarct in the left posterior putamen (*). *cca* common carotid artery, *eca* external carotid artery, *ica* internal carotid artery, *mca* middle cerebral artery, *sca* subclavian artery

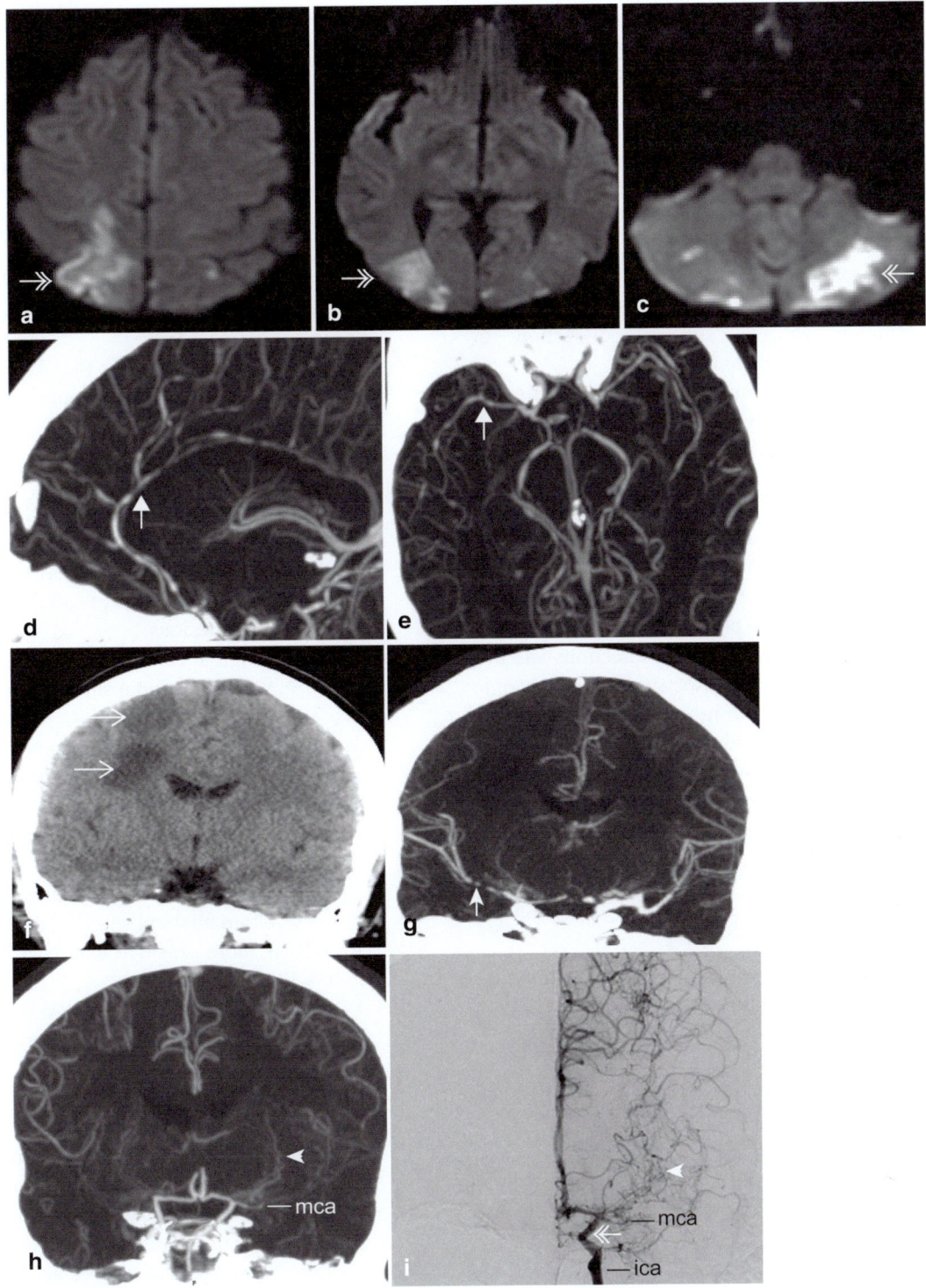

Fig. 5.12 Intracranial vasculopathies. (**a–e**) Reversible vasoconstriction syndrome (RCVS). 55-year-old female patient with recurrent thunderclap headaches who presented with left greater than right-sided weakness. (**a–c**) Axial DWI images show multifocal areas of diffusion restriction throughout both cerebral and cerebellar hemispheres, consistent with acute multifocal, multi-territorial infarcts (white double arrows ⇒). (**d**) Sagittal and (**e**) axial CTA head images show diffuse multifocal stenoses of the intracranial cerebral arteries with "string of beads" or "sausage string" appearance (white closed arrow →). (**f**, **g**) Varicella Zoster vasculitis. 30-year-old female with HIV infection, acute left upper extremity weakness and facial numbness. (**f**) Noncontrast-enhanced CT head shows two hypodense areas involving the right superior frontal gyrus and corona radiata, consistent with acute to subacute infarcts (open white arrow →). (**g**) Coronal CTA head shows multifocal severe stenoses in both proximal MCAs and ACAs (white arrow →). (**h**) Moyamoya disease. Coronal CTA head of a patient with Moyamoya disease demonstrates mild tapering of both distal intracranial ICAs, prominent lenticulostriate arteries (white arrowhead) bilaterally, occlusion of the proximal M1 branch of the right MCA, and severe stenosis of the M1 branch of the left MCA. (**i**) Diagnostic cerebral angiogram better delineates the prominent lenticulostriate arteries (white arrowhead), in keeping with the puff of smoke pattern (moyamoya) and mild tapering of both ICAs (white double arrow ⇒). *ica* internal carotid artery, *mca* middle cerebral artery

- Non-atherosclerotic vasculopathies [70]—further subdivided into extracranial and intracranial vasculopathies (with or without abnormal circle of Willis (COW)).
  - Extracranial vasculopathies:
    - Arterial dissection (tear in the intimal layer of an artery with an intramural thrombus) (Fig. 5.10) cause ~15% of ischemic strokes in young adults.
      - Most commonly in the extracranial ICA near the skull base or in the V3 vertebral artery segments, either through occlusion of the true lumen at the site of dissection or thromboembolism.
      - Etiologies: trauma, connective tissue disease, fibromuscular dysplasia (FMD), iatrogenic.
    - Carotid web, FMD, radiation vasculopathy, large vessel vasculitis (Takayasu arteritis, giant cell arteritis) (Fig. 5.11).
  - Intracranial vasculopathies (Fig. 5.12):
    - With abnormal COW.
      - Cerebral vasculitis.
        - Can occur as primary central nervous system angiitis (PACNS), infectious vasculitis, vasculitis associated with systemic disease, drug-induced vasculitis, malignancy-induced vasculitis.
        - Pathophysiology: vessel wall inflammation → luminal narrowing → thromboembolism → ischemic stroke or parenchymal hemorrhage.
      - Others: RCVS, Moyamoya vasculopathy, radiation vasculopathy.
    - With normal COW.
      - Cerebral amyloid angiopathy, CADASIL, certain vasculitides (Susac syndrome), others.
- Prothrombotic disorders.
  - Implicated in both arterial ischemic events and CVT.
  - Can be genetic or acquired.
    - Important acquired causes: antiphospholipid syndrome, oral contraceptive, pregnancy and puerperium, malignancy, systemic inflammatory diseases, COVID-19 infection (or following COVID-19 vaccination).
- Cerebral venous thrombosis [26].
  - Prothrombotic condition in ~85% of cases.
  - Local factors implicated in remaining cases.
    - Infections: Otomastoiditis, sinusitis.
    - Trauma: Skull fractures extending into dural sinus.
  - In most patients with CVT, multiple venous sinuses are involved.
    - Superior sagittal sinus, transverse sinus, and sigmoid sinus are the most frequently involved.
  - Sequelae:
    - Parenchymal edema and hemorrhage are common.
  - Imaging.
    - NCCT: Often first imaging modality used in the investigation.
      - Moderate sensitivity (41–73%), high specificity (97–100%) in diagnosing CVT [71].
      - "Cord sign."
        - Hyperdense occluded sinus in acute to subacute CVT.
        - Low-to-moderate sensitivity (25–56%).
    - Subcortical hypodense foci in areas that are not in the distribution of arterial territories (30–40%).
    - Parenchymal hemorrhage (30–35%).
    - Location of lesions.
      - Parasagittal cerebral hemispheric.
        - Superior sagittal sinus thrombosis.
        - May be bilateral.
      - Temporo-occipital and cerebellar.
        - Transverse sinus thrombosis, may extend into vein of Labbé.
      - Thalami, basal ganglia, internal capsule.
        - Thrombosis of internal cerebral veins, vein of Galen, or straight sinus.
        - Often bilateral.
    - MRI is more sensitive than NCCT at detecting CVT.
      - T2*-weighed GRE or SWI sequences are 90% sensitive at detecting venous thrombosis [26].
      - Areas of vasogenic edema with elevated diffusion, combined with areas of cytotoxic edema with restricted diffusion.
      - Hyperintense sinus (T1W) and absent flow void (T2W) in acute venous thrombosis.
        - Signal intensity depends on the age of the thrombus and evolves according to different stages of hemoglobin breakdown.
    - Both CT venography and 3D phase contrast MR venography are highly sensitive and specific in diagnosing CVT [72, 73]. Insufficient evidence to select which modality is more accurate [73].

5 Stroke

Stroke Mimics

- Entities that are associated with cortical or white matter diffusion restriction and mimic stroke on imaging [74, 75].
- Approximately 20% of patients who present with stroke symptoms do not have an AIS.
- Imaging findings: Nonvascular distribution and absence of vascular occlusion.
- Common stroke mimics (Table 5.4).
  - Seizures.
    - Approximately one-third of stroke mimics.
    - Cortical restricted diffusion, cortical vasogenic edema, and gyral enhancement can occur.
    - Status epilepticus.
      - Restricted diffusion in the cortex and thalamus [76].
  - Tumors.
    - About 10% of stroke mimics.
    - Metastases with restricted diffusion—non small cell lung cancer.
    - Primary tumors with restricted diffusion—lymphoma and medulloblastoma.
    - Unlike acute stroke, tumors have enhancement and persistent surrounding vasogenic edema.
  - Migraine.
    - About 10% of stroke mimics.
    - Cortical restricted diffusion reported in hemiplegic migraine [77].
- Uncommon stroke mimics.
  - Herpes simplex encephalitis.
    - Bilateral, asymmetric involvement of mesial temporal and inferior frontal lobes, insula and cingulate gyri (limbic structures).
    - Cortical restricted diffusion, gyral swelling, and subcortical FLAIR hyperintensities.
  - Transient global amnesia [78].
    - Small, punctate hippocampal lesions with restricted diffusion in >60% of cases.
    - Left> right; bilateral in ~30%.
  - Hypoxic-ischemic injury.
    - Bilateral, symmetric restricted diffusion involving cortex (especially peri Rolandic and occipital cortex) and deep gray nuclei.
    - Delayed post hypoxic leukoencephalopathy—diffuse white matter involvement with restricted diffusion.
  - Hyperammonemia and hepatic encephalopathy.
    - Bilateral, symmetric restricted diffusion affecting mainly the cingulate and insular cerebral cortex, and thalami.
    - Diffuse pattern of cortical restricted diffusion indicates poor prognosis in hepatic encephalopathy [79].
  - Creutzfeldt-Jakob disease (CJD).
    - Bilateral, symmetric, or asymmetric restricted diffusion.
    - Absence of gyral swelling.
    - Affects mainly cingulate, precuneus, angular, parahippocampal, superior and middle frontal gyri, insula, and deep gray nuclei.
    - Pulvinar sign with variant CJD.
  - MELAS [80].
    - Stroke-like lesions in a nonarterial distribution.
    - Most common sites—primary visual cortex, middle-third of the primary somatosensory cortex, and primary auditory cortex.
    - Multiple, frequently bilateral lesions in various stages of evolution.
    - Symmetric pattern of lesions in about half of cases.
  - Posterior reversible encephalopathy syndrome (PRES) [81, 82].
    - Focal or confluent T2/FLAIR hyperintense areas of vasogenic edema secondary to dysfunction of cerebral autoregulation or endothelial injury.
    - Most commonly associated with hypertension, eclampsia, cytotoxic or immunosuppressive drugs, e.g., cyclosporin or tacrolimus.
    - Most common sites: subcortical and deep white matter in the posterior cerebral hemispheres, less commonly in the brainstem, cerebellum or superior frontal lobes with relative sparing of the cortical gray matter, calcarine, and paramedian occipital lobes.
    - Shares same pathophysiology of cerebrovascular dysregulation and may coexist with RCVS [83, 84]. In these cases, intracranial hemorrhage, beaded appearance of focal vasoconstriction, and focal areas of restricted diffusion may be present superimposed on areas with facilitated diffusion.
  - Other lesions with restricted diffusion:
    - Hypoglycemia: T2 hyperintensity and restricted diffusion in cortex, the posterior limb of the internal capsule, the corona radiata, the centrum semiovale, the hippocampi and basal ganglia.
    - Acute methotrexate toxicity: T2 hyperintensity and restricted diffusion in the corona radiata and centrum semiovale.
    - Metronidazole toxicity: T2 hyperintensity and restricted diffusion in the dentate nuclei, midbrain, medulla, and pons.
    - Heroin-induced leukoencephalopathy: T2 hyperintensity and restricted diffusion in cortex, the poste-

rior limb of the internal capsule, the corona radiata, the centrum semiovale, the hippocampi, and basal ganglia.
- Nonketotic hyperglycemia: Unilateral basal ganglia lesion with T1 and T2 hyperintensity and restricted diffusion.
- Wernicke's encephalopathy: T2 hyperintensity and restricted diffusion in the mamillary bodies, hypothalamus, dorsomedial thalami, tectum, and periaqueductal gray matter.

References

1. Saini V, Guada L, Yavagal DR. Global epidemiology of stroke and access to acute ischemic stroke interventions. Neurology. 2021;97(20 Suppl 2):S6–S16. https://doi.org/10.1212/WNL.0000000000012781.
2. Kleindorfer DO, Towfighi A, Chaturvedi S, Cockroft KM, Gutierrez J, Lombardi-Hill D, et al. 2021 guideline for the prevention of stroke in patients with stroke and transient ischemic attack: a guideline from the American Heart Association/American Stroke Association. Stroke. 2021;52(7):e364–467. https://doi.org/10.1161/STR.0000000000000375.
3. Powers WJ, Rabinstein AA, Ackerson T, Adeoye OM, Bambakidis NC, Becker K, et al. Guidelines for the early management of patients with acute ischemic stroke: 2019 update to the 2018 guidelines for the early management of acute ischemic stroke: a guideline for healthcare professionals from the American Heart Association/American Stroke Association. Stroke. 2019;50(12):e344–418. https://doi.org/10.1161/STR.0000000000000211.
4. de Oliveira EP, Fiebach JB, Vagal A, Schaefer PW, Aviv RI. Controversies in imaging of patients with acute ischemic stroke: AJR expert panel narrative review. AJR Am J Roentgenol. 2021;217(5):1027–37. https://doi.org/10.2214/AJR.21.25846.
5. Liebeskind DS, Saber H, Bhuva P, Xiang B, Yoo AJ, Jadhav AP, et al. Serial ASPECTS in the DAWN Trial: infarct evolution and clinical impact. Stroke. 2021;52(10):3318–24. https://doi.org/10.1161/STROKEAHA.120.033477.
6. Sacco RL, Kasner SE, Broderick JP, Caplan LR, Connors JJ, Culebras A, et al. An updated definition of stroke for the 21st century: a statement for healthcare professionals from the American Heart Association/American Stroke Association. Stroke. 2013;44(7):2064–89. https://doi.org/10.1161/STR.0b013e318296aeca.
7. George PM, Steinberg GK. Novel stroke therapeutics: unraveling stroke pathophysiology and its impact on clinical treatments. Neuron. 2015;87(2):297–309. https://doi.org/10.1016/j.neuron.2015.05.041.
8. Kanekar SG, Zacharia T, Roller R. Imaging of stroke: part 2, pathophysiology at the molecular and cellular levels and corresponding imaging changes. AJR Am J Roentgenol. 2012;198(1):63–74. https://doi.org/10.2214/AJR.10.7312.
9. Liebeskind DS, Juttler E, Shapovalov Y, Yegin A, Landen J, Jauch EC. Cerebral edema associated with large hemispheric infarction. Stroke. 2019;50(9):2619–25. https://doi.org/10.1161/STROKEAHA.118.024766.
10. Randomised trial of endarterectomy for recently symptomatic carotid stenosis: final results of the MRC European Carotid Surgery Trial (ECST). Lancet. 1998;351(9113):1379–1387.
11. North American Symptomatic Carotid Endarterectomy Trial Collaborators, Barnett HJM, Taylor DW, Haynes RB, Sackett DL, Peerless SJ, et al. Beneficial effect of carotid endarterectomy in symptomatic patients with high-grade carotid stenosis. N Engl J Med. 1991;325(7):445–53. https://doi.org/10.1056/NEJM199108153250701.
12. Johansson E, Fox AJ. Carotid near-occlusion: a comprehensive review, part 1-definition, terminology, and diagnosis. AJNR Am J Neuroradiol. 2016;37(1):2–10. https://doi.org/10.3174/ajnr.A4432.
13. Grossberg JA, Haussen DC, Cardoso FB, Rebello LC, Bouslama M, Anderson AM, et al. Cervical carotid pseudo-occlusions and false dissections: intracranial occlusions masquerading as extracranial occlusions. Stroke. 2017;48(3):774–7. https://doi.org/10.1161/STROKEAHA.116.015427.
14. Kappelhof M, Marquering HA, Berkhemer OA, Borst J, van der Lugt A, van Zwam WH, et al. Accuracy of CT angiography for differentiating pseudo-occlusion from true occlusion or high-grade stenosis of the extracranial ICA in acute ischemic stroke: a retrospective MR CLEAN substudy. AJNR Am J Neuroradiol. 2018;39(5):892–8. https://doi.org/10.3174/ajnr.A5601.
15. Dimmick SJ, Faulder KC. Normal variants of the cerebral circulation at multidetector CT angiography. Radiographics. 2009;29(4):1027–43. https://doi.org/10.1148/rg.294085730.
16. Shapiro M, Becske T, Riina HA, Raz E, Zumofen D, Jafar JJ, et al. Toward an endovascular internal carotid artery classification system. AJNR Am J Neuroradiol. 2014;35(2):230–6. https://doi.org/10.3174/ajnr.A3666.
17. Goyal M, Menon BK, Krings T, Patil S, Qazi E, McTaggart RA, et al. What constitutes the M1 segment of the middle cerebral artery? J Neurointerv Surg. 2016;8(12):1273–7. https://doi.org/10.1136/neurintsurg-2015-012191.
18. Shapiro M, Raz E, Nossek E, Chancellor B, Ishida K, Nelson PK. Neuroanatomy of the middle cerebral artery: implications for thrombectomy. J Neurointerv Surg. 2020;12(8):768–73. https://doi.org/10.1136/neurintsurg-2019-015782.
19. Tanriover N, Kucukyuruk B, Ulu MO, Isler C, Sam B, Abuzayed B, et al. Microsurgical anatomy of the cisternal anterior choroidal artery with special emphasis on the preoptic and postoptic subdivisions. J Neurosurg. 2014;120(5):1217–28. https://doi.org/10.3171/2014.1.JNS131325.
20. Wiesmann M, Yousry I, Seelos KC, Yousry TA. Identification and anatomic description of the anterior choroidal artery by use of 3D-TOF source and 3D-CISS MR imaging. AJNR Am J Neuroradiol. 2001;22(2):305–10.
21. Takahashi S, Suga T, Kawata Y, Sakamoto K. Anterior choroidal artery: angiographic analysis of variations and anomalies. AJNR Am J Neuroradiol. 1990;11(4):719–29.
22. Hindenes LB, Haberg AK, Johnsen LH, Mathiesen EB, Robben D, Vangberg TR. Variations in the Circle of Willis in a large population sample using 3D TOF angiography: the Tromso study. PLoS One. 2020;15(11):e0241373. https://doi.org/10.1371/journal.pone.0241373.
23. Novakovic-White R, Corona JM, White JA. Posterior circulation ischemia in the endovascular era. Neurology. 2021;97(20 Suppl 2):S158–69. https://doi.org/10.1212/WNL.0000000000012808.
24. Tatu L, Moulin T, Bogousslavsky J, Duvernoy H. Arterial territories of the human brain: cerebral hemispheres. Neurology. 1998;50(6):1699–708. https://doi.org/10.1212/wnl.50.6.1699.
25. Kaesmacher J, Kaesmacher M, Berndt M, Maegerlein C, Monch S, Wunderlich S, et al. Early thrombectomy protects the internal capsule in patients with proximal middle cerebral artery occlusion. Stroke. 2021;52(5):1570–9. https://doi.org/10.1161/STROKEAHA.120.031977.
26. Canedo-Antelo M, Baleato-Gonzalez S, Mosqueira AJ, Casas-Martinez J, Oleaga L, Vilanova JC, et al. Radiologic clues to cerebral venous thrombosis. Radiographics. 2019;39(6):1611–28. https://doi.org/10.1148/rg.2019190015.

27. Berge E, Whiteley W, Audebert H, De Marchis GM, Fonseca AC, Padiglioni C, et al. European Stroke Organisation (ESO) guidelines on intravenous thrombolysis for acute ischaemic stroke. Eur Stroke J 2021;6(1):I-LXII. doi: https://doi.org/10.1177/2396987321989865.
28. Campbell BCV, Mitchell PJ, Churilov L, Yassi N, Kleinig TJ, Dowling RJ, et al. Tenecteplase versus alteplase before thrombectomy for ischemic stroke. N Engl J Med. 2018;378(17):1573–82. https://doi.org/10.1056/NEJMoa1716405.
29. Lees KR, Bluhmki E, von Kummer R, Brott TG, Toni D, Grotta JC, et al. Time to treatment with intravenous alteplase and outcome in stroke: an updated pooled analysis of ECASS, ATLANTIS, NINDS, and EPITHET trials. Lancet. 2010;375(9727):1695–703. https://doi.org/10.1016/S0140-6736(10)60491-6.
30. Thomalla G, Simonsen CZ, Boutitie F, Andersen G, Berthezene Y, Cheng B, et al. MRI-guided thrombolysis for stroke with unknown time of onset. N Engl J Med. 2018;379(7):611–22. https://doi.org/10.1056/NEJMoa1804355.
31. Ma H, Campbell BCV, Parsons MW, Churilov L, Levi CR, Hsu C, et al. Thrombolysis guided by perfusion imaging up to 9 hours after onset of stroke. N Engl J Med. 2019;380(19):1795–803. https://doi.org/10.1056/NEJMoa1813046.
32. Nogueira RG, Jadhav AP, Haussen DC, Bonafe A, Budzik RF, Bhuva P, et al. Thrombectomy 6 to 24 hours after stroke with a mismatch between deficit and infarct. N Engl J Med. 2018;378(1):11–21. https://doi.org/10.1056/NEJMoa1706442.
33. Albers GW, Marks MP, Kemp S, Christensen S, Tsai JP, Ortega-Gutierrez S, et al. Thrombectomy for stroke at 6 to 16 hours with selection by perfusion imaging. N Engl J Med. 2018;378(8):708–18. https://doi.org/10.1056/NEJMoa1713973.
34. Potter CA, Vagal AS, Goyal M, Nunez DB, Leslie-Mazwi TM, Lev MH. CT for treatment selection in acute ischemic stroke: a code stroke primer. Radiographics. 2019;39(6):1717–38. https://doi.org/10.1148/rg.2019190142.
35. Hart RG, Diener HC, Coutts SB, Easton JD, Granger CB, O'Donnell MJ, et al. Embolic strokes of undetermined source: the case for a new clinical construct. Lancet Neurol. 2014;13(4):429–38. https://doi.org/10.1016/S1474-4422(13)70310-7.
36. Perry JJ, Stiell IG, Sivilotti ML, Bullard MJ, Emond M, Symington C, et al. Sensitivity of computed tomography performed within six hours of onset of headache for diagnosis of subarachnoid haemorrhage: prospective cohort study. BMJ. 2011;343:d4277. https://doi.org/10.1136/bmj.d4277.
37. Latchaw RE, Alberts MJ, Lev MH, Connors JJ, Harbaugh RE, Higashida RT, et al. Recommendations for imaging of acute ischemic stroke: a scientific statement from the American Heart Association. Stroke. 2009;40(11):3646–78. https://doi.org/10.1161/STROKEAHA.108.192616.
38. Goldmakher GV, Camargo EC, Furie KL, Singhal AB, Roccatagliata L, Halpern EF, et al. Hyperdense basilar artery sign on unenhanced CT predicts thrombus and outcome in acute posterior circulation stroke. Stroke. 2009;40(1):134–9. https://doi.org/10.1161/STROKEAHA.108.516690.
39. O'Brien P, Sellar RJ, Wardlaw JM. Fogging on T2-weighted MR after acute ischaemic stroke: how often might this occur and what are the implications? Neuroradiology. 2004;46(8):635–41. https://doi.org/10.1007/s00234-004-1230-2.
40. Honig A, Percy J, Sepehry AA, Gomez AG, Field TS, Benavente OR. Hemorrhagic transformation in acute ischemic stroke: a quantitative systematic review. J Clin Med. 2022;11(5):1162. https://doi.org/10.3390/jcm11051162.
41. Puntonet J, Richard ME, Edjlali M, Ben Hassen W, Legrand L, Benzakoun J, et al. Imaging findings after mechanical thrombectomy in acute ischemic stroke. Stroke. 2019;50(6):1618–25. https://doi.org/10.1161/STROKEAHA.118.024754.
42. von Kummer R, Broderick JP, Campbell BC, Demchuk A, Goyal M, Hill MD, et al. The Heidelberg bleeding classification: classification of bleeding events after ischemic stroke and reperfusion therapy. Stroke. 2015;46(10):2981–6. https://doi.org/10.1161/STROKEAHA.115.010049.
43. Payabvash S, Qureshi MH, Khan SM, Khan M, Majidi S, Pawar S, et al. Differentiating intraparenchymal hemorrhage from contrast extravasation on post-procedural noncontrast CT scan in acute ischemic stroke patients undergoing endovascular treatment. Neuroradiology. 2014;56(9):737–44. https://doi.org/10.1007/s00234-014-1381-8.
44. Edlow BL, Hurwitz S, Edlow JA. Diagnosis of DWI-negative acute ischemic stroke: a meta-analysis. Neurology. 2017;89(3):256–62. https://doi.org/10.1212/WNL.0000000000004120.
45. Shono K, Satomi J, Tada Y, Kanematsu Y, Yamamoto N, Izumi Y, et al. Optimal timing of diffusion-weighted imaging to avoid false-negative findings in patients with transient ischemic attack. Stroke. 2017;48(7):1990–2. https://doi.org/10.1161/STROKEAHA.117.014576.
46. Allen LM, Hasso AN, Handwerker J, Farid H. Sequence-specific MR imaging findings that are useful in dating ischemic stroke. Radiographics. 2012;32(5):1285–97; discussion 97–9. https://doi.org/10.1148/rg.325115760.
47. Schaefer PW, Grant PE, Gonzalez RG. Diffusion-weighted MR imaging of the brain. Radiology. 2000;217(2):331–45. https://doi.org/10.1148/radiology.217.2.r00nv24331.
48. Allibert R, Billon Grand C, Vuillier F, Cattin F, Muzard E, Biondi A, et al. Advantages of susceptibility-weighted magnetic resonance sequences in the visualization of intravascular thrombi in acute ischemic stroke. Int J Stroke. 2014;9(8):980–4. https://doi.org/10.1111/ijs.12373.
49. Mittal S, Wu Z, Neelavalli J, Haacke EM. Susceptibility-weighted imaging: technical aspects and clinical applications, part 2. AJNR Am J Neuroradiol. 2009;30(2):232–52. https://doi.org/10.3174/ajnr.A1461.
50. Radbruch A, Mucke J, Schweser F, Deistung A, Ringleb PA, Ziener CH, et al. Comparison of susceptibility weighted imaging and TOF-angiography for the detection of thrombi in acute stroke. PLoS One. 2013;8(5):e63459. https://doi.org/10.1371/journal.pone.0063459.
51. Darwish EAF, Abdelhameed-El-Nouby M, Geneidy E. Mapping the ischemic penumbra and predicting stroke progression in acute ischemic stroke: the overlooked role of susceptibility weighted imaging. Insights Imaging. 2020;11(1):6. https://doi.org/10.1186/s13244-019-0810-y.
52. Taoka T, Fukusumi A, Miyasaka T, Kawai H, Nakane T, Kichikawa K, et al. Structure of the medullary veins of the cerebral hemisphere and related disorders. Radiographics. 2017;37(1):281–97. https://doi.org/10.1148/rg.2017160061.
53. Demeestere J, Wouters A, Christensen S, Lemmens R, Lansberg MG. Review of perfusion imaging in acute ischemic stroke: from time to tissue. Stroke. 2020;51(3):1017–24. https://doi.org/10.1161/STROKEAHA.119.028337.
54. van Seeters T, Biessels GJ, Kappelle LJ, van der Schaaf IC, Dankbaar JW, Horsch AD, et al. The prognostic value of CT angiography and CT perfusion in acute ischemic stroke. Cerebrovasc Dis. 2015;40(5–6):258–69. https://doi.org/10.1159/000441088.
55. Campbell BCV, Lansberg MG, Broderick JP, Derdeyn CP, Khatri P, Sarraj A, et al. Acute stroke imaging research roadmap IV: imaging selection and outcomes in acute stroke clinical trials and practice. Stroke. 2021;52(8):2723–33. https://doi.org/10.1161/STROKEAHA.121.035132.
56. Copen WA, Schaefer PW, Wu O. MR perfusion imaging in acute ischemic stroke. Neuroimaging Clin N Am. 2011;21(2):259–83, x. https://doi.org/10.1016/j.nic.2011.02.007.
57. Iutaka T, de Freitas MB, Omar SS, Scortegagna FA, Nael K, Nunes RH, et al. Arterial spin labeling: techniques, clinical applications, and interpretation. Radiographics. 2023;43(1):e220088. https://doi.org/10.1148/rg.220088.

58. Schaefer PW, Barak ER, Kamalian S, Gharai LR, Schwamm L, Gonzalez RG, et al. Quantitative assessment of core/penumbra mismatch in acute stroke: CT and MR perfusion imaging are strongly correlated when sufficient brain volume is imaged. Stroke. 2008;39(11):2986–92. https://doi.org/10.1161/STROKEAHA.107.513358.
59. Mandell DM, Mossa-Basha M, Qiao Y, Hess CP, Hui F, Matouk C, et al. Intracranial vessel wall MRI: principles and expert consensus recommendations of the American Society of Neuroradiology. AJNR Am J Neuroradiol. 2017;38(2):218–29. https://doi.org/10.3174/ajnr.A4893.
60. Schaafsma JD, Rawal S, Coutinho JM, Rasheedi J, Mikulis DJ, Jaigobin C, et al. Diagnostic impact of intracranial vessel wall MRI in 205 patients with ischemic stroke or TIA. AJNR Am J Neuroradiol. 2019;40(10):1701–6. https://doi.org/10.3174/ajnr.A6202.
61. Tan HW, Chen X, Maingard J, Barras CD, Logan C, Thijs V, et al. Intracranial vessel wall imaging with magnetic resonance imaging: current techniques and applications. World Neurosurg. 2018;112:186–98. https://doi.org/10.1016/j.wneu.2018.01.083.
62. Wintermark M, Albers GW, Broderick JP, Demchuk AM, Fiebach JB, Fiehler J, et al. Acute stroke imaging research roadmap II. Stroke. 2013;44(9):2628–39. https://doi.org/10.1161/STROKEAHA.113.002015.
63. LeCouffe NE, Kappelhof M, Treurniet KM, Lingsma HF, Zhang G, van den Wijngaard IR, et al. 2B, 2C, or 3: what should be the angiographic target for endovascular treatment in ischemic stroke? Stroke. 2020;51(6):1790–6. https://doi.org/10.1161/STROKEAHA.119.028891.
64. Campbell BCV, De Silva DA, Macleod MR, Coutts SB, Schwamm LH, Davis SM, et al. Ischaemic stroke. Nat Rev Dis Primers. 2019;5(1):70. https://doi.org/10.1038/s41572-019-0118-8.
65. Campbell BCV, Khatri P. Stroke. Lancet. 2020;396(10244):129–42. https://doi.org/10.1016/S0140-6736(20)31179-X.
66. Adams HP Jr, Biller J. Classification of subtypes of ischemic stroke: history of the trial of org 10172 in acute stroke treatment classification. Stroke. 2015;46(5):e114–7. https://doi.org/10.1161/STROKEAHA.114.007773.
67. Mangla R, Kolar B, Almast J, Ekholm SE. Border zone infarcts: pathophysiologic and imaging characteristics. Radiographics. 2011;31(5):1201–14. https://doi.org/10.1148/rg.315105014.
68. Regenhardt RW, Das AS, Lo EH, Caplan LR. Advances in understanding the pathophysiology of lacunar stroke: a review. JAMA Neurol. 2018;75(10):1273–81. https://doi.org/10.1001/jamaneurol.2018.1073.
69. Kamel H, Healey JS. Cardioembolic stroke. Circ Res. 2017;120(3):514–26. https://doi.org/10.1161/CIRCRESAHA.116.308407.
70. McCarty JL, Leung LY, Peterson RB, Sitton CW, Sarraj A, Riascos RF, et al. Ischemic infarction in young adults: a review for radiologists. Radiographics. 2019;39(6):1629–48. https://doi.org/10.1148/rg.2019190033.
71. Buyck PJ, Zuurbier SM, Garcia-Esperon C, Barboza MA, Costa P, Escudero I, et al. Diagnostic accuracy of noncontrast CT imaging markers in cerebral venous thrombosis. Neurology. 2019;92(8):e841–51. https://doi.org/10.1212/WNL.0000000000006959.
72. Saposnik G, Barinagarrementeria F, Brown RD Jr, Bushnell CD, Cucchiara B, Cushman M, et al. Diagnosis and management of cerebral venous thrombosis: a statement for healthcare professionals from the American Heart Association/American Stroke Association. Stroke. 2011;42(4):1158–92. https://doi.org/10.1161/STR.0b013e31820a8364.
73. van Dam LF, van Walderveen MAA, Kroft LJM, Kruyt ND, Wermer MJH, van Osch MJP, et al. Current imaging modalities for diagnosing cerebral vein thrombosis—a critical review. Thromb Res. 2020;189:132–9. https://doi.org/10.1016/j.thromres.2020.03.011.
74. Pai V, Sitoh YY, Purohit B. Gyriform restricted diffusion in adults: looking beyond thrombo-occlusions. Insights Imaging. 2020;11(1):20. https://doi.org/10.1186/s13244-019-0829-0.
75. Prodi E, Danieli L, Manno C, Pagnamenta A, Pravata E, Roccatagliata L, et al. Stroke mimics in the acute setting: role of multimodal CT protocol. AJNR Am J Neuroradiol. 2022;43(2):216–22. https://doi.org/10.3174/ajnr.A7379.
76. Cole AJ. Status epilepticus and periictal imaging. Epilepsia. 2004;45(Suppl 4):72–7. https://doi.org/10.1111/j.0013-9580.2004.04014.x.
77. Thaler AI, Kim BD, Fara MG. Teaching neuroimages: magnetic resonance perfusion and diffusion findings in hemiplegic migraine. Neurology. 2020;95(12):554–5. https://doi.org/10.1212/WNL.0000000000010249.
78. Choi BS, Kim JH, Jung C, Kim SY. High-resolution diffusion-weighted imaging increases lesion detectability in patients with transient global amnesia. AJNR Am J Neuroradiol. 2012;33(9):1771–4. https://doi.org/10.3174/ajnr.A3072.
79. McKinney AM, Lohman BD, Sarikaya B, Uhlmann E, Spanbauer J, Singewald T, et al. Acute hepatic encephalopathy: diffusion-weighted and fluid-attenuated inversion recovery findings, and correlation with plasma ammonia level and clinical outcome. AJNR Am J Neuroradiol. 2010;31(8):1471–9. https://doi.org/10.3174/ajnr.A2112.
80. Bhatia KD, Krishnan P, Kortman H, Klostranec J, Krings T. Acute cortical lesions in MELAS syndrome: anatomic distribution, symmetry, and evolution. AJNR Am J Neuroradiol. 2020;41(1):167–73. https://doi.org/10.3174/ajnr.A6325.
81. Bartynski WS. Posterior reversible encephalopathy syndrome, part 2: controversies surrounding pathophysiology of vasogenic edema. AJNR Am J Neuroradiol. 2008;29(6):1043–9. https://doi.org/10.3174/ajnr.A0929.
82. Bartynski WS. Posterior reversible encephalopathy syndrome, part 1: fundamental imaging and clinical features. AJNR Am J Neuroradiol. 2008;29(6):1036–42. https://doi.org/10.3174/ajnr.A0928.
83. Singhal AB. Posterior reversible encephalopathy syndrome and reversible cerebral vasoconstriction syndrome as syndromes of cerebrovascular dysregulation. Continuum (Minneap Minn). 2021;27(5):1301–20. https://doi.org/10.1212/CON.0000000000001037.
84. Singhal AB, Hajj-Ali RA, Topcuoglu MA, Fok J, Bena J, Yang D, et al. Reversible cerebral vasoconstriction syndromes: analysis of 139 cases. Arch Neurol. 2011;68(8):1005–12. https://doi.org/10.1001/archneurol.2011.68.

Intracranial Hemorrhage

Eric K. van Staalduinen and Tarik F. Massoud

Imaging Features of Intracranial Hemorrhage

ICH ON CT

- CT is usually the first modality in the assessment of ICH, as it is accurate, fast, and widely available.
- Sensitivity depends on numerous factors, including the amount of blood, its hematocrit, its protein concentration (Hb), and the time since intracranial hemorrhage (ICH).
- It follows a predictable pattern and time course (Fig. 6.1):
  - Beginning as a smooth, hyperdense focus (relative to brain parenchyma).
  - A hypodense halo of edema may be visualized 1–3 days later, with maximal mass effect around day 5.
  - As the clot concentrates, it may become more attenuated (brighter on CT).
  - As the clot resorbs, its margins become indistinct with centripetal density reduction.
  - Fluid levels may be seen in the first 1–2 days and ring enhancement may occur between 3 days and 3 weeks.
  - Blood products usually become isodense at 3–7 days and are seldom visible beyond 7 weeks.
  - A linear, hypodense scar is often evident after 3–7 months.
- Important signs to know include the *swirl*, *black hole*, and *spot signs* (Fig. 6.2).
  - *Swirl sign* refers to the heterogeneous noncontrast appearance of extravasating blood in a hematoma. It is thought to represent fresh, unclotted blood (which is of lower attenuation than the clotted blood surrounding it) and is associated with hematoma expansion.
  - *Black Hole sign* also refers to the noncontrast appearance of fresh, unclotted blood in a hematoma, and is defined as a hypoattenuated area (the black hole) encapsulated within the hyperattenuating hematoma. Its presence is also associated with hematoma expansion.
- *Spot sign* refers to the CTA appearance of contrast extravasation within a hematoma. It also predicts hematoma expansion and is associated with high rates of early clinical deterioration, high mortality, more severe clinical presentation, and decompression into the intraventricular space [1].

ICH ON MRI

- MRI has been shown to be more sensitive than CT in the detection of intracranial hemorrhage [2], although it is often not the first modality used owing to limited access, costs, and logistics.
- The appearance of ICH depends primarily on hematoma age and the pulse sequences used for characterization, as blood products evolve in a predictable manner and time course (Figs. 6.3, 6.6, and 6.8).
- The classically described appearances are outlined by age, biochemical form, and T1/T2 signal characteristics (Table 6.1).
- Gradient echo (GRE) and susceptibility weighted (SWI) sequences are primarily affected by hemoglobin oxygenation state, such that paramagnetic effects of deoxyhemoglobin, methemoglobin, and hemosiderin result in signal loss.

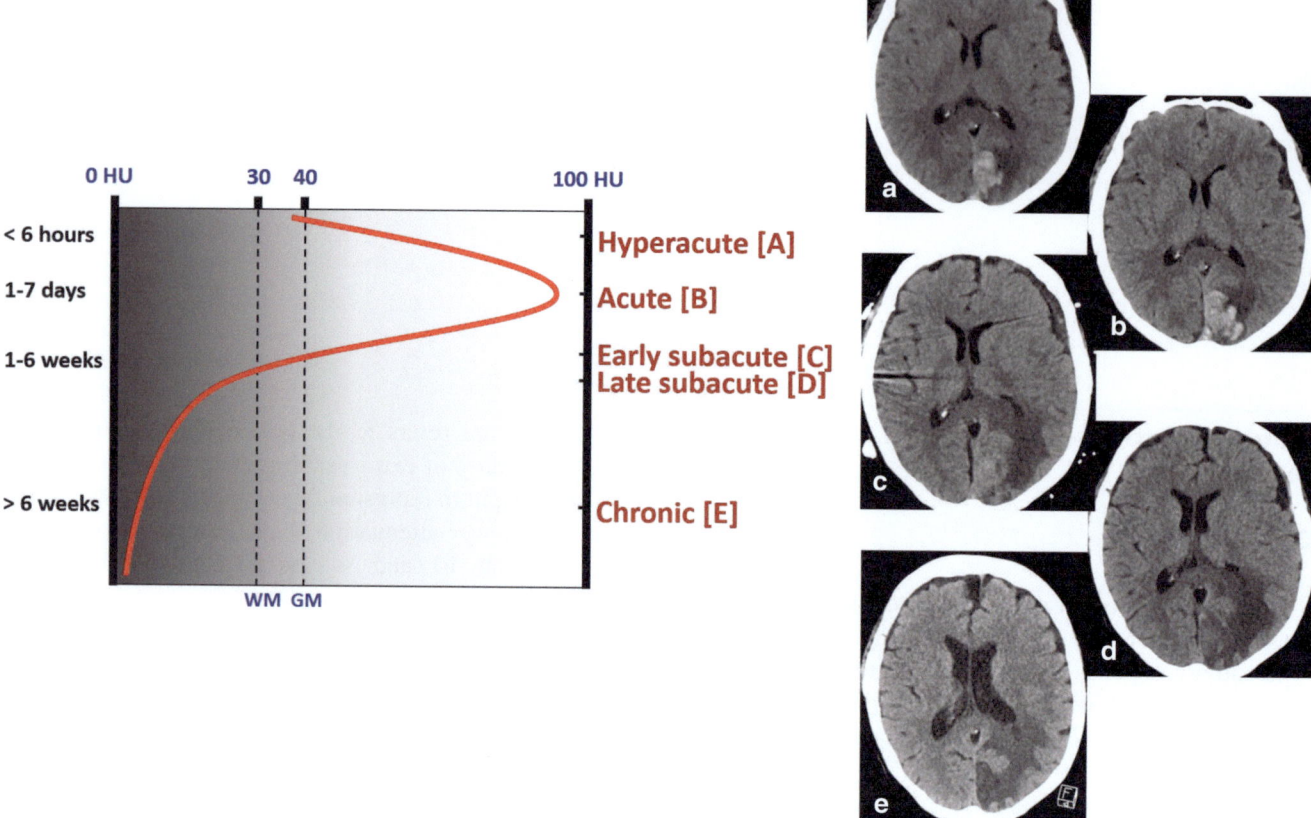

Fig. 6.1 Intracranial hemorrhage on CT. The expected change in density over time is graphed in image **a**. Images B-E demonstrate the evolution of a hemorrhagic venous infarct in the left cuneus (medial occipital lobe), including hyperacute (**b**), acute (**c**), early subacute (**d**), and late subacute (**e**) stages. The keen observer will note a hyperdense and expanded superior sagittal sinus (orange arrows), in keeping with venous sinus thrombosis

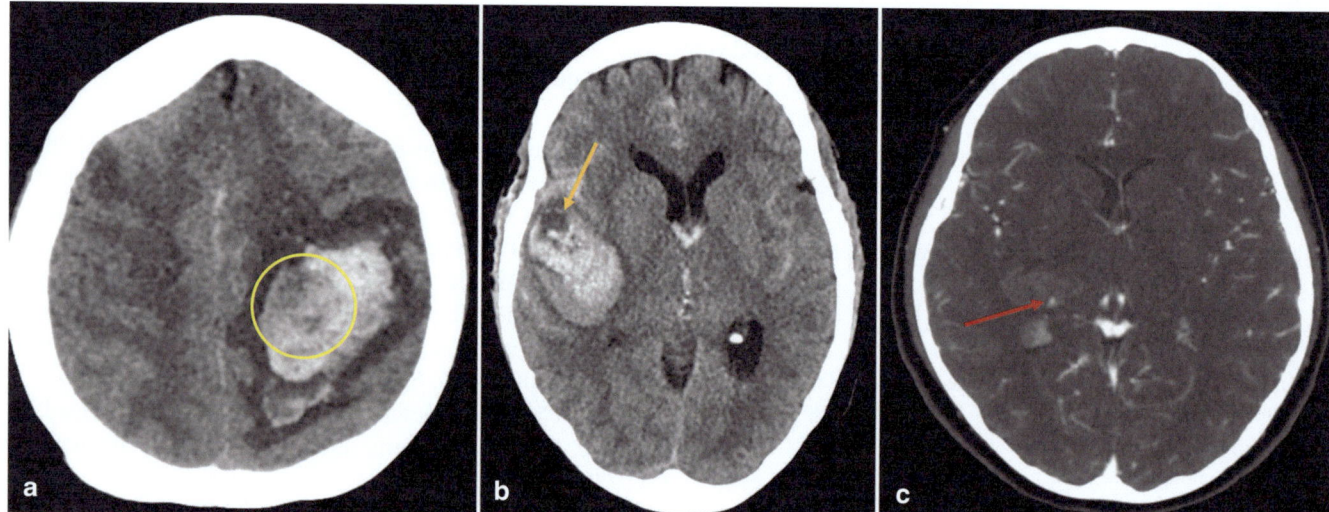

Fig. 6.2 *Swirl*, *black hole*, and *spot* **signs.** Images (**a**) and (**b**) demonstrate the *Swirl* (yellow circle) and *Black Hole* (orange arrow) signs on noncontrast CT, both of which are associated with early hematoma expansion. Image (**c**) demonstrates the *Spot* (red arrow) sign on CT angiography, which is an angiographic correlate that is also associated with hematoma expansion. There are also intraventricular blood products in the right occipital horn

6 Intracranial Hemorrhage

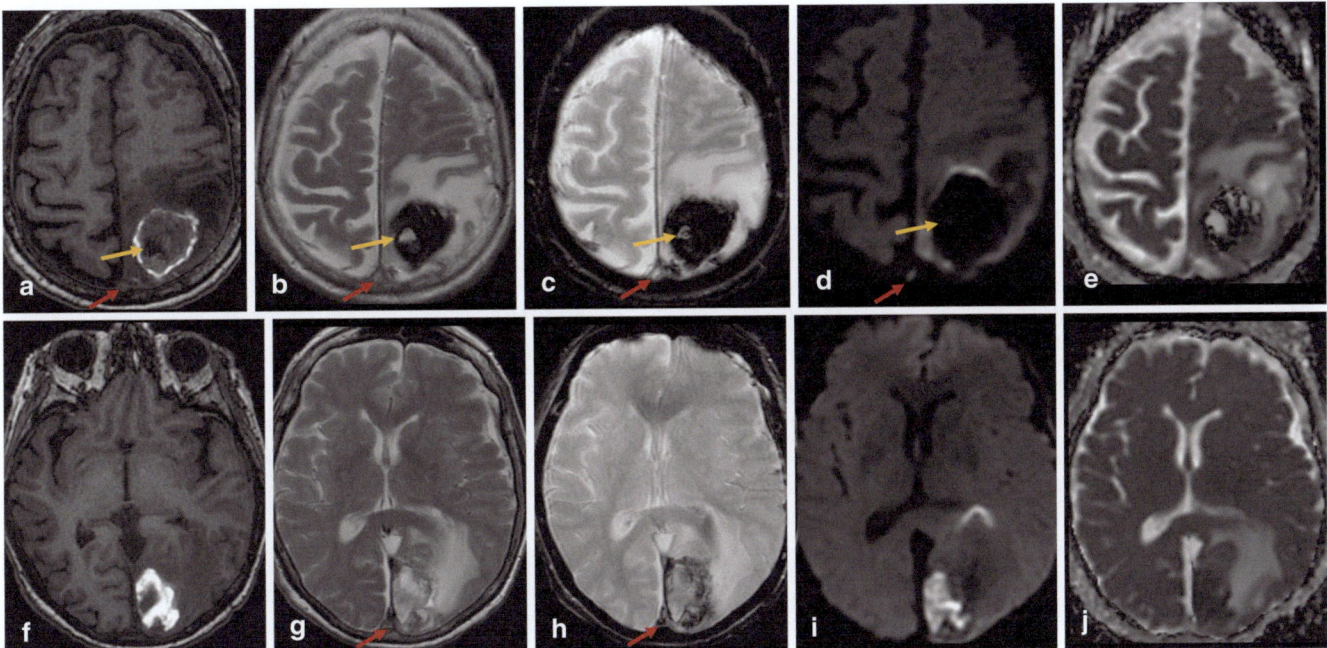

Fig. 6.3 Intracranial hemorrhage on MRI. Acute (**a–e**) left parietal intraparenchymal hematoma and late subacute (**f–j**) hemorrhagic venous infarct in the left cuneus (medial occipital lobe) in this patient with venous sinus thrombosis. T1 (**a, f**), T2 (**b, g**), GRE (**c, h**), Trace DWI (**d, i**), and ADC (**e, j**) sequences demonstrate the classically described characteristics of intracranial blood products, as summarized in Table 6.1. Note is made of moderate perilesional edema surrounding the areas of hemorrhage as well as the signal abnormality in the superior sagittal sinus (red arrows), in keeping with sinus thrombosis. A fluid-level is also visualized in the left parietal hematoma with hyperacute blood products (orange arrows), consistent with fresh unclotted blood

Table 6.1 Appearance of intracranial hemorrhage on noncontrast CT and MRI by age and biochemical form

Age	Phase of blood (biochemical form)	NCCT	T1 signal	T2 signal
Hyperacute (immediately–first several hours)	Oxyhemoglobin	Smooth, hyperdense	Hypo- or Isointense	Hyperintense
Acute (hours–several days)	Deoxyhemoglobin	Hyperdense with fluid levels	Iso- or mildly hypointense	Hypointense with hyperintense rim
Early subacute (first several days)	Methemoglobin intracellular	Less dense with increasing peripheral edema and mass effect	Hyperintense	Hypointense
Late subacute (several days–months)	Methemoglobin extracellular	Isodense with or without ring-like enhancement	Hyperintense	Hyperintense
Chronic (months–indefinitely)	Hemosiderin and ferritin	Iso- or hypodense	Hypointense	Hypointense

- o Notably however, recently extravasated (hyperacute) blood products contain significant amounts of central diamagnetic oxyhemoglobin surrounded by a rim of paramagnetic deoxyhemoglobin, resulting in an iso- or hyperintense central core and peripheral hypointense rim on GRE images [3, 4].
- With DWI, the trace (or B1000) images tend to follow the T2 appearance (bright on hyperacute and late subacute phases), while the corresponding ADC maps are typically hypointense at all stages, except for the chronic phase, where there are increased ADC values.
- These imaging features are present regardless of location (e.g., intracerebral, subdural, intraventricular, etc.).

Locations of ICH

EXTRA-AXIAL HEMORRHAGE

Epidural (or Extradural) Hemorrhage (EDH)

- Refers to blood products located between the inner table of the skull and the outer layer of dura mater (Fig. e6.1. All electronic images (Figs. e6.1–e6.8) can be found in this chapter's website on SpringerLink: https://doi.org/10.1007/978-3-031-55124-6_6).
- Well-visualized on both CT and MRI.

- Limited by adjacent sutures, classically resulting in a "biconvex" or "lenticular" shape (Fig. 6.4).
- May be arterial or venous in origin; caused by laceration of vessels running along the inner table (classically a middle meningeal artery), often secondary to an associated skull fracture in the setting of trauma.
- Often characterized clinically by a lucid interval, representing an asymptomatic period of time between the injury and the mass effect secondary to accumulation of blood products in the epidural space.
- Mass effect from epidural hematomas may result in significant brain displacement (e.g., midline, subfalcine, or transtentorial herniation), which may rapidly progress to obtundation or death (please see head trauma Chap. 8 for a more detailed discussion of herniation patterns), thus requiring urgent operative evacuation or close clinical monitoring.
- Younger patients are more commonly affected owing to higher prevalence of traumatic injury as well as less adherent dura.
- May demonstrate peripheral enhancement or calcification in the chronic setting.
- Venous extradural hematomas represent an uncommon subtype, whereby tearing of dural venous sinuses results in the accumulation of blood products in characteristic locations (vertex, anterior middle cranial fossa, posterior fossa) (Figs. e6.2 and 6.5c).
  - Anterior middle cranial fossa extradural hemorrhages classically do not enlarge and are usually managed conservatively.

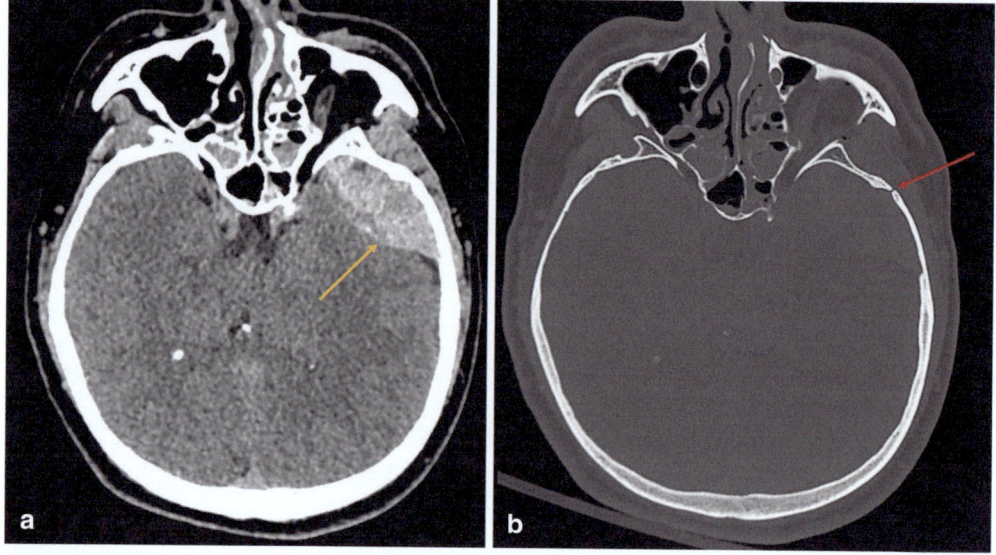

Fig. 6.4 Acute epidural hematoma. Axial CT images in soft tissue (**a**) and bone (**b**) kernel demonstrate an acute epidural hematoma along the left temporal convexity (orange arrow) with an associated skull fracture (red arrow)

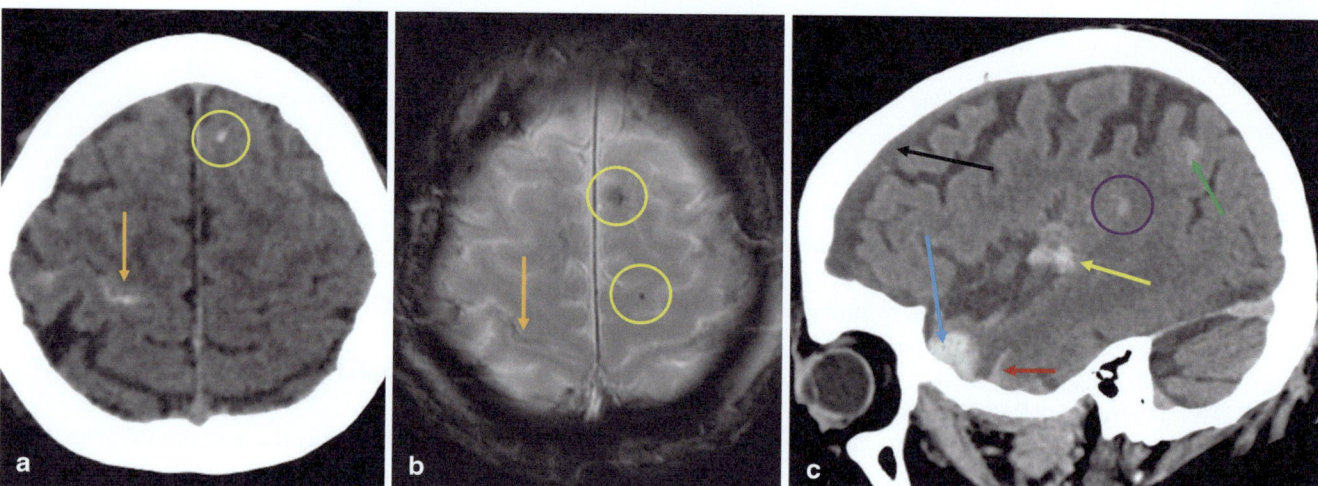

Fig. 6.5 Multicompartmental traumatic intracranial hemorrhage. Axial noncontrast CT (**a**) and corresponding GRE (**b**) MR images demonstrate acute subarachnoid blood products in the right central sulcus (orange arrows). Foci of hemorrhagic axonal injury are also seen in the left frontal lobe (yellow circles). Sagittal post-contrast CT image (**c**) in a different patient demonstrates multicompartmental intracranial blood products, including subarachnoid hemorrhage in temporal (red arrow) and parietal sulci (green arrow), as well as the sylvian fissure (yellow arrow). Additional injuries include a small parietal focus of hemorrhagic axonal injury (purple circle), a small acute on chronic subdural hematoma (white arrow), and a venous epidural hematoma along the anterior middle cranial fossa (blue arrow)

Subdural Hemorrhage (SDH)

- Refers to blood products in the potential space between the dura and arachnoid mater of the meninges (Figs. e6.1, e6.3, and 6.5c).
- Seen in patients of all ages, most commonly in the setting of trauma (non-accidental injury in infants, motor vehicle accidents in young adults, and falls in the elderly).
- Additional, less common causes include glutaric aciduria type I and intracranial hypotension.
- Most commonly caused by tearing of bridging veins that cross the subdural space.
- Extent is not limited by bony sutures since location is deep to the dura mater; however, it is limited by dural reflections (falx cerebri and tentorium cerebri).
- Classically described as a "crescentic" shape along the cerebral convexities. A small SDH collection is sometimes referred to as a "smear" SDH.
- Less likely to be acutely symptomatic owing to the slower growth rate caused by venous injury and increased lateral extent permitted by the subdural space.
- Subdural hematomas become covered by a thin membrane along its inner aspect and a thicker outer membrane containing capillaries and arterioles (which are prone to leakage and hematoma re-bleeding/expansion).
- May see fluid-fluid levels in the setting of re-bleed (acute on chronic).
- Chronic subdural hematomas may resemble CSF hygromas.

Subarachnoid Hemorrhage (SAH)

- Refers to the presence of blood products (arterial or venous) in the subarachnoid space overlying the brain parenchyma (Figs. e6.1, e6.2c, e6.3b, 6.5, and 6.9).
- Typically distributes in the cerebral sulci overlying the brain at the vertex in the setting of trauma and in the basal cisterns in the setting of aneurysm rupture.
- Clinically presents with thunderclap headache, photophobia, meningismus, and/or collapse.
- May be identified on CT as abnormal hyperdensity in the subarachnoid space.
- May be identified on MRI as hyperintense signal abnormality overlying the cerebral sulci on FLAIR and hypointense susceptibility blooming on GRE and/or SWI sequences, although hyperacute blood products may not demonstrate blooming on GRE sequences.
- The combination of FLAIR and SWI MRI sequences has been shown to be superior to CT in the detection of acute SAH [5].
- Perimesencephalic SAH (typically with small-volume blood in the interpeduncular fossa) is a less common distinct pattern, which often demonstrates a normal cerebral angiogram and is favored to be venous in origin.

INTRACEREBRAL HEMORRHAGE

Lobar Hemorrhage

- Primary lobar hemorrhage is most commonly seen in the elderly in the setting of amyloid angiopathy (Fig. e6.4).
- In younger patients, it may be seen in the setting of an underlying lesion, such as tumor or vascular malformation, or in the setting of venous sinus thrombosis, venous infarction, or a coagulopathy (Figs. 6.1, 6.2, 6.3, 6.9a, e6.7b, and e6.8c).
- Blood products are often located superficially within a lobe but may extend into the adjacent subarachnoid spaces.

Basal Ganglia Hemorrhage

- Most commonly secondary to poorly controlled hypertension (Fig. 6.6).
- Hemorrhage may extend into the ventricles.

Pontine Hemorrhage

- Usually owing to hypertension.
- Other causes include vascular malformations, tumors, and Duret hemorrhages in the setting of downward transtentorial herniation (Fig. e6.5).

Cerebellar Hemorrhage

- Usually owing to hypertension, although can also be seen in the setting of tumor and vascular malformation.
- May obstruct or extend into the fourth ventricle and subarachnoid spaces.

Intraventricular Hemorrhage (IVH)

- Primary intraventricular hemorrhage is uncommon but may be seen with vascular malformations and tumors.
- Blood products are heavier than CSF, so they pool dependently; most often visualized in the occipital horns (Figs. 6.2c, 6.8, and e6.4a). Look carefully for small-volume hemorrhage in this location.
- Large volumes of blood can form a cast, potentially resulting in obstructive hydrocephalus.

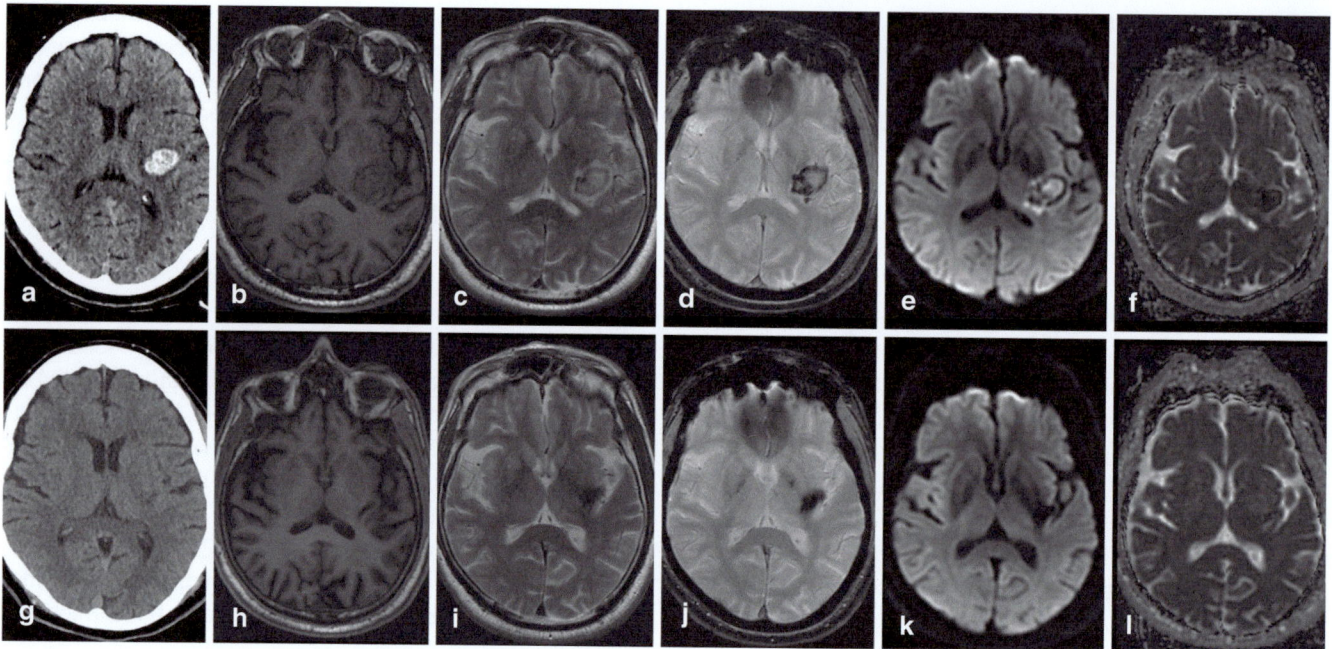

Fig. 6.6 Basal ganglia hypertensive hemorrhage. Axial CT and MR images demonstrate a hypertensive hemorrhage in the left basal ganglia in the hyperacute (**a–f**) and chronic (**g–l**) stages. Noncontrast CT (**a, g**) and T1 (**b, h**), T2 (**c, i**), GRE (**d, j**), Trace DWI (**e, k**), and ADC (**f, l**) MR images show the classic imaging appearances, as summarized in Fig. 6.4. Of note, hyperacute blood products are hyperintense on GRE (**d**), while the signal on Trace DWI (**e, k**) follows the T2 (**c, i**) signal intensity

Etiologies of ICH

TRAUMA

- May result in numerous forms of ICH, including SAH, EDH, and SDH as well as hemorrhagic parenchymal contusions and cerebral microhemorrhages, which often represent hemorrhagic axonal injury in the traumatic setting (Figs. 6.4, 6.5, and 6.7).
- Hemorrhagic parenchymal contusions are often visualized in the anterior (poles) and posterior temporal lobes, as well as the anterior (poles) and inferior frontal lobes in the setting of trauma. These locations are characteristic, as the brain impacts the adjacent skull in a "coup" and "contre-coup" pattern owing to significant traumatic forces (Fig. 6.7).
- Hemorrhagic axonal injury may be occult on CT and appears as hypointense susceptibility blooming on GRE and SWI sequences. It often occurs at gray-white matter junctions and the burden and distribution has been correlated to patient outcome, with involvement of the posterior body and splenium of corpus callosum, corona radiata, and dorsolateral upper brainstem portending a poorer prognosis [6] (Figs. 6.5a, b and 6.7b).
- Intracerebral hemorrhage volume ≥ 30 cm^3, infratentorial origin, lower Glasgow Coma Scale score, presence of intraventricular blood products, and age ≥ 80 years are considered independent variables for 30-day mortality [7].

HYPERTENSION

- Poorly controlled hypertension may result in ICH involving the basal ganglia (80%), pons (10%), and cerebellum (10%) (Fig. 6.6).
- Most commonly seen in patients in their sixth and seventh decades of life.
- Charcot-Bouchard microaneurysms are prone to rupture in the setting of hypertension, increasing risk of SAH.
- Serial imaging is often performed to assess for interval hematoma expansion or worsening mass effect, both of which could prompt clinical management strategies.

CEREBRAL AMYLOID ANGIOPATHY (CAA)

- Classically affects normotensive elderly individuals and is secondary to beta-amyloid deposition within the walls of small and medium-sized arteries, leading to wall weakening.
- This results in classic imaging features, including large, lobar parenchymal hematomas, predominantly peripheral cerebral microhemorrhages, and convexity SAH.
- Parenchymal hemorrhage secondary to amyloid usually involves the subcortical white matter and spares the basal ganglia, brainstem, and posterior fossa (Fig. e6.4).
- Convexity SAH can result in transient focal neurological symptoms (or "amyloid spells"), which is likely

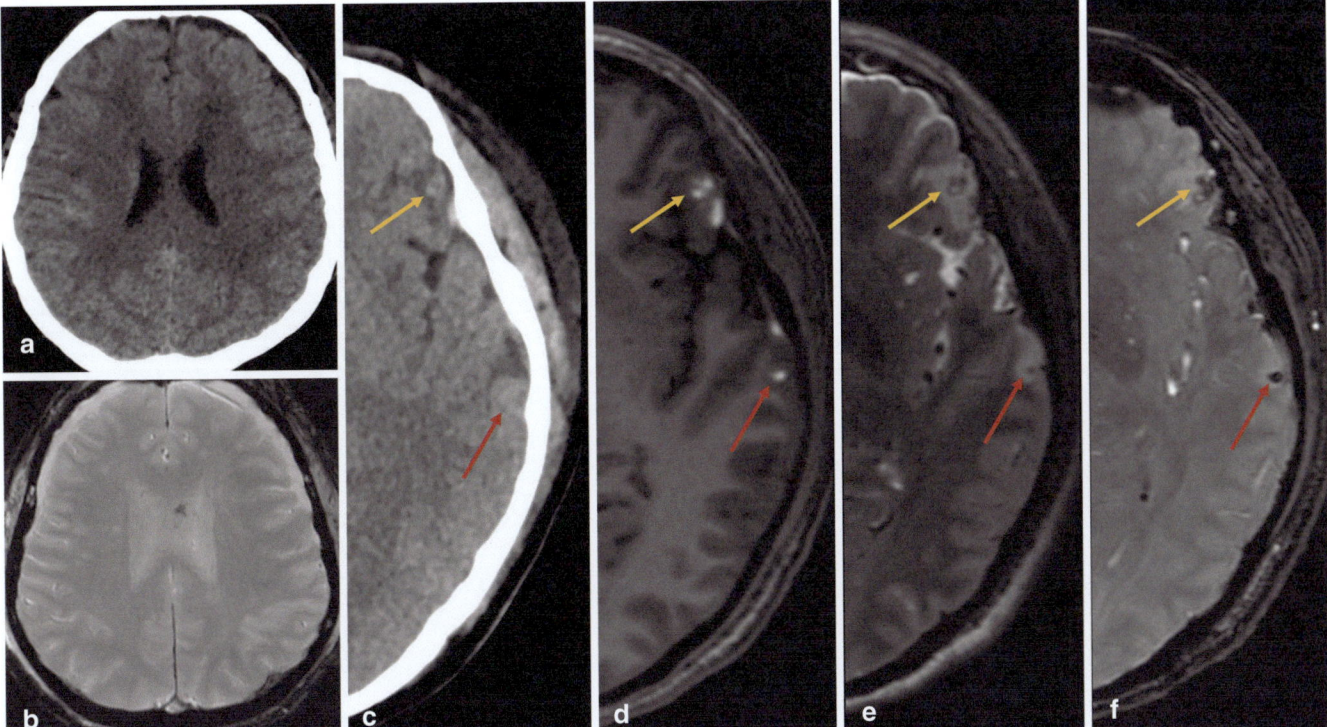

Fig. 6.7 Traumatic brain injury. Axial noncontrast CT (**a**) and GRE (**b**) MR images demonstrate hemorrhagic axonal injury in the corpus callosum. CT and MR images in a different patient demonstrate hemorrhagic parenchymal contusions in the left frontal operculum (orange arrows) and lateral temporal lobe (red arrows) on CT (**c**) as well as T1 (**d**), T2 (**e**), and SWAN (**f**) MR sequences

related to blood products in and around the central sulcus (Fig. e6.6).
- Superficial siderosis refers to the presence of hemosiderin on the brain (pial) surface and results from persistent or recurrent SAH (Fig. e6.6).
- Inflammatory CAA is an uncommon variant, which tends to affect younger patients (≥40 years) and often presents with rapidly progressive cognitive decline, seizures, headaches, and stroke-like symptoms.
  - Imaging features demonstrate areas of asymmetric T2/FLAIR signal abnormality in the subcortical white matter (representing vasogenic edema), and up to half of patients may demonstrate leptomeningeal contrast enhancement.
  - Differential diagnostic considerations include amyloid-related imaging abnormalities (ARIA), infections such as progressive multifocal leukoencephalopathy (PML), and vascular pathologies such as posterior reversible encephalopathy syndrome (PRES) or primary CNS vasculitis.
- With FDA approval of the drug Aduhelm (aducanumab) in 2021 for the treatment of Alzheimer's disease, amyloid-related imaging abnormalities (ARIA) are an entity to be aware of; specifically, ARIA-E (edema) and ARIA-H (hemorrhage), which can mimic CAA.

ARTERIOVENOUS MALFORMATIONS (AVM)

- AVMs are vascular lesions characterized by abnormal arteriovenous shunting through a nidus of dysplastic cerebral arteries and veins (Fig. 6.8).
- They are prone to rupture and most commonly result in intraparenchymal hemorrhage (IPH), although IVH and SAH are also commonly observed.
- Imaging techniques useful for identification and classification include noncontrast head CT, CTA, MRI, MRA, and digital subtraction angiography (DSA). Additionally, arterial spin labeling (ASL) is a valuable MR perfusion technique capable of detecting arteriovenous shunting and is particularly useful in evaluating for the early venous drainage seen in AVMs.
- Risk factors for hemorrhage include deep venous drainage, intranidal aneurysms, elevated feeding artery pressures, and stenosis of the draining vein(s). These imaging features may be difficult to appreciate on CT or MR imaging and are more fully characterized on DSA.
- The Spetzler-Martin Grading scale is used to characterize AVMs by size, eloquence of adjacent brain, and venous drainage in order to predict the morbidity and mortality risks of surgery.

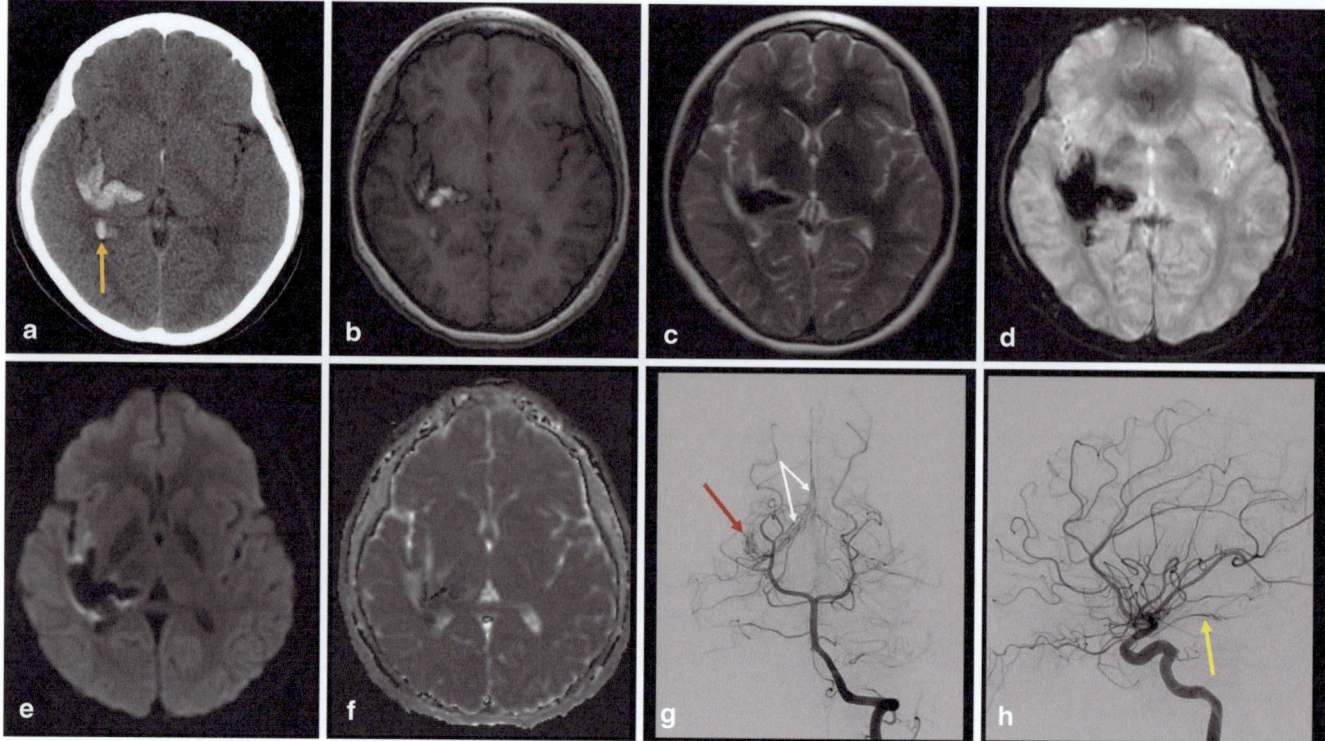

Fig. 6.8 Ruptured cerebral arteriovenous malformation. Axial noncontrast CT image (**a**) demonstrates acute intraparenchymal blood products centered in the right posterolateral thalamus with extension into the posterior insular region and right occipital horn (orange arrow). T1 (**b**), T2 (**c**), GRE (**d**), Trace DWI (**e**), and ADC (**f**) MR images obtained a few days later show early subacute blood products. Digital subtraction angiography (**g** and **h**) depicts an underlying AVM (red arrow) with supply via posterior choroidal and anterior choroidal (yellow arrow) branches. Note the early venous drainage into the right basal vein of Rosenthal and the straight sinus (white arrows)

DURAL ARTERIOVENOUS FISTULAE (DAVF)

- DAVFs are vascular lesions characterized by direct fistulous connections between dural or cerebral arteries and dural venous sinuses or cortical veins (Fig. e6.7).
- In contrast to AVMs, DAVF lack a vascular nidus and are hypothesized to be acquired lesions secondary to trauma or dural venous sinus thrombosis.
- The clinical presentation is varied, including tinnitus, cranial nerve deficits, and signs of increased intracranial pressure.
- A ruptured DAVF often presents with IPH in an unusual location or SAH and is seen as hyperdense blood products on noncontrast CT.
- MRI is useful in the assessment of suspected DAVF, particularly the ASL perfusion sequence, which is able to assess for arteriovenous shunting (identified by the presence of abnormally increased venous ASL signal).
- DSA remains the gold standard for fully characterizing DAVF, as it is able to assess for patterns of venous outflow from the fistula. This allows for grading via the Cognard and Borden systems and helps predict the risk of future hemorrhage and rupture.

CORTICAL VENOUS OR VENOUS SINUS THROMBOSIS

- These may be clinically confusing entities, often presenting with headaches.
- Risk factors include hormonal imbalance (e.g., elevated estrogen in the setting of oral contraceptive pills) and other prothrombotic states (including dehydration, factor deficiencies, and genetic mutations) as well as skull base infections and sepsis. Local injury secondary to trauma or compression in the setting of adjacent tumor are also risk factors.
- Imaging demonstrates signs of venous hypertension, including areas of edema, infarction, and/or hemorrhage. When hemorrhages are present, they are often near gray-white matter junctions and do not conform to arterial distributions. The odd location of the bleed(s) should alert the radiologist to the possibility of cortical venous or venous sinus thrombosis.
- Important signs to know include the *cord, dense vein, delta,* and *empty delta* signs (Figs. 6.1c and e6.8).
  - *Cord* sign refers to cordlike hyperattenuation of a dural venous sinus on noncontrast CT images owing to dural venous sinus thrombosis. It is most commonly seen in the transverse sinus.

- o *Dense vein* sign refers to the noncontrast CT appearance of hyperattenuating thrombus with a cortical vein or dural venous sinus. When located in the superior sagittal sinus, it is referred to as a *delta* or *dense triangle* sign, owing to its triangular shape resembling the uppercase form of the Greek letter delta (Δ) (Fig. e6.8a).
- o *Empty delta* sign refers to the triangular filling defect of a thrombosed superior sagittal sinus on post-contrast CT images. A similar appearance can also be seen in the transverse sinuses on coronal or sagittal images (Fig. e6.8b).
- Note that a *pseudo-delta* sign may be seen when the post-contrast filling defect in the sinus may be owing to other entities such as arachnoid granulations or fat deposits, and not thrombus. Moreover, this sign has also been described on noncontrast CT (and also in the absence of thrombus) as an apparent hyperdense triangle surrounding the low density of the superior sagittal sinus owing to: (1) adjacent extra-axial interhemispheric subdural hemorrhage or subarachnoid hemorrhage; (2) with increased attenuation of normal dura surrounding the SSS owing to dural or arachnoid granulation calcification; and (3) as an optical illusion when there is increased conspicuity of the normal dura next to surrounding relatively hypodense diffuse cerebral edema.
- Deep cerebral venous thromboses can result in unusual patterns of injury, including bilateral thalamic infarctions.

COAGULOPATHY

- Coagulation disorders may be acquired or congenital and may result in acute ICH involving any location.
- There are numerous acquired causes, including medications such as aspirin, anticoagulants, or thrombolytic therapy, as well as coagulopathy secondary to malignancy. Thrombocytopenia may also result in ICH, including immune thrombocytopenic purpura (ITP) and thrombocytopenia induced by drugs, alcohol, and liver or kidney disease.
- Congenital causes are less common, but include hemophilia A, hemophilia B, and von Willebrand disease, among others.

CEREBRAL ANEURYSMS

- Cerebral aneurysms are focal outpouchings arising from arteries, representing sites of arterial wall weakening that are prone to rupture.
- Commonly described types include saccular (or berry) and fusiform aneurysms, although pseudoaneurysms in the setting of dissection and mycotic aneurysms also occur.
- Saccular aneurysms are often seen in the circle of Willis, most commonly at the junction of the anterior cerebral and the anterior communicating arteries, the posterior communicating artery, the middle cerebral artery bifurcation, carotid terminus, and basilar tip.
- Aneurysm rupture classically presents with sudden onset of the worst headache of a patient's life, which is caused by SAH and irritation of the dura mater.
- Unruptured aneurysms may also present with headache, cranial neuropathies (including visual disturbances and oculomotor palsy), epilepsy, or even cerebral infarction.
- The Hunt and Hess classification is a clinical grading system used to help determine the risk of surgical mortality in patients admitted with aneurysmal SAH (aSAH). It is not intended to be used in patients with SAH secondary to other causes, including trauma, vascular malformations, and vasculitis.
- Noncontrast head CT is excellent for detecting acute SAH in the setting of aneurysm rupture, with blood products often visualized in the basal cisterns closest to the site of ruptured aneurysm. Blood products may also extend into the brain parenchyma or the ventricles (Fig. 6.9).
- The Modified Fisher Grading Scale is a radiographic tool used to describe the volume and distribution of hemorrhage and predict the risk of clinical vasospasm and delayed cerebral ischemia following aSAH.
- CT, MR, and catheter-angiography (DSA) are used to identify the ruptured aneurysm, help determine the most appropriate treatment strategy, and screen for additional unruptured aneurysms (Fig. 6.9).

TUMORS

- Hemorrhagic tumors may present with headache, altered mental status, or seizure.
- Almost all primary neoplasms may demonstrate hemorrhage. Additional tumors include pituitary lesions and even cavernous malformations.
- Several metastases are prone to hemorrhage, including renal, thyroid, melanoma, and choriocarcinoma. Breast and lung metastases are other common metastases, which may also present with hemorrhage.
- It is not uncommon to see hemorrhage or petechial blood products in and around metastases following radiation therapy.

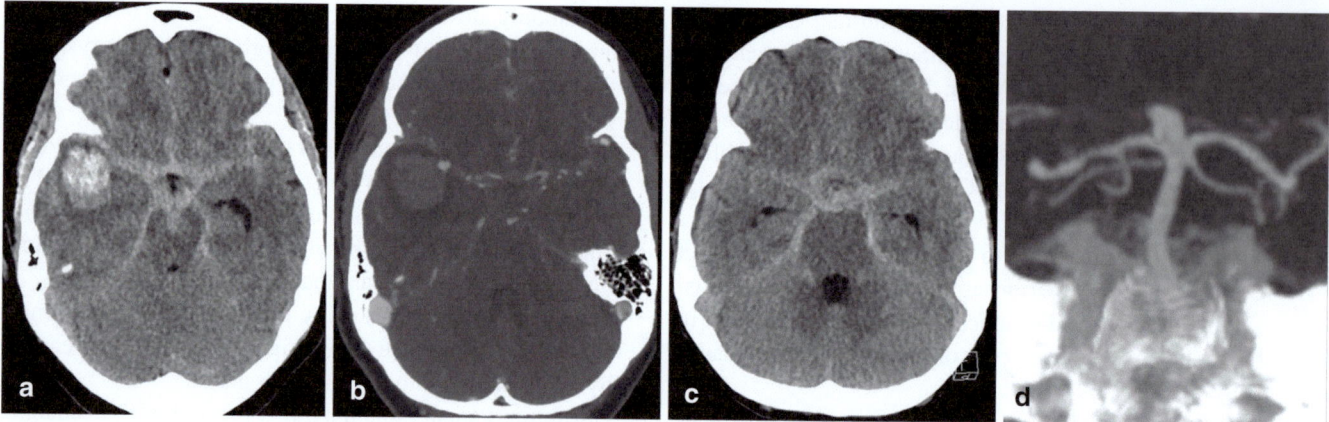

Fig. 6.9 Ruptured cerebral aneurysms. Axial noncontrast CT (**a**) image demonstrates diffuse subarachnoid hemorrhage throughout the basal cisterns with intraparenchymal extension into the right temporal lobe. Subsequent CT angiogram (**b**) demonstrates a large right middle cerebral artery (MCA) bifurcation aneurysm. Axial noncontrast CT (**c**) and coronal CT angiogram (**d**) images in a different patient also demonstrate diffuse subarachnoid hemorrhage throughout the basal cisterns with a large basilar tip aneurysm

HEMORRHAGIC CONVERSION OF ISCHEMIC INFARCTION

- Hemorrhagic transformation (HT) is a common complication following recanalization of an ischemic infarct, and often occurs secondary to disruption of the blood–brain barrier.
- HT increases stroke morbidity and mortality, with most instances occurring within 24 h of thrombolysis or within 3–4 days following infarction.
- A spectrum of HT is graded according to the Heidelberg Bleeding Classification, including small scattered petechiae along the infarct margin (HI1), confluent petechial hemorrhage within the infarcted tissue (HI2), parenchymal hematoma involving <30% of the infarcted tissue without substantive mass effect (PH1), and parenchymal hematoma involving ≥30% of the infarcted tissue with obvious mass effect (PH2).
- PH2 is usually the only form of clinical significance.
- HT can be seen on noncontrast CT, although evaluation may be limited and challenging secondary to iodinated contrast "staining" from the cerebral angiogram that is often performed during the treatment of these patients. Because of this, dual-energy CT (DECT) is an emerging technique used to help distinguish iodinated contrast from blood products in and around the infarct bed.
- HT is also readily appreciated on MRI owing to the sensitivity of GRE and SWI sequences for detecting blood products (Fig. 6.10).

VASCULITIS OR VASCULOPATHY

- Cerebral arterial vasculitis may occasionally present with small-volume convexity SAH, headaches, and neurological deficits.
- This can be seen on CT as hyperdensity within the cerebral sulci and on MRI as sulcal signal abnormality on FLAIR (hyperintense) and GRE (hypointense) sequences.
- Convexity SAH in the absence of trauma and obvious abnormality on CTA or MRA should be followed by DSA to evaluate for signs of vasculitis (subtle beading and luminal irregularities, often in distal branches beyond the resolution of CTA and MRA).

Clinical Pearls and Caveats

- Describe ICH location, size, shape, density/intensity, age, local effect, and global effect.
- Six easy to miss hemorrhages are: (1) tiny SAH at the vertex or in sulci, (2) in dependent occipital horns, (3) in the interpeduncular fossa, (4) in pre-brainstem cisterns, (5) small or smear SDHs, and (6) hemorrhages that are isodense or isointense. These are sometimes challenging to detect.
- When clearing an examination for ICH, one should always use thin sections and multiplanar reformations. Coronal images are especially useful for identifying blood products along the falx and tentorial leaflets while sagittal reformations are useful for confirming hemorrhage location (e.g., within a sulcus).
- The accurate identification of intracranial blood products greatly impacts patient care, as numerous systems and scores are used for prognostic assessment and the identification of blood products in additional locations can change patient management strategies (e.g., the addition of IVH in the setting of aSAH).

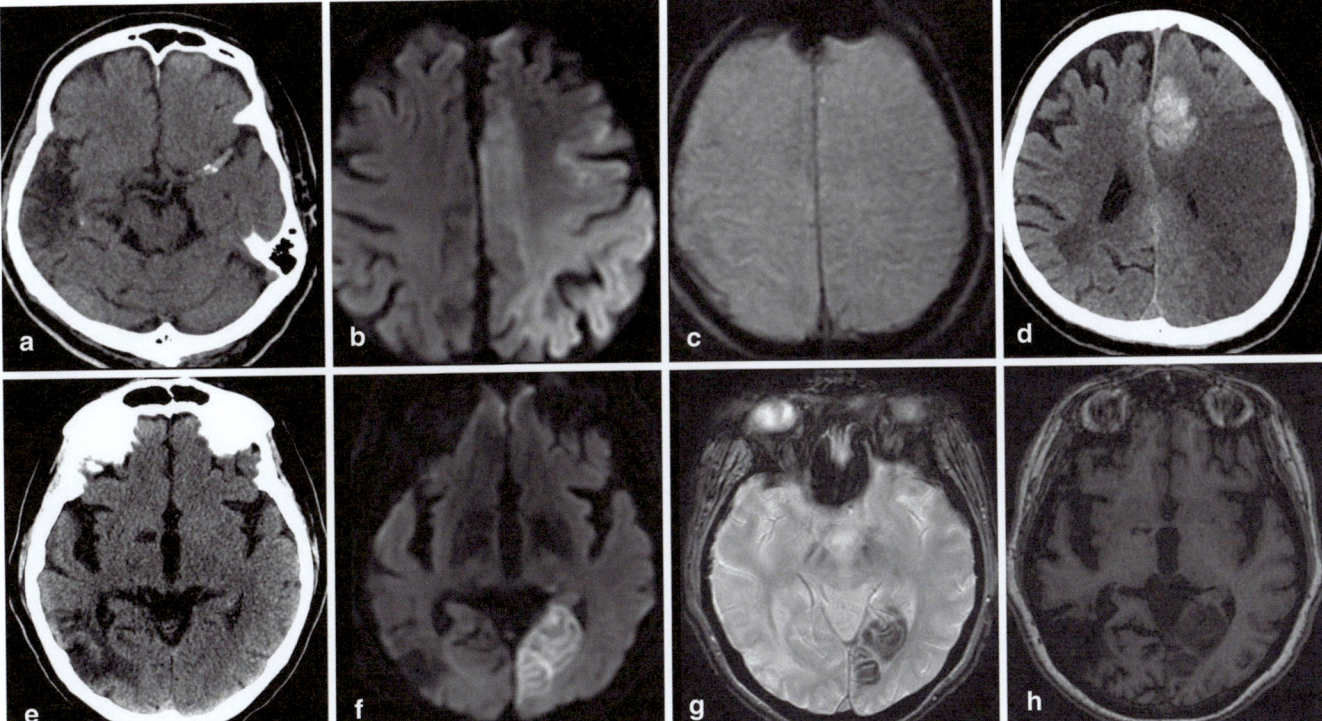

Fig. 6.10 Hemorrhagic conversion of ischemic infarcts. Axial noncontrast CT (**a**) demonstrates a dense M1 segment of the left middle cerebral artery (MCA), consistent with thrombus. A chronic right MCA territory infarct is also seen. Same-day Trace DWI (**b**) and GRE (**c**) MR images demonstrate a large area of infarction involving the left MCA and ACA territories without hemorrhage. Noncontrast head CT (**d**) the following day demonstrates an acute parenchymal hematoma in the left anterior cingulate gyrus with mass effect, consistent with PH2 hemorrhagic transformation. Axial noncontrast CT (**e**) in a different patient demonstrates loss of gray-white matter differentiation in the left posterior cerebral artery (PCA) territory along the medial occipital lobe, consistent with acute infarction. Same-day Trace DWI (**f**), GRE (**g**), and T1 (**h**) MR images demonstrate acute infarction with confluent petechial hemorrhage, consistent with HI2 hemorrhagic transformation. Chronic right PCA territory and right basal ganglia lacunar infarcts are also visualized

References

1. Goldstein JN, Fazen LE, Snider R, Schwab K, Greenberg SM, Smith EE, et al. Contrast extravasation on CT CME angiography predicts hematoma expansion in intracerebral hemorrhage. Neurology. 2007;68:889–94.
2. Orrison WW, Gentry LR, Stimac GK, Tarrel RM. Blinded comparison of cranial CT and MR in closed head injury evaluation. AJNR Am J Neuroradiol. 1994;15(2):351–6.
3. Linfante I, Llinas RH, Caplan LR, Warach S. MRI features of intracerebral hemorrhage within 2 hours from symptom onset. Stroke. 1999;30(11):2263–7.
4. Saad AF, Chaudhari R, Fischbein NJ, Wintermark M. Intracranial hemorrhage imaging. Semin Ultrasound CT MRI. 2018;39(5):441–56.
5. Verma RK, Kottke R, Andereggen L, Weisstanner C, Zubler C, Gralla J, et al. Detecting subarachnoid hemorrhage: comparison of combined FLAIR/SWI versus CT. Eur J Radiol. 2013;82(9):1539–45.
6. Kampfl A, Schmutzhard E, Franz G, Pfausler B, Haring H-P, Ulmer H, et al. Prediction of recovery from post-traumatic vegetative state with cerebral magnetic-resonance imaging. Lancet. 1998;351(9118):1763–7.
7. Hemphill JC, Bonovich DC, Besmertis L, Manley GT, Johnston SC. The ICH score: a simple, reliable grading scale for intracerebral hemorrhage. Stroke. 2001;32(4):891–7.

Intracranial Aneurysms and Vascular Malformations: Imaging Findings and Clinical Considerations

Justin E. Vranic and Javier M. Romero

SUBARACHNOID HEMORRHAGE (SAH)

TRAUMATIC SAH (tSAH)

- Occurs in up to 11% of traumatic brain injuries [1].
- Traumatic injury to the small bridging cortical vessels along the pia and arachnoid leptomeninges crossing the subarachnoid space results in tSAH.
- tSAH is often more focal and superficial when compared to aneurysmal SAH (aSAH), layering within sulci adjacent to areas of hemorrhagic contusion [2].
- tSAH is frequently encountered along the anterior and inferior surfaces of the frontal and temporal lobes.
- Hemorrhagic brain contusions are a common concomitant injury, occurring in over 40% of patients with blunt or nonpenetrating head injuries [3].
- These injuries occur as the brain decelerates upon impact with the calvarium and commonly develop along the inferior frontal and anterior and lateral temporal lobes where impact occurs with the floor of the anterior cranial fossa, the sphenoid wings, and the petrous ridges, respectively [2].

Supplementary Information The online version contains supplementary material available at https://doi.org/10.1007/978-3-031-55124-6_7.

J. E. Vranic (✉)
Division of Neuroradiology, Department of Radiology, Massachusetts General Hospital, Boston, MA, USA

Department of Neurosurgery, Massachusetts General Hospital, Boston, MA, USA
e-mail: Jvranic@hms.harvard.edu

J. M. Romero
Division of Neuroradiology, Department of Radiology, Massachusetts General Hospital, Boston, MA, USA
e-mail: JMROMERO@mgh.harvard.edu

ANEURYSMAL SAH (aSAH)

- Saccular aneurysm rupture commonly results in aSAH layering predominantly within the basal cisterns (Fig. 7.1).
- The distribution of cisternal SAH can help with aneurysm localization.
- aSAH predominantly within the interhemispheric fissure is suggestive of an anterior communicating (ACOM) artery aneurysm.
- aSAH within the Sylvian fissure is suggestive of a middle cerebral artery (MCA) bifurcation (Fig. e7.3. All electronic images (Figs. e7.1–e7.8) can be found in this chapter's website on SpringerLink: https://doi.org/10.1007/978-3-031-55124-6_7), posterior communicating (PCOM) artery, or internal carotid artery (ICA) terminus aneurysm.
- aSAH within the prepontine and interpeduncular cisterns is suggestive of a basilar tip aneurysm.
- aSAH within the premedullary and prepontine cisterns is suggestive of a PICA origin aneurysm.
- aSAH with intraventricular extension is frequently related to anterior communicating artery and tip of the basilar artery aneurysms.
- Identification of intraventricular extension of aSAH is important as this increases the risk of developing obstructive hydrocephalus and/or vasospasm [4].
- Mycotic aneurysms typically arise from distal arterial branches and therefore more commonly manifest as sulcal convexity SAH [5].

> **NONCONTRAST HEAD CT REPORT IMPRESSION PEARLS**
>
> - Distribution of SAH within the basal cisterns.
> - Presence of intraventricular extension of blood.
> - Evidence of developing hydrocephalus.
> - Presence of intraparenchymal hemorrhage.

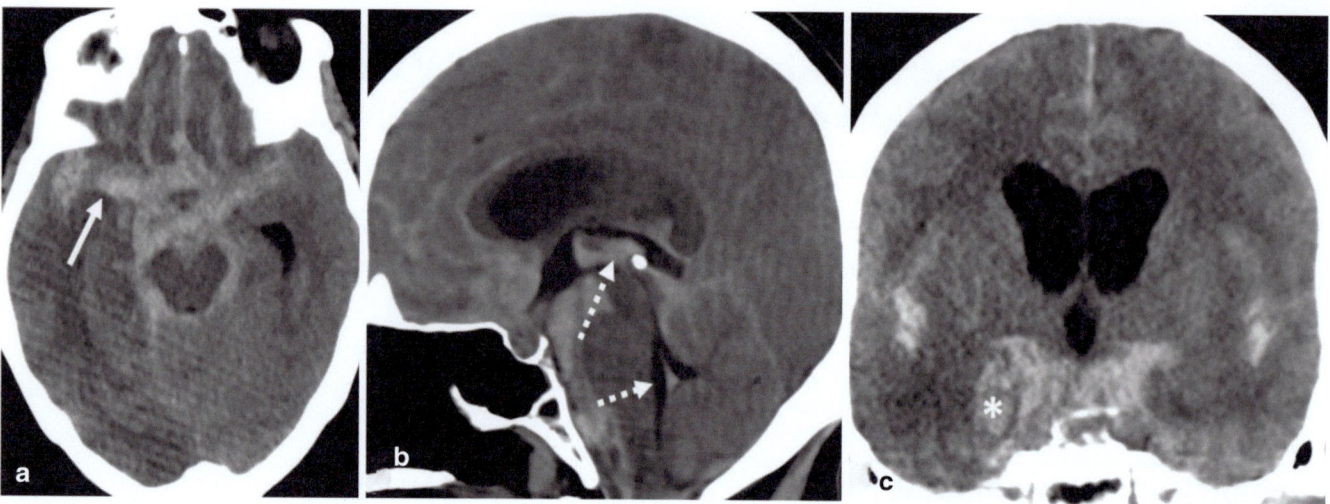

Fig. 7.1 Noncontrast head CT demonstrating aSAH. (**a**) Thick clot layering within the basal cisterns with an asymmetric volume layering within the right suprasellar cistern and Sylvian fissure (solid white arrow) suggestive of a ruptured right posterior communicating artery (PCOM) aneurysm. (**b**) Hemorrhage extends into the third and fourth ventricles (dashed white arrows). (**c**) Small intraparenchymal hemorrhage within the right mesial temporal lobe (white asterisk), which can be seen in the setting of a ruptured PCOM aneurysm

INTRACRANIAL ANEURYSMS

Intracranial aneurysms are acquired arterial lesions characterized by abnormal outpouching of the vessel wall. They are most commonly located at arterial branch points, as the intracranial artery courses through the subarachnoid space. Their morphologies can be varied ranging from saccular berry aneurysms, segmental fusiform aneurysms (Fig. e7.1), and small dissecting/blister aneurysms. These vascular lesions are of clinical significance due to the association of rupture with poor patient outcomes [6].

EPIDEMIOLOGY

- The prevalence of intracranial saccular aneurysms in the general population is estimated to be 0.5–3% [7].
- 80–85% of aneurysms are located in the anterior circulation [8]. Table 7.1 demonstrates the distribution of aneurysms within the intracranial circulation.
- 20–30% of patients with an intracranial aneurysm will ultimately be found to have multiple intracranial aneurysms [9].
- Women are three times more likely than men to harbor unruptured intracranial aneurysms [10].

Table 7.1 Intracranial aneurysm distribution

Location	N	%
ICA (supraclinoid)	815	22
MCA	669	18
Acom	485	13
BA	232	7
ICA (paraclinoid)	247	7
ACA	262	7
Pcom	258	7
ICA (cavernous)	234	6

ACA anterior cerebral artery, *Acom* anterior communicating artery, *BA* basilar artery, *IA* intracranial aneurysm, *ICA* internal carotid artery, *MCA* middle cerebral artery, *Pcom* posterior communicating artery [12]

- The frequency of unruptured intracranial aneurysms is believed to peak in the fifth to sixth decades of life [11].

RISK FACTORS FOR INTRACRANIAL ANEURYSM RUPTURE

- Aneurysm size (measured from center of the neck plane to the aneurysm dome) is one of the most important predictors of rupture [13] with the International Study of Unruptured Intracranial Aneurysm trial reporting a negligible annual risk of rupture in aneurysms less than 7 mm in size and increasing rupture risks for larger aneurysms [14].

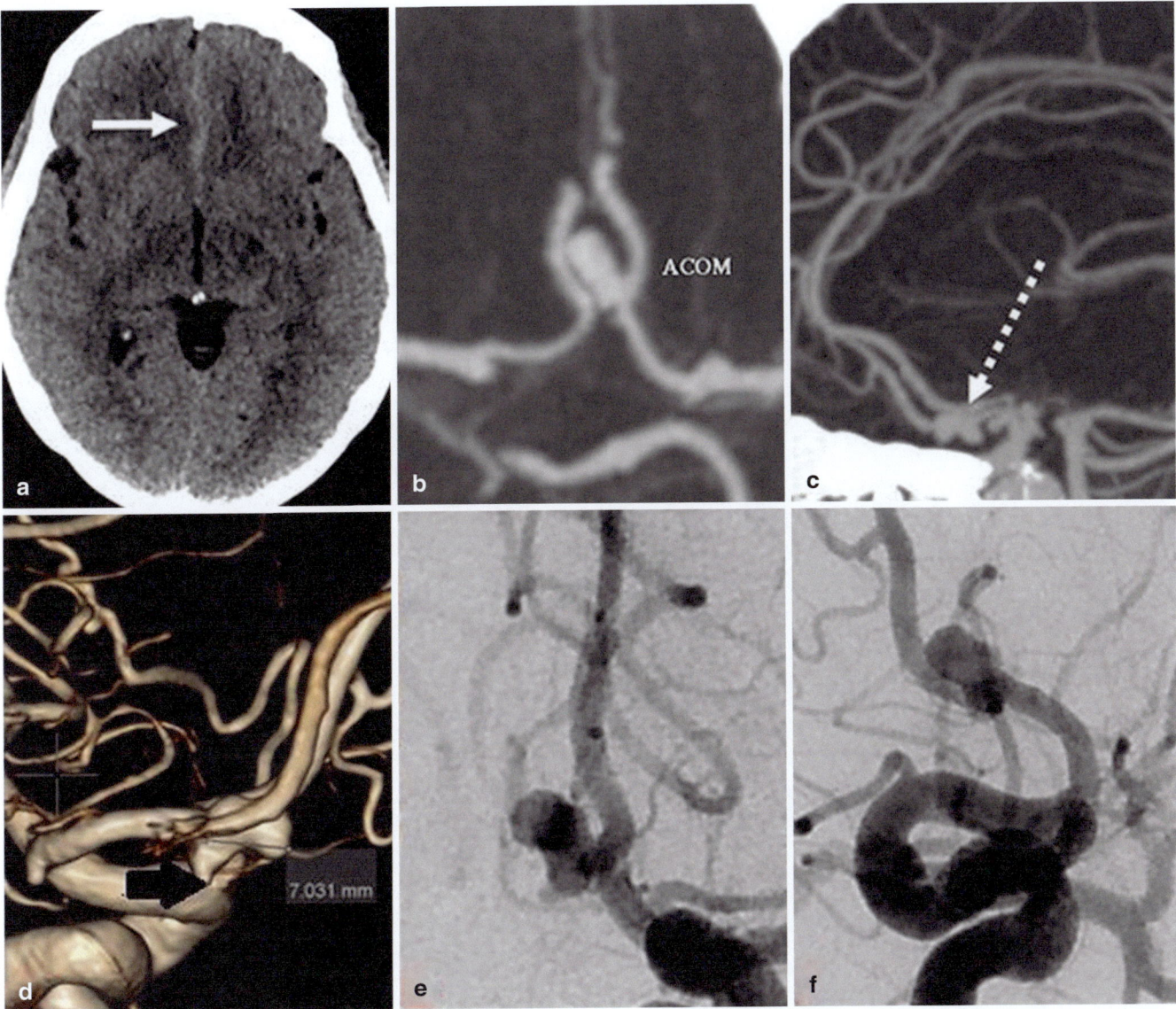

Fig. 7.2 (**a**) Noncontrast head CT demonstrating SAH within the anterior interhemispheric fissure suggestive of a ruptured anterior communicating (ACOM) artery aneurysm. (**b**, **c**) CTA demonstrating an anteroinferiorly projecting, multilobulated saccular ACOM aneurysm (dashed white arrow) that is supplied by a dominant left A1 segment. (**d**) 3D reconstructions acquired from catheter angiography demonstrates a small secondary bleb (Black arrow) along the inferior margin of the aneurysm that was the likely site of rupture. (**e**, **f**) Catheter angiogram working projections demonstrating the multilobulated morphology of the aneurysm and its narrow neck

- However, up to 30% of ruptured aneurysms are <5 mm in size suggesting other factors may also play an important role in influencing rupture risk [15].
- Irregular morphology is strongly and independently associated with aneurysm rupture, irrespective of aneurysm size and location [16].
- The presence of multiple lobulations, daughter sacs, or irregular margins along the aneurysm sac are strong predictors of rupture (Figs. 7.2 and e7.2) [17, 18].
- Aneurysm location influences rupture risk with aneurysms involving the anterior communicating artery, posterior communicating artery, and posterior circulation being at increased risk of rupture relative to other locations within the intracranial circulation [19].
- The PHASES risk score attempts to predict aneurysm rupture risk using a combination of clinical (age, race, history of prior aneurysm rupture, and presence of hypertension), morphologic (aneurysm size), and anatomic (aneurysm location) variables [19].
- A higher PHASES score corresponds to a higher risk of future aneurysm rupture.

IMAGING

- CTA and MRA routinely identify incidental unruptured aneurysms within the intracranial circulation.
- Given their noninvasive nature and relative ease of acquisition, CTA and MRA are well-suited for intracranial aneurysm screening in individuals at increased risk for aneurysm development.
- CTA and MRA allow for easy identification of aneurysm location; care should be taken to accurately identify the anatomic location of intracranial aneurysms as this will influence treatment decisions.
- Small aneurysms (≤2–3 mm in size) may be missed with MRA [20].
- Aneurysm dome diameter, dome height, and neck diameter are important morphological features that should be assessed on CTA and MRA as these morphological features aid with rupture risk stratification and influence treatment decisions.
- Both CTA and MRA can readily demonstrate branch vessels arising from intracranial aneurysms.
- The relationship of branch vessels to the aneurysm dome is important in treatment planning (Fig. 7.3), and whenever possible, the radiologist should comment on whether

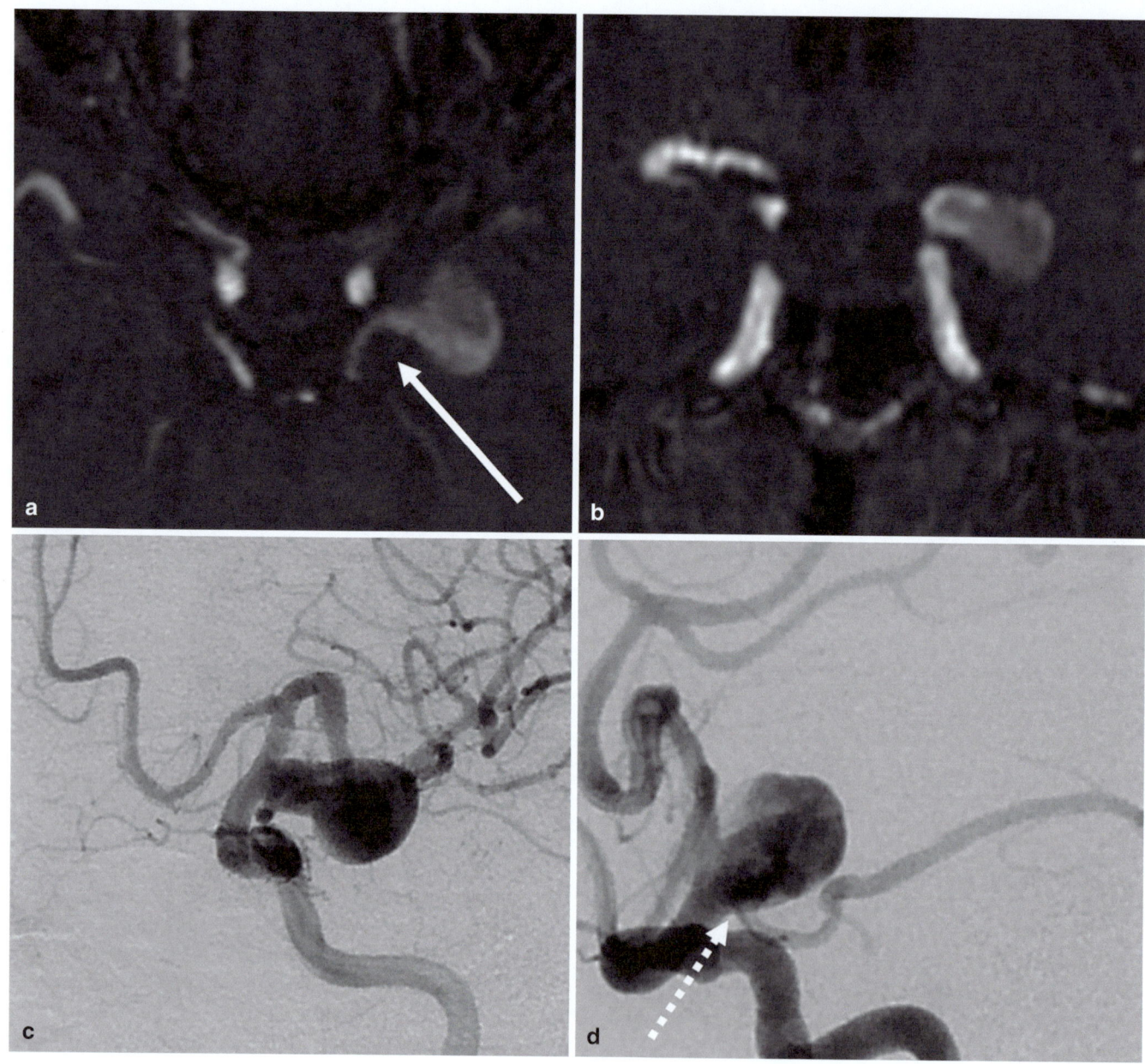

Fig. 7.3 (**a, b**) 3D-TOF-MRA demonstrating an inferolaterally projecting, unruptured, saccular PCOM aneurysm with a prominent posterior communicating artery arising from its neck (solid white arrow). Slow flow within the aneurysm dome results in diminished flow-related signal on 3D-TOF-MRA. (**c, d**) Catheter angiogram confirming a large saccular PCOM aneurysm. Once again, a prominent PCOM artery arises from the aneurysm neck (dashed white arrow)

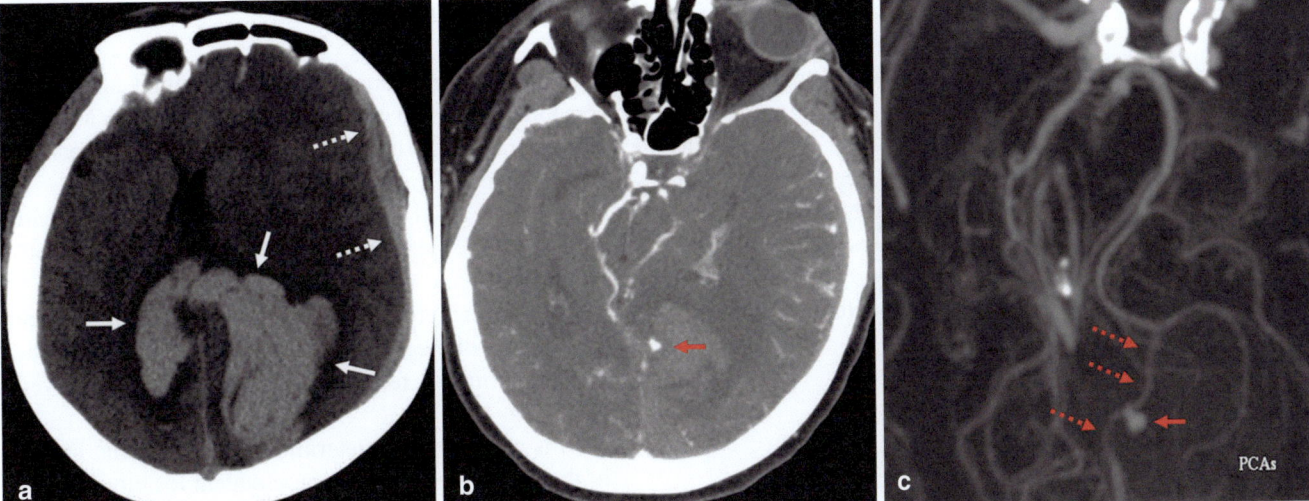

Fig. 7.4 (**a**) Noncontrast head CT demonstrating a large left occipital intraparenchymal hematoma (solid white arrows), which dissects across midline through the splenium of the corpus callosum as well as into the subdural space along the left cerebral convexity (dashed white arrows). (**b**) CTA demonstrates an abnormal globular focus of contrast along the medial border of the intraparenchymal hematoma (red arrow). (**c**) Axial CTA MIP images demonstrate a small, irregular mycotic aneurysm arising from a small cortical branch of the left PCA (dashed red arrows)

an aneurysm-associated branch vessel arises from the aneurysm dome, neck, or the adjacent parent vessel.
- The presence of aneurysm dome lobulations, daughter sacs, and/or other contour irregularities must be identified and conveyed in the radiology report as these morphological characteristics are associated with an increased risk of rupture.
- Although saccular aneurysms commonly develop at arterial branch points in the Circle of Willis, infectious mycotic aneurysms frequently develop in small distal arterial branches (Fig. 7.4) making careful review of the distal arterial tree important, particularly for patients with known bacteremia.
- Digital subtraction angiography (DSA) remains the gold standard imaging test for the assessment of intracranial aneurysms and post flow diverter treatment (Fig. e7.4).
- In addition to providing necessary diagnostic information about aneurysm morphology and location, catheter angiography allows for potential endovascular intervention (Fig. e7.5).
- DSA should be considered for all aneurysms whose size approaches 7 mm and treatment may be warranted [21] or for patients who present with atraumatic SAH in a distribution suspicious for an aneurysmal bleed who do not show evidence of an underlying aneurysm on CTA or MRA.

> **CT AND MR ANGIOGRAM REPORT IMPRESSION PEARLS**
> - Aneurysm location within the intracranial circulation.
> - Aneurysm size including maximum dome diameter, maximum dome height, and aneurysm neck diameter.
> - The presence of aneurysm-associated branch vessels and their location (i.e., arising from the dome, neck, or adjacent parent vessel).
> - The presence of multiple lobulations, daughter sacs, or aneurysm sac irregularity.

INTRACRANIAL ARTERIOVENOUS MALFORMATIONS

Intracranial arteriovenous malformations (AVM) are congenital vascular anomalies of the brain that result from the maldevelopment of intervening capillary networks between cerebral arteries and veins. This maldevelopment results in an abnormal tangle of parenchymal vessels referred to as a nidus with direct connection between the cerebral arteries and veins. Rapid arteriovenous shunting of blood through the nidus is characteristic of these lesions [22].

EPIDEMIOLOGY

- Autopsy series have suggested an AVM prevalence of 4–5% in the general population [23].
- Prospective population-based surveys have reported AVM detection rates of 1.34 per 100,000 person years with 60–70% of AVMs diagnosed before hemorrhage [24].
- First time, acute AVM hemorrhage rates are estimated at 0.51 per 100,000 person years [24].
- AVMs commonly present in young adults (mean age: 35 ± 18 years) [24].

CLINICAL PRESENTATION

- Symptomatic presentations of intracranial AVMs include headache, seizure, focal neurologic deficits, and spontaneous intracranial hemorrhage [25].
- Spontaneous intracranial hemorrhage is the most common clinical presentation, occurring in at least 50% of patients with AVMs [24, 26–28].
- Seizures occur in approximately 30–35% of patients [29–31].
- Headache is the presenting symptom in approximately 15% of patients [25].
- Nonhemorrhagic focal neurologic deficits are relatively rare with slowly progressive neurologic deficits occurring in approximately 4–8% of patients [32–36].

NATURAL HISTORY

- The average annual hemorrhage risk is estimated to be 2–4% [29, 37–39].
- Hemorrhage risk increases to approximately 6–18% for the first year following a bleeding event before gradually return to its baseline risk level [25].
- Up to 15% of intracranial AVMs may experience asymptomatic hemorrhage [40].
- Approximately 13% of patients die as a result of AVM hemorrhage [40].
- The long-term annual mortality rate associated with AVMs is 1–1.5% [39, 41].
- The long-term morbidity rate associated with AVMs is estimated to be 10–30% [42].
- Risk factors for AVM hemorrhage include history of prior hemorrhage [43], exclusive deep venous drainage [44], the presence of a single draining vein [45], and the presence of intranidal aneurysms [46].

IMAGING CHARACTERISTICS

- CT and MRI are frequently used as initial noninvasive screening studies to evaluate for intracranial AVMs.
- Noncontrast CT is useful for the detection of intracranial hemorrhage.
- CTA can be used to identify the AVM nidus, potential feeding arteries, draining veins, and the presence of intranidal aneurysms or venous ectasia (Fig. e7.6).
- MRI/MRA can provide information regarding the angioarchitecture of the AVM including the location and size of the AVM nidus, feeding arteries, and draining veins (Fig. 7.5).
- MRI is also useful in determining the anatomic location of the AVM (eloquent vs. non-eloquent locations) as well as assessing for underlying parenchymal abnormalities such as vasogenic edema secondary to venous congestion.
- Catheter angiography remains the gold standard imaging test for defining the AVM angioarchitecture and flow dynamics through the lesion [47].
- The Spetzler-Martin grading ranges from grade I to V. The system utilizes AVM location and morphological features to predict the risk of morbidity and mortality associated with operative treatment (Table 7.2) [48] and much of this information can be obtained from CTA/MRA. The higher the grade of the AVM, the higher the associated morbidity and mortality, a grade VI was added for diffuse nidus arteriovenous malformations, which were considered inoperable.

> **CT AND MR ANGIOGRAM REPORT IMPRESSION PEARLS**
> - Anatomic location of the AVM nidus with attention paid to eloquent locations (i.e., sensorimotor cortex, language areas, visual cortex, hypothalamus, thalamus, internal capsule, brainstem, cerebellar peduncles, deep cerebellar nuclei).
> - Nidus size in centimeters.
> - Feeding arteries supplying the AVM nidus.
> - Venous drainage from the AVM nidus with attention paid to possible deep drainage through the internal cerebral veins, basal veins, or precentral cerebellar vein.
> - The presence of intranidal aneurysms or focal venous ectasia, which can serve as an AVM rupture point.

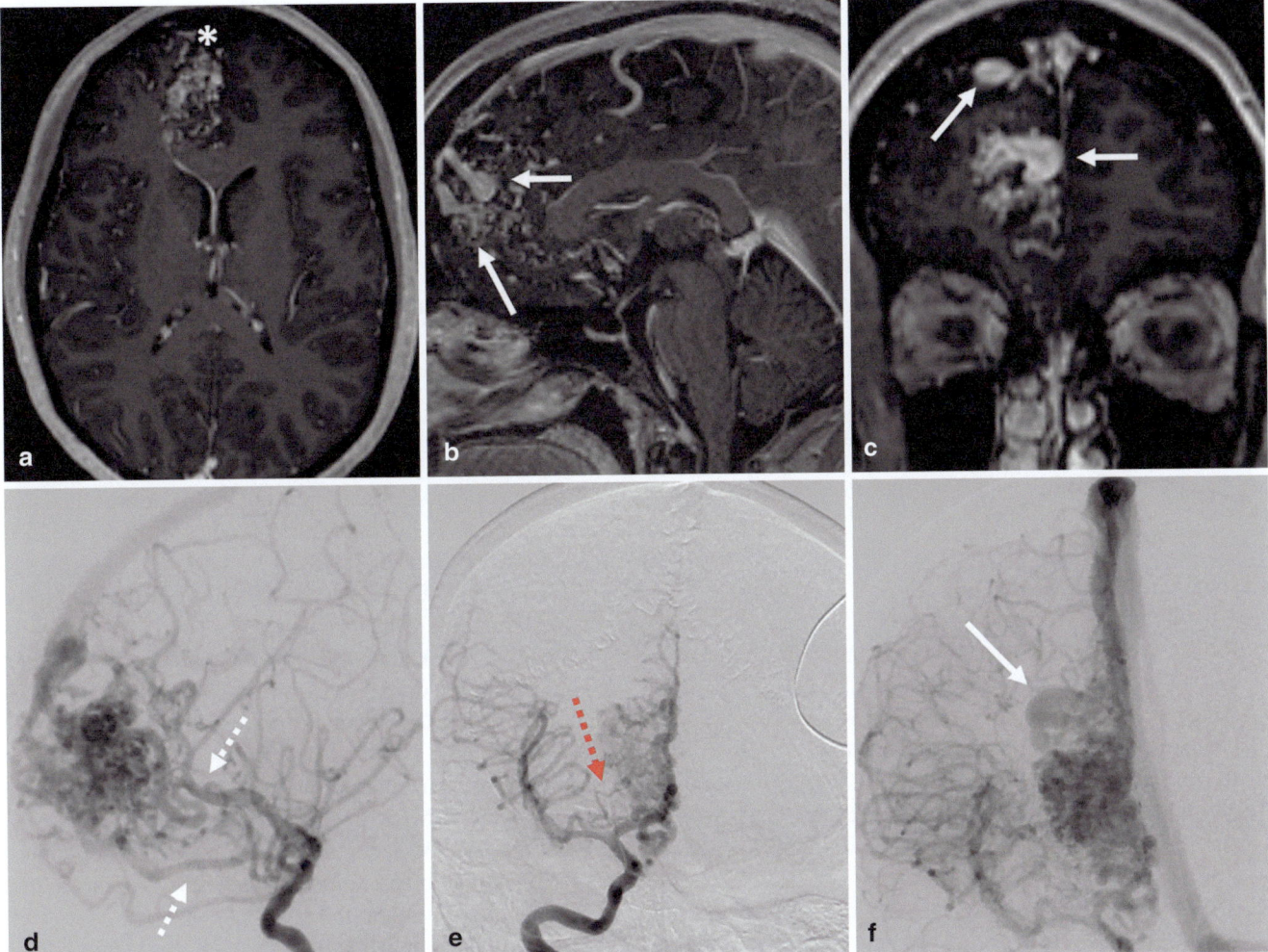

Fig. 7.5 (a) Postcontrast MPRAGE demonstrating an unruptured right frontal AVM draining into the superior sagittal sinus (asterisk). The AVM nidus is of moderate size with a diameter >3 cm but <6 cm. (**b, c**) Multiple dilated cortical veins with superficial venous drainage into the superior sagittal sinus (solid white arrows). (**d**) Lateral projection from catheter angiography demonstrating multiple hypertrophied anterior cerebral artery (ACA) branches (dashed white arrow) supplying the AVM nidus. (**e**) A hypertrophied lenticulostriate artery (dashed red arrow) also supplies the AVM nidus. (**f**) A dilated cortical vein is again visualized draining the AVM nidus superficially into the superior sagittal sinus (solid white arrow)

DURAL ARTERIOVENOUS FISTULAE

Dural arteriovenous fistulae (dAVF) are shunting vascular lesions characterized by abnormal communications between meningeal arteries and the dural venous sinuses within the dural leaflets and/or subarachnoid veins. They are differentiated from intracranial AVMs by their lack of a parenchymal nidus, the fact that meningeal arteries supply them, and their acquired nature [49]. It is hypothesized that dAVFs arise from progressive stenosis and/or occlusion of a dural venous sinus [50]. As pressures rise in the dural sinus, meningeal arteries develop fistulous connections with the sinus or adjacent cortical veins resulting in a complex network of venous channels through which arteriovenous shunting occurs [49, 51].

EPIDEMIOLOGY

- Account for 10–15% of all intracranial vascular malformations [52].
  - dAVFs represent 6% of supratentorial vascular malformations [52].
  - dAVFs represent 35% of infratentorial vascular malformations [52].
- Detection rates range from approximately 0.15–0.30 dAVFs per 100,000 people per year [26, 53].
- These lesions most commonly affect middle aged and elderly patients (i.e., 5th–sixth decades of life) [54].
- There is no obvious sex predilection for the development of dAVFs [49].

Table 7.2 Spetzler-Martin grading system for intracranial arteriovenous malformations

AVM characteristic	Number of points assigned
Nidus size	
Small (<3 cm)	1
Medium (3–6 cm)	2
Large (>6 cm)	3
Venous drainage	
Superficial	0
Component of deep drainage	1
Location	
Non-eloquent	0
Eloquent	1

[a] Adapted from Spetzler et al. [48]
[b] Deep venous drainage constitutes venous egress through the internal cerebral veins, basal veins, or precentral cerebellar vein
[c] Eloquent regions of brain parenchyma include the sensorimotor cortex, language areas, visual cortex, hypothalamus, thalamus, internal capsule, brainstem, cerebellar peduncles, and deep cerebellar nuclei

CLINICAL PRESENTATION

- Patient symptoms are dependent upon the dAVF location and the pattern of venous drainage.
- Antegrade drainage into a dural sinus may present with headaches, pulsatile tinnitus, and bruits [55].
- Retrograde drainage into a dural sinus results in elevation of venous and intracranial pressure and can produce severe headaches, papilledema, and progressive cognitive decline [55].
- dAVFs with cortical venous drainage may present with intracranial hemorrhage or nonhemorrhagic neurologic deficits including seizures, cranial nerve palsies, dementia, Parkinsonism, and cerebellar dysfunction [55].

NATURAL HISTORY

- dAVFs with shunting exclusively into a dural sinus have a benign natural history and rarely cause intracranial hemorrhage or nonhemorrhagic neurologic deficits.
- dAVFs without cortical venous drainage have the potential to develop cortical venous drainage with an annual conversion rate of 0.8% [56].
- Conversion to cortical venous drainage typically presents with new or recurrent neurological symptoms [50].
- dAVFs with cortical venous drainage have an annual hemorrhage rate of 8.1%, nonhemorrhagic neurologic deficit rate of 6.9%, and a combined adverse neurological event rate of 15% [57].
- These lesions with cortical venous drainage have an annual mortality rate of 10.4% [57].

IMAGING CHARACTERISTICS

- Noncontrast CT is useful for the detection of intracranial hemorrhage.
- Hemorrhage location may be distant from the site of fistulous connection.
- CTA may demonstrate hypertrophied ECA branches that supply a dAVF, including the presence of hypertrophied transosseous arterial branches.
- CTA may also show early opacification of a dural sinus or underlying dural sinus occlusion.
- Care must be taken to assess for asymmetrically enlarged and/or ectatic cortical veins given their association with intracranial hemorrhage and nonhemorrhagic focal neurologic deficits.
- Flow voids from enlarged, arterialized veins may be visualized on T2W MRI.
- Postcontrast T1W sequences may show dilated leptomeningeal and medullary veins, venous ectasia, parenchymal enhancement, and/or dural sinus occlusion.
- T2/FLAIR imaging may demonstrate vasogenic edema and high signal of the leptomeninges secondary to venous congestion.
- 3D-TOF-MRA may demonstrate hypertrophied ECA branches as well as arterialized flow within dural sinuses and/or cortical veins (Fig. 7.6).
- DSA remains the gold standard imaging modality for the evaluation of dAVF angioarchitecture, number and location of fistulae, presence or absence of cortical venous drainage, and the presence of venous ectasia [55] (Fig. e7.6).
- Multiple dAVF classification systems have been developed to risk stratify these lesions. These classification systems are based on dAVF venous drainage patterns on DSA (Table 7.3) [58, 59].

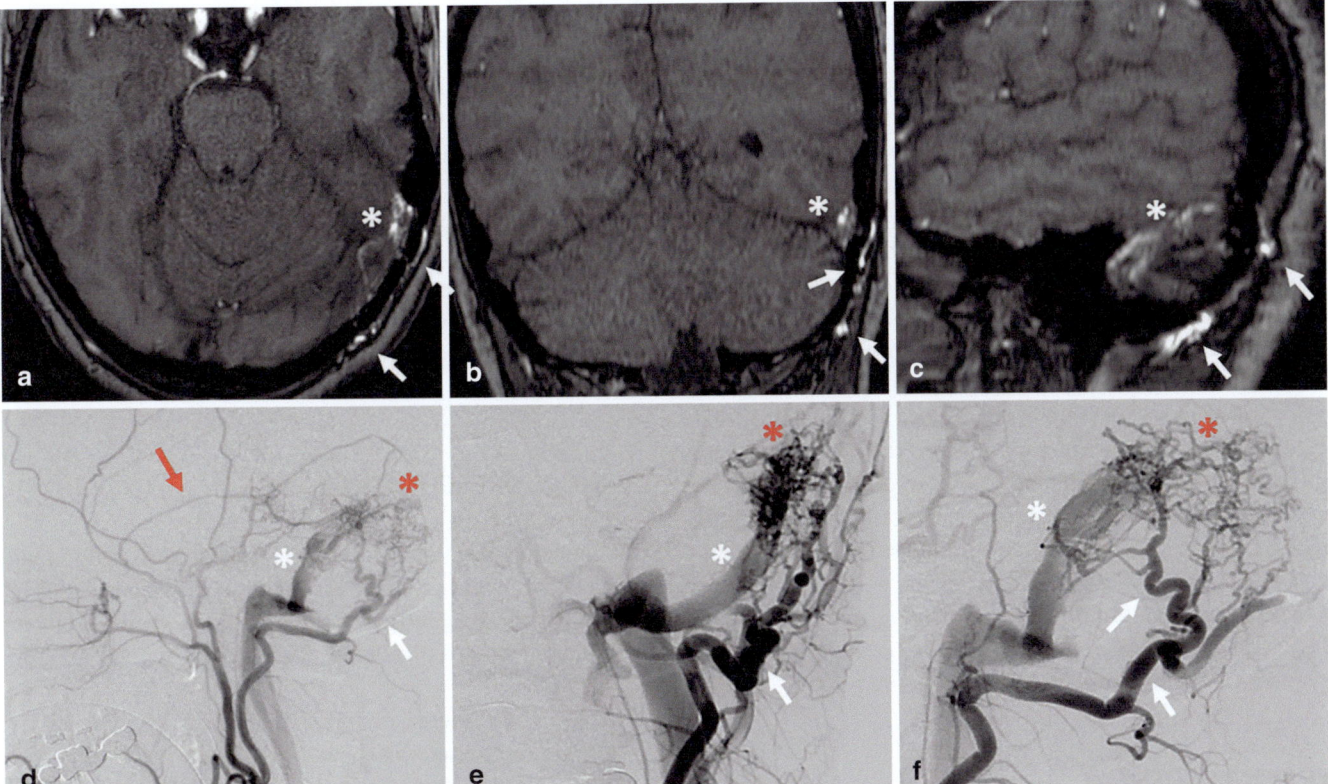

Fig. 7.6 (a–c) 3D-TOF-MRA demonstrates an enlarged left occipital artery with multiple serpiginous transosseous arterial branches (solid white arrows). There is arterialized flow within the left transverse and sigmoid sinus (white asterisk). (d) Selective catheter angiography in the left external carotid artery (ECA) shows brisk arteriovenous shunting into the distal left transverse sinus (white asterisk). Arterial flow is supplied predominantly by a hypertrophied left occipital artery (solid white arrow) with a minor contribution from the petrous branch of the left middle meningeal artery (MMA; solid red arrow). There is a prominent network of serpiginous arterial branches along the left transverse and sigmoid sinus (red asterisk). (e, f) Selective catheter angiography performed in the left occipital artery again demonstrating abnormal arteriovenous shunting consistent with a Borden/Cognard type I dAVF

Table 7.3 The Borden and Cognard classification systems of dural arteriovenous fistulae

Borden class	Venous drainage pattern	Cognard class	Venous drainage pattern
I	Antegrade flow into dural sinus, meningeal veins, or spinal epidural veins	I	Antegrade flow into dural sinus without cortical venous drainage or reflux
		IIa	Retrograde flow (reflux) into a dural sinus without cortical venous drainage or reflux
II	Drainage into dural sinus, meningeal veins, or spinal epidural veins with retrograde flow (reflux) into normal cortical veins	IIb	Antegrade flow into a dural sinus with reflux into cortical veins
		IIa + b	Retrograde flow into a dural sinus with reflux into cortical veins
III	Direct drainage into cortical veins or into an isolated segment of the venous sinus	III	Direct drainage into a cortical vein without venous ectasia (Fig. e7.7)
		IV	Direct drainage into a cortical vein with venous ectasia (Fig. e7.8)
		V	Spinal perimedullary venous drainage

[a] DAVF classification adapted from Borden et al. [58] and Cognard et al. [59]

CAROTICOCAVERNOUS FISTULAE

Caroticocavernous fistulae (CCF) are acquired arteriovenous malformations that shunt blood from the carotid artery into the cavernous sinus. These shunting vascular lesions may be the result of a defect in the cavernous segment of the ICA directly shunting arterial blood into the adjacent cavernous sinus or from ICA and/or ECA branch vessels indirectly shunting blood into the cavernous sinus with variable paths of egress out of the cavernous sinus through the superior and inferior petrosal sinuses, superior and inferior ophthalmic veins, intercavernous (circular) sinus into the contralateral sphenoid sinus, sphenoparietal sinus, superficial middle cerebral vein, and/or emissary veins of the pterygoid plexus [60]. As flow through the cavernous sinus increases, so too does the pressure it experiences resulting in a myriad of clinical symptoms. The underlying etiologies for CCF are highly variable. Direct fistulae are more likely to be the result of head and/or facial trauma. Indirect fistulae are more likely to be nontraumatic in nature with underlying venous thrombosis potentially precipitating their formation [60].

EPIDEMIOLOGY

- Traumatic CCFs account for approximately 75% of all CCFs [61, 62].
  - The ICA may be directly torn by either a bone fracture or an applied shear force during a high-energy trauma [60].
  - Alternatively, a sudden increase in intraluminal pressure with concurrent distal artery compression may rupture the ICA wall during trauma [63].
  - Occur in up to 0.2% of patients with craniocerebral trauma [63].
  - Occur in up to 4% of patients with skull base fractures [64].
  - Bilateral CCFs are encountered in 1–2% of patients with posttraumatic CCFs [64].
  - Direct CCFs account for the majority of posttraumatic CCFs.

> **CT AND MR ANGIOGRAM REPORT IMPRESSION PEARLS**
> - The anatomic location of the dAVF.
> - The presence of intracranial hemorrhage or evidence of venous congestion.
> - Arterial supply to the fistula.
> - Evidence of arteriovenous shunting into and/or ectasia of cortical veins.
> - Dural sinus occlusion.

- Spontaneous CCFs account for approximately 15–30% of all CCFs.
  - Elderly, female patients are predisposed to developing spontaneous CCFs [60].
  - Connective tissue disorders such as fibromuscular dysplasia [65], Ehlers-Danlos syndrome [66], and pseudoxanthoma elasticum [67] are risk factors for spontaneous CCF formation.
  - Venous thrombosis or increases in venous sinus pressure are hypothesized to promote CCF formation by causing microscopic breaks in dural vessels to the cavernous sinus [60, 61, 68].

CLINICAL PRESENTATION

- Clinical symptoms are dependent upon the predominant routes of fistula drainage through the cavernous sinus.
- Anterior drainage through the ophthalmic veins produces orbital venous congestion with orbital symptoms [69] including:
  - Proptosis (increased intraorbital pressure).
  - Pain (increased intraocular pressure).
  - Impaired vision (ischemic retinopathy and/or optic neuropathy).
  - Chemosis.
  - Subconjunctival hemorrhage.
- Posterior drainage can produce cranial nerve palsies [70].
- Lateral drainage into the sphenoparietal sinus can produce cortical venous hypertension resulting in focal neurological deficits and/or intracranial hemorrhage [68].
- Direct CCFs typically demonstrate a more rapid onset and escalation in the severity of symptoms, with vision loss reported in up to 50% of patients and intracranial hemorrhage reported in approximately 5% of patients [69].
- Indirect CCFs tend to demonstrate a more insidious clinical course with relapsing and remitting symptoms [69].

IMAGING CHARACTERISTICS

- CT/CTA and/or MRI/MRA may serve as a useful, noninvasive screening test when there is clinical suspicion for a CCF.
- Indirect signs of an underlying CCF on CT and/or MRI include proptosis, enlargement of the extraocular muscles, and asymmetric enlargement/bulging of the cavernous sinus.
- CTA/MRA may demonstrate early enhancement and dilation of the cavernous sinus, ophthalmic veins, facial veins, pial veins, underlying venous thrombosis, and/or enlarge-

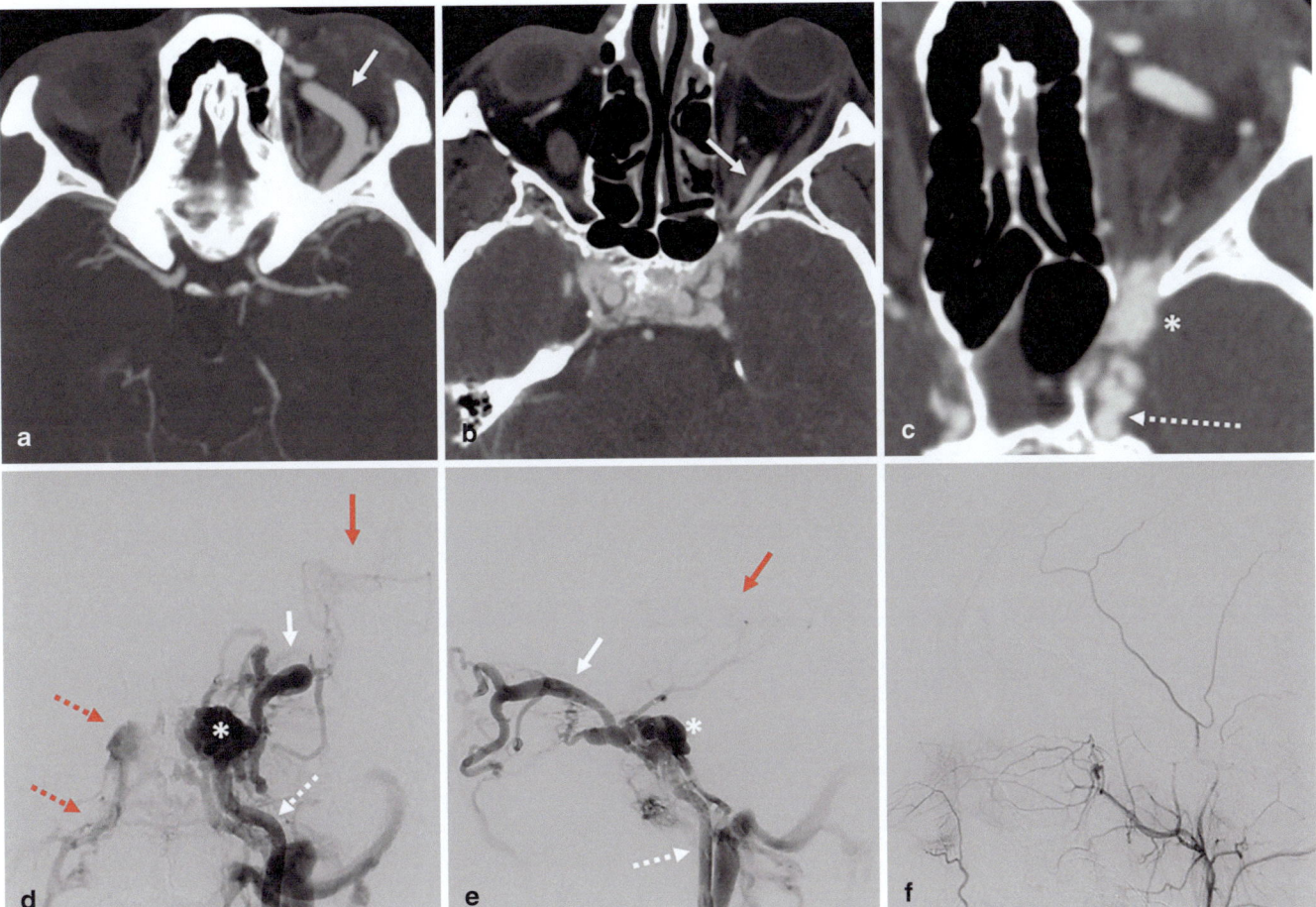

Fig. 7.7 (a–c) Axial CTA images demonstrated dilated left superior and inferior ophthalmic veins (solid white arrows) with asymmetric enlargement and enhancement of the left cavernous sinus that extends into the left orbital apex (white asterisk). The proximal left cavernous ICA segment is indistinguishable from the adjacent sinusoids of the left cavernous sinus (dashed white arrow), suspicious for a direct CCF (Barrow Type A). (d, e) Selective catheter angiography of the left ICA (dashed white arrows) demonstrates rapid shunting of contrast through a defect in the proximal cavernous ICA into the adjacent cavernous sinus (white asterisk) with egress into the right cavernous sinus (dashed red arrows) and a dilated left superior ophthalmic vein (solid white arrow). Note the diminished antegrade flow provided by the left ICA into the left MCA (solid red arrow) due to the fistula. (f) Selective catheter angiography of the left ECA failed to show any abnormal arteriovenous shunting to the cavernous sinus from branches of the ECA, confirming a Barrow Type A CCF

ment of branch arteries arising from the ICA and/or ECA (Fig. 7.7).
- Flow-sensitive MR sequences such as 3D-TOF-MRA and arterial spin labeling (ASL) may demonstrate increased flow-related signal within the cavernous sinus and/or its routes of venous drainage (Fig. 7.8).
- The absence of imaging findings on CT/MRI does not exclude the diagnosis of CCF, however. If clinical suspicion for a CCF is high, DSA should be pursued despite normal CT/MRI findings [60].
- DSA is the gold standard imaging study for the detection and evaluation of CCFs, allowing for in-depth assessment of the angioarchitecture and flow dynamics through the lesion.
- The Barrow classification system [61] attempts to classify CCFs based on their arterial supply (Table 7.4) and aids with treatment decisions.

> **CT AND MR ANGIOGRAM REPORT IMPRESSION PEARLS**
> - The presence of early enhancement and asymmetric enlargement of the cavernous sinus.
> - The presence of early enhancement and enlargement of the ophthalmic veins and/or cortical veins.
> - Potential arterial supply to the fistula, including from branches of the ECA.
> - Evidence of venous thrombosis, including within the cavernous sinus or ophthalmic veins.

CEREBRAL CAVERNOUS MALFORMATIONS

Cavernous malformations are congenital vascular lesions composed of compact sinusoidal vessels without intervening

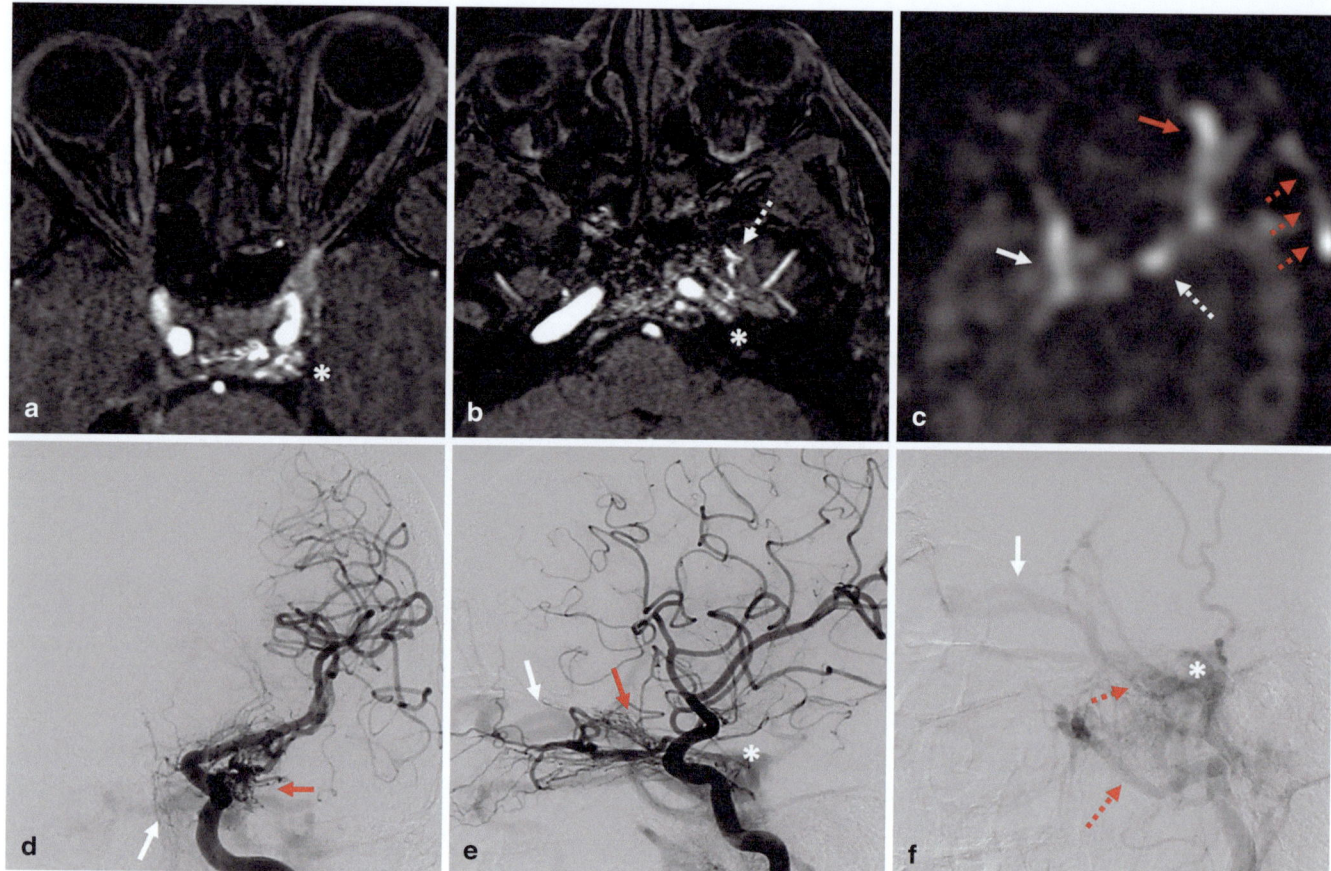

Fig. 7.8 (**a**) 3D-TOF-MRA demonstrates asymmetric signal hyperintensity within the left cavernous (white asterisk) sinus suspicious for arterialized flow. (**b**) 3D-TOF-MRA again demonstrates asymmetric signal hyperintensity within the left cavernous sinus extending inferiorly into the clival venous plexus (white asterisk). A hypertrophied accessory meningeal artery is visualized extending through the left foramen ovale and coursing toward the left cavernous sinus (dashed white arrow). (**c**) Arterial spin labeling (ASL) shows rapid arteriovenous shunting through the left cavernous sinus (dashed white arrow) into the right cavernous sinus (solid white arrow) and left superior ophthalmic vein (solid red arrow), which subsequently drains into the left facial vein (dashed red arrows). (**d, e**) Selective catheter angiography of the left ICA shows significant arteriovenous shunting through the inferolateral trunk (solid red arrows) into the left cavernous sinus (white asterisk) with egress through the intercavernous sinus and left superior ophthalmic vein (solid white arrows). (**f**) Selective catheter angiography of the left ECA show hypertrophied internal maxillary and middle meningeal arteries (dashed red arrows) shunting into the left cavernous sinus (white asterisk) with reflux into the left superior ophthalmic vein (solid white arrow). Involvement of ICA and ECA branches is consistent with a Barrow Type D CCF

Table 7.4 Barrow classification system for caroticocavernous fistulae

Barrow grade	Direct vs. indirect	Arterial supply
A	Direct	Cavernous ICA
B	Indirect	ICA branches (i.e., MHT, ILT)
C	Indirect	ECA branches
D	Indirect	ICA + ECA branches

MHT meningohypophyseal trunk, *ILT* inferolateral trunk
[a] Table based on the work of Barrow et al. [61]

normal brain parenchymal. At surgery, these lesions are well-circumscribed yet unencapsulated. They may contain internal cysts with blood products in various stages of degradation, explaining the variable T1W- and T2W-imaging characteristics observed with MRI. The brain parenchyma surrounding these lesions may be gliotic and is commonly stained with hemosiderin from prior hemorrhage events [71].

EPIDEMIOLOGY

- Estimated prevalence of 0.2–0.5% in autopsy and MRI studies [72–75].
- Incidence of 0.43 diagnoses per 100,000 people per year [76].
- Peak incidence of presentation is in the third-fourth decades of life without a gender preponderance [75, 77].
- There is a bimodal distribution of pediatric presentations with children presenting as infant and toddlers (0–3 years of age) and early adolescence (12–16 years of age) [78, 79].
- 50–80% of cases are sporadic without evidence of a cavernous malformation family history [74, 75].

- Approximately 75% of all patients with multiple cavernous malformations will have a familial cavernous malformation syndrome [80].
  - Confirmed by genetic testing for mutations in 1 of 3 genes (CCM1, CCM2, or CCM3) [81].

CLINICAL PRESENTATION

- Patient presentation is dependent upon the anatomic location of the cavernous malformation.
- Seizure (50%), intracranial hemorrhage (25%), and focal neurological deficits without evidence of hemorrhage (25%) are the most common forms of lesion presentation [82].
- The average 5-year risk for intracranial hemorrhage is estimated to be 15.8% (13.7–17.9%) overall [83].
- Risk factors for future hemorrhage include an initial presentation with hemorrhage and a location within the brainstem [83].
- Symptoms may be caused by low-pressure hemorrhages that exert mass effect on the surrounding brain parenchyma [71] or recurrent microhemorrhages, perilesional gliosis, and/or inflammation [84].

IMAGING CHARACTERISTICS

- Cavernous malformations often appear as a cluster of well-defined, rounded hyperdensities on noncontrast CT.
- Intra-lesional calcifications may be present and are best appreciated with CT imaging [85].
- Subtle enhancement may be appreciated on postcontrast CT and MR imaging [71].
- Cavernous malformations have a distinctive "popcorn" appearance on MRI with significant susceptibility effect appreciated on SWI/GRE sequences [86, 87].
- T1W- and T2W-signal characteristics are variable and reflect the composition of blood products within the lesion (Fig. 7.9).
- An intrinsically T1W and T2W hypointense rim surrounding the lesion is frequently observed and corresponds to hemosiderin deposition within the surrounding brain parenchyma.
- Mild T2/FLAIR hyperintensity may be observed in the surrounding brain parenchyma secondary to reactive gliosis.
- More prominent T2/FLAIR hyperintensity may be observed in the surrounding brain parenchyma following a recent bleeding event and is reflective of reactive vasogenic edema.
- 10–15% of cavernous malformations have an associated developmental venous anomaly (DVA). Postcontrast CT and MR imaging will show enhancing radial veins draining into a main collecting vein (Fig. 7.10) [88].

CT AND MR ANGIOGRAM REPORT IMPRESSION PEARLS
- The anatomic location of the cavernous malformation.
- Evidence of acute hemorrhage and reactive vasogenic edema.
- The size of the cavernous malformation.
- The presence of an associated developmental venous anomaly.

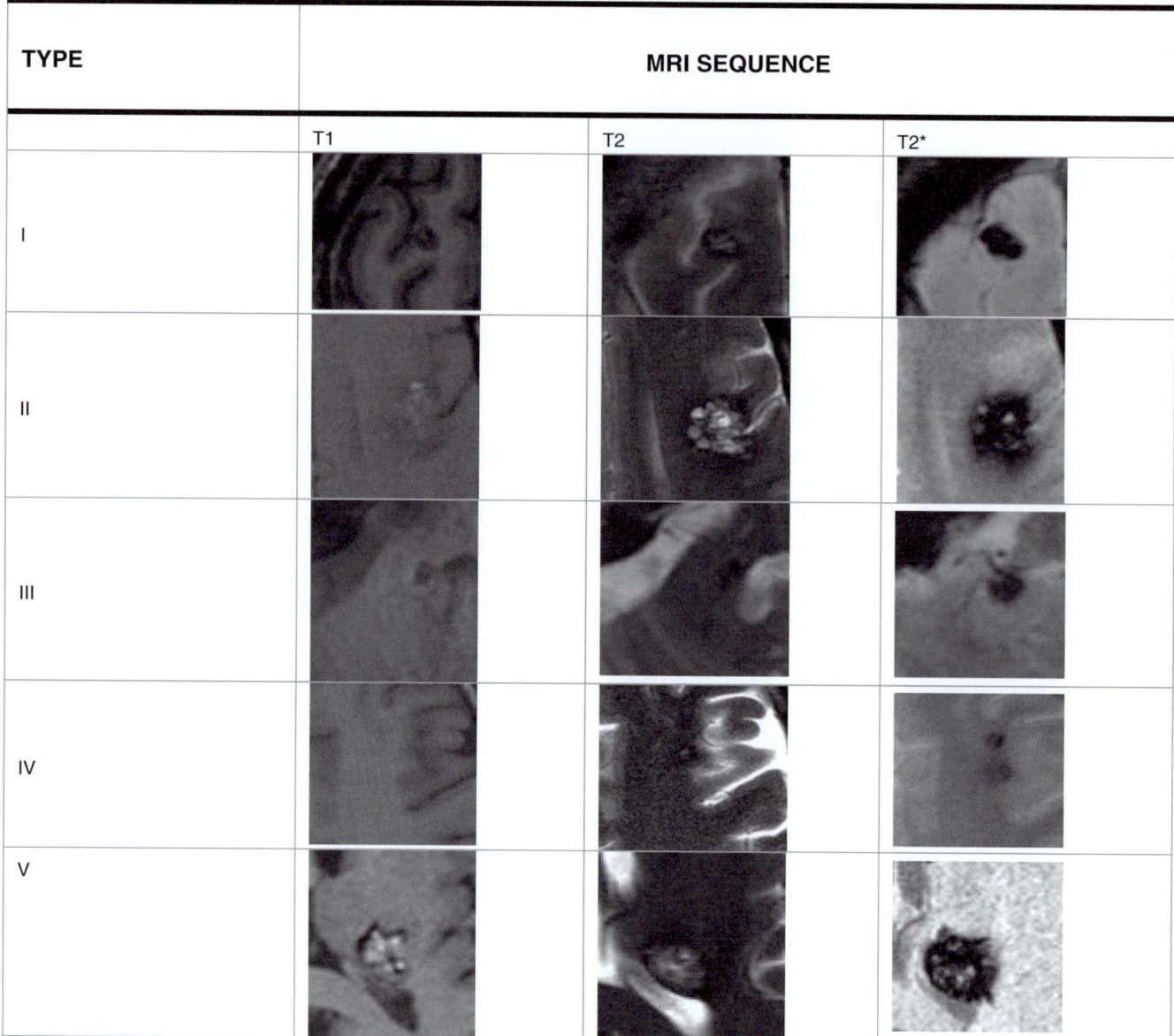

Fig. 7.9 MRI signal characteristics of cavernous malformations based on the Zabramski classification [74]

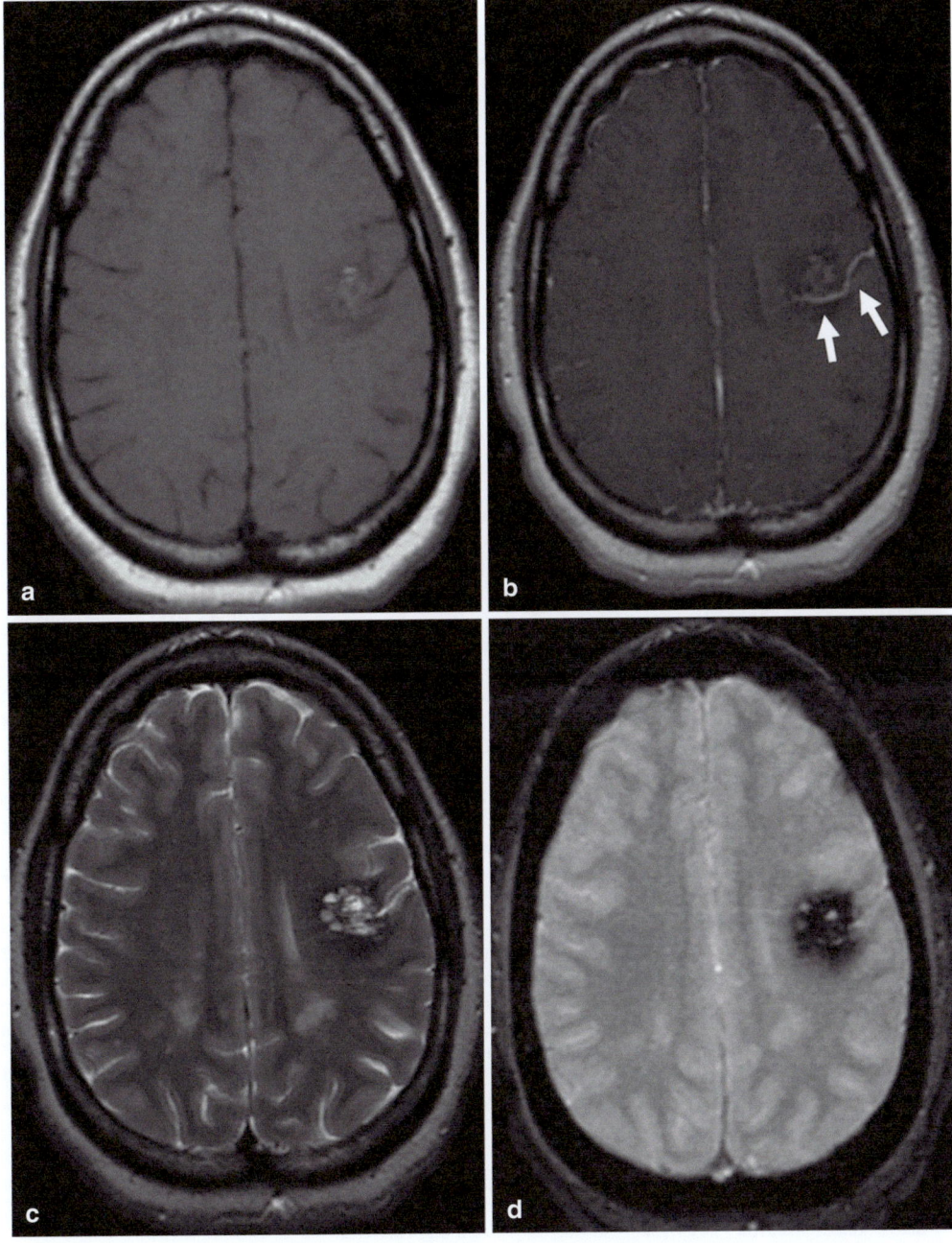

Fig. 7.10 (a) T1W pre-contrast image demonstrates an intrinsically T1 hyperintense lesion with a subtle hypointense rim within the left frontal lobe. (b) T1W postcontrast imaging with an associated developmental venous anomaly along the posterior margin of the lesion (solid white arrows). (c) T2W imaging shows a lobulated T2 hyperintense lesion with thin, hypointense internal septations and a thin, hypointense rim about the lesion. There is no associated vasogenic edema. (d) GRE imaging with susceptibility intralesional susceptibility. These are hallmark imaging features of a cavernous malformation

References

1. Greene KA, Marciano FF, Johnson BA, Jacobowitz R, Spetzler RF, Harrington TR. Impact of traumatic subarachnoid hemorrhage on outcome in nonpenetrating head injury. Part I: a proposed computerized tomography grading scale. J Neurosurg. 1995;83(3):445–52. https://doi.org/10.3171/jns.1995.83.3.0445.
2. Young RJ, Destian S. Imaging of traumatic intracranial hemorrhage. Neuroimaging Clin N Am. 2002;12(2):189–204. https://doi.org/10.1016/s1052-5149(02)00003-5.
3. Gentry LR, Godersky JC, Thompson B. MR imaging of head trauma: review of the distribution and radiopathologic features of traumatic lesions. AJR Am J Roentgenol. 1988;150(3):663–72. https://doi.org/10.2214/ajr.150.3.663.
4. Claassen J, Bernardini GL, Kreiter K, et al. Effect of cisternal and ventricular blood on risk of delayed cerebral ischemia after subarachnoid hemorrhage: the Fisher scale revisited. Stroke. 2001;32(9):2012–20. https://doi.org/10.1161/hs0901.095677.
5. Saad AF, Chaudhari R, Fischbein NJ, Wintermark M. Intracranial hemorrhage imaging. Semin Ultrasound CT MR. 2018;39(5):441–56. https://doi.org/10.1053/j.sult.2018.01.003.
6. Schievink WI. Intracranial aneurysms. N Engl J Med. 1997;336(1):28–40. https://doi.org/10.1056/NEJM199701023360106.
7. Winn HR, Jane JA Sr, Taylor J, Kaiser D, Britz GW. Prevalence of asymptomatic incidental aneurysms: review of 4568 arteriograms. J Neurosurg. 2002;96(1):43–9. https://doi.org/10.3171/jns.2002.96.1.0043.
8. Kassell NF, Torner JC, Jane JA, Haley EC Jr, Adams HP. The international cooperative study on the timing of aneurysm surgery. Part

2: surgical results. J Neurosurg. 1990;73(1):37–47. https://doi.org/10.3171/jns.1990.73.1.0037.
9. Rinne J, Hernesniemi J, Puranen M, Saari T. Multiple intracranial aneurysms in a defined population: prospective angiographic and clinical study. Neurosurgery. 1994;35(5):803–8. https://doi.org/10.1227/00006123-199411000-00001.
10. International Study of Unruptured Intracranial Aneurysms Investigators. Unruptured intracranial aneurysms—risk of rupture and risks of surgical intervention. N Engl J Med. 1998;339(24):1725–33. https://doi.org/10.1056/NEJM199812103392401.
11. Malhotra A, Wu X, Gandhi D. Management of unruptured intracranial aneurysms. Neuroimaging Clin N Am. 2021;31(2):139–46. https://doi.org/10.1016/j.nic.2021.02.001.
12. Heit JJ, Gonzalez RG, Sabbag D, et al. Detection and characterization of intracranial aneurysms: a 10-year multidetector CT angiography experience in a large center. J Neurointerv Surg. 2016;8(11):1168–72. https://doi.org/10.1136/neurintsurg-2015-012082.
13. Thompson BG, Brown RD Jr, Amin-Hanjani S, et al. Guidelines for the management of patients with unruptured intracranial aneurysms: a guideline for healthcare professionals from the American Heart Association/American Stroke Association. Stroke. 2015;46(8):2368–400. https://doi.org/10.1161/STR.0000000000000070.
14. Wiebers DO, Whisnant JP, Huston J 3rd, et al. Unruptured intracranial aneurysms: natural history, clinical outcome, and risks of surgical and endovascular treatment. Lancet. 2003;362(9378):103–10. https://doi.org/10.1016/s0140-6736(03)13860-3.
15. Wong GK, Teoh J, Chan EK, Ng SC, Poon WS. Intracranial aneurysm size responsible for spontaneous subarachnoid haemorrhage. Br J Neurosurg. 2013;27(1):34–9. https://doi.org/10.3109/02688697.2012.709559.
16. Lindgren AE, Koivisto T, Bjorkman J, et al. Irregular shape of intracranial aneurysm indicates rupture risk irrespective of size in a population-based cohort. Stroke. 2016;47(5):1219–26. https://doi.org/10.1161/STROKEAHA.115.012404.
17. Abboud T, Rustom J, Bester M, et al. Morphology of ruptured and unruptured intracranial aneurysms. World Neurosurg. 2017;99:610–7. https://doi.org/10.1016/j.wneu.2016.12.053.
18. Mehan WA Jr, Romero JM, Hirsch JA, et al. Unruptured intracranial aneurysms conservatively followed with serial CT angiography: could morphology and growth predict rupture? J Neurointerv Surg. 2014;6(10):761–6. https://doi.org/10.1136/neurintsurg-2013-010944.
19. Greving JP, Wermer MJ, Brown RD Jr, et al. Development of the PHASES score for prediction of risk of rupture of intracranial aneurysms: a pooled analysis of six prospective cohort studies. Lancet Neurol. 2014;13(1):59–66. https://doi.org/10.1016/S1474-4422(13)70263-1.
20. Burns JD, Huston J 3rd, Layton KF, Piepgras DG, Brown RD Jr. Intracranial aneurysm enlargement on serial magnetic resonance angiography: frequency and risk factors. Stroke. 2009;40(2):406–11. https://doi.org/10.1161/STROKEAHA.108.519165.
21. Gondar R, Gautschi OP, Cuony J, et al. Unruptured intracranial aneurysm follow-up and treatment after morphological change is safe: observational study and systematic review. J Neurol Neurosurg Psychiatry. 2016;87(12):1277–82. https://doi.org/10.1136/jnnp-2016-313584.
22. Friedlander RM. Clinical practice. Arteriovenous malformations of the brain. N Engl J Med. 2007;356(26):2704–12. https://doi.org/10.1056/NEJMcp067192.
23. McCormick WF, Rosenfield DB. Massive brain hemorrhage: a review of 144 cases and an examination of their causes. Stroke. 1973;4(6):946–54. https://doi.org/10.1161/01.str.4.6.946.
24. Stapf C, Mast H, Sciacca RR, et al. The New York Islands AVM study: design, study progress, and initial results. Stroke. 2003;34(5):e29–33. https://doi.org/10.1161/01.STR.0000068784.36838.19.
25. Strozyk D, Nogueira RG, Lavine SD. Endovascular treatment of intracranial arteriovenous malformation. Neurosurg Clin N Am. 2009;20(4):399–418. https://doi.org/10.1016/j.nec.2009.07.004.
26. Brown RD Jr, Wiebers DO, Torner JC, O'Fallon WM. Incidence and prevalence of intracranial vascular malformations in Olmsted County, Minnesota, 1965 to 1992. Neurology. 1996;46(4):949–52. https://doi.org/10.1212/wnl.46.4.949.
27. Kupersmith MJ, Vargas ME, Yashar A, et al. Occipital arteriovenous malformations: visual disturbances and presentation. Neurology. 1996;46(4):953–7. https://doi.org/10.1212/wnl.46.4.953.
28. Lobato RD, Rivas JJ, Gomez PA, Cabrera A, Sarabia R, Lamas E. Comparison of the clinical presentation of symptomatic arteriovenous malformations (angiographically visualized) and occult vascular malformations. Neurosurgery. 1992;31(3):391–6; discussion 396–7. https://doi.org/10.1227/00006123-199209000-00001.
29. Brown RD Jr, Wiebers DO, Forbes G, et al. The natural history of unruptured intracranial arteriovenous malformations. J Neurosurg. 1988;68(3):352–7. https://doi.org/10.3171/jns.1988.68.3.0352.
30. Mast H, Mohr JP, Osipov A, et al. 'Steal' is an unestablished mechanism for the clinical presentation of cerebral arteriovenous malformations. Stroke. 1995;26(7):1215–20. https://doi.org/10.1161/01.str.26.7.1215.
31. Wilkins RH. Natural history of intracranial vascular malformations: a review. Neurosurgery. 1985;16(3):421–30. https://doi.org/10.1227/00006123-198503000-00026.
32. ApSimon HT, Reef H, Phadke RV, Popovic EA. A population-based study of brain arteriovenous malformation: long-term treatment outcomes. Stroke. 2002;33(12):2794–800. https://doi.org/10.1161/01.str.0000043674.99741.9b.
33. Halim AX, Johnston SC, Singh V, et al. Longitudinal risk of intracranial hemorrhage in patients with arteriovenous malformation of the brain within a defined population. Stroke. 2004;35(7):1697–702. https://doi.org/10.1161/01.STR.0000130988.44824.29.
34. Hillman J. Population-based analysis of arteriovenous malformation treatment. J Neurosurg. 2001;95(4):633–7. https://doi.org/10.3171/jns.2001.95.4.0633.
35. Hofmeister C, Stapf C, Hartmann A, et al. Demographic, morphological, and clinical characteristics of 1289 patients with brain arteriovenous malformation. Stroke. 2000;31(6):1307–10. https://doi.org/10.1161/01.str.31.6.1307.
36. Khaw AV, Mohr JP, Sciacca RR, et al. Association of infratentorial brain arteriovenous malformations with hemorrhage at initial presentation. Stroke. 2004;35(3):660–3. https://doi.org/10.1161/01.STR.0000117093.59726.F9.
37. Aminoff MJ. Treatment of unruptured cerebral arteriovenous malformations. Neurology. 1987;37(5):815–9. https://doi.org/10.1212/wnl.37.5.815.
38. Jane JA, Kassell NF, Torner JC, Winn HR. The natural history of aneurysms and arteriovenous malformations. J Neurosurg. 1985;62(3):321–3. https://doi.org/10.3171/jns.1985.62.3.0321.
39. Ondra SL, Troupp H, George ED, Schwab K. The natural history of symptomatic arteriovenous malformations of the brain: a 24-year follow-up assessment. J Neurosurg. 1990;73(3):387–91. https://doi.org/10.3171/jns.1990.73.3.0387.
40. Krayenbuehl H, Siebenmann R. Small vascular malformations as a cause of primary intracerebral hemorrhage. J Neurosurg. 1965;22:7–20. https://doi.org/10.3171/jns.1965.22.1.0007.
41. Hartmann A, Mast H, Mohr JP, et al. Morbidity of intracranial hemorrhage in patients with cerebral arteriovenous malformation. Stroke. 1998;29(5):931–4. https://doi.org/10.1161/01.str.29.5.931.
42. Itoyama Y, Uemura S, Ushio Y, et al. Natural course of unoperated intracranial arteriovenous malformations: study of 50 cases. J Neurosurg. 1989;71(6):805–9. https://doi.org/10.3171/jns.1989.71.6.0805.

43. Mast H, Young WL, Koennecke HC, et al. Risk of spontaneous haemorrhage after diagnosis of cerebral arteriovenous malformation. Lancet. 1997;350(9084):1065–8. https://doi.org/10.1016/s0140-6736(97)05390-7.
44. Langer DJ, Lasner TM, Hurst RW, Flamm ES, Zager EL, King JT Jr. Hypertension, small size, and deep venous drainage are associated with risk of hemorrhagic presentation of cerebral arteriovenous malformations. Neurosurgery. 1998;42(3):481–6; discussion 487–9. https://doi.org/10.1097/00006123-199803000-00008.
45. Pollock BE, Flickinger JC, Lunsford LD, Bissonette DJ, Kondziolka D. Factors that predict the bleeding risk of cerebral arteriovenous malformations. Stroke. 1996;27(1):1–6. https://doi.org/10.1161/01.str.27.1.1.
46. Redekop G, TerBrugge K, Montanera W, Willinsky R. Arterial aneurysms associated with cerebral arteriovenous malformations: classification, incidence, and risk of hemorrhage. J Neurosurg. 1998;89(4):539–46. https://doi.org/10.3171/jns.1998.89.4.0539.
47. Turjman F, Massoud TF, Vinuela F, Sayre JW, Guglielmi G, Duckwiler G. Aneurysms related to cerebral arteriovenous malformations: superselective angiographic assessment in 58 patients. AJNR Am J Neuroradiol. 1994;15(9):1601–5.
48. Spetzler RF, Martin NA. A proposed grading system for arteriovenous malformations. J Neurosurg. 1986;65(4):476–83. https://doi.org/10.3171/jns.1986.65.4.0476.
49. Gandhi D, Chen J, Pearl M, Huang J, Gemmete JJ, Kathuria S. Intracranial dural arteriovenous fistulas: classification, imaging findings, and treatment. AJNR Am J Neuroradiol. 2012;33(6):1007–13. https://doi.org/10.3174/ajnr.A2798.
50. Reynolds MR, Lanzino G, Zipfel GJ. Intracranial dural arteriovenous fistulae. Stroke. 2017;48(5):1424–31. https://doi.org/10.1161/STROKEAHA.116.012784.
51. Kojima T, Miyachi S, Sahara Y, et al. The relationship between venous hypertension and expression of vascular endothelial growth factor: hemodynamic and immunohistochemical examinations in a rat venous hypertension model. Surg Neurol. 2007;68(3):277–84; discussion 284. https://doi.org/10.1016/j.surneu.2006.10.075.
52. Newton TH, Cronqvist S. Involvement of dural arteries in intracranial arteriovenous malformations. Radiology. 1969;93(5):1071–8. https://doi.org/10.1148/93.5.1071.
53. Satomi J, Satoh K. [Epidemiology and etiology of dural arteriovenous fistula]. Brain Nerve. 2008;60(8):883–886.
54. Brown RD Jr, Wiebers DO, Nichols DA. Intracranial dural arteriovenous fistulae: angiographic predictors of intracranial hemorrhage and clinical outcome in nonsurgical patients. J Neurosurg. 1994;81(4):531–8. https://doi.org/10.3171/jns.1994.81.4.0531.
55. Elhammady MS, Ambekar S, Heros RC. Epidemiology, clinical presentation, diagnostic evaluation, and prognosis of cerebral dural arteriovenous fistulas. Handb Clin Neurol. 2017;143:99–105. https://doi.org/10.1016/B978-0-444-63640-9.00009-6.
56. Shah MN, Botros JA, Pilgram TK, et al. Borden-Shucart type I dural arteriovenous fistulas: clinical course including risk of conversion to higher-grade fistulas. J Neurosurg. 2012;117(3):539–45. https://doi.org/10.3171/2012.5.JNS111257.
57. van Dijk JM, terBrugge KG, Willinsky RA, Wallace MC. Clinical course of cranial dural arteriovenous fistulas with long-term persistent cortical venous reflux. Stroke. 2002;33(5):1233–6. https://doi.org/10.1161/01.str.0000014772.02908.44.
58. Borden JA, Wu JK, Shucart WA. A proposed classification for spinal and cranial dural arteriovenous fistulous malformations and implications for treatment. J Neurosurg. 1995;82(2):166–79. https://doi.org/10.3171/jns.1995.82.2.0166.
59. Cognard C, Gobin YP, Pierot L, et al. Cerebral dural arteriovenous fistulas: clinical and angiographic correlation with a revised classification of venous drainage. Radiology. 1995;194(3):671–80. https://doi.org/10.1148/radiology.194.3.7862961.
60. Ellis JA, Goldstein H, Connolly ES Jr, Meyers PM. Carotid-cavernous fistulas. Neurosurg Focus. 2012;32(5):E9. https://doi.org/10.3171/2012.2.FOCUS1223.
61. Barrow DL, Spector RH, Braun IF, Landman JA, Tindall SC, Tindall GT. Classification and treatment of spontaneous carotid-cavernous sinus fistulas. J Neurosurg. 1985;62(2):248–56. https://doi.org/10.3171/jns.1985.62.2.0248.
62. Debrun GM, Vinuela F, Fox AJ, Davis KR, Ahn HS. Indications for treatment and classification of 132 carotid-cavernous fistulas. Neurosurgery. 1988;22(2):285–9. https://doi.org/10.1227/00006123-198802000-00001.
63. Helmke K, Kruger O, Laas R. The direct carotid cavernous fistula: a clinical, pathoanatomical, and physical study. Acta Neurochir (Wien). 1994;127(1–2):1–5. https://doi.org/10.1007/BF01808537.
64. Liang W, Xiaofeng Y, Weiguo L, Wusi Q, Gang S, Xuesheng Z. Traumatic carotid cavernous fistula accompanying basilar skull fracture: a study on the incidence of traumatic carotid cavernous fistula in the patients with basilar skull fracture and the prognostic analysis about traumatic carotid cavernous fistula. J Trauma. 2007;63(5):1014–20; discussion 1020. https://doi.org/10.1097/TA.0b013e318154c9fb.
65. Hirai T, Korogi Y, Goto K, Ogata N, Sakamoto Y, Takahashi M. Carotid-cavernous sinus fistula and aneurysmal rupture associated with fibromuscular dysplasia. A case report. Acta Radiol. 1996;37(1):49–51. https://doi.org/10.1177/02841851960371P110.
66. Farley MK, Clark RD, Fallor MK, Geggel HS, Heckenlively JR. Spontaneous carotid-cavernous fistula and the Ehlers-Danlos syndromes. Ophthalmology. 1983;90(11):1337–42. https://doi.org/10.1016/s0161-6420(83)34384-0.
67. Rios-Montenegro EN, Behrens MM, Hoyt WF. Pseudoxanthoma elasticum. Association with bilateral carotid rete mirabile and unilateral carotid-cavernous sinus fistula. Arch Neurol. 1972;26(2):151–5. https://doi.org/10.1001/archneur.1972.00490080069007.
68. Ringer AJ, Salud L, Tomsick TA. Carotid cavernous fistulas: anatomy, classification, and treatment. Neurosurg Clin N Am. 2005;16(2):279–95, viii. https://doi.org/10.1016/j.nec.2004.08.004.
69. Zanaty M, Chalouhi N, Tjoumakaris SI, Hasan D, Rosenwasser RH, Jabbour P. Endovascular treatment of carotid-cavernous fistulas. Neurosurg Clin N Am. 2014;25(3):551–63. https://doi.org/10.1016/j.nec.2014.04.011.
70. Stiebel-Kalish H, Setton A, Nimii Y, et al. Cavernous sinus dural arteriovenous malformations: patterns of venous drainage are related to clinical signs and symptoms. Ophthalmology. 2002;109(9):1685–91. https://doi.org/10.1016/s0161-6420(02)01166-1.
71. Smith ER, Scott RM. Cavernous malformations. Neurosurg Clin N Am. 2010;21(3):483–90. https://doi.org/10.1016/j.nec.2010.03.003.
72. Barnes B, Cawley CM, Barrow DL. Intracerebral hemorrhage secondary to vascular lesions. Neurosurg Clin N Am. 2002;13(3):289–97, v. https://doi.org/10.1016/s1042-3680(02)00015-3.
73. Hang Z, Shi Y, Wei Y. [A pathological analysis of 180 cases of vascular malformation of brain]. Zhonghua Bing Li Xue Za Zhi. 1996;25(3):135–138.
74. Zabramski JM, Wascher TM, Spetzler RF, et al. The natural history of familial cavernous malformations: results of an ongoing study. J Neurosurg. 1994;80(3):422–32. https://doi.org/10.3171/jns.1994.80.3.0422.
75. Gault J, Sarin H, Awadallah NA, Shenkar R, Awad IA. Pathobiology of human cerebrovascular malformations: basic mechanisms and clinical relevance. Neurosurgery. 2004;55(1):1–16; discussion 16–7.
76. Al-Shahi R, Bhattacharya JJ, Currie DG, et al. Prospective, population-based detection of intracranial vascular malformations in adults: the Scottish Intracranial Vascular Malformation Study (SIVMS). Stroke. 2003;34(5):1163–9. https://doi.org/10.1161/01.STR.0000069018.90456.C9.

77. Baumann SB, Noll DC, Kondziolka DS, et al. Comparison of functional magnetic resonance imaging with positron emission tomography and magnetoencephalography to identify the motor cortex in a patient with an arteriovenous malformation. J Image Guid Surg. 1995;1(4):191–7. https://doi.org/10.1002/(SICI)1522-712X(1995)1:4<191::AID-IGS1>3.0.CO;2-5.
78. Mottolese C, Hermier M, Stan H, et al. Central nervous system cavernomas in the pediatric age group. Neurosurg Rev. 2001;24(2–3):55–71; discussion 72–3. https://doi.org/10.1007/pl00014581.
79. Fortuna A, Ferrante L, Mastronardi L, Acqui M, d'Addetta R. Cerebral cavernous angioma in children. Childs Nerv Syst. 1989;5(4):201–7. https://doi.org/10.1007/BF00271020.
80. Labauge P, Laberge S, Brunereau L, Levy C, Tournier-Lasserve E. Hereditary cerebral cavernous angiomas: clinical and genetic features in 57 French families. Societe Francaise de Neurochirurgie. Lancet. 1998;352(9144):1892–7. https://doi.org/10.1016/s0140-6736(98)03011-6.
81. Akers A, Al-Shahi Salman R, Awad IA, et al. Synopsis of guidelines for the clinical management of cerebral cavernous malformations: consensus recommendations based on systematic literature review by the Angioma Alliance Scientific Advisory Board Clinical Experts Panel. Neurosurgery. 2017;80(5):665–80. https://doi.org/10.1093/neuros/nyx091.
82. Al-Shahi Salman R, Hall JM, Horne MA, et al. Untreated clinical course of cerebral cavernous malformations: a prospective, population-based cohort study. Lancet Neurol. 2012;11(3):217–24. https://doi.org/10.1016/s1474-4422(12)70004-2.
83. Horne MA, Flemming KD, Su IC, et al. Clinical course of untreated cerebral cavernous malformations: a meta-analysis of individual patient data. Lancet Neurol. 2016;15(2):166–73. https://doi.org/10.1016/S1474-4422(15)00303-8.
84. Washington CW, McCoy KE, Zipfel GJ. Update on the natural history of cavernous malformations and factors predicting aggressive clinical presentation. Neurosurg Focus. 2010;29(3):E7. https://doi.org/10.3171/2010.5.FOCUS10149.
85. Bartlett JE, Kishore PR. Intracranial cavernous angioma. AJR Am J Roentgenol. 1977;128(4):653–6. https://doi.org/10.2214/ajr.128.4.653.
86. Rigamonti D, Drayer BP, Johnson PC, Hadley MN, Zabramski J, Spetzler RF. The MRI appearance of cavernous malformations (angiomas). J Neurosurg. 1987;67(4):518–24. https://doi.org/10.3171/jns.1987.67.4.0518.
87. Imakita S, Nishimura T, Yamada N, et al. Cerebral vascular malformations: applications of magnetic resonance imaging to differential diagnosis. Neuroradiology. 1989;31(4):320–5. https://doi.org/10.1007/BF00344175.
88. San Millan Ruiz D, Delavelle J, Yilmaz H, et al. Parenchymal abnormalities associated with developmental venous anomalies. Neuroradiology. 2007;49(12):987–95. https://doi.org/10.1007/s00234-007-0279-0.

Head Trauma

Sara G. Tedla, Tarik F. Massoud, and Elizabeth Tong

TRAUMA

- Imaging plays a critically important role in the detection of head injuries and their complications. This information is time-sensitive and has a high impact on patient management and outcome.
- Findings such as intracranial hemorrhage, herniation, hydrocephalus, and fractures should be communicated as soon as possible.
- In the setting of moderate (GCS 9–12), or severe (GCS 3–8) acute head trauma, initial imaging with a noncontrast head CT is usually appropriate [1].
- For mild acute head trauma (GCS 13–15), imaging may be obtained in selective patients based on clinical decision rules (taking into account age, loss of consciousnesses, symptoms, intoxication, coagulopathy, etc.) [2, 3].
- In cases of suspected intracranial vascular injury, a CT angiogram of the head and neck with contrast is warranted [1].
- Subtle subdural hematomas may be more visible when wider CT window settings (150–200 HU, "blood window") are utilized, compared to the narrow window settings (75–100 HU) used to evaluate brain parenchyma.
- While CT is considered the first-line imaging modality, MRI is useful when there are persistent neurologic deficits that remain unexplained after CT, especially in the subacute or chronic phase [1]. Furthermore, in subacute or chronic head trauma with unexplained cognitive/neurologic deficits, initial imaging with a noncontrast CT or MRI is usually appropriate [1].

CALVARIAL FRACTURES

- CT is the most sensitive imaging technique for detection of skull fractures.
- 1 mm thick slices or less are ideal for detecting fractures on CT. 3D reconstructions can be helpful when evaluating fractures.
- Fractures are described by the bones involved, displacement, morphology, and characteristics of the osseous fragments if present (Table 8.1, Figs. 8.1, 8.2, 8.3, and e8.1. All electronic images (Figs. e8.1–e8.6) can be found in this chapter's website on SpringerLink: https://doi.org/10.1007/978-3-031-55124-6_8).
- Assess involvement of cranial foramina, fissures, or canals when a fracture occurs. These are locations vulnerable to vessel and cranial nerve injury, such as dissection, pseudoaneurysm, thrombosis, carotid-cavernous fistula, or rarely, arterial, venous, or nerve transection [5].
- Look for associated intracranial hemorrhage, brain injury, overlying scalp contusion (non-hemorrhagic swelling vs. hemorrhagic) and laceration.

Table 8.1 Most common types of calvarial fractures

Fracture	Description
Linear	Lucent well-delineated linear fracture
Diastatic	Fracture of a cranial suture or synchondrosis, which is widened
Comminuted	More than two osseous fragments related to a fracture
Depressed	Osseous fragments are displaced inwardly. Surgical management is considered when fragments are 5 mm below the normal inner skull table
Elevated	Osseous fragments are displaced superficial to the skull
Compound	Open fracture that communicates with the outside environment

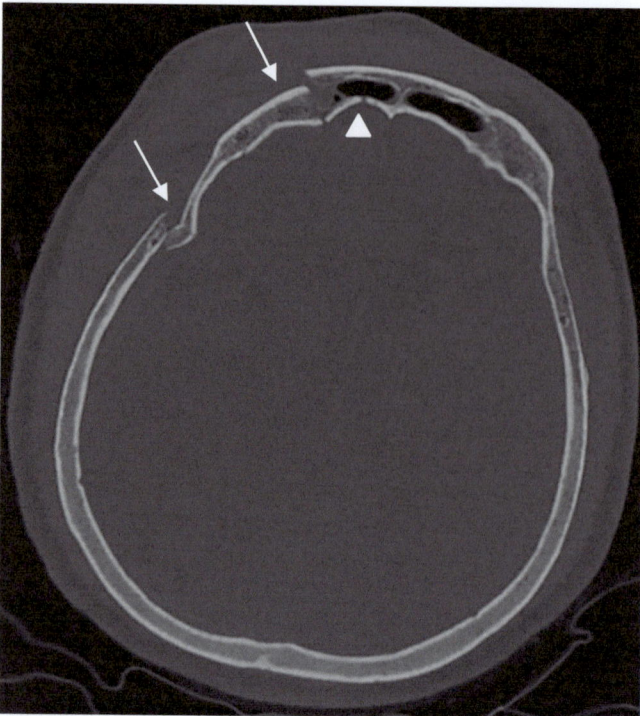

Fig. 8.1 Depressed and linear skull fractures. Right frontal depressed skull fracture (arrow). Fracture fragment displaced below the normal calvarial contour. Tiny linear right frontal inner table fracture extending into the right frontal sinus (arrowhead) is important to mention, as it may lead to intracranial infection

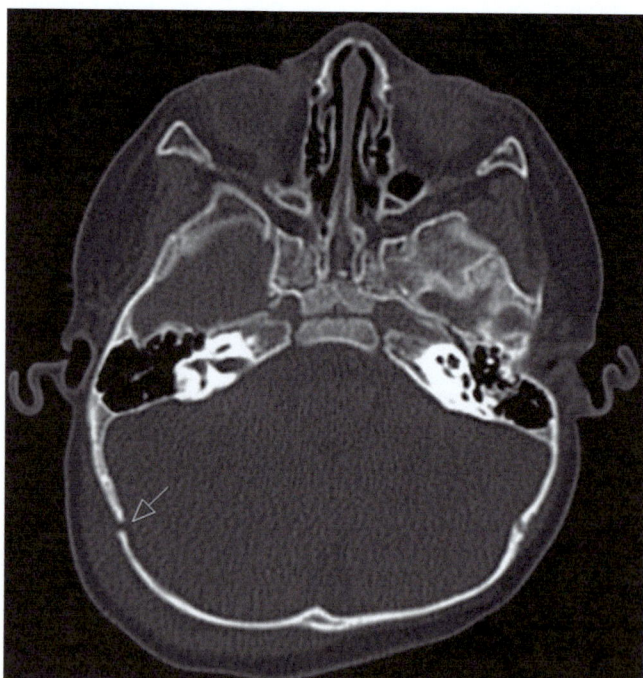

Fig. 8.2 Diastatic skull fracture. Widening of the right lambdoid suture due to a diastatic fracture (arrow). Also note the overlying scalp hematoma

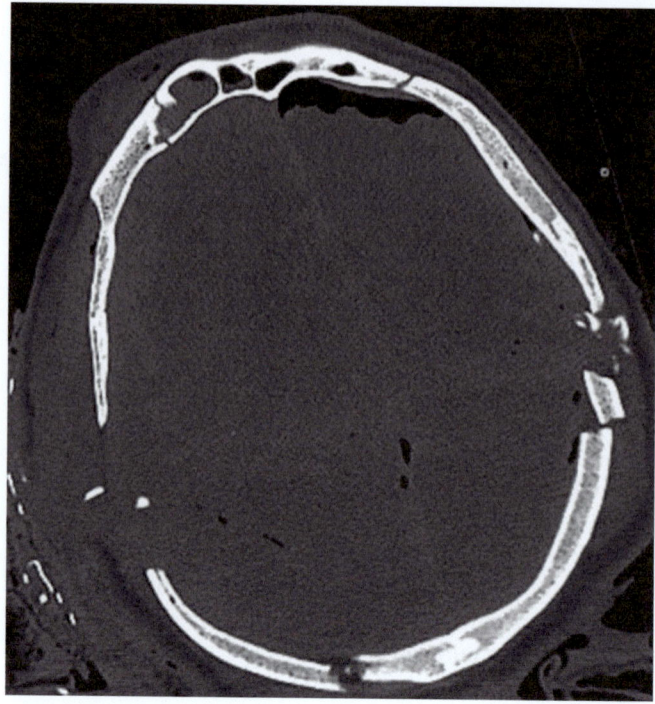

Fig. 8.3 Complex calvarial fractures. Fatal gunshot wound to the head causing bilateral comminuted compound fractures with elevated and depressed components. Bifrontal and right posterior parietal linear fractures are also present, along with pneumocephalus, intracranial hemorrhage, scalp contusions, and subcutaneous emphysema. Entry wound on the left is smaller and more regular. Greater damage is usually seen away from the entry wound, which is more irregular [4], as seen on the right

- Fracture complications include, but are not limited to, hemorrhage, parenchymal damage, CSF leak, vascular injury, dural venous sinus thrombosis, infection, seizures, and growing fractures.
- Rarely, a *growing fracture*, also known as a posttraumatic leptomeningeal cyst, can occur (Fig. e8.1).
    - The fracture enlarges slowly over time and can progress months to years after the inciting trauma.
    - Craniocerebral erosion is present rarely.
    - The underlying brain and arachnoid herniate through the defect.
    - Usually, encephalomalacia is present.

Please refer to Chap. 36 for discussion and examples of facial and skull base fractures.

EXTRACRANIAL INJURY

- Scalp:
    - Cephalohematoma: Subperiosteal hematoma *limited by sutures* (Fig. 8.4). Usually unilateral, but can be bilateral, and often related to birth trauma.
    - Subgaleal hematoma: Hematoma between the galea aponeurosis and periosteum, which *crosses sutures*

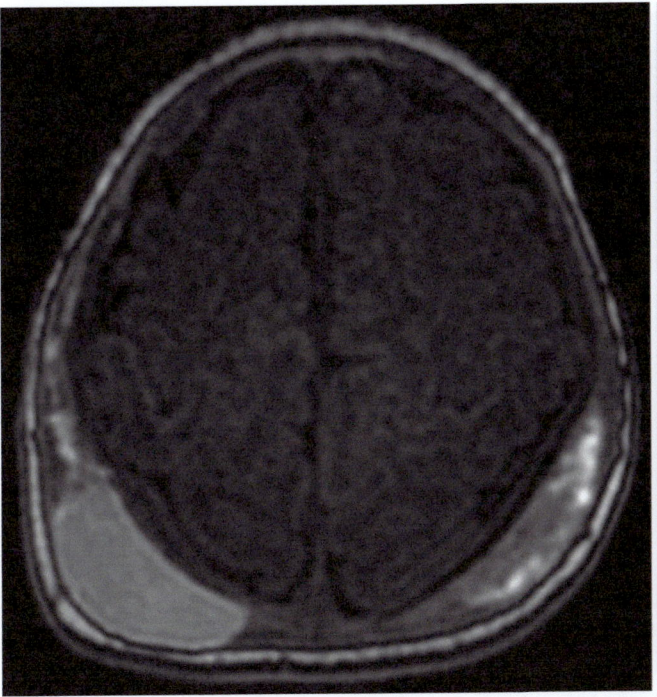
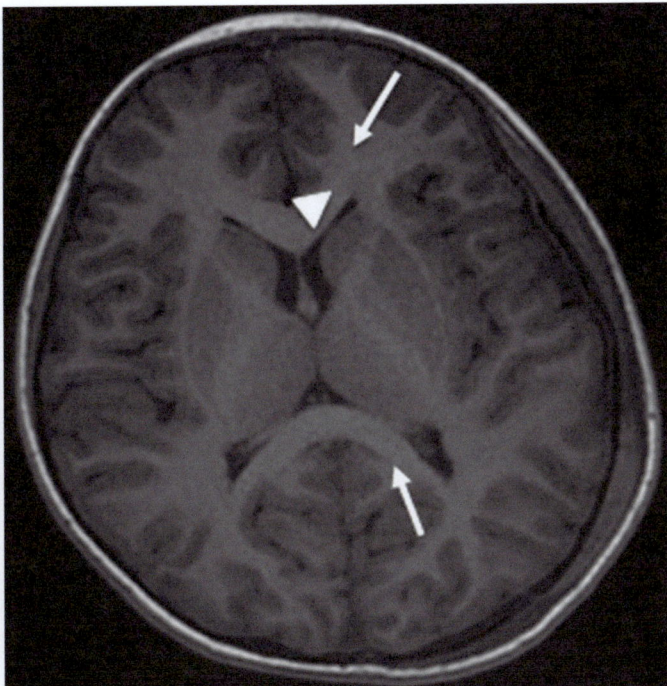

Fig. 8.4 Scalp hematomas. Left image: Bilateral cephalohematomas on axial T1 image. Right cephalohematoma is more homogeneous. Left cephalohematoma is more heterogeneous with more intrinsic T1 hyperintensities. Note the cephalohematomas are limited by sutures. Right image: Left parietal and temporal scalp subgaleal hematoma (arrow) that crosses sutures. Left temporal extra axial hemorrhage is also noted (arrowhead)

(Fig. 8.4). Usually related to head trauma and birth trauma.
 o Caput succedaneum: Hematoma in the subcutaneous tissues, external to the galea aponeurosis, which *crosses sutures*. Often related to birth trauma (Fig. e8.2).
 o Always look for a subjacent fracture and any intracranial injury.

TRAUMATIC HEMORRHAGE

Please refer to Chap. 6 'Intracranial Hemorrhage' for more detailed discussion and examples.

- Extra axial:
  o Epidural or extradural hemorrhage (EDH): Biconvex or lentiform collection of blood between the calvarial inner table and dura (Fig. 8.5). EDH is commonly associated with calvarial fractures. The most common source of bleeding is the middle meningeal artery. Arterial EDHs are *limited by sutures* but can *cross dural attachments*. Venous EDH can occur from injury to dural venous sinuses.
  o Subdural hemorrhage (SDH): Crescentic collection of blood between the dura and arachnoid that can layer along the convexities, falx, or tentorium (Fig. 8.5). Usually owing to tearing of the bridging veins in the setting of trauma. SDH does *cross sutures* but is *limited by dural attachments, such as the falx cerebri, tentorium, and falx cerebelli*.
  o Subdural hygroma: Crescentic collection of CSF owing to damage of the arachnoid, often from trauma or surgery. The collection will follow CSF attenuation on CT and CSF intensity on all MRI sequences (Fig. e8.3).
  o Subarachnoid hemorrhage (SAH): Collection of blood between the arachnoid and pia, which layers in the cerebral sulci and basal cisterns (Fig. 8.6). Trauma is the most common cause of SAH.
- Intraparenchymal:
  o Hemorrhagic contusion: Head trauma causes the brain to impact the inner table of the calvarium, resulting in hemorrhage and edema. This can occur in any location; however, the most common sites are:
    • Anterior-inferior frontal lobes (frontal poles).
    • Anterior-inferior temporal lobes (temporal poles).
    • Coup and contrecoup pattern: Injury at the first site of impact (coup) and 180° away from the initial site of impact (contrecoup) (Fig. 8.6).
  o Diffuse axonal injury (DAI): a.k.a. traumatic axonal injury (TAI). DAI is caused by shearing forces from sudden changes in acceleration and deceleration. DAI is multifocal and may be hemorrhagic or non-hemorrhagic [6]. Most common locations include the

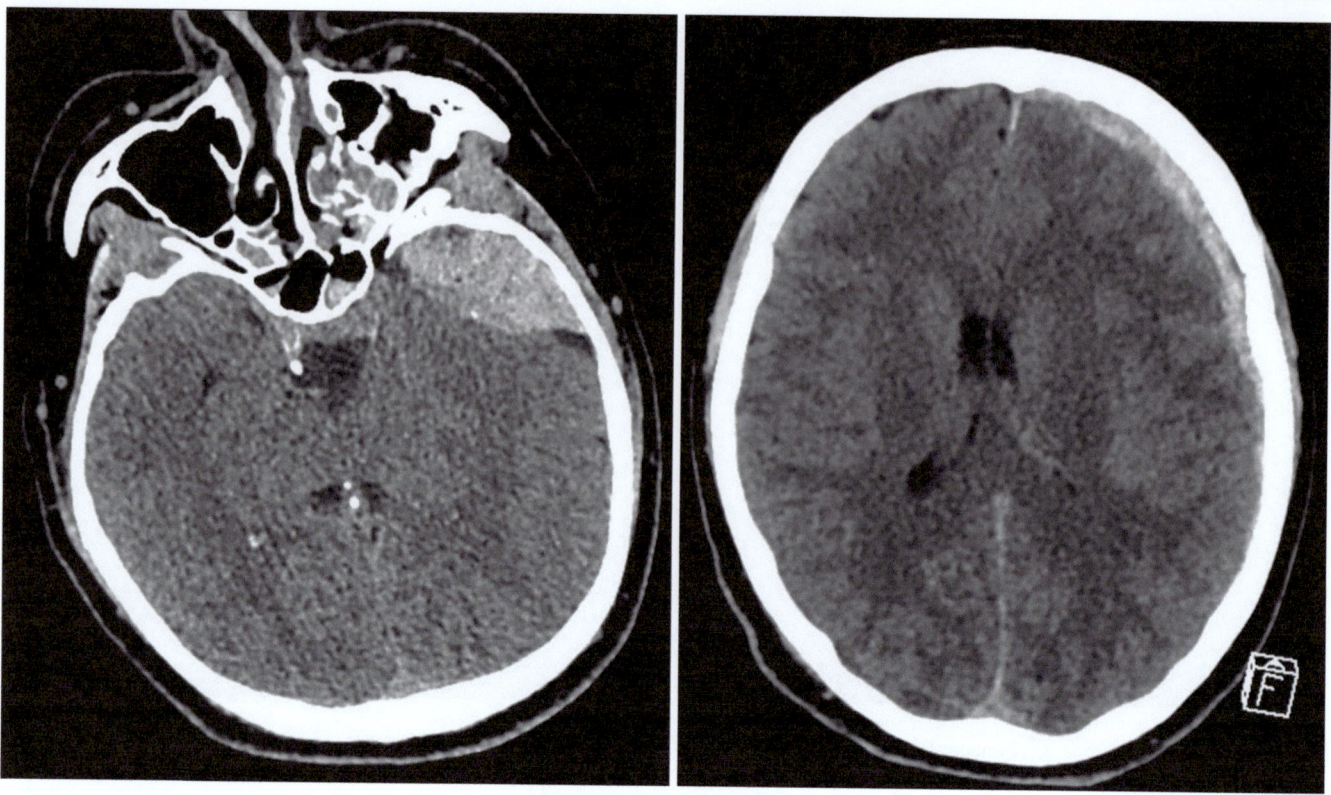

Fig. 8.5 Epidural vs. subdural hemorrhage. Left image: A biconvex-shaped left temporal epidural hematoma with local mass effect. Right image: A left frontoparietal subdural hematoma, which is limited by the anterior falx

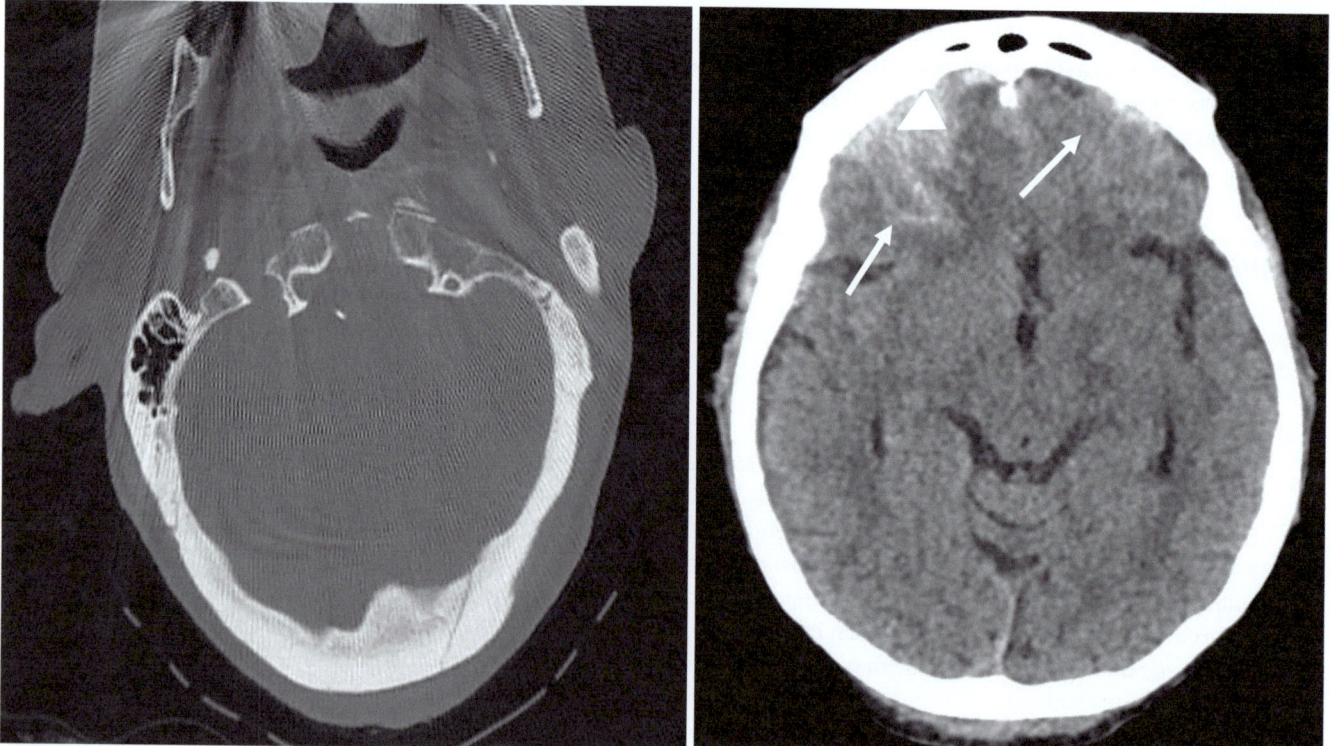

Fig. 8.6 Coup/contrecoup hemorrhagic contusion. Left image: Left occipital linear nondisplaced fracture, representing the site of impact (coup). Right image: Right frontal hemorrhagic contusion at contrecoup location (arrowhead), right greater than left subarachnoid hemorrhage (arrows), and partially seen subdural hematomas along the right frontotemporal convexity and posterior falx. Also note the edema in the bifrontal lobes, and occipital scalp hematoma

8 Head Trauma

gray-white junction, corpus callosum, brainstem, and cerebellum. The imaging findings are:
- Punctate hemorrhage might be present on CT (Fig. 8.7). However, CT is not sensitive and often appears normal.
- Multifocal hypointensities (hematomas) on GRE/SWI and hyperintensities on FLAIR, with or without diffusion restriction (Fig. 8.7).
- Gunshot wounds are often complex traumatic injuries. Damage from penetration, shear force, and heat damage

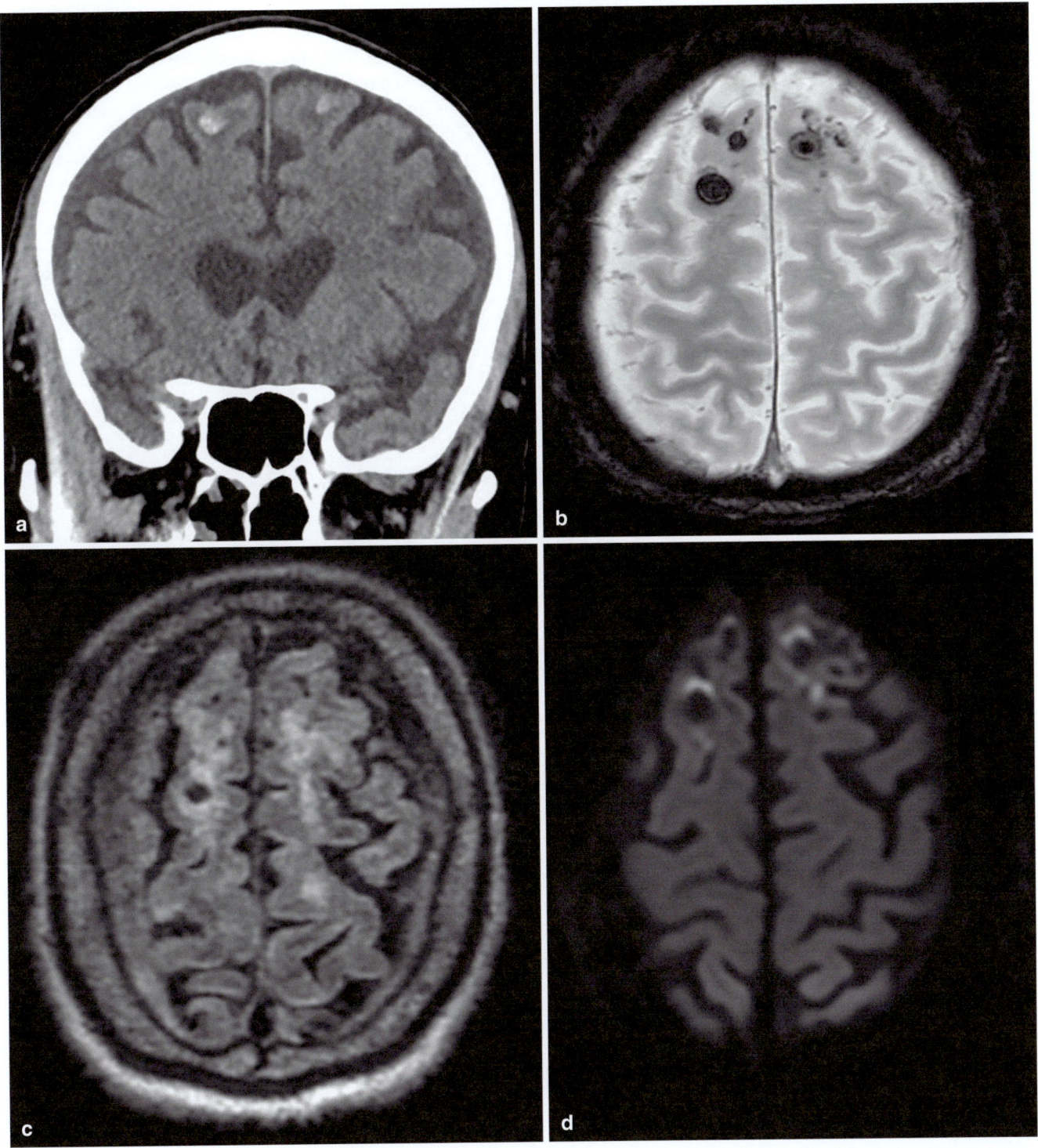

Fig. 8.7 Diffuse axonal injury. (**a**) CT Head with bilateral frontal gray-white matter junction and subcortical hemorrhage. Also note the bilateral subdural hematomas. MRI images: (**b**) GRE, (**c**) FLAIR, and (**d**) DWI, demonstrate greater extent of diffuse axonal injury. The bilateral frontoparietal convexity subdural hematomas are best seen on FLAIR

can be seen along the projectile. Entry wounds are generally smaller and more regular than exit wounds. Greater damage is usually seen away from the entry wound. Exit wounds are more irregular and often have an outward beveling of the bone (Fig. 8.3) [4].
- Intraventricular: In the setting of trauma, intraventricular hemorrhage (IVH) is usually owing to the extension of intraparenchymal and/or extra-axial blood. IVH can be subtle with only a trace amount of dependent blood present, or it can be large. Hydrocephalus is a serious complication, requiring prompt attention and possible intervention.

NONACCIDENTAL TRAUMA (NAT)

- NAT should be considered when injuries are disproportionate to the history provided.
- Head injury in pediatric patients suspected of NAT may be caused by direct impact or repeated shaking.
- Subdural hematomas are most common. Blood products with variable ages and multiple skull fractures are highly suggestive of NAT (Fig. 8.8). Other imaging findings can include scalp hematoma, cerebral edema, ischemia, subdural hygroma, intracranial hemorrhage, venous injury with or without thrombosis, or DAI.
- If NAT is suspected, a radiographic skeletal survey should be obtained to evaluate for other injuries.

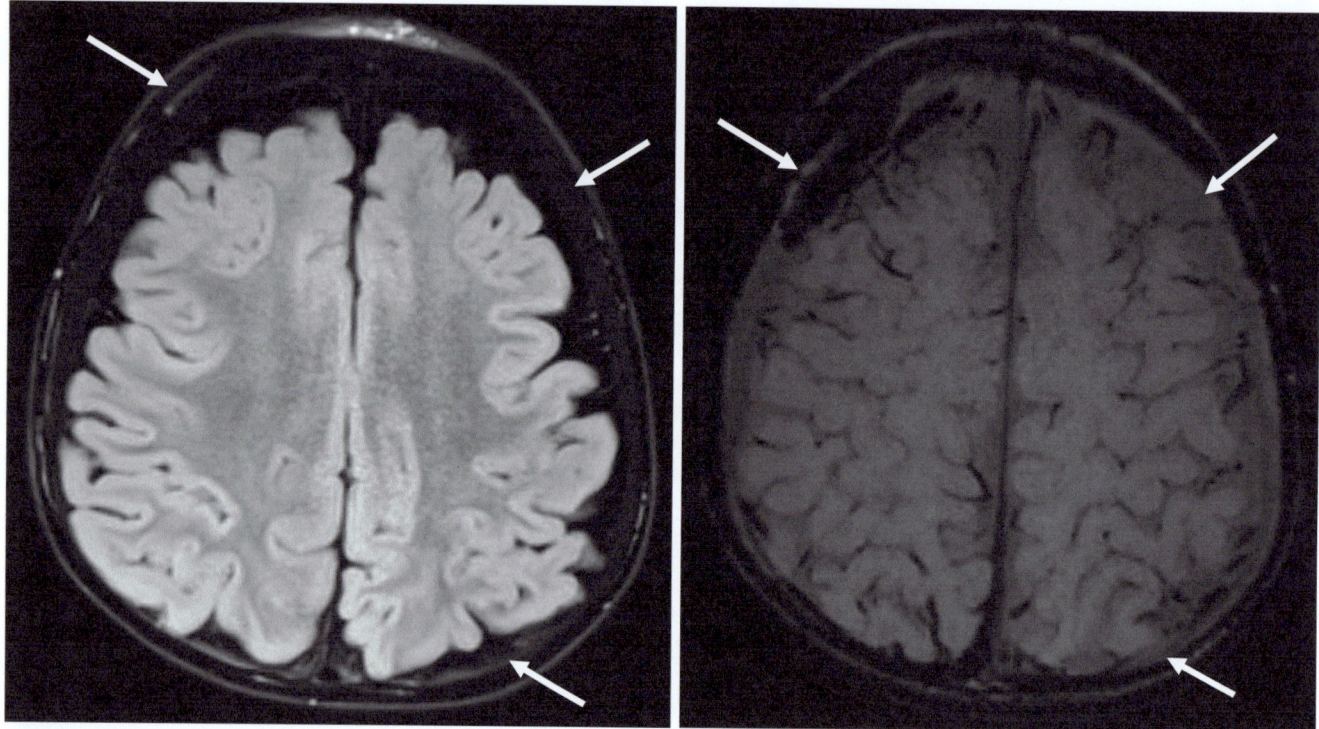

Fig. 8.8 Nonaccidental trauma. Left image: FLAIR. Right image: SWI. MRI images demonstrate bilateral subdural hematomas (arrows) in a toddler with blood products of variable ages. Findings should raise suspicion for NAT

ACUTE EFFECTS AND LONG-TERM SEQUELAE OF HEAD TRAUMA

- Hemorrhage or cerebral edema from trauma can cause local mass effect, effacement of the sulci, and/or more global mass effects due to increased intracranial pressure resulting in brain herniations (Fig. 8.9).
- Types of brain herniation [7]:
  (a) Extracranial herniation: Brain parenchyma herniates through a skull fracture or bone defect (e.g., craniectomy).
  (b) Subfalcine herniation (midline shift): Cingulate gyrus herniates under the falx. Complications may include ACA territory infarcts.
  (c) Transalar (transsphenoidal) herniation:
     o Downward: Frontal lobe is inferiorly and posteriorly displaced over the sphenoid wing. Complications may include MCA territory infarcts.
     o Upward: Temporal lobe is superiorly and anteriorly displaced over the sphenoid ridge. Complications may include ACA or MCA territory infarcts.
  (d) Uncal/Transtentorial herniation:
     o Downward: The medial temporal lobe/uncus is displaced inferiorly and medially through tentorial incisura. The midbrain and pons can also be inferiorly displaced. Some high-yield complications to be aware of are noted in Table 8.2.
     o Upward: The cerebellum is superiorly displaced through the tentorial incisura. Complications may include hydrocephalus.
  (e) Central herniation: Inferior displacement of the pons, midbrain, and diencephalon. Central herniation usually occurs with downward transtentorial herniation. When severe, this can lead to altered consciousness, abnormal posturing, coma, and death.
  (f) Tonsillar herniation: The cerebellar tonsils are inferiorly displaced through the foramen magnum. Complications may include hydrocephalus and PICA infarcts.

Table 8.2 Complications of central and downward transtentorial herniation [7]

Complication	
3rd cranial nerve palsy	Compression of the ipsilateral third cranial nerve causes ptosis, dilated pupil, and the globe being fixed in the "down and out" position
Kernohan notch	Contralateral cerebral peduncle is indented by the tentorium, resulting in ipsilateral hemiplegia. This is a false localizing sign, as the symptoms are discordant with the lesion laterality
Duret hemorrhage	Bleeding in the midbrain or pons from damage to the perforating branches of the basilar artery
Infarct	Occlusion of the PCA or basilar penetrating arteries
Hydrocephalus	Compression of the cerebral aqueduct

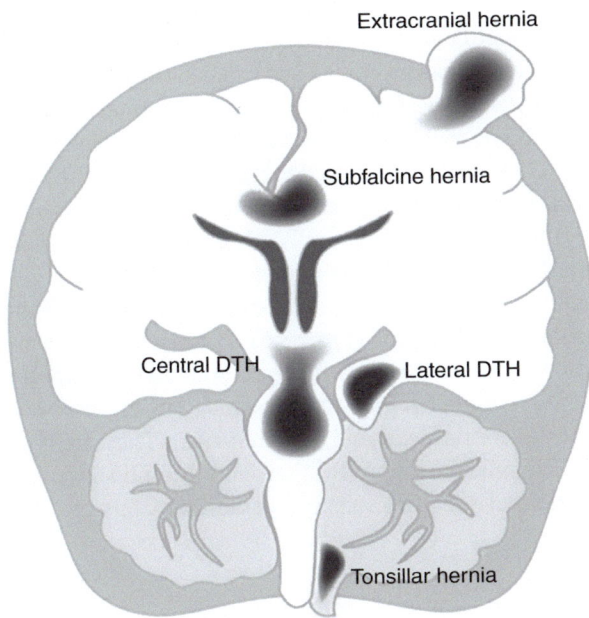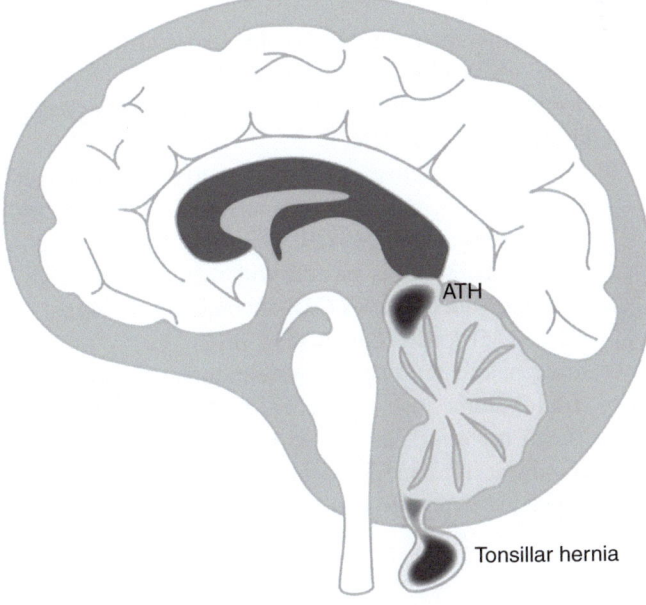

Fig. 8.9 Types of brain herniation [7]. *DTH* descending transtentorial herniation, *ATH* ascending transtentorial herniation

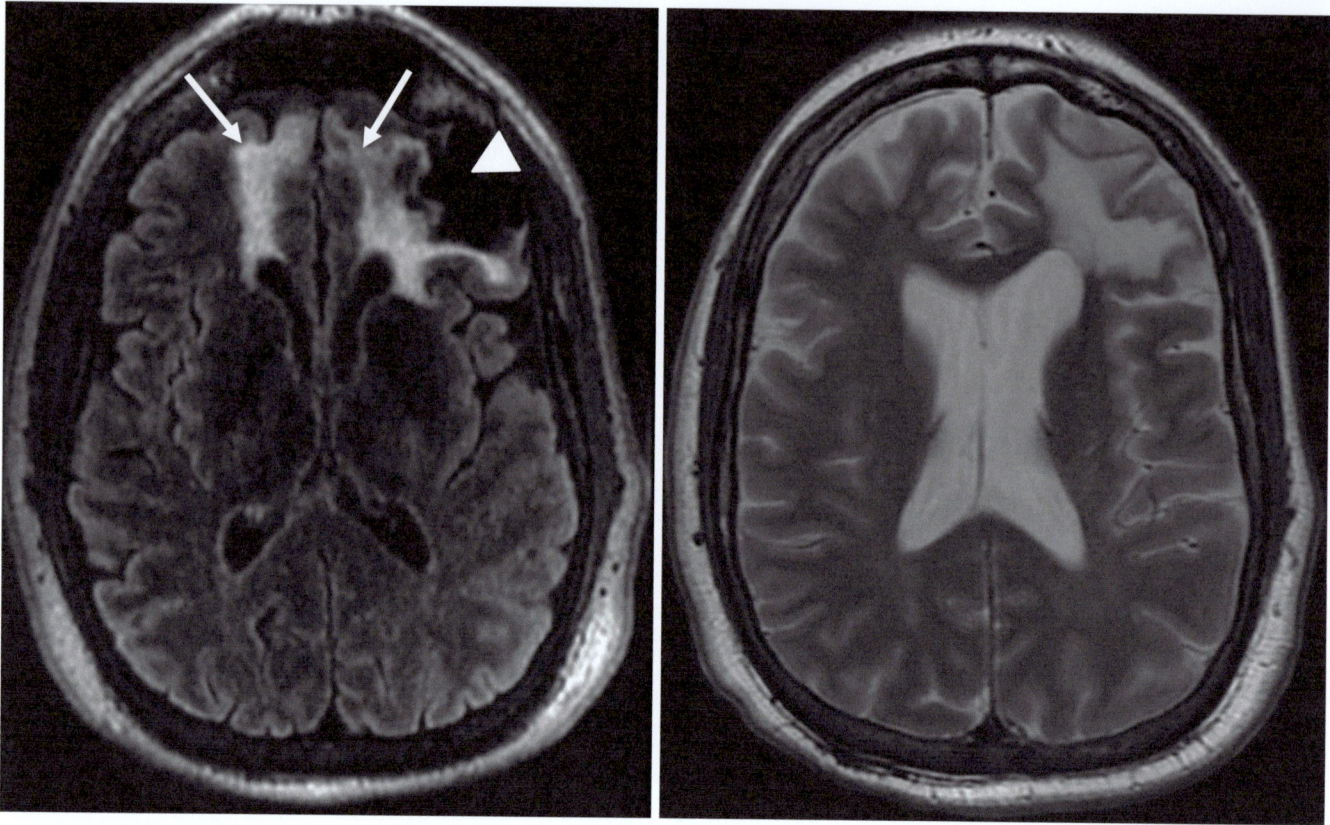

Fig. 8.10 Sequelae of traumatic brain injury. Left image: FLAIR demonstrates bilateral frontal lobe gliosis (arrow) and left frontal lobe encephalomalacia (arrowhead). Right image: T2 shows mild ex-vacuo dilatation of the left lateral ventricle frontal horn

LONG-TERM SEQUELAE

- Fractures may heal with deformity, especially when the nasal or orbital bones are involved.
- Injury to the brain may lead to irreversible damage with unique imaging features.
    - Glial cells are activated in response to an insult, resulting in gliosis, which is hypoattenuating on CT, and hyperintense on T2/FLAIR (Fig. 8.10).
    - Damaged brain cells may die with resultant encephalomalacia, which follows CSF attenuation and signal on CT and MRI, respectively (Fig. 8.10).
    - Encephalomalacia and gliosis can both be present.
    - Brain volume loss often coexists with ex-vacuo dilation of the ventricles and extra-axial spaces.
    - Hemosiderin staining from chronic blood products, which are hypointense on T1, T2, and GRE/SWI.

RARE COMPLICATIONS

- Acute injury or rare transection of cranial nerves may lead to transient or permanent cranial nerve deficit (Fig. e8.4) [5].
- Caroticocavernous fistulas (CCF) are abnormal communications between the carotid artery and the cavernous sinus. They are classified as direct or indirect CCF. Direct CCF are often caused by trauma (Fig. e8.5). Patients usually present with proptosis, pulsatile exophthalmos, visual change, chemosis, or subconjunctival hemorrhage.
- Pseudoaneurysms of intracranial arteries are rare traumatic vascular complications (Fig. e8.6). Pseudoaneurysms are abnormal outpouchings, which are bounded only by the tunica adventitia (as opposed to bounded by all three layers of the arterial wall in true aneurysms). They are typically irregular in shape. Rupture and thromboembolism are potential complications of pseudoaneurysms.

- Skull base CSF leaks result from head trauma in 80–90% of cases [8]. They occur in 1–3% patients after closed head injury. In 80% of patients, the leak manifests as CSF rhinorrhea or otorrhea within 48 h of injury, but most resolve spontaneous.

References

1. Shih R, Burns J, Utukuri P, et al. ACR appropriateness criteria head trauma: 2021 update. J Am Coll Radiol. 2021;18:S13–36.
2. Haydel M, Preston C, DeBlieux P. Indications for computed tomography in patients with minor head injury. N Engl J Med. 2000;343:100–5.
3. Stiell IG, Wells GA, Vandemheen K, et al. The Canadian CT head rule for patients with minor head injury. Lancet. 2001;357:1391–6.
4. Wilson A. Gunshot injuries: what does a radiologist need to know? Radiographics. 1999;19(5):1358–68.
5. Adams A. Imaging of skull base trauma: fracture patterns and soft tissue injuries. Neuroimaging Clin N Am. 2021;31(4):599–620.
6. Bruggeman GF, Haitsma IK, Dirven CM, Volovici V. Traumatic axonal injury (TAI): definitions, pathophysiology and imaging—a narrative review. Acta Neurochir. 2020;163:31–44.
7. Riveros Gilardi B, Muñoz López JI, Hernández Villegas AC, Garay Mora JA, Rico Rodríguez OC, Chávez Appendini R, De la Mora MM, Higuera Calleja JA. Types of cerebral herniation and their imaging features. Radiographics. 2019;39:1598–610.
8. Scoffings DJ. Imaging of acquired skull base cerebrospinal fluid leaks. Neuroimaging Clin N Am. 2021;31(4):509–22.

Post-operative Appearances

Francis Scott, Tarik F. Massoud, and Tomasz Matys

POST-OPERATIVE CRANIUM

BURR HOLES

- A burr hole is a small defect through the inner and outer tables of the calvarium formed using a surgical drill.
- This is a commonly used technique to provide intracranial access while causing minimal trauma to the scalp and cranium.
- Indications include:
  o Drainage of subdural hematoma.
  o Insertion of invasive devices, such as ventricular drainage catheters and intracranial pressure monitoring probes.
  o Access for stereotactic brain biopsy.
  o Enabling craniotomy bone flap formation.

EXPECTED APPEARANCES

- Recent burr holes are filled with fluid and may demonstrate an air fluid-level (Fig. 9.1).
- Over time, fluid is resorbed and enhancing granulation tissue forms at the burr hole margins—please note that an enhancing burr hole can mimic a skull lesion, particularly at MRI (see Fig. e9.1. All electronic images (Figs. e9.1–e9.15) can be found in this chapter's website on SpringerLink: https://doi.org/10.1007/978-3-031-55124-6_9).
- Over time, the scalp can retract into the burr hole defect, producing an undesirable cosmetic result (Fig. 9.1).
- Different strategies to prevent this include the use of burr hole covers and packing of the burr hole with synthetic polymers or bone graft material.

COMPLICATIONS

- "Plunging" injury:
  o The surgical drill may rarely breach the dura resulting in localized injury to the subjacent brain (see Fig. e9.2).
  o This is a rare complication with modern surgical drills, which are designed to stop automatically once the inner table is breached.
- Burr hole pseudomeningocele:
  o A localized collection of CSF overlying the burr hole can progressively enlarge, resulting in focal bulging of the scalp.

CRANIOTOMY

- Craniotomy involves removal of a bone flap from the calvarium, which is then replaced prior to surgical closure.
- This is required to provide adequate exposure for more invasive neurosurgical procedures.
- According to the intended surgical approach, a variety of different craniotomies can be performed, named after where they are located in the cranium (Fig. 9.2):
  o Pterional.

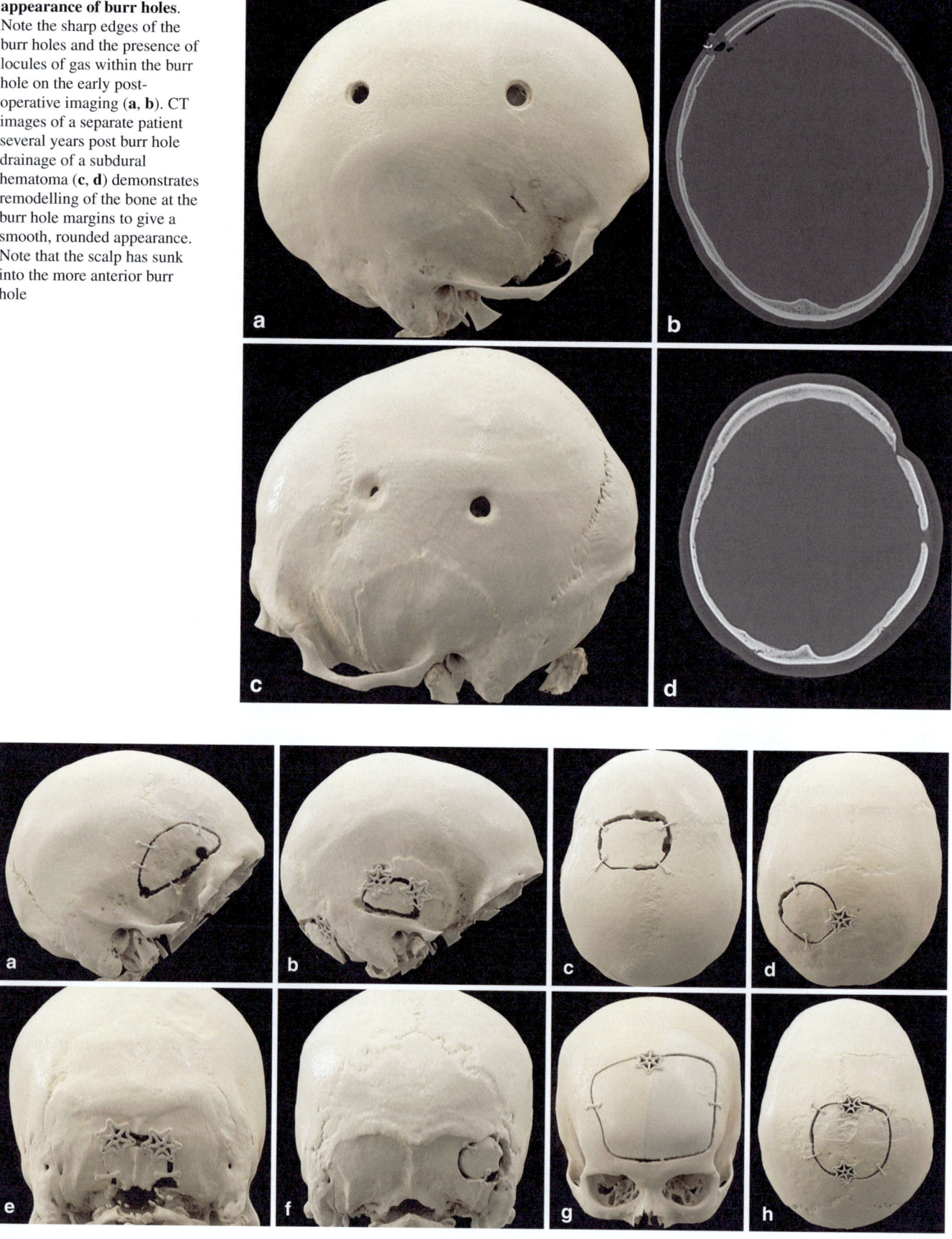

Fig. 9.1 Acute and chronic appearance of burr holes. Note the sharp edges of the burr holes and the presence of locules of gas within the burr hole on the early post-operative imaging (**a, b**). CT images of a separate patient several years post burr hole drainage of a subdural hematoma (**c, d**) demonstrates remodelling of the bone at the burr hole margins to give a smooth, rounded appearance. Note that the scalp has sunk into the more anterior burr hole

Fig. 9.2 Eight different craniotomy approaches. Surfaced rendered reconstructions demonstrate different craniotomy approaches—right pterional (**a**), right subtemporal (**b**), left anterior parasagittal (**c**), left posterior parasagittal (**d**), suboccipital (**e**), right retrosigmoid (**f**), bifrontal (**g**) and biparietal (**h**). Panel **b** also demonstrates a previous suboccipital craniotomy

- o Subtemporal.
- o Anterior parasagittal.
- o Posterior parasagittal.
- o Suboccipital.
- o Retrosigmoid.
- o Bifrontal.
- o Biparietal.
- Mini-craniotomies also may be performed for minimally invasive endoscopic neurosurgery (see Fig. e9.3).

EXPECTED APPEARANCES

- In the early post-operative phase, the bone flap should have sharp margins and be well-approximated to the adjacent bone.
- Fixation plates, screws or wires may be used to secure the bone flap.
- Small extradural and subgaleal fluid collections adjacent to the bone flap containing fluid, blood products and gas are almost invariably seen.
- Over time, fluid collections should resolve and the margins of the bone flap become more rounded and less sharply defined owing to bone remodelling.
- Bone flaps are devascularized and may demonstrate foci of sclerosis or resorption, as well as reduced enhancement compared to normal calvarial bone.

COMPLICATIONS

- Bone flap resorption:
  - o Extensive resorption of the bone flap can occasionally result in detachment from fixation plates.
  - o In severe cases this may even permit herniation of brain tissue.
  - o Cranioplasty is the definitive treatment.
- Bone flap infection (see Fig. e9.4):
  - o As described above, poorly defined lysis or sclerosis is a non-specific feature in a longstanding bone flap.
  - o This should raise concern of infection if it develops in the early post-operative period or is otherwise rapidly progressive.
  - o New inflammatory changes in the adjacent scalp or associated collections should also raise suspicion for bone flap infection.

CRANIECTOMY

- Craniectomy involves removal or a bone flap, which is not subsequently replaced.
- Indications include:
  - o Decompressive surgery for uncontrolled intracranial hypertension.
  - o Removal of infected bone flap.
  - o Removal of bone infiltrated by tumor.
  - o Posterior fossa surgery, to reduce mass effect associated with post-operative swelling.

EXPECTED APPEARANCES

- After early post-operative fluid collections resolve, the galea aponeurotica and dura become fused with intervening scar tissue to form a *meningogaleal complex* (Fig. 9.3).
- The *meningogaleal complex* should be 2–6 mm in thickness, smooth and homogeneously enhancing.
- Following suboccipital craniectomy, a pseudomeningocele of variable size is usually seen.
- As with a craniotomy, the margins of the craniectomy will become rounded over time owing to bone remodelling (Fig. 9.3).

COMPLICATIONS

- Extracranial herniation:
  - o Some degree of herniation of brain tissue beyond the craniectomy margins is frequently seen, particularly for decompressive craniectomy.
  - o However, with a relatively small craniectomy defect deformation of the herniated brain tissue can produce a "mushroom cap" appearance.
  - o This can result in venous ischaemia and infarction of herniated tissue.
- External brain tamponade:
  - o Rarely, a pressurized subgaleal fluid collection may accumulate within the craniectomy defect.
  - o This can cause compression of the underlying brain parenchyma and contralateral midline shift.
  - o This is a neurosurgical emergency requiring decompression of the subgaleal collection.
- Sinking skin flap syndrome (a.k.a. syndrome of the trephined, Fig. 9.4):
  - o This is a late complication of craniectomy resulting from atmospheric pressure exceeding intracranial pressure.
  - o It produces symptoms of headache, fatigue and seizures, accompanied with progressive depression of the skin flap overlying the craniectomy defect.
  - o Mass effect on the underlying brain produces paradoxical herniation to the contralateral side.
  - o CSF drainage or lumbar puncture can precipitate acute neurologic deterioration.
  - o This is a neurosurgical emergency when presenting with disabling neurologic deficits, and cranioplasty is the definitive treatment.

Fig. 9.3 Early and late post-operative appearances following decompressive craniectomy. CT performed 1 day following right decompressive craniectomy for a large acute right MCA territory infarct demonstrates a bulging of edematous brain tissue through the craniectomy defect (**a**), which has sharp bony margins (**b**). CT performed 1 year later demonstrates mature encephalomalacia with an overlying smooth meningogaleal complex (**c**) and remodelling of the bone at the craniectomy margins (**d**)

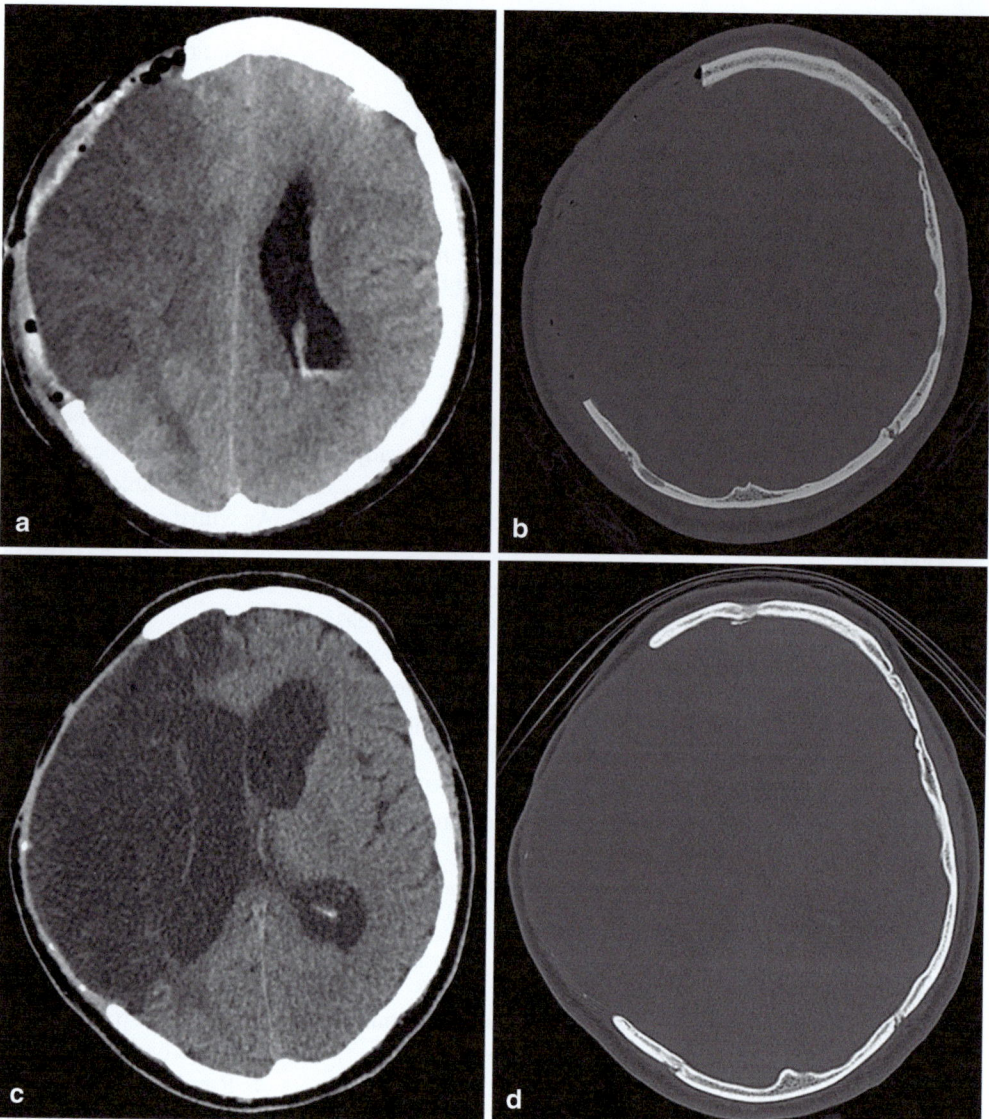

CRANIOPLASTY

- Cranioplasty is the surgical repair of a cranial defect, which may be post-surgical, traumatic or congenital.
- This can be performed for cosmetic reasons, but also to restore mechanisms that allow regulation of intracranial pressure, such as in patients with sinking skin flap syndrome.
- Acrylic cranioplasty (see Fig. e9.5):
  o Methyl methacrylate (MMA) is most commonly used, which has an attenuation of approximately 100 HU.
  o Plates may be preformed or they may be moulded intraoperatively—in the latter case the plate can contain small gas bubbles.
- Titanium cranioplasty (Fig. 9.5):
  o A titanium mesh or plate can be moulded to restore the outer contour of the skull, and it can be used in combination with MMA.
  o This causes similar beam hardening effects as the normal calvarium with minimal streak artefact.

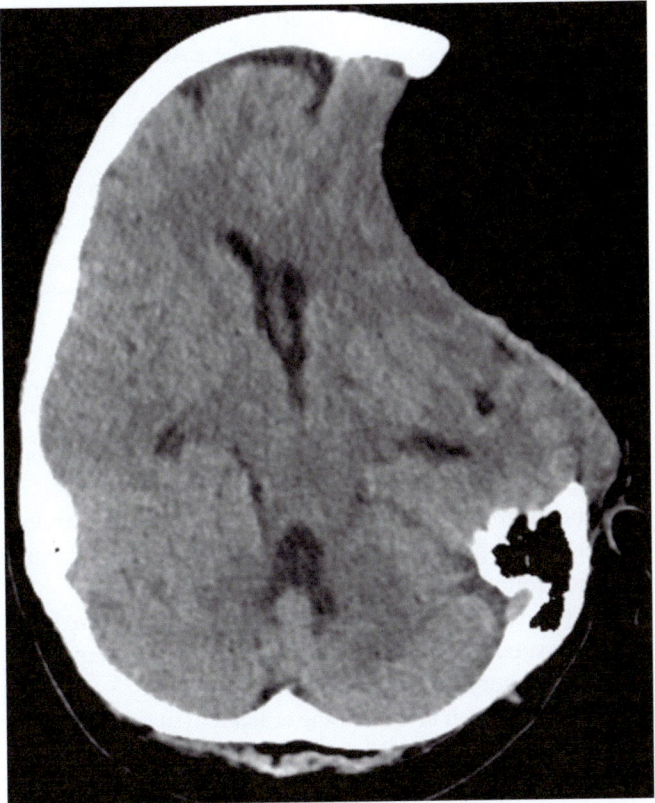

Fig. 9.4 Sinking skin flap syndrome. A patient presented with progressive indrawing of the scalp at the site of a previous left decompressive craniectomy. CT demonstrates marked depression of the left frontal scalp with mass effect on the underlying brain and paradoxical herniation to the contralateral side

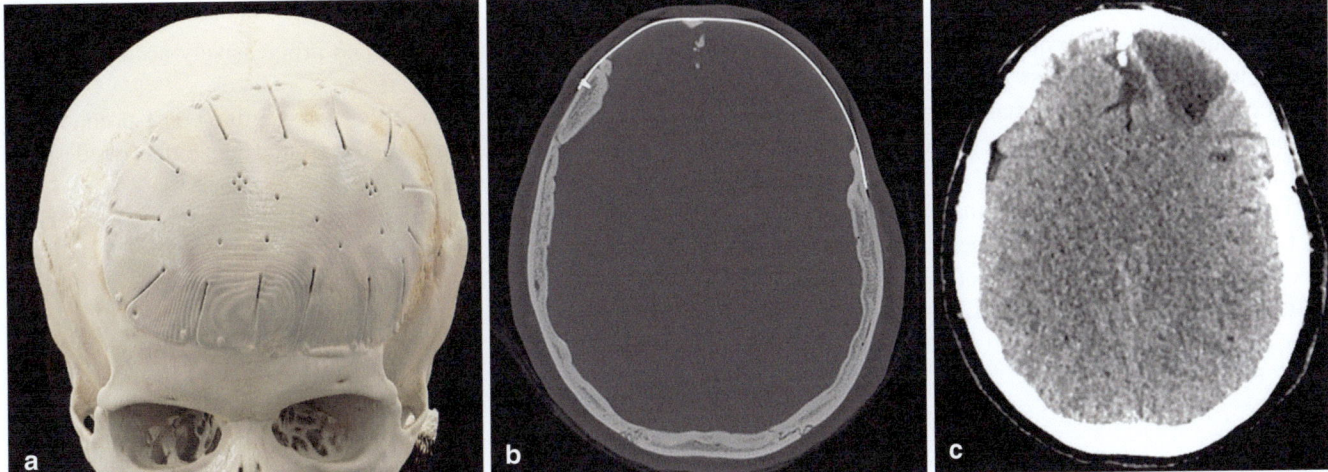

Fig. 9.5 Bifrontal titanium plate cranioplasty. Surface rendered (**a**), bone kernel (**b**) and brain kernel (**c**) reconstructions in a patient with a bifrontal titanium plate cranioplasty. Note that there is no resulting streak artefact, but beam hardening artefact results in subtle apparent hyperattenuation of the cortex adjacent to the cranioplasty plate

OTHER SURGICAL APPROACHES

TRANS-SPHENOIDAL

- This transnasal or endonasal endoscopic approach (EEA) is commonly used for resecting pituitary tumours and other sellar and parasellar lesions.
- Fat, fascia and a septonasal flap are typically grafted into the skull base defect, which reduces over time.
- There is usually inflammatory mucosal thickening in the sphenoid sinus, which may persist indefinitely.
- Enhancing granulation tissue at the site of surgery is expected to slowly involute, enabling it to be distinguished from residual tumor.

TRANS-LABYRINTHINE

- This approach is used for resecting large cerebellopontine angle tumors and tumors within the lateral internal auditory canal and inner ear that are not accessible from a retrocochlear approach.
- It involves complete mastoidectomy and labyrinthectomy (resection of the inner ear) and therefore results in permanent hearing loss.
- The surgical defect is packed with grafted fat, which may demonstrate thin peripheral enhancement on initial follow-up imaging.

MASTOIDECTOMY

- Mastoidectomy is frequently performed for infectious and inflammatory disease of the middle ear and mastoid air cells, such that prior mastoidectomy may be encountered as an incidental finding in patients undergoing neuroimaging for other reasons.
- There are four main types of mastoidectomy:
  - Simple—Resection of superficial cortex of mastoid process, with preservation of the air cells.
  - Canal wall up—Resection of mastoid air cells with preservation of the posterior wall of the external auditory canal (EAC).
  - Canal wall down—Resection of mastoid air cells including the posterior wall of the EAC, resulting in a mastoidectomy bowl that communicates with the middle ear cavity. This may be obliterated by filling with grafted fat or other packing material.
  - Radical—Resection of the ossicles in addition to canal wall down mastoidectomy.

PNEUMOCEPHALUS

- Pneumocephalus refers to intracranial air, which can arise in any anatomical compartment.
- Asymptomatic small bubbles of air confined to intracranial veins may be seen after peripheral venepuncture.
- Some degree of pneumocephalus is almost invariably seen in all patients imaged in the early post-operative period following neurosurgery.
- Most commonly, a small volume of extra-axial (predominantly subdural) pneumocephalus is seen adjacent to the site of surgery (Fig. 9.6).
- If there has been breach of the arachnoid mater, subarachnoid or intraventricular pneumocephalus (pneumoventricle) may be seen, which is often distant from the site of surgery.
- Following surgery to the skull base, an enlarging volume of subarachnoid pneumocephalus should be regarded as suspicious for ongoing CSF leak (see Fig. e9.6).

TENSION PNEUMOCEPHALUS

- Rarely, extra-axial air can progressively accumulate due to a one-way valve effect.
- This results in compression of the brain producing a peaked appearance of the frontal lobes described as the "Mount Fuji sign" (Fig. 9.6).
- This is a neurosurgical emergency that may require urgent surgical decompression.
- Rarely, tension pneumoventricle can also occur.

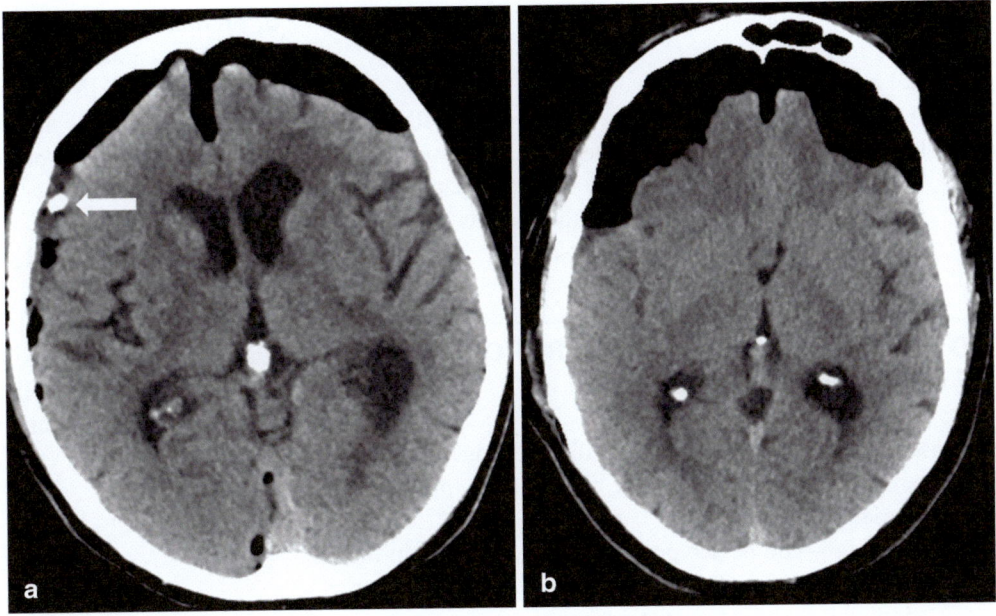

Fig. 9.6 Expected post-operative pneumocephalus versus tension pneumocephalus. (a) Post-operative CT following burr hole drainage of bilateral chronic subdural hematomas demonstrates subdural pneumocephalus overlying both frontal lobes. Note a right-sided subdural drain (white arrow). (b) Post-operative CT in another patient with neurological deterioration demonstrates a large volume of subdural pneumocephalus that compresses the frontal lobes to give the "Mount Fuji sign" of tension pneumocephalus

POST-OPERATIVE BRAIN

STEREOTACTIC BIOPSY

- Following biopsy a small amount of edema is seen along the biopsy tract, and there may be a small volume of hemorrhage.
- Linear contrast enhancement may develop along the biopsy tract after 48 h.
- These findings can help to determine the site of biopsy to confirm that the intended target has been sampled.

SURGICAL RESECTION

- The early post-operative resection cavity contains a variable amount of fluid and blood products.
  - Hyperdense surgical material including hemostatic agents, synthetic dural grafts and chemotherapy wafers may mimic post-operative hematoma.
- The appearances of the adjacent brain tissue depend on the presence of residual tumor although there is usually some edema at the resection margins.
- Enhancing granulation tissue forms at the resection margins after approximately 3 days.
  - For this reason, early post-operative imaging to assess for any residual enhancing tumor should be performed within 48 h of surgery.
- Small foci of restricted diffusion are frequently seen in the parenchyma adjacent to the resection cavity on early post-operative MRI, representing localized parenchymal injury. This may be owing to parenchymal manipulation or retraction (see Fig. e9.7).
  - These may demonstrate enhancement on follow-up examinations within the first few months, similar to evolution of infarcts, and should not be confused for recurrent tumor.
- Over time, the resection cavity will contract, surrounding edema will resolve and hypodense/T2 hyperintense gliosis will form at the resection margins, associated with volume loss in the surrounding brain tissue (see Fig. e9.7).
  - Progressive increase in edema adjacent to the surgical site should raise suspicion of post-operative infection or recurrent tumor.

LOBECTOMY AND HEMISPHERECTOMY

- Temporal lobectomy is the most common type of surgery for temporal lobe epilepsy.
- Frontal lobectomy may be performed for limited lesions, such as tumor, contusions and hematoma but extensive frontal lobe resection may be used to treat intractable epilepsy.
- Hemispherectomy is also rarely used for the treatment of intractable epilepsy.
- It may be total (anatomical) or partial (functional, involving complete disconnection of the affected hemisphere).
- Total hemispherectomy:
  - In the immediate post-operative period, the surgical cavity fills with fluid within a few days.
  - Contralateral shift of the remaining hemisphere can develop.

- Synthetic dura may be sutured in the midline to prevent this.
- Partial hemispherectomy:
  - A variable proportion of the hemisphere will have been resected, depending on the surgical approach.
  - The residual portions of the resected hemisphere undergo accelerated atrophy in the months following surgery.

NOTE ON MRI SAFETY CONSIDERATIONS OF CATHETERS AND DEVICES

- Based on the outcome of MRI safety testing, the FDA classifies implanted devices into one of three categories:
  - MR safe—The device poses no safety hazards in the MR environment. The patient can be scanned with no additional scanning restrictions.
  - MR conditional—The device may enter the MRI scanner room but only under specific conditions. The patient should not be scanned unless the device is confirmed as MR conditional and the conditions for safe use are met.
  - MR unsafe—The device should not enter the MRI scanner room. Patients with MR unsafe devices should not be scanned.

VENTRICULAR CATHETERS

- Ventricular drainage catheters are used to treat hydrocephalus and other disorders that benefit from CSF drainage, such as idiopathic intracranial hypertension.
- Two approaches are commonly used for insertion, both of which are intended to avoid areas of eloquent cortex:
  - Frontal approach—via Kocher's point, 11 cm posterior to the nasion, 3 cm lateral to the midline and at least 1 cm anterior to the coronal suture.
  - Parieto-occipital approach—via Keen's point, 3 cm superior and 3 cm posterior to the pinna.

EXTERNAL VENTRICULAR DRAIN (Fig. 9.7)

- Comprises a simple plastic drainage catheter, usually attached to a drainage bag.
- Used to temporarily relieve ventricular obstruction such as that caused by meningitis or following surgery to the posterior fossa.
- Most are MR safe.

OMMAYA RESERVOIR

- Comprises a reservoir implanted into the subcutaneous tissues of the scalp attached to a ventricular catheter.
- Used for the administration of intrathecal chemotherapy, to avoid repeated lumbar punctures.
- Depending on composition, these may be MR safe or MR conditional.

VENTRICULOPERITONEAL SHUNT (Fig. 9.8)

- Comprises a ventricular catheter, valve and a distal catheter that is tunneled subcutaneously with its tip draining into the peritoneal cavity
- Familiarity with the appearance of these components is essential to ensure that any radiolucent component is not misinterpreted as a shunt fracture.

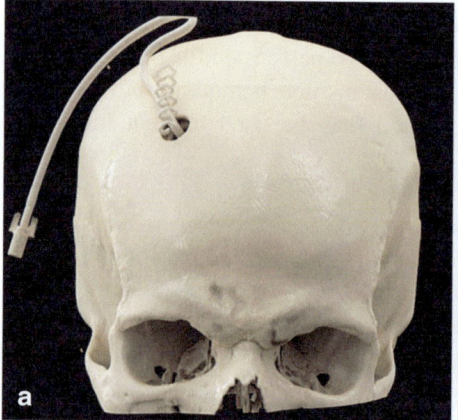
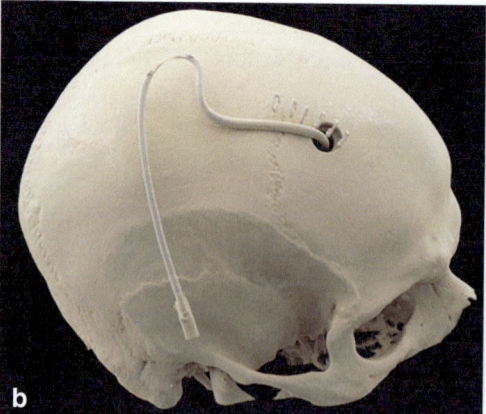
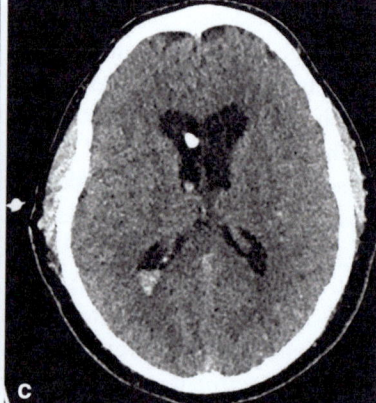

Fig. 9.7 Right frontal approach external ventricular drain. Surface rendered reconstructions (**a**, **b**) and axial unenhanced CT (**c**) demonstrates satisfactory positioning of the EVD, which is inserted via Kocher's point with its tip within the frontal horn of the right lateral ventricle

Fig. 9.8 Right parietal approach VP shunt. Surface rendered reconstruction (**a**) and unenhanced CT (**b**) demonstrates satisfactory positioning of a right parietal approach ventriculoperitoneal shunt catheter, which has its tip within the body of the right lateral ventricle. The right lateral ventricle is slit-like and there is a small volume of chronic subdural hematoma at the left frontal convexity, suggesting CSF overdrainage

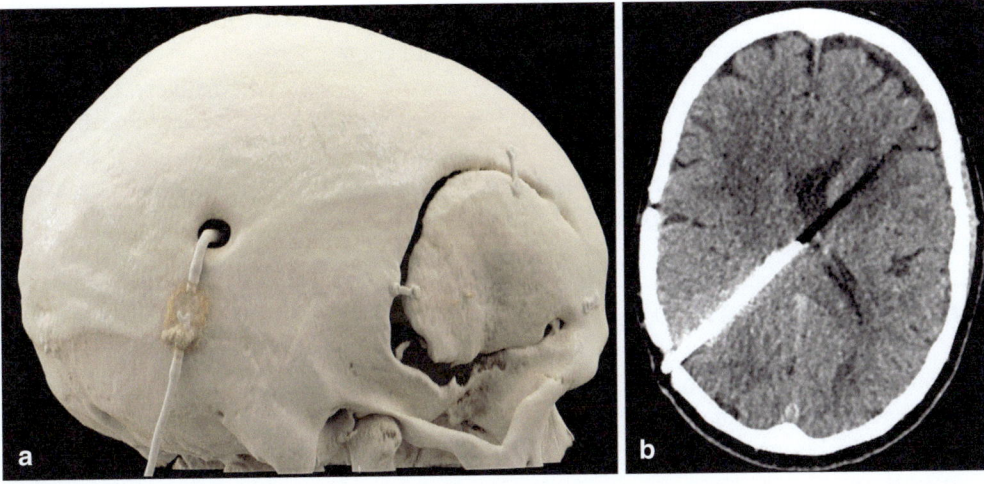

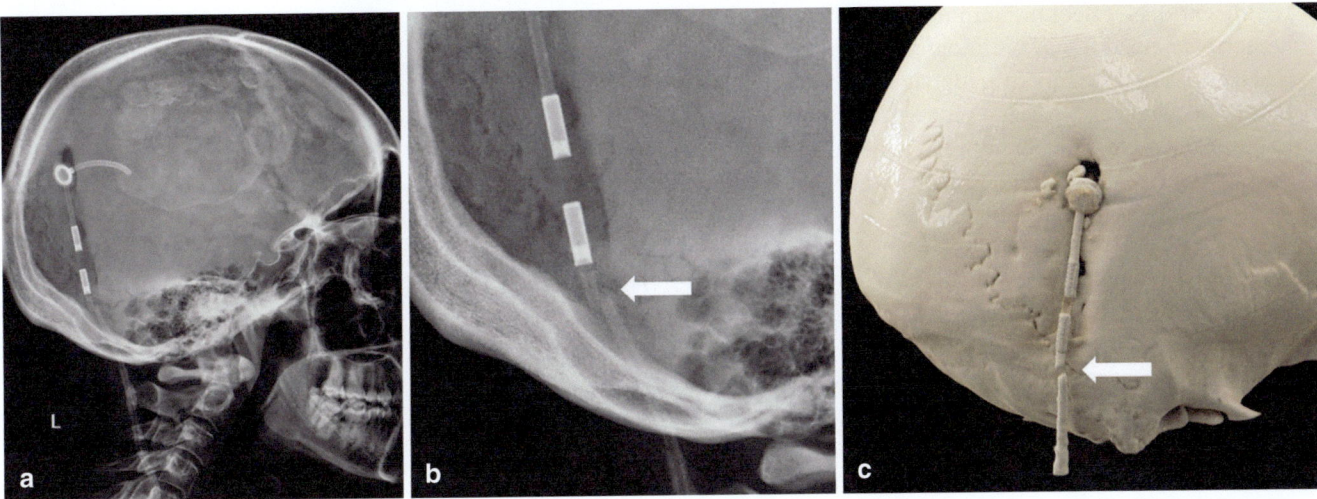

Fig. 9.9 VP shunt fracture. A lateral skull radiograph performed as part of a shunt series (**a**) demonstrates abnormal discontinuity in the extracranial shunt tubing (white arrow in magnified image **b**). A surface rendered reconstruction from a CT confirms shunt fracture (white arrow, **c**)

- Modern VP shunts have programmable valves that allow the settings to be adjusted non-invasively—these are MR conditional up to 3 T.
- Patients with programmable shunts should always have valve settings confirmed following MRI to ensure that they have not been inadvertently altered.

OTHER SHUNT CATHETERS

- Ventricular shunts may also drain into the right atrium (ventriculoatrial, VA) or pleural space (ventriculopleural, VPL).
- These are less commonly used in modern neurosurgical practice.

COMPLICATIONS

- Infection:
  o Usually detected by analysis of a CSF sample obtained from the catheter.
  o May produce little in the way of imaging findings.
  o Severe cases can produce features of ventriculitis or cerebral abscess formation.
- Obstruction (see Fig. e9.8):
  o Imaging demonstrates deteriorating hydrocephalus despite an appropriately sited catheter.
- Shunt fracture (Fig. 9.9):
  o May occur anywhere along the course of the catheter.
  o In addition to head CT, a radiographic shunt series is used to examine the entire extracranial course of the shunt catheter.

- CSF overdrainage (Fig. 9.8):
  - May produce symptoms of headache, nausea and vomiting or seizures.
  - Imaging demonstrates collapsed (slit) ventricles with features of intracranial hypotension (dural thickening and enhancement, subdural collections or subdural hematomas and brain sagging).

SUBDURAL DRAINS AND DEVICES

- Chronic subdural hematoma (CSDH) is a common cause of neurologic impairment, particularly in elderly patients.
- CSDH can be managed conservatively but may require neurosurgical evacuation.
- Surgery is considered for large CSDH (>10 mm in depth), significant mass effect (>5 mm midline shift) or repeated hemorrhage resulting in neurologic deterioration.
- CSDH are evacuated by irrigation of the hematoma via a burr hole, which also permits access to the subdural space to break down any membranes that may have formed.
- Several devices can be used to reduce rates of hematoma recurrence following surgical evacuation.

SUBDURAL DRAIN (See Fig. e9.9)

- A plastic drainage catheter inserted into the subdural space via the burr hole, which is usually removed after approximately 48 h.
- Most drainage catheters contain no metallic components and are MR safe.

SUBPERIOSTEAL/SUBGALEAL DRAIN

- Alternatively, a drainage catheter may be placed under the scalp overlying the burr hole, either in the subgaleal or subperiosteal space.
- As above, most drainage catheters are MR safe.

SUBDURAL EVACUATING PORT SYSTEM (SEPS™) (See Fig. e9.10)

- An alternative approach to burr hole evacuation is SEPS—a stainless steel evacuating port that is inserted into the diploic space overlying the hematoma.
- Insertion can be performed at the bedside under local anesthesia which may be preferable in elderly patients with comorbidities.
- It has a distinctive appearance at CT and should not be mistaken for an intracranial pressure monitoring bolt.
- This device is MR unsafe.

VASCULAR DEVICES

ANEURYSM CLIPS (See Fig. 9.10)

- Surgical clipping is used for the treatment of intracranial aneurysms.
- Occlusion of the aneurysm neck is the objective of surgery.
- Aneurysm clips are small hinged metallic clips that may be straight or curved.

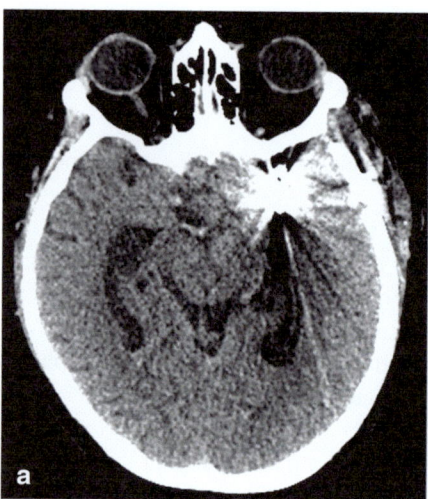
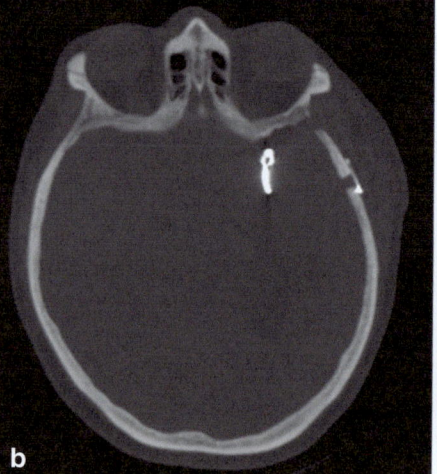
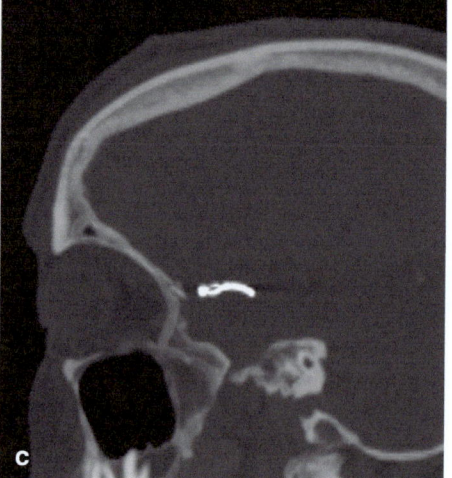

Fig. 9.10 Left internal carotid artery aneurysm clip. Unenhanced CT performed following surgical clipping of an aneurysm at the origin of the left anterior choroidal artery demonstrates extensive streak artefact centered on the left Sylvian fissure (**a**). Bone reconstructions in the axial (**b**) and sagittal (**c**) planes demonstrate the hinged aneurysm clip, which in this case is curved

9 Post-operative Appearances

- They produce streak artefact that will limit assessment of structures in the immediate vicinity of the clip.
- Modern aneurysm clips are MRI-conditional, but historically (over 30 years ago) MR unsafe stainless steel clips were used.
- It is therefore essential to confirm the device used prior to performing MRI.

EMBOLISATION COILS (See Fig. e9.11)

- Endovascular coiling is the most commonly used treatment for intracranial aneurysms.
- Complete exclusion of the aneurysm from the circulation is the objective of treatment.
- On follow-up imaging, coil compaction can result in filling of the aneurysm neck.
- Coils produce streak artefact that can limit assessment of adjacent structures, particularly for larger aneurysms, which limits the value of CTA in aneurysm follow-up.
- MRA is a validated technique for the follow-up of coiled aneurysms for the detection of recurrences.
- DSA is the gold-standard technique to confirm aneurysm recurrence, which can also enable planning of any required neurointervention.
- All devices are MR conditional up to 3 T.

ARTERIAL STENTS (See Fig. e9.12)

- Uncovered arterial stents have a number of intracranial applications.
- Self-expanding stents can be used for the treatment of intracranial arterial stenosis.
- Flow-diverting stents can be used to treat dissecting pseudoaneurysms and wide-necked aneurysms.
- Stents can also be used to assist in aneurysm coiling.
- CTA/MRA is used to confirm stent patency, to monitor for in-stent stenosis and (if relevant) to assess for aneurysm thrombosis.
- Most devices are MR conditional up to 3 T.

ENDOSACCULAR FLOW DISRUPTION DEVICES

- In recent years, new embolisation systems have been developed that involve deployment of a device within the sac of the aneurysm.
- These are particularly advantageous for the treatment of wide-necked bifurcation aneurysms, which are challenging to treat with conventional endovascular methods.
- The WEB device (Woven EndoBridge, MicroVention/Terumo) is currently the only FDA-approved device in this class.
- It is composed of a nitinol/platinum mesh and has a distinctive spherical/cylindrical morphology (see Fig. e9.13).
- The WEB device is MR conditional up to 3 T.

VENOUS STENTS (See Fig. e9.14)

- Venous sinus stents are used to treat symptomatic venous stenosis, including stenosis of the transverse sinuses in idiopathic intracranial hypertension.
- Potential long-term complications include in-stent stenosis and delayed stent thrombosis.
- Most devices are MR conditional up to 3 T.

LIQUID EMBOLIC AGENTS

- Liquid embolic agents such as Onyx (and other copolymers) and cyanoacrylate glue are used for the embolisation of arteriovenous malformations/fistulas and/or tumours.
- They contain tantalum powder to enable angiographic visualization and provide a vascular cast of the embolized tissue on follow-up imaging.
- This highly radiopaque material tends to produce extensive streak artefact, which can impair assessment on any follow-up CT.
- Most agents are MR conditional up to 3 T.

OTHER IMPLANTED DEVICES

INVASIVE INTRACRANIAL PRESSURE MONITORING

- Patients managed in a neuro-critical care setting may require invasive monitoring of intracranial pressure.
- This involves insertion of a pressure transducer into the substance of the brain via a frontal burr hole.
- CT can be used to confirm appropriate device positioning, as readings will be unreliable if the device is coiled within the burr hole or sited within abnormal brain tissue/hematoma.
- Complications of insertion include hemorrhage and infection.
- Most are MR conditional, but fiber optic transducer systems are MR unsafe.

- At some centers additional devices may be inserted alongside an ICP probe including probes for monitoring of intracranial oxygen levels and temperature, and microdialysis catheters for interstitial fluid sampling.

INVASIVE ELECTROENCEPHALOGRAPHY (EEG) MONITORING

- Invasive EEG monitoring is used to provide the most accurate localization of the seizure focus, which may be required prior to epilepsy surgery.
- Several approaches can be used:
  - Subdural electrode strips inserted via burr holes.
  - Depth electrodes inserted into the brain parenchyma.
  - Epidural peg electrodes inserted via small burr holes.
  - Electrode strips abutting the mesial temporal lobes inserted via the foramen ovale.
- Most devices are MR unsafe.

DEEP BRAIN STIMULATION (DBS) ELECTRODES
(See Fig. e9.15)

- Deep brain stimulation using implanted electrodes is a surgical technique used for the treatment of movement disorders refractory to medical management, particularly Parkinson's disease. There are also other emerging indications.
- The subthalamic nucleus (STN) and globus pallidus internus (GPi) are the most commonly used targets.
- Post-operative imaging is used to confirm satisfactory electrode positioning and also to exclude any operative complications, such as intra- or extra-axial hemorrhage, or air near the electrode tip. Discontinuity of extracranial extension leads may occur long-term.
- All modern DBS systems are MR conditional (with strict requirements), but many older systems are MR unsafe.

FIDUCIAL MARKERS

- External fiducial markers applied to the scalp are temporary and used for imaging co-registration for frame-based (as opposed to frameless) stereotactic neurosurgery.
- Edematous/inflammatory changes in bilateral temporalis muscles may be seen if imaging is obtained soon after removal of fiducials.
- Fiducial markers may also be embedded in the skull for repeated use for radiotherapy targeting.
- Rarely, a marker may penetrate through the inner table of the skull—injury to dural vessels can result in epidural hematoma particularly if the marker tip is near the course of the middle meningeal artery in its groove.
- Most fiducial markers are MR conditional up to 3 T.

Further Reading

1. Ginat DT, Westesson PLA, editors. Atlas of postsurgical neuroradiology. Berlin: Springer; 2012.
2. Sinclair AG, Scoffings DJ. Imaging of the post-operative cranium. Radiographics. 2010;30(2):461–82.
3. De Almeida AN, Marino R Jr, Aguiar PH, Jacobsen TM. Hemispherectomy: a schematic review of the current techniques. Neurosurg Rev. 2006;29(2):97–102; discussion 102.
4. Shellock FG, Woods TO, Crues JV 3rd. MR labeling information for implants and devices: explanation of terminology. Radiology. 2009;253(1):26–30.
5. Morone PJ, Dewan MC, Zuckerman SL, Tubbs RS, Singer RJ. Craniometrics and ventricular access: a review of Kocher's, Kaufman's, Paine's, Menovksy's, Tubbs', Keen's, Frazier's, Dandy's, and Sanchez's points. Oper Neurosurg (Hagerstown). 2020;18(5):461–9.
6. Soleman J, Kamenova M, Lutz K, Guzman R, Fandino J, Mariani L. Drain insertion in chronic subdural hematoma: an international survey of practice. World Neurosurg. 2017;104:528–36.
7. Soleman J, Lutz K, Schaedelin S, Kamenova M, Guzman R, Mariani L, Fandino J. Subperiosteal vs subdural drain after Burr-hole drainage of chronic subdural hematoma: a randomized clinical trial (cSDH-drain-trial). Neurosurgery. 2019;85(5):E825–34.
8. Lollis SS, Wolak ML, Mamourian AC. Imaging characteristics of the subdural evacuating port system, a new bedside therapy for subacute/chronic subdural hematoma. AJNR Am J Neuroradiol. 2006;27(1):74–5.
9. Soize S, Gawlitza M, Raoult H, Pierot L. Imaging follow-up of intracranial aneurysms treated by endovascular means: why, when, and how? Stroke. 2016;47(5):1407–12.
10. Dmytriw AA, Salem MM, Yang VXD, Krings T, Pereira VM, Moore JM, Thomas AJ. Endosaccular flow disruption: a new frontier in endovascular aneurysm management. Neurosurgery. 2020;86(2):170–81.
11. Stuart RM, Schmidt M, Kurtz P, Waziri A, Helbok R, Mayer SA, Lee K, Badjatia N, Hirsch LJ, Connolly ES, Claassen J. Intracranial multimodal monitoring for acute brain injury: a single institution review of current practices. Neurocrit Care. 2010;12(2):188–98.
12. Shah AK, Mittal S. Invasive electroencephalography monitoring: indications and presurgical planning. Ann Indian Acad Neurol. 2014;17(Suppl 1):S89–94.
13. Lozano AM, Lipsman N, Bergman H, Brown P, Chabardes S, Chang JW, Matthews K, McIntyre CC, Schlaepfer TE, Schulder M, Temel Y, Volkmann J, Krauss JK. Deep brain stimulation: current challenges and future directions. Nat Rev Neurol. 2019;15(3):148–60.

Congenital and Neonatal Infections

Pamela Nguyen

- Congenital infections are infections acquired while the fetus is developing in utero.
- Neonatal infections are infections acquired during the intrapartum period, or in the first days to weeks following birth.
- Risk of damage to the brain differs significantly from those acquired in utero and perinatally, to those acquired in later childhood and adulthood.
- Infections acquired early in pregnancy, in the first and second trimesters, can interfere with normal brain development and lead to migrational abnormalities, cortical disorganization, and altered white matter myelination [1].
- Infections may be caused by a variety of bacteria, viruses, fungi, or parasites.
- The TORCH acronym denotes a group of pathogens with strong CNS tropism and present with similar clinical presentations, which includes Toxoplasmosis, Other (Syphilis), Rubella, Cytomegalovirus (CMV), Herpes simplex virus (HSV 1 & 2).
- The "Other" in TORCH has recently expanded to include HIV, enteroviruses, Varicella-Zoster virus, parvovirus B19, and Zika virus.

Cytomegalovirus

- Cytomegalovirus (CMV) is a member of the *Herpesviridae* family, and is the most common intrauterine infection in the United States.
- It has a prevalence of 0.48–1.3% in the USA [2].
- Risk of fetal infection is higher in women who initially acquire the virus during pregnancy (primary) than in those who acquired it prior to becoming pregnant (secondary or reactivation).

- Transmission of the virus to the fetus occurs across the placenta.
- CMV is neurotropic and replicates in the ependyma, germinal matrix, and capillary endothelium.
- Approximately 10% of infected infants are symptomatic at birth, and this is termed congenital CMV disease.
- Symptomatic infants have a high risk of developing epilepsy, neurodevelopmental delay, cerebral palsy, chorioretinitis with subsequent vision impairment, and sensorineural hearing loss.
- Among those who are asymptomatic, up to 25% still develop sequelae by age 2, such as sensorineural hearing loss.
- Prenatally the diagnosis is made by amniocentesis; Postnatally, diagnosis is made by polymerase chain reaction analysis detecting CMV DNA in the blood, urine, or saliva within the first 3 weeks of life.
- Early recognition is important because treatment with ganciclovir in the first 30 days after birth has been shown to improve long-term audiologic and neurodevelopmental outcomes [2].

Imaging

- Neuroimaging is important for diagnosis of congenital CMV infection especially in infants and children who were asymptomatic at birth and for whom serologic results from the first 3 weeks of life are unavailable.
- Imaging findings may also be used to help predict neurologic outcomes in patients with symptomatic congenital CMV infection.
- Intracranial calcification is the most frequently reported imaging finding in congenital CMV infection, occurring in 35–70% pf patients; calcifications may be thick and chunky or fine and punctate; calcifications can occasionally be detected in head ultrasound exam, are usually easily detected on noncontrast CT exam, but MR imaging

P. Nguyen (✉)
Columbia University Irving Medical Center, New York, NY, USA
e-mail: pn2295@cumc.columbia.edu

may be more sensitive for detecting fine and punctate calcifications.
- Calcification occurs in a variety of locations including periventricular regions and within the basal ganglia and brain parenchyma. In congenital CMV infection, the most common pattern is thick and chunky calcifications and periventricular in location (Fig. 10.1).
- A variety of migrational abnormalities have been reported and may be present in as many as 10% of patients.
- Lissencephaly, pachygyria, and diffuse or focal polymicrogyria are the most common migrational abnormalities, and occasionally schizencephaly can be seen with late second trimester infections (Fig. 10.2).
- White matter abnormalities occur in as many as 22% of patients and represents areas of myelin delay or destruction; a pattern of white matter signal abnormality in a predominantly posterior distribution, with sparing of the subcortical and periventricular white matter, is the common pattern (Fig. 10.3).
- Periventricular cysts can occur in and around the ventricular system secondary to necrosis or hemorrhage of the germinal matrix. In congenital CMV, cysts have been described most commonly in the anterior temporal lobes in association with white matter abnormalities (Fig. 10.4).
- Cerebral and cerebellar atrophy can manifest as microcephaly and ventriculomegaly and occurs in as many as 27% of patients and is associated with poor neurologic outcome (Fig. 10.2).

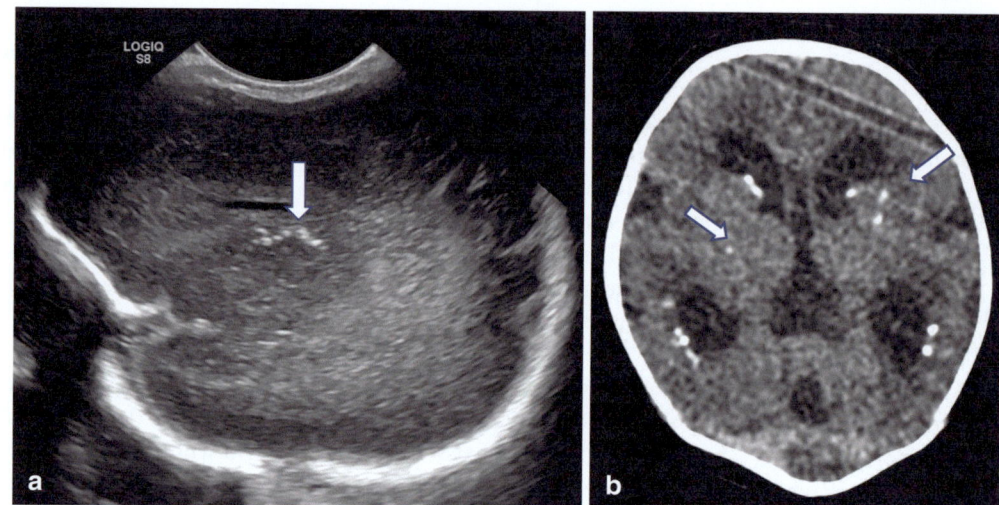

Fig. 10.1 Congenital CMV. (**a**) Head ultrasound shows clustered punctate echogenic foci with mild posterior shadowing in the periventricular white matter consistent with calcifications (arrow). (**b**) Noncontrast axial head CT shows coarse calcifications in the bilateral basal ganglia and periventricular white matter (arrows)

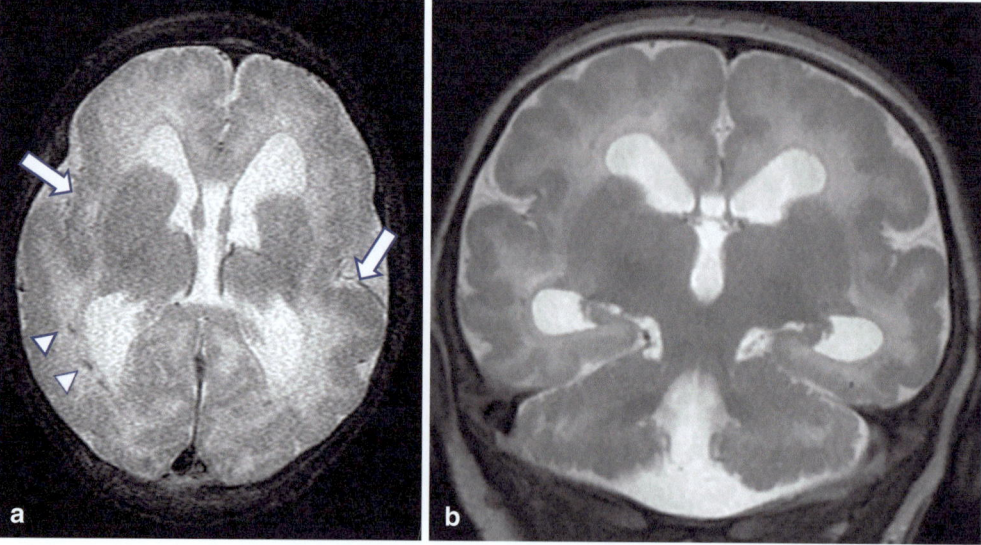

Fig. 10.2 Congenital CMV. (**a**) Axial T2 weighted image shows diffuse abnormal thickening of the cortex which shows a lumpy bumpy appearance compatible with polymicrogyria (arrows); note also the periventricular calcifications in the right periatrial white matter (arrowheads). (**b**) Coronal T2 weighted image shows the polymicrogyria also involves the cerebellar hemispheres, which are atrophic

Fig. 10.3 Congenital CMV. (a) Axial T2 weighted image shows abnormal T2 prolongation in the bilateral parietal periventricular white matter (arrows). (b) Axial T2 weighted image in the same patient showing concurrent presence of polymicrogyria in the left frontal and bilateral temporal lobes (arrows)

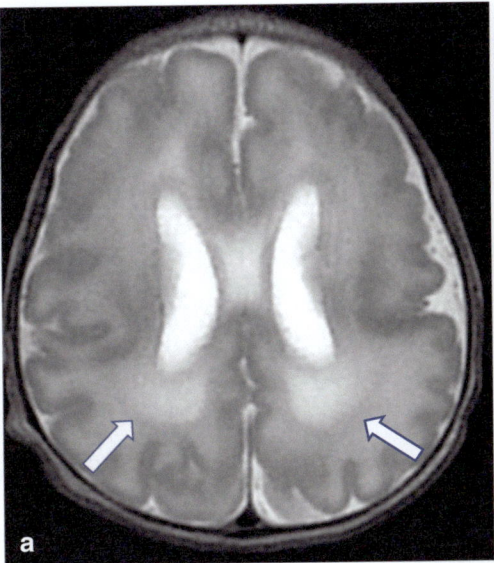
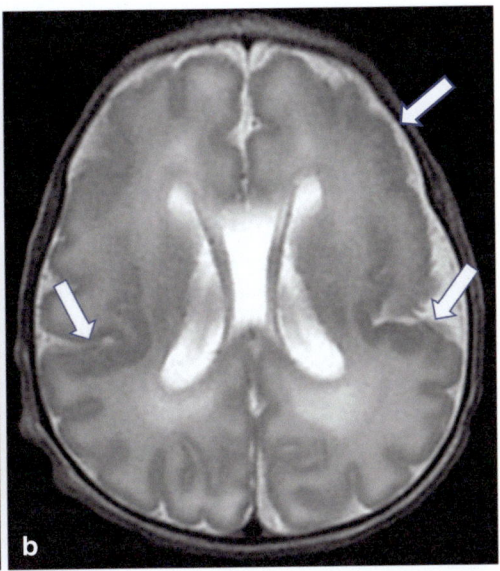

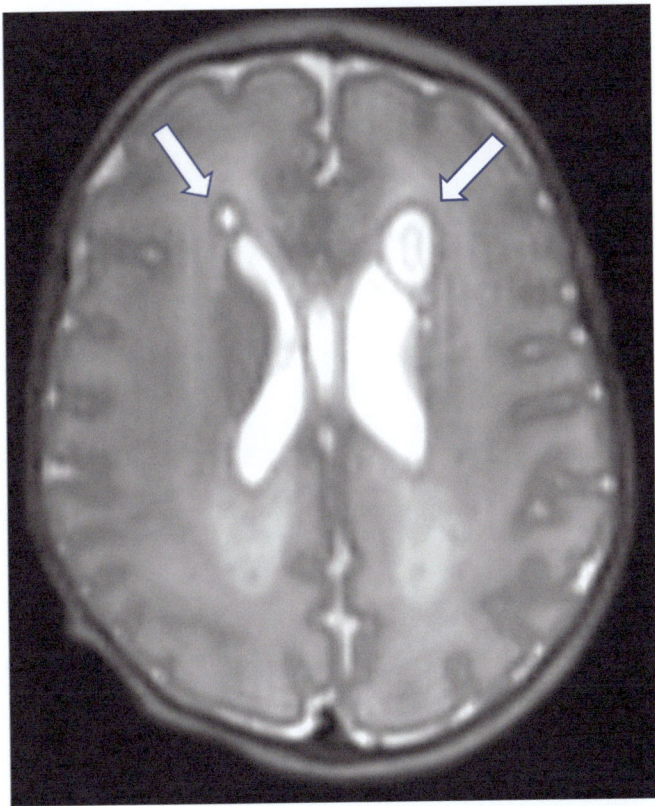

Fig. 10.4 Congenital CMV. Axial T2 weighted image shows two large areas of cystic encephalomalacia in the bilateral frontal periventricular white matter secondary to necrosis (arrows). White matter abnormalities are also present posteriorly in parietal periventricular white matter

Toxoplasmosis

- Toxoplasmosis is the second most common congenital infection after CMV and is caused by *Toxoplasma gondii*, a protozoan parasite [1].
- Transmission to humans occurs by ingestion of undercooked meat containing the parasite's cysts, contaminated vegetable, and contact with cat feces.
- The parasite enters the fetus through the placental barrier after primary maternal infection and diagnosis is by fetal and maternal serology.
- Infection is often asymptomatic in immunocompetent hosts, with disease occurring in the settings of immunosuppression or congenital infections.
- Congenital infections range from 1 in 10,000 births in the USA to 1 in 1000 births in endemic areas.
- The risk of fetal transmission increases as gestational age increases, but severity of disease decreases.
- Infants with symptomatic infection have a clinical profile similar to that of congenital CMV disease.

Imaging

- Majority of infants (70–90%) have a subclinical infection with normal routine neonatal examination prompting no imaging.
- Classic triad of chorioretinitis, hydrocephalus, and intracranial calcifications occurs in fewer than 10% of cases.
- Calcifications are seen in the basal ganglia, periventricular, corticomedullary junction, and cortex (Fig. 10.5).
- Cortical and white matter destruction with cyst formation is seen in more severe cases (Fig. 10.6).
- Migrational abnormalities are less common than in congenital CMV.
- Other organ systems are affected including hepatosplenomegaly, jaundice, seizures, lymphadenopathy, abnormal CSF, and anemia.

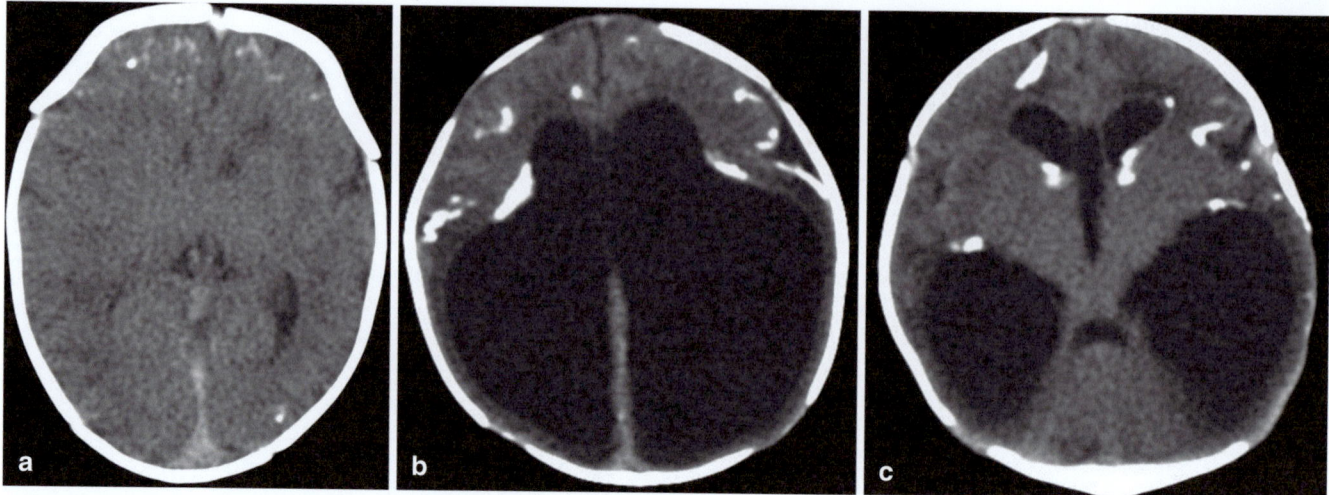

Fig. 10.5 Congenital toxoplasmosis. (**a**) Noncontrast axial CT shows coarse and punctate calcifications in the cortex and corticomedullary junction. (**b**, **c**) Serial noncontrast head CT images showing coarse calcifications in the bilateral basal ganglia, periventricular and corticomedullary junction and severe hydrocephalus

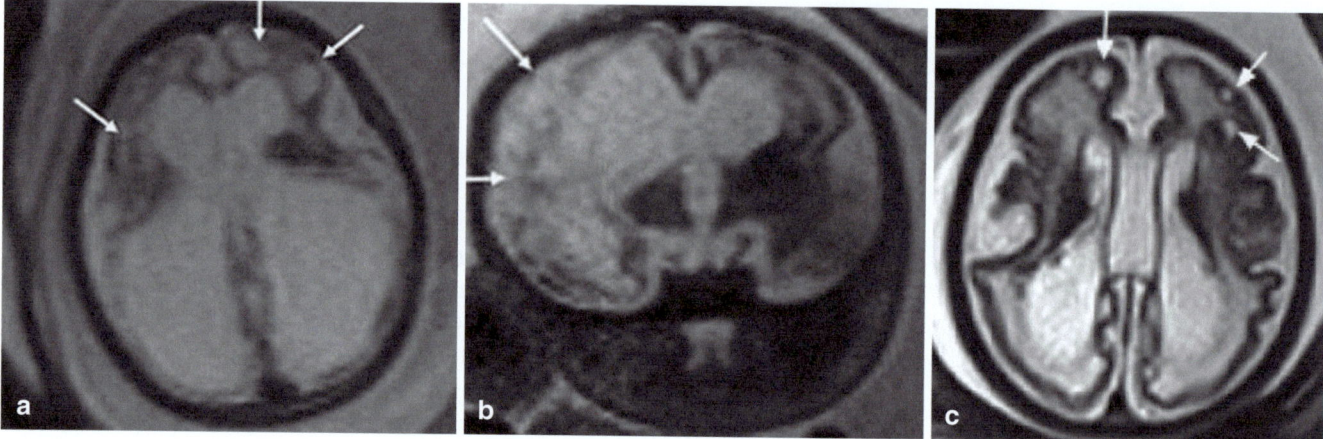

Fig. 10.6 Congenital toxoplasmosis. (**a**, **b**) Axial T2 weighted image from a 32 week fetal MRI shows diffuse, severe white matter destruction with areas of cyst formation (arrows), and ventriculomegaly. (**c**) Axial T2 weighted image shows diffuse white matter destruction and volume loss, subcortical cyst formation and ventriculomegaly

Herpes Simplex Virus

- HSV-1 and HSV-2 are members of the *Herpesviridae* family; the virus's neurotropism is reflected in their tendency to establish latency in neural ganglia and, when reactivated, spread to the CNS in a retrograde manner along the nerves or by diffusion across endothelial cells of cerebral vessels.
- Congenital symptomatic herpes infections are caused by Herpes simplex virus 1 (HSV-1) and Herpes simplex virus 2 (HSV-2), with HSV-2 being the major cause of neonatal herpes meningitis and encephalitis [3].
- Neonatal herpes infection is rare with a prevalence of 1 in 3000 to 10,000 births in the USA [4].
- The most common route of transmission, up to 85%, is in the perinatal period from contact of the fetus with the infected maternal genital tract, with intrauterine infection being extremely rare (<5% of cases).
- Neonatal HSV usually presents in the first 3 weeks after birth and is grouped into three clinical forms: localized to the skin, eyes, and mouth (SEM); central nervous system disease with or without skin involvement, and disseminated disease.
- Disseminated disease may involve the CNS along with multiple other organ systems including the liver, adrenals, GI tract, and skin, eyes, and mouth. If left untreated, disease of the SEM can progress to disseminated disease.

- Up to 50% of infected infants will have CNS disease, which can present with meningitis, encephalitis, seizures, lethargy, irritability, tremors, poor feeding, and temperature liability.

Imaging

- Intrauterine infection can show calcifications, ventriculomegaly, encephalomalacia, and microcephaly.
- Early on, imaging may be normal, especially on ultrasound evaluation.
- Appearance differs greatly from older children and adults. Unlike in older children where the limbic and paralimbic cortex are predominantly involved, neonatal herpes has a more variable, multifocal appearance [1].
- Within the first week of infection, MRI might demonstrate patchy edema and multifocal diffusion restriction in the deep and periventricular white matter, with or without hemorrhage (Fig. 10.7).
- After the initial week diffusion imaging becomes less useful and severe parenchymal destruction rapidly develops, evidenced by subsequent diffuse cystic encephalomalacia, cortical thinning, atrophy, scattered calcifications, and ventricular enlargement (Fig. 10.8).
- Neonatal HSV encephalitis can occasionally involve the brain stem and cerebellum; patchy parenchymal enhancement may also be seen.

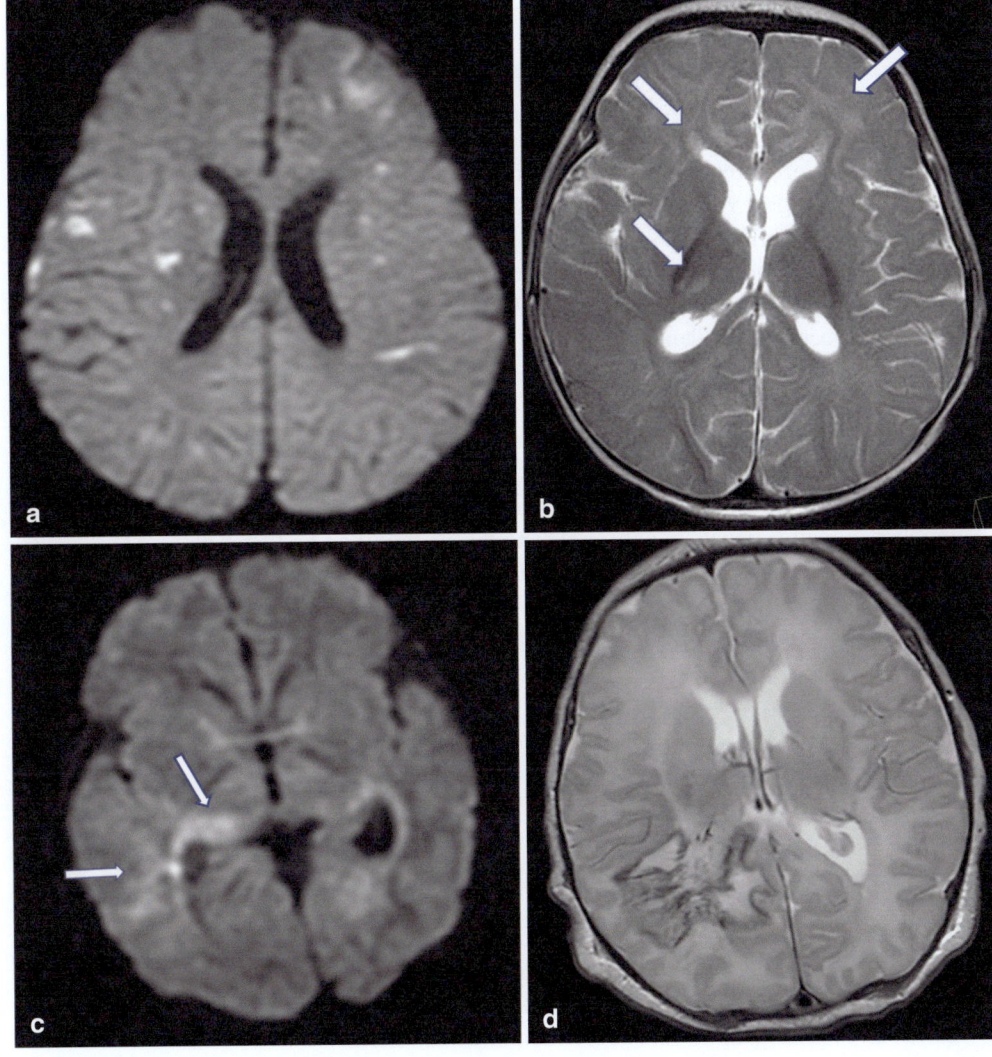

Fig. 10.7 Congenital HSV. (**a**) Axial DWI image shows multifocal restricted diffusion predominantly in the deep white matter. (**b**) Axial T2 weighted image shows confluent areas and patchy discrete foci of edema (arrows). (**c**) Axial DWI image shows patchy areas of diffusion restriction in the right thalamus and right temporal and parietal periventricular white matter (arrows). (**d**) Axial T2 weighted image at the same level shows associated hemorrhage in the area of diffusion restriction

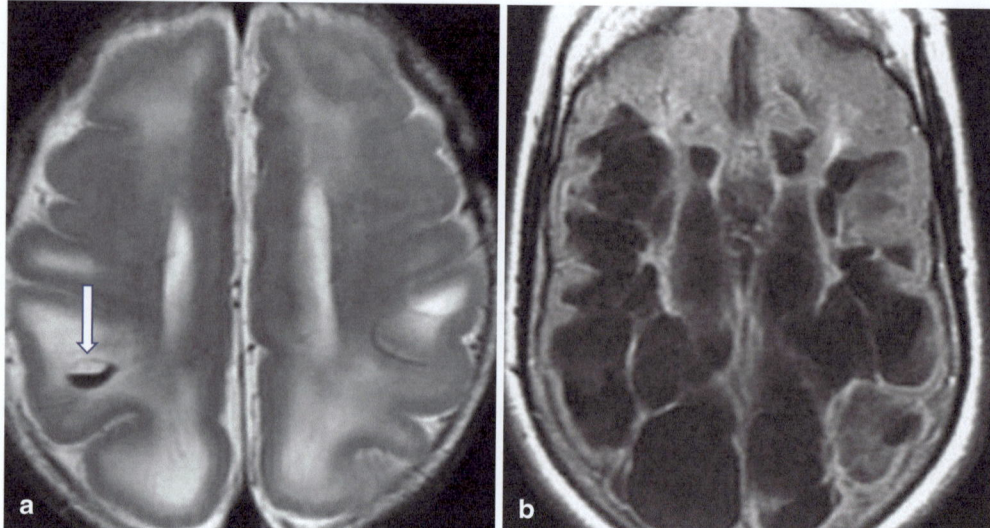

Fig. 10.8 Congenital HSV. (**a**) Axial T2 weighted image shows extensive edema and evolving encephalomalacia with a small focus of hemorrhage seen in the right parietal lobe (arrow). (**b**) Axial FLAIR image shows late stage severe parenchymal destruction with cortical thinning and ventricular enlargement

HIV

- The incidence of perinatal HIV is dramatically decreasing in the USA; in 2015 in the USA only 53 infants were diagnosed with perinatal HIV infection [1].
- Transmission can occur during pregnancy, labor, delivery, or with breast feeding; most perinatal HIV infections are thought to occur during delivery.
- Infants with congenital HIV are often asymptomatic at birth.
- When symptomatic most infants present with diffuse encephalopathy secondary to direct effects of HIV virus infection and immune mediators; other symptoms include lymphadenopathy, hepatomegaly, oral candidiasis, failure to thrive and developmental delay, typically develop after 3 months.
- Neurologic symptoms from HIV encephalitis include spasticity, extremity weakness, microcephalus, and seizures; if left untreated, severe developmental delay and milestone regression develop, and there are high mortality rates, with most children dying by age 5.

Imaging

- The most frequently encountered imaging findings are parenchymal calcifications and global atrophy (Fig. 10.9).
- Calcifications favor the frontal lobe subcortical white matter and basal ganglia and are commonly identified with in utero infection; the burden of calcification positively correlates with viral load.

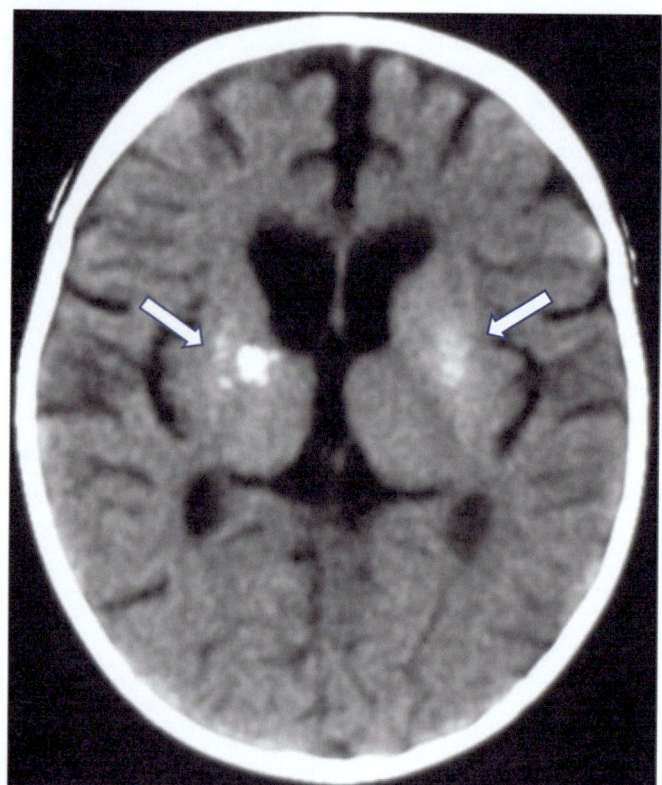

Fig. 10.9 Congenital HIV. Noncontrast axial head CT in a 3 year old child with history of congenital HIV shows global cerebral atrophy and bilateral basal ganglia calcifications (arrows)

Varicella

- Congenital varicella syndrome is caused by Varicella Zoster virus, a member of the Herpesvirus family, and is also extremely rare since the establishment of immunization in 1995 [1].
- Varicella-Zoster can be transmitted in utero, perinatally or postnatally to the infant.
- The in utero transmission rate is low, with a risk of 2% if the infection occurs before 20 weeks' gestation.
- Varicella infections may present with low birth weight due to intrauterine growth retardation.
- Characteristic cicatricial skin scarring might be seen at birth, usually occurring on one or more of the arms or legs, which may be malformed or hypoplastic.
- Ocular defects and gastrointestinal abnormalities might also be present.
- Neurologic sequelae include microcephaly or macrocephaly with hydrocephalus, seizures, and developmental delay including varying degrees of mental retardation.

Imaging

- Brain imaging is nonspecific and not well-defined, possibly reflecting variability secondary to gestational age of infection [5].
- Early infection can result in lobar destruction and basal ganglia necrosis.
- Infection can result in a vasculopathy resulting in arterial infarcts (Fig. 10.10).
- Other brain MRI findings include cerebellar hypoplasia/aplasia, polymicrogyria, and hydrocephalus (Fig. 10.11).

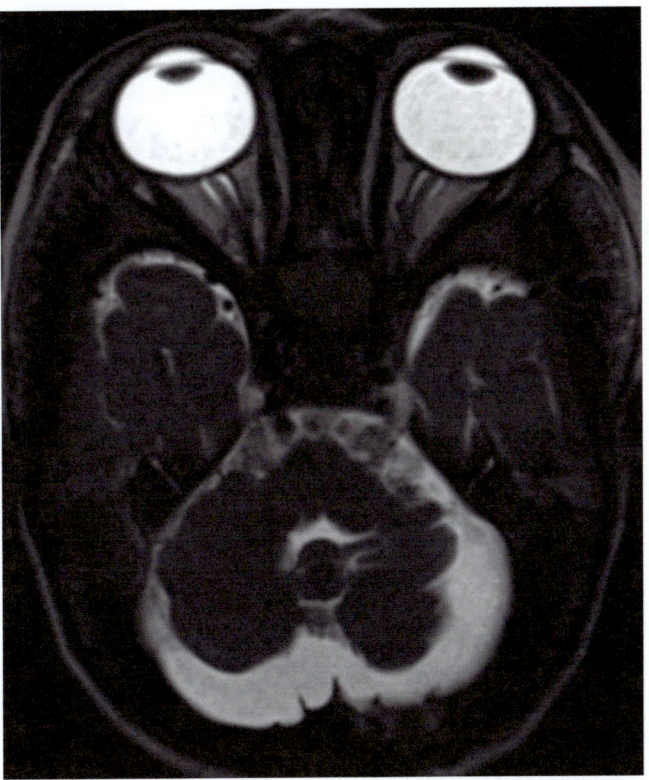

Fig. 10.11 Axial T2 MRI showing bilateral cerebellar hypoplasia in an infant with positive Varicella IgG

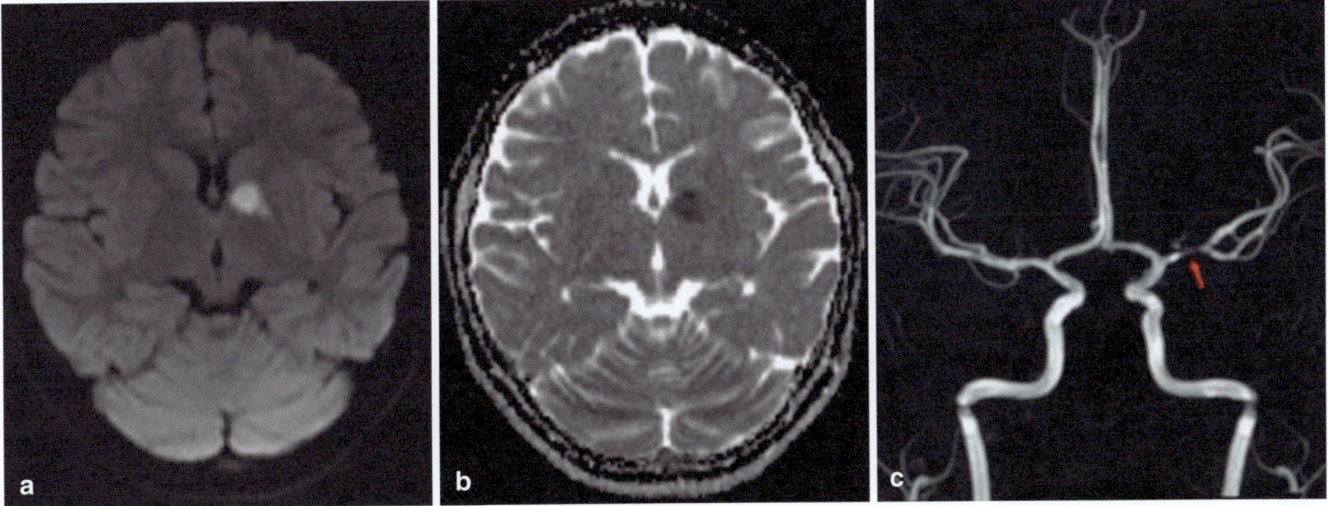

Fig. 10.10 Post-varicella arteriopathy with acute ischemic stroke. (**a**) Axial DWI with (**b**) ADC map showing acute infarct in the left basal ganglia. (**c**) Time of flight MRA showing focal narrowing of the left middle cerebral artery M1 segment secondary to an inflammatory arteriopathy (arrow)

Rubella

- Congenital rubella syndrome (CRS) is caused by the rubella virus; Rubella virus is the only member of the genus Ribivirus, a family of the Togaviridae viruses.
- Congenital rubella syndrome (CRS) is extremely rare in developed countries since the establishment of vaccination programs; the last US epidemic was in the 1960s [1].
- Transmission is via the blood-placental barrier during maternal viremia and has the highest risk of congenital defects when infection occurs in the first 10 weeks of gestation, with fetal damage in up to 90% of infected fetuses.
- Fetuses can show intrauterine growth retardation, hepatosplenomegaly, and postnatally a classic "blueberry muffin" rash is often described, a reflection of extramedullary hematopoiesis.
- Hearing loss, cataracts, glaucoma, cardiac disease, and mental and motor retardation are the most frequently encountered sequelae.
- No direct therapy exists and survivors sometimes develop microcephaly and learning disabilities, presumably the sequelae of meningoencephalitis and vasculitis.

Imaging

- Brain imaging is not specific and has a wide range of appearances [6].
- White matter gliosis or demyelination have been described and seen as patchy frontal predominant white matter hypointensities on CT, and T2 and FLAIR hyperintensities on MRI Brain, similar to that of CMV (Fig. 10.12).
- Periventricular and basal ganglia calcifications, ventriculomegaly and cystic encephalomalacia have also been described, usually without a lobar predominance (Fig. 10.12).
- Early infections, before 10 weeks, and lead to near total brain destruction and microcephaly.

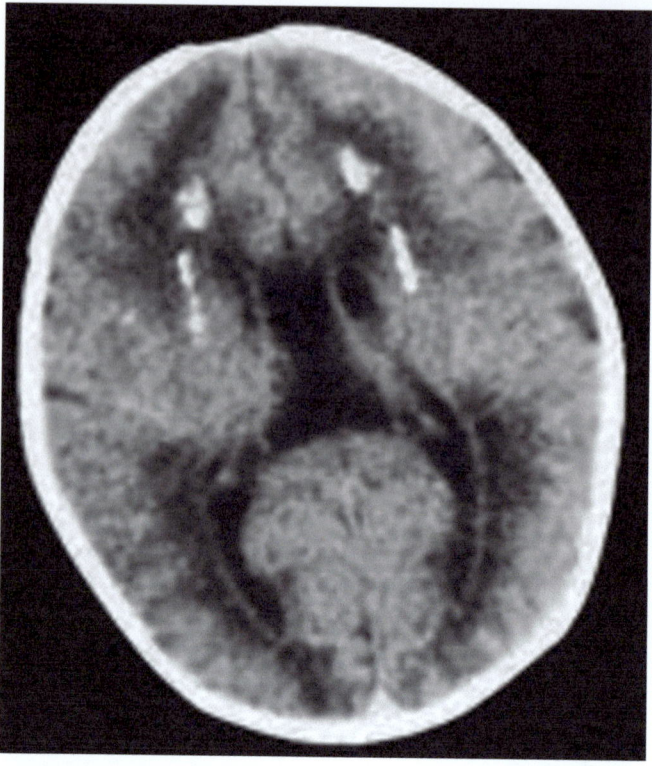

Fig. 10.12 Axial noncontrast head CT of a 2 year old child with history of congenital Rubella showing confluent bilateral white matter hypoattenuation and periventricular calcifications

Enterovirus

- Enteroviruses are a group of viruses that mostly infect humans from the gastrointestinal tract and cause mild symptoms; however several enteroviruses exhibit neurotropism and can invade the central nervous system resulting in various neurological illnesses.
- Of the numerous enteroviruses, Coxsackie B and echovirus are the most common causes of aseptic viral meningitis, often occurring in children [7].

Fig. 10.13 Axial DWI images in 6 week old infant with signs and symptoms of meningoencephalitis and a maternal history of viral illness several weeks prior to delivery, with an enterovirus isolated by CSF culture showing multifocal white matter restricted diffusion

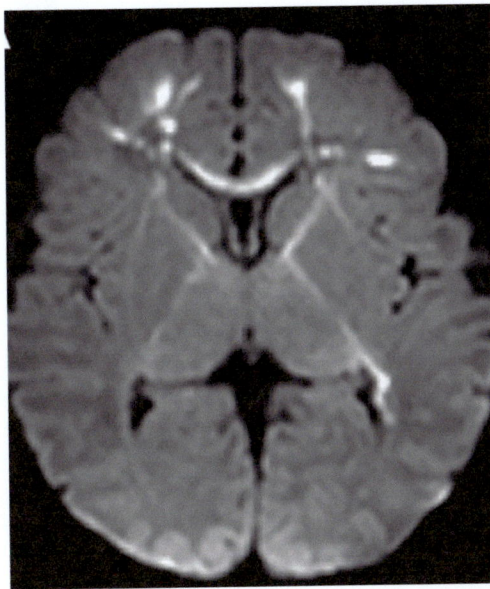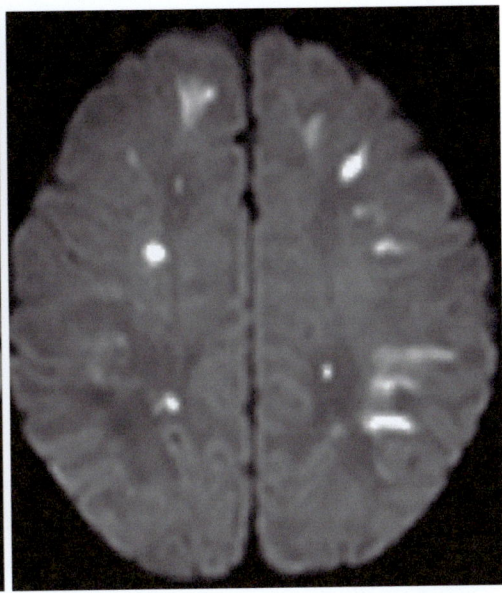

- Acquisition of the virus can sometimes be difficult to ascertain, but maternal illness in the 2 weeks preceding delivery (59–80% of cases in the literature) suggests that the mother is the likely source of infection.
- The route of transmission is either transplacental or from inhalation or swallowing of cervical secretions or feces during delivery.
- Onset of illness at birth is associated with more severe illness and increased mortality, and includes meningitis and meningoencephalitis, cardiomyopathy, and coagulopathy; whereas later onset with 4–14 days post-delivery is associated with milder illness.

Imaging

- Aseptic meningitis in Coxsackie infection is similar to that seen with Herpes simplex meningoencephalitis in that meningeal enhancement is rare.
- Coxsackie B virus has been shown to affect some specific regions: the anterior horn cells of the spinal cord, the medulla and pons, and the cerebellum.
- The most consistently involved structure has been the inferior olivary nucleus.
- Multifocal white matter injury with or without associated hemorrhage may be seen, and may show associated restricted diffusion (Fig. 10.13).

References

1. Neuberger I, Garcia J, Meyers ML, Feygin T, Bulas DI, Mirsky DM. Imaging of congenital central nervous system infections. Pediatr Radiol. 2018;48(4):513–23. https://doi.org/10.1007/s00247-018-4092-1.
2. Fink KR, Thapa MM, Ishak GE, Pruthi S. Neuroimaging of pediatric central nervous system cytomegalovirus infection. Radiographics. 2010;30(7):1779–96. https://doi.org/10.1148/rg.307105043.
3. Leonard JR, Moran CJ, Cross DT, Wippold FJ, Schlesinger Y, Storch GA. MR imaging of herpes simplex type 1 encephalitis in infants and young children: a separate pattern of findings. AJR Am J Roentgenol. 2000;174(6):1651–5. https://doi.org/10.2214/ajr.174.6.1741651.
4. Flagg EW, Weinstock H. Incidence of neonatal herpes simplex virus infections in the United States, 2006. Pediatrics. 2011;127(1):e1–8. https://doi.org/10.1542/peds.2010-0134.
5. Mustonen K, Mustakangas P, Valanne L, Professor MH, Koskiniemi M. Congenital varicella-zoster virus infection after maternal subclinical infection: clinical and neuropathological findings. J Perinatol. 2001;21(2):141–6. https://doi.org/10.1038/sj.jp.7200508.
6. Schneider JF, Hanquinet S, Severino M, Rossi A. MR imaging of neonatal brain infections. Magn Reson Imaging Clin N Am. 2011;19(4):761–75; vii–viii. https://doi.org/10.1016/j.mric.2011.08.013.
7. Bryant PA, Tingay D, Dargaville PA, Starr M, Curtis N. Neonatal coxsackie B virus infection-a treatable disease? Eur J Pediatr. 2004;163(4–5):223–8. https://doi.org/10.1007/s00431-004-1408-y.

Brain Infections

Rosaura Suazo Aguero and Rafael Rojas

Introduction

Infections of the central nervous system (CNS) remain an important cause of morbidity and mortality. Bacterial, viral, parasitic, and fungal pathogens are different microorganisms that affect the brain, spinal cord, or meninges [1]. This chapter discusses the most relevant imaging features related to bacterial, viral, fungal, and parasitic infections.

BACTERIAL AND MYCOBACTERIAL INFECTIONS OF THE BRAIN

Introduction

Bacterial CNS infection is a life-threatening condition. It requires prompt diagnosis and specific treatment because of high mortality and morbidity [2]. In some cases, despite adequate treatment, major complications and sequela can occur. The gold standard in diagnosing bacterial CNS infections is cerebrospinal fluid (CSF) analysis; however imaging is often easier and faster to obtain and can noninvasively allow rapid diagnosis, raise suspicion for specific pathogens, and monitor treatment response [3]. The following subsections discuss the different presentations in bacterial CNS infections.

R. S. Aguero
Tufts Medical Center, Boston, MA, USA
e-mail: rsuazoag@bidmc.harvard.edu

R. Rojas (✉)
Neuroradiology Section, Radiology Department, Harvard Medical School, Beth Israel Deaconess Medical Center, Boston, MA, USA
e-mail: rrojas3@bidmc.harvard.edu

Bacterial Meningitis

- Meningitis (aka pyogenic meningitis or leptomeningitis) involves the diffuse inflammation of the pia mater and arachnoid [2].
- Common causative organisms of meningitis include *group B streptococcus, and Escherichia coli* (newborns), *Haemophilus influenzae* (children younger than 7 years), *Neisseria meningitidis* (older children and adolescents), and *Streptococcus pneumoniae* (leading cause of bacterial meningitis in adults) [1, 4].
- Bacteria may reach the meninges by hematogenous dissemination from distant infection (most common), direct implantation, usually traumatic (e.g., following a lumbar puncture), and local extension (e.g., sinusitis, otitis, mastoiditis, orbital cellulitis, or infected tooth) [4].
- The classic clinical features of meningitis include headache, neck stiffness, high fever, photophobia, followed by mental status changes. Nausea and vomiting, signs of increased intracranial pressure, and nerve palsy are other symptoms that can be seen [5, 6].

Imaging Patterns

- Cross-sectional imaging is not specific for the diagnosis of meningitis [1].
- Non-contrast CT: subtle swelling and effacement of sulcus with slight hyperattenuation [7, 8].
- Postcontrast CT: leptomeningeal enhancement, secondary to inflammatory breakdown of the blood–brain barrier [8].
- Fluid-attenuated inversion recovery (FLAIR) sequence have been reported to be the most sensitive magnetic resonance (MR) technique for the detection of meningeal diseases. Postcontrast 3D T2-FLAIR has been reported to be superior to postcontrast 3D T1-weighted MR imaging [2].
- The nulling of the CSF signal due to the inversion time facilitates an optimized delineation of hyperintense pathology

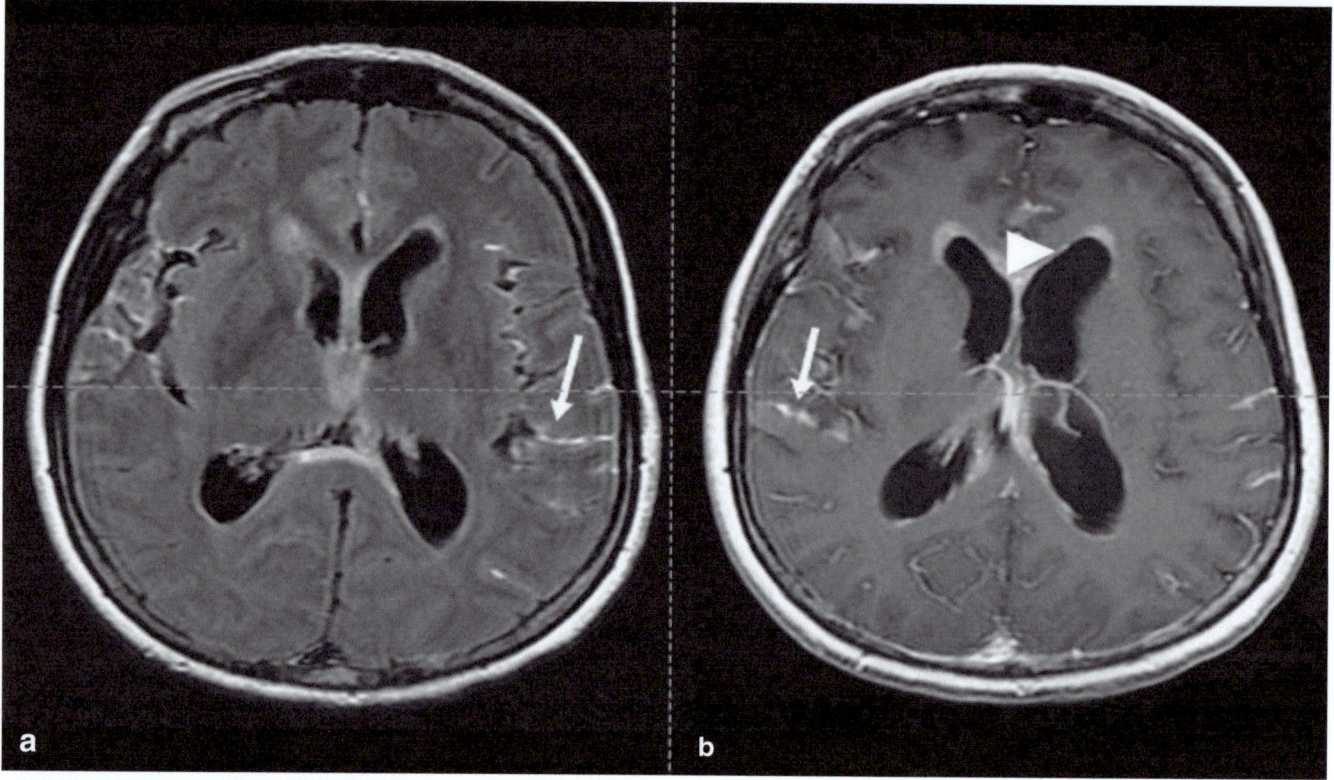

Fig. 11.1 Bacterial meningitis (*Streptococcus pneumoniae* meningitis). (a) Axial FLAIR image demonstrate high signal intensity in the subarachnoid spaces due to high proteinaceous material content within the cerebrospinal fluid (white arrow). (b) Axial T1 post intravenous gadolinium contrast demonstrates sulcal enhancement after contrast administration. There is also periventricular enhancement consistent with ependymitis (white arrow head)

adjacent to the CSF in the sulcal and leptomeningeal space while the T1 shortening in FLAIR sequences is responsible for the highly sensitive delineation of pathologic contrast enhancement following application of gadolinium [3].
- High signal intensity in the subarachnoid spaces seen on FLAIR sequences is due to high proteinaceous material content within the cerebrospinal fluid [2] (Fig. 11.1a).
- Postcontrast sequences demonstrate linear enhancement of the meninges in basal cisterns, sylvian fissure region, and deep within the cortical sulci [2] (Fig. 11.1b).
- In acute meningitis, leptomeningeal enhancement is preferentially located over the cerebral convexity, whereas in chronic meningitis enhancement is most prominent in the basal cisterns [4].
- Contents of purulent meningitis are responsible for areas of restricted diffusion within the CSF spaces on diffusion-weighted imaging (DWI) sequences, specifically in the cortical sulci and in the perivascular spaces or Virchow-Robin spaces (VRS's) [2].
- Ischemic infarctions can be seen in pneumococcal meningitis, commonly located in the corpus callosum and genu of the internal capsule [2].
- Acute pneumococcal meningitis may be accompanied by immunological parainfectious processes, such as acute demyelinating encephalomyelitis (ADEM), cerebral vasculitis, or acute necrotizing hemorrhagic encephalomyelitis [2].

Cerebritis and Brain Abscess

- Cerebritis refers to pyogenic nonencapsulated inflammation of the brain parenchyma and leads to abscess formation if untreated [1].
- It may arise by contiguous infection of the meninges, hematogenous spread of infection or direct extension into the brain [1].
- The early parenchymal infection starts as a cerebritis and then progresses through four stages to form an abscess: early cerebritis (first to third day), late cerebritis with central necrosis formation (fourth to the ninth day), early encapsulation (tenth to the 13th day), and late capsule stage or mature abscess (14th day and forward) [5, 7].
- Brain abscess is a focal, intracerebral infection that begin with a localized region of cerebritis, evolving into a discrete collection of pus surrounded by a well-vascularized capsule [5].

- Commonly located at the gray matter–white matter junction, mostly in the frontal and temporal lobes [9].
- The most common organisms involved in brain abscesses include Staphylococcus and Streptococcus species [5].
- Clinical manifestations include seizures, nausea, headache, and vomiting. Focal neurologic signs depend on the region of brain involved [2].

Imaging Patterns

- Early cerebritis stage:
  - Noncontrast CT: area of ill-defined low attenuation.
  - Postcontrast CT: variable pattern of contrast enhancement ranging from no enhancement to nodular or ring-like enhancement.
  - MR: nonspecific poorly defined hyperintensity on T2-weighted sequence that is isointense to mildly hypointense on T1-weighted images, with ill-defined enhancement [5, 7].
- Late cerebritis stage:
  - Noncontrast CT: poorly defined low-attenuation edema.
  - Postcontrast CT: thick ringlike or nodular enhancement that is stable or increases on delayed images.
  - MR: The low T1-weighted signal becomes better demarcated with high T2 signal, both in the cavity and surrounding parenchyma [5, 7].
- Early and late encapsulation stages:
  - Noncontrast CT: the pus containing central region appears as a well-defined area of low attenuation with a subtle surrounding capsule ring.
  - Postcontrast CT: ring enhancement is seen. The medial or ventricular wall of the abscess cavity may be thinner than the lateral wall, attributed to differences in capsule blood supply.
  - MR: necrotic center of a mature brain abscess includes fluid hyperintense relative to CSF and hypointense relative to white matter on the T1-weighted sequence. On T2-weighted and FLAIR sequences, the fluid in the abscess cavity is iso- to hyperintense to CSF and gray matter. The abscess capsule, a smooth circumferential ring is iso- to hyperintense to white matter on the T1 sequence, iso- to hypointense on the T2-weighted sequence and enhances on postcontrast images. Vasogenic edema surrounding the abscess cavity is characterized by surrounding hypointensity on the T1-weighted sequence and hyperintensity on the T2-weighted sequence. The central nonenhancing region of an abscess usually demonstrates restricted diffusion, this finding is very useful to narrow the diagnosis in an abscess formation. Figure 11.2 demonstrates the different stages of cerebritis and abscess formation.
  - On susceptibility-weighted MR imaging (SWI), pyogenic brain abscesses demonstrate the "dual-rim sign," defined as two concentric rims surrounding the central cavity at the lesion margins, with the outer one hypointense and the inner one hyperintense relative to the cavity contents.
  - MR spectroscopy (MRS): necrotic centers lack the normal brain metabolites of N-acetyl aspartate (NAA), choline, and creatine. Elevated levels of cytosolic

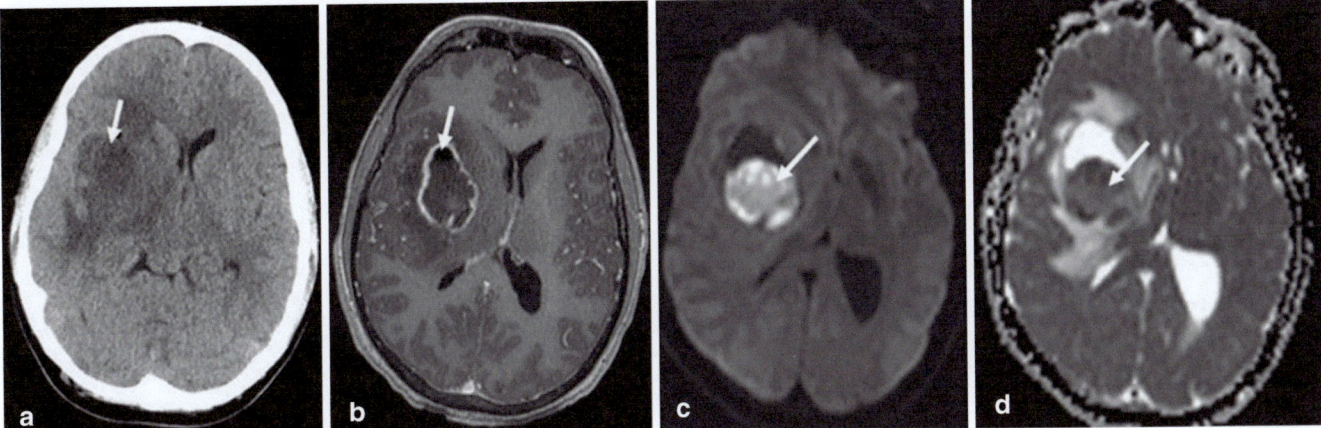

Fig. 11.2 Cerebral abscess. (**a**) Early stage, CT axial image without contrast, showing an ill-defined subcortical area of vasogenic edema, and moderate mass effect causing narrowing of the right lateral ventricle (white arrow). (**b**) late encapsulation stage axial postcontrast T1-weighted image in the encapsulation stage demonstrates a right subcortical ring enhancing lesion with underlying necrotic changes surrounded by vasogenic edema (white arrow). Please note that the differential diagnosis for a brain abscess is broad and may mimic a tumor or metastasis, among other entities such as resolving hematoma, tumefactive demyelinating lesions. (**c**) MRI axial diffusion DWI, and (**d**) MRI axial apparent diffusion coefficient (ADC) maps demonstrate restricted diffusion (white arrows), helping to narrow the differential diagnosis for an abscess formation

amino acids and lactate with or without acetate and succinate are identified. Disappearance of the elevated peaks of amino acids has been documented during successful treatment of brain abscesses.
- MR Perfusion: brain abscess demonstrates low relative cerebral blood volume (rCBV), while necrotic brain tumors have elevated rCBV [1–3, 5, 7, 9].
- Differential diagnoses include abscesses of other etiologies, high-grade primary central nervous system (CNS) neoplasm, metastasis, infarct, hematoma, thrombosed giant aneurysm, radiation necrosis, and demyelinating disease [2].
- Imaging features favoring abscess include:
  - 2–7 mm continuous smooth thin rim of enhancement.
  - T2 hyperintense rim.
  - thinning along the medial wall. 29

Ventriculitis

- Ventriculitis is an inflammation of the ependyma of the ventricular system with accumulation of suppurative fluid in the ventricles.
- It has been variably referred to as ependymitis, intraventricular abscess, ventricular empyema, and pyocephalus.
- Possible routes of intraventricular infectious spread include direct implantation secondary to trauma or neurosurgical procedures, contiguous extension, such as rupture of a brain abscess and extension into the ventricles and hematogenous spread to the subependyma or the choroid plexus.
- The pathogens that most frequently cause pyogenic ventriculitis are gram-negative bacteria and Staphylococcus species.
- Clinical signs and symptoms may be subtle, and the course can be indolent [1, 6–8, 10].

Imaging Patterns

- Noncontrast CT: increased ventricular density, with fluid-debris levels in the dependent portions of the ventricles, corresponding to the intraventricular pus, with possible loculation and even resulting in hydrocephalus. The walls of the ventricle are usually thickened from concurrent ependymitis. Periventricular cerebral edema usually causes low density of the parenchyma.
- Postcontrast CT: enhancement of the ventricular walls and enhancement within any juxta ventricular cerebritis or abscess.
- MR: dependent debris with air-fluid levels on T2-weighted and FLAIR sequences, ependymal thickening and enhancement, hydrocephalus, periventricular hyperintensity from the hydrocephalus and/or periventricular inflammation, and leptomeningeal signal abnormality and enhancement reflecting concurrent meningitis. Restricted diffusion is seen in the dependent purulent intraventricular fluid with ADC values significantly lower than in the white matter (Fig. 11.3) [1, 6–8, 10].

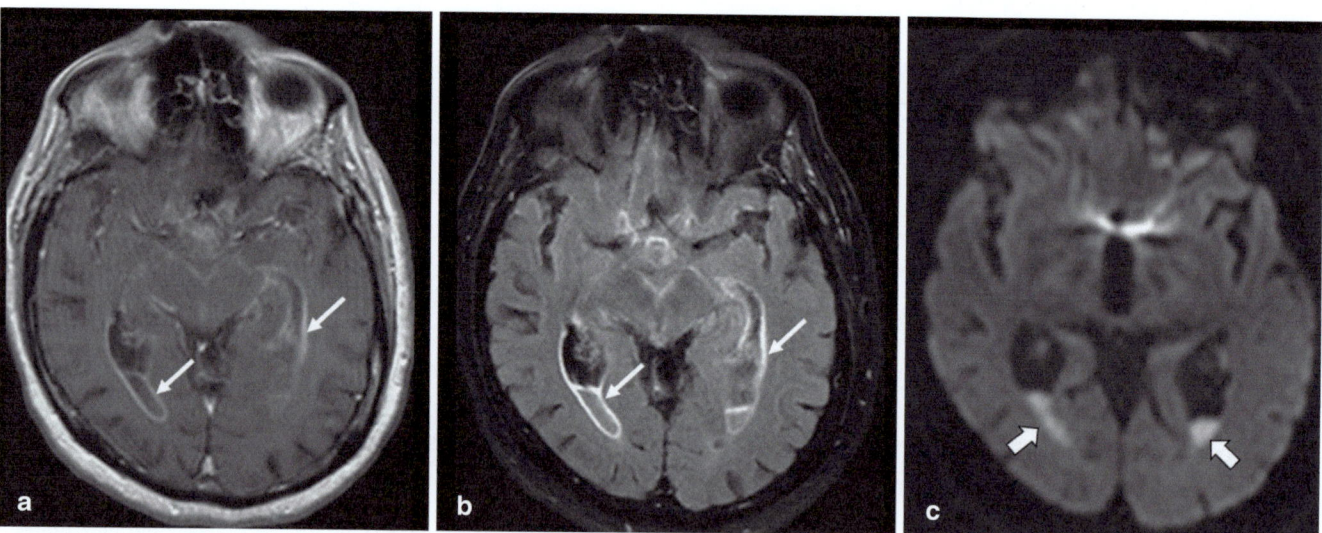

Fig. 11.3 Ventriculitis. (**a**) Axial T1 and (**b**) axial FLAIR MRI images with intravenous gadolinium contrast at the level of the midbrain, demonstrate subependymal enhancement surrounding the occipital horns of the lateral ventricles (white arrows), and bilateral fluid levels layering in the occipital ventricular horns bilaterally, (**c**) axial MRI diffusion-weighted image (DWI), demonstrates restricted diffusion in the occipital ventricular horns bilaterally, which is characteristic of ventriculitis and purulent intraventricular material (white arrows)

11 Brain Infections

Empyema

- Extra fluid may collect in the subdural and epidural spaces. These fluid collections can be found over the convexities or inter-hemispherically.
- Usually caused by retrograde thrombophlebitis via the skull emissary veins from an infected area nearby [1, 8, 10, 11].

Imaging Patterns

- CT: epidural empyema characteristically appears as lenticular and subdural empyema as crescentic-shaped fluid collections slightly denser than cerebrospinal fluid.
- MR: higher signal than cerebrospinal fluid on T1-weighted and FLAIR images because of higher concentrations of proteins. On enhanced T1-weighted images, the verge of empyema also enhanced. On DWI, the empyema shows higher signal and low ADC values like in an abscess (Fig. 11.4) [1, 8, 10, 11].

Tuberculosis

- CNS Tuberculosis (TB) involvement is a serious manifestation of chronic infection and includes meningitis, intracranial tuberculoma, abscess, vasculitis, ischemia and spinal tuberculous arachnoiditis [5].
- CNS infection usually occurs secondary to hematogenous spread from distant pulmonary infection or less frequently via contiguous spread from adjacent bone infection [2, 12].
- Tuberculomas are the most common intracranial lesions that develop from deep seated tubercles acquired during bacillaemia [5, 9].
- Patients typically present with classic meningitis symptoms, stiff neck, confusion, fevers, headache, lethargy, and meningismus [2, 12].

Tuberculous meningitis

- Tuberculous meningitis is mostly due to the hematogenous spread of *Mycobacterium tuberculosis* [13, 14].
- It can also occur secondary to extension and/or rupture of a subpial or subependymal focus into the subarachnoid spaces or into the ventricular system [13, 14].

Imaging Patterns

- Noncontrast CT: obliteration of the basal cisterns by isodense or mildly hyperdense exudates [13, 14].
- Postcontrast CT: enhancing exudate in the basal cisterns and leptomeningeal enhancement [7, 14, 15].
- MR: FLAIR hyperintense subarachnoid spaces and cisterns at the base of the brain (interpeduncular fossa, suprasellar, peri mesencephalic, and pontine cisterns). Intense leptomeningeal enhancement on postcontrast T1WI or postcontrast FLAIR. High signal within the brain parenchyma on T2WI and FLAIR secondary to edema [2, 7, 13, 15].
- Chronic tuberculous infection may cause pachymeningitis, with focal or diffuse dural thickening [2].
- Possible complications include progressive hydrocephalus (communicating and non-communicating), vasculitis, infarction, and cranial neuropathies [2, 12, 15].
- The differential diagnosis of tuberculous meningitis includes nontuberculous bacterial meningitis, sarcoidosis, and neoplastic meningitis[2] (Figs. 11.5 and 11.6).

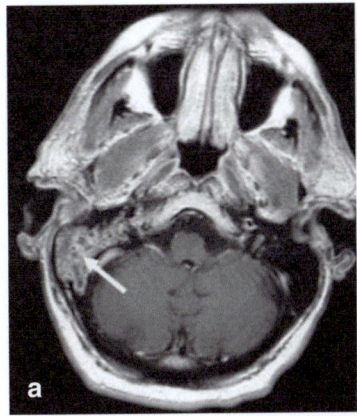
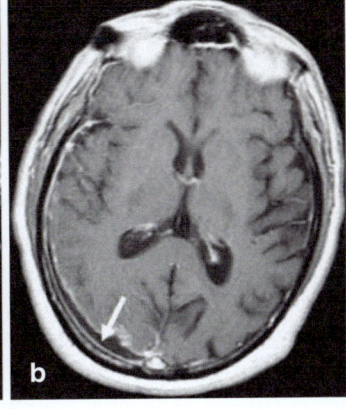
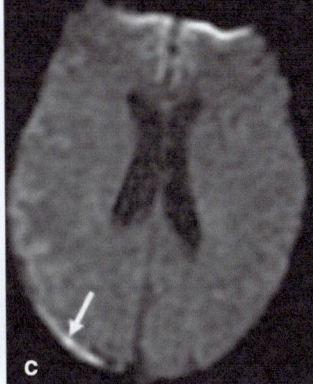
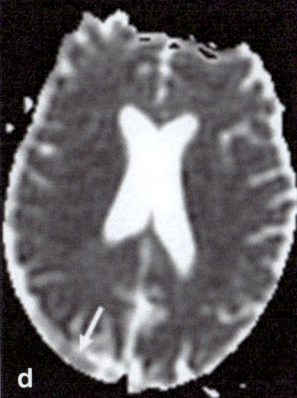

Fig. 11.4 Empyema. Right otomastoiditis producing a right temporo-occipital empyema. (**a**) MRI axial T1 post gadolinium intravenous contrast image demonstrates almost complete opacification of the right mastoid air cells, consistent with otomastoiditis (white arrow). (**b**) MRI axial T1 post gadolinium intravenous contrast demonstrating an extra-axial subdural fluid collection (white arrow). (**c**) MRI axial diffusion DWI, and (**d**) MRI axial apparent diffusion coefficient (ADC) maps demonstrate restricted diffusion within the right subdural collection (white arrows), which is characteristic of empyema and differentiates it from a simple subdural collection

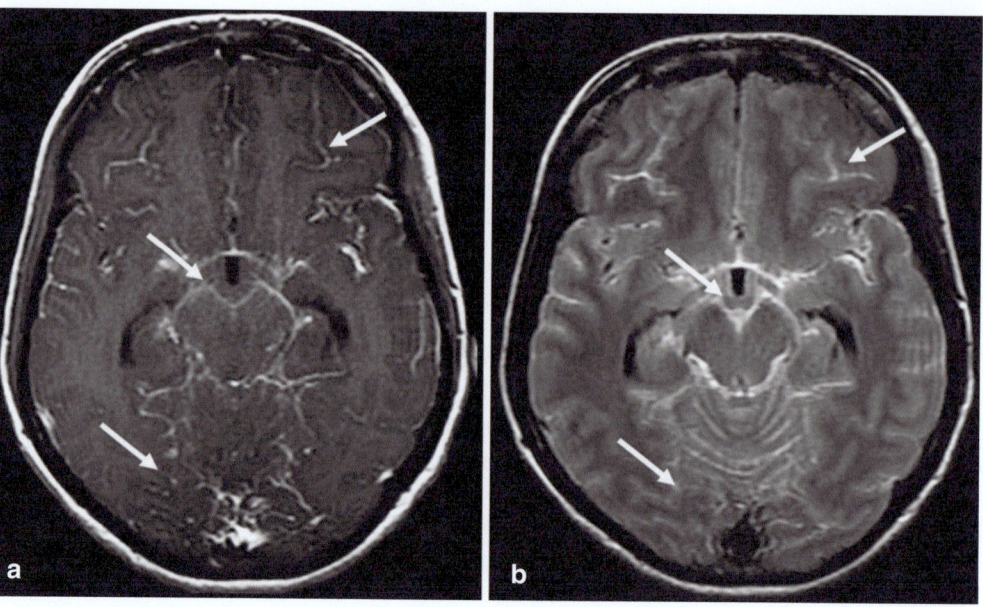

Fig. 11.5 Tuberculosis meningitis. (**a**) Axial T1 postcontrast MRI demonstrates subtle diffuse enhancement of the peri-mesencephalic cisterns and mild enhancement in the subarachnoid spaces of the right cerebellar folia, and left frontal lobe (white arrows). (**b**) Axial postcontrast FLAIR images show similar pattern of subtle enhancement in the same areas (white arrows), consistent with tuberculous meningitis

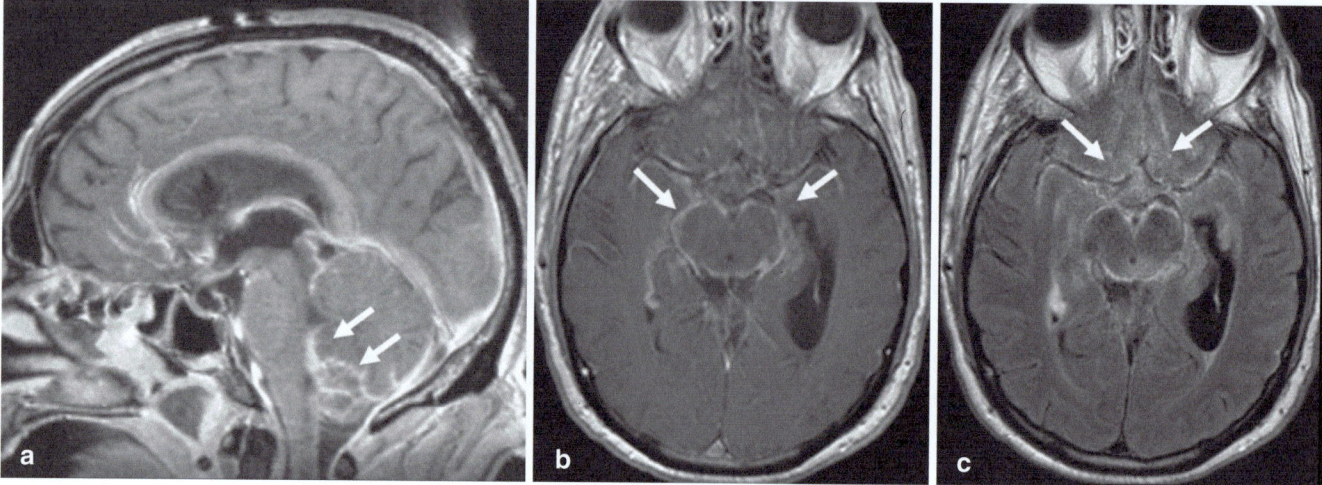

Fig. 11.6 Tuberculosis meningitis. (**a**) Sagittal postcontrast T1W image demonstrates diffuse enhancement (white arrows), in the posterior fossa. (**b**) Axial postcontrast T1W image shows significant enhancement in the peri-mesencephalic cisterns. (**c**) Axial postcontrast FLAIR image shows significant enhancement in the subarachnoid space of the basal frontal regions. These findings were consistent with tuberculous meningitis

Parenchymal Tuberculosis

Tuberculoma

- Tuberculous granuloma (tuberculoma) is the most common parenchymal form of CNS TB and can be solitary or multiple focal brain lesions [2, 16].
- Common locations include the corticomedullary junction, the basal ganglia, and the cerebellum [2, 16].
- Intraventricular tuberculomas are mostly reported in children and are extremely rare in adults [2].
- The mature tuberculoma is composed of a necrotic caseous center surrounded by a capsule [13].

Imaging Patterns

- Noncontrast CT: isodense, hyperdense, or of mixed density. Sometimes healed tuberculomas appear as calcified foci on nonenhanced CT, for example, calcification in the basal cisterns [13, 16].
- Postcontrast CT: pattern of ring-like enhancement or, less likely, as an area of nodular or irregular nonhomogeneous enhancement. A central nidus of calcification with surrounding ring-like enhancement, known as the target sign, suggests the diagnosis [5, 7, 13].
- MR: mixed, predominantly low signal intensity lesion with a central zone of high signal intensity (caseating

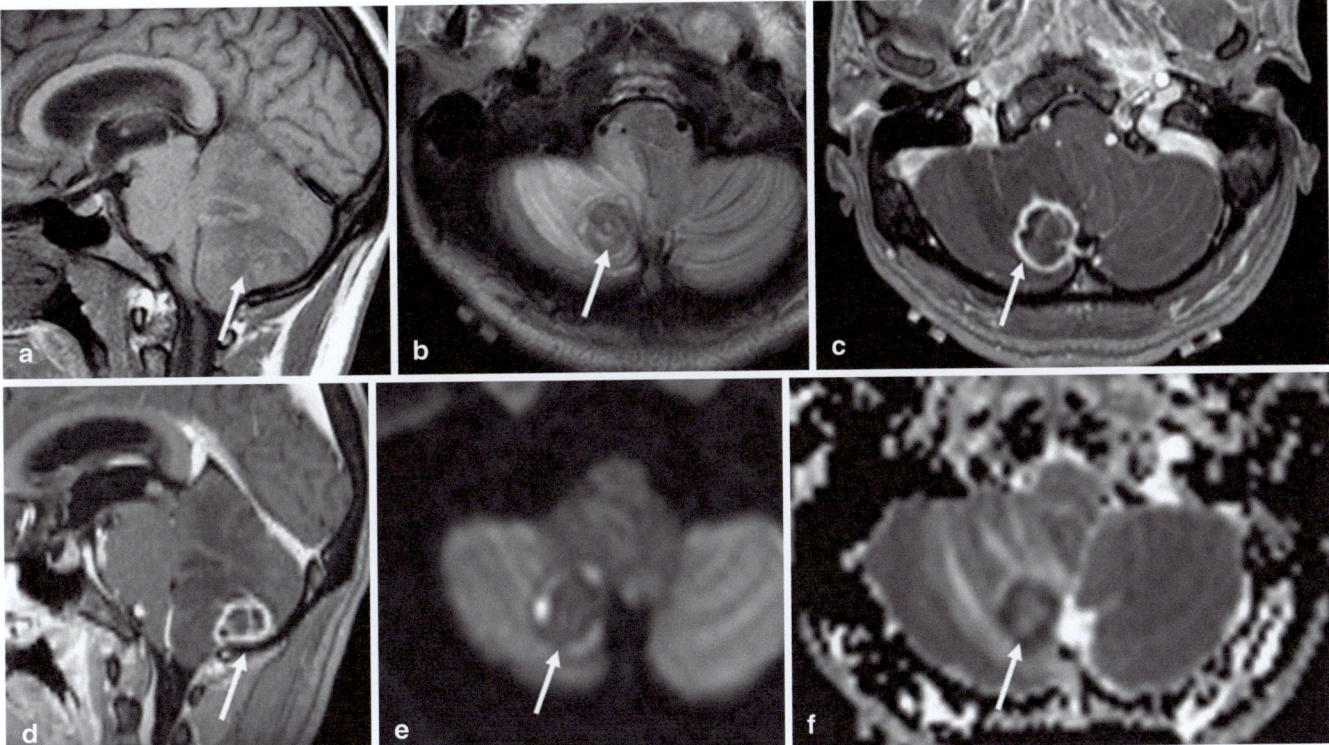

Fig. 11.7 Tuberculoma. (**a**) Precontrast sagittal T1-weighted MRI image of the posterior fossa demonstrates an ill-defined area of low signal in the cerebellum. (**b**) Axial T2-weighted image demonstrates low signal on T2 (arrow), (which is characteristic for solid caseation), surrounded by vasogenic edema in the right cerebellar hemisphere. Axial (**c**) and sagittal (**d**) T1 postcontrast images demonstrate slightly irregular ring enhancement pattern of this lesion with peripheral restricted diffusion on DWI (**e**) and ADC maps (**f**)

necrosis) and surrounding high signal intensity edema on T2-weighted or FLAIR images. Postcontrast MR images usually show a pattern of ring-like enhancement. These lesions may be single or multiple. Noncaseating granulomas are usually hypointense to isointense on T1-weighted and hyperintense on T2-weighted images. Homogeneous enhancement is seen after administration of contrast media. On DWI, caseating tuberculomas with a T2 high-signal-intensity center (lipid) show restricted diffusion and cannot be differentiated from bacterial abscesses, whereas caseating tuberculomas with a T2-low-signal-intensity (solid) center have elevated diffusion. The iso- to hypointensity in T1- and T2-weighed images is characteristic of solid caseation [2, 5, 7, 9, 16] (Fig. 11.7).
- MR Spectroscopy: lipid level peaks in lesions with a T2 hypointense center, whereas those with heterogeneous appearance reveal a choline peak in addition to lipid.[2]

Cerebritis and Abscess

- Parenchymal tuberculosis may occur with or without accompanying meningitis.
- Tuberculosis cerebritis or abscess may have an appearance similar to that of pyogenic bacterial infection.
- Tuberculous abscess is rare and is characterized by a central area of liquefaction with pus. It may be solitary or multiple and is frequently multiloculated [13].

Imaging Patterns

- CT: tuberculous abscess is hypodense with peripheral edema and mass effect [13].
- MR: focal tuberculous cerebritis is very rare, with T1 hypointense and T2 hyperintense signal with patchy enhancement on postcontrast images. TB abscesses are solitary, multiloculated masses, usually >3 cm in diameter, with central necrosis demonstrating increased T2 signal with thick enhancement and perilesional edema with mass effect. There is restricted diffusion on DWI with associated low apparent diffusion coefficient (ADC) values [5, 7, 13, 17].
- MR spectroscopy: lipid, lactate, and phosphoserine peaks without evidence of cytosolic amino acids.[2, 3]

Miliary Tuberculosis

- Miliary tuberculosis is seen mostly in severely immunocompromised patients.

- Usually associated with meningeal involvement or extracranial primary sites.
- The lesions are usually located at the corticomedullary junctions (hematogenous spread) [2, 18].

Imaging Patterns

- CT: occasionally small hypodensities.
- MR: tiny (2–3 mm in diameter) scattered lesions that may be invisible or seen as T2 hypointense lesions on noncontrast MR sequences. Postcontrast T1-weighted MR images show numerous, round, small, homogeneous, enhancing (usually ring enhancement) lesions. Invisible lesions that may or may not enhance can be clearly visible on magnetization transfer spin echo T1-weighted imaging [2, 18, 19].

Tuberculous Encephalopathy

- Typically seen in children.
- Clinical presentation may include seizures, stupor, and coma with no signs of meningeal irritation or focal neurological deficit [2, 13].

Imaging Patterns

- Cerebral edema, unilateral or bilateral.
- CT: Hypodensity.
- MR: Hyperintensity on T2-weighted images [2, 13].

Calvarial Tuberculosis

- Rare, commonly involves the frontal and parietal bones, followed by the occipital and sphenoid bones [2, 13].

Imaging Patterns

- CT: Bone destruction.
- MR: Bone marrow signal abnormality with enhancing soft tissue masses [2, 13].

VIRAL AND PRION INFECTIONS OF THE BRAIN

Introduction

Viral infections involving the CNS may result in a wide variety of agents and can take the form of meningitis, encephalitis, encephalomyelitis, and encephalomyeloradiculitis (spinal cord and nerve roots). In humans, viruses may gain access via bodily fluids (saliva, blood, urine, feces, semen, and mucosal secretions). Cerebrospinal fluid (CSF) exam is invariably performed and serves a dual purpose of excluding a nonviral infection. CSF profile in viral meningitis reflects lymphocyte predominant pleocytosis (25–500 cells/μL) with normal to mildly elevated protein (20–80 mg/dL) and normal glucose. Neuroimaging findings in viral CNS infections is nonspecific, in certain cases it may be suggestive of some pathogens but often have considerable overlap among various microorganisms [20, 21].

In 1982, prions were described as particles lacking nucleic acid and therefore not reported as virus. Prions produce characteristic neuroimaging findings that are distinct from those seen in most viral infections [21].

Human Herpesvirus

- Human Herpesvirus (HHVs) represent a large group of DNA viruses categorized by molecular features.
- α viruses are represented by herpes simplex virus type 1 (HSV-1) and type 2 (HSV-2), B virus, and varicella zoster virus.
- β viruses include cytomegaloviruses, HHV-6, and HHV-7.
- γ viruses include Epstein-Barr virus and HHV-8.
- Herpes simplex is the most common cause of viral encephalitis (mainly by HSV-1 in adults and HSV-2 in neonates) that can occur secondary to neuronal transmission or by hematogenous spread.
- Patients can present with focal neurologic deficits, seizures, headache, and fever.
- Herpes simplex encephalitis (HSE) typically affects the limbic system, specifically the medial temporal lobe (unilateral more frequent bilateral), but also the insular cortex, cingulate and orbital surface of the frontal lobes [2, 7, 17, 20–22].

Imaging Patterns

HSV-1

- Noncontrast CT: normal findings within the first 72 h. Afterward, low attenuation and mass effect in the affected areas. Occasionally, hemorrhage can be seen [5].
- Postcontrast CT: patchy or gyriform enhancement and sulcal effacement of the temporal lobes in the late acute and/or subacute stage of HSE [5].
- MR: Typically, there is sparing of the deep gray nuclei.
  ○ Acute phase: nonenhancing T1-hypointense and T2WI/FLAIR hyperintense lesions characteristically including both the cortex and white matter of the affected regions. DWI is the most sensitive sequence for detecting restricted diffusion involving the medial and inferior aspects of temporal lobe, cingulate gyrus, and insula.

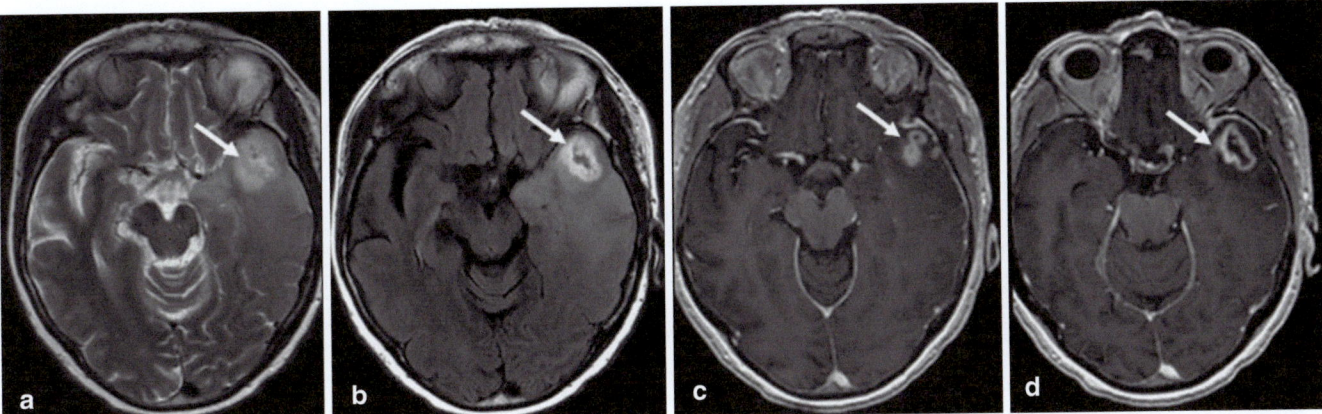

Fig. 11.8 Herpes encephalitis. (a) Axial T2-weighted MR image showing high signal intensity within the left temporal lobe with small internal foci of low signal (white arrow), (b) Axial FLAIR image demonstrates extensive vasogenic edema (arrow) and narrowing of the left peri-mesencephalic cistern, causing mild uncal herniation. (c, d) Axial T1 post-gadolinium intravenous contrast images, demonstrate regions of nodular enhancement and a ring-enhancing lesion in the left temporal lobe (white arrows)

- o Subacute phase: cortical swelling with loss of the gray-white junction. Parenchymal or leptomeningeal enhancement can be seen with patchy or gyriform pattern [2] (Fig. 11.8).
- Susceptibility artifact in gradient echo sequences is secondary to hemorrhage [7, 22].
- MR perfusion: increased rCBV and relative cerebral blood flow (rCBF).
- MR spectroscopy: may show a decreased NAA peak and/or increased lactate peak [9].
- Differential diagnoses include acute ischemia/infarction, status epilepticus, autoimmune limbic encephalitis, and diffuse infiltrating glioma [20].

HSV-2

- MR: parenchymal T2 hyperintensities with restricted diffusion and variable contrast enhancement [2, 20].
- Multifocal involvement of supratentorial gray and white matter, thalami, basal ganglia, and the posterior fossa with areas of restricted diffusion and hemorrhage progressing to parenchymal or gyral calcifications, cystic encephalomalacia, and atrophy [20].

Cytomegalovirus

- Most common congenital encephalitis and also affecting immunosuppressed adults [23].
- CNS manifestations include parenchymal necrosis, calcifications, volume loss, migrational anomalies, ventriculomegaly, microcephaly, and white matter disease [20].
- Focal neurologic signs include nystagmus, ataxia, and cranial nerve palsies [7].
- Congenital cytomegalovirus infection is discussed in Chap. 10.

Imaging Patterns

- CT: periventricular hyperdensities (coarse calcifications).
- MR: calcifications as blooming artifact in gradient echo images.
- Migrational anomalies include lissencephaly, pachygyria, polymicrogyria, or schizencephaly.
- White matter changes, predominantly posterior/parietal white matter T2 prolongation with sparing of the immediately periventricular white matter and associated with anterior temporal cysts.
- Hemorrhage and necrosis may occur [2, 7, 20, 21].

Polyomavirus or John Cunningham Virus (JC Virus)

- Reactivation causes Progressive Multifocal Encephalopathy (PML), which is progressive demyelination of the white matter seen in immunocompromised patients, most commonly in acquired immunodeficiency syndrome (AIDS).
- PML may present with focal neurological symptoms such as muscle weakness, sensory deficit, hemianopia, cognitive dysfunction, aphasia, coordination, and/or gait difficulties and seizures.
- Bilateral, asymmetric periventricular and subcortical white matter lesions, including the subcortical U fibers, usually in the frontal and parieto-occipital regions.
- In late stages, there may be involvement of the basal ganglia, thalamus, brainstem, and cerebellar gray matter [5, 8, 17, 20].

Imaging Patterns

- CT: nonenhancing asymmetric periventricular and subcortical white matter hypodensities, with no mass effect.
- MR: subcortical white matter lesions with high signal on FLAIR and T2WI, very low signal on T1WI, no or minimal peripheral contrast enhancement. Peripheral patchy restricted diffusion on DWI.
- Punctate T2 hyperintensities, and the presence of SWI hypointensities within the adjacent gray matter, can suggest the diagnosis.
- MR spectroscopy: increased choline and myo-inositol, decreased NAA, and presence of lactate and lipid peaks [2, 5, 8, 17, 20].
- PML–immune reconstitution inflammatory syndrome (PML-IRIS): begins 1 week to 2 years after establishment of immune surveillance consisting of paradoxical deterioration, with transient clinical worsening. MR images demonstrate development of edema and transient contrast enhancement at the sites of previously documented PML lesions [2, 7] (Fig. 11.9).

Coronavirus

- Since December 2019, an outbreak of coronavirus 2019 (COVID 19) has rapidly spread around the world to become a pandemic.
- Severe respiratory illness is the predominant presentation; however, it has been reported to affect multiple organ systems, including the CNS.

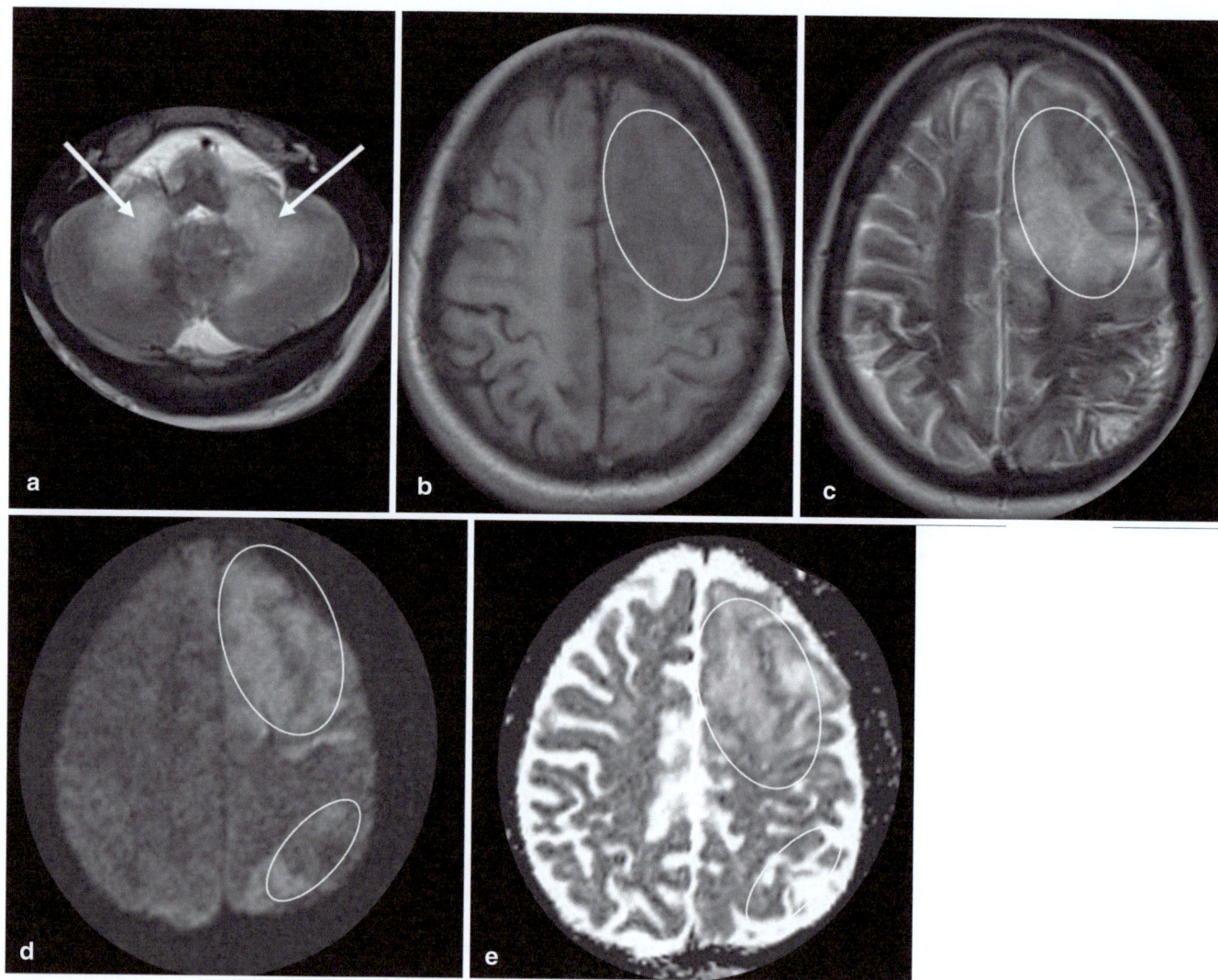

Fig. 11.9 Progressive multifocal encephalopathy, immune reconstitution inflammatory syndrome (**PML-IRIS**). (**a**) Axial T2-weighted image shows bilateral areas of high signal in the middle cerebellar peduncles (white arrows). Axial T1- (**b**) and axial T2- (**c**) weighted images demonstrate edema and mild effacement of the sulci on the left with no mass effect (white ellipsoids). DWI (**d**) and ADC maps (**e**) demonstrate high signal intensity on both sequences consistent with T2 shine through effect, indicating that there is no restricted diffusion

- Neurologic involvement is frequently secondary to direct viral effects, para-infectious immune response to the virus, postinfectious delayed immune response, and/or complications of prolonged hospitalization.
- COVID 19 neurologic manifestations are nonspecific and may include headache, agitation, confusion, paresthesia, generalized muscle weakness, delirium, and altered mental status [24–27].

Imaging Patterns

- Variety of neuroimaging features (Fig. 11.10), including:
  o Ischemic infarcts (large vessel, small vessel, and watershed infarcts), frequently with hemorrhagic transformation.
  o Intracranial hemorrhage (ICH) in non-hypertension-associated locations (lobar, cortical, and/or subarachnoid) and microbleeds (callosal and juxtacortical).
  o Cerebral venous and sinus thrombosis (CVST): sigmoid and transverse sinus thrombosis as well as involvement of the deep cerebral veins.
  o Leukoencephalopathy: nonspecific finding demonstrating symmetric confluent white matter T2 hyperintensity and restricted diffusion, with relative sparing of juxtacortical and infratentorial white matter.
  o Posterior reversal encephalopathy syndrome (PRES): vasogenic edema, manifested by hyperintensity on FLAIR images in occipital lobes, posterior temporal lobes, and the cerebellar hemispheres.

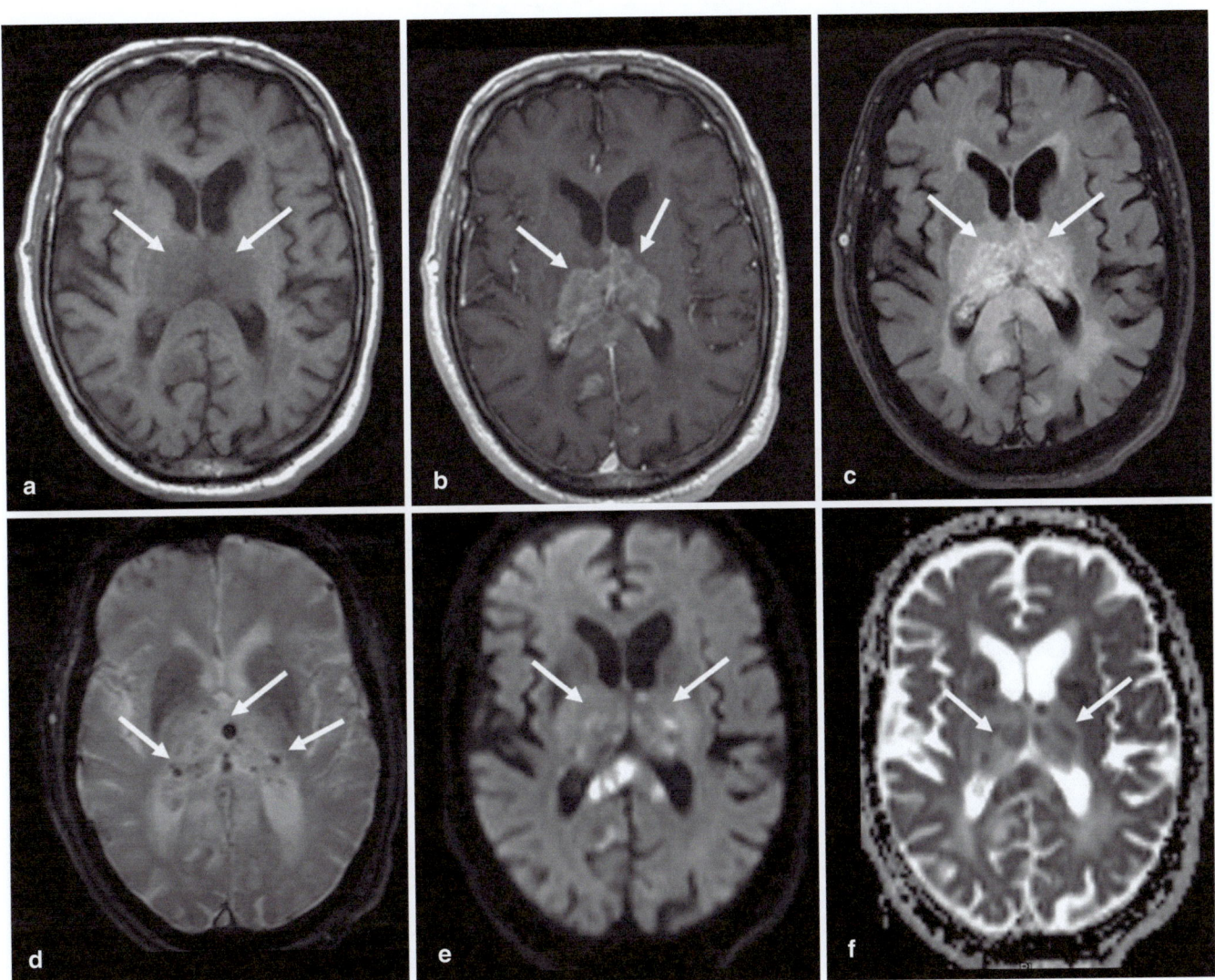

Fig. 11.10 Coronavirus 2019 (COVID 19), unvaccinated. (**a**) Precontrast axial T1-weighted image demonstrates edematous thalami (white arrows), with significant enhancement after intravenous contrast administration (**b**, white arrows) and increased signal on FLAIR images (**c**, white arrows), with superimposed microhemorrhages seen as areas of magnetic susceptibility on the axial gradient echo sequence (**d**), suggestive of acute hemorrhagic encephalopathy in the setting of known viral infection (COVID-19 infection). Axial DWI (**e**) and axial ADC map (**f**) demonstrate foci of acute ischemic changes involving the thalami and splenium of the corpus callosum

- Meningitis/Encephalitis: ranging from restricted diffusion and FLAIR hyperintensity in mesial temporal lobe and hippocampus to mild encephalitis with a reversible splenial callosal lesion. Leptomeningeal enhancement can be seen. Acute hemorrhagic necrotizing encephalopathy has been reported. Lesions appear hypoattenuating on CT images, and hyperintense on FLAIR/T2 WI with internal hemorrhage on MRI. Contrast-enhanced images may show rim enhancement.
- Corpus callosum involvement including cytotoxic lesions, manifested as multiple or focal areas of hyperintensity on FLAIR and DWI associated with microhemorrhages on SWI.
- Demyelination: symmetric and confluent T2 hyperintensities across the subcortical white matter, with restricted diffusion, sparing the deep gray matter structures as well as the juxtacortical white matter and the infratentorial regions.
- Olfactory pathway and cranial nerve involvement: bilateral olfactory bulb FLAIR signal hyperintensities, edema, and subtle contrast enhancement are hypothesized to be secondary to anosmia/hyposmia, frequent manifestation in patients with COVID 19 infection. Additional cranial involvement has been reported including optic neuritis and optic nerve enhancement.
- Myelitis: isolated or multifocal hyperintense lesions on STIR or T2 W in the cervical and thoracic cord [24–27].

Prions

- The most common human prion disease is subacute spongiform encephalopathy or Creutzfeldt-Jakob disease (CJD).
- Can be inherited, sporadic, acquired, and in a new variant form.
- CJD presents as rapidly progressive dementia with a "classic triad" of rapidly progressive cognitive dysfunction, myoclonus, and periodic slow-wave complexes (PSWCs) on electroencephalogram (EEG).
- The differential diagnosis frequently includes Alzheimer disease and autoimmune encephalopathy.
- Brain biopsy is the gold standard for diagnosis of CJD [8, 21].

Imaging Patterns

- CT: imaging findings are not evident until late disease stages when brain atrophy is seen.
- MR: gray matter changes in early stage disease (less than 4 months from symptom onset). Bilateral symmetric T2/FLAIR hyperintensities in the basal ganglia, posterior thalamus (Pulvinar sign), posterior medial thalamus (Hockey stick sign), and cerebral cortex with no contrast enhancement (Fig. 11.11).
- Gray matter signal abnormality in cortical regions on DWI and FLAIR images. On FLAIR conspicuous lesions can be present.

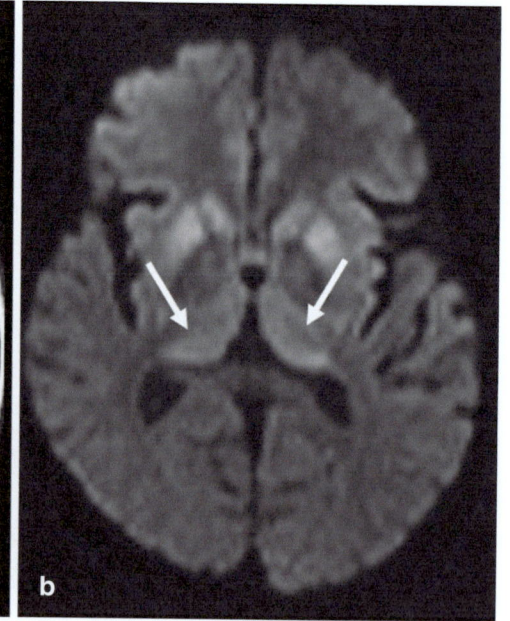

Fig. 11.11 Creutzfeldt-Jakob disease. (a) Axial FLAIR image demonstrates bilateral symmetric FLAIR hyperintensities in the basal ganglia and posterior thalamus (Pulvinar sign), also known as posterior medial thalamus "Hockey stick sign" (white arrows) with hyperintensity on the DWI image (b)

- DWI hyperintensity is persistent over many weeks with a predilection for involvement of the striatum, spreading from the caudate nucleus to the anterior putamen to the posterior putamen.
- Arterial spin labeling (ASL)-perfusion MRI: reduction of blood flow in the cerebral cortex and basal ganglia.
- MR spectroscopy: decrease in NAA, but the finding is nonspecific and has limited value [8, 21].

PARASITIC INFECTIONS OF THE BRAIN

Introduction

Parasitic diseases affecting the CNS cause significant morbidity and mortality worldwide. Cysticercosis is the most common CNS parasitic infection, followed by other less frequent infections including toxoplasmosis, echinococcosis, and schistosomiasis. These infections most commonly affect developing countries and immunosuppressed people, including HIV positive patients. Neuroimaging studies play a critical role in the diagnosis and management of these patients [1, 2, 7].

Neurocysticercosis

- Neurocysticercosis (NC) is a parasitic infection of the CNS caused by the larval form of the pork tapeworm *Taenia solium*.
- NC occurs when humans become intermediate hosts in the life cycle of *T. solium* by ingesting its eggs directly from a taenia carrier or, less often, by contaminated food.
- NC CNS locations include: parenchymal (brain or cord), extra parenchymal (ventricular system or subarachnoid space), and mixed forms.
- Parenchymal NC may manifest as seizures, headache, motor deficits, and cognitive impairment secondary to inflammation.
- Extra parenchymal NC symptoms are more frequently related to the mass effect due to parasitic obstruction of CSF drainage pathways including intracranial hypertension, cranial nerve abnormalities, meningitis, and hydrocephalus [1, 2, 4, 7].

Imaging Patterns

Parenchymal Stages

- Noncystic NC: asymptomatic with negative imaging findings.
- Vesicular stage: thin-walled cyst (5–20 mm) or a cluster of cysts (racemose form), frequently found at the subarachnoid space near the gray matter–white matter junction or in the basal ganglia, cerebellum, brainstem, cisterns, or ventricular system. It is possible to find the scolex (2–4 mm) as a nodular structure (cyst with a dot). Little or no edema is noted.
  - CT: hypodense nonenhancing cysts.
  - MR: isointense to CSF nonenhancing lesions. Scolex may characteristically show restricted diffusion or blooming on gradient echo or SWI sequences.
- Colloidal vesicular stage: the larva degenerates, the scolex disintegrates and produces an inflammatory reaction.
  - CT: intense perilesional edema, enhancing capsule.
  - MRI: perilesional edema in T2- and FLAIR-weighted images (diffuse encephalitis). Ringlike pattern of enhancement is often evident at postcontrast T1-weighted imaging.
- Granular-nodular stage: partial involution of inflammatory reaction with a granulomatous nodule that will later calcify. The lesion size reduces, the capsule thickens, with resolving perilesional edema and surrounding gliosis (Fig. 11.12).
- Nodular calcified stage: granulomatous lesion that has involuted and completely calcified (inactive and final stage).
- The differential diagnosis includes gliomas, cavernous malformations, and echinococcal cysts [1, 2, 5, 7–9].

Extra Parenchymal Stages

- The identification of cisternal and intraventricular cysts can be challenging due to the cyst's fluid component appearing similar to the subarachnoid space.
- Neuroimaging mainly relies on indirect signs such as local asymmetric enlargement of the ventricle, compression of the choroid plexus, or obstructive hydrocephalus.
- The fourth ventricle is the most common location for intraventricular cysticercosis.
- Bruns' syndrome: Intermittent or positional CSF obstruction caused by mobile intraventricular cyst leading to acute and transient increase in intracranial pressure with relapsing/remitting symptoms.
- Racemose NC appear as a cluster of cysts usually lacking scolex and located in suprasellar, sylvian, peri mesencephalic, and other basal cisterns, potentially causing ventriculitis and obstructive hydrocephalus.
- The differential diagnosis includes choroid plexus cyst, ependymal cyst, and colloidal cyst [1, 2, 5, 7–9].

Vasculitis

- NC complication: segmental narrowing, beaded appearance, or abrupt vascular obstruction is depicted at CT angiography or three-dimensional time-of-flight (3D-TOF) MR angiography.

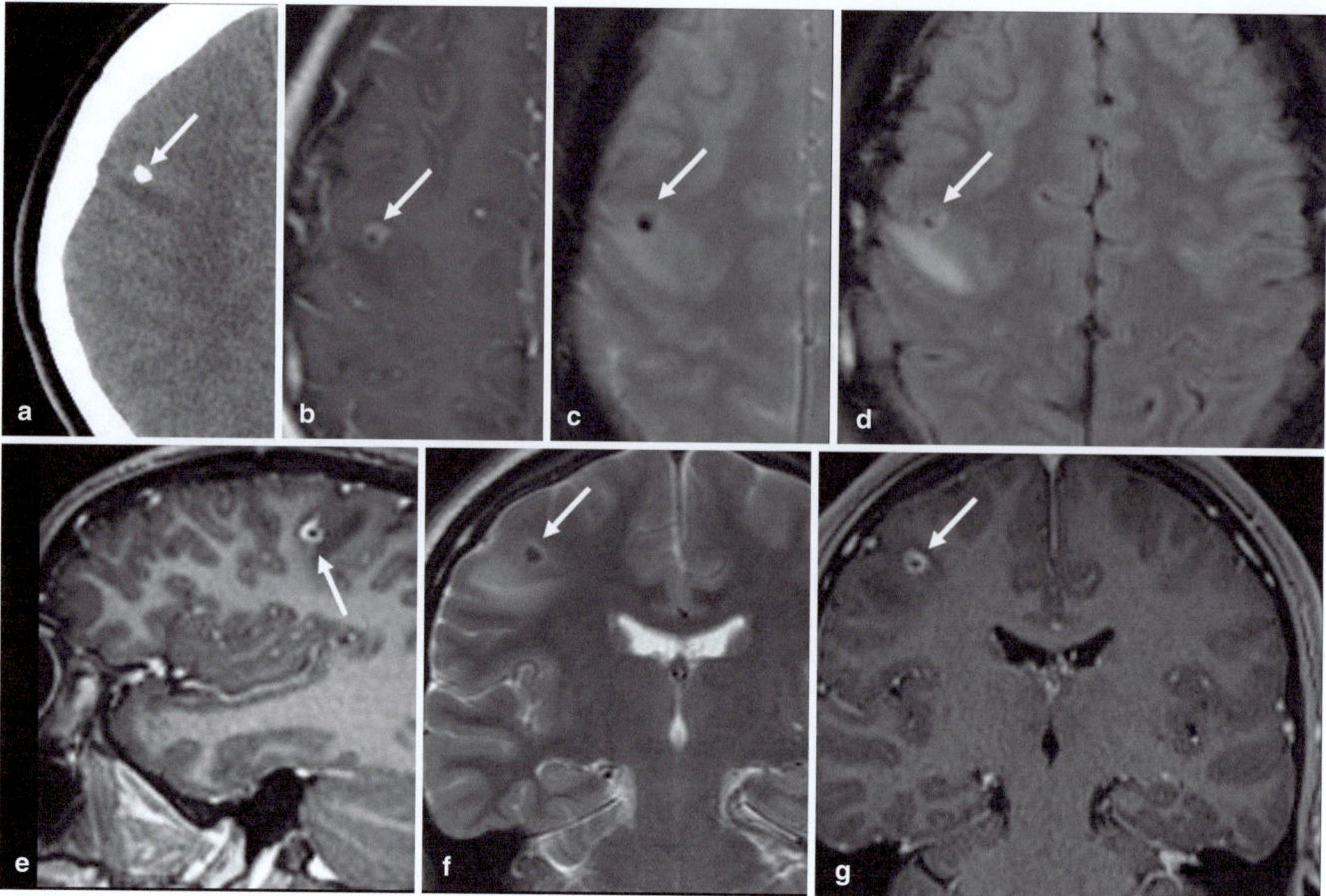

Fig. 11.12 Neurocysticercosis Granular-nodular stage. (**a**) Axial non-contrast head CT image showing a punctate calcified lesion in the right frontal lobe, with mild underlying vasogenic edema (white arrow), (**b, e, g**) axial, sagittal and coronal MRI T1 images after intravenous contrast administration showing ring enhancement pattern surrounded the calcified granuloma seen on the prior CT, axial magnetic susceptibility (**c**) and axial FLAIR (**d**) images show the calcified granuloma and better assessment of the vasogenic edema (**f** coronal T2)

- Tram track appearance (concentric pattern of wall enhancement) of the vessel walls.
- Brain infarction (when present) may be indistinguishable from other causes of ischemic vascular events [2].

Toxoplasmosis

- Toxoplasmosis results from *Toxoplasma gondii*, an intracellular protozoan parasite [1].
- It is usually an asymptomatic infection in immunocompetent hosts, but may become reactivated in immunocompromised patients and is the most common opportunistic infection in acquired immunodeficiency syndrome (AIDS) patients [9].
- Congenital disease is transmitted transplacentally affecting the fetal brain and manifesting with seizures, microcephaly, and chorioretinitis [7].
- Acquired cerebral toxoplasmosis is secondary to consumption of oocysts from contaminated food or water [1].
- Susceptible immunocompromised patients present with fever, headaches, confusion, seizure, and Toxoplasmosis encephalitis [2, 7].

Imaging Patterns

- Multifocal lesions, frequently located in the basal ganglia, cerebral cortex, brain stem, and cerebellum [1, 2, 4].

Early Stage

- Noncontrast CT: encephalitis and meningitis with multiple irregular, asymmetric low-density areas located in the corticomedullary junction and the basal ganglia.
- Postcontrast CT: linear and ring-like enhancing focal masses.
- MRI: bilateral, multiple, irregular, and asymmetric hypointensity on T1WI and hyperintensity on T2WI (coagulative necrosis).

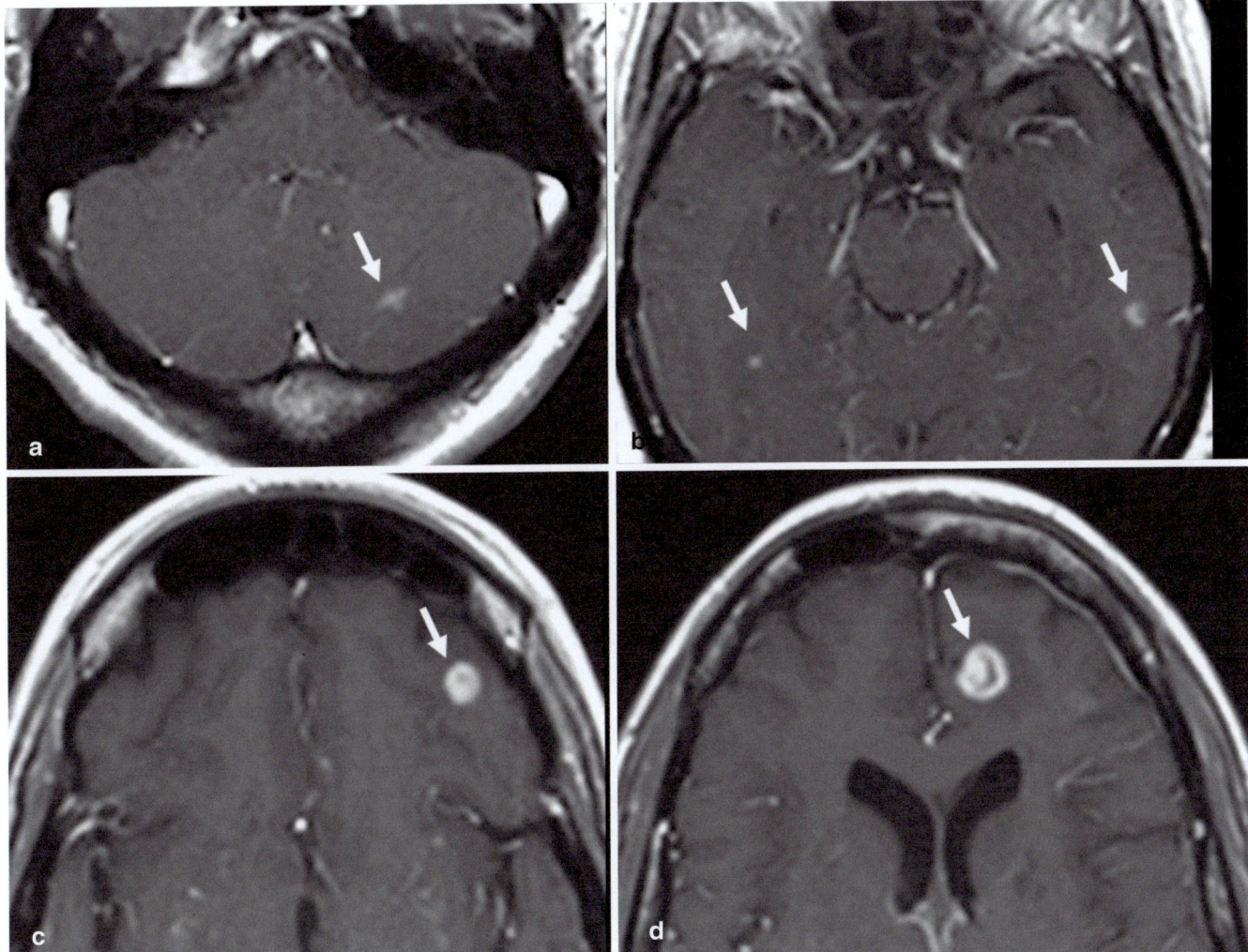

Fig. 11.13 Toxoplasmosis. 49-year-old male with history HIV and seizures, multiple axial brain MRI images in T1-weighted images after the intravenous administration of gadolinium contrast (**a**) enhancing focus on the left cerebellar hemisphere (white arrow), (**b**) supratentorial image demonstrate two small foci of enhancement on the temporal lobes (white arrow), (**c, d**) demonstrate the so-called target sign on the left frontal lobe (white arrows), as a central area of enhancement surrounded by a ring of enchantment (white arrow)

- o Granuloma: nodular mass with extensive perifocal edema and significant mass effect with nodular or curvilinear enhancement.
- o Eccentric target sign: ring-shaped zone of peripheral enhancement with a small eccentric nodule along the wall.
- o Concentric target sign: alternating concentric layers of T2-weighted hypointensities (hemorrhage) and hyperintensities (necrosis with edema (Fig. 11.13).
- Differential diagnosis includes primary central nervous system lymphoma (PCNSL), fungal infection, tuberculosis and cytomegalovirus infection. Specifically, differentiating lymphoma from CNS Toxoplasmosis can be challenging and metabolic imaging (thallium-201 brain SPECT, FDG-PET) can be useful (lymphoma is positive, whereas toxoplasmosis is not) [1, 2, 5, 7, 9, 11].

Final Stage

- Congenital Toxoplasmosis: microcephaly, neuronal migration disorder, and atelencephalia and hydrocephalus.
- Multiple nodular or curvilineal calcifications [7].

FUNGAL INFECTIONS OF THE BRAIN

Introduction

Fungal infections of the CNS are very rare in the general population and predominantly affect immunocompromised people, frequently acting as an opportunistic infection resulting from hematogenous dissemination. There are behavioral similarities to mycobacteria, which also produce granulomatous inflammation. Fungal pathogens can be divided into yeast, mold, and dimorphic fungus, which influence pathophysiology and neuroimaging patterns. Given the lack of inflammatory response, neuroradiological findings are often nonspecific [1, 2, 11, 28]. Although almost any fungus may cause encephalitis, cryptococcal meningoencephalitis is most frequently seen, followed by aspergillosis. Cerebral candidiasis is usually preceded by a systemic candida infection and is frequently catheter related [9, 28].

Cryptococcus

- Cryptococcal meningitis is the most common fungal disease of the CNS.
- It is an airborne disease with the primary focus in the lungs, from which secondary systemic dissemination occurs via hematogenous spread.
- CNS cryptococcal infection commonly presents with meningitis (subacute or chronic) or meningoencephalitis as well as cryptococcomas and gelatinous pseudocysts. In immunocompetent patients, it can manifest as solid or abscess-like lesions.
- Chronic meningitis is present with periods of remission and relapses.
- At the onset, patients usually present with headaches, nausea, vomiting, visual impairment, and papilledema; followed by a later stage of neck stiffness, fever, personality changes, seizures, cranial nerve palsies, and hydrocephalus.
- Diagnosed by India ink staining of the CSF film and positive cryptococcal antigen titer in CSF or blood [1, 5, 7, 9, 11, 28].

Imaging Patterns (Fig. 11.14)

- CT: Ranges from normal to nonspecific findings, ventricular dilation is commonly seen.
- MR: ill-defined T2 high-signal-intensity changes in the basal ganglia described as the "hazy brain base."
- High signal intensity of the subarachnoid spaces on FLAIR images.
- Leptomeningeal enhancement may be smooth or thick, nodular and irregular or asymmetric, where postcontrast FLAIR images have the highest sensitivity and specificity.
- Hydrocephalus can also be present.
- Dilation of the Virchow-Robin spaces up to 2–3 mm. If they measure >3 mm they become gelatinous pseudocysts. Both are seen as nonenhancing CSF signal cystic lesions in the basal ganglia, midbrain peduncles, and dentate nucleus, producing a "soap bubble appearance."
- Cryptococcomas are nodular or ring-like enhancing intraparenchymal or intraventricular lesions, occasionally involving the choroid plexus with postcontrast enhancement [1, 5, 7, 9, 11, 28].

Aspergillus

- Cerebral aspergillosis may originate from hematogenous dissemination from a distant pulmonary infection, contiguous spread from a paranasal sinus or orbital infection (rhino-cerebral disease), or direct traumatic implantation, producing meningitis and meningoencephalitis among highly compromised hosts.
- CNS aspergillosis may present with fever, seizures, headache, alteration of mental status, CNS depression, and may even present with stroke-like symptoms.
- It is diagnosed on direct examinations and culture of aspirates/swabs/biopsy material [1, 2, 5, 7, 9].

Imaging Patterns

- CT: imaging findings are nonspecific and usually subtle, with varying densities and minimal mass effect, poor contrast enhancement, and no ring formation.
- MR: nonspecific findings, lesions may show areas of isointense or low signal intensity on T2WI.
- Several patterns of cerebral aspergillosis, including edematous, hemorrhagic, and solid enhancing lesions (aspergilloma or "tumoral form") as well as abscess-like ring-like enhancing lesions and infarction-like lesions.
- Fungal abscesses commonly demonstrate a very thin rim of peripheral enhancement ("weak ring" enhancement). On SWI, they have a prominent, thick, black rim, or central susceptibility effects due to hemorrhage (Fig. 11.4).
- Dural enhancement is usually seen in lesions adjacent to infected paranasal sinuses.
- Cortical and subcortical infarction with or without hemorrhage can be seen secondary to fungal infiltration of the vessel wall and thrombosis as well as fungal mycotic aneurysms.
- Involvement of the corpus callosum, thalami, basal ganglia, and other perforator artery territories are suggestive of aspergillus infection in immunocompromised patients.
- MR spectroscopy: peaks similar to those seen in bacterial abscesses including amino acids, lipids and lactate peaks.
- MR perfusion: decreased rCBV (Fig. 11.15) [1, 2, 5, 9].

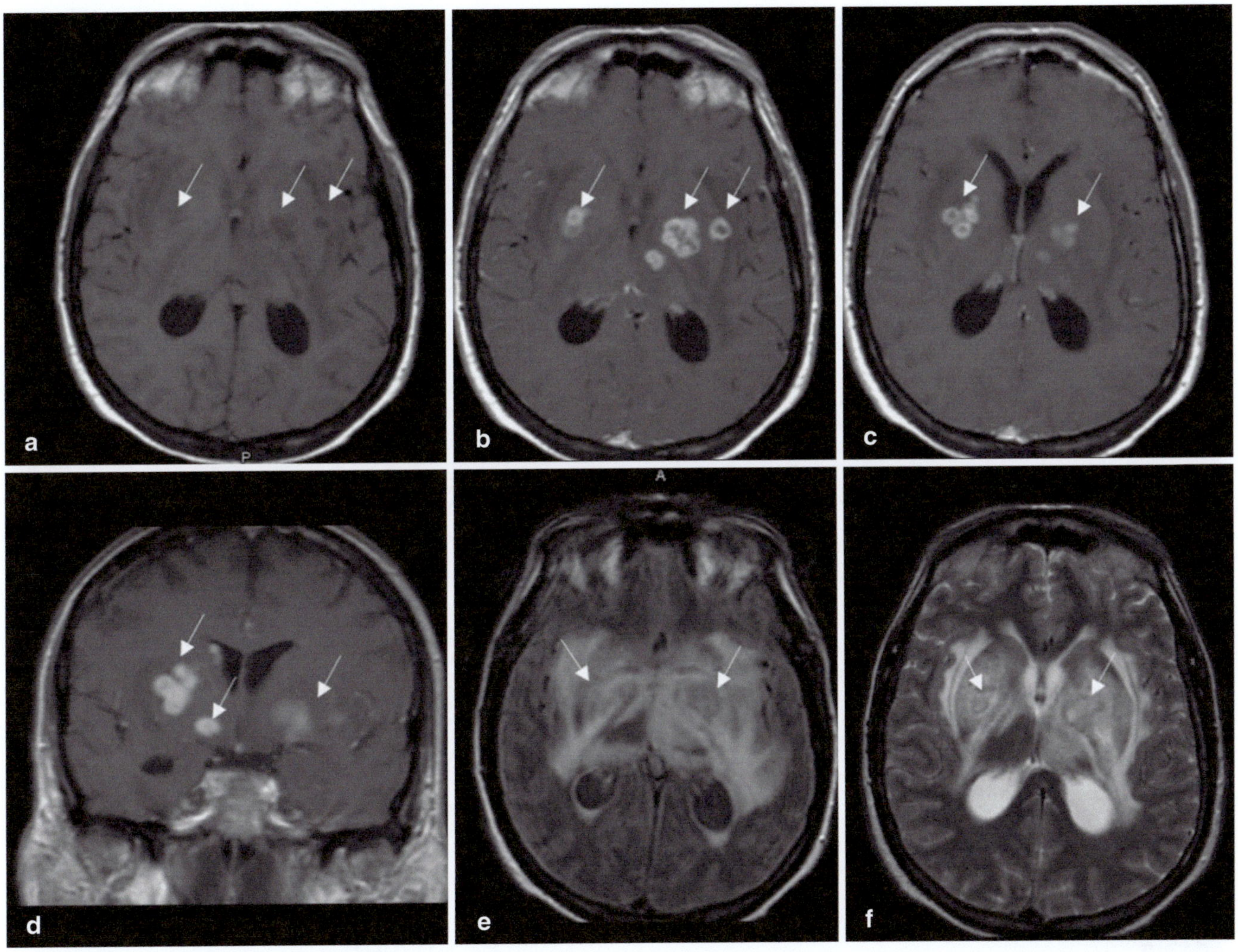

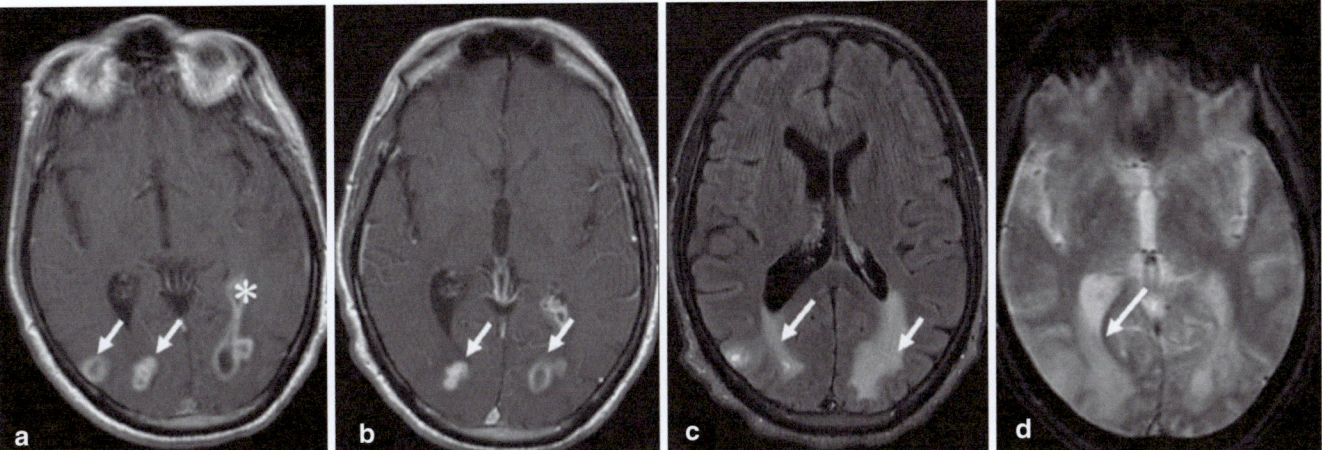

Fig. 11.14 CNS cryptococcal infection. (**a**) Precontrast axial T1-weighted image demonstrates edematous changes in the bilateral basal ganglia, left greater than right with underlying foci of low signal (white arrows), (**b**, **c** axial, and **d** coronal) images after the intravenous administration of Gadolinium contrast demonstrate ring, and nodular enhancement of this lesions (white arrows). (**e**, **f**) Axial T2-weighted images demonstrate significant vasogenic edema in the basal ganglia with dilation of the Virchow-Robin spaces suggestive of gelatinous pseudocysts (white arrows)

Fig. 11.15 Cerebral aspergillosis infection. (**a**, **b**) Postcontrast axial T1-weighted images demonstrate bilateral rim enhancing lesions in the occipital lobes and left subependymal region of the left occipital ventricular horn (white arrows and white asterisk), (**c**) Axial T2-weighted image demonstrate significant vasogenic edema posterior to the occipital ventricular horns and occipital lobes bilaterally (white arrows), (**d**) Axial magnetic susceptibility image demonstrate low signal in the medial aspect in the right subependymal region

References

1. Shih RY, Koeller KK. Bacterial, fungal, and parasitic infections of the central nervous system: radiologic-pathologic correlation and historical perspectives. Radiographics. 2015;35:1141–69.
2. Barkhof F, Thurnher MM. Infectious brain disease. In: Clinical neuroradiology. Springer Nature Switzerland AG; 2019. pp. 599–691.
3. Saberi A, Roudbary S, Ghayeghran A, Kazemi S, Hosseininezhad M. Review paper: diagnosis of meningitis caused by pathogenic microorganisms using magnetic resonance imaging: a systematic review. Basic Clin Neurosci. 2018;9(2):73–86.
4. Mohan S, Jain KK. Imaging of meningitis and ventriculitis. Neuroimaging Clin N Am. 2012;22(4):557–83.
5. Foerster BR, Thurnher MM, Malani PN, Petrou M, Sundgren PC, Thurnher MM, Petrou M. Intracranial infections: clinical and imaging characteristics. Acta Radiol. 2007;48(8):875–89.
6. Thurnher MM. Meningitis and ventriculitis. In: Imaging of the brain. 2016. pp. 865–876.
7. Gao B, Law M. Infections of CNS. In: Imaging of CNS infections and neuroimmunology. Springer Nature Singapore; 2019. pp. 37–121.
8. Abdalkader M, Xie J, Cervantes-arslanian A, Takahashi C, Mian AZ. Imaging of intracranial infections. Semin Neurol. 2019;39:322–33.
9. Cuvinciuc V, Vargas MI, Haller S. Diagnosing infection of the CNS with MRI. Imaging Med. 2011;3:689–710.
10. Hughes DC, Raghavan A, Mordekar SR, Griffiths PD, Connolly DJA. Role of imaging in the diagnosis of acute bacterial meningitis and its complications. Postgrad Med J. 2010;86:478–85.
11. Kastrup O, Wanke I, Maschke M. Neuroimaging of infections. NeuroRx. 2005;2:324–32.
12. Etlik Ö, Evirgen Ö, Bay A, Yılmaz N. Original Article. Radiologic and clinical findings in tuberculosis. Eur J Gen Med. 2004;1(2):19–24.
13. Taheri MS, Karimi MA, Haghighatkhah H, Pourghorban R, Samadian M, Kasmaei HD. Central nervous system tuberculosis: an imaging-focused review of a reemerging disease. Radiol Res Pract. 2015;2015:202806.
14. Andres MM, Uy JAU, Reyes-paguia MP Basal cistern enhancement pattern on CT imaging. 2016. pp. 1–9.
15. Modi M, Sharma K, Prabhakar S, Goyal MK, Takkar A, Sharma N, Lal V. Clinical and radiological predictors of outcome in tubercular meningitis: a prospective study of 209 patients. Clin Neurol Neurosurg. 2017;161:29–34.
16. Id SD, Hermawan R, Van Laarhoven A, Immaculata S, Achmad H, Ruslami R, Van Crevel R. Brain MRI findings in relation to clinical characteristics and outcome of tuberculous meningitis. PLoS One. 2020;15:e0241974.
17. Bertrand A, Leclercq D, Martinez-Almoyna L, Stahl JP, Debroucker T, Bertrand A, Stahl JP. MR imaging of adult acute infectious encephalitis. Elsevier Masson; 2017. https://doi.org/10.1016/j.medmal.2017.01.002.
18. Burrill J, Williams FCJ, Bain FG, Conder FG, Hine FAL, Rakesh R. Tuberculosis: a radiologic review. Radiographics. 2007;27:1255–74.
19. Andronikou S, Govender N, Ramdass A. MRI appearances of tuberculous meningitis in HIV-infected children: a paradoxically protective mechanism? Imaging Med. 2012;4:359–66.
20. Maller VV, Bathla G, Moritani T, Helton KJ. Imaging in viral infections of the central nervous system: can images speak for an acutely ill brain? Emerg Radiol. 2017;24:287–300.
21. Shih RY, Koeller KK. Viral and prion infections of the central nervous system: radiologic-pathologic correlation. Radiographics. 2017;37:199–233.
22. Granerod J, Davies NWS, Mukonoweshuro W, Mehta A, Das K, Lim M, Brown DWG. Neuroimaging in encephalitis: analysis of imaging findings and interobserver agreement. Clin Radiol. 2016;71:1050–8.
23. Jayaraman K, Rangasami R, Chandrasekharan A. Magnetic resonance imaging findings in viral encephalitis: a pictorial essay. J Neurosci Rural Pract. 2019;9:556–60.
24. Ladopoulos T, Zand R, Shahjouei S, Chang JJ, Motte J, Charles J, Krogias C. COVID-19: neuroimaging features of a pandemic. J Neuroimaging. 2021;31:228–43.
25. Mahammedi A, Gaskill M, Bachir S, Gasparotti R. Imaging of neurologic disease in hospitalized patients with COVID-19: an Italian multicenter retrospective. Radiology. 2020;297:E270–3.
26. Poyiadji N, Shahin G, Noujaim D, Stone M, Patel S, Griffith B. COVID-19—associated acute hemorrhagic necrotizing encephalopathy: imaging features. Radiology. 2020;5:26–7.
27. Rasmussen C, Niculescu I. COVID-19 and involvement of the corpus callosum: potential effect of the cytokine storm? AJNR Am J Neuroradiol. 2020;41:1625–8.
28. Patir R, Borkar SA. Management of tuberculous and fungal infections of the nervous system. Management of tuberculous infections. In: Schmidek and Sweet: operative neurosurgical techniques, 2-vol set, 7th ed. 2021. pp. 1548–1591.

Noninfectious Inflammatory Processes

Derek Hsu and Ranliang Hu

Chemical Meningitis

- An aseptic meningitis is most often caused by the release of fat from a ruptured dermoid cyst or rarely from a chemical irritant such as intrathecal contrast or medications.
- Dermoid cyst is a rare primary midline intracranial tumor, which typically presents in the second to third decade of life [1].
- Most common symptoms include headache and seizure [2].
- Treatment includes complete surgical resection of the dermoid cyst, possible ventricular shunt placement to manage hydrocephalus, or conservative management if no clinical symptoms.

Imaging

- CT
  - Dermoid cyst appears as a unilocular, well-delineated, hypodense (fat density) mass with or without capsular calcifications.
  - Scattered fat density in the cerebral sulci and ventricles in an anti-dependent fashion are seen in dermoid cyst rupture.
- MRI
  - A dermoid cyst is a nonenhancing, T1- and T2-hyperintense cystic lesion, which demonstrates fat suppression (Fig. 12.1).
  - Fatty droplets within the ventricles and/or sulci are highly suggestive of a ruptured dermoid cyst (Fig. 12.2).
  - Extensive pachymeningeal and leptomeningeal enhancement can be seen in an aseptic chemical meningitis as a result of dermoid cyst rupture (Fig. 12.3).

D. Hsu · R. Hu (✉)
Department of Radiology and Imaging Sciences, Emory University School of Medicine, Atlanta, GA, USA
e-mail: derek.evan.hsu@emory.edu; ranliang.hu@emory.edu

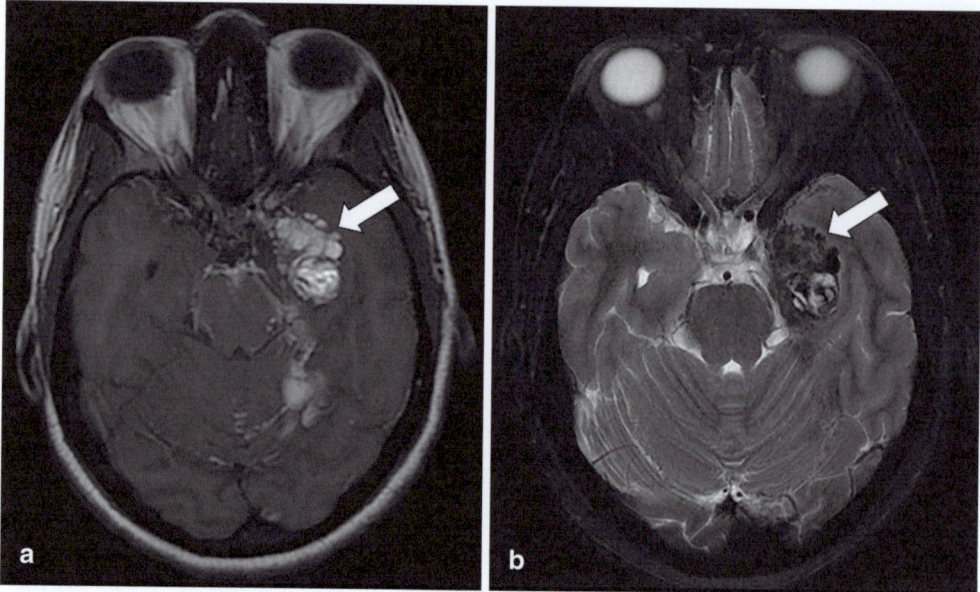

Fig. 12.1 Dermoid cyst. (**a**) In the left medial temporal lobe, there is a T1-hyperintense lesion, which abuts the left cavernous sinus (arrow). (**b**) The lesion demonstrates signal dropout with fat suppression (arrow), compatible with fatty components

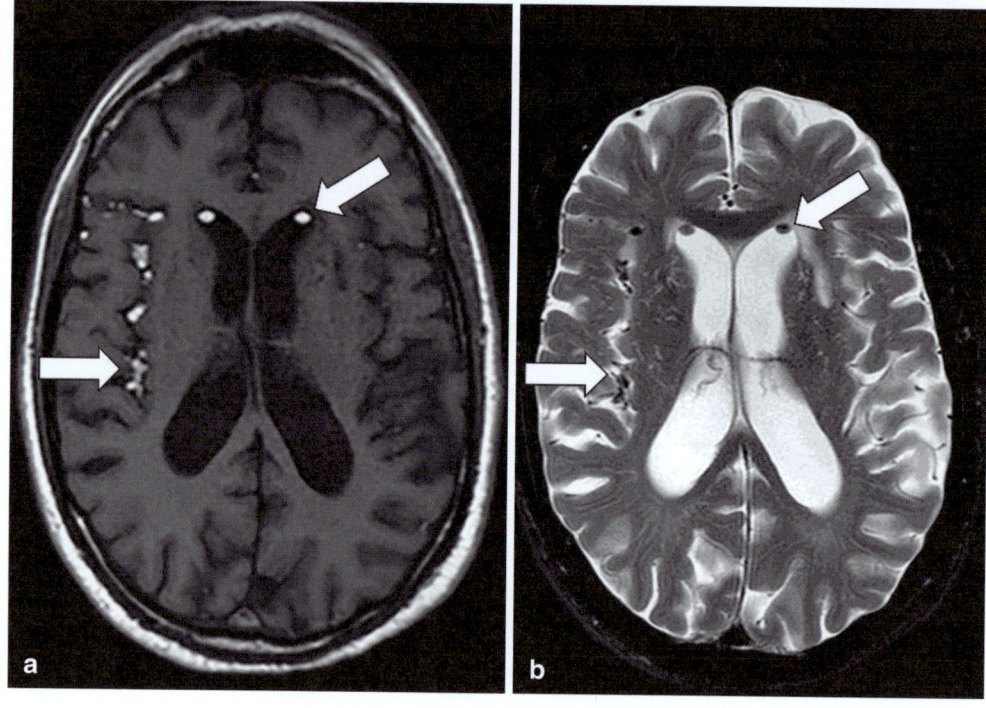

Fig. 12.2 Dermoid cyst rupture. (**a**) Scattered T1-hyperintense foci are seen within the bilateral frontal horns of the lateral ventricles and along the right sylvian fissure (arrows). (**b**) These foci within the ventricles and right sylvian fissure demonstrate signal dropout on fat-suppression imaging (arrows), confirming the presence of fat

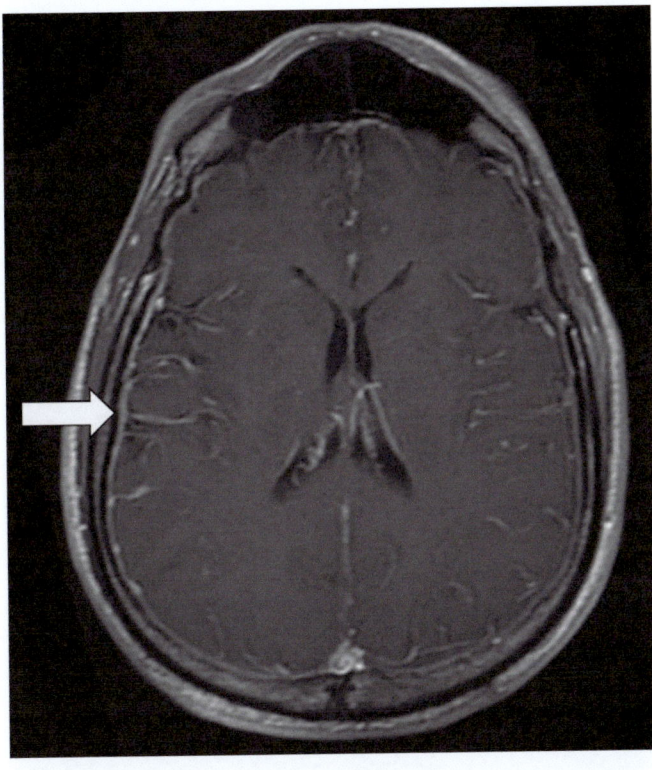

Fig. 12.3 Aseptic chemical meningitis. Contrast-enhanced T1-weighted imaging with contrast demonstrates diffuse pachymeningeal and leptomeningeal enhancement, compatible with a chemical meningitis

Limbic Encephalitis

- Limbic encephalitis (LE) is a legacy term often used interchangeably with autoimmune encephalitis, commonly referring to antibody-mediated brain inflammation involving the limbic system and beyond. It can have both paraneoplastic and non-paraneoplastic causes [3].
- Patients typically present with memory loss, cognitive dysfunction, dementia, psychological features (anxiety, depression, hallucinations), or seizures.
- LE may be categorized by the location of the neuronal antigen: group I (intracellular) or group II (cell surface) [4].
  - Group I antibodies are more closely associated with underlying malignancy.
    - Anti-Hu: small cell lung cancer.
    - Anti-Ma/Ta: testicular germ cell tumor.
    - Anti-Yo: breast and ovarian cancer.
  - Group II antibodies.
    - *N*-methyl-D-aspartate receptor (NMDA-R) and voltage-gated potassium channels (VGKC): thymoma, teratoma, and Hodgkin lymphoma.
- Treatment of the primary tumor may improve neurologic symptoms. Additional immunotherapy may be used such as IV steroids, plasma exchange, and IV immunoglobulins.

Imaging

- CT
  - Majority are normal on CT; rarely will there be hypodensity of the mesial temporal lobes and other limbic regions.
- MRI
  - MRI may be normal or subtly abnormal in some patients, especially early in the disease. When involved, T2/FLAIR hyperintensity and swelling will be mostly seen in the mesial temporal lobes, cingulate, frontobasal, and insular regions (Fig. 12.4).
    - Often bilateral but can be unilateral.
    - May have subtle enhancement.
    - Progression of disease will result in eventual atrophy and sclerosis of involved structures.
  - Herpes encephalitis can have overlapping findings and must be covered for and excluded clinically, especially when hemorrhage is present.
  - Systemic imaging such as CT of chest, abdomen, and pelvis and pelvic/scrotal ultrasound may be useful for workup of a primary neoplasm.

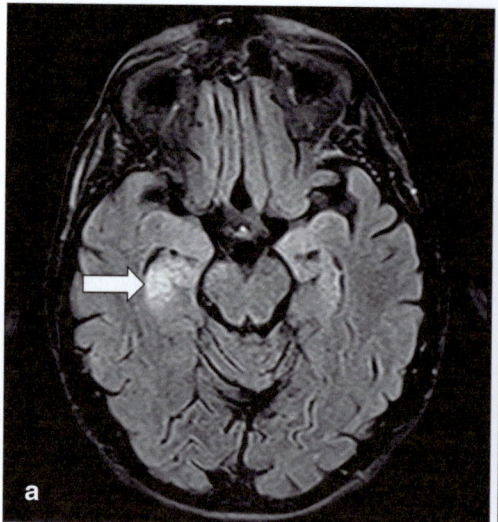 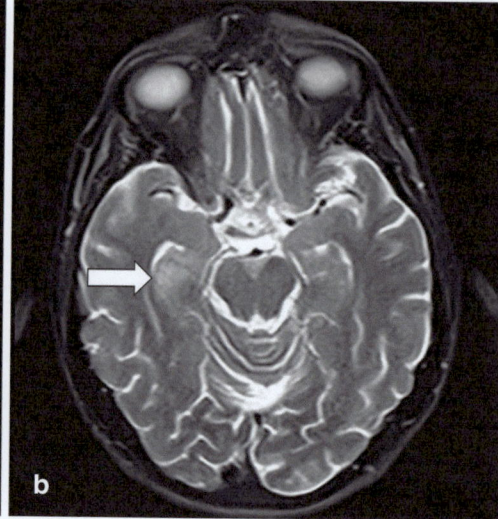

Fig. 12.4 Limbic encephalitis. Axial (**a**) FLAIR and (**b**) T2-weighted imaging demonstrate hyperintensity of the bilateral right greater than left mesial temporal lobes (arrows), compatible with limbic encephalitis. Patient was discovered to have a small cell lung cancer

Lymphocytic Hypophysitis

- Lymphocytic hypophysitis (LH) is a rare, self-limiting autoimmune/inflammatory process of the pituitary infundibulum and/or pituitary gland, resulting in pituitary dysfunction. LH is also known as adenohypophysitis and primary hypophysitis.
- There is a strong female predominance, with M:F of 1:9. Most commonly seen in peripartum or early postpartum women who present with a headache, vision changes, and neuroendocrine deficiencies [5].
- Etiology of primary LH is likely autoimmune. Immune checkpoint inhibitors such as ipilimumab can also induce a secondary autoimmune hypophysitis. Other causes of hypophysitis include granulomatous diseases and IgG4-related inflammation [5, 6].
- Treatments typically include high-dose steroids and hormone replacement therapy for neuroendocrine deficiencies.

Imaging

- MRI
  - Enlargement of the pituitary infundibulum (>2 mm in thickness and loss of the typical "top to bottom" tapering) with or without pituitary gland enlargement.
  - Intense homogeneous enhancement due to infiltration into the anterior pituitary gland (Fig. 12.5).
  - Loss of posterior pituitary gland "bright spot" on T1 imaging (75% of cases).
  - LH may mimic a pituitary adenoma as imaging characteristics can be similar, although the latter should not thicken the pituitary stalk.

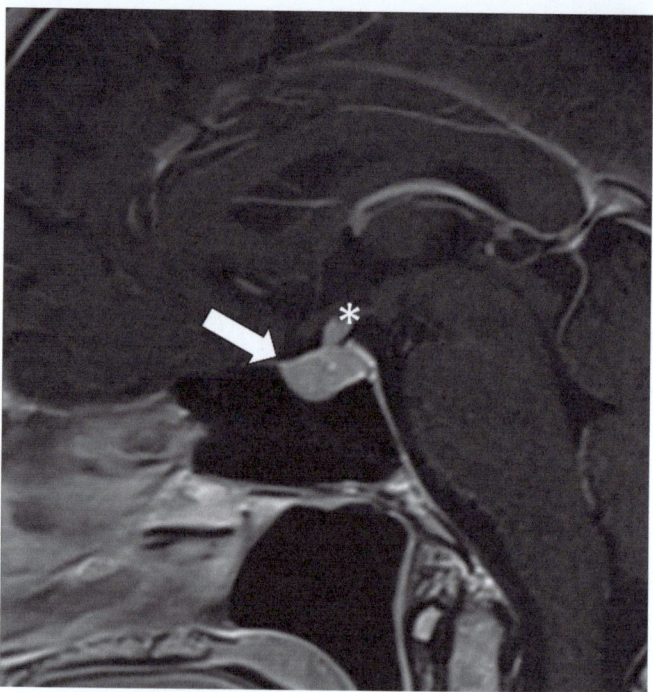

Fig. 12.5 Lymphocytic hypophysitis. (**a**) Sagittal postcontrast T1-weighted imaging demonstrates homogeneous enlargement of the pituitary gland (arrow) and pituitary infundibulum (*) with associated enhancement

Sarcoidosis

- A chronic multisystem, noncaseating granulomatous inflammatory process with reported neurological involvement in 5–10% of cases.
- Majority (80–90%) of patients presenting with neurosarcoidosis also have systemic involvement.

- Central and peripheral nervous system can be involved, including the dura, leptomeninges, spinal cord, brain parenchyma, and perivascular spaces.
- More common in African Americans and females in the fourth and fifth decade of life.
- Neurological presentation can be protean but often include a basilar meningitis or cranial nerve palsy [7].
- Heerfordt syndrome, a clinical variant of sarcoidosis, includes facial nerve palsy, fever, parotid gland enlargement, and uveitis [8].
- Treatment includes high-dose corticosteroids and immunosuppressive therapy.

Imaging

- MRI
    - Multifocal, multi-spatial CNS nodular lesions with surrounding edema and predilection for the base of the brain ("basilar meningitis").
        - T1-isointense/T2-hypointense and avidly enhancing (Figs. 12.6 and 12.7).
    - Nodular leptomeningeal and/or pachymeningeal enhancement.
    - Diffuse or focal enhancement along dilated medullary veins, resulting from perivascular inflammation (Fig. 12.8).

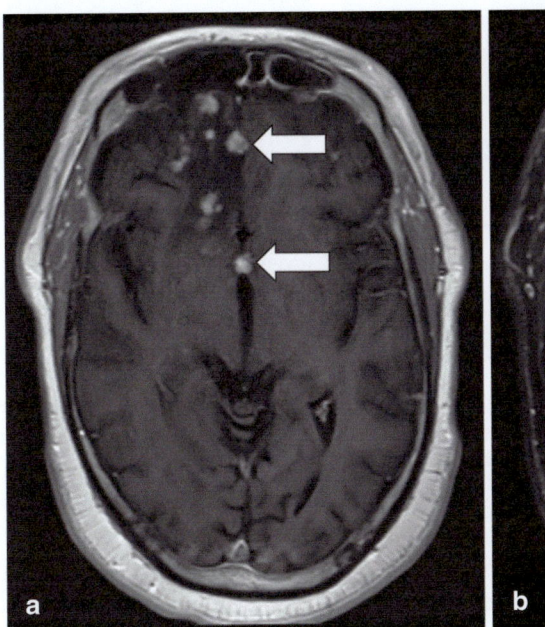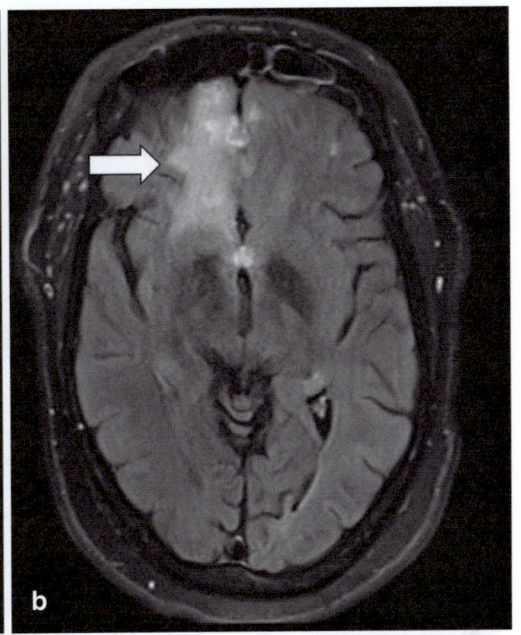

Fig. 12.6 Sarcoidosis. (**a**) Axial postcontrast T1-weighted imaging demonstrate parenchymal and leptomeningeal nodular enhancement (arrows) in the anterior cranial fossa with associated (**b**) FLAIR signal (arrow)

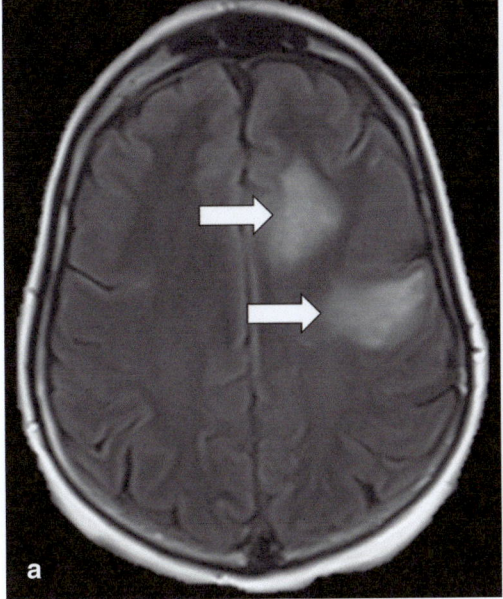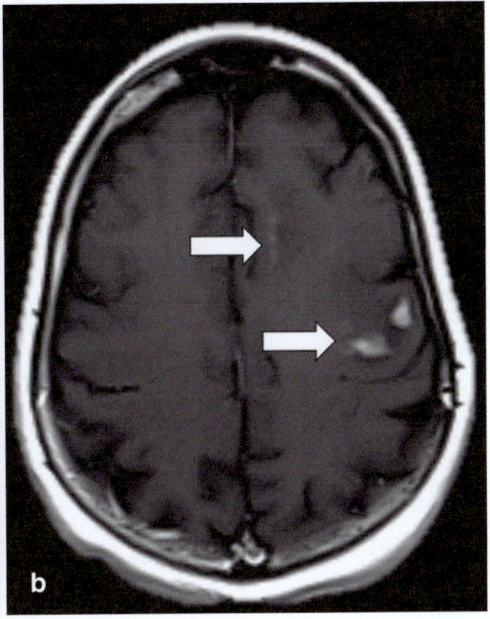

Fig. 12.7 Sarcoidosis with parenchymal involvement. (**a**) Axial T2/FLAIR signal abnormality is seen within the left superior and middle frontal gyrus white matter (arrows) with associated (**b**) underlying ill-defined and stippled enhancement (arrows)

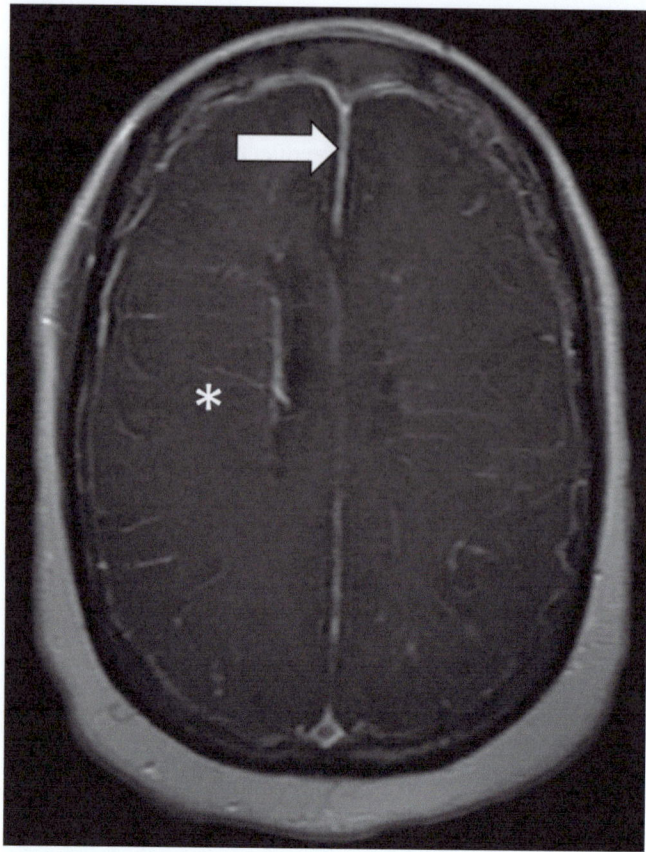

Fig. 12.8 Sarcoidosis with meningeal involvement. Axial postcontrast T1-weighted images demonstrate diffuse dural thickening with uniform enhancement (arrow) and prominent medullary veins (*)

○ CNS sarcoidosis often associated with abnormal chest x-ray (~90%, hilar adenopathy) and elevated serum ACE levels.

Histiocytosis

- Langerhans cell histiocytosis (LCH) is a clonal neoplastic proliferation of eosinophils and Langerhans cells, often associated with BRAFV600E mutation [9].
- Commonly seen in children with a third of cases presenting in adulthood and a 2:1 male to female predominance.

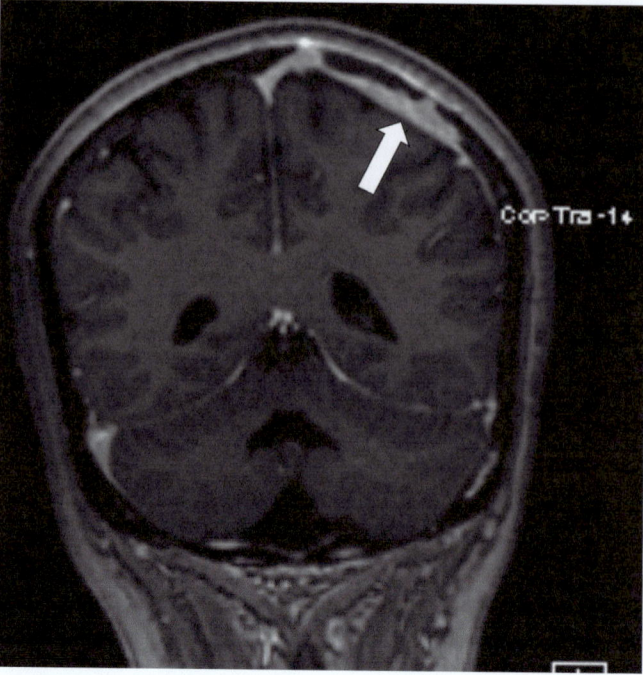

Fig. 12.9 Osseous histiocytosis. On postcontrast coronal T1-weighted imaging, there is a homogeneously enhancing soft tissue mass involving the left parietal calvarium. This is the most common site of bony involvement

- The calvarium is the most common bony site and typically presents with pain at the site of lesion [10].
- The pituitary infundibulum is the most common site of CNS involvement and presents with visual disturbances or central diabetes insipidus [10].
- Treatment varies including conservative/observation, excision/curettage, and radiation/chemotherapy.

Imaging

- CT
  ○ Sharply marginated lytic calvarial lesion with "beveled" edges and soft tissue mass on CT.
- MRI
  ○ Homogeneously enhancing soft tissue mass involving the calvarium, mastoids, or orbits (Fig. 12.9).

12 Noninfectious Inflammatory Processes

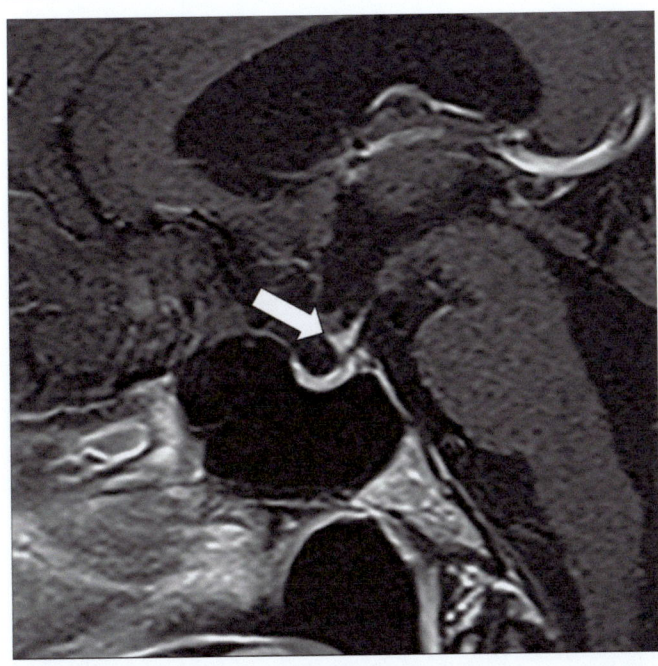

Fig. 12.10 CNS histiocytosis. On sagittal postcontrast T1-weighted imaging, there is a thickened and enhancing pituitary infundibulum. This is the most common site of CNS involvement

- Thickened, enhancing pituitary infundibulum (Fig. 12.10).
- Enhancing, slightly T2 hyperintense mass, which may involve the choroid plexus, leptomeninges, basal ganglia.

Amyloid-Related Inflammation

- Cerebral amyloid angiopathy-related inflammation (CAA-RI) is a spectrum disorder distinguished from classic cerebral amyloid angiopathy (CAA) by the presence of inflammatory response to deposits of beta-amyloid in small and medium-sized cerebral vessels [11].
- Pathologic spectrum include inflammatory cerebral amyloid (perivascular inflammation) and amyloid β-related angiitis (vessel wall inflammation), not distinguishable by conventional imaging [12].
- Typically presents with new onset headache, progressive neurologic deficit, or seizures in the elderly (~60 years old, younger than classic CAA) [12].
- Treatment includes steroids with or without immunosuppressants.

Imaging

- CT
  - Multifocal asymmetric juxtacortical and subcortical white matter hypoattenuation (Fig. 12.11a).
- MRI
  - Multifocal asymmetric juxtacortical and subcortical white matter T2/FLAIR hyperintensity without significant mass effect (Fig. 12.11b).
  - Chronic microhemorrhages in 90% of cases, helps in diagnosis but not required (Fig. 12.11c).
  - Low cerebral blood volume (CBV) on MR perfusion differentiates from neoplastic disorders (Fig. 12.11d).

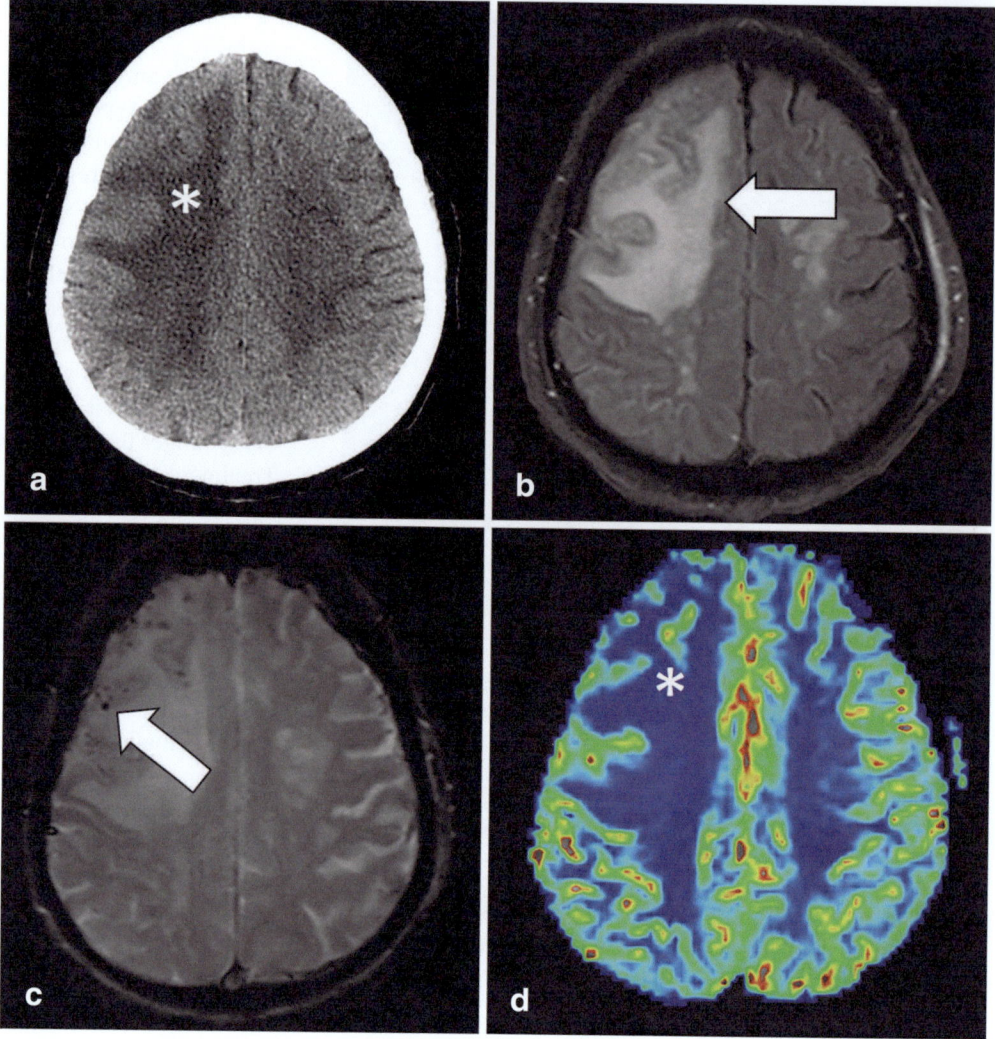

Fig. 12.11 Cerebral amyloid angiopathy-related inflammation (CAA-RI). (**a**) On noncontrast head CT, there is a focal hypodensity in the right front lobe (*). (**b**) Axial T2-weighted FLAIR imaging demonstrates increased signal corresponding with CT hypodensity with (**c**) foci of susceptibility signal loss on GRE, compatible with chronic microhemorrhages. (**d**) Perfusion MRI demonstrates corresponding area of hypoperfusion

Anti-MOG Encephalomyelitis

- A rare autoimmune inflammatory disorder that targets myelin oligodendrocyte glycoprotein (MOG), which is thought to have a role in microtubule stability and complement activation cascade [13].
- Depending on age, presentation may vary. Children typically present with acute disseminated encephalomyelitis like symptoms while adults typically present with bilateral optic neuritis [14].
- Treatments include steroids, plasma exchange, or intravenous immunoglobulin [15].

Imaging

- MRI (Fig. 12.12)
  - Long segment involvement (>50%) of the bilateral optic nerves, typically the anterior segment, unlike neuromyelitis optica (NMO), which typically affects the chiasm and optic tracts.
  - Edematous and tortuous optic nerve.
  - Enhancement of the perioptic nerve sheath and surrounding orbital fat.

Fig. 12.12 Anti-MOG encephalomyelitis with optic nerve involvement. (**a**) Axial fat saturation T2-weighted imaging demonstrates increased hazy T2-signal in the anterior optic nerves (arrows). (**b**) Coronal postcontrast, fat saturation T1-weighted imaging demonstrates avid enhancement of the bilateral optic nerves (arrows)

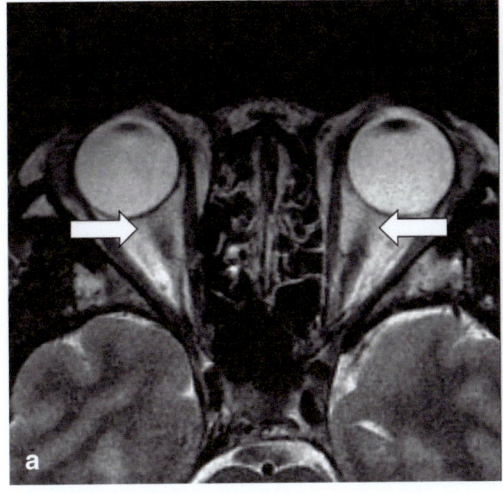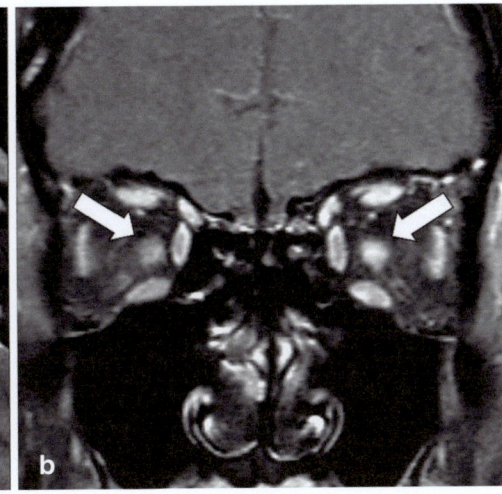

References

1. Orakcioglu B, et al. Intracranial dermoid cysts: variations of radiological and clinical features. Acta Neurochir. 2008;150(12):1227–34. discussion 1234
2. Liu JK, et al. Ruptured intracranial dermoid cysts: clinical, radiographic, and surgical features. Neurosurgery. 2008;62(2):377–84; discussion 384
3. da Rocha AJ, et al. Recognizing autoimmune-mediated encephalitis in the differential diagnosis of limbic disorders. AJNR Am J Neuroradiol. 2015;36(12):2196–205.
4. Kelley BP, et al. Autoimmune encephalitis: pathophysiology and imaging review of an overlooked diagnosis. AJNR Am J Neuroradiol. 2017;38(6):1070–8.
5. Caranci F, et al. Imaging findings in hypophysitis: a review. Radiol Med. 2020;125(3):319–28.
6. Chodakiewitz Y, et al. Ipilimumab treatment associated pituitary hypophysitis: clinical presentation and imaging diagnosis. Clin Neurol Neurosurg. 2014;125:125–30.
7. Smith JK, Matheus MG, Castillo M. Imaging manifestations of neurosarcoidosis. AJR Am J Roentgenol. 2004;182(2):289–95.
8. Ganeshan D, et al. Sarcoidosis from head to toe: what the radiologist needs to know. Radiographics. 2018;38(4):1180–200.
9. Park H, et al. Imaging of Histiocytosis in the era of genomic medicine. Radiographics. 2019;39(1):95–114.
10. Zaveri J, et al. More than just Langerhans cell histiocytosis: a radiologic review of histiocytic disorders. Radiographics. 2014;34(7):2008–24.
11. Martucci M, et al. Cerebral amyloid angiopathy-related inflammation: imaging findings and clinical outcome. Neuroradiology. 2014;56(4):283–9.
12. Moussaddy A, et al. Inflammatory cerebral amyloid angiopathy, amyloid-β–related angiitis, and primary angiitis of the central nervous system. Stroke. 2015;46(9):e210–3.
13. Denève M, et al. MRI features of demyelinating disease associated with anti-MOG antibodies in adults. J Neuroradiol. 2019;46(5):312–8.
14. Shahriari M, et al. MOGAD: how it differs from and resembles other neuroinflammatory disorders. AJR Am J Roentgenol. 2021;216(4):1031–9.
15. Salama S, et al. MOG antibody-associated encephalomyelitis/encephalitis. Mult Scler. 2019;25(11):1427–33.

Inherited Metabolic Disorders

Sara Fardin and Neel Madan

INTRODUCTION

- Inherited metabolic disorders (IMD) are a large group of rare genetic disorders characterized by a disorder of enzyme activity, leading to either reduced ability to synthesize essential compounds or the accumulation of substances that are either toxic or interfere with normal cellular function.
- Can be inherited or sporadic mutations.
- Can be classified by affected organelle, metabolites that accumulate, or using an image-based approach.
- Whole-exome sequencing along with technological advancements in molecular techniques have greatly increased the number of known IMDs, and improved diagnosis and treatment.
- Therapies are only beneficial early in the disease course, emphasizing the need for a speedy diagnosis.
- Imaging modalities, most importantly magnetic resonance imaging (MRI), keeps its central place in diagnosis [1].
  - Initial step is determining whether the process involves the white matter, gray matter, or both.
  - For those predominantly involving the white matter, further categorized as dysmyelination (white matter doesn't form normally), demyelination (normal myelin with subsequent myelin breakdown), and hypomyelination (normal myelination, but delayed and/or incomplete) [2].
- This chapter will cover the most common IMDs.

ADRENOLEUKODYSTROPHY

- A peroxisomal disorder that affects the white matter of the central nervous system, adrenal cortex, and testes [3, 4].
- Caused by a deficiency of a single enzyme, acyl-CoA synthetase, which breaks down the very long chain fatty acids (VLCFAs); if deficient, VLCFAs accumulate in tissue and plasma, which result in severe inflammatory demyelination in white matter.
- Diagnosis is made by detecting increased VLCFAs concentrations in plasma and cultured skin fibroblasts.
- Presentation will depend on the phenotype.
- Most common forms:
  - Classic X-linked adrenoleukodystrophy (X-ALD).
    - Severe form, which almost exclusively involves boys at 5–12 years.
    - Presents with impaired learning, ataxia, visual troubles, adrenal insufficiency, seizures.
  - Adrenomyeloneuropathy (AMN).
    - Milder adult spinocerebellar form, with cerebral involvement in up to 50%.
    - Usually presents with incontinence, ataxia, paresthesia.
  - X-ALD and AMN account for 80% of cases.
- Imaging (Fig. 13.1):
  - Most common findings of X-ALD:
    - Symmetric white matter demyelination occurs in a posterior predominant pattern, with involvement of the peri-trigonal regions and crossing the splenium of the corpus callosum.
    - As disease progresses, it extends more laterally and anteriorly; subcortical U fibers are spared in the early phase but involved later.
    - Can have atypical presentations in 10–15% of cases.
    - Imaging findings considered in terms of different zones of demyelination:

S. Fardin
Massachusetts General Hospital, Boston, MA, USA

N. Madan (✉)
Tufts University School of Medicine, Boston, MA, USA

© The Author(s), under exclusive license to Springer Nature Switzerland AG 2024
B. A. Vachha et al. (eds.), *What Radiology Residents Need to Know: Neuroradiology*, What Radiology Residents Need to Know,
https://doi.org/10.1007/978-3-031-55124-6_13

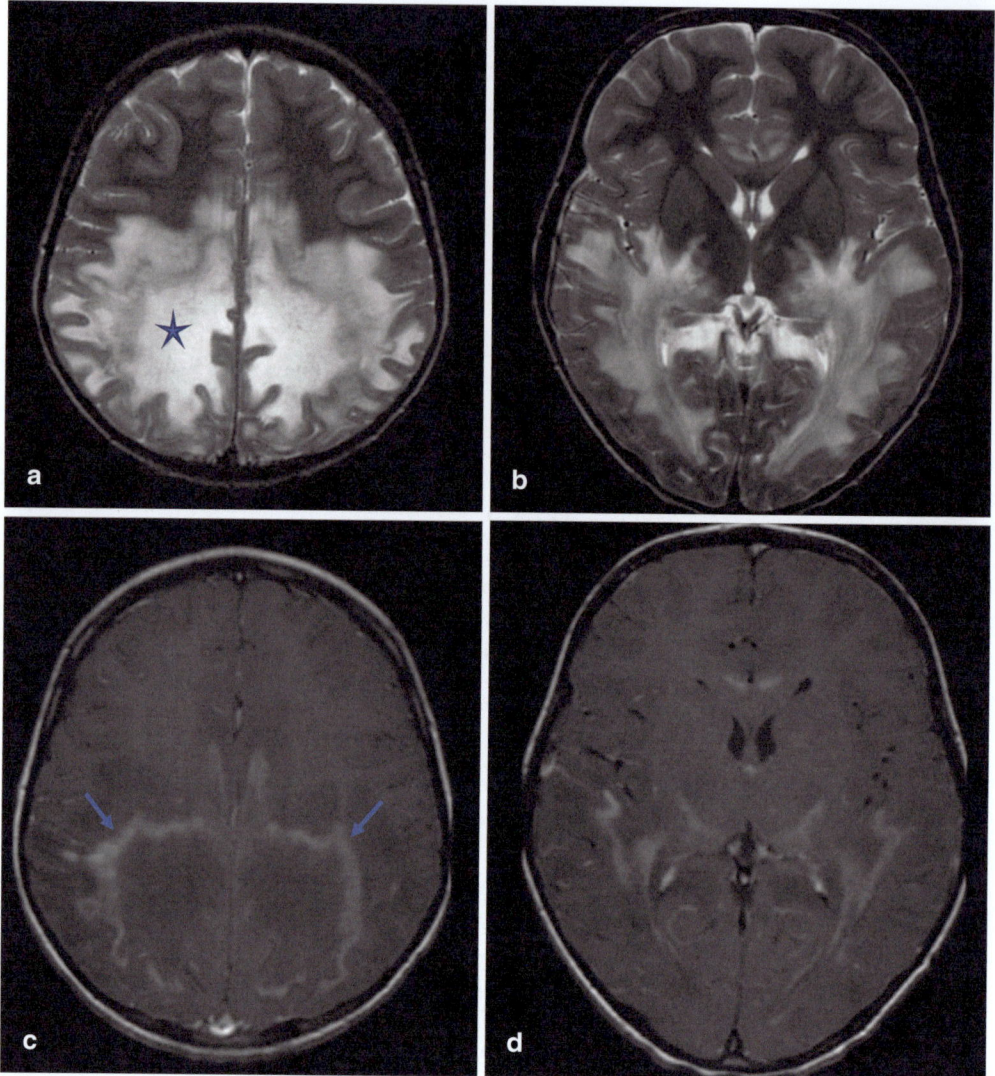

Fig. 13.1 X-linked adrenoleukodystrophy. Axial T2 (**a**) and (**b**) as well as axial T1 postcontrast (**c**) and (**d**) MRI images show confluent T2 hyperintensity of the white matter with a posterior predominance, with the central region of burnt out disease demonstrating more T1 hypointensity and T2 hyperintensity (Blue star), with the intermediate zone demonstrating a front of enhancement (Blue arrows)

- Central (inner) region represents irreversible gliosis and scarring.
  - ♦ Moderately hypointense on T1-weighted MR imaging.
  - ♦ Markedly hyperintense on T2-weighted imaging.
- Intermediate zone representing active inflammation and breakdown in the blood–brain barrier.
  - ♦ Isointense to hypointense at T2.
  - ♦ Enhances after intravenous administration of contrast material.
  - ♦ May have restricted diffusion.
- Peripheral (outer zone) representing the leading edge of active demyelination.
  - ♦ Moderately hyperintense on T2-weighted MR imaging.
  - ♦ No enhancement.
- ○ Adrenomyeloneuropathy:
  - Typically spares cerebral hemispheres.
  - Predominant involvement in cerebellum, corticospinal tracts, spinal cord with T2 hyperintensity, without enhancement.
- Progressive disease.
- Treatment includes dietary intake of Lorenzo's oil (mixture of triolein and trierucin), bone marrow transplantation, and/or hematopoietic stem cell therapy.

METACHROMATIC LEUKODYSTROPHY

- Autosomal recessive leukodystrophy and lysosomal storage disorder, caused by an inborn error of metabolism in the arylsulfatase A enzyme [4, 5].
- Enzyme necessary for normal metabolism of sphingolipid sulfatide, an important constituent of the myelin sheath. If deficient, sulfatides accumulate in various tissues including brain, peripheral nerves, kidneys, liver, and gallbladder.

13 Inherited Metabolic Disorders

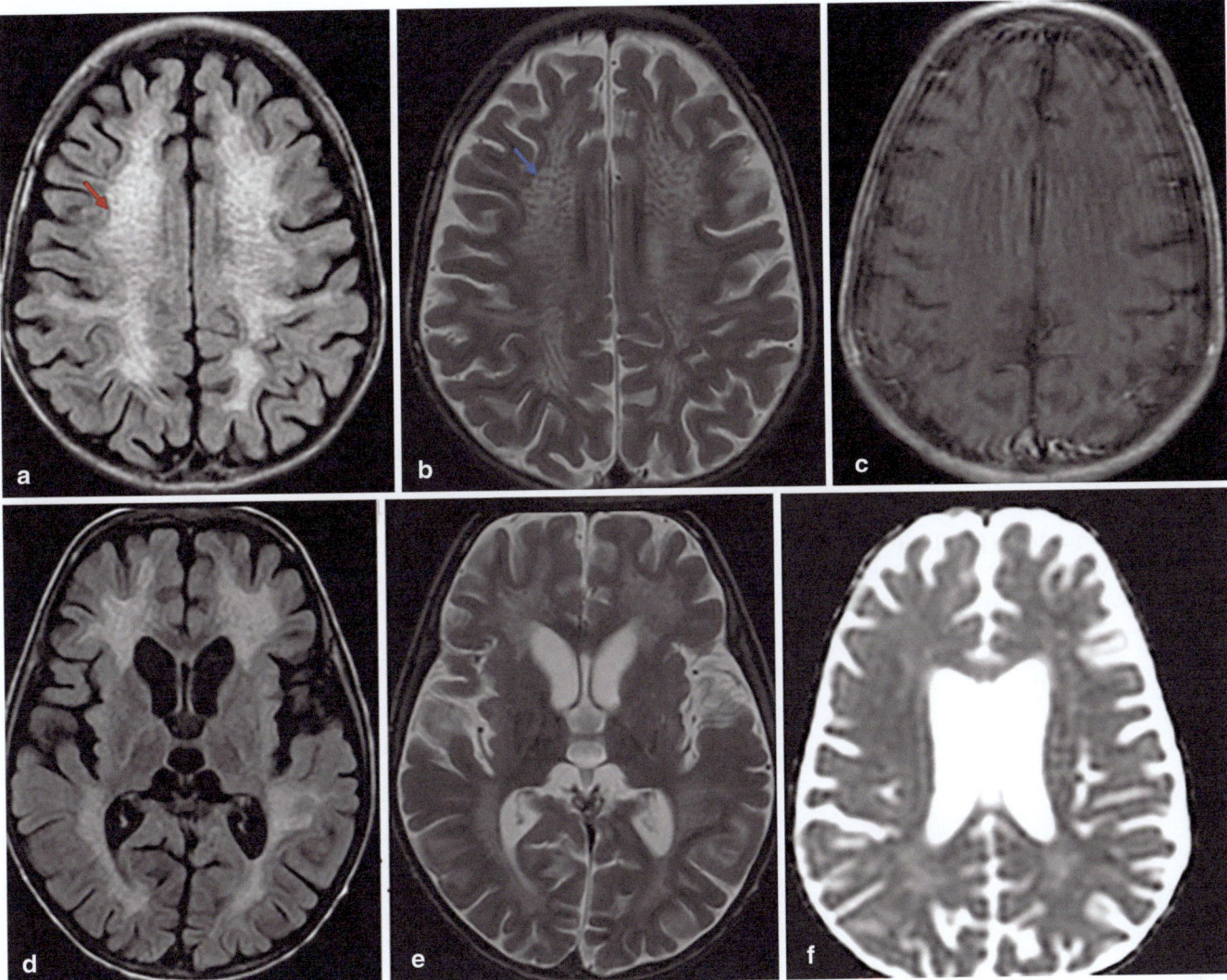

Fig. 13.2 Metachromatic leukodystrophy. Axial FLAIR (**a**) and (**d**), axial T2 (**b**) and (**e**), axial T1 postcontrast (**c**), and ADC map (**f**), demonstrate confluent T2/FLAIR hyperintensity involving the periventricular and deep white matter, with sparing of the subcortical U fibers (Red Arrow), as well as a "tigroid" appearance in the centrum semiovale (Blue Arrow). There is sparing of the corpus callosum, without restricted diffusion or abnormal enhancement

- Diagnosed biochemically on the basis of an abnormally low level of arylsulfatase A in peripheral blood leukocytes and in urine.
- Three clinical forms: late infantile, juvenile, and adult metachromatic leukodystrophy (MLD).
- All forms involve a progressive deterioration of neurodevelopment and neurocognitive function.
- Late infantile MLD accounts for >50% and manifests in children between 12 and 18 months of age, characterized by gait abnormality, muscle rigidity, loss of vision, impaired swallowing, and convulsions.
- Imaging (Fig. 13.2):
  - Confluent butterfly-shaped high T2 signal in periventricular white matter and corpus callosum.
  - Affected areas may show hypointense stripes and dots within the demyelinated white matter giving a "tigroid" or "leopard skin" appearance representing sparing of perivenular myelin.
  - Subcortical U fibers and cerebellum spared in early phase but involved later.
  - No white matter enhancement but cranial nerve enhancement has been reported.
- Treatment options include hematopoietic stem cell transplantation. Enzyme replacement and gene therapy is experimental.

ALEXANDER DISEASE

- De novo dominant mutation in the GFAP gene, which encodes glial fibrillary acidic protein [4, 6].
- Results in deposition of Rosenthal fibers, which contain large, abnormal GFAP, which affects astrocyte function.
- Classically, three clinical subgroups are recognized—infantile, juvenile, and adult, though more recently separated into Type I and Type II.
  - Type I:
    - Age of onset by age 4.
    - Characterized by early onset of macrocephaly, developmental delay (psychomotor retardation), and seizures with development of spasticity, ataxia, as well as bulbar and pseudobulbar signs.
    - Death occurs within 2–3 years.
  - Type II:
    - Any age, but typically after 4 years of age.
    - Slow cognitive decline, with progressive bulbar/pseudobulbar symptoms, ataxia, and spasticity.
    - Symptoms and disease course can be indistinguishable from those of other disorders, including multiple sclerosis.
- Imaging (Fig. 13.3):
  - Infantile:
    - Large head.
    - Characteristic symmetric bifrontal T2 hyperintensity, with a T1 hypointense, T2 hyperintense rim around the frontal horns, with enhancement.
    - Caudate and anterior putamen involvement, with T2 hyperintensity, enlargement, and rim of enhancement.
    - Subcortical U fibers involved early in disease course.
  - Juvenile/Adult:
    - Cerebellar, brainstem, and upper cervical cord involvement with T2 hyperintensity, and enhancement.
- No current treatment; symptomatic and supportive treatment only.

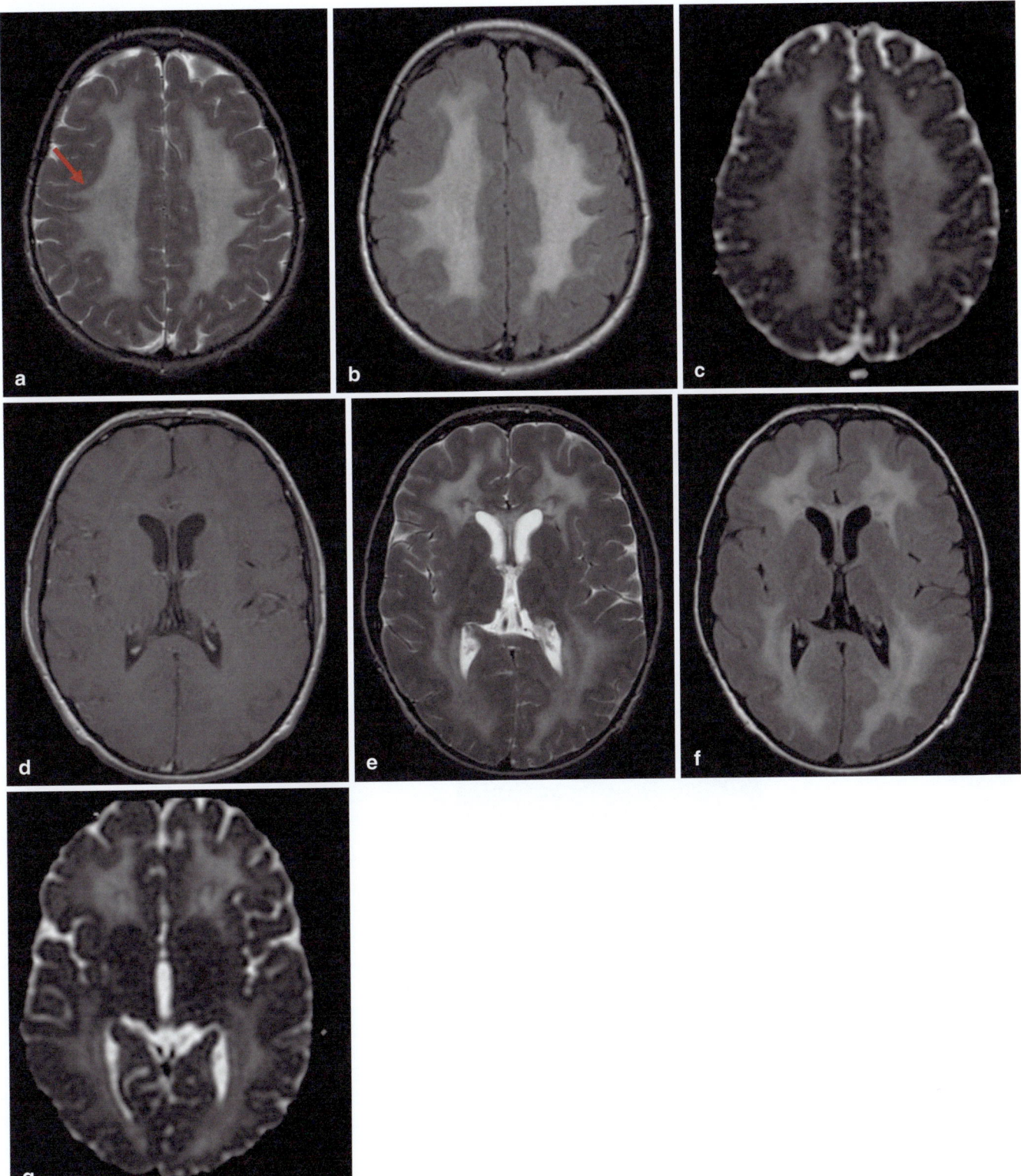

Fig. 13.3 Alexander disease. Axial T2 (**a**) and (**e**), axial FLAIR (**b**) and (**f**), axial ADC (**c**) and (**g**) and axial T1 postcontrast (**d**) MRI sequences demonstrate confluent T2/FLAIR hyperintensity throughout the white matter, with corresponding facilitated diffusion, with sparing of subcortical U-fibers (red arrow), and without enhancement

CANAVAN DISEASE

- Autosomal recessive spongiform leukodystrophy caused by a deficiency of N-acetylaspartylase, which results in an accumulation of *N*-acetylaspartate acid (NAA) in the urine, plasma, and brain [4, 6].
- Results in intramyelinic edema and myelin damage.
- Three clinical variants:
  o Congenital: Presents within a few days of life with profound hypotonia with poor head control; rapidly fatal.
  o Infantile: Presents at 3–6 months of life with hypotonia, megalencephaly, and seizures with death at 1–2 years of age.
  o Juvenile: Begins at 4–5 years of age, with slow progressive neurodegenerative disorder.
- Most common in Ashkenazi Jews.
- Imaging (Fig. 13.4):
  o Confluent T2/FLAIR hyperintensity throughout the white matter, with involvement of the globi pallidi.
  o Subcortical U-fibers involved early, with swollen gyri.
  o Eventually diffuse volume loss with expansion of extra-axial spaces.
  o Involvement of supratentorial and infratentorial white matter, deep gray nuclei, as well as cortex.
  o MR spectroscopy (MRS) shows markedly elevated NAA, diagnostic of Canavan Disease.
- No current treatment; symptomatic and supportive treatment only.

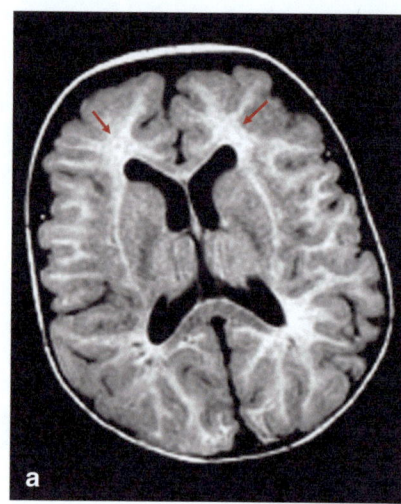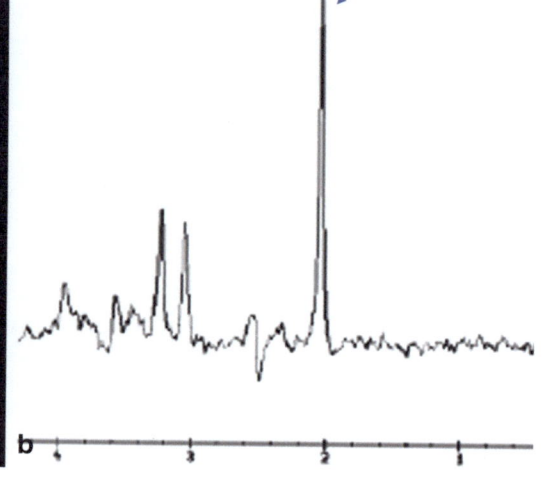

Fig. 13.4 Canavan disease. Axial FLAIR MRI (**a**) demonstrates characteristic extensive FLAIR hyperintensity (red arrows) throughout the white matter, with some enlargement of the ventricles reflecting volume loss. MR Spectroscopy (**b**) shows characteristic marked elevation of NAA (Blue arrow)

13 Inherited Metabolic Disorders

GLOBOID CELL LEUKODYSTROPHY (KRABBE DISEASE)

- Progressive autosomal recessive lysosomal storage disorder caused by a deficiency of the enzyme galactocerebroside β-galactosidase that degrades cerebroside, a normal constituent of myelin, which then accumulates in the lysosomes of macrophages within the white matter of CNS and PNS, forming the globoid cells characteristic of the disease [4, 6].
- Diagnosis is made by demonstrating a deficiency of the enzyme in peripheral blood leukocytes.
- Infantile form:
  - Most common (90% of cases), usually presenting under 7 months, with extreme irritability and feeding difficulties, spasticity, seizures, and regression.
  - Female predominance (80%).
  - Rapidly progressive and fatal.
- Late-onset form: Occurs at 18 months or later, with impaired control of voluntary movements and spastic paraparesis, progressive vision loss, and polyneuropathy.
- Imaging (Fig. 13.5):
  - CT Findings: Symmetric hyperdensity reflecting calcification in thalami, basal ganglia, corona radiata, cerebellum, and dentate nuclei, with periventricular white matter hypodensity.

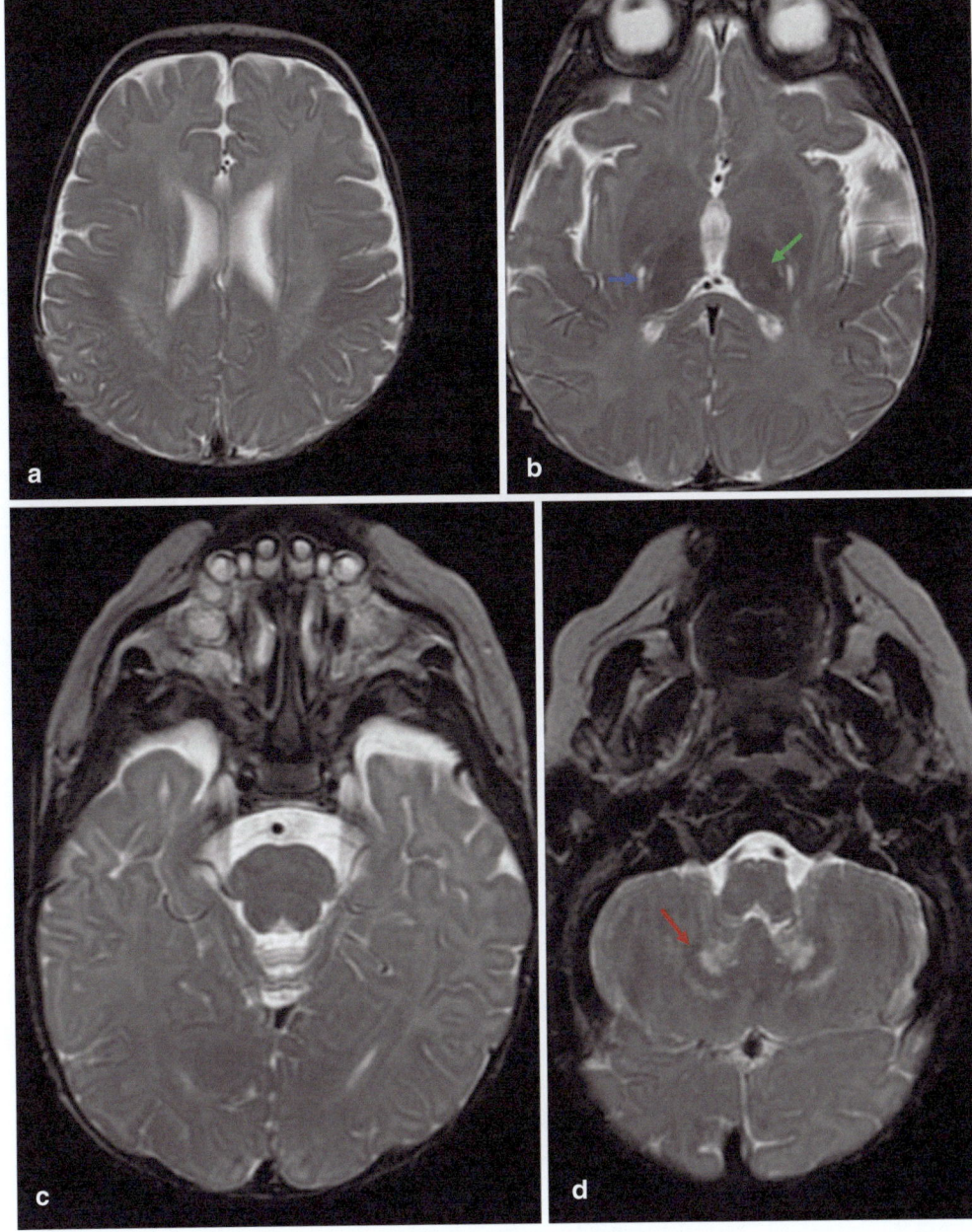

Fig. 13.5 Globoid cell leukodystrophy (Krabbe disease). Krabbe in a 4-month-old with multiple axial T2 images (**a–d**) showing early increased T2 signal in the posterior limbs of the internal capsule (blue arrow) and cerebellar white matter with characteristic "halo" around the dentate nuclei (red arrow), and T2 hypointensity of the thalami (green arrow)

- MRI:
  - T2 hyperintensity involving the corticospinal tracts and deep periventricular white matter, initially sparing subcortical U-fibers.
  - T2 hypointensity/susceptibility in regions of calcification including thalami and basal ganglia.
  - Cerebellar findings early in disease, with "halo" or ring-like T1 hypointensity and T2 hyperintensity surrounding dentate nuclei.
  - May show enhancement of cranial nerves as well as enhancement and thickening of cauda equina nerve roots.
- Treatment with hematopoietic stem cell transplantation may be helpful.

PELIZAEUS-MERZBACHER DISEASE

- X-linked leukodystrophy, which is due to abnormality of a gene encoding two primary components of myelin [4, 6].
- Hypomyelinating disorder due to variations in PLP1.
- Traditionally divided into two subtypes:
  - Classic form:
    - Usually presents in the first year of life with nystagmus, delayed motor, and cognitive milestones, and ataxia.
    - Usually live until late adolescence or early adulthood.
  - Connatal form:
    - More severe and rare.
    - Usually presents at birth or in early infancy with nystagmus, extrapyramidal hyperkinesia, spasticity, optic atrophy, and seizure.
    - Death usually occurs in early childhood.
- Imaging (Fig. 13.6):
  - Low signal intensity white matter on CT scan.
  - It appears as a lack of myelination as opposed to myelin destruction on MRI. Thus, diffuse T2 hyperintensity of white matter with either complete absence of myelination in severe cases, or rests of myelination including around perivascular spaces.
  - Progressive white matter and cerebellar volume loss.
- Treatment is supportive, with death in early childhood.

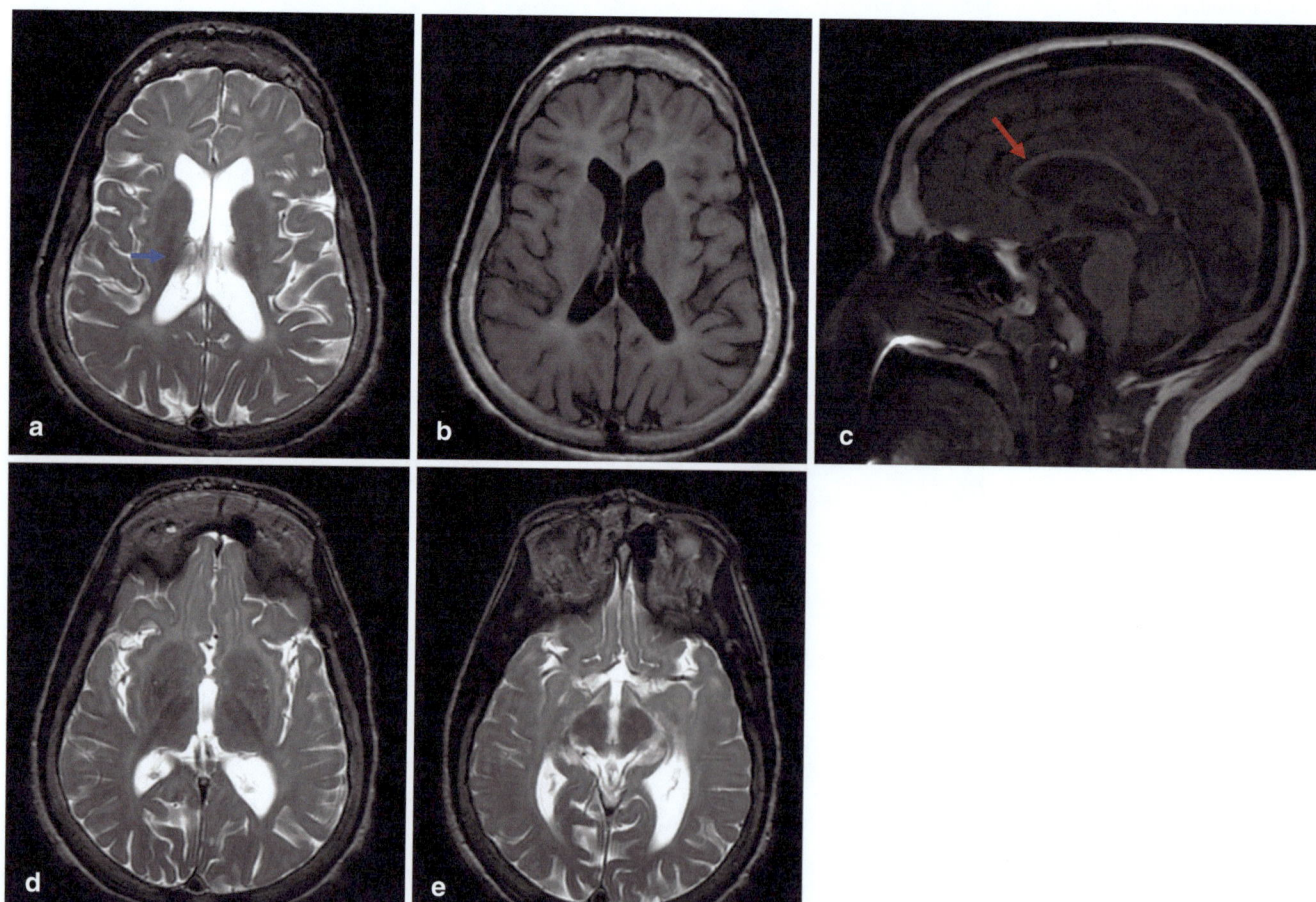

Fig. 13.6 Pelizaeus-Merzbacher disease. Axial T2 (**a, d, e**), axial FLAIR (**b**), and sagittal T1 (**c**) MRI images demonstrate a hypomyelination pattern, with overall delayed myelination. Regions with some myelination include the posterior limb of the internal capsule (blue arrow) and the thin corpus callosum (red arrow)

References

1. Barkovich AJ. An approach to MRI of metabolic disorders in children. J Neuroradiol J Neuroradiol. 2007;34(2):75–88. https://doi.org/10.1016/j.neurad.2007.01.125.
2. Resende LL, de Paiva ARB, Kok F, da Costa LC, Lucato LT. Adult leukodystrophies: a step-by-step diagnostic approach. Radiogr Rev Publ Radiol Soc N Am Inc. 2019;39(1):153–68. https://doi.org/10.1148/rg.2019180081.
3. Siddiqui S, Pawar G, Hogg JP. MRI in X-linked adrenoleukodystrophy. Neurology. 2015;84(2):211. https://doi.org/10.1212/WNL.0000000000001122.
4. van der Knaap MS. Magnetic resonance of myelination and myelin disorders. 3rd ed. New York: Springer; 2005.
5. Chauhan NS, Sharma M, Bhardwaj A. Classical case of late-infantile form of metachromatic leukodystrophy. J Neurosci Rural Pract. 2016;7(3):473–5. https://doi.org/10.4103/0976-3147.181482.
6. van der Knaap MS, Schiffmann R, Mochel F, Wolf NI. Diagnosis, prognosis, and treatment of leukodystrophies. Lancet Neurol. 2019;18(10):962–72. https://doi.org/10.1016/S1474-4422(19)30143-7.

Demyelinating Diseases

Komal Manzoor, Behroze A. Vachha, and Susie Y. Huang

Demyelinating disorders can be classified into:

- Primary demyelinating diseases.
- Secondary demyelinating diseases.

Primary Demyelinating Diseases

Multiple Sclerosis (MS)

- Most common acquired demyelinating and inflammatory disease of the central nervous system.
- Affects females more than males (3:1 ratio) between the ages of 20 and 50.
- Prevalence of MS varies with geographic location. Occurs most often in temperate climates.
- Several causative factors have been implicated, including autoimmune reaction, prior infection, e.g., Epstein-Barr virus, and genetic factors (HLA associations).
- Variable clinical course, with relapsing-remitting subtype being the most common, followed by primary and secondary progressive MS.
- Typical presenting symptoms: double vision, weakness, numbness, tingling, and gait disturbances.
- With disease progression, there may be loss of bowel/bladder function, blindness, paralysis, and dementia.
- The McDonald criteria specify that the diagnosis of MS is made based on demonstrating dissemination of lesions in space and time [1].

- *Dissemination in space* can be shown on MRI with presence of ≥1 T2 hyperintense lesion in at least two of the following four locations: periventricular, juxtacortical, infratentorial, and spinal cord.
- *Dissemination in time* can be demonstrated on MRI with either a new T2 or gadolinium-enhancing lesion on a follow-up MRI with reference to a baseline scan, or simultaneous presence of gadolinium-enhancing and nonenhancing lesions on a single scan.
- 2017 revised McDonald criteria include cortical lesions as evidence of dissemination in space and CSF oligoclonal bands as evidence of dissemination in time [2].

Imaging Findings

- MS plaques can occur anywhere in the central nervous system with a greater predilection for the following areas: periventricular white matter (85%) (Fig. 14.1), callososeptal interface, subcortical white matter, internal capsule, optic nerves and visual pathways, brainstem, middle cerebellar peduncles, and cervical spinal cord.
- Burden of T1 hypointense lesions "T1 black holes" correlate with clinical disability better than volume of T2 hyperintense lesions.
- Enhancement is variable and typically transient, seen during active demyelination.
- Demyelinating lesions are characterized by incomplete rim of enhancement with the advancing front of active demyelination facing the white matter and an open border of non-enhancement pointing toward the gray matter (open rim sign) (Fig. 14.1).
- In the acute phase, lesions may demonstrate restricted diffusion, which is thought to reflect cytotoxic edema related to intense inflammation.
- Central atrophy and atrophy of the corpus callosum indicate severe disease and correlate with cognitive symptoms.

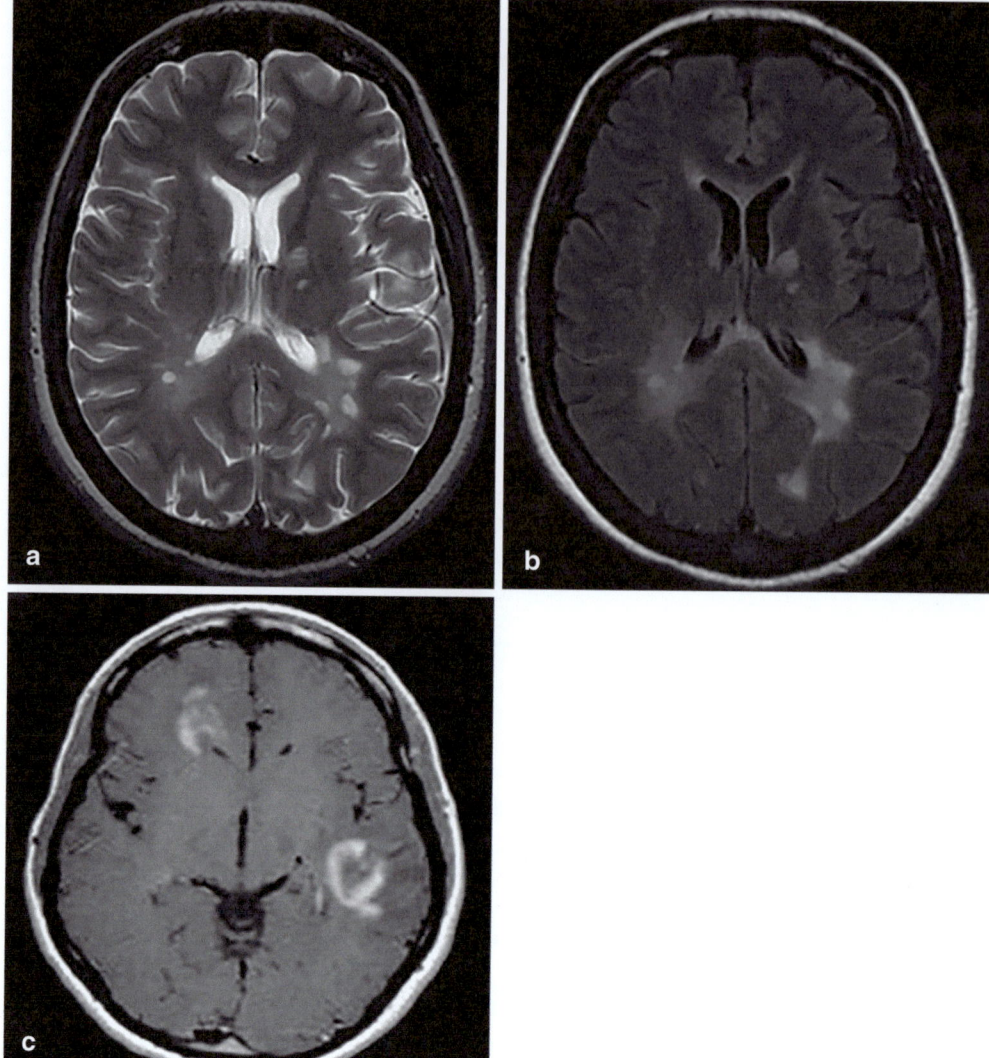

Fig. 14.1 Multiple sclerosis lesions. (**a**) Axial T2 and (**b**) FLAIR images demonstrating T2-hyperintense lesions in the bilateral periventricular white matter and genu of the left internal capsule. (**c**) Open rim sign. Axial T1-weighted postcontrast image demonstrating incomplete rim-enhancing lesions in the periventricular white matter, consistent with active demyelinating lesions

- Cortical lesions are a key component of MS pathology and play a major role in disease progression.
- There are three types of cortical lesions detected on MRI: leukocortical, intracortical, and subpial.
- Cortical lesions can be detected on 3 T using double IR (inversion recovery) and phase-sensitive IR sequences.
- 7T MRI has high sensitivity for detection of cortical lesion.
- Ependymal dot-dash sign: an early imaging sign of MS on FLAIR images. When these lesions propagate centrifugally along the medullary veins and are arranged perpendicular to the lateral ventricles extending radially outward (best seen on parasagittal images), they are termed Dawson's fingers (Fig. 14.2).

Tumefactive MS

- Clinical and imaging features help in differentiating demyelinating disease from a tumor (see Table 14.1).
- Demyelinating lesions typically have minimal mass effect for the size and extent of the lesion (Fig. 14.3).

Spine Imaging in MS

- Lesions in the spinal cord are seen in 50–60% of MS patients on imaging studies.
- Typically involve no more than 1–2 contiguous spinal levels and less than ½ of the cord cross-sectional area (Fig. 14.4).
- In early MS, predilection for the cervical spinal cord that become more evenly distributed along the thoracic spine and conus with advancing disease.
- MS plaques occur preferentially in the dorsolateral spinal cord and do not respect boundaries between specific tracts or between gray and white matter.
- Elongated poorly marginated T2 hyperintense intramedullary lesions.
- Spinal cord may be normal in size or enlarged.

14 Demyelinating Diseases

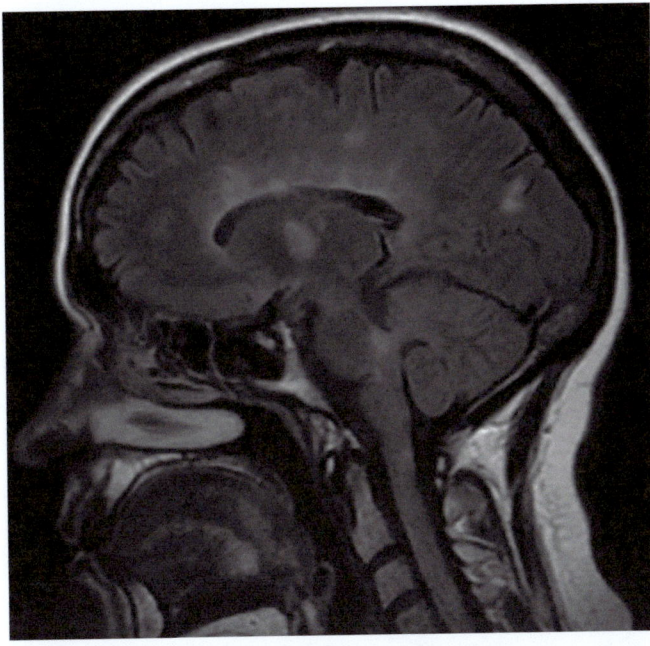

Fig. 14.2 Dawson's fingers. Sagittal FLAIR image demonstrating T2/FLAIR hyperintense lesions radiating perpendicular to the lateral ventricles

- Active lesions may enhance.
- Enhancing MS lesions can be indistinguishable from neoplastic or other inflammatory lesions, particularly when the cord is enlarged.
- Clinical correlation and often serial scanning are necessary to make diagnosis, especially in cases where MRI of the brain is normal.

Differential Diagnosis of MS

- ADEM (Acute disseminated encephalomyelitis).
- Lyme disease.
- Vasculitis.
- Hypertension and chronic ischemic white matter lesions.
- Migraine.
- Diffuse axonal injury.

Other MS Variants

- Charcot (Classic form), which is present in majority of cases.
- Balo concentric sclerosis: A histologic MS lesion with alternating concentric regions of demyelination and normal brain. This variant of MS has little mass effect with peripheral medial enhancement "advancing enhancement" (Fig. 14.5).
- Schilder (Diffuse sclerosis): Acute rapidly progressive form of MS with bilateral relatively symmetric demyelination. Commonly seen in childhood and often involves the centrum semiovale and occipital lobes.
- Marburg: Virulent form of acute MS. Can be preceded by fever and rapidly progresses to immobility and death.

Table 14.1 Features of tumefactive MS versus tumor

Tumefactive MS	Tumor
Typically occurs in younger patients	Occurs across all age groups, most commonly in older patients
Symptoms disseminated in space and time	Symptoms worsen progressively over time and are localized to affected brain areas
Presence of other white matter lesions separate from mass	Typically solitary unless metastatic disease is suspected
Little mass effect for the size of the lesion	Marked associated mass effect

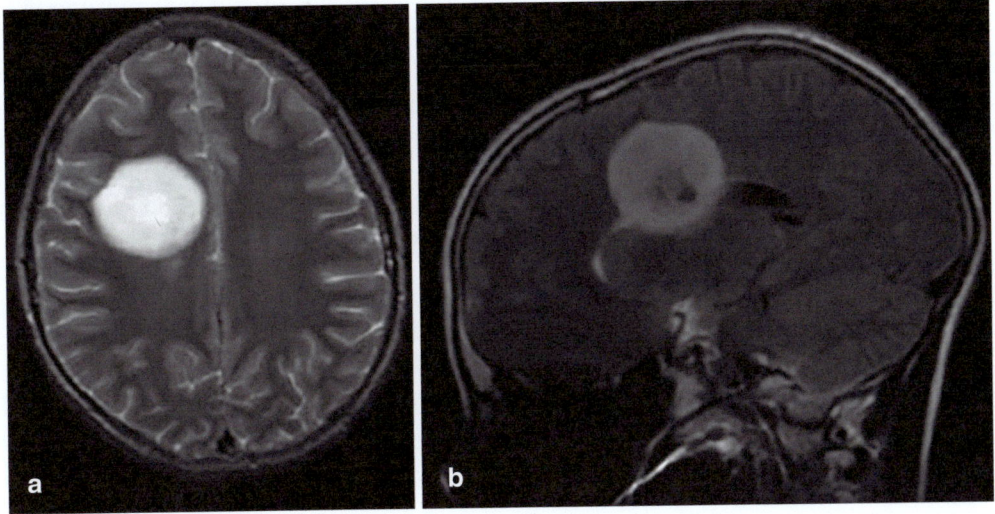

Fig. 14.3 Tumefactive MS. (**a**) Axial T2 and (**b**) sagittal FLAIR images demonstrate a large round T2 hyperintense mass-like lesion. Notice that the lesion has relatively little mass effect for the size of the lesion

Fig. 14.4 Cervical spine lesions in MS. (**a**) Sagittal T2 and (**b**) STIR images demonstrate multiple short segment T2 hyperintense lesions in the cervical spinal cord, most prominent at the level of C4–C6

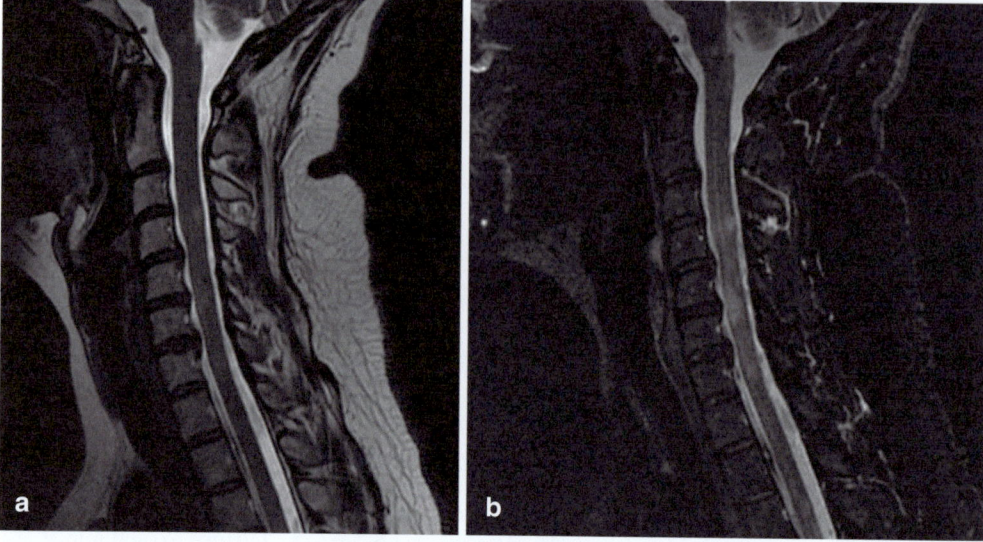

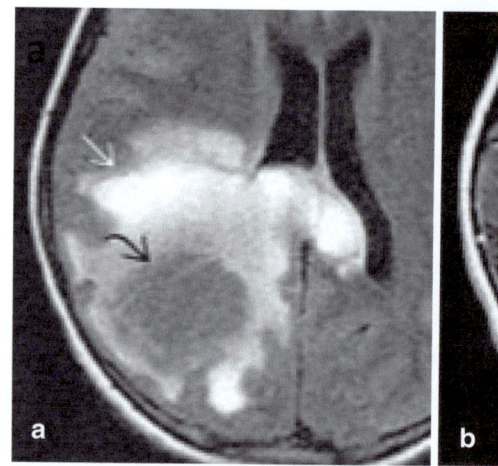
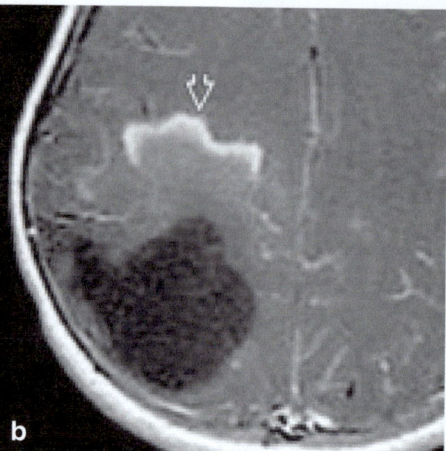
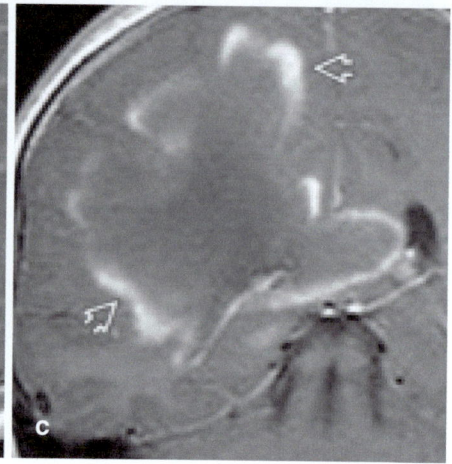

Fig. 14.5 Balo concentric sclerosis. (**a**) Axial FLAIR and (**b**) axial and (**c**) coronal postcontrast T1-weighted images demonstrate a central FLAIR and T1 hypointense mass in the right parieto-occipital region with extensive surrounding T2/FLAIR hyperintensity and ill-defined enhancement at the edge of the lesion

Optic Neuritis in MS

- Inflammation of the optic nerve.
- Many disease processes can be associated with optic neuritis, most common being demyelinating disease such as MS and neuromyelitis optica.
- Often the first presenting sign of MS.
- In older patients, ischemic optic neuropathy is the main differential diagnosis.

Imaging

- MS usually involves one optic nerve. Bilateral involvement is rare in MS.
- Abnormal enhancement of optic nerve on contrast-enhanced MRI.
- Appears as T2/STIR hyperintensity in the optic nerve.
- Active inflammation is associated with enhancement in the optic nerve.
- Extent of nerve involvement on imaging correlates with the visual impairment and prognosis.
- In chronic cases, optic nerve becomes atrophic.
- Optic nerve involvement in MS is more focal as compared to NMO and MOG in which it is more extensive.

Other Neuroinflammatory Demyelinating Diseases

Neuromyelitis Optica (NMO)

- B-cell-mediated antibody response against aquaporin-4 (AQP-4) water channels.
- Diagnosis can be made with demonstration of serum NMO-IgG antibodies: 90% specific, 70–75% sensitive.

14 Demyelinating Diseases

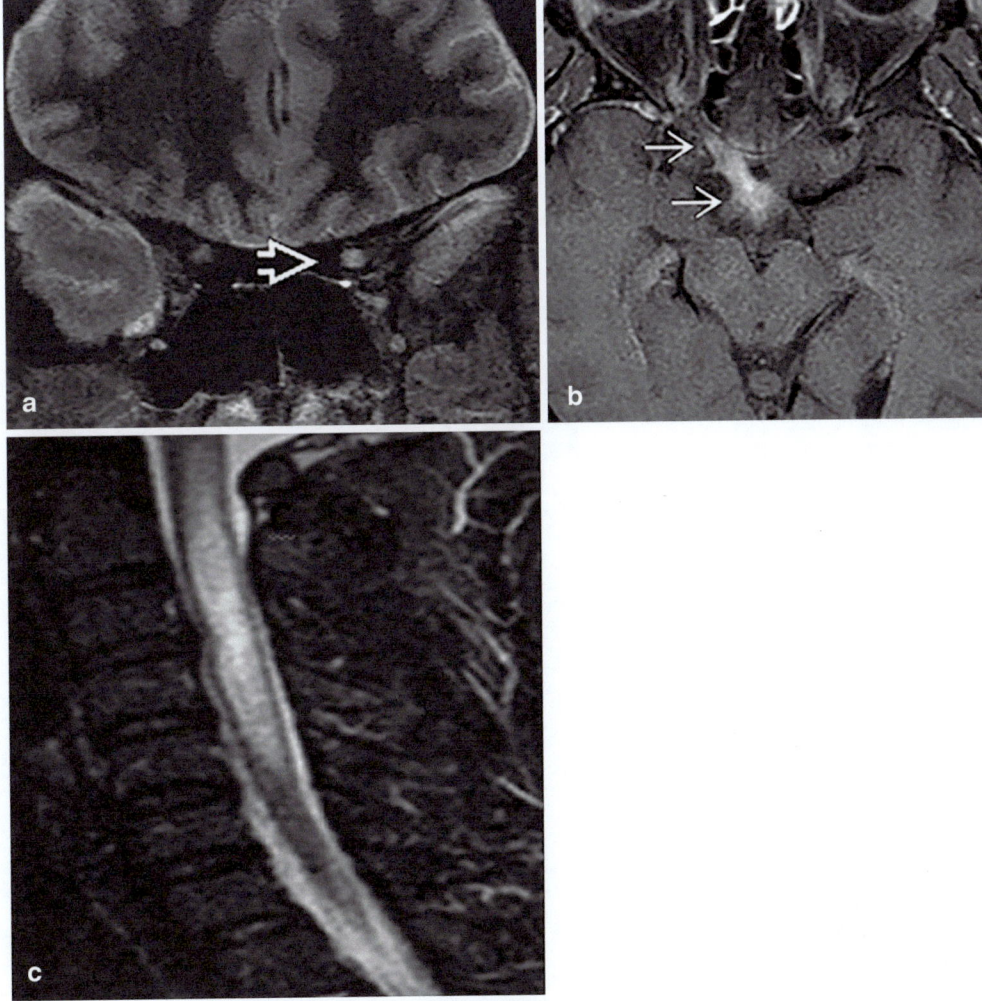

Fig. 14.6 Neuromyelitis optica. (**a**) Coronal STIR image showing T2/STIR hyperintensity and enlargement of the left optic nerve. There is also subtle T2/STIR hyperintensity in the right optic nerve. (**b**) Axial T1-weighted postcontrast image demonstrating enhancement of the right optic nerve and optic chiasm. (**c**) Sagittal T2 image showing longitudinally extensive T2 hyperintensity extending from C2 to C5

Imaging

- Bilateral optic nerve involvement in 50% cases of NMO (Fig. 14.6).
- Lesions involving the optic chiasm on MRI are more specific for NMO.
- Brain MRI may be normal or may show hyperintense lesions in areas with greater expression of AQP-4 [3].
- Transverse myelitis involves the cervical and thoracic spinal cord most commonly with long-segment lesions spanning more than three spinal segments (Fig. 14.6).
- Lesions are hypointense on T1 and hyperintense on T2-weighted images.
- With the progression of disease, spinal cord becomes atrophic.

Susac Syndrome

- Retinocochleocerebral vasculopathy, a multisystem immune-mediated microvascular occlusive endotheliopathy [4].
- More common in females than males with ages 20–40.
- Classic clinical triad:
  - Acute or subacute encephalopathy with or without migraine.
  - Sensorineural hearing loss.
  - Branch retinal artery occlusions.

Imaging

- On T2/FLAIR, punctate white matter hyperintensities are seen in >90% of cases (Fig. 14.7).
- Involvement of corpus callosum (80%) with lesions in the middle of corpus callosum rather than at the callososeptal interface, in distinction to MS.
- Basal ganglia lesions (70%).
- Variable enhancement can be seen, usually punctate.
- White matter lesions represent small infarcts due to occlusive endotheliopathy and often demonstrate restricted diffusion.

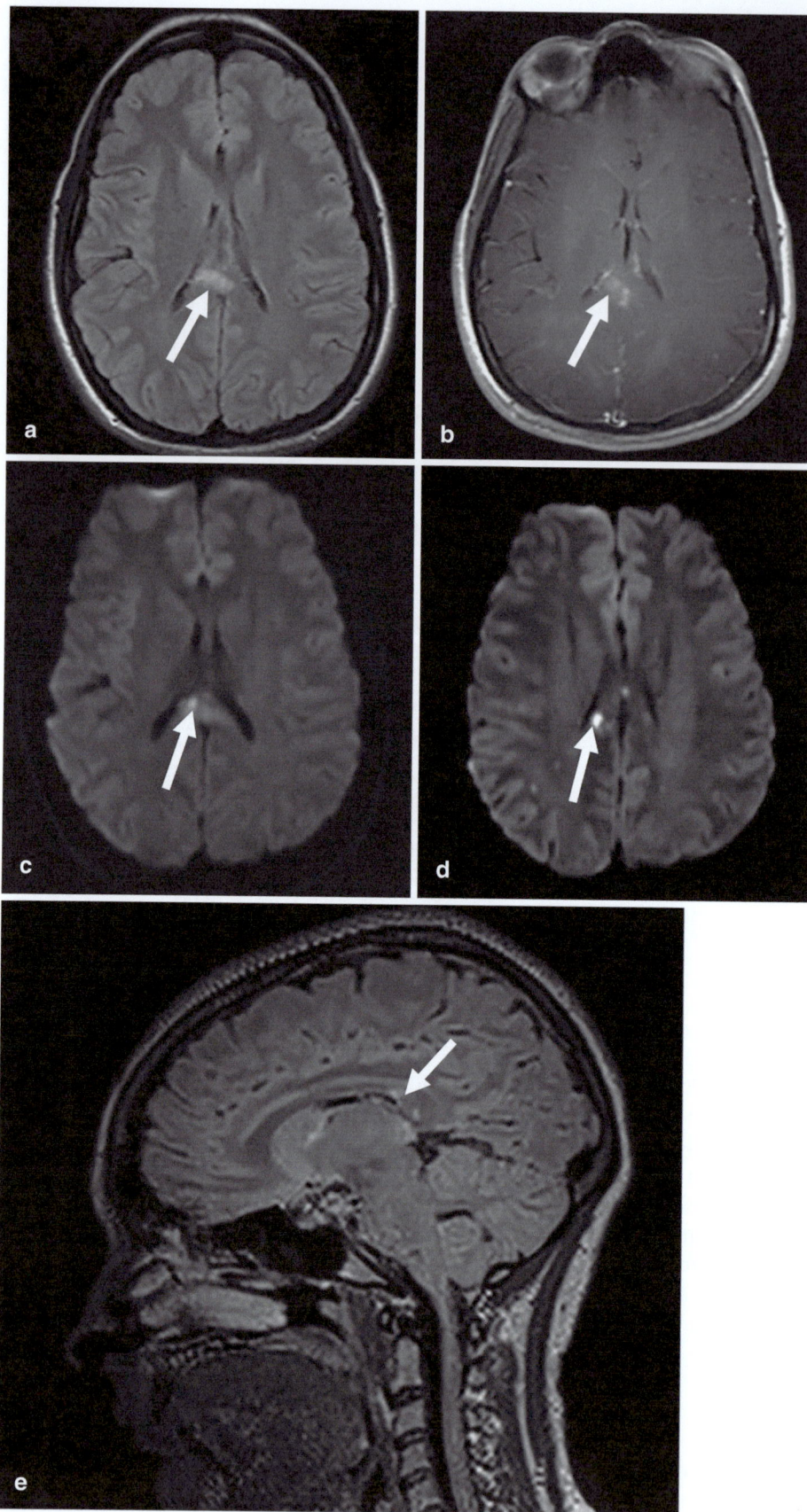

Fig. 14.7 Susac syndrome. (**a**) Axial FLAIR image demonstrates a T2/FLAIR hyperintense lesion in the central splenium of the corpus callosum. (**b**) Axial T1-weighted postcontrast image shows punctate enhancement within the lesion in the splenium of the corpus callosum. (**c**) Axial diffusion-weighted image shows restricted diffusion in the splenial lesion and (**d**) additional punctate foci of restricted diffusion in the posterior body of the corpus callosum corresponding to additional ischemic lesions related to occlusive endotheliopathy. (**e**) Sagittal FLAIR image demonstrating a punctate T2/FLAIR hyperintense lesion in the posterior body/splenium of the corpus callosum

14 Demyelinating Diseases

Secondary Demyelinating Diseases

Acute Disseminated Encephalomyelitis (ADEM)

- Immune-mediated demyelinating disease related to an antecedent viral infection or vaccination [5].
- Most commonly associated with measles, also with chickenpox, rubella, mumps, and other viral agents.
- Clinically can present as focal neurologic deficits typically within 2–3 weeks following a viral illness.
- Both clinically and on MRI, ADEM may appear identical to the initial presentation of MS.
- The diagnosis is usually made by history and CSF, which may demonstrate increase in white cells with a lymphocytic predominance and increased myelin basic protein.
- Follows a monophasic course. Follow-up MRI demonstrating regression of lesions and enhancement is helpful in distinguishing MS from ADEM.

Imaging

- Predominantly involves white matter with basal ganglia involvement in up to 50% of cases.
- Most lesions are located in the subcortical white matter with asymmetric involvement of both cerebral hemispheres (Fig. 14.8).
- Lesions are identical in age and demonstrate similar phase of enhancement.
- Hemorrhage indicates worse prognosis.
- Lesions usually regress.

Progressive Multifocal Leukoencephalopathy

- A demyelinating disease caused by JC virus infecting the oligodendrocytes.
- Associated with an immunosuppressed state, e.g., HIV, organ transplant patients.

Imaging

- PML lesions can occur anywhere in the brain with a greater predilection for the parieto-occipital region, thalamus, basal ganglia, and corpus callosum.
- Appears initially as a focal region of low intensity on T1-weighted imaging and high intensity on T2-weighted imaging, which progresses in extent and can be accompanied by cortical atrophy.
- See Chap. 11 for a further description of PML.

Cerebral Autosomal Dominant Arteriopathy with Subcortical Infarcts and Leukoencephalopathy (CADASIL)

- Autosomal dominant inherited arteriopathy of small and medium size vessels [4].
- Caused by a point mutation on chromosome 19 (NOTCH3 gene).
- Usually presents in fourth to fifth decades with subcortical dementia.
- Early presentation includes migraines, transient ischemic attacks, and strokes.
- Diagnosis is usually made by skin biopsy or genetic testing.

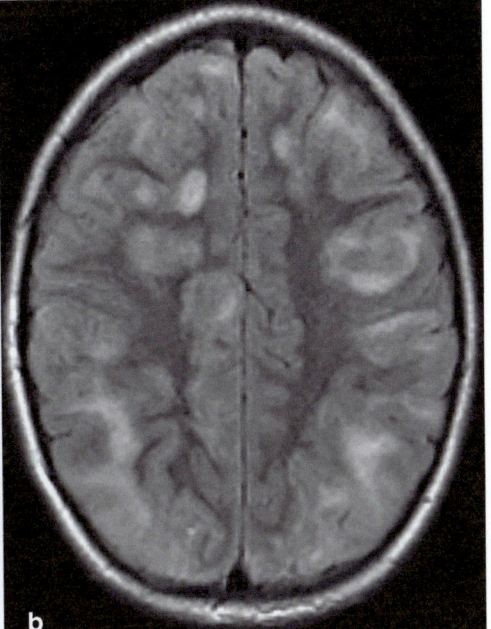

Fig. 14.8 ADEM. 8-year-old male with ataxia and change in mental status. (**a**) and (**b**) Axial FLAIR images show multiple patchy T2/FLAIR hyperintense lesions predominantly in the subcortical white matter distributed asymmetrically throughout the cerebral hemispheres

Imaging

- Symmetric, confluent high signal on T2-weighted images (Fig. 14.9).
- Predominantly involves the frontal, temporal, and insular regions.
- Anterior temporal lobe and external capsule involvement have high sensitivity and specificity for CADASIL.
- Patients often present with lacunar infarcts in the setting of widespread white matter disease.

Binswanger Disease (Subcortical Arteriosclerotic Encephalopathy)

- Commonly associated with HTN (98% of pts).
- Affects both older men and women of ages >50.
- Can present initially as stroke followed by declining mental status, seizures, psychiatric disturbances, and gait abnormalities.

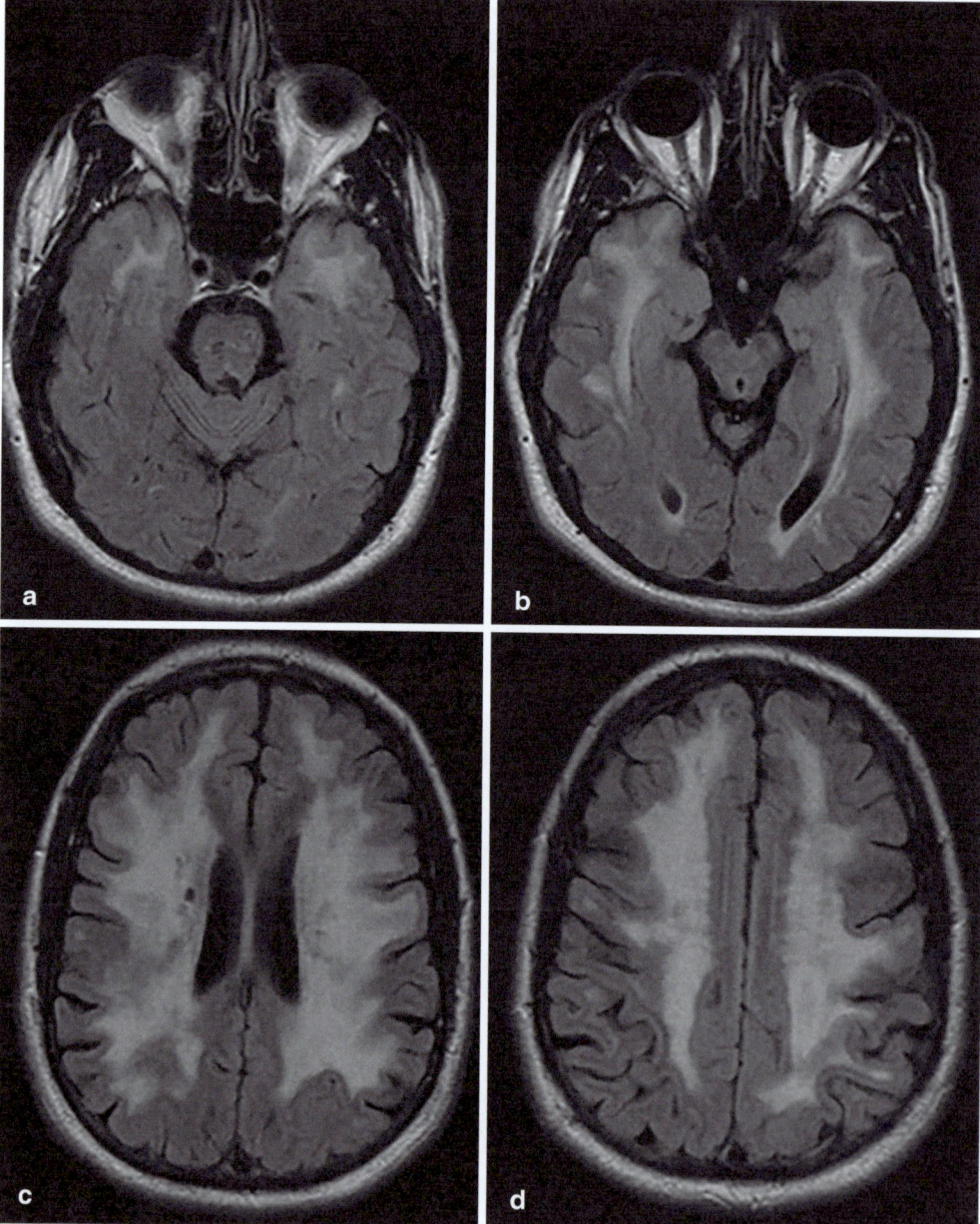

Fig. 14.9 CADASIL. (**a**) and (**b**) Axial FLAIR images show extensive symmetric confluent T2/FLAIR hyperintensity in the bilateral anterior temporal lobes, (**c**) bilateral corona radiata with scattered white matter lacunar infarcts, and (**d**) bilateral centrum semiovale

Fig. 14.10 PRES. (**a**) and (**b**) Axial FLAIR images show extensive symmetric confluent T2/FLAIR hyperintensity in the bilateral occipital and posterior temporal lobes

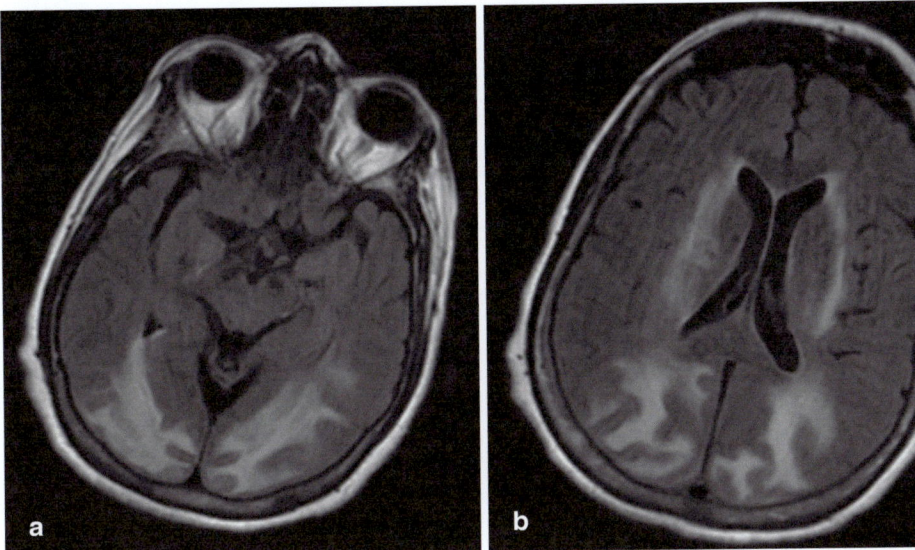

Imaging

- Diffuse, confluent white matter involvement and lacunar infarcts.
- Subcortical U fibers are spared because of dual blood supply from the involved medullary arteries and uninvolved cortical arteries.
- High T2 signal intensity in the white matter of the frontal, parietal, and occipital regions.

Posterior Reversible Encephalopathy Syndrome (PRES)

- Disorder of cerebrovascular autoregulation with multiple etiologies, most of which cause acute hypertension.
- Predilection for posterior circulation, which is sparsely innervated by sympathetic nerves and unable to autoregulate in response to acute changes in blood pressure.
- Etiologies include: severe hypertension, preeclampsia/eclampsia, uremic encephalopathy, and drug toxicity (e.g., cyclosporin, tacrolimus, cisplatin).
- Clinical symptoms include altered mental status, headache, blurred vision, seizures, and focal neurologic deficits.

Imaging

- Parietal-occipital T2 hyperintense cortical and subcortical white matter lesions (Fig. 14.10) [6].
- Lesions occasionally show enhancement.
- Lesions do not typically show restricted diffusion in the reversible phase. Restricted diffusion indicates presence of underlying cerebral ischemia.
- Lesions may be accompanied by hemorrhage in a minority of cases.
- Involvement of the cerebellum, basal ganglia, brainstem, and deep white matter can occur but is less common (atypical PRES).
- Symptoms and radiologic findings may be reversible with the treatment of hypertension.

References

1. Polman CH, Reingold SC, Banwell B, Clanet M, Cohen JA, Filippi M, Fujihara K, Havrdova E, Hutchinson M, Kappos L, Lublin FD, Montalban X, O'Connor P, Sandberg-Wollheim M, Thompson AJ, Waubant E, Weinshenker B, Wolinsky JS. Diagnostic criteria for multiple sclerosis: 2010 revisions to the McDonald criteria. Ann Neurol. 2011;69(2):292–302. https://doi.org/10.1002/ana.22366.
2. Thompson AJ, Banwell BL, Barkhof F, Carroll WM, Coetzee T, Comi G, Correale J, Fazekas F, Filippi M, Freedman MS, Fujihara K, Galetta SL, Hartung HP, Kappos L, Lublin FD, Marrie RA, Miller AE, Miller DH, Montalban X, Mowry EM, Sorensen PS, Tintore M, Traboulsee AL, Trojano M, Uitdehaag BMJ, Vukusic S, Waubant E, Weinshenker BG, Reingold SC, Cohen JA. Diagnosis of multiple sclerosis: 2017 revisions of the McDonald criteria. Lancet Neurol. 2018;17(2):162–73. https://doi.org/10.1016/S1474-4422(17)30470-2.
3. Kim HJ, Paul F, Lana-Peixoto MA, Tenembaum S, Asgari N, Palace J, Klawiter EC, Sato DK, de Seze J, Wuerfel J, Banwell BL, Villoslada P, Saiz A, Fujihara K, Kim SH, Guthy-Jackson Charitable Foundation NMOICC, Biorepository. MRI characteristics of neuromyelitis optica spectrum disorder: an international update. Neurology. 2015;84(11):1165–73. https://doi.org/10.1212/WNL.0000000000001367.
4. Sarbu N, Shih RY, Jones RV, Horkayne-Szakaly I, Oleaga L, Smirniotopoulos JG. White matter diseases with radiologic-pathologic correlation. Radiographics. 2016;36(5):1426–47. https://doi.org/10.1148/rg.2016160031.
5. Ryan M, Ibrahim M, Parmar HA. Secondary demyelination disorders and destruction of white matter. Radiol Clin North Am. 2014;52(2):337–54. https://doi.org/10.1016/j.rcl.2013.11.007.
6. Bartynski WS, Boardman JF. Distinct imaging patterns and lesion distribution in posterior reversible encephalopathy syndrome. AJNR Am J Neuroradiol. 2007;28(7):1320–7. https://doi.org/10.3174/ajnr.A0549.

Tumors and Tumor-Like Lesions

15

Susie Yi Huang, Raymond Y. Huang, and Behroze A. Vachha

Introduction

In this chapter, we utilize the most recent (fifth) edition of the World Health Organization (WHO) Classification of Tumors of the Central Nervous System (CNS) published in 2021, which builds upon the fourth edition by incorporating molecular biomarkers into CNS tumor classification [1]. This chapter is not intended as a comprehensive reference for all CNS tumors; rather, we present the imaging patterns of a select number of CNS neoplasms that residents are expected to be familiar with. The chapter is organized with the overarching categories of tumors, groups of tumor types, and under these groups, the individual tumor types as outlined under the latest 2021 WHO Classification of CNS tumors. Some CNS neoplasms are presented in other chapters throughout this text. For example, chordomas and chondrosarcomas are covered in Chap. 33. Tumors of the cerebellopontine angle are covered in Chap. 34, while the sellar and suprasellar regions are covered in Chap. 35.

Supplementary Information The online version contains supplementary material available at https://doi.org/10.1007/978-3-031-55124-6_15.

S. Y. Huang
Department of Radiology, Division of Neuroradiology, Massachusetts General Hospital, Boston, MA, USA
e-mail: susie.huang@mgh.harvard.edu

R. Y. Huang
Department of Radiology, Division of Neuroradiology, Brigham and Womens Hospital, Boston, MA, USA
e-mail: ryhuang@bwh.harvard.edu

B. A. Vachha (✉)
Department of Radiology, Division of Neuroradiology, UMass Chan Medical School/UMass Memorial Medical Center, Worcester, MA, USA
e-mail: Behroze.Vachha@umassmemorial.org

GLIOMAS, GLIONEURAL TUMORS, AND NEURONAL TUMORS

Adult-type Diffuse Gliomas

- The 2021 WHO Classification of Tumors of the CNS [1] simplifies the classification of adult-type diffuse gliomas into three types:
    - Astrocytoma, isocitrate dehydrogenase (IDH) mutant, and demonstrated absence of 1p/19q co-deletion.
    - Oligodendroglioma, IDH-mutant, and 1p/19q co-deleted.
    - Glioblastoma, IDH-wildtype.
- IDH-mutant diffuse gliomas harbor mutations in IDH1 or IDH2.
- Importantly, a grade 4 IDH-mutant astrocytoma is no longer called a glioblastoma.
- Glioblastoma must be IDH-wildtype and is considered a separate entity.
- Consider magnetic resonance imaging (MRI) with contrast with the addition of perfusion-weighted sequences to assist with further characterization (i.e., grade, progression of tumor vs. pseudo-progression status post treatment).

Astrocytoma, IDH-Mutant

- CNS WHO grades 2, 3, and 4 [1].
- The median age at diagnosis is 36 years for grades 2 and 3 while the median age at diagnosis is 38 years for grade 4 IDH-mutant astrocytomas [2].

Imaging Patterns

- The majority of IDH mutant astrocytomas are supratentorial but can occur anywhere including the brainstem.
- On MRI the tumor may appear as a well-circumscribed lesion, which is homogeneously hyperintense on

T2-weighted imaging. On fluid-attenuated inversion recovery (FLAIR) images the majority of the tumor appears relatively hypointense except for a thin hyperintense rim. This is called the T2-FLAIR mismatch sign (Fig. 15.1a, b) [3–6].
- The T2-FLAIR mismatch sign has high specificity (100%, 95% CI, 88–100%) and high interobserver agreement for the prediction of IDH-mutant non-codeleted astrocytomas. However, the sign demonstrates low sensitivity (42%, 95% CI, 28–58%), and a few studies with false positive cases have been reported [7].
- Enhancement of tumor depends on tumor grade: CNS WHO grade 2 lesions show little or no enhancement (Fig. 15.1c); WHO grade 3,4 lesions show increased enhancement and necrosis within the enhancing mass usually suggests grade 4 lesion [8].
- Diffusion-weighted imaging (DWI) shows no restriction for grade 2 tumors.
- On perfusion-weighted imaging, rCBV or plasma volume increases with increasing tumor grade (Fig. 15.1d) [9].
- MR spectroscopy can show 2-hydroxyglutarate (2HG) at 2.25 ppm, which indicates presence of the IDH mutation [10].

Main Differential Considerations

- *Glioblastoma, IDH-wildtype* presents as a lesion with a necrotic center and thick, irregular enhancement. Grade 4

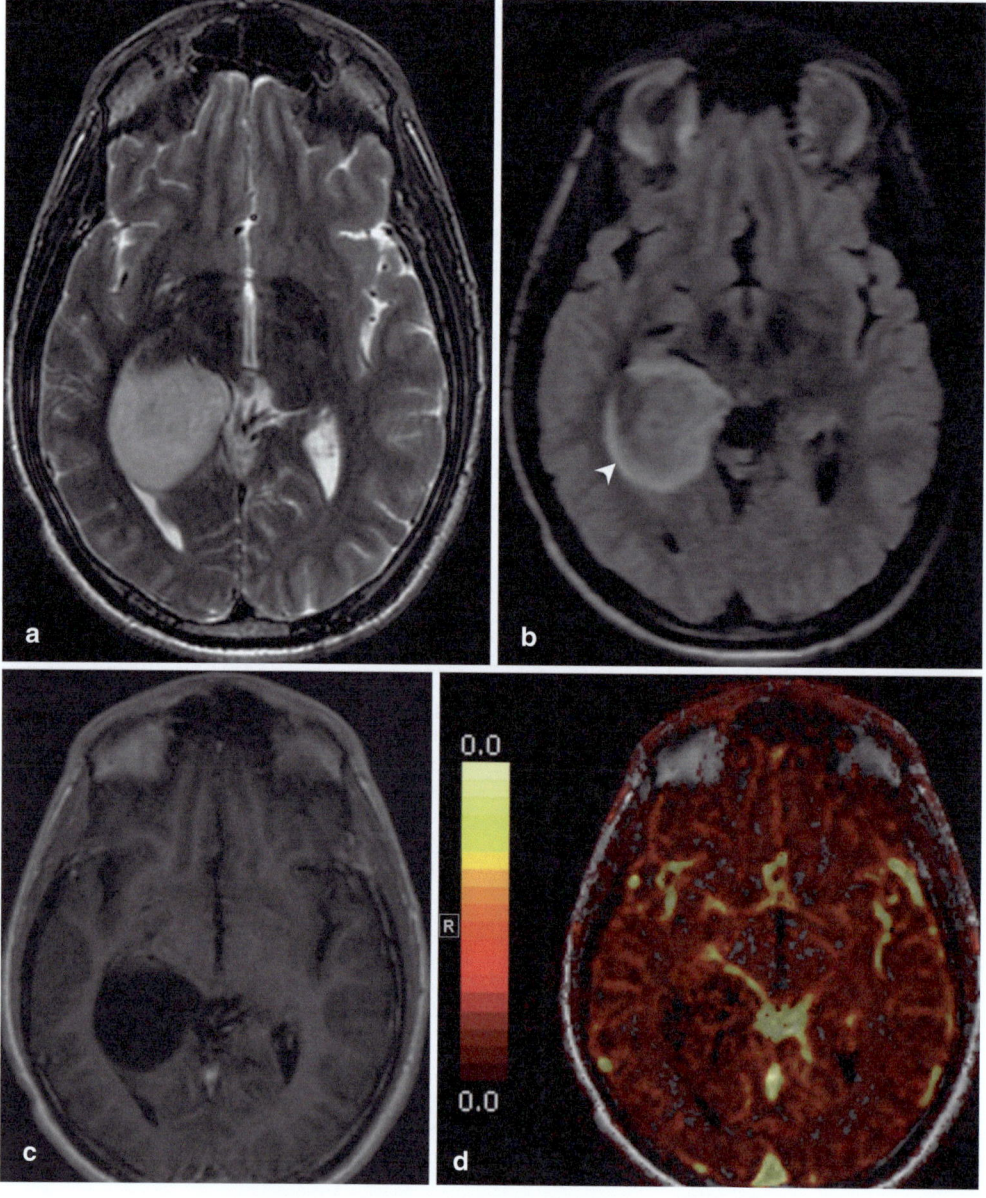

Fig. 15.1 IDH-mutant, 1p19q non-co-deleted astrocytoma. (**a**) Axial T2-weighted MRI demonstrates a homogeneously T2 hyperintense mass lesion in the right medial temporal lobe. (**b**) Axial FLAIR image demonstrates iso- to hypo-intense signal within the majority of the lesion with a peripheral hyperintense rim (arrowhead). This is consistent with the T2-FLAIR mismatch sign, which is highly specific for IDH-mutant, 1p19q non-co-deleted astrocytoma. The lesion does not demonstrate enhancement (**c**) or focal hyperperfusion (**d**), suggesting a low grade tumor

IDH mutant astrocytoma may be indistinguishable from glioblastoma by imaging features alone [11].
- *Oligodendroglioma* is a poorly circumscribed (remember astrocytoma is often well-circumscribed), cortically and subcortically based mass with gyriform calcifications [12–14].

Oligodendroglioma, IDH Mutant, and 1p/19q Co-Deleted

- CNS WHO grade 2 or 3 [1, 6].
- The median age of diagnosis is 44 years and this is rare in children [2].
- The most common presentation is seizure due to cortical involvement [15].

Imaging Patterns [6, 12–14]

- Oligodendroglioma is most commonly found in the frontal lobe followed by the temporal lobe.
- It typically appears as a poorly circumscribed, cortical/subcortical mass lesion with the majority showing gyriform calcification on CT (Fig. 15.2a, b).
- On MRI it shows blooming on T2* gradient recalled echo (T2*GRE) or susceptibility-weighted images (SWI) due to calcification and is heterogeneously hyperintense on T2/FLAIR (Fig. 15.2c).
- Enhancement of the lesion depends on the grade and ranges from none to mild (grade 2; Fig. 15.2d) to moderate (grade 3).

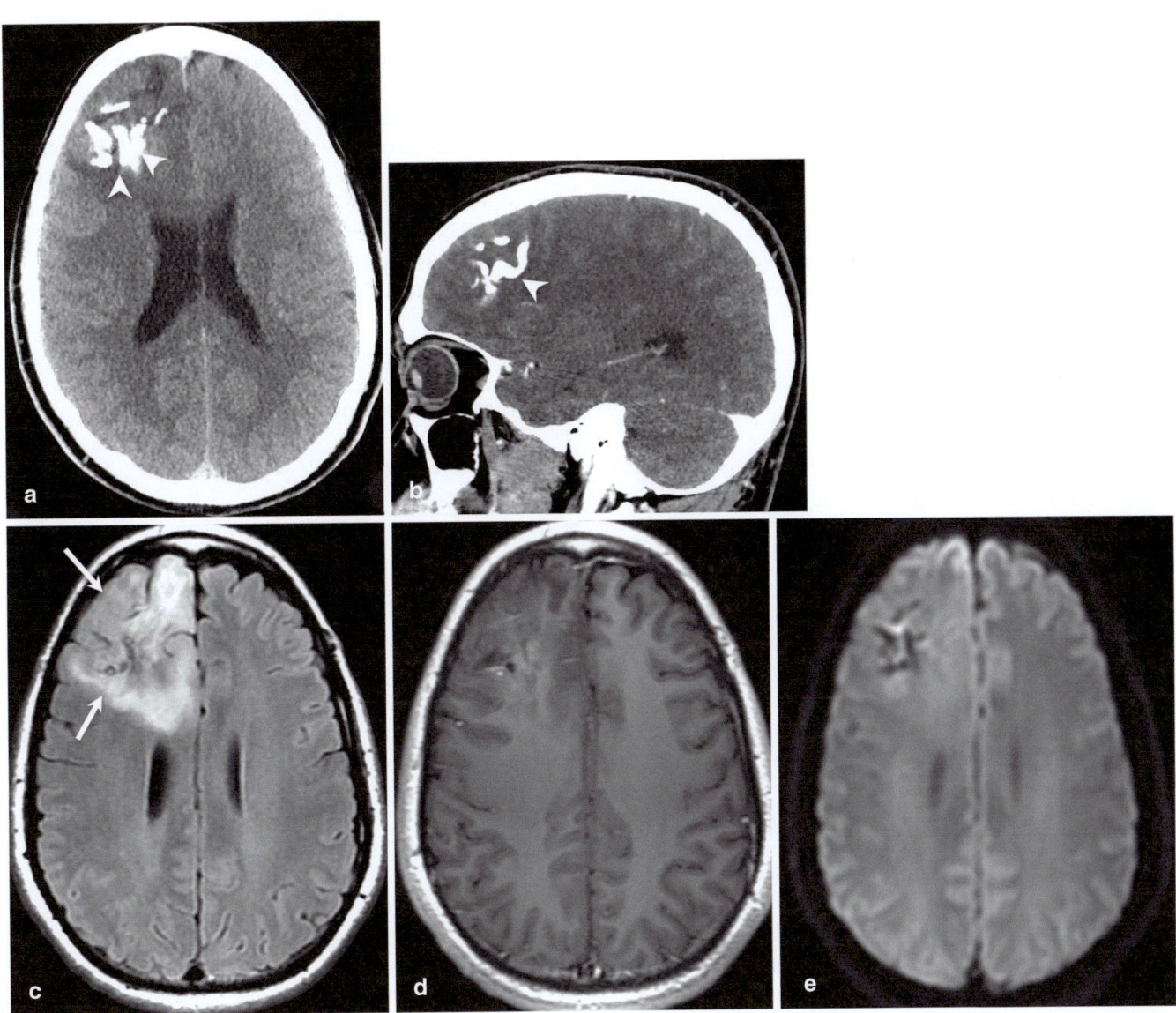

Fig. 15.2 Oligodendroglioma. (**a**) Axial and (**b**) Sagittal CT demonstrates a hypodense right frontal lesion with gyriform calcifications (arrowheads). (**c**) Axial FLAIR image in the same patient shows a hyperintense infiltrative mass expanding the gyrus (arrows). (**d**) Axial T1WI C+ images show minimal heterogeneous enhancement and no restricted diffusion on DWI (**e**)

- Restricted diffusion within the lesion is typically absent (Fig. 15.2e) for grade 2 oligodendroglioma.

Main Differential Considerations

- *IDH mutant Astrocytoma* is a well-circumscribed lesion that is rarely calcified and the T2/FLAIR mismatch sign is common [5].
- Consider other cortical-based lesions (see below) all of which are more commonly seen in the temporal lobe and are seen in children or young adults. Additional specific differences include:
  - *Ganglioglioma* is a well-circumscribed cystic mass lesion with enhancing mural nodule [16].
  - *Dysembryoplastic neuroepithelial tumor (DNET)* appears as a cortically based tumor with bubbly appearance [17].
  - *Pleomorphic xanthoastrocytoma* appears as a cystic lesion with enhancing mural nodule touching the pial surface [18].

Glioblastoma, IDH-Wildtype

- IDH-wildtype glioblastomas are diffuse gliomas with IDH-wildtype mutation, either with histological features of microvascular proliferation or necrosis, or molecular features of telomerase reverse transcriptase (TERT) promoter mutation, epidermal growth factor receptor (EGFR) gene amplification, or + 7/−10 chromosome copy number changes [6].
- CNS WHO grade 4 [1].
- Viable neoplasms usually extend well beyond the visualized radiological margins.

Imaging Patterns [6, 11, 19–21]

- Glioblastomas are usually located within the white matter of cerebral hemispheres and rarely involve the brainstem and cerebellum. The term "Butterfly glioblastoma" is used to describe transcallosal glioblastoma (think of lymphoma and demyelinating disorders in the differential).
- On MRI the lesion demonstrates central necrosis with surrounding irregular, thick heterogeneous enhancement (Fig. 15.3a), heterogeneous diffusion restriction (Fig. 15.3b), and blooming susceptibility artifacts on T2*GRE/SWI due to intralesional hemorrhagic products of different ages (Fig. 15.3c).
- There is extensive peritumoral T2/FLAIR signal intensity, which usually represents a combination of tumor and vasogenic edema (Fig. 15.3d).
- On perfusion-weighted imaging there is elevated relative cerebral blood volume (rCBV) or plasma volume (Vp) within the viable components (Fig. 15.3e).

Main Differential Considerations

- *IDH-mutant Astrocytoma* is usually seen at a younger age and T2/FLAIR mismatch is common. Grade 4 IDH-mutant astrocytoma can be indistinguishable from glioblastoma by imaging features alone [6, 11].
- *Metastatic disease* usually presents with multiple lesions at the gray-white matter junction. Solitary metastasis can be difficult to distinguish from glioblastoma, however often a primary cancer is already known [20].
- *Tumefactive variant of demyelinating disease* in the corpus callosum can mimic butterfly glioblastoma but it has less mass effect compared to the size of the lesion. There is usually incomplete "C-shaped" or "horse-shoe"-shaped peripheral enhancement with the open segment facing the cortical surface [22].
- *Primary CNS lymphoma* may be transcallosal or periventricular in location, T2 iso- to hypointense, more homogeneously enhancing than glioblastoma and shows more homogeneous restricted diffusion [23].
- *Abscess* shows a thin rim of peripheral enhancement compared to the more thick, irregular enhancement seen in glioblastoma. The early capsule stage of abscess formation has a characteristic T2 hypointense rim. There is intense central diffusion restriction whereas glioblastoma often shows more heterogeneous restricted diffusion [24].

Circumscribed Astrocytic Gliomas

Pilocytic Astrocytoma

- This is the most common primary benign brain neoplasm in children with peak incidence between 5 and 14 years [25].
- CNS WHO grade 1 [1].
- The most common location is the posterior fossa (cerebellum) followed by the optic pathway/hypothalamus. The supratentorial location is rare and usually seen in adults.
- Optic pathway/hypothalamus location may be associated with Neurofibromatosis Type 1 (syndromic) or may be sporadic [26].

Imaging Patterns [27–30]

- In the posterior fossa:
  - This is seen as a cystic/solid mass isodense to gray matter with variable enhancement on CT (lack of hyperdensity helps differentiate pilocytic astrocytoma from medulloblastoma).
  - On MRI the typical appearance is that of a cystic mass with heterogeneously enhancing mural nodule

15 Tumors and Tumor-Like Lesions

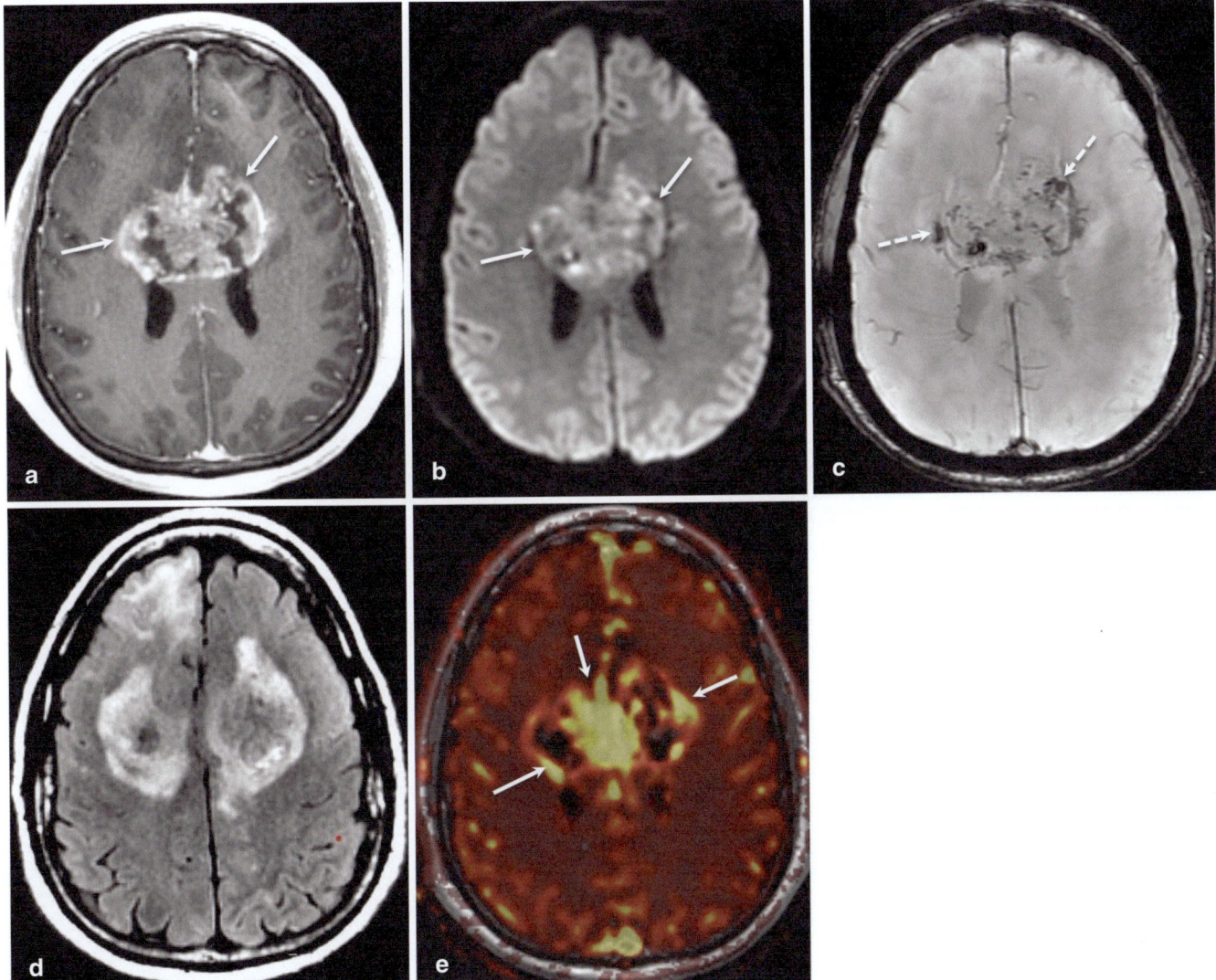

Fig. 15.3 Glioblastoma. (**a**) Axial T1-weighted postcontrast and (**b**) DWI images demonstrate a heterogeneously enhancing, diffusion restricted transcallosal mass lesion (solid arrows) with regions of necrosis. (**c**) SWI demonstrates intralesional blooming artifact suggesting hemorrhagic products of varying ages (dashed arrows). (**d**) Axial FLAIR image demonstrates extensive surrounding signal abnormality, likely reflecting a combination of nonenhancing tumor and vasogenic edema. (**e**) There is focal hyperperfusion in the enhancing component of the lesion, consistent with a high grade tumor (solid arrows)

(Fig. 15.4a, b). Occasionally the cyst wall may enhance. Remember, that absence of the cystic component does not exclude the diagnosis of pilocytic astrocytoma.
  o There is no restricted diffusion and higher apparent diffusion coefficient (ADC) compared to medulloblastoma.
  o There is none to minimal surrounding edema.
- Optic Pathway:
  o The syndromic subtype shows variable T2 hyperintensity and variable enhancement with diffuse enlargement along the optic pathway.
  o The sporadic subtype shows moderate to intense enhancement and may present as a fusiform mass along optic pathway.

Main Differential Considerations

- Posterior fossa tumors:
  o *Medulloblastoma* is usually seen in a younger aged patient with a midline mass that is hyperdense on CT and shows restricted diffusion (lower ADC values) on MRI [31, 32].

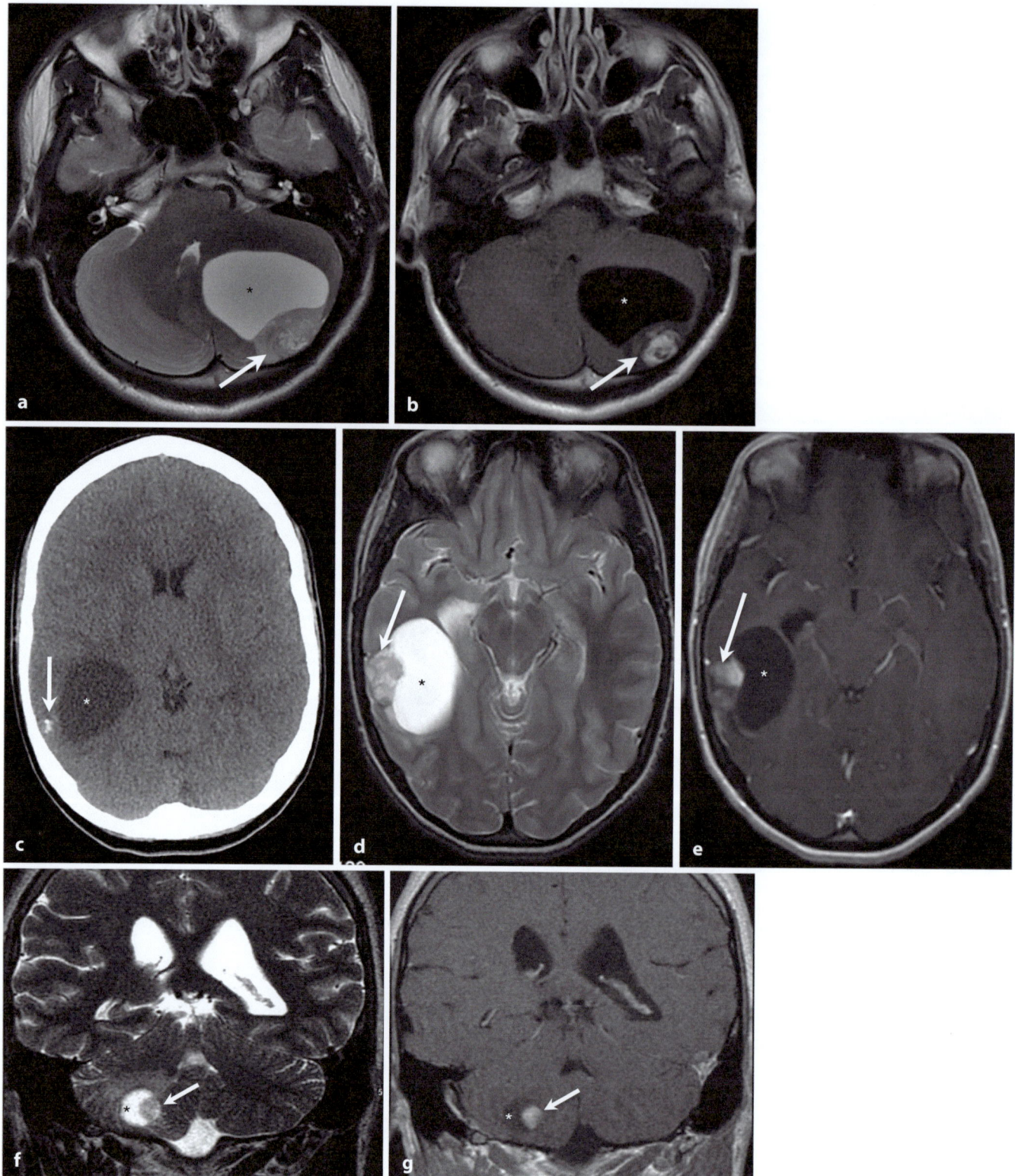

Fig. 15.4 Cystic tumors with a mural nodule. (**a**, **b**) Pilocytic astrocytoma. (**a**) Axial T2W and (**b**) axial T1-weighted postcontrast images demonstrate a mass lesion with cystic components (asterisk) and enhancing mural nodule (arrow) in the posterior fossa in a young child, consistent with pilocytic astrocytoma. (**c–e**) Ganglioglioma. (**c**) Axial CT shows a large cystic mass (asterisk) in the right temporal lobe with a solid nodule that demonstrates internal calcification (arrow). (**d**) Axial T2-weighted image shows a large cyst (asterisk) with a solid nodule (arrow). (E) Axial T1-weighted postcontrast images show enhancement within the solid nodule (arrow). (**f**, **g**) Hemangioblastoma. (**f**) Coronal T2W and (**g**) Coronal T1-weighted postcontrast images in an elderly patient show a cerebellar cystic mass lesion (asterisk) with an enhancing mural nodule (arrow)

- ○ *Ependymoma* appears as a heterogeneous mass with calcification, hemorrhagic and cystic components that fills and squeezes out of fourth ventricle foramina [31, 33].
- ○ *Hemangioblastoma* appears as a cystic mass with enhancing mural nodule in the cerebellum and is more commonly seen in adults [34].
- Optic pathway location:
  - ○ *Optic pathway pilomyxoid astrocytoma* is a more aggressive and bulky appearing mass with more T2/FLAIR hyperintensity compared to optic pathway pilocytic astrocytoma [29].
  - ○ *Optic nerve sheath meningioma* shows tram-track calcification/enhancement. In the pediatric age group this is often associated with NF2 while optic pathway pilocytic astrocytoma is associated with NF1 [30].
  - ○ *Optic neuritis* usually presents with an acute onset of symptoms compared to the more indolent presentation of optic pathway gliomas and shows minimal to no nerve enlargement.

Pleomorphic Xantoastrocytoma (PXA)

- CNS WHO grades 2 and 3 [1].
- Usually seen in children and young adults.
- This lesion presents with seizures due to cortical involvement.

Imaging Patterns [18, 35, 36]

- This is a peripherally located mass with involvement of cortex and meninges usually located in the temporal lobes followed by frontal and parietal lobes.
- The most common finding is a cystic mass with an enhancing mural nodule that touches the pial surface (Fig. e15.1).
- (All electronic images (Figs. e15.1–e15.8) can be found on this chapter's website on SpringerLink: https://doi.org/10.1007/978-3-031-55124-6_15)
- There is enhancement of the adjacent meninges with associated "pial tail" that can mimic a dural tail.
- There is minimal surrounding edema for grade 2 PXA.

Main Differential Considerations

- Consider supratentorial tumors that present as cystic masses with enhancing mural nodule (ganglioglioma, pilocytic astrocytoma, and hemangioblastoma) and other cortical-based masses (oligodendroglioma, DNET, ganglioglioma, and pilocytic astrocytoma). None of these masses show an enhancing pial tail as is seen in PXA.

Additionally, DNET and oligodendroglioma may remodel the calvarium.

Subependymal Giant Cell Astrocytoma (SEGA)

- CNS WHO grade 1 [1].
- The majority of SEGAs are associated with tuberous sclerosis complex although occasionally these can arise in the absence of tuberous sclerosis and are called "solitary SEGA" [37, 38].
- These are typically seen between 5 and 15 years of age but can occur earlier. Children may present with symptoms related to obstructive hydrocephalus due to mass lesion at the foramen of Monro.
- MRI brain with contrast every 1–2 years is recommended to follow SEGA [37, 39].
- Complete surgical resection is usually curative. More recently, mammalian target of rapamycin inhibitors (mTORi) have become known to effectively reduce the size of SEGAs [40].

Imaging Patterns [41, 42]

- This is seen as an enhancing mass lesion ≥1 cm in the lateral ventricle near the foramen of Monro (Fig. 15.5).
- This is associated with other CNS imaging findings related to tuberous sclerosis including cortical tubers, subependymal nodules (SEN), and white matter radial bands.
- SEN versus SEGAS:
  - ○ SENs arise along the lateral ventricles at the caudothalamic groove. SEGAs may arise from SENs but are almost always near the foramen of Monro.
  - ○ SEN are usually small (<1 cm) and remain unchanged in size over serial imaging while SEGAs are slowly growing and usually ≥1 cm.
- The common teaching is that a large SEN near the foramen of Monro should be followed with serial imaging to rule out development of SEGA.

Main Differential Considerations

- *Choroid Plexus Papilloma* appears as an avidly enhancing cauliflower-like intraventricular mass usually in the atrium of the lateral ventricle in children [43].
- *Subependymoma* is usually in the frontal horn of lateral ventricle or inferior fourth ventricle and is seen in middle-aged or older adults [44].
- *Central Neurocytoma* is a multicystic mass in a young adult, usually in the anterior part of the lateral ventricle and attached to the septum pellucidum [35].

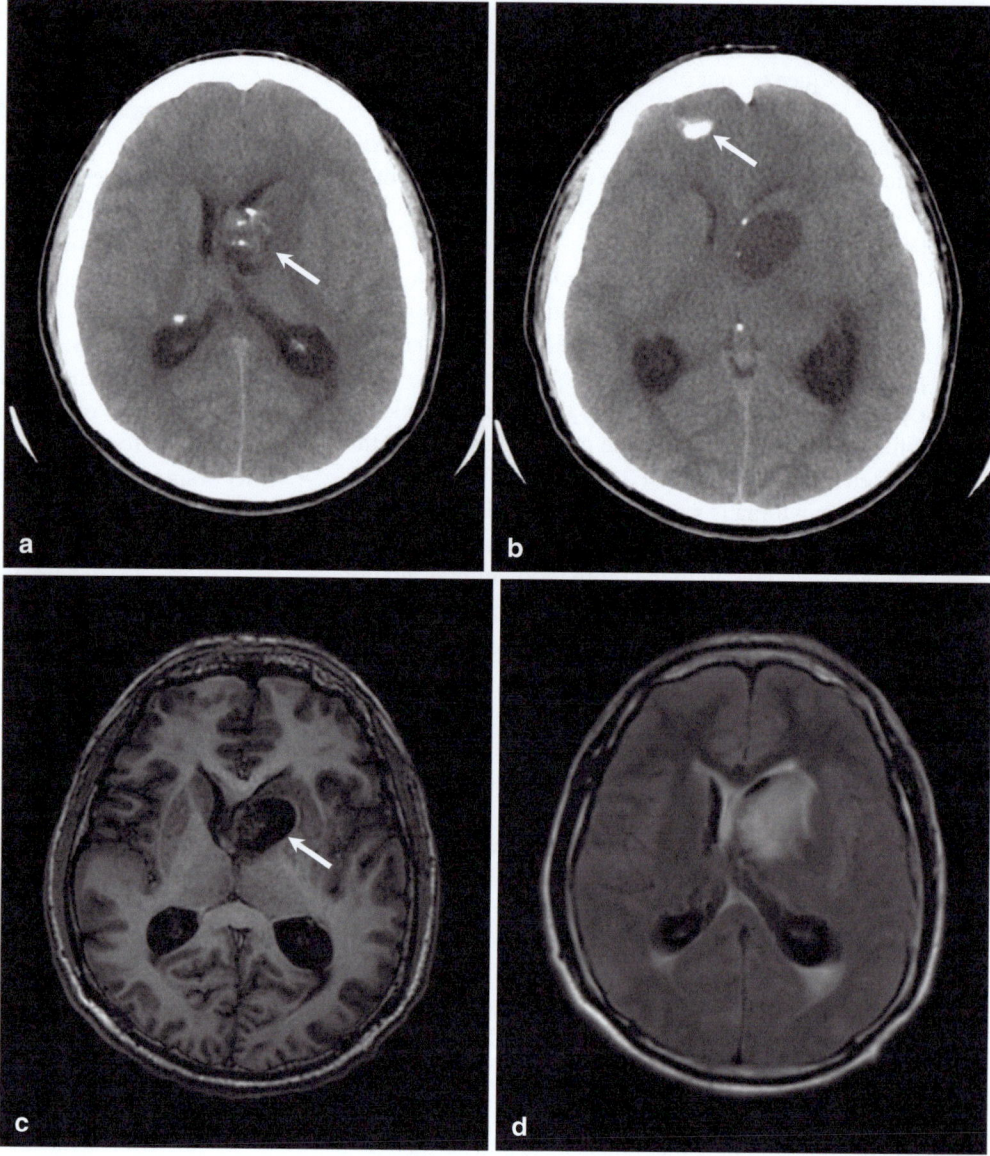

Fig. 15.5 Subependymal giant cell astrocytoma. (**a**) Axial noncontrast CT image demonstrates a partially calcified cystic and solid mass in the left lateral ventricle at the level of the foramen of Monro (solid arrow). (**b**) Axial noncontrast CT image at the level of the caudate head demonstrates a calcified cortical tuber in the right frontal lobe (dashed arrow) in this patient with tuberous sclerosis. (**c**) Axial noncontrast T1-weighted image shows a partially cystic and solid mass obstructing the foramen of Monro (solid arrow). (**d**) Axial FLAIR image shows T2/FLAIR hyperintensity within the mass and obstructive hydrocephalus with transependymal flow of CSF

Glioneural and Neuronal Tumors

Ganglioglioma

- CNS WHO grade 1 [1].
- These typically occur in children and young adults and can cause temporal lobe epilepsy [45].

Imaging Patterns [16, 35, 46]

- Ganglioglioma involves the cortex and is most commonly located in the temporal lobe followed by the frontal and parietal lobes.
- It is most commonly seen as a well-circumscribed cystic mass with an enhancing mural nodule often with calcifications seen in 50% cases (Fig. 15.4c–e).
- Occasionally, however, it can present as a solidly enhancing tumor or as an infiltrating poorly defined mass.
- It is rarely associated with leptomeningeal enhancement.
- There is usually no surrounding edema in typical gangliogliomas.
- These frequently coexist with focal cortical dysplasia.

Main Differential Considerations

- Similar to PXA, consider tumors that present as cystic masses with enhancing mural nodule (PXA, pilocytic astrocytoma, and hemangioblastoma) and other cortical-based masses (oligodendroglioma, DNET, PXA, and pilocytic astrocytoma).

Dysembryoplastic Neuroepithelial Tumor (DNET)

- CNS WHO grade 1 [1].
- This occurs in children and young adults aged 10–30 years of age with a slight male predominance noted.
- It arises from dysplastic cells in germinal matrix that follow the migratory path of neurons toward the cortex and presents with longstanding partial complex seizures [47].

Imaging Patterns [17, 35, 47]

- These are most commonly seen in the mesial temporal lobe followed by the frontal lobe; less frequently these are seen in the caudate nucleus and septum pellucidum.
- DNET appears as an intracortical, circumscribed, pseudocystic, "bubbly," septated appearing mass lesion that points toward the ventricle in a wedge-shaped configuration.
- On T2/FLAIR it is strongly hyperintense (Fig. 15.6a, b), and on FLAIR it can show a hyperintense rim.
- Usually it shows no enhancement (Fig. 15.6c, d), with 20–30% lesions demonstrating punctate or ring enhancement.
- Calcification is seen in 20–30%.
- There is minimal to no mass effect.
- These lesions may be associated with osseous remodeling.
- They frequently coexist with focal cortical dysplasia.

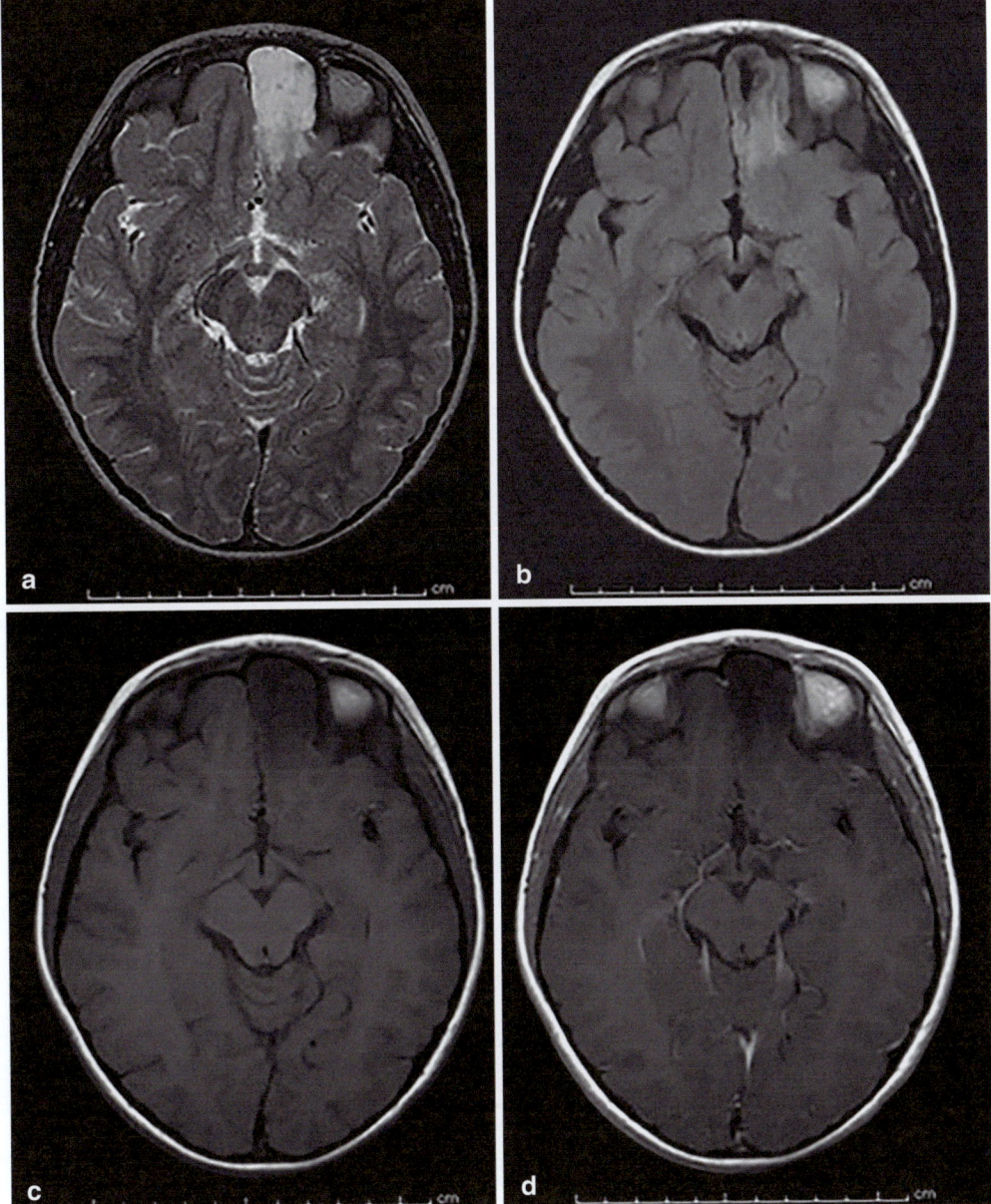

Fig. 15.6 DNET. (a) Axial T2-weighted and (b) axial FLAIR image shows a wedge-shaped T2/FLAIR hyperintense cortically based mass in the left inferior frontal lobe. (c) Axial noncontrast T1W and (D) axial T1-weighted postcontrast images show absence of enhancement

Main Differential Considerations

- *Focal cortical dysplasia Type II* is nonenhancing and may have blurred margins at the cortical-subcortical junction [48].
- *Ganglioglioma* is a cystic mass with an enhancing nodule and with calcification commonly present [16].
- *Pleomorphic xanthoastryctoma* shows intense enhancement, often with a pial tail [36].
- *Multinodular and vacuolating neuronal tumor* appears as small T2/FLAIR hyperintense nodules along the deep margin of the cortex or are subcortical in location [49].

Central Neurocytoma

- CNS WHO grade 2 [1].
- These are seen in young adults (20–40 years old) and usually present with symptoms of increased intracranial pressure, such as headache, visual disturbances, and mental status changes [50].
- Rarely these have been associated with sudden death due to acute ventricular obstruction.

Imaging Patterns [35]

- This is typically located in the anterior part of the lateral ventricle usually attached to the septum pellucidum near the foramen of Monro and can sometimes extend into the third ventricle.
- On CT, it is a hyperdense, circumscribed solid and cystic mass with calcification.
- On MRI it appears as a T1 isointense, T2 hyperintense, moderately enhancing multicystic mass with "bubbly" appearance (Fig. 15.7) although occasionally it can be entirely solid.
- It is commonly associated with obstructive hydrocephalus and transependymal flow of CSF.

Main Differential Considerations

- *Meningioma* appears as a homogeneously enhancing, slightly T2 hypointense solid mass, which usually occurs in an older age group [51].
- *Subependymoma* usually occurs in older patients and appears as a faint or nonenhancing mass in the fourth ventricle and less commonly in the lateral ventricle [35, 44].
- *Ependymoma* shows prominent enhancement with more solid components and is more commonly in the fourth ventricle [51].
- *SEGA* is usually found in patients with tuberous sclerosis [42].
- *Intraventricular metastases* are usually seen in an older age group and in most cases a primary tumor is already known.

Extraventricular Neurocytoma

- CNS WHO grade 2 [1].

Imaging Patterns [35, 52]

- This occurs outside the ventricular system in the brain parenchyma usually in the frontal and parietal lobes and

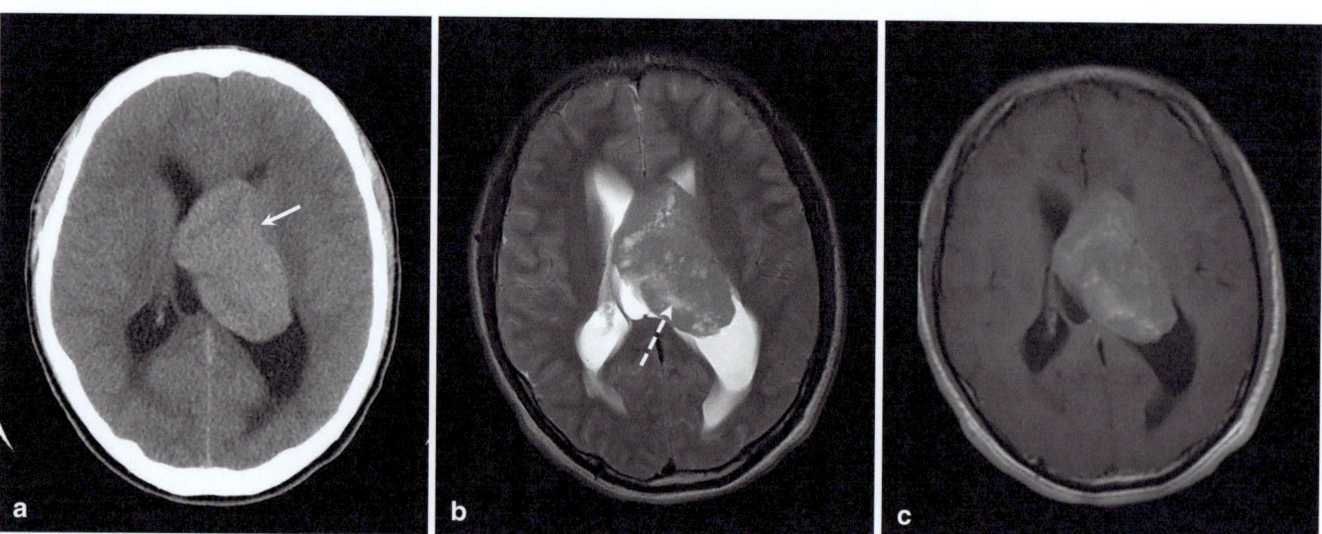

Fig. 15.7 Central neurocytoma. (**a**) Axial CT image shows a hyperdense mass centered in the left lateral ventricle (solid arrow). (**b**) Axial T2-weighted image demonstrates multiple internal T2 hyperintense foci suggestive of cystic areas (dashed arrow). (**c**) The mass is T1 isointense to gray matter and enhances heterogeneously

is seen as a solid and cystic mass with calcification in 10–15% cases with or without enhancement.

Main Differential Considerations

- *Oligodendroglioma* presents as a cortical-based mass often with calcification in the frontal lobe [13, 14]. Extraventricular neurocytoma occasionally involves the cortex but is usually located in the deep white matter.
- *Ganglioglioma* appears as a cystic and solid mass usually located in the temporal lobe more than in the frontal and parietal lobes [16].
- *Pilocytic astrocytoma* is usually located in the posterior fossa or if it is located supratentorially, then the hypothalamus/optic pathway is involved [29].
- *Glioblastoma* is usually seen in an older patient and is more aggressive looking [11].

Gangliocytoma

- CNS WHO grade 1 [1].
- This is a rare slow-growing tumor of ganglion cells that occurs primarily in children and often presents with seizures.

Imaging Patterns [35]

- On CT it appears as a hyperdense mass.
- There is little mass effect and no surrounding edema.
- It can present with calcifications and cyst formation.
- The solid components enhance.

Main Differential Considerations

- *Ganglioglioma* is seen as a cystic mass with solid enhancing mural nodule [16].

- *Focal cortical displasia* shows no enhancement [48].
- *DNET* appears as a bubbly multicystic mass [17].

Dysplastic Cerebellar Gangliocytoma (Lhermitte-Duclos Disease)

- The exact pathogenesis is unknown. It is thought to be a hamartomatous lesion versus true tumor.
- It is usually seen in children and young adults and may present with subtle cerebellar signs or obstructive hydrocephalus when large.
- It is associated with Cowden syndrome and with PTEN (Phosphatase and TENsin homolog deleted on chromosome 10) mutation in adults [53].

Imaging Patterns [35]

- This is commonly a solitary lesion located within the cerebellum.
- There is thickening of the cerebellar folia with increased T2 signal intensity.
- A characteristic imaging appearance is that of striated, tigroid, or corduroy appearance on MRI (Fig. 15.8).

Multinodular and Vacuolating Neuronal Tumor (MVNT)

- CNS WHO grade 1 [1].
- This is seen in young and middle-aged adults.

Imaging Patterns [49]

- It is usually located along the deep margin of the cortex and subcortical region and is seen as a small, well-circumscribed cluster of T2/FLAIR hyperintense nodules with minimal to no enhancement and no mass effect.

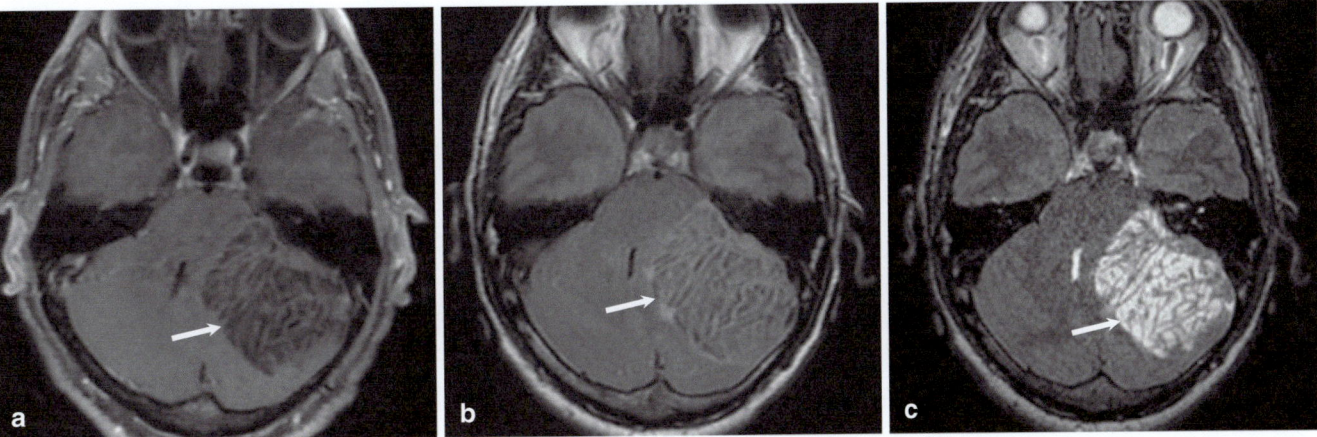

Fig. 15.8 Dysplastic cerebellar gangliocytoma (Lhermitte-Duclos disease). (**a**) Axial postcontrast T1-weighted image shows a T1 hypointense nonenhancing mass in the left cerebellar hemisphere (arrow). Axial FLAIR (**b**) and T2-weighted (**c**) images demonstrate thickened FLAIR/T2 hyperintense cortical striations (arrows)

Main Differential Considerations

- *Focal cortical displasia* shows no enhancement and follows gray matter signal on all sequences [48].
- *DNET* appears as a bubbly multicystic mass with involvement of the cortex [17].

Ependymal Tumors

- Based on location, these are now divided into Posterior Fossa Ependymomas, Supratentorial Ependymomas (not discussed), Spinal Ependymomas (discussed in Chap. 24) and Subependymomas.

Posterior Fossa Ependymoma

- This accounts for 2/3 of all cases of CNS ependymomas.
- CNS WHO grade 2 or 3 [1].
- There are two distinct subtypes based on methylation: Subtype A, which occurs primarily in infants and young children and the less common subtype B, which primarily occurs in adolescents and young adults. Group A has a poor prognosis [54].
- Remember to request MR imaging of spine if you see posterior fossa ependymoma for complete staging.

Imaging Patterns [27, 28, 31, 33, 55]

- This is a posterior fossa mass with a propensity to fill the body or inferior fourth ventricle (floor) and extend/squeeze through the foramina of Luschka and Magendie into the adjacent basal cisterns. For this reason they are called "toothpaste" or "plastic" tumors (Fig. 15.9).
- It is an iso- to hypodense mass in the inferior fourth ventricle with coarse calcifications and cysts on CT.
- There is heterogeneous enhancement on CT and MRI (Fig. 15.9a).
- On MRI it appears as T2 hyperintense cysts (Fig. 15.9b). Calcifications are seen as T1 hyperintense, T2 hypointense foci with blooming on GRE/SWI (Fig. 15.9c).
- There is no diffusion restriction (Fig. 15.9d). Remember, medulloblastomas show restricted diffusion.
- The sagittal images help distinguish if it arises from the floor (ependymoma) versus roof (medulloblastoma) of the fourth ventricle.

Main Differential Considerations

- Other posterior fossa lesions:
  - *Medulloblastoma* usually arises from the roof of the fourth ventricle, shows restricted diffusion/low ADC on MRI and hyperattenuation on noncontrast CT [31, 33].
  - *Posterior Fossa Pilocytic Astrocytoma* is usually off-midline arising from the cerebellar parenchyma and presents as a cystic mass lesion with enhancing mural nodule [29].
  - *Hemangioblastoma* appears as a cystic mass with enhancing mural nodule. In younger patients this is often associated with von Hippel Lindau.
  - *Metastases* is usually seen in adults and usually the primary is known.
- *Choroid Plexus Papilloma* can be seen as an enhancing frond-like tumor in the fourth ventricle but usually this location is more common in adults [43].

Subependymoma

- CNS WHO grade 1 [1].
- This is usually seen in a middle-aged to elderly male [44].

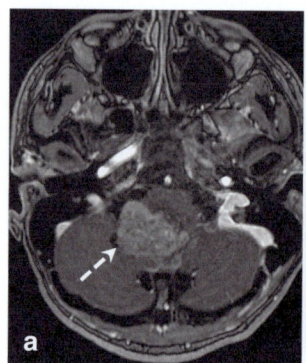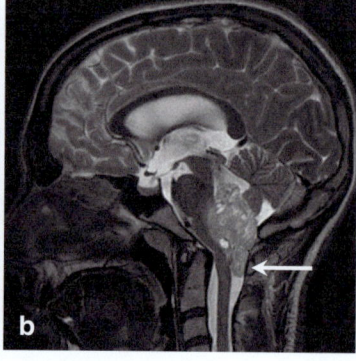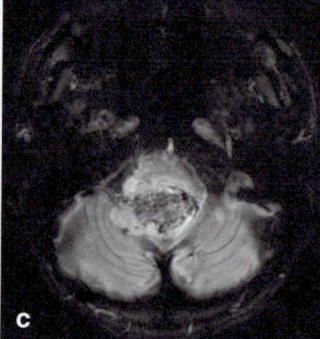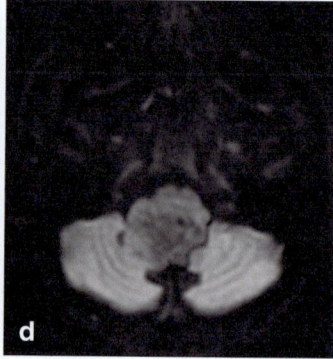

Fig. 15.9 Ependymoma. (**a**) Axial T1-weighted postcontrast image demonstrates a heterogeneously enhancing lesion in the inferior fourth ventricle that extends through the right foramen of Luschka (dashed arrow). (**b**) Sagittal T2W image in the same patient shows the mass contains cystic components, expands the fourth ventricle with mass effect on the brainstem and cerebellum and extends inferiorly through the foramen of Magendie into the cisterna magna (solid arrow). (**c**) Axial SWI demonstrates blooming artifact probably due to calcifications and hemorrhagic products. (**d**). Axial DWI demonstrates no restricted diffusion

- It is recommended that these be followed with serial imaging if the patient is asymptomatic and surgical resection if symptomatic (usually curative).

Imaging Patterns (Fig. e15.2) [35, 44, 56]

- This is located in the fourth ventricle more than the lateral ventricle.
- On CT, this is seen as an iso- to hypodense mass usually in inferior fourth ventricle with coarse calcifications and cysts.
- On MRI subependymoma appears as a T2/FLAIR hyperintense mass with mild to no enhancement in the ventricle.

Main Differential Considerations

- *Ependymoma* is seen in a younger patient with a heterogeneous enhancing mass in the fourth ventricle [55].
- *Choroid Plexus Papilloma* should be part of the differential when subependymoma is present in the fourth ventricle [43].
- *Central Neurocytoma* is seen as a bubbly appearing enhancing mass in the anterior part of the lateral ventricle attached to septum pellucidum [35].
- *Metastases* usually have a primary source that is known.

CHOROID PLEXUS TUMORS

- Choroid Plexus tumors are classified as:
  o Choroid plexus papilloma (CPP; CNS WHO grade 1).
  o Atypical choroid plexus papilloma (AtypCPP; CNS WHO grade 2).
  o Choroid plexus carcinoma (CPCa; CNS WHO grade 3) [1].
- Imaging cannot reliably distinguish between the three different subtypes [43, 57].
- These are usually seen in young children and are rarely seen in adults [43, 57].
- They are associated with Aicardi and Li Fraumeni syndromes [58].

Imaging Patterns [33, 43, 57]

- The most common location for CPP is the atrium of the lateral ventricle in children while the fourth ventricle is the most common location in adults. The most common location for CPCa is mainly the lateral ventricle.
- These present as heterogeneously enhancing lobulated, mass lesions with frond-like surface projections (cauliflower appearance).
- Calcification and intralesional flow voids may be seen.
- CPCa often extends beyond the borders of the ventricle and invades the adjacent brain parenchyma.
- Figure 15.10 demonstrates CPP (a–c) and CPCa (d–f).

Main Differential Considerations

- *Choroid Plexus Tumor Subtypes* should always be included in the differential as it is difficult to reliably distinguish between the three different tumor subtypes by imaging alone, although CPCa is more likely to invade the brain [35, 57].
- *Medulloblastoma* can be seen in the fourth ventricle but is more well-defined and rounded than choroid plexus papilloma, which is more lobulated [33].
- *Ependymoma* is located in the fourth ventricle in children and is more heterogeneously enhancing with cystic/necrotic changes and calcifications compared to CPP [55]. Usually CPP in children is more commonly seen in the lateral ventricle and much less commonly in the fourth ventricle.
- *Meningioma* appears as an enhancing mass lesion usually in the trigone of the lateral ventricle and is mainly seen in older adults [59].
- *Intraventricular metastases* are uncommon in the pediatric population and the primary is often known.
- *Subependymoma* is usually seen as a nonenhancing or minimally enhancing mass lesion in the lateral or fourth ventricle in a middle-aged or older adult [44].

EMBRYONAL TUMORS

Medulloblastoma

- Medulloblastoma is the most common malignant posterior fossa tumor of childhood.
- CNS WHO grade 4 [1].
- This is a primitive neuroectodermal tumor involving the cerebellum with considerable biological heterogeneity.
- It arises from multipotential embryonic cells located along the roof of the fourth ventricle and posterior medullary velum that migrate laterally and upward to form the cerebellum.
- At least four molecular subgroups have been identified arising from separate cytogenetic pathways, including the Sonic hedgehog (SHH), Wingless (WNT) pathways, non-WNT/non-SHH Group 3, and WNT/non-SHH Group 4 [60].
- Desmoplastic/nodular histopathologic subtype refers to the presence of collagenous connective tissue and is

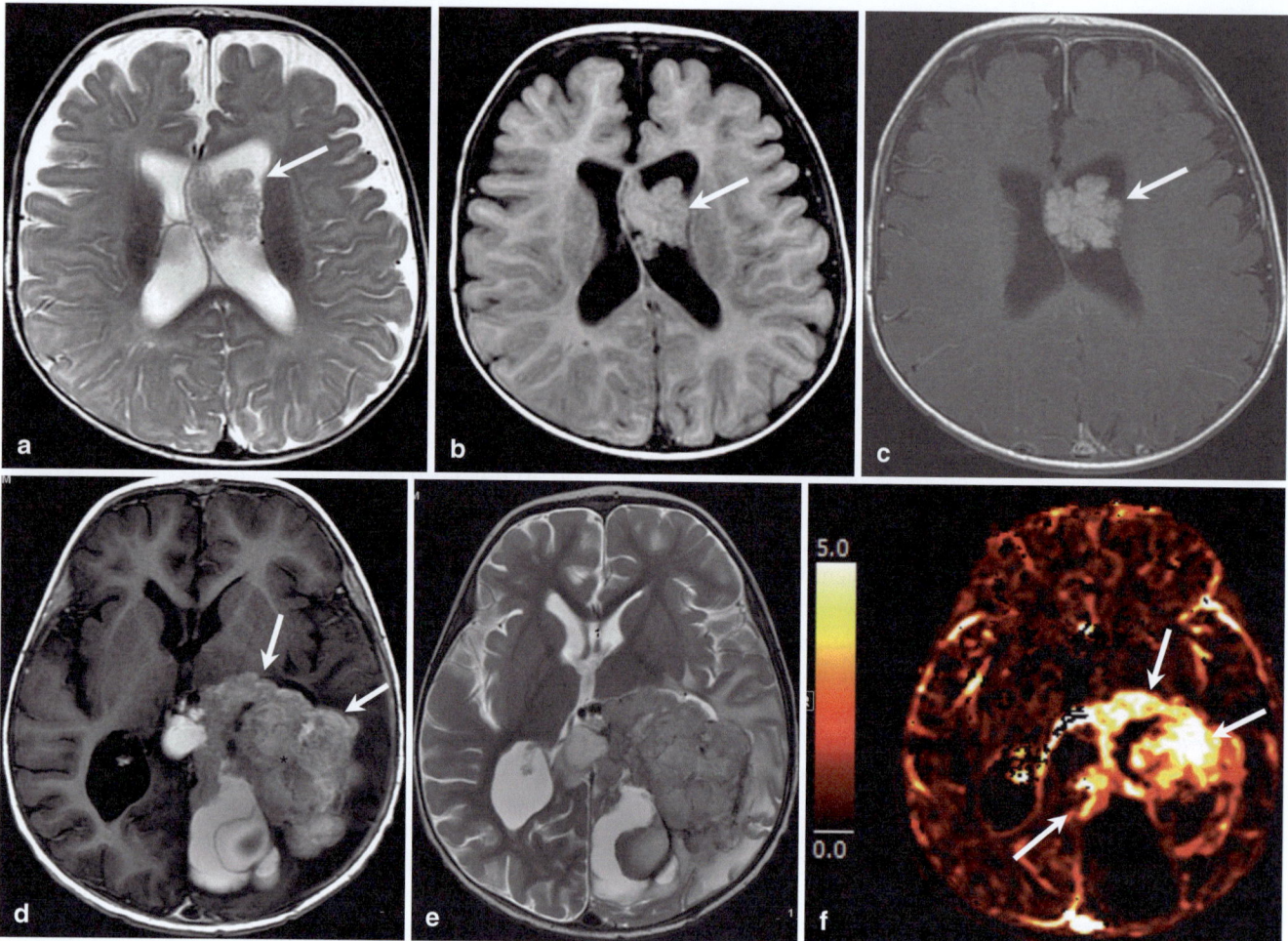

Fig. 15.10 Choroid plexus tumors. (a–c) Choroid plexus papilloma. (a) Axial T2W and (b) axial T1W image shows a heterogeneously T2 hyperintense, T1 isointense mass lesion (arrows) confined within the body of the left lateral ventricle with robust homogeneous enhancement on the axial T1-weighted postcontrast image (C; arrow). Note the frond-like projections characteristic of choroid plexus papilloma. (d-f) Choroid plexus carcinoma. (d) Axial T1-weighted postcontrast image demonstrates a heterogeneously enhancing lobulated mass lesion with "cauliflower-like" appearance centered in the atrium of the left lateral ventricle (asterisk) with extensive invasion of the adjacent brain parenchyma (arrows). (e) Axial T2-weighted image in the same patient shows the mass is heterogeneous in signal intensity with cystic and solid components. (f) Axial perfusion-weighted images demonstrate elevated plasma volume in the solid enhancing components of the lesion (arrows)

linked to the SHH molecular group, typically seen in adolescents and young adults.
- Imaging of the entire neuroaxis is recommended to rule out leptomeningeal seeding [61].

Imaging Patterns [28, 31, 33, 61]

- The classic appearance is that of a midline posterior fossa mass extending into the fourth ventricle (Non-WNT/non-SHH groups 3 and 4 usually but can be any type). It can be seen along the cerebellar peduncle/cerebellopontine angle (WNT type usually) or cerebellar hemisphere (SHH type usually).
- On CT, the mass is hyperdense reflecting high cellularity (Fig. 15.11a).
- On MRI, medulloblastoma is heterogeneously T2 hypointense (Fig. 15.11b), enhancing (Fig. 15.11c) and typically shows restricted diffusion due to high cellular density (Fig. 15.11d, e).
- Desmoplastic/nodular medulloblastoma is more often located in the cerebellar hemisphere rather than along the midline (Fig. e15.3).
- Leptomeningeal metastatic spread can be seen as enhancement over the brain and spinal cord and is referred to as "Zuckerguss" literally translating as sugar icing or sugar coating.

15 Tumors and Tumor-Like Lesions

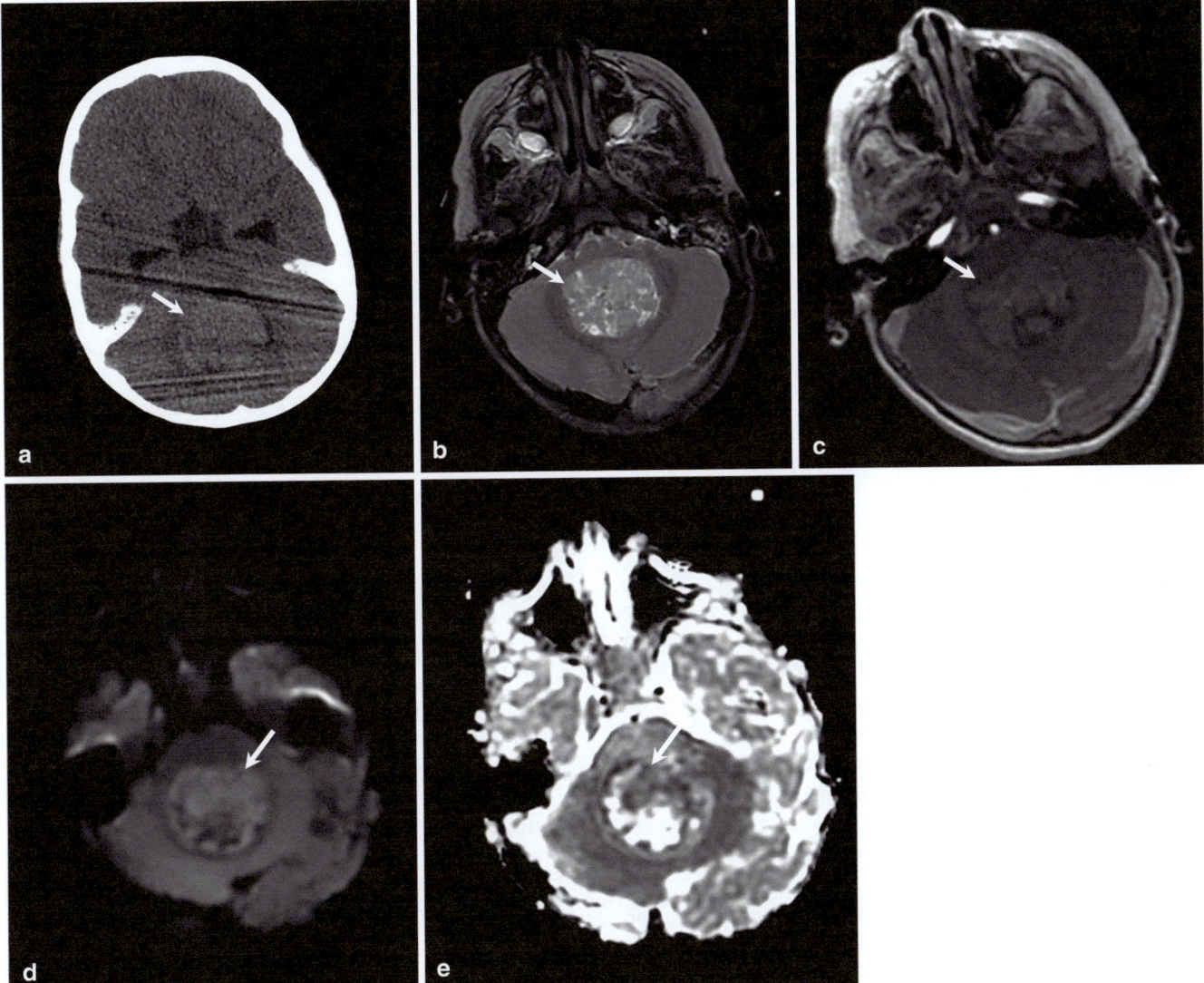

Fig. 15.11 Medulloblastoma. (**a**) Axial CT image demonstrates a hyperdense mass centered in the fourth ventricle (arrow). (**b**) Axial T2-weighted image shows a heterogeneously T2 hypointense mass (arrow) with (**c**) mild enhancement on T1-weighted postcontrast imaging. The mass demonstrates restricted diffusion indicative of high cellularity (arrows) on axial DWI (**d**) and ADC maps (**e**)

Main Differential Considerations

- *Ependymoma* is said to arise from the floor while medulloblastoma arises from the roof of the fourth ventricle. Ependymoma is more heterogeneous in appearance and "toothpaste"-like, filling the fourth ventricle and squeezing through its foramina into the adjacent cisterns. It shows increased diffusivity (higher ADC) than medulloblastoma [55].
- *Atypical teratoid/rhabdoid tumor* is indistinguishable by imaging, but is typically seen in patients younger than 3 years of age [33].
- *Cerebellar pilocytic astrocytoma* is usually seen in older children and presents as a cerebellar hemispheric lesion with cyst and enhancing nodule [29].
- *Choroid plexus papilloma* is much less common in the fourth ventricle in this age group and demonstrates avid frond-like enhancement [43].
- *Brainstem glioma* that extends into the fourth ventricle can be confusing but the center of the tumor usually suggests that it originates from the brainstem.

Other CNS Embryonal Tumors

- These are rare tumors that make up 5% of all childhood brain tumors.
- CNS WHO grade 4 [1].
- They were formerly known as supratentorial primitive neuroectodermal tumors (PNETs) and are now classified as embryonal tumors with multilayered rosettes (ETMR)

in the 2021 WHO classification if C19MC amplification or *DICER1* mutations are present and as atypical teratoid/rhabdoid tumors (Fig. e15.4) if *SMARCB1* or *SMARCA4* mutations are present [62].

Imaging Patterns [33]

- On MRI this appears as a heterogeneously T1 and T2 hyperintense mass with restricted diffusion and heterogeneous enhancement.
- Cysts or hemorrhage are common and these contain calcifications.
- It is recommended that the spine is imaged to identify subarachnoid spread.

PINEAL TUMORS

- Pineal parenchymal tumors are divided into pineocytomas (CNS WHO Grade 1), pineal parenchymal tumors of intermediate differentiation (CNS WHO Grades 2 and 3), papillary tumor of the pineal region (CNS WHO grade 2 and 3), pineoblastoma (CNS WHO Grade 4), and Desmoplastic myxoid tumor of the pineal region [1].
- Due to the location of these tumors, they usually present with headache due to hydrocephalus secondary to obstruction of the Aqueduct of Sylvius and paralysis of upward gaze (Parinaud's syndrome) due to mass effect on the tectum of the midbrain [63, 64].
- Pineoblastomas are mostly seen in children while the other pineal parenchymal tumors affect adults.
- The common teaching is that pineal parenchymal tumors peripherally displace existing pineal calcifications, i.e., they show "exploded calcifications" on imaging whereas germ cell tumors surround or "engulf" the calcified pineal gland.

Pineoblastoma

- Pineoblastoma may be seen in patients with retinoblastoma (trilateral retinoblastoma) [65].
- CSF dissemination is common so imaging of the entire neuroaxis is recommended [33, 64, 66].

Imaging Patterns [33, 64, 66]

- On CT, pineoblastoma appears as a hyperdense pineal mass with peripheral calcifications (Fig. e15.5).
- On MRI, it typically appears as a T2 iso- to hypointense, heterogeneously enhancing pineal region mass (Fig. e15.5b, c) with cystic/necrotic and solid components and peripheral blooming on susceptibility-weighted imaging. Solid components may show restricted diffusion.

Main Differential Considerations

- *Pineocytoma* is usually seen in an older patient with a more well-circumscribed homogeneously enhancing mass [67].
- *Germinoma and Other Germ Cell Tumors (GCT)* can occur in the pineal region. Germinoma is typically seen in a young male patient and appears as a hyperdense mass on CT. The mass appears to surround the calcified pineal gland whereas in pineal parenchymal tumors calcification is usually peripheral. However, often the two can be indistinguishable on imaging. Teratoma can be seen in this region and has a heterogeneous appearance but intralesional fat can help suggest the diagnosis [68, 69].
- *Pineal region meningioma* appears as an enhancing mass with dural tail usually seen in middle-aged females. The common teaching is that a tentorial meningioma in the pineal region depresses the internal cerebral veins while pineal gland tumors usually elevate the internal cerebral veins [70].
- *Metastases* in the pineal region can occur but this is an uncommon location and the primary is usually known.

Pineocytoma

- This is a slow growing tumor in adults with good prognosis.

Imaging Patterns [35, 63, 67, 71]

- On CT, pineocytoma is seen as a well-circumscribed iso- to hypodense pineal region enhancing mass with peripheral calcifications.
- On MRI, this appears as a well-circumscribed, homogeneously enhancing pineal region mass with areas of blooming at the periphery on susceptibility-weighted imaging consistent with calcifications.
- Cystic changes may be present.

Main Differential Considerations

- *Benign Pineal Cyst* shows minimal to no enhancement and is usually less than 1 cm but can be difficult to distinguish from pineocytoma by imaging [67].
- *Pineal Parenchymal Tumor of Intermediate Differentiation* is usually seen in older patients with a more aggressive appearing pineal lesion [67].
- *Pineoblastoma* is seen in a younger patient with heterogeneous mass lesion [66].

- *Germinoma and other GCTs* (see explanation above).
- *Meningioma* (see explanation above).

MENINGEAL TUMORS

Meningioma

- Meningioma is the most common extra-axial tumor and arises from menigothelial arachnoid cap cells [35].
- It is divided into three groups based on WHO grade and likelihood of recurrence: typical (grade 1), atypical (grade 2), and anaplastic (grade 3) [1].
- Approximately half have inactivation of the NF2 gene and are commonly seen in neurofibromatosis type 2 [72].
- They can be induced by prior radiation therapy, with onset years after treatment [73].

Imaging Patterns [35, 74]

- Meningiomas can be seen anywhere including along convexities, falcine, sphenoid wing, cavernous, clinoid, optic sheath, tuberculum, planum sphenoidale, olfactory, petroclival, tentorial, torcular, CPA, intraventricular, and foramen magnum.
- On CT, meningiomas present as a hyperdense extra-axial mass. There is associated reactive hyperostosis.
- They may show calcifications on CT or T2*-weighted imaging.
- On MRI they are T1 isointense, T2 variable signal intensity, homogeneously enhancing mass lesions with a dural tail (Fig. 15.12a, b).
- CSF cleft between the tumor and brain is commonly seen on T2W imaging (Fig. 15.12c).

Main Differential Considerations

- *Dural metastasis* may be indistinguishable on imaging, however usually the primary is known and these may be multifocal. The most common primary malignancies that can cause dural metastases are breast, prostate, and lung cancer [74].
- *Granulomas such as sarcoid and tuberculosis* should be included in the differential. Tuberculosis usually involves basal meninges and there is usually bone erosion instead of hyperostosis [74].
- *Idiopathic Hypertrophic Pachymeningitis* is often IgG4-related disease [74].
- *Dural-based lymphoma* shows no calcification or hyperostosis [74].
- *Solitary fibrous tumor* is often more aggressive in appearance, with bone destruction instead of hyperostosis, but can be indistinguishable from meningioma [75].

MESENCHYMAL, NONMENINGOTHELIAL TUMORS

Solitary Fibrous Tumor

- This was previously called Solitary Fibrous Tumor/Hemangiopericytoma and now is just called Solitary Fibrous Tumor.
- WHO 2021 classification: Mesenchymal, nonmeningothelial, soft tissue, fibroblastic, and myofibroblastic tumor; CNS WHO grades 1, 2, and 3 [1].

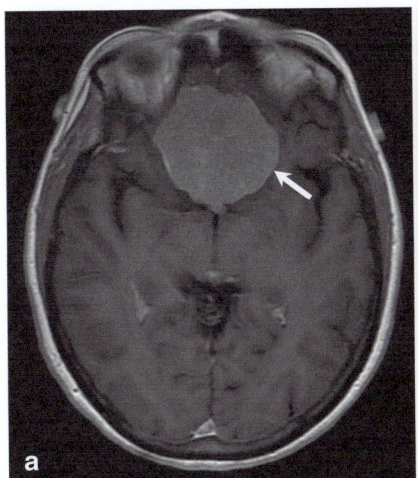 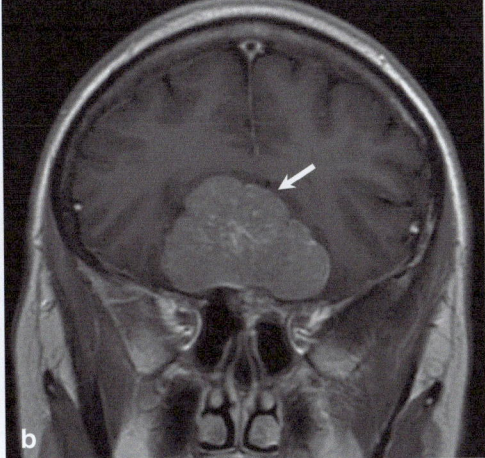 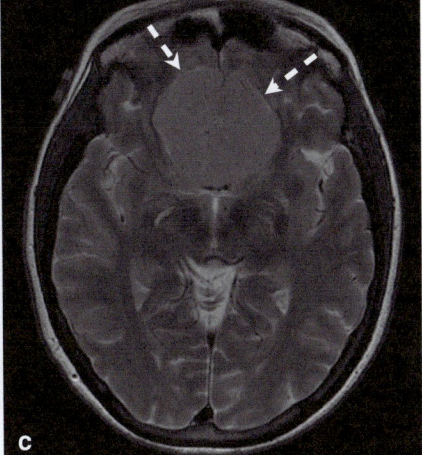

Fig. 15.12 Meningioma. (**a**) Axial and (**b**) coronal T1-weighted post-contrast MR image demonstrates a homogeneously enhancing extra-axial mass lesion overlying the planum sphenoidale. (**c**) Axial T2-weighted image demonstrates a subtle T2 hyperintense rim surrounding the mass (dashed arrows) representing CSF cleft

Imaging Patterns [75, 76]

- This usually involves the occipital region.
- On CT, it appears as a hyperdense extra-axial mass with cystic/necrotic regions.
- There may be skull erosion but no hyperostosis or calcification/mineralization is noted (which helps to distinguish it from meningioma).
- On MRI, solitary fibrous tumor typically appears as a heterogeneously enhancing, extra-axial mass lesion (Fig. e15.6) with patches of hypointense and hyperintense T2 signal intensity.
- Prominent flow voids may be present.

Main Differential Considerations

- *Meningioma* often has calcifications and hyperostosis, which are absent in solitary fibrous tumor. Solitary fibrous tumor can show osseous erosions and prominent flow voids [74].
- *Dural metastasis* typically presents as multiple lesions with the primary tumor often known [74].
- *Lymphoma* has no flow voids and skull erosion is uncommon.

Hemangioblastoma

- Hemangioblastoma is the most common *primary* intra-axial neoplasm of the posterior fossa in adults.
- CNS WHO grade 1 [1].
- It can be sporadic or seen in patients with Von Hippel Lindau disease (vHL).
- vHL-associated hemangioblastomas are typically multiple and present at a younger age (mean age 29 years) while the sporadic form is commonly solitary and seen in older patients (mean age 47 years) [77].

Imaging Patterns [34, 35]

- The most common site is the posterior fossa (mainly cerebellum). Extracerebellar sites such as spine, supratentorial, and retina are also seen in patients with vHL-associated hemangioblastoma even though the cerebellum still remains the most common location even in vHL.
- Hemangioblastomas typically appear as a cystic mass with enhancing mural nodule (Fig. 15.4f, g).
- Solid tumor with enhancement is less commonly seen.
- There is usually no surrounding edema.

Main Differential Considerations

- *Pilocytic astrocytoma* is usually a solitary cystic mass with enhancing mural nodule in the posterior fossa in a child or young adult [29].
- *Metastasis* is usually more solid than cystic and usually multiple rather than solitary. They also much more commonly show surrounding edema.

Remember that the most common intra-axial neoplasm in the posterior fossa in middle aged to older adults is metastasis while the most common *primary* intra-axial neoplasm in the posterior fossa in middle aged to older adults is hemangioblastoma!

HEMATOLYMPHOID TUMORS

Primary CNS Lymphoma

- Primary CNS lymphoma is lymphoma confined to the CNS without systemic spread [78].
- Most are diffuse large B-cell lymphoma [78].
- By contrast, secondary CNS lymphoma usually affects skull, leptomeninges, and dura more commonly than the parenchyma.

Imaging Patterns [23, 79, 80]

- The majority are supratentorial and often cross the corpus callosum or involve the periventricular white matter contacting the ependymal surface (Fig. e15.7).
- The high cellularity of primary CNS lymphoma results in it appearing as a hyperdense lesion on CT and hypointense on T2-weighted imaging with restricted diffusion on MRI.
- Hemorrhage and/or central necrosis with ring enhancement may be seen in immunocompromised patients on both CT and MRI while there is usually homogeneous intense enhancement in the immunocompetent patient.
- On perfusion weighted imaging, rCBV is lower than high grade glioma.
- There is increased hypermetabolic avidity on FDG PET and Thallium SPECT.

Main Differential Considerations

- *Acquired toxoplasmosis* appears as ring-enhancing mass lesions often in the basal ganglia region without ependymal involvement. These may be difficult to differentiate from lymphoma in immunocompromised patients

on MRI. Short interval follow-up MRI post anti-toxoplasmosis treatment will show improvement if toxoplasmosis and no improvement if lymphoma. Additionally, on FDG PET-CT and Thallium SPECT, toxoplasmosis lesions are hypometabolic while lymphoma lesions are hypermetabolic [23].
- *Glioblastoma,* especially butterfly glioma involving the corpus callosum, shows more heterogeneous enhancement and higher mean apparent diffusion coefficient (ADC) than primary CNS lymphoma [19].
- Demyelinating disease in the corpus callosum will show incomplete enhancement with the open segment toward the cortex [22].
- *Secondary lymphoma* more commonly affects the skull, leptomeninges and dura than the parenchyma.

GERM CELL TUMORS

Germinoma

- Germinoma is the most common intracranial germ cell tumor that predominantly occurs in young males with peak age of 10–12 years [68, 81].
- Extragonadal germ cell tumors are thought to arise from mismigrated and maldifferentiated primordial germ cells [82].
- In the pineal region, patients may present with Parinaud syndrome (paralysis of upward gaze and abnormal convergence) [81, 82].
- Headache due to hydrocephalus from invasion or compression of the midbrain tectum (and aqueduct) is another common presentation [81, 82].
- Diabetes insipidus can occur with germinomas in the pineal, suprasellar, and basal ganglia region and should raise concern for a germinoma in a young male [82].
- Lumbar puncture and imaging of the entire neuraxis are indicated as CSF dissemination and invasion of the adjacent brain are common [68, 82].

Imaging Patterns [68, 81, 82]

- Germinoma occurs in the pineal region, along the third ventricle and less commonly in the suprasellar region.
- It typically appears as a well-defined hyperdense mass on CT.
- The classic teaching is that germinoma "engulfs" the pineal gland and stimulates calcification resulting in central calcifications Fig. e15.8a).
- On MRI it is T1 and T2 isointense to slightly hyperintense to gray matter and demonstrates avid enhancement (Fig. e15.8b).
- It invades the adjacent brain parenchyma with associated edema (Fig. e15.8c) and may show restricted diffusion (Fig. e15.8d).

Main Differential Considerations

- *Pineoblastoma* appears as a large heterogeneously enhancing mass lesion with peripheral calcifications [66].
- *Pineoctyoma* is usually seen in an older age group than germinoma [67].
- *Teratoma and other germ cell tumors* can occur in the pineal region. Presence of intralesional fat can help suggest the diagnosis of teratoma [69].
- Also don't forget to include other pineal region masses such as metastases, meningioma, and astrocytoma in the differential.

Teratoma

- These are uncommon intracranial tumors.
- They are classified into three types: mature, immature, and mature with somatic malignancy [83].
- They may be intra- or extra-axial tumors, with intra-axial tumors occurring in young children and fetuses, and extra-axial tumors presenting in children and young adults.
- Intra-axial teratomas may present as very large intracranial tumors producing macrocephaly.
- Extra-axial teratomas occur most commonly in the pineal region and suprasellar region and often result in obstructive hydrocephalus.
- They are associated with elevated serum alpha-fetal protein and carcinoembryonic antigen.

Imaging Patterns [69, 83]

- These are seen as heterogeneously T1 and T2 hyperintense cystic and solid mass lesions.
- Presence of intralesional fat can help distinguish a teratoma from other masses.
- They often contain hemorrhage or calcification.
- Solid components usually enhance.

Main Differential Considerations

- *Germinoma* has central calcifications. Teratoma is more heterogeneous in appearance and usually shows presence of intralesional fat [68].
- *Pineal parenchyal tumors such as pineoblastoma* typically appear as pineal masses with peripheral calcifications [66].

- Other nongerminomatous cell tumors should also be considered in the differential.
- *Dermoid* has fat intensity, shows minimal to no enhancement and can occasionally rupture with T1 hyperintense fat intensity seen in the cisterns and subarachnoid spaces [84].
- *Lipoma* is a fat intensity lesion without soft tissue components [69].

METASTASES

- The most common primary cancers to cause brain metastases are lung cancer, breast cancer, and melanoma but any primary can cause brain metastases.
- They can be parenchymal or extraxial (pachymeningeal).
- For parenchymal metastases, the common teaching is that they are at the gray-white junction.
- Some metastases including those secondary to lung cancer may be very small, may not have surrounding edema and therefore can be missed if contrast is not given.
- Breast cancer metastasis to the eye can cause enophthalmos.

TUMOR MIMICS

- Various nonneoplastic entities can mimic primary or metastatic brain tumors.
- Common tumor mimics are discussed in this section.

Abscess

- Cerebral abscess can be difficult to distinguish from metastatic disease or primary neoplasm.
- Some features that can help distinguish abscess from other ring-enhancing lesions:
  - Usually, abscess has a thin enhancing rim compared to the thick irregular enhancing rim of glioblastoma.
  - They show the dual rim sign on susceptibility-weighted imaging (hypointense outer rim representing fibrocollagenous abscess capsule and hyperintense inner rim representing a zone of granulation tissue between the necrotic core and capsule) [85].
  - Restricted diffusion of abscess cavity contents is often seen in pyogenic abscesses; however abscesses imaged after initiation of treatment or in immunocompromised hosts may not show strong restricted diffusion [24].
  - MR spectroscopy shows elevated amino acids, acetate, aspartate, and succinate peaks in the abscess cavity.

Demyelinating Process

- Tumefactive demyelinating lesions can show mass effect and edema, however disproportionately less when compared with tumors of the same size [24].
- Enhancement usually is an incomplete ring with the incomplete segment facing the cortex.

Subacute Arterial Infarction

- This is usually restricted to a single vascular territory and enhancement is usually gyriform.

Radiation Necrosis

- This is typically seen as irregular, feather-like enhancement, often with central necrosis and surrounding edema.
- Perfusion imaging can help discriminate between radiation necrosis and tumor with tumor showing hyperperfusion and radiation necrosis showing hypoperfusion [86].

RAPID REVIEW

Tumors with cystic mass and enhancing mural nodule
• Pilocytic astrocytoma
• Ganglioglioma
• Pleomorphic xanthoastrocytoma
• Hemangioblastoma
Posterior fossa masses
In children:
• Medulloblastoma
• Posterior fossa pilocytic astrocytoma
• Ependymoma
• Hemangioblastoma
In adults:
• Metastasis
• Hemangioblastoma
• Medulloblastoma
Cortical-based lesions
• Oligodendroglioma
• Pilocytic astrocytoma
• Ganglioglioma
• Pleomorphic xanthoastrocytoma
• DNET

Transcallosal lesions
- Glioblastoma
- Lymphoma
- Tumefactive demyelinating disease

Pineal region mass lesions
- Pineocytoma
- Pineal tumor of intermediate differentiation
- Pineoblastoma
- Germinoma
- Teratoma
- Astrocytoma
- Meningioma
- Metastases

Hemorrhagic metastases
- Melanoma
- Thyroid carcinoma (papillary)
- Choriocarcinoma
- Renal cell carcinoma
- Lung cancer[a]
- Breast cancer[a]

[a] Less commonly present as hemorrhagic metastases but are included here because of their high prevalence

References

1. Louis DN, Perry A, Wesseling P, et al. The 2021 WHO classification of tumors of the central nervous system: a summary. Neuro-Oncology. 2021;23(8):1231–51.
2. Molinaro AM, Taylor JW, Wiencke JK, Wrensch MR. Genetic and molecular epidemiology of adult diffuse glioma. Nat Rev Neurol. 2019;15(7):405–17.
3. Deguchi S, Oishi T, Mitsuya K, et al. Clinicopathological analysis of T2-FLAIR mismatch sign in lower-grade gliomas. Sci Rep. 2020;10(1):10113.
4. Juratli TA, Tummala SS, Riedl A, et al. Radiographic assessment of contrast enhancement and T2/FLAIR mismatch sign in lower grade gliomas: correlation with molecular groups. J Neuro-Oncol. 2019;141(2):327–35.
5. Patel SH, Poisson LM, Brat DJ, et al. T2-FLAIR mismatch, an imaging biomarker for IDH and 1p/19q status in lower-grade gliomas: a TCGA/TCIA project. Clin Cancer Res. 2017;23(20):6078–85.
6. Vagvala S, Guenette JP, Jaimes C, Huang RY. Imaging diagnosis and treatment selection for brain tumors in the era of molecular therapeutics. Cancer Imaging. 2022;22(1):19.
7. Park SI, Suh CH, Guenette JP, Huang RY, Kim HS. The T2-FLAIR mismatch sign as a predictor of IDH-mutant, 1p/19q-noncodeleted lower-grade gliomas: a systematic review and diagnostic meta-analysis. Eur Radiol. 2021;31(7):5289–99.
8. Joyner DA, Garrett J, Batchala PP, et al. MRI features predict tumor grade in isocitrate dehydrogenase (IDH)-mutant astrocytoma and oligodendroglioma. Neuroradiology. 2023;65(1):121–9.
9. Yang X, Xing Z, She D, et al. Grading of IDH-mutant astrocytoma using diffusion, susceptibility and perfusion-weighted imaging. BMC Med Imaging. 2022;22(1):105.
10. Bhandari A, Sharma C, Ibrahim M, Riggs M, Jones R, Lasocki A. The role of 2-hydroxyglutarate magnetic resonance spectroscopy for the determination of isocitrate dehydrogenase status in lower grade gliomas versus glioblastoma: a systematic review and meta-analysis of diagnostic test accuracy. Neuroradiology. 2021;63(11):1823–30.
11. Salzman K. Glioblastoma. In: Osborn AG, Salzman K, Jhaveri M, editors. Diagnostic imaging brain. Philadelphia, PA: Elsevier; 2016. p. 442–5.
12. Johnson DR, Diehn FE, Giannini C, et al. Genetically defined oligodendroglioma is characterized by indistinct tumor borders at MRI. AJNR Am J Neuroradiol. 2017;38(4):678–84.
13. Lasocki A, Gaillard F, Gorelik A, Gonzales M. MRI features can predict 1p/19q status in intracranial gliomas. AJNR Am J Neuroradiol. 2018;39(4):687–92.
14. Saito T, Muragaki Y, Maruyama T, et al. Calcification on CT is a simple and valuable preoperative indicator of 1p/19q loss of heterozygosity in supratentorial brain tumors that are suspected grade II and III gliomas. Brain Tumor Pathol. 2016;33(3):175–82.
15. Engelhard HH. Current diagnosis and treatment of oligodendroglioma. Neurosurg Focus. 2002;12(2):E2.
16. Salzman K. Ganglioglioma. In: Osborn AG, Salzman K, Jhaveri M, editors. Diagnostic imaging brain. Philadelphia, PA: Elsevier; 2016. p. 502–5.
17. Salzman K, Loevner L. DNET. In: Osborn AG, Salzman K, Jhaveri M, editors. Diagnostic imaging brain. Philadelphia, PA: Elsevier; 2016. p. 510–3.
18. Shaikh N, Brahmbhatt N, Kruser TJ, et al. Pleomorphic xanthoastrocytoma: a brief review. CNS Oncol. 2019;8(3):CNS39.
19. Aftab K, Aamir FB, Mallick S, et al. Radiomics for precision medicine in glioblastoma. J Neuro-Oncol. 2022;156(2):217–31.
20. Aparici-Robles F, Davidhi A, Carot-Sierra JM, et al. Glioblastoma versus solitary brain metastasis: MRI differentiation using the edema perfusion gradient. J Neuroimaging. 2022;32(1):127–33.
21. van Dijken BRJ, van Laar PJ, Smits M, Dankbaar JW, Enting RH, van der Hoorn A. Perfusion MRI in treatment evaluation of glioblastomas: clinical relevance of current and future techniques. J Magn Reson Imaging. 2019;49(1):11–22.
22. Suh CH, Kim HS, Jung SC, Choi CG, Kim SJ. MRI findings in tumefactive demyelinating lesions: a systematic review and meta-analysis. AJNR Am J Neuroradiol. 2018;39(9):1643–9.
23. Salzman K, Primary CNS, Lymphoma. In: Osborn AG, Salzman K, Jhaveri M, editors. Diagnostic imaging brain. Philadelphia, PA: Elsevier; 2016. p. 566–9.
24. Donahue JH, Patel SH, Fadul CE, Mukherjee S. Imaging mimics of brain tumors. Radiol Clin North Am. 2021;59(3):457–70.
25. Tabash MA. Characteristics, survival and incidence rates and trends of pilocytic astrocytoma in children in the United States; SEER-based analysis. J Neurol Sci. 2019;400:148–52.
26. Kinori M, Armarnik S, Listernick R, Charrow J, Zeid JL. Neurofibromatosis type 1-associated optic pathway glioma in children: a follow-up of 10 years or more. Am J Ophthalmol. 2021;221:91–6.
27. Alves C, Lobel U, Martin-Saavedra JS, et al. A diagnostic algorithm for posterior fossa tumors in children: a validation study. AJNR Am J Neuroradiol. 2021;42(5):961–8.
28. Kerleroux B, Cottier JP, Janot K, Listrat A, Sirinelli D, Morel B. Posterior fossa tumors in children: radiological tips & tricks in the age of genomic tumor classification and advance MR technology. J Neuroradiol. 2020;47(1):46–53.
29. Salzman K, Ho C. Pilocytic astrocytoma. In: Osborn AG, Salzman K, Jhaveri M, editors. Diagnostic imaging brain. Philadelphia, PA: Elsevier; 2016. p. 452–5.
30. Joseph AK, Guerin JB, Eckel LJ, et al. Imaging findings of pediatric orbital masses and tumor mimics. Radiographics. 2022;42(3):880–97.
31. D'Arco F, Khan F, Mankad K, Ganau M, Caro-Dominguez P, Bisdas S. Differential diagnosis of posterior fossa tumours in children: new insights. Pediatr Radiol. 2018;48(13):1955–63.
32. Kurokawa R, Kurokawa M, Baba A, et al. Differentiation of pilocytic astrocytoma, medulloblastoma, and hemangioblastoma on diffusion-weighted and dynamic susceptibility contrast perfusion MRI. Medicine (Baltimore). 2022;101(44):e31708.

33. Zimmerman R, Bilaniuk L. Pediatric brain tumors. In: Atlas S, editor. Magnetic resonance imaging of the brain and spine. 5th ed. Philadelphia, PA: Wolters Kluver; 2017. p. 430–83.
34. Salzman K, Rees J. Hemangioblastoma. In: Osborn AG, Salzman K, Jhaveri M, editors. Diagnostic imaging brain. Philadelphia, PA: Elsevier; 2016. p. 558–61.
35. Telles R, D'Amore F, Jayaram M, et al. Adult brain tumors. In: Atlas S, editor. Magnetic resonance imaging of the brain and spine. 5th ed. Philadelphia, PA: Wolters Kluver; 2017. p. 303–429.
36. Salzman K. Pleomorphic xanthoastrocytoma. In: Osborn AG, Salzman K, Jhaveri M, editors. Diagnostic imaging brain. Philadelphia, PA: Elsevier; 2016. p. 460–4.
37. Barnett JR, Freedman JH, Zheng H, Thiele EA, Caruso P. Growth curves of subependymal giant cell tumors in tuberous sclerosis complex. AJNR Am J Neuroradiol. 2021;42(10):1891–7.
38. O'Rawe M, Chandran AS, Joshi S, Simonin A, Dyke JM, Lee S. A case of subependymal giant cell astrocytoma without tuberous sclerosis complex and review of the literature. Childs Nerv Syst. 2021;37(4):1381–5.
39. Krueger DA, Northrup H, International Tuberous Sclerosis Complex Consensus G. Tuberous sclerosis complex surveillance and management: recommendations of the 2012 international tuberous sclerosis complex consensus conference. Pediatr Neurol. 2013;49(4):255–65.
40. Weidman DR, Palasamudram S, Zak M, et al. The effect of mTOR inhibition on obstructive hydrocephalus in patients with tuberous sclerosis complex (TSC) related subependymal giant cell astrocytoma (SEGA). J Neuro-Oncol. 2020;147(3):731–6.
41. Gaillard AL, Crombe A, Jecko V, et al. Magnetic resonance imaging diagnosis of subependymal giant cell astrocytomas in follow-up of children with tuberous sclerosis complex: should we always use contrast enhancement? Pediatr Radiol. 2020;50(10):1397–408.
42. Osborn A, Rees J. Subependymal giant cell astrocytoma. In: Osborn AG, Salzman K, Jhaveri M, editors. Diagnostic imaging brain. Philadelphia, PA: Elsevier; 2016. p. 464–7.
43. Osborn A, Ho C. Typical choroid plexus papilloma. In: Osborn AG, Karen S, Miral J, editors. Diagnostic imaging brain. Philadelphia, PA: Elsevier; 2016. p. 494–7.
44. Salzman K. Subependymoma. In: Osborn AG, Salzman K, Jhaveri M, editors. Diagnostic imaging brain. Philadelphia, PA: Elsevier; 2016. p. 490–3.
45. Giulioni M, Marucci G, Martinoni M, et al. Epilepsy associated tumors: review article. World J Clin Cases. 2014;2(11):623–41.
46. Abdel Razek AAK, Elsebaie NA, Zamora C, Castillo M. Imaging of neuronal and mixed Glioneuronal tumors. J Comput Assist Tomogr. 2020;44(3):356–69.
47. Phi JH, Kim SH. Dysembryoplastic neuroepithelial tumor: a benign but complex tumor of the cerebral cortex. Brain Tumor Res Treat. 2022;10(3):144–50.
48. Urbach H, Kellner E, Kremers N, Blumcke I, Demerath T. MRI of focal cortical dysplasia. Neuroradiology. 2022;64(3):443–52.
49. Nunes RH, Hsu CC, da Rocha AJ, et al. Multinodular and vacuolating neuronal tumor of the cerebrum: a new "leave me alone" lesion with a characteristic imaging pattern. AJNR Am J Neuroradiol. 2017;38(10):1899–904.
50. Lee SJ, Bui TT, Chen CH, et al. Central neurocytoma: a review of clinical management and histopathologic features. Brain Tumor Res Treat. 2016;4(2):49–57.
51. Smith AB, Smirniotopoulos JG, Horkanyne-Szakaly I. From the radiologic pathology archives: intraventricular neoplasms: radiologic-pathologic correlation. Radiographics. 2013;33(1):21–43.
52. Romano N, Federici M, Castaldi A. Imaging of extraventricular neurocytoma: a systematic literature review. Radiol Med. 2020;125(10):961–70.
53. Jiang T, Wang J, Du J, et al. Lhermitte-duclos disease (dysplastic gangliocytoma of the cerebellum) and Cowden syndrome: clinical experience from a single institution with long-term follow-up. World Neurosurg. 2017;104:398–406.
54. Zapotocky M, Beera K, Adamski J, et al. Survival and functional outcomes of molecularly defined childhood posterior fossa ependymoma: cure at a cost. Cancer. 2019;125(11):1867–76.
55. Osborn A, Thurnher M. Infratentorial ependymoma. In: Osborn AG, Salzman K, Jhaveri M, editors. Diagnostic imaging brain. Philadelphia, PA: Elsevier; 2016. p. 482–5.
56. Haider AS, El Ahmadieh TY, Haider M, et al. Imaging characteristics of 4th ventricle subependymoma. Neuroradiology. 2022;64(9):1795–800.
57. Osborn A, Ho C. Choroid plexus carcinoma. In: Osborn AG, Salzman K, Jhaveri M, editors. Diagnostic imaging brain. Philadelphia, PA: Elsevier; 2016. p. 498–501.
58. Thomas C, Metrock K, Kordes U, Hasselblatt M, Dhall G. Epigenetics impacts upon prognosis and clinical management of choroid plexus tumors. J Neuro-Oncol. 2020;148(1):39–45.
59. Smith AB, Horkanyne-Szakaly I, Schroeder JW, Rushing EJ. From the radiologic pathology archives: mass lesions of the dura: beyond meningioma-radiologic-pathologic correlation. Radiographics. 2014;34(2):295–312.
60. Jaju A, Yeom KW, Ryan ME. MR imaging of pediatric brain tumors. Diagnostics (Basel). 2022;12(4):961.
61. Osborn A, Thurnher M. Medulloblastoma. In: Osborn AG, Salzman K, Jhaveri M, editors. Diagnostic imaging brain. Philadelphia, PA: Elsevier; 2016. p. 536–9.
62. Li BK, Al-Karmi S, Huang A, Bouffet E. Pediatric embryonal brain tumors in the molecular era. Expert Rev Mol Diagn. 2020;20(3):293–303.
63. Lombardi G, Poliani PL, Manara R, et al. Diagnosis and treatment of pineal region tumors in adults: a EURACAN overview. Cancers (Basel). 2022;14(15):3646.
64. Tamrazi B, Nelson M, Bluml S. Pineal region masses in pediatric patients. Neuroimaging Clin N Am. 2017;27(1):85–97.
65. de Jong MC, Shaikh F, Gallie B, et al. Asynchronous pineoblastoma is more likely after early diagnosis of retinoblastoma: a meta-analysis. Acta Ophthalmol. 2022;100(1):e47–52.
66. Osborn A, Loevner L. Pineoblastoma. In: Osborn AG, Karen S, Miral J, editors. Diagnostic imaging brain. Philadelphia, PA: Elsevier; 2016. p. 530–3.
67. Salzman K, Loevner L. Pineocytomas. In: Osborn AG, Salzman K, Jhaveri M, editors. Diagnostic imaging brain. Philadelphia, PA: Elsevier; 2016. p. 524–7.
68. Osborn A, Thurnher M. Germinoma. In: Osborn AG, Salzman K, Jhaveri M, editors. Diagnostic imaging brain. Philadelphia, PA: Elsevier; 2016. p. 578–81.
69. Osborn A, Thurnher M. Teratoma. In: Osborn AG, Salzman K, Jhaveri M, editors. Diagnostic imaging brain. Philadelphia, PA: Elsevier; 2016. p. 582–5.
70. Lensing FD, Abele TA, Sivakumar W, Taussky P, Shah LM, Salzman KL. Pineal region masses-imaging findings and surgical approaches. Curr Probl Diagn Radiol. 2015;44(1):76–87.
71. Hsieh CC, Chen JS. Radiotherapy after endoscopic biopsy in an adult with pineocytoma, the rare brain tumor in an adult: a case report and literature review. Int Med Case Rep J. 2022;15:307–11.
72. Bachir S, Shah S, Shapiro S, et al. Neurofibromatosis type 2 (NF2) and the implications for vestibular schwannoma and meningioma pathogenesis. Int J Mol Sci. 2021;22(2):690.
73. Morgenstern PF, Shah K, Dunkel IJ, et al. Meningioma after radiotherapy for malignancy. J Clin Neurosci. 2016;30:93–7.
74. Lyndon D, Lansley JA, Evanson J, Krishnan AS. Dural masses: meningiomas and their mimics. Insights Imaging. 2019;10(1):11.

75. Salzman K. Hemangiopericytoma. In: Osborn AG, Salzman K, Jhaveri M, editors. Diagnostic imaging brain. Philadelphia, PA: Elsevier; 2016. p. 562–5.
76. Chen T, Jiang B, Zheng Y, et al. Differentiating intracranial solitary fibrous tumor/hemangiopericytoma from meningioma using diffusion-weighted imaging and susceptibility-weighted imaging. Neuroradiology. 2020;62(2):175–84.
77. Yoda RA, Cimino PJ. Neuropathologic features of central nervous system hemangioblastoma. J Pathol Transl Med. 2022;56(3):115–25.
78. Grommes C, DeAngelis LM. Primary CNS lymphoma. J Clin Oncol. 2017;35(21):2410–8.
79. Chiavazza C, Pellerino A, Ferrio F, Cistaro A, Soffietti R, Ruda R. Primary CNS lymphomas: challenges in diagnosis and monitoring. Biomed Res Int. 2018;2018:3606970.
80. Jimenez de la Pena MD, Vicente LG, Alonso RC, Cabero SF, Suarez AM, de Vega VM. The multiple faces of nervous system lymphoma. Atypical magnetic resonance imaging features and contribution of the advanced imaging. Curr Probl Diagn Radiol. 2017;46(2):136–45.
81. Favero G, Bonomini F, Rezzani R. Pineal gland tumors: a review. Cancers (Basel). 2021;13(7):1547.
82. Lim EA, Alves C, Picariello S, et al. Neuroimaging of paediatric pineal, sellar and suprasellar tumours: a guide to differential diagnosis. Childs Nerv Syst. 2022;38(1):33–50.
83. Abdelmuhdi AS, Almazam AE, Dissi NA, Albastaki UM, Pierre-Jerome C. Intracranial teratoma: imaging, intraoperative, and pathologic features: AIRP best cases in radiologic-pathologic correlation. Radiographics. 2017;37(5):1506–11.
84. Liu JK, Gottfried ON, Salzman KL, Schmidt RH, Couldwell WT. Ruptured intracranial dermoid cysts: clinical, radiographic, and surgical features. Neurosurgery. 2008;62(2):377–84; discussion 384
85. Toh CH, Wei KC, Chang CN, et al. Differentiation of pyogenic brain abscesses from necrotic glioblastomas with use of susceptibility-weighted imaging. AJNR Am J Neuroradiol. 2012;33(8):1534–8.
86. Nael K, Bauer AH, Hormigo A, et al. Multiparametric MRI for differentiation of radiation necrosis from recurrent tumor in patients with treated glioblastoma. AJR Am J Roentgenol. 2018;210(1):18–23.

Toxic and Metabolic Diseases of the CNS

Harry Subramanian and Amit Mahajan

Introduction

Metabolic abnormalities affecting the brain usually present with generalized nonspecific symptoms manifesting as alteration of the sensorium, ranging from mild confusion to coma. This is distinct from disorders with stroke-like symptoms, which usually present with unilateral neurological deficits.

The differential diagnosis is broad, and initial work-up often seeks to exclude catastrophic events such as traumatic injury, stroke, or infection. Once these causes have been excluded, an evaluation for toxic-metabolic etiologies, including electrolyte abnormalities, drug intoxication, hypoxemia, and hyperammonemia, usually ensues.

While magnetic resonance imaging (MRI) is usually not a first-line imaging modality, specific MRI findings can be helpful in narrowing the differential diagnosis and providing information on the extent of disease involvement. Additionally, MRI can be very helpful in comatose patients or those who cannot provide a reliable neurologic exam. As toxic-metabolic encephalopathy may be reversible depending on the cause, timely diagnosis can help the referring clinician initiate early treatment to prevent further and/or permanent neurologic damage.

Brain Metabolism

The human brain is highly dependent upon oxygen and glucose for metabolism, and lack of either of them can lead to neuronal injury and cause cortical swelling and necrosis. The gray matter is more susceptible to these insults, considering that the neuronal cell bodies are located predominantly in the cortical layers. Optimal ionic concentrations are essential for brain homeostasis. Hence, derangements in these can produce profound functional and pathological consequences, which may become detectable on imaging.

Imaging Appearances of Metabolic Disorders

Severe metabolic disorders can produce nonspecific imaging appearances with overlapping imaging characteristics. However, in less severe cases, various regions of the brain parenchyma can be selectively involved, thus producing distinctive patterns, which can help formulate a differential diagnosis. We will describe these patterns that can assist the reader develop a short list of plausible diagnoses, which can assist in diagnosis and management. Correlation with clinical history and findings is essential in less clear cases. Most findings described here are better seen on MRI; however, if severe enough, these may be seen on CT as well.

Supplementary Information The online version contains supplementary material available at https://doi.org/10.1007/978-3-031-55124-6_16.

H. Subramanian
Department of Radiology and Biomedical Imaging,
New Haven, CT, USA

A. Mahajan (✉)
Yale University School of Medicine, New Haven, CT, USA
e-mail: amit.mahajan@yale.edu

Differential Diagnosis Based Upon Predominant Brain Site Involvement

Cerebral Cortex
- Hypoxic-ischemic Encephalopathy.
- Hypoglycemic encephalopathy.
- Hepatic encephalopathy.

Deep White Matter
- Hypernatremia.
- Posterior reversible encephalopathy syndrome (PRES).
- Heroin-induced Inhalational leukoencephalopathy.
- Methotrexate toxicity.

Brainstem
- Osmotic myelinolysis.
- Wernicke encephalopathy.

Basal Ganglia
- Carbon monoxide toxicity.
- Wilson's disease.
- Methanol toxicity.
- Chemotherapy-associated PRES.
- Parathyroid dysfunction disorder.
- Uremic encephalopathy.
- Diabetic striatopathy.

Cerebellum
- Maple syrup urine disease.
- Metronidazole toxicity.

Corpus Callosum
- Marchiafava-Bignami disease.

Predominant Cortical Involvement

Hypoxic-Ischemic Encephalopathy

- Sequela of hypoxia leads to cytotoxic (intracellular) edema.
- Etiologies include cardiac arrest, near-drowning, asphyxiation, and respiratory arrest.
- Regions of high metabolic demand are most sensitive: basal ganglia, thalami, and occipital and perirolandic cortices.

Imaging Findings [1, 2]

- Diffuse gray matter restricted diffusion and T2 and FLAIR hyperintensity due to swelling of the injured gray matter (Fig. 16.1).

Hypoglycemic Encephalopathy

- Imbalance between the supply and consumption of glucose.
- Clinical manifestations include seizures, altered mental status, and coma.

Imaging Findings [3, 4]

- Symmetric T2 and FLAIR hyperintensity and restricted diffusion in the temporal and parieto-occipital cortex (Fig. e16.1).
- (All electronic images (Figs. e16.1–e16.10) can be found on this chapter's website on SpringerLink: https://doi.org/10.1007/978-3-031-55124-6_16)
- Basal ganglia may also be involved.
- Sparing of white matter, thalami, and cerebellum.
  - Thalamic and cerebellar involvement may suggest hypoxic-ischemic injury.

Hepatic Encephalopathy (Hyperammonemia)

- Acute stage: Result of reduced clearance of nitrogenous wastes from the blood stream due to liver failure and/or portosystemic shunting.
  - Suspected intracerebral accumulation of glutamine, resulting in increased intracellular osmolarity and cerebral edema, intracranial hypertension, and hypoperfusion.
- Chronic stage: Associated with manganese deposition in the basal ganglia (manganese is predominantly cleared by hepatobiliary excretion).

Imaging Findings in Acute Disease [2, 5–7]

- Diffuse edema and T2 hyperintensity, most frequently involving the cingulate gyri, thalami, and insular cortex, with relative sparing of the perirolandic and occipital cortex and the white matter (Fig. 16.2).
- MR spectroscopy can demonstrate a rise in the glutamine and glutamate peaks with reductions in choline and myo-inositol peaks.

Imaging Findings in Chronic Disease [2, 5]

- T1 hyperintensity in the basal ganglia, midbrain, and white matter (Fig. e16.2).
  - Likely due to the deposition of manganese.
- Cerebral atrophy as well as diffuse mild edema.

16 Toxic and Metabolic Diseases of the CNS

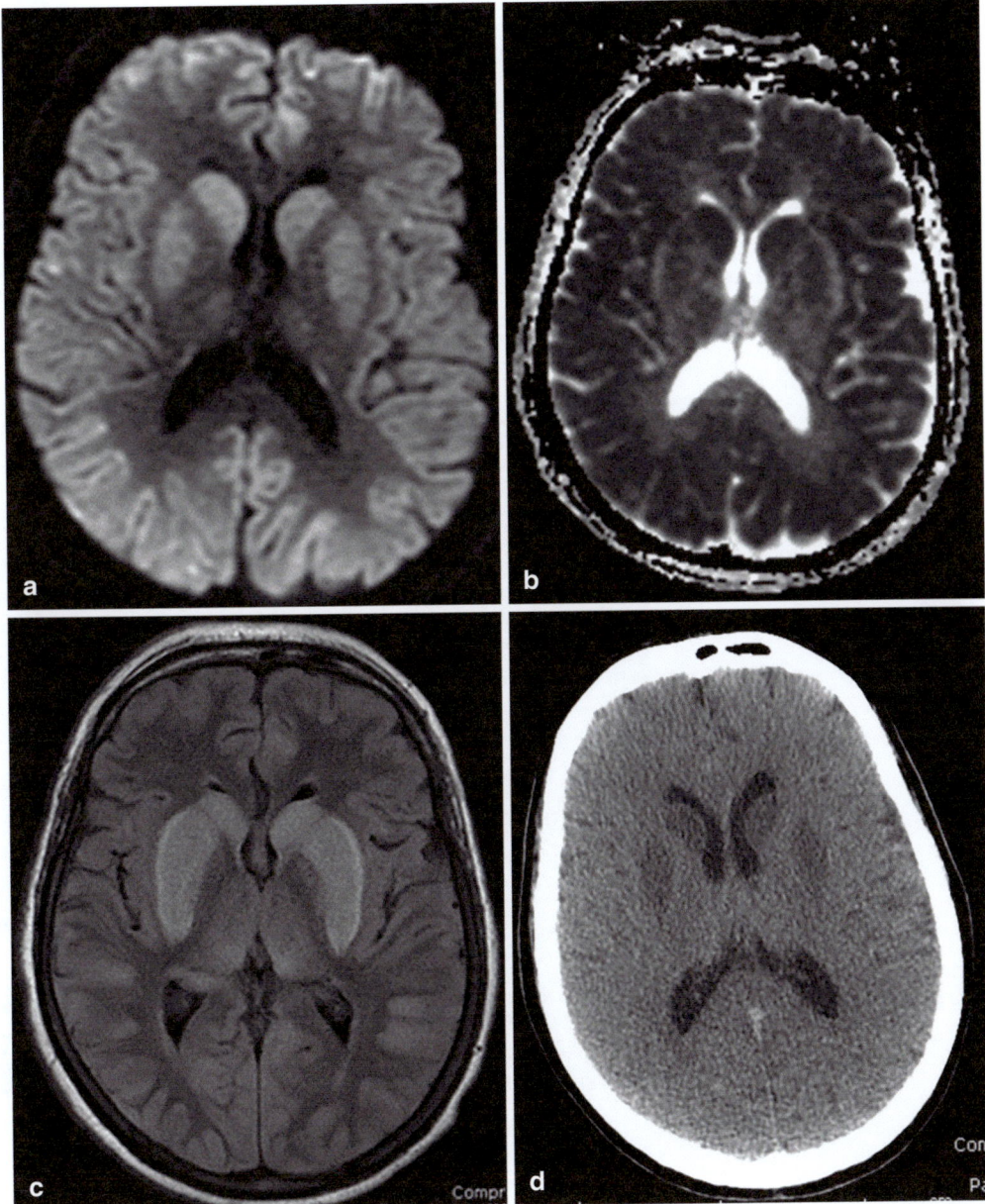

Fig. 16.1 Hypoxic ischemic encephalopathy. A 55-year-old female who was found unconscious. (**a**) Diffusion-weighted image demonstrates symmetric, bilateral high signal intensity in the hemispheric gray matter, basal ganglia, and insular region, (**b**) with corresponding low signal on the ADC map image. (**c**) FLAIR image demonstrates increased signal in these regions. (**d**) Concurrent CT head demonstrates hypodensity in the basal ganglia with loss of gray–white differentiation in the cerebral cortex

Predominant Deep White Matter Involvement

Hypernatremia

- Related to loss of free water within the body. Numerous causes include diarrhea, vomiting, hypodipsia, and renal, adrenal, or hypothalamic dysfunction in the setting of trauma, stroke, or brain tumors.
- Osmotic shift of water from the brain into the bloodstream can result in intracranial hemorrhage from vascular shear injury.
- Compensatory generation of idiogenic osmolytes that retain water within the cells increases susceptibility to cerebral edema if hypernatremia is corrected too rapidly.

Imaging Findings [2, 8–10]

- Restricted diffusion as well as T2 and FLAIR hyperintensity within the cerebral white matter (Fig. e16.3).
- Cortex is spared.
- Basal ganglia and thalamic signal changes are also possible.

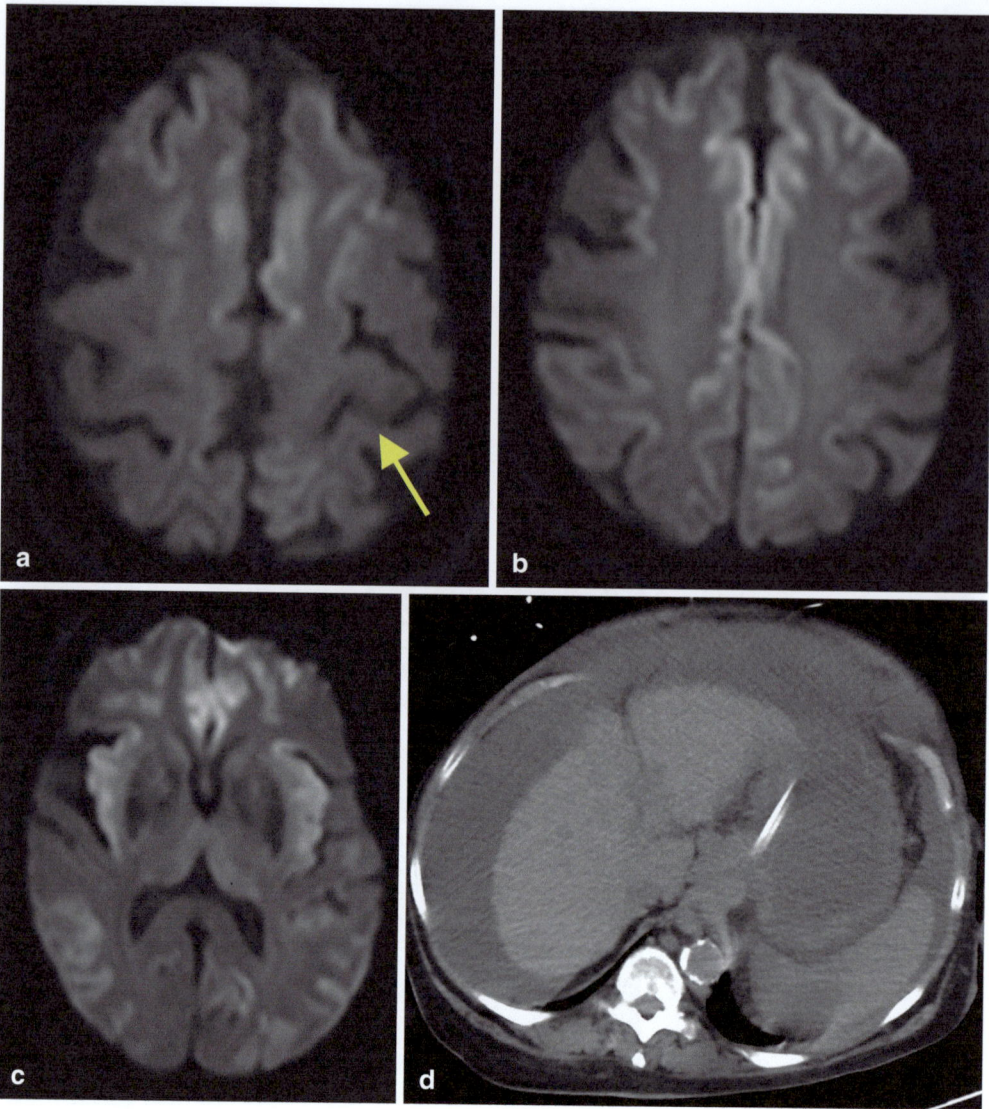

Fig. 16.2 Hepatic encephalopathy (acute hyperammonemia). A 74-year-old female with a history of alcoholic cirrhosis who presented obtunded with decompensated cirrhosis. (**a–c**) Diffusion-weighted images demonstrate restricted diffusion in the frontal, parietal, temporal, insular, and cingulate cortices, with sparing of the peri-rolandic (arrow) and occipital cortices (ADC map not shown). (**d**) CT of the abdomen demonstrates a shrunken cirrhotic liver with ascites, consistent with decompensated liver disease

- Hemorrhage (can be petechial, extra-axial, or secondary to venous thrombosis) appears as a low signal on susceptibility-weighted and gradient echo sequences.
- Subdural effusions.
- Irregular enhancement on contrast-enhanced images due to disruption of the blood–brain barrier.

Posterior Reversible Encephalopathy Syndrome (PRES)

- Reversible subcortical vasogenic edema with acute neurologic symptoms including seizure, headache, and altered mental status.
- Suspected mechanism: Disordered cerebrovascular autoregulation in the setting of hypertension and endothelial injury.

Imaging Findings [11, 12]

- Bilateral asymmetric vasogenic edema in the subcortical white matter (Fig. e16.4).
  - Parieto-occipital pattern is most common.
  - Superior frontal sulcus, holohemispheric watershed, cerebellum, basal ganglia, and brainstem patterns may also be seen.
- No restricted diffusion or enhancement on postcontrast images.

Opioid-Induced Leukoencephalopathy

- Inhaled heroin produces a toxic leukoencephalopathy with a nonlinear progression that includes a latent period prior to onset as well as progression for up to 6 months after cessation of heroin use.
- In contrast, injected heroin most commonly presents with bilateral globus pallidus stroke, with an appearance similar to carbon monoxide poisoning.

Imaging Findings [13–16]

- Confluent bilateral symmetric T2 and FLAIR hyperintensity and restricted diffusion in the supratentorial and infratentorial white matter (Fig. 16.3).
    - Most commonly involving the posterior limb of the internal capsule.
    - Anterior limb of the internal capsule and subcortical U fibers are spared.
- Basal ganglia and cerebellar dentate nuclei are spared.

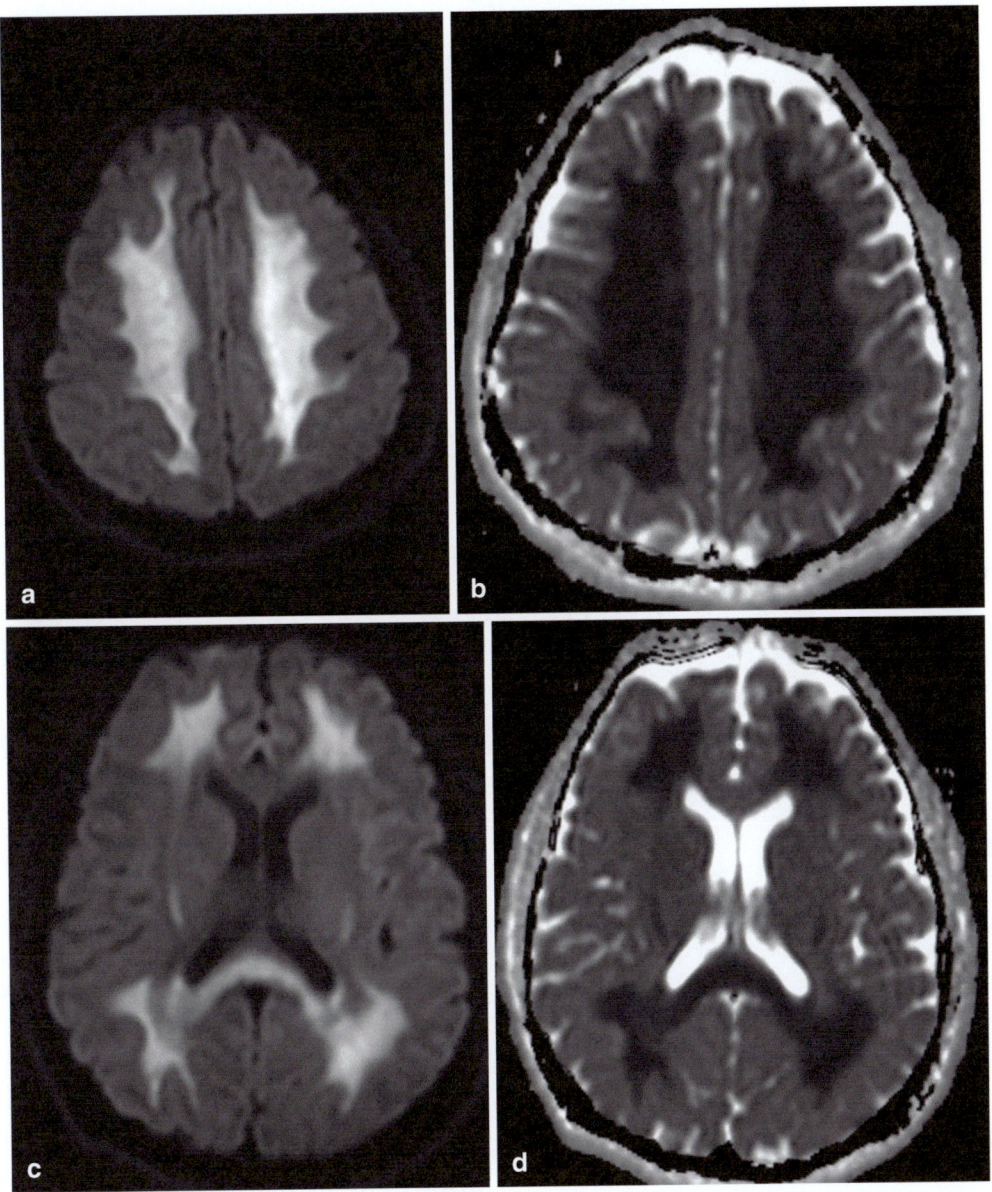

Fig. 16.3 Opioid-induced leukoencephalopathy. A 29-year-old male who was found unconscious after an opioid and cocaine overdose. (**a**) and (**c**) Axial diffusion-weighted and (**b**) and (**d**) corresponding ADC images demonstrate diffuse confluent restricted diffusion in the deep white matter of the bilateral frontal, parietal, and temporal lobes with sparing of the subcortical U fibers with additional involvement of the splenium of the corpus callosum. (**e–h**) Axial FLAIR images demonstrate confluent hyperintensity in these areas

Fig. 16.3 (continued)

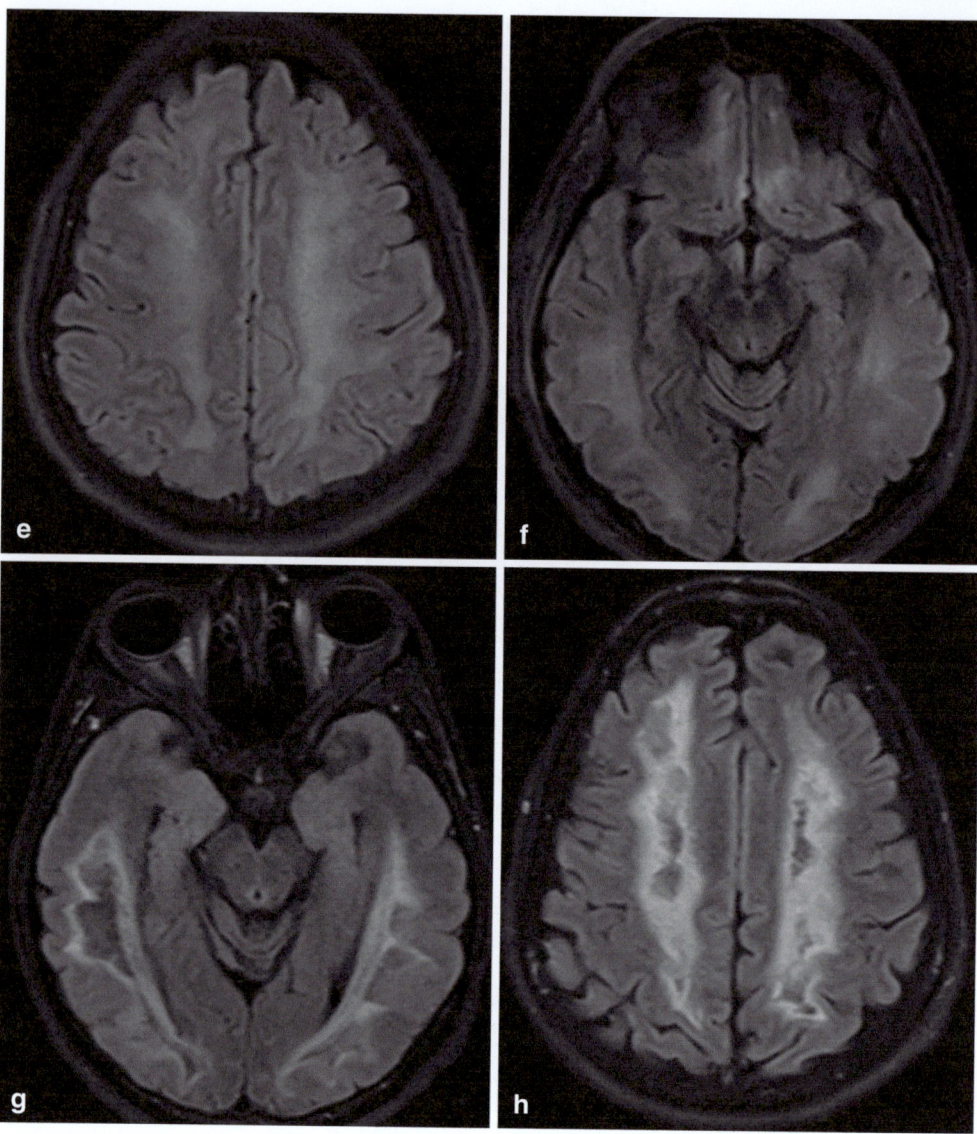

Methotrexate Toxicity

- Methotrexate is a chemotherapeutic agent associated with CNS toxicity at high doses and with intrathecal administration.
- Other chemotherapeutic agents may have a similar effect, including cyclosporine, 5-fluorouracil, and fludarabine.

Imaging Findings [17–19]

- Toxic leukoencephalopathy is most common and can occur usually days after administration.
  - Bilateral asymmetric T2 and FLAIR hyperintensity and restricted diffusion across multiple vascular territories, involving the centrum semiovale and sparing the subcortical U fibers (Fig. e16.5).
- Disseminated necrotizing encephalopathy is a rare complication of intrathecal methotrexate when combined with whole-brain radiation therapy.
  - Diffuse T2 hyperintensity in the white matter with hypointense hemorrhagic foci that display peripheral or solid enhancement (tumor-like).
- Subacute combined degeneration may be seen in the setting of vitamin B12 deficiency.

Brainstem Involvement

Osmotic Myelinolysis

- Classically the result of rapid correction of hyponatremia and also associated with psychogenic polydipsia and malnutrition.

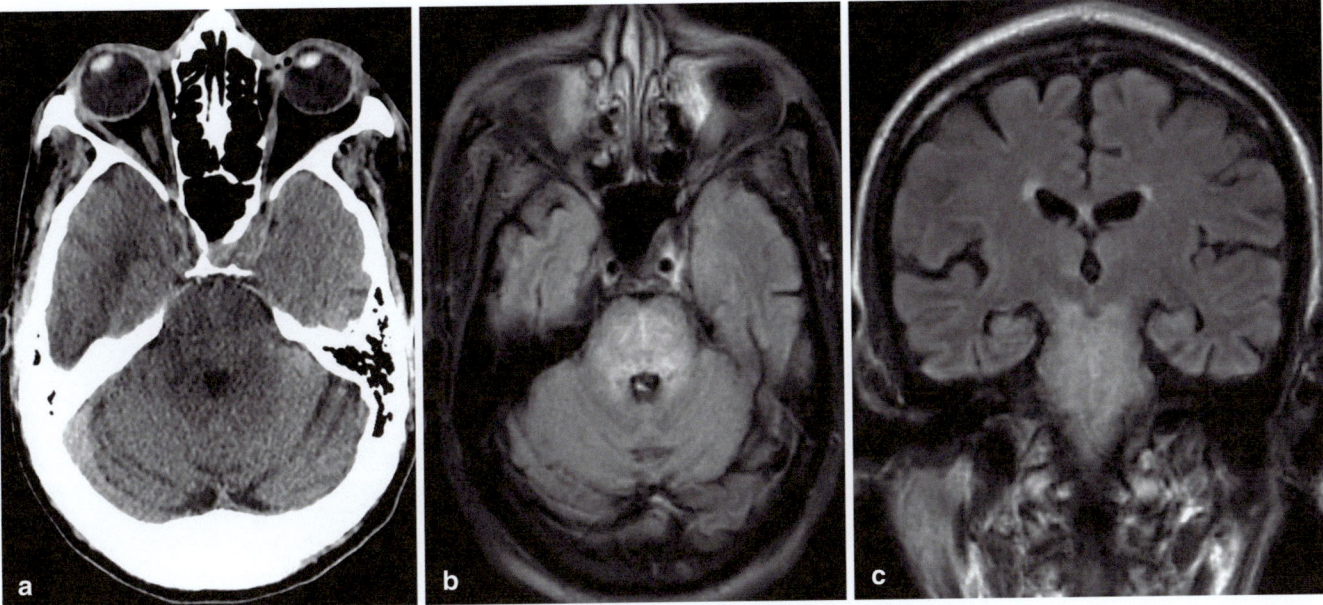

Fig. 16.4 Osmotic myelinolysis. A 56-year-old male with a history of alcohol use who presented to the emergency room with lethargy. (**a**) Initial non-contrast head CT reveals hypodensity and enlargement of the pons. (**b**) Axial and (**c**) coronal FLAIR images demonstrate diffuse enlargement and hyperintensity of the pons, with some peripheral sparing

- Most commonly occurs as central pontine myelinolysis, but can also be extrapontine. The most common extrapontine location is the cerebellar folia.
- Symptoms are nonspecific but include dysarthria and dysphagia, with an overlap of symptoms between pontine hemorrhage, infarction, and glioma.

Imaging Findings [2]

- Pontine hypodensity on CT.
- Symmetric T2 and FLAIR hyperintensity in the central pons, often sparing the outer rim (Fig. 16.4).
- Restricted diffusion in the acute phase.
- Peripheral enhancement of the affected area on contrast-enhanced MRI.
- Necrosis and cavitation in severe cases.

Wernicke Encephalopathy

- Sequela of thiamine (vitamin B1) deficiency. Most commonly resulting from malnutrition in the setting of chronic alcohol use, but also seen after gastrointestinal surgery, with prolonged vomiting, or malnutrition of any cause.
- Clinical triad of ocular symptoms (nystagmus, gaze palsies), ataxia, and altered mental status, only present in 16–38% of patients.

Imaging Findings [20, 21]

- T2 hyperintensity in the medial thalami and periventricular regions of the third ventricle.
  - Mammillary bodies, tectal plate, and periaqueductal gray matter are also symmetrically affected (Fig. 16.5).
- Involvement of the mammillary bodies is more commonly seen in alcoholics, and enhancement of these structures may be the only sign of Wernicke encephalopathy in these patients.
- Less common MRI findings include abnormalities of the cerebellum, cranial nerve nuclei, red nuclei, corpus callosum, and cerebral cortex. These atypical findings are seen in non-alcoholic patients.

Basal Ganglia Involvement

Carbon Monoxide Toxicity

- Carbon monoxide (CO) is a colorless, tasteless, and odorless gas, which binds to hemoglobin with greater affinity than oxygen and reduces the oxygen-carrying capacity of the blood.
- Sources of CO include cigarette smoking, motor vehicle exhaust, and faulty heaters and furnaces.
- Symptoms of CO poisoning result from hypoxic injury, are nonspecific, and include headache, nausea, vomiting, and weakness, as well as cognitive deficits or coma.

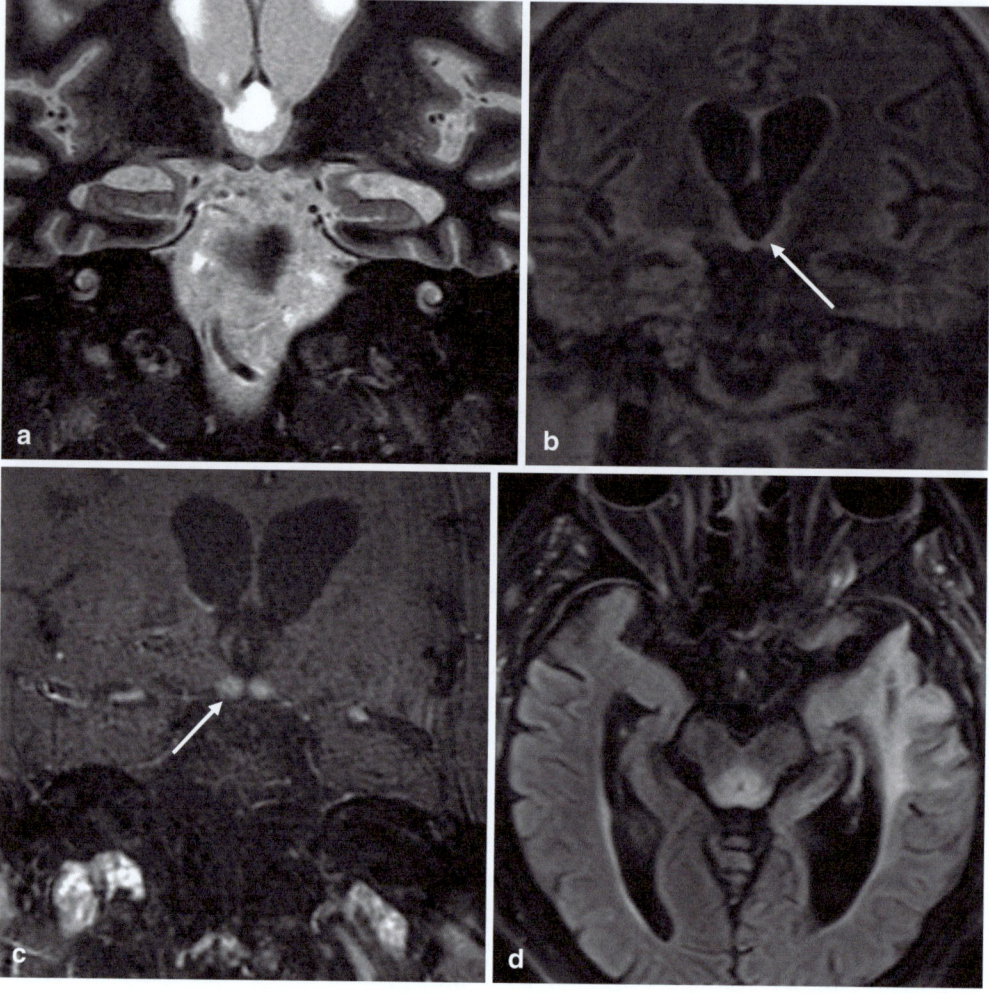

Fig. 16.5 Wernicke Encephalopathy. A 51-year-old male with a history of alcohol use, altered mental status, and low thiamine levels. (**a**) Coronal T2 and (**b**) Coronal FLAIR images demonstrate increased signal in the mammillary bodies (**b**, arrow). (**c**) Postcontrast MPRAGE image showing postcontrast enhancement of the mammillary bodies. (**d**) Axial FLAIR image from another patient with Wernicke's disease showing increased T2 signal abnormality in the periacqueductal gray in the midbrain

Imaging Findings [6, 22]

- Edema and necrosis of the globus pallidus (bilateral and symmetric).
  - T1 hypointense and T2 hyperintense, restricted diffusion, and low signal on susceptibility-weighted images if there is hemorrhage (Fig. e16.6).
- Thalamus, caudate, putamen, and cerebral white matter can also be affected.
- Delayed leukoencephalopathy in the subacute phase.

Wilson's Disease

- Inherited autosomal recessive defect in copper transport and metabolism, leading to accumulation of copper in tissues.
- Copper accumulation does not lead to brain signal abnormality.
- Acute decompensations lead to histopathologic findings of spongiform degeneration, cavitation, and atrophy in the basal ganglia, thalami, and brainstem.
- Findings are felt to be related to oxidative damage following excessive copper deposition.

Imaging Findings [23–25]

- T2 hyperintensity in the basal ganglia, as well as midbrain and pons (Fig. 16.6).
- T1 hyperintense lesions in the basal ganglia reflect hepatic disease.
- "Face of the giant panda" sign on MRI consists of T2 hyperintensity in the tegmentum, normal signal in the substantia nigra and red nuclei, and T2 hypointensity in the superior colliculus (Fig. e16.7). This may also be seen in the dorsal pons.

Methanol Toxicity

- Methanol is a component of solvents or adulterated alcoholic drinks, which can be ingested or inhaled.

Imaging Findings [26, 27]

- Bilateral hemorrhagic necrosis of the putamina (Fig. e16.8) [28].
  - Hyperattenuation on CT.

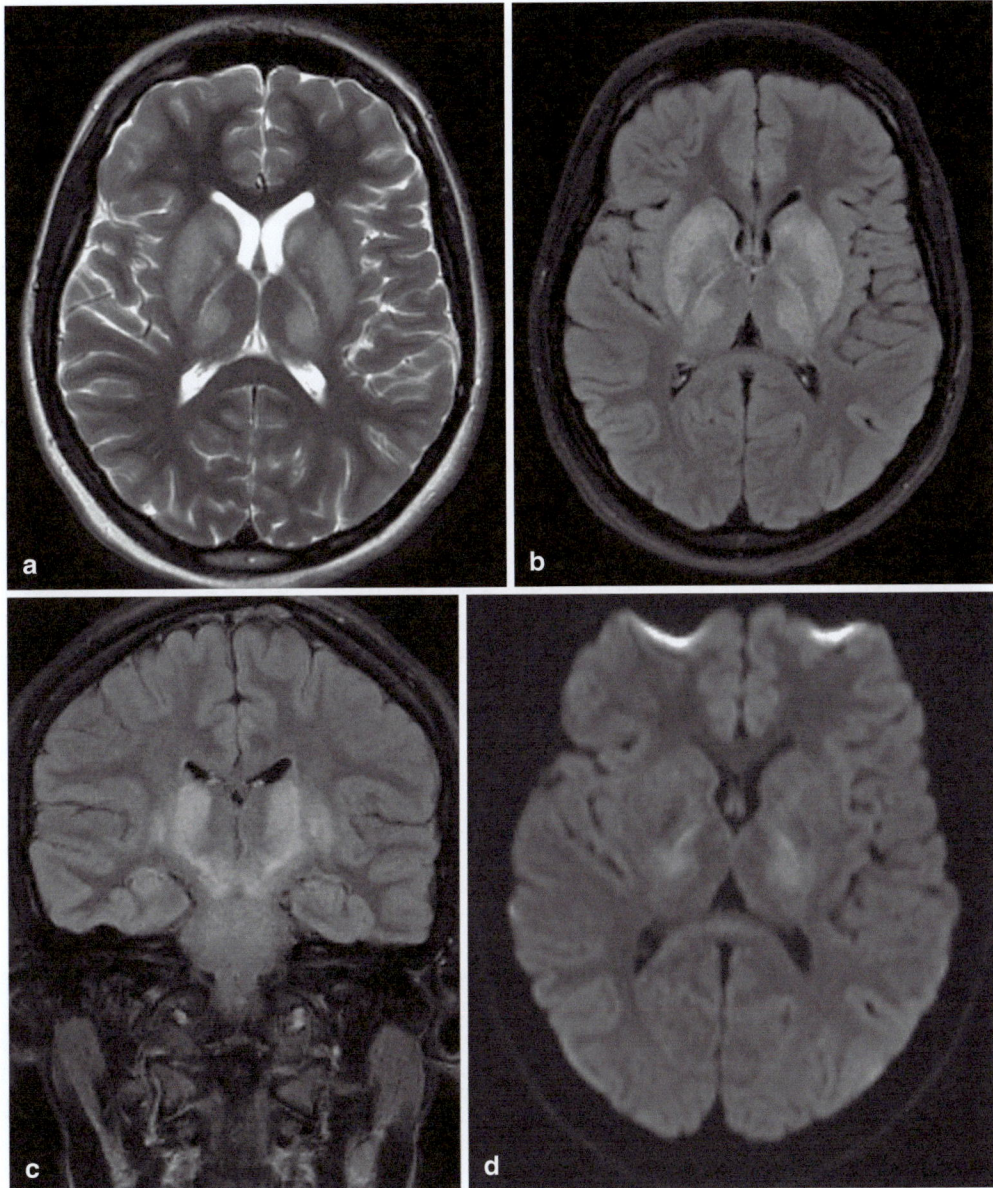

Fig. 16.6 Wilson's disease. A 14-year-old female with a history of Wilson's disease and altered mental status. (**a**) Axial T2-weighted, (**b**) axial FLAIR, and (**c**) coronal FLAIR images demonstrate bilateral, symmetric hyperintense signal within the basal ganglia, thalami, and along the corticospinal tracts. (**d**) Axial diffusion-weighted image demonstrates restricted diffusion in this region (ADC map not shown)

- o T2 and FLAIR hyperintensity, restricted diffusion, and low signal on susceptibility-weighted images.
- o Reduced N-acetyl aspartate and elevated lactate peaks on MR spectroscopy.

Chemotherapy-Associated PRES

- Atypical PRES when compared with traditional presentation.
- Symmetric involvement of unusual sites with enhancement postcontrast [29].

Parathyroid Dysfunction Disorder

- Dysfunction of calcium metabolism.

Imaging Findings [30]

- Bilateral and symmetric calcium deposition in the basal ganglia, thalamus, subcortical white matter, and cerebellar dentate nuclei.
  - o Blooming artifacts on T2* and susceptibility-weighted images.
  - o Hyperdensity on CT in the above-mentioned areas.

Fahr's Disease

- Genetic disease of idiopathic basal ganglia calcifications.
- Similar pattern to parathyroid dysfunction but without laboratory anomalies (Fig. e16.9).

Uremic Encephalopathy

- Accumulation of uremic toxins in the setting of acute or chronic renal failure.
- Clinical manifestations include tremor, asterixis, myoclonus, seizure, and altered mental status.

Imaging Findings [31, 32]

- Bilateral symmetric T2 and FLAIR hyperintensity in the basal ganglia is the most common.
- "Lentiform fork" sign is characterized by T2 and FLAIR hyperintensity in the white matter surrounding the lentiform nuclei (internal capsule, external capsule, and medullary lamina; Fig. 16.7).
- Other patterns include a PRES-like appearance or white matter acute toxic leukoencephalopathy.

Diabetic Striatopathy

- Hyperglycemia-induced hemichorea-hemiballismus.

Imaging Findings [33, 34]

- Unilateral T1 hyperintensity in the striatum with correlate hyperdensity on CT (Fig. e16.10) [35].

Cerebellum Involvement

Maple Syrup Urine Disease

- Rare autosomal recessive inborn error of metabolism due to a defect in the catabolism of branched-chain amino acids (BCAAs; leucine, isoleucine, and valine).
- Presents in the first week of life with lethargy, vomiting, irritability, poor feeding, and neurologic deterioration, with a characteristic maple syrup smell of the urine.
- Treatment consists of lifelong dietary restriction of BCAA. Orthotopic liver transplantation is curative.

Imaging Findings [36–38]

- Diffuse mild edema with more localized intense edema (so-called MSUD edema) involving the cerebellar white matter, posterior brainstem, cerebral peduncles, posterior limb of the internal capsule, and posterior centrum semiovale (Fig. 16.8). These regions are myelinated or myelinating at birth.

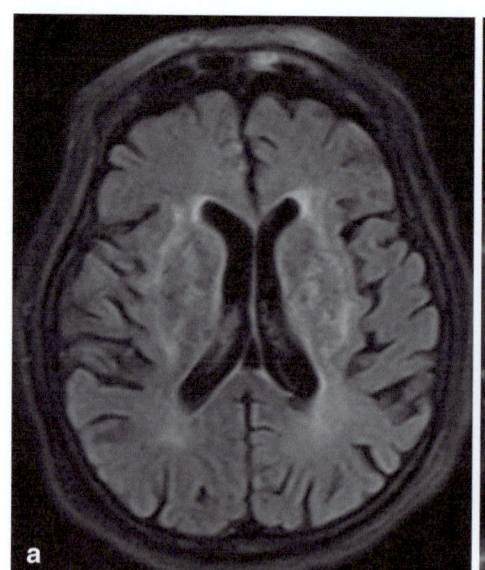 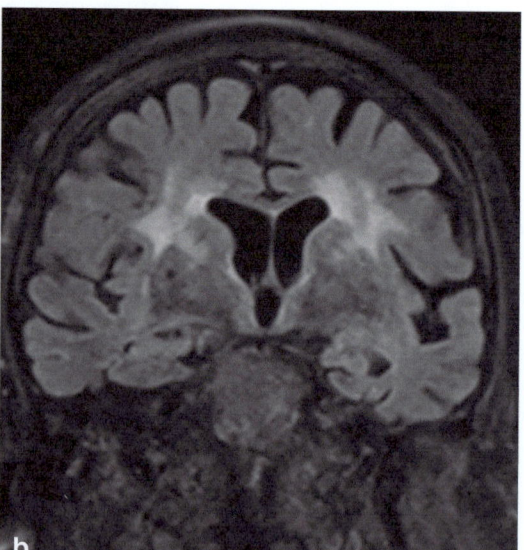

Fig. 16.7 Uremic encephalopathy. A 78-year-old female who presented with septic shock and renal failure. (**a**) Axial and (**b**) coronal FLAIR images show increased signal within the internal capsule and external capsule bilaterally ("lentiform fork" sign)

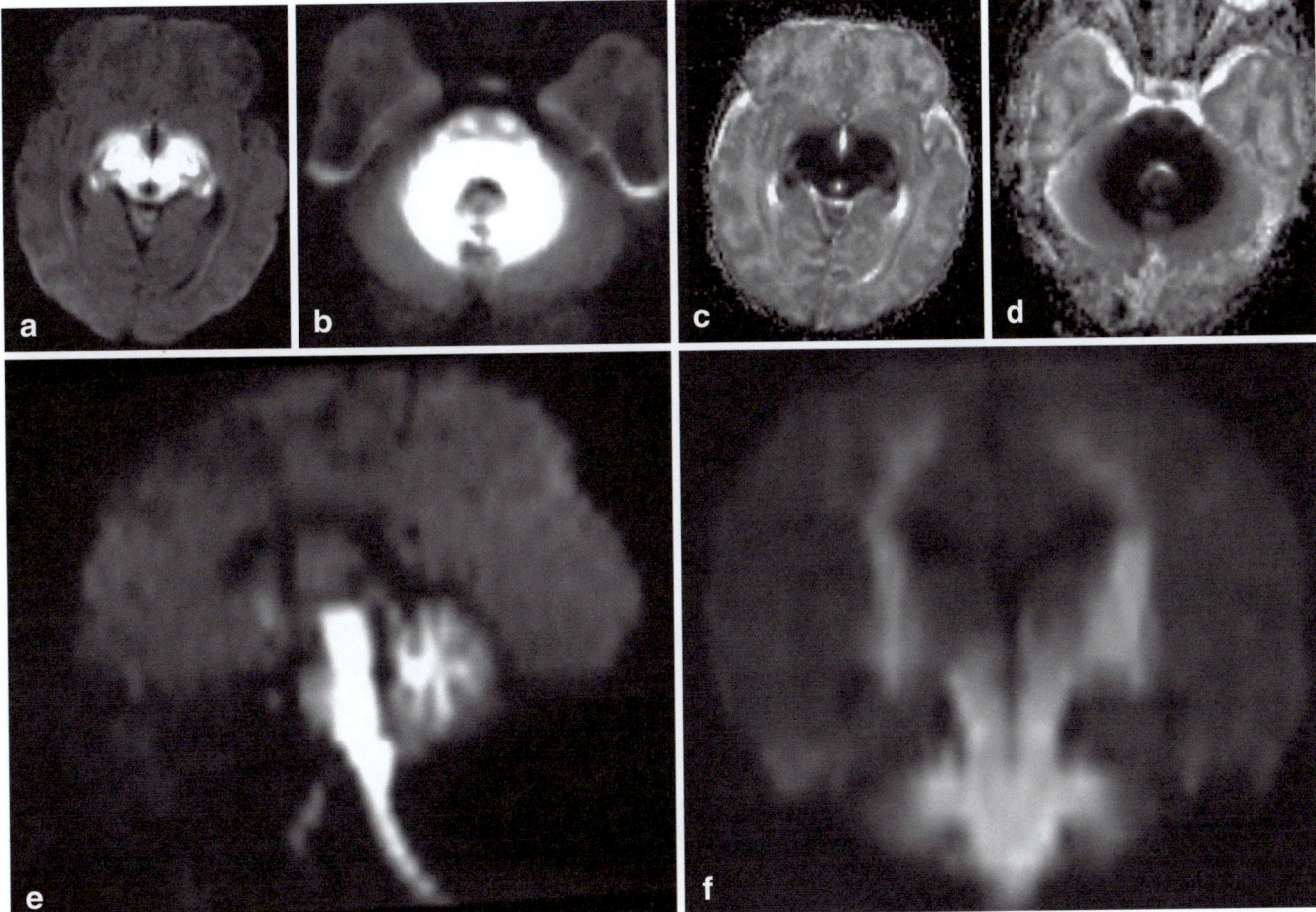

Fig. 16.8 Maple syrup urine disease. An 8-day-old female with feeding difficulties and lethargy. (**a**) and (**b**) Axial diffusion-weighted images, and (**c**) and (**d**) corresponding ADC images, demonstrate intense restricted diffusion within the cerebellum, brainstem, midbrain, and pyramidal tracts. This is also demonstrated on (**e**) sagittal and (**f**) coronal diffusion-weighted images

- Restricted diffusion is the most sensitive acute finding.
- Following the acute phase, varying degrees of brain damage are seen depending on when treatment is initiated. In untreated cases, there is spongiform degeneration of the white matter most pronounced near the gray matter–white matter junction.

Metronidazole Toxicity

- Metronidazole is a nitroimidazole antibiotic commonly used for anaerobic and protozoal infections, as well as chronic therapy in patients with Crohn's disease.
- Has good cellular penetration and is believed to enter the cerebrospinal fluid and central nervous system easily.
- When administered in excess of 2 g/day, it can produce peripheral neuropathies and cerebellar dysfunction, likely due to axonal swelling rather than demyelination due to reversibility on drug discontinuation.

Imaging Findings [39, 40]

- T2 hyperintensity in the dentate nuclei of the cerebellum is the most common (Fig. 16.9).
  - Other affected areas may include the tectum, red nucleus, periaqueductal gray matter, dorsal pons, dorsal medulla, and corpus callosum.
  - Involvement is bilateral and symmetric.
- No enhancement on postcontrast images.
- Reversible after drug discontinuation.

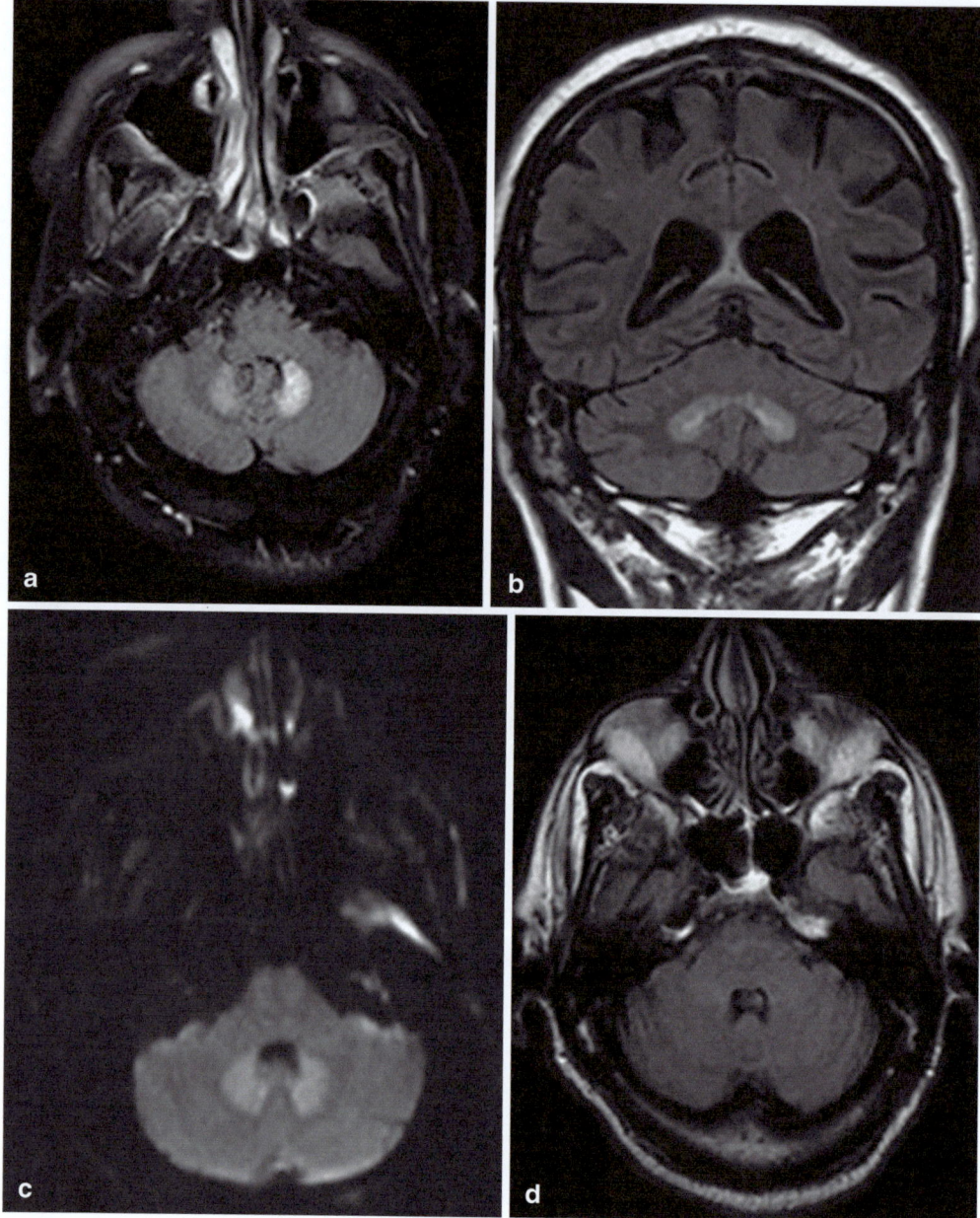

Fig. 16.9 Metronidazole toxicity. A 67-year-old male with stroke-like symptoms and cerebellar signs, receiving metronidazole for *Clostridium difficile* colitis. (**a**) Axial and (**b**) coronal FLAIR images show symmetric, increased signal within the dentate nuclei of the cerebellum. (**c**) Axial diffusion-weighted image demonstrates restricted diffusion in this region (ADC map not shown). (**d**) Axial FLAIR image of a follow-up MR performed 6 months after therapy demonstrates resolution of findings

Corpus Callosum Involvement

Marchiafava-Bignami Disease

- Osmotic demyelination and necrosis of the corpus callosum.
- Setting of chronic alcohol use or vitamin B complex deficiency.
- Type A is acute and characterized by seizures and coma, involvement of the entire corpus callosum, and rapid progression to death within days.
- Type B is chronic and characterized by mild encephalopathy and focal lesions in the corpus callosum.

Imaging Findings [41, 42]

- T2 and FLAIR hyperintensity in the corpus callosum (Fig. 16.10), most commonly with selective involvement of the middle layers ("sandwich sign").
- Type B typically manifests initially in the genu and frontoparietal cortex followed by the splenium.
  - Chronic findings include curvilinear T1 hypointensity in the central corpus callosum.
- Acute lesions may show enhancement on postcontrast images, and no restricted diffusion.
- Reduction of callosal fibers on DTI.

Fig. 16.10 Marchiafava-Bignami disease. A 60-year-old male with a history of chronic alcohol use. Axial (**a**) and (**b**) coronal FLAIR images demonstrate increased signal throughout the corpus callosum. (**c**) and (**d**) Axial diffusion-weighted images demonstrate corresponding restricted diffusion in this region (ADC map not shown). (**e**) Sagittal T1-weighted image demonstrates the splitting of the corpus callosum (arrows)

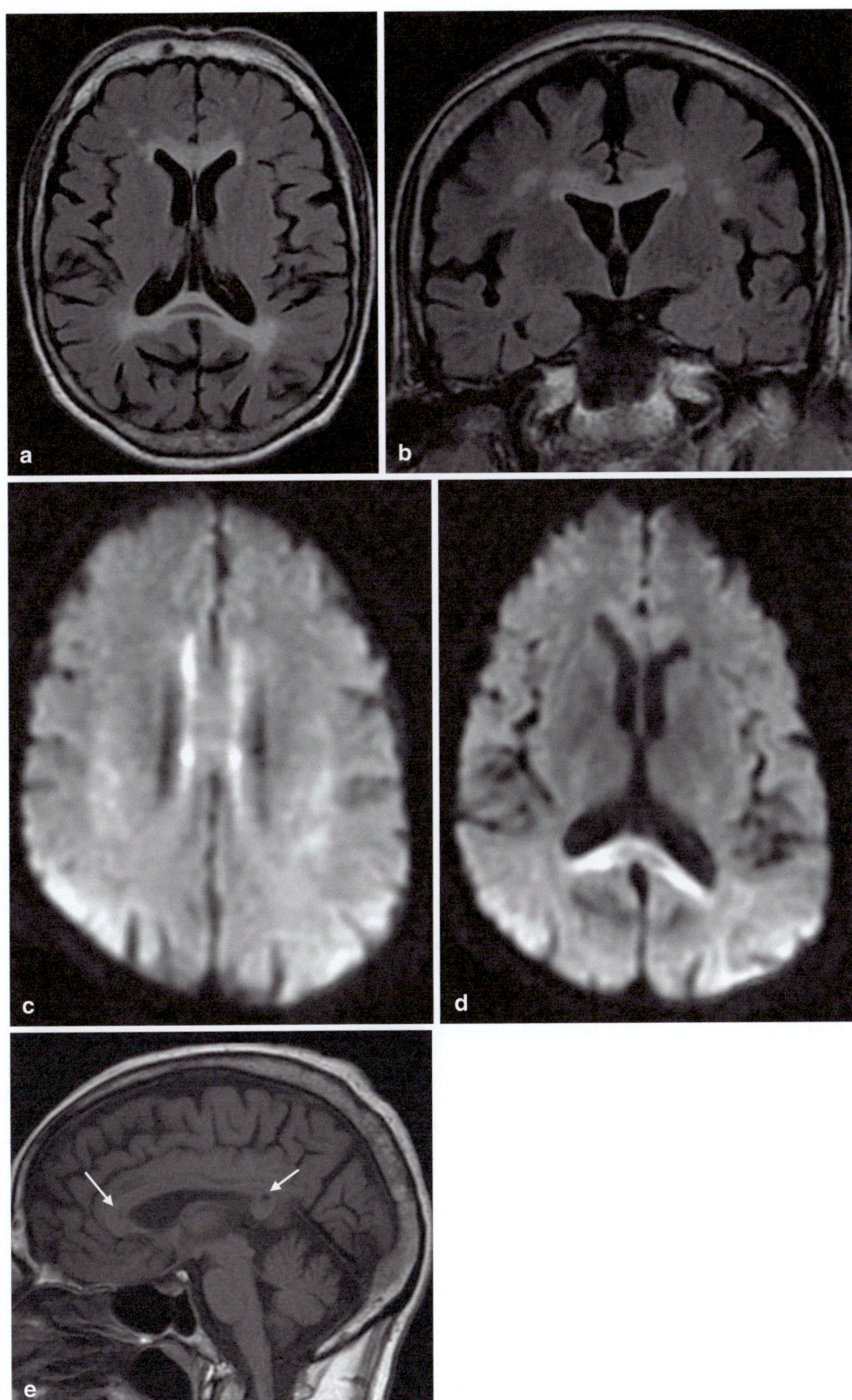

References

1. Huang BY, Castillo M. Hypoxic-ischemic brain injury: imaging findings from birth to adulthood. Radiographics. 2008;28:417–39; quiz 617
2. Van der Knaap MS, Valk J, Barkhof F. Magnetic resonance of myelination and myelin disorders. 3rd ed. Berlin/New York: Springer; 2005.
3. Osborn A, Hedlund G, Salzman K. Toxic, metabolic, degenerative and CSF disorders. Philadelphia, PA: Elsevier; 2017.
4. Kang EG, Jeon SJ, Choi SS, Song CJ, Yu IK. Diffusion MR imaging of hypoglycemic encephalopathy. AJNR Am J Neuroradiol. 2010;31:559–64.
5. Rovira A, Alonso J, Cordoba J. MR imaging findings in hepatic encephalopathy. AJNR Am J Neuroradiol. 2008;29:1612–21.
6. Sharma P, Eesa M, Scott JN. Toxic and acquired metabolic encephalopathies: MRI appearance. AJR Am J Roentgenol. 2009;193:879–86.
7. Takanashi J, Barkovich AJ, Cheng SF, Kostiner D, Baker JC, Packman S. Brain MR imaging in acute hyperammonemic encephalopathy arising from late-onset ornithine transcarbamylase deficiency. AJNR Am J Neuroradiol. 2003;24:390–3.
8. Adrogue HJ, Madias NE. Hypernatremia. N Engl J Med. 2000;342:1493–9.
9. Hartfield DS, Loewy JA, Yager JY. Transient thalamic changes on MRI in a child with hypernatremia. Pediatr Neurol. 1999;20:60–2.
10. Ozdemir H, Kabakus N, Kurt AN, Artas H. Bilateral symmetrical hypodensities in the thalamus in a child with severe hypernatraemia. Pediatr Radiol. 2005;35:449–50.
11. Bartynski WS, Boardman JF. Distinct imaging patterns and lesion distribution in posterior reversible encephalopathy syndrome. AJNR Am J Neuroradiol. 2007;28:1320–7.
12. Fugate JE, Rabinstein AA. Posterior reversible encephalopathy syndrome: clinical and radiological manifestations, pathophysiology, and outstanding questions. Lancet Neurol. 2015;14:914–25.
13. Geibprasert S, Gallucci M, Krings T. Addictive illegal drugs: structural neuroimaging. AJNR Am J Neuroradiol. 2010;31:803–8.
14. Keogh CF, Andrews GT, Spacey SD, Forkheim KE, Graeb DA. Neuroimaging features of heroin inhalation toxicity: "chasing the dragon". AJR Am J Roentgenol. 2003;180:847–50.
15. Tamrazi B, Almast J. Your brain on drugs: imaging of drug-related changes in the central nervous system. Radiographics. 2012;32:701–19.
16. de Oliveira AM, Paulino MV, Vieira APF, et al. Imaging patterns of toxic and metabolic brain disorders. Radiographics. 2019;39:1672–95.
17. Inaba H, Khan RB, Laningham FH, Crews KR, Pui CH, Daw NC. Clinical and radiological characteristics of methotrexate-induced acute encephalopathy in pediatric patients with cancer. Ann Oncol. 2008;19:178–84.
18. Kim JY, Kim ST, Nam DH, Lee JI, Park K, Kong DS. Leukoencephalopathy and disseminated necrotizing leukoencephalopathy following intrathecal methotrexate chemotherapy and radiation therapy for central nerve system lymphoma or leukemia. J Korean Neurosurg Soc. 2011;50:304–10.
19. Reddick WE, Glass JO, Helton KJ, et al. Prevalence of leukoencephalopathy in children treated for acute lymphoblastic leukemia with high-dose methotrexate. AJNR Am J Neuroradiol. 2005;26:1263–9.
20. Zuccoli G, Gallucci M, Capellades J, et al. Wernicke encephalopathy: MR findings at clinical presentation in twenty-six alcoholic and nonalcoholic patients. AJNR Am J Neuroradiol. 2007;28:1328–31.
21. Zuccoli G, Pipitone N. Neuroimaging findings in acute Wernicke's encephalopathy: review of the literature. AJR Am J Roentgenol. 2009;192:501–8.
22. O'Donnell P, Buxton PJ, Pitkin A, Jarvis LJ. The magnetic resonance imaging appearances of the brain in acute carbon monoxide poisoning. Clin Radiol. 2000;55:273–80.
23. Jacobs DA, Markowitz CE, Liebeskind DS, Galetta SL. The "double panda sign" in Wilson's disease. Neurology. 2003;61:969.
24. Kim TJ, Kim IO, Kim WS, et al. MR imaging of the brain in Wilson disease of childhood: findings before and after treatment with clinical correlation. AJNR Am J Neuroradiol. 2006;27:1373–8.
25. Singh P, Ahluwalia A, Saggar K, Grewal CS. Wilson's disease: MRI features. J Pediatr Neurosci. 2011;6:27–8.
26. Blanco M, Casado R, Vazquez F, Pumar JM. CT and MR imaging findings in methanol intoxication. AJNR Am J Neuroradiol. 2006;27:452–4.
27. Hegde AN, Mohan S, Lath N, Lim CC. Differential diagnosis for bilateral abnormalities of the basal ganglia and thalamus. Radiographics. 2011;31:5–30.
28. Sefidbakht S, Rasekhi AR, Kamali K, et al. Methanol poisoning: acute MR and CT findings in nine patients. Neuroradiology. 2007;49:427–35.
29. McKinney AM, Short J, Truwit CL, et al. Posterior reversible encephalopathy syndrome: incidence of atypical regions of involvement and imaging findings. AJR Am J Roentgenol. 2007;189:904–12.
30. Shoback DM, Bilezikian JP, Costa AG, et al. Presentation of hypoparathyroidism: etiologies and clinical features. J Clin Endocrinol Metab. 2016;101:2300–12.
31. Kim DM, Lee IH, Song CJ. Uremic encephalopathy: MR imaging findings and clinical correlation. AJNR Am J Neuroradiol. 2016;37:1604–9.
32. Kumar G, Goyal MK. Lentiform Fork sign: a unique MRI picture. Is metabolic acidosis responsible? Clin Neurol Neurosurg. 2010;112:805–12.
33. Bathla G, Policeni B, Agarwal A. Neuroimaging in patients with abnormal blood glucose levels. AJNR Am J Neuroradiol. 2014;35:833–40.
34. Lai PH, Tien RD, Chang MH, et al. Chorea-ballismus with nonketotic hyperglycemia in primary diabetes mellitus. AJNR Am J Neuroradiol. 1996;17:1057–64.
35. Ottaviani S, Arecco A, Boschetti M, et al. Prevalence of diabetic striatopathy and predictive role of glycated hemoglobin level. Neurol Sci. 2022;43:6059–65.
36. Cavalleri F, Berardi A, Burlina AB, Ferrari F, Mavilla L. Diffusion-weighted MRI of maple syrup urine disease encephalopathy. Neuroradiology. 2002;44:499–502.
37. Parmar H, Sitoh YY, Ho L. Maple syrup urine disease: diffusion-weighted and diffusion-tensor magnetic resonance imaging findings. J Comput Assist Tomogr. 2004;28:93–7.
38. Strauss KA, Puffenberger EG, Carson VJ. In: Adam MP, Ardinger HH, Pagon RA, et al., editors. Maple syrup urine disease. Seattle, WA: GeneReviews((R)); 1993.
39. Kim E, Na DG, Kim EY, Kim JH, Son KR, Chang KH. MR imaging of metronidazole-induced encephalopathy: lesion distribution and diffusion-weighted imaging findings. AJNR Am J Neuroradiol. 2007;28:1652–8.
40. Kim H, Kim YW, Kim SR, Park IS, Jo KW. Metronidazole-induced encephalopathy in a patient with infectious colitis: a case report. J Med Case Rep. 2011;5:63.
41. Arbelaez A, Pajon A, Castillo M. Acute marchiafava-bignami disease: MR findings in two patients. AJNR Am J Neuroradiol. 2003;24:1955–7.
42. Tung CS, Wu SL, Tsou JC, Hsu SP, Kuo HC, Tsui HW. Marchiafava-Bignami disease with widespread lesions and complete recovery. AJNR Am J Neuroradiol. 2010;31:1506–7.

Neurodegenerative Disorders

Johannes H. Decker, Max Wintermark, and Michael Zeineh

INTRODUCTION

- A large group of acquired and inherited disorders whose etiology are incompletely understood, are difficult to diagnose, and have limited treatment options, but with a unifying feature of gradual synaptic and neuronal loss producing cognitive symptoms.
- The clinical presentations of these disorders are associated with characteristic patterns of neuronal degeneration, such as tau, amyloid-beta (Aβ), and α-synuclein aggregates.
- The following sections will feature the common and several less common neurodegenerative disorders and highlight distinguishing imaging features.
- Overlap of both clinical and imaging manifestations of these disorders often limits definitive diagnosis on an imaging basis, with imaging used to exclude other disorders, and to some extent distinguish between the different neurodegenerative disorders.
- A further complication is the growing evidence that co-pathology of multiple neurodegenerative disorders may be more common than a single, pure neurodegenerative disorder in aging individuals [1, 2].
- Of note, multiple classification schemes exist based on clinical presentation, pathology, and imaging, and disorders will be highlighted that appear in multiple categories.

NORMAL AGING

- Natural neuronal degeneration causes diffuse brain atrophy that increases with age.
- Approximately 5% volume loss per decade after 40 which accelerates later in life [3].
- Volume loss manifests as increased ventricle size, particularly in the body of the lateral ventricles, and increased sulcal size with greater separation between gyri (Fig. 17.1).
- Increased age is also associated with white matter changes that are typically attributed to microvascular ischemic disease from hypertension and diabetes.
- When in excess, these may contribute to the clinical entity of vascular dementia, or reduce cognitive reserve and predispose to clinical symptoms from other neurodegenerative pathology.
- Typical age-related volume loss is often superimposed on vascular disease and neurodegenerative diseases as all increase in prevalence and burden with age.

Supplementary Information The online version contains supplementary material available at https://doi.org/10.1007/978-3-031-55124-6_17.

J. H. Decker · M. Wintermark · M. Zeineh (✉)
Division of Neuroimaging and Neurointervention, Stanford University School of Medicine, Stanford, CA, USA
e-mail: jhdecker@stanford.edu; mzeineh@stanford.edu

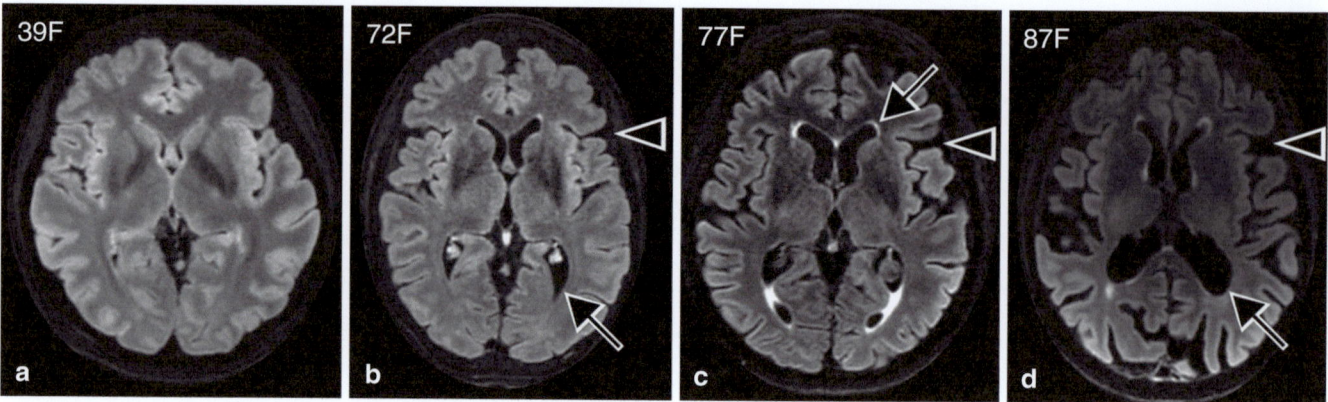

Fig. 17.1 Natural aging of the brain. Axial T2-FLAIR-weighted images of the brain showing normal brain volume for age. (**a**) A 39-year-old female with narrow sulci and ventricles. (**b**) A 72-year-old female with mild volume loss exhibited by mildly increased ventricle size (arrow) and sulcal widening (arrowhead). (**c**) A 77-year-old male with moderately widened ventricles (arrow) and sulci. (**d**) An 87-year-old female with markedly widened ventricles (arrow) and sulci (arrowhead). Few foci of T2 hyperintensity in the white matter, including periventricular regions, are considered normal and are expected to increase with age

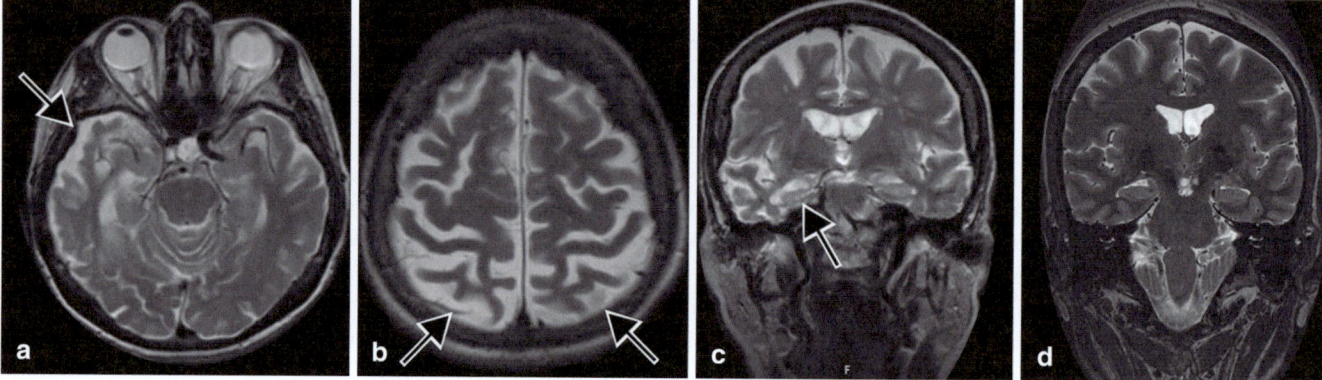

Fig. 17.2 Morphologic changes of Alzheimer dementia (AD). (**a**) and (**b**) Axial and (**C**) coronal T2-weighted images of a 77-year-old female with AD. Note the predominant atrophy (arrows) of the temporal lobes (**a**), parietal lobes (**b**), and mesial temporal cortex/hippocampus (**C**). (**d**) Coronal T2-weighted image of a 53-year-old female with normal hippocampal volumes

ALZHEIMER DISEASE (AD)

- The most common neurodegenerative disorder resulting in progressive dementia and which increases in prevalence with age (12.5% over age 65 years, 50% over age 85 years) [4].
- AD is primarily sporadic though 10% of cases are familial and present early in life.
- The etiology of neurodegeneration is unknown [5, 6], but Aβ plaques are required for the pathological diagnosis, and there is a strong correlation with neuropathological aggregates of Tau-filled neurofibrillary tangles.
- Imaging plays a primary role in excluding other diagnoses that cause dementia such as masses, normal pressure hydrocephalus, and other cortical dementias.
- Classic imaging findings of AD are pronounced bilateral parietal, temporal, and hippocampal atrophy (Fig. 17.2), though these findings are nonspecific as they can be seen in frontotemporal lobar degeneration (FTLD) and limbic-predominant age-related TDP-43 encephalopathy (LATE).
- While classic involvement is medial temporal, and later involvement of the remainder of the neocortex and brainstem, AD can present in two other patterns: hippocampal predominant, or involvement of other neocortical areas (logopenic primary progressive aphasia, posterior cortical atrophy) [7]—see the section on other cortical dementias.
- Multiple PET tracers have been used to assess AD, with FDG-PET showing areas of abnormal glucose metabo-

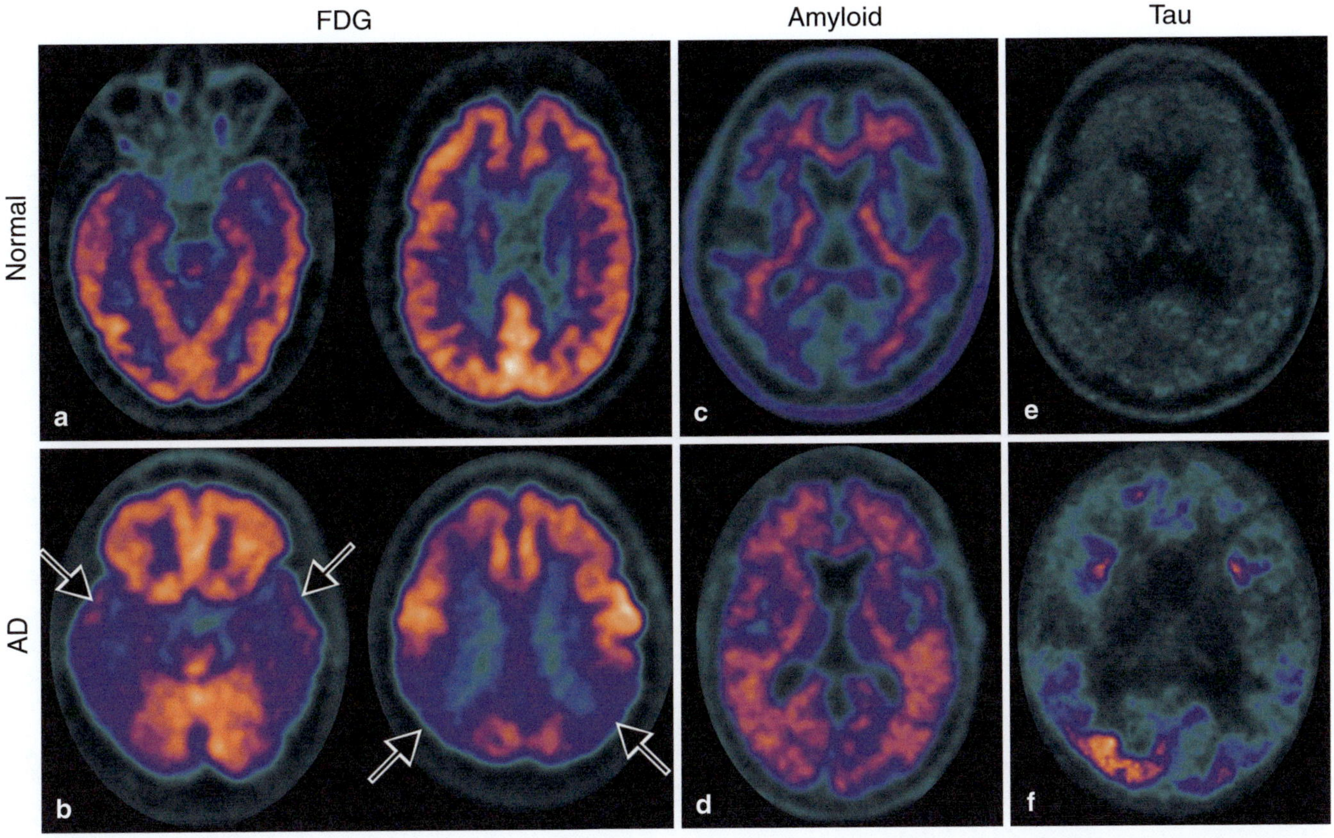

Fig. 17.3 PET imaging in Alzheimer dementia (AD). (**a**) FDG-PET exam showing symmetric glucose metabolism in a 59-year-old male without AD. (**b**) FDG-PET exam highlighting temporal and most-importantly parietal lobe hypometabolism in an 80-year-old male with AD (arrows). (**c**) Amyvid-PET exam showing sharp demarcation between gray and white matter, with no uptake in the cortex, in a 70-year-old male without AD. (**d**) Amyvid-PET exam highlighting diffuse tracer uptake in gray and white matter (with loss of the sharp gray–white demarcation) in a 58-year-old amyloid-positive male with AD. (**e**) F18-GTP1 tau-PET exam without uptake in the brain in a 79-year-old female without AD. (**f**) F18-MK-6240 tau-PET exam with multifocal radiotracer uptake in the cortex in a 78-year-old male with AD

lism, amyloid tracers localizing to abnormal Aβ plaque accumulation, and tau tracers localizing to neurofibrillary tangles (Fig. 17.3).
- Imaging with amyloid/tau tracers (FDA-approved forms exist for both) can show abnormalities that precede (in the case of amyloid) and correlate with (in the case of tau) clinical manifestations of the disease.
- Aducanumab is an FDA-approved anti-amyloid passive immunotherapy; such Aβ-immunotherapy can result in so-called amyloid-related imaging abnormalities related to edema (ARIA-E) and microhemorrhages (ARIA-H), which are thought to reflect the breakdown of the blood–brain barrier associated with amyloid clearance [8] (Fig. e17.1).

(All electronic images (Figs. e17.1–e17.4) can be found on this chapter's website on SpringerLink: https://doi.org/10.1007/978-3-031-55124-6_17)

OTHER CORTICAL DEMENTIAS

- This section reviews other less common cortical-predominant disorders that result in dementia, namely, dementia with Lewy bodies (DLB), several subtypes of FTLD, and posterior cerebral atrophy (PCA).
- DLB classically presents with dementia, visual hallucinations, and parkinsonism (see the Parkinson Plus section), but variable presentation complicates the distinction from AD.
- DLB imaging findings are nonspecific with temporal and parietal atrophy and hypometabolism, though DLB can in theory be distinguished from AD if the occipital cortex is involved (Fig. e17.2) and if the DaTscan is positive (see the PD section).
- FTD (frontotemporal dementia) and the pathological counterpart FTLD (frontotemporal lobar degeneration)

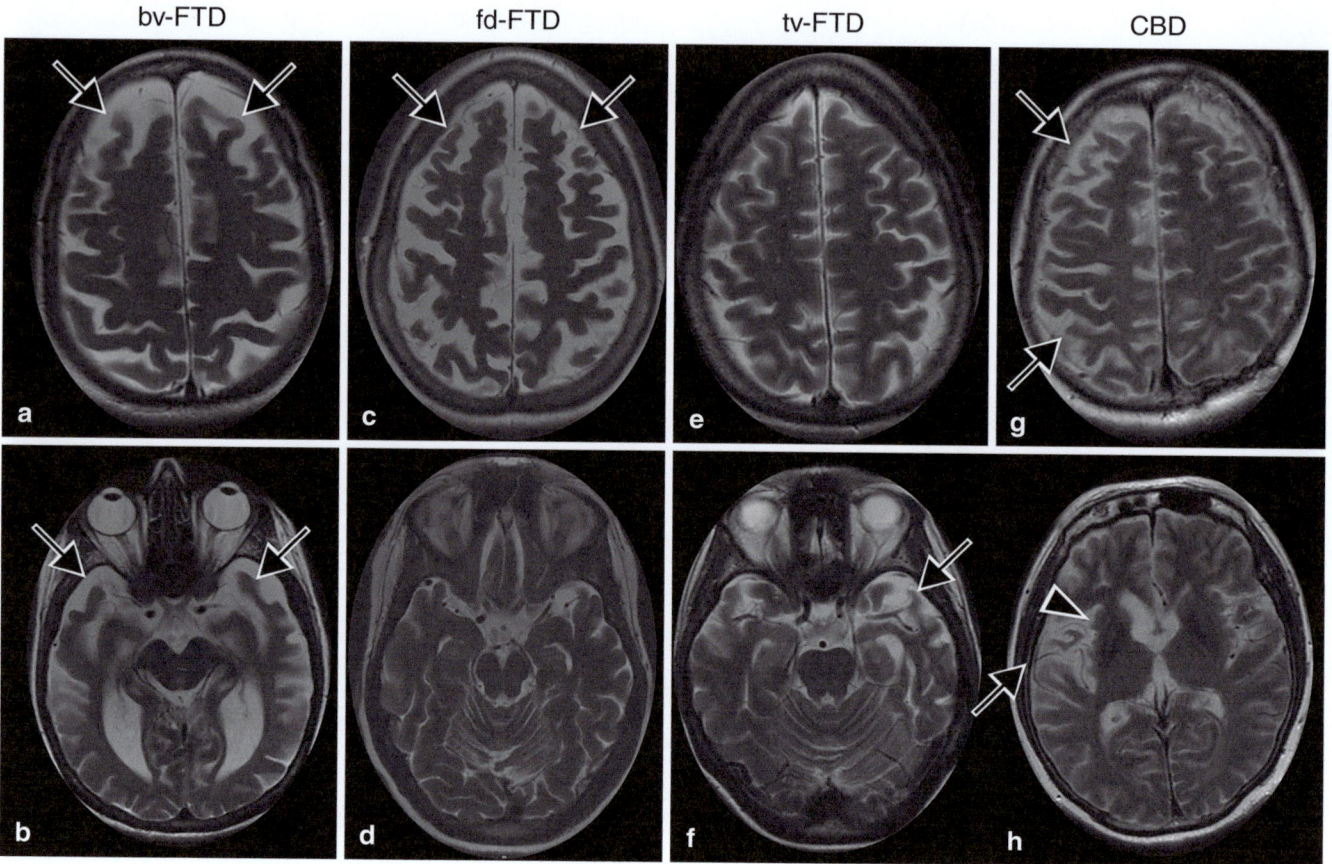

Fig. 17.4 Morphological changes in FTD on axial T2-weighted images. (**a, b**) A 64-year-old female with bv-FTD (behavioral variant—FTD, synonymous with Pick's disease) with atrophy in the bilateral frontal and temporal lobes (arrows). (**c, d**) A 50-year-old female with atrophy in the bilateral frontal lobes (arrows) and sparing of the temporal lobes, suspicious for an fd-FTD (frontal dominant—FTD), though unconfirmed. (**e, f**) A 58-year-old-female with tv-FTD (temporal variant—FTD) with asymmetric atrophy in the left temporal lobe (arrow) and sparing of the frontal lobes. (**g, h**) A 67-year-old female with CBD (corticobasilar degeneration) with asymmetric atrophy of the frontal lobe, temporal lobe, and motor strip (arrows) as well as the basal ganglia (arrowhead)

are a group of proteinopathies causing dementia, with subtypes identified by the most prominent symptoms.
- FTD imaging findings are predominant frontal and/or temporal atrophy [9] (Fig. 17.4) and hypometabolism on FDG-PET imaging [10] (Fig. e17.3).
    - Behavioral variant FTD (bvFTD, Pick's disease, or simply FTD) is the most common FTD and presents clinically with behavioral symptoms; imaging shows frontal and temporal atrophy and hypometabolism.
    - Frontal dominant FTD (fd-FTD) shows frontal hypometabolism and atrophy with sparing of the temporal lobes and can be seen in cases of progressive supranuclear palsy (PSP) (see the Parkinson Plus section).
    - Primary progressive aphasia (PPA, PPA-FTD, or temporal variant FTD) has three variants depending on the aspect of language affected (semantic, logopenic, or nonfluent/agrammatic); imaging shows temporal atrophy and hypometabolism.
        - Note that logopenic PPA is considered a subtype of AD.
    - Corticobasal degeneration (CBD) is classically described with "alien limb" and parkinsonism with asymmetric motor strip and basal ganglia atrophy [11].
    - Amyotrophic lateral sclerosis (ALS-FTD) was classically described as a pure motor disorder, but recent pathologic and genetic overlaps of ALS and FTD, as well as approximately 50% of ALS patients showing cognitive decline, indicate that these may be on a continuum of the same disease [12, 13] (see the ALS section).
- PCA is an uncommon subtype of AD that spares the temporal lobe, centers on the parietal and occipital lobes, and can mimic the occipital lobe predominant hypometabolism seen in DLB, though without DaTscan findings [7] (Fig. e17.2).

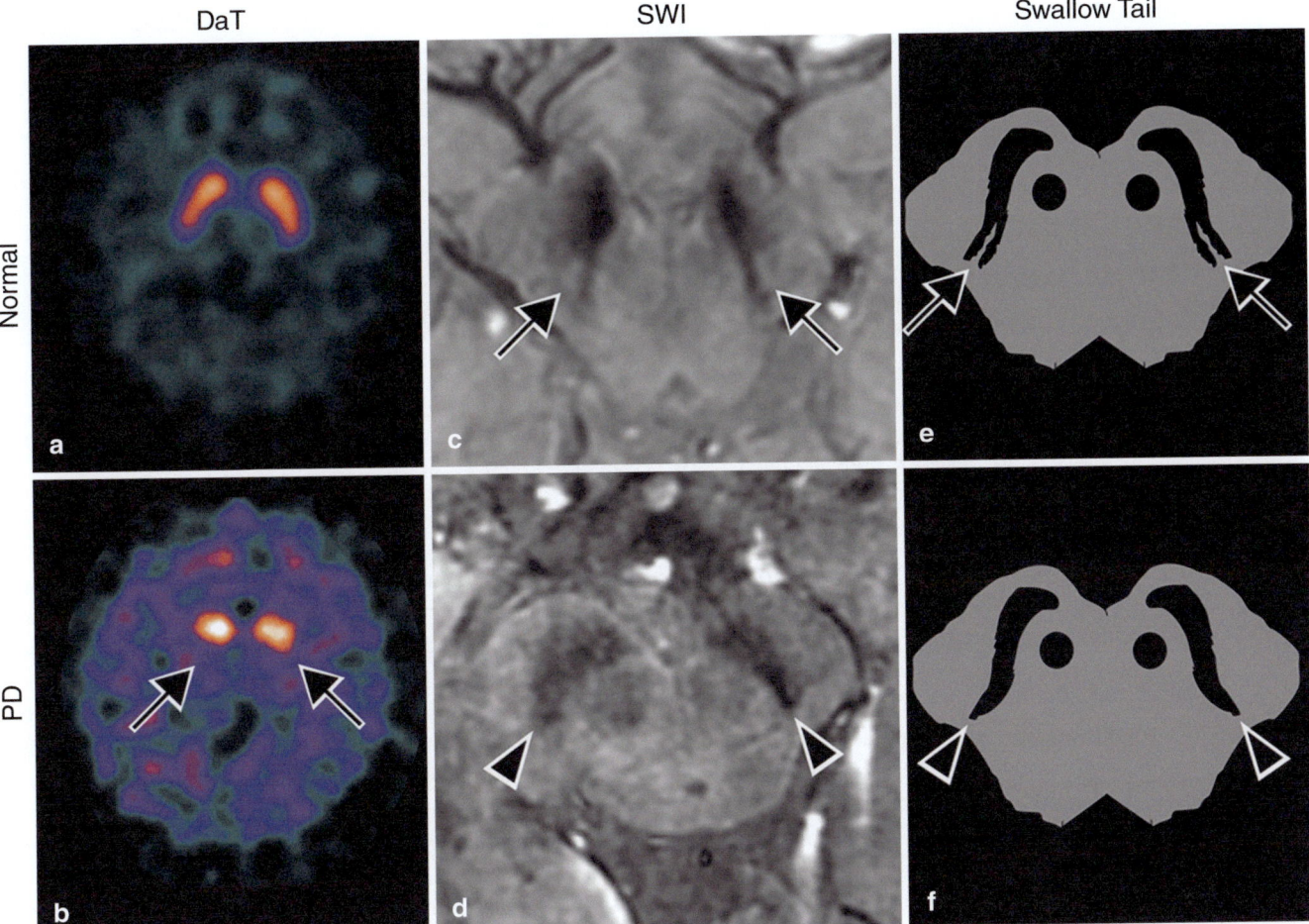

Fig. 17.5 PD imaging findings. I-123 DaTscan SPECT images show (**a**) normal tracer uptake in the bilateral caudate and putamen of a 73-year-old female without PD and (**b**) abnormal loss of tracer uptake in the bilateral putamen (arrows) in a 79-year-old male with PD. (**c**) Axial SWI image of the midbrain in a 41-year-old female shows a normally hyperintense nigrosome between two hypointense iron-rich portions of the posterolateral substania nigra—the *"swallow tail"* sign (arrows). (**d**) Axial SWI image in a 52-year-old female with PD that shows the loss of the *swallow tail* sign (arrowheads). Illustration depicting the *swallow tail* (arrows; **e**) and its loss (arrowheads; **f**)

PARKINSON DISEASE (PD)

- PD is the second most common neurodegenerative disorder after AD, with progressive motor symptoms of tremor, bradykinesia, and rigidity, and variable cognitive symptoms including dementia (PDD—Parkinson disease dementia).
- The etiology is α-synuclein aggregate-related neuronal loss in the substantia nigra [14].
- Imaging helps distinguish PD from drug-related parkinsonism with findings of decreased tracer uptake in the putamen on DaTscan, and a classic loss of the *"swallow tail"* in the midbrain on susceptibility-weighted imaging (SWI) (Fig. 17.5); note that identification of the swallow tail sign requires thin section 3T susceptibility imaging and is absent in other parkinsonian syndromes as well and thus is not specific for PD.

PARKINSON-Plus SYNDROMES

- A group of disorders with additional clinical and imaging findings beyond that of PD.
- In DLB (Dementia with Lewy bodies), cognitive symptoms develop before parkinsonism (note this pattern is reversed in PDD (Parkinson Disease Dementia)) [15].
- DLB is an α-synucleinopathy with cortical atrophy and hypometabolism (similar to the PCA subtype of AD) (see the section on Other Cortical Dementias).
- PSP (progressive supranuclear palsy or PSP-FTD) is a tauopathy that presents with cognitive changes including dementia, parkinsonism, and vertical gaze palsy.
- PSP imaging findings include frontal predominant atrophy and hypometabolism (see the section on Other Cortical Dementias) as well as midbrain atrophy and flat-

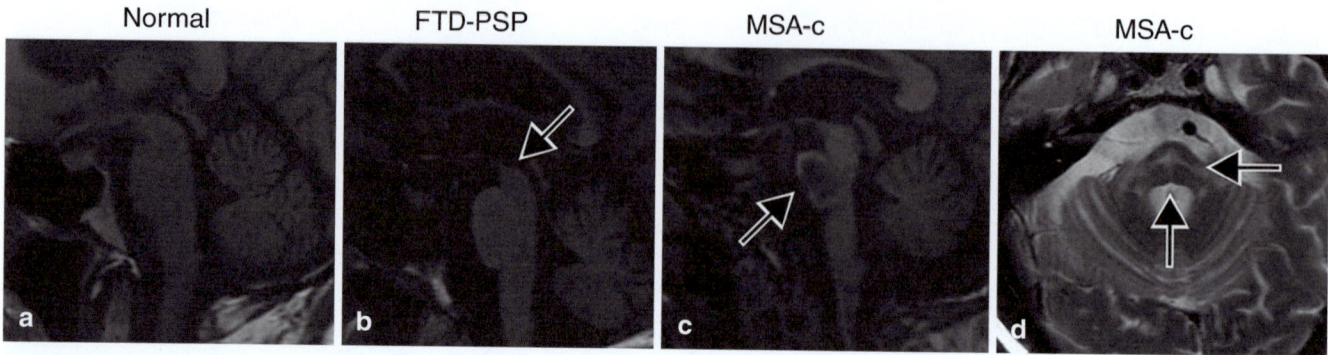

Fig. 17.6 Morphological findings of PSP and MSA. Sagittal T1-weighted images centered on the brainstem in (**a**) a 74-year-old female without PSP and (**b**) an 86-year-old male with PSP showing midbrain atrophy resulting in the *"hummingbird"* sign (arrow). (**c**) Sagittal T1-weighted image of a 66-year-old female with MSA-c showing pontine atrophy (arrow) and (**d**) axial T2-weighted image showing atrophy of selective pontine fibers—the *"hot cross bun"* sign (arrows)

tening resulting in the classic *"hummingbird"* sign (Fig. 17.6).
- MSA (multiple systems atrophy) is an α-synucleinopathy resulting in autonomic failure and variable parkinsonism or cerebellar ataxia, designating the two subtypes [16].
  - MSA-p (parkinsonism) shows putamen atrophy and iron deposition, with characteristic FLAIR signal abnormality along the outer putamen margin.
  - MSA-c (cerebellar, olivopontocerebellar degeneration) shows selective atrophy of the transverse cerebellopontine fibers and pontine raphe resulting in the *"hot cross bun"* sign [17].
  - Neither of these findings are sensitive or specific for MSA [18].
- CBD (corticobasal degeneration) (see the section on Other Cortical Dementias).

NEURODEGENERATIVE DISORDERS OF THE BASAL GANGLIA (BG)

- Multiple neurodegenerative disorders involve a classic pattern of deep brain nuclei involvement within the basal ganglia, though imaging findings may overlap between them and with non-neurodegenerative disorders involving the BG [19] and must be viewed in the appropriate clinical context.
- Nonspecific mild mineralization of the globus pallidus occurs with increasing age, starting in the 20 s [20].
- Fahr disease/syndrome presents clinically with nonspecific motor and cognitive symptoms secondary to marked bilateral calcification of the BG, thalami, and subcortical white matter [19] (Fig. 17.7).
- NBIA (neurodegeneration with brain iron accumulation) is a heterogeneous group of neurodegenerative disorders that present clinically with extra-pyramidal symptoms and dystonia and with imaging showing elevated iron accumulation in the globus pallidus and other deep brain nuclei [21].
  - PKAN (pantothenate kinase-associated neurodegeneration; previously known as Hallervorden-Spatz) is the most common NBIA subtype and has the classic imaging finding of *"eye of the tiger"* in which there is a central area of T2 hyperintensity surrounded by T2 hypointensity in the globus pallidus.
- Wilson disease (hepatolenticular degeneration) is a multisystem disease owing to copper deposition with extrapyramidal symptoms from basal ganglia involvement, which can present as T2 hyperintensity in the putamen during the acute phase of disease (Fig. e17.4) [19].
- HD (Huntington disease; Huntington chorea) presents clinically with chorea and neuropsychiatric symptoms secondary to neuronal loss in the subthalamic nucleus.
- The classic imaging finding of HD is caudate head atrophy with atrophy of other deep brain nuclei reported by voxel-based morphometry [22, 23].

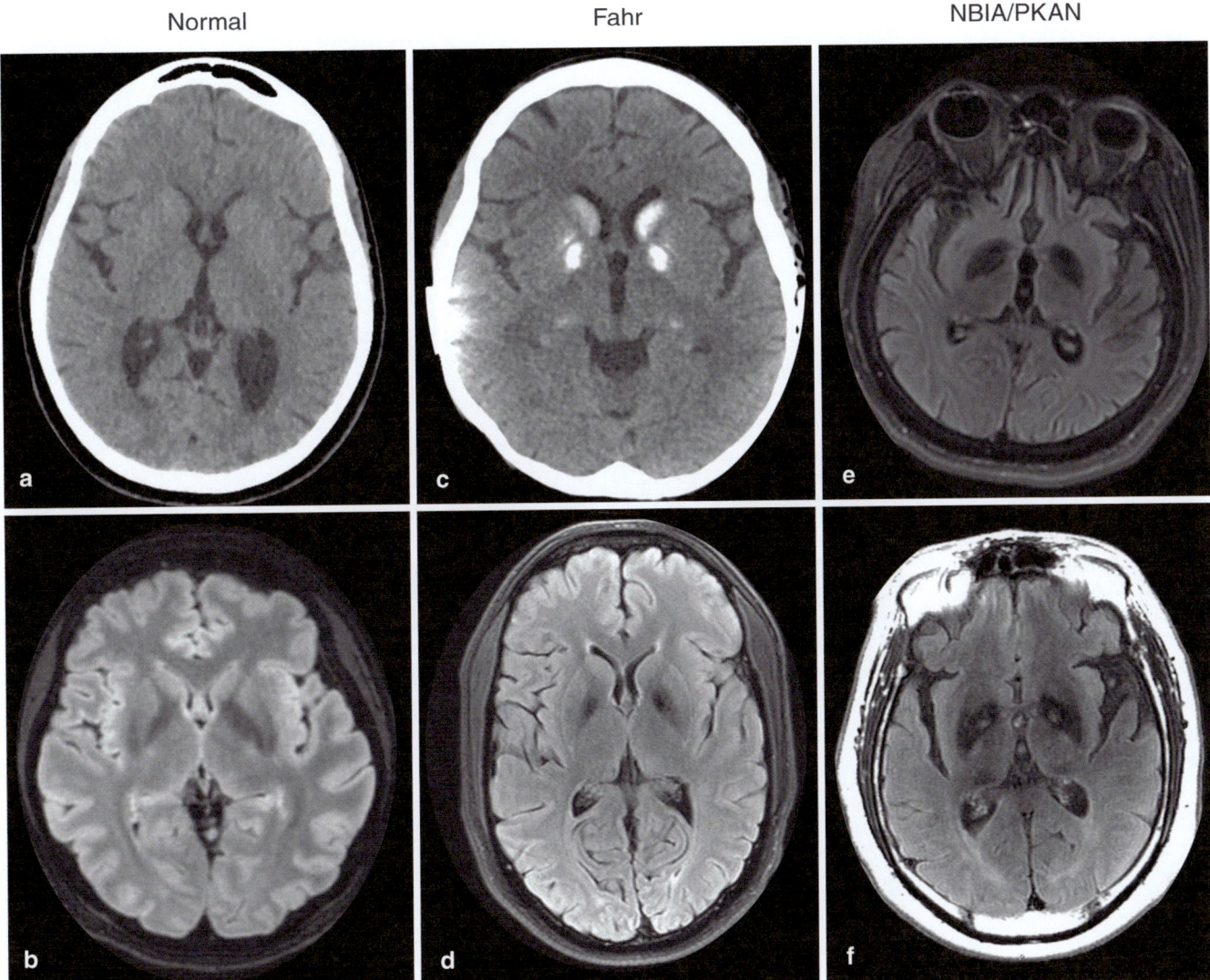

Fig. 17.7 Imaging of neurodegenerative disorders of the basal ganglia. (**a**) Axial CT in a 45-year-old female and (**b**) T2-FLAIR-weighted MR in a 39-year-old female without abnormal imaging findings. (**c**) Axial CT in a 44-year-old female with Fahr disease shows bilateral globus pallidus and caudate calcification. (**d**) Axial T2-FLAIR-weighted MR of a 51-year-old male with Fahr disease shows symmetric globus pallidus hypointensity. (**e**) Axial T2-FLAIR-weighted images of a 26-year-old female with NBIA (neurodegeneration with brain iron accumulation) showing symmetric globus pallidus hypointensity, and (**f**) a 64-year-old male with the PKAN (pantothenate kinase-associated neurodegeneration) subtype of NBIA showing characteristic central T2-hyperintensity surrounded by hypointensity—the *"eye of the tiger"* sign

AMYOTROPHIC LATERAL SCLEROSIS (ALS; LOU GEHRIG DISEASE)

- The third most common neurodegenerative disorder, causing progressive motor neuron degeneration that leads to weakness and eventual respiratory failure.
- ALS and an FTD subtype are considered a spectrum of diseases given the common TDP-43-aggregate associated neurodegeneration and a common genetic mutation in familial cases [13].
- Conventional imaging is primarily used to exclude other diseases, though imaging can occasionally show T2-hyperintensity along the corticospinal tracts or increased susceptibility along the motor cortex [24] (Fig. 17.8).

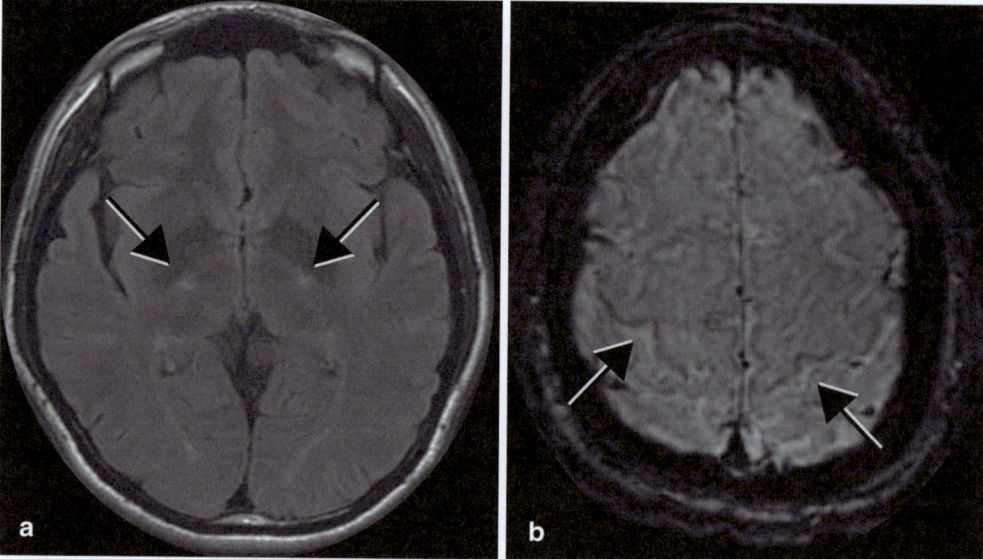

Fig. 17.8 Imaging findings in ALS. (**a**) Axial T2-FLAIR-weighted image of a 44-year-old male with ALS shows T2-FLAIR hyperintensity along the corticospinal tracts in the posterior limb of the internal capsule (arrows). (**b**) Axial SWI image of a 64-year-old male patient with ALS shows increased susceptibility artifact in the primary motor cortex bilaterally (arrows)

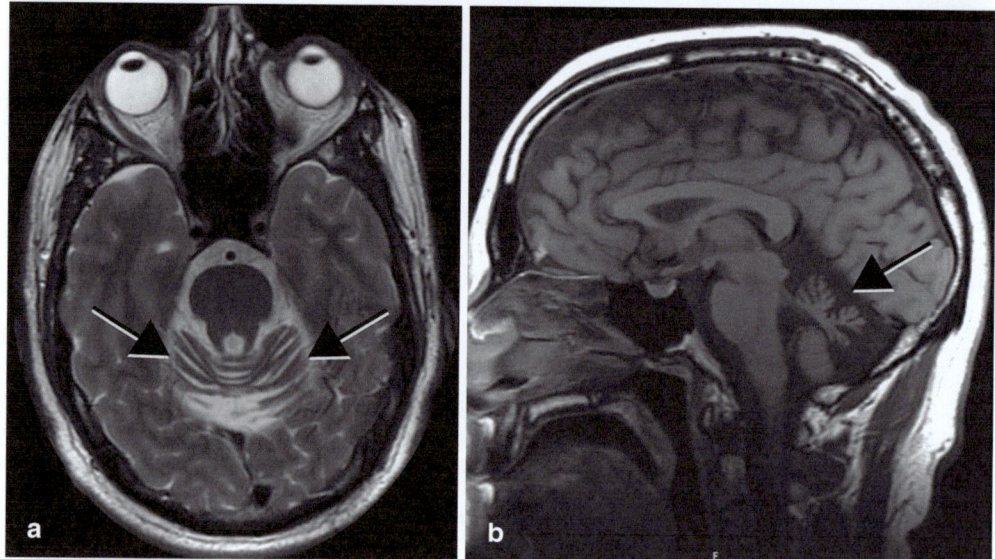

Fig. 17.9 Cerebellar atrophy. (**a**) Axial T2-weighted and (**b**) sagittal T1-weighted images in a 44-year-old male with cerebellar ataxia show marked cerebellar atrophy (arrows) with relatively preserved cerebral parenchymal volume

CEREBELLAR DEGENERATION

- Numerous neurodegenerative disorders present clinically with cerebellar ataxia.
- These have a variable age of onset and severity but frequently present with cerebellar predominant atrophy (Fig. 17.9).
- Freidrich's ataxia is the most common progressive ataxia of childhood but does not have imaging findings on conventional imaging [25].
- The spinocerebellar ataxias are a diverse set of autosomal dominant disorders with imaging ranging from exclusive cerebellar atrophy to no visible cerebellar atrophy [26].
- MSA-c (see the section on Parkinson Plus) classically presents with cerebellar and pontine atrophy.
- Fragile-X syndrome presents clinically with cerebellar ataxia with imaging showing T2 hyperintensity in the middle cerebellar peduncles and generalized atrophy.
- Of note, ataxia and cerebellar atrophy can also result from chronic alcohol use.

INBORN ERRORS OF METABOLISM

- Heterogeneous group of individually rare genetic disorders related to the toxic accumulation or deficiency of specific metabolic products.
- Early-onset disorders present with acute encephalopathy and life-threatening episodes, while late-onset disorders have more management options [27].

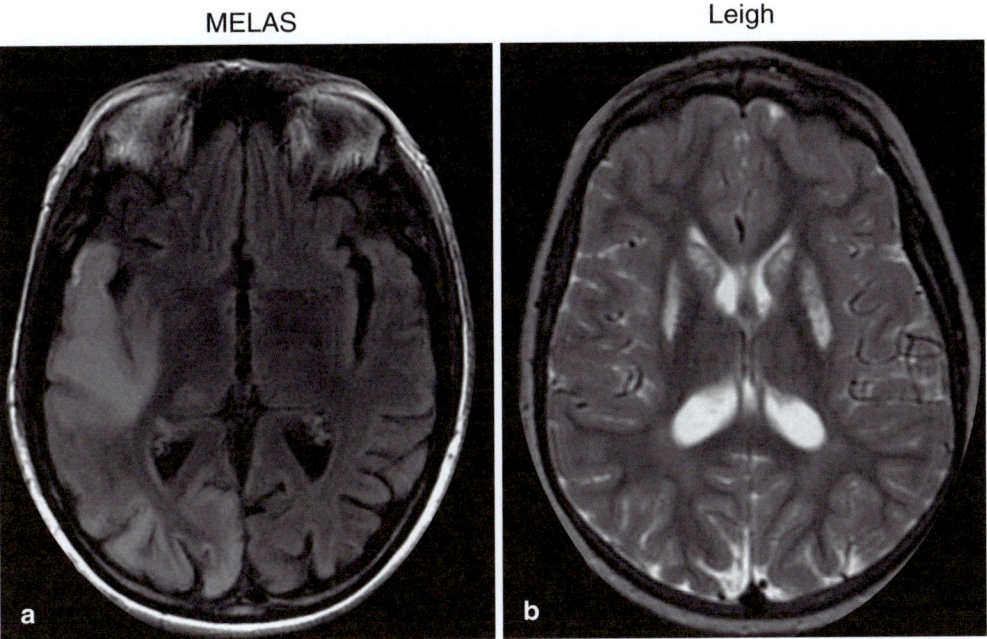

Fig. 17.10 Imaging of MELAS and Leigh syndromes. (**a**) Axial T2-FLAIR-weighted image in a 44-year-old female with MELAS experiencing a stroke-like episode with edema in the temporal lobe and occipital cortex, crossing vascular boundaries. (**b**) Axial T2-weighted image of a 5-year-old female with Leigh syndrome, showing marked hyperintensity in the bilateral caudate and putamen

- These are covered in Chap. 16—Toxic and Metabolic Disorders—including the lysosomal storage diseases such as Tay Sachs, and mucopolysaccharidoses such as Hurler.
- Below is a description of two mitochondrial disorders, MELAS and Leigh syndrome.
- MELAS (mitochondrial encephalopathy with lactic acidosis and stroke-like episodes) is a mitochondrial disorder inherited along the maternal line and presents with imaging findings matching those of stroke, though not in a vascular distribution (Fig. 17.10).
- Leigh syndrome (SNE—subacute necrotizing encephalomyelopathy) is another mitochondrial disorder with varied clinical and imaging presentation related to chronic energy deprivation, with imaging abnormalities typically seen in the putamen and brainstem [28].

References

1. McAleese KE, Colloby SJ, Thomas AJ, Al-Sarraj S, Ansorge O, Neal J, Roncaroli F, Love S, Francis PT, Attems J. Concomitant neurodegenerative pathologies contribute to the transition from mild cognitive impairment to dementia. Alzheimers Dement. 2021;17:1121–33.
2. Robinson JL, Lee EB, Xie SX, et al. Neurodegenerative disease concomitant proteinopathies are prevalent, age-related and APOE4-associated. Brain. 2018;141:2181–93.
3. Peters R. Ageing and the brain. Postgrad Med J. 2006;82:84–8.
4. Jack CR. Alzheimer disease: new concepts on its neurobiology and the clinical role imaging will play. Radiology. 2012;263:344–61.
5. Jevtic S, Sengar AS, Salter MW, McLaurin JA. The role of the immune system in Alzheimer disease: etiology and treatment. Ageing Res Rev. 2017;40:84–94.
6. Ashraf GM, Tarasov VV, Makhmutova A, Chubarev VN, Avila-Rodriguez M, Bachurin SO, Aliev G. The possibility of an infectious etiology of Alzheimer disease. Mol Neurobiol. 2019;56:4479–91.
7. Whitwell JL, Graff-Radford J, Tosakulwong N, et al. Imaging correlations of tau, amyloid, metabolism, and atrophy in typical and atypical Alzheimer's disease. Alzheimers Dement. 2018;14:1005–14.
8. Sperling RA, Jack CR, Black SE, et al. Amyloid-related imaging abnormalities in amyloid-modifying therapeutic trials: recommendations from the Alzheimer's association research roundtable workgroup. Alzheimers Dement. 2011;7:367–85.
9. Kitagaki H, Mori E, Yamaji S, Ishii K, Hirono N, Kobashi S, Hata Y. Frontotemporal dementia and Alzheimer disease: evaluation of cortical atrophy with automated hemispheric surface display generated with MR images. Radiology. 1998;208:431–9.
10. Brown RKJ, Bohnen NI, Wong KK, Minoshima S, Frey KA. Brain PET in suspected dementia: patterns of altered FDG metabolism. Radiographics. 2014;34:684–701.
11. Hassan A, Whitwell JL, Boeve BF, Jack CR, Parisi JE, Dickson DW, Josephs KA. Symmetric corticobasal degeneration (S-CBD). Park Relat Disord. 2010;16:208–14.
12. Lomen-Hoerth C, Murphy J, Langmore S, Kramer JH, Olney RK, Miller B. Are amyotrophic lateral sclerosis patients cognitively normal? Neurology. 2003;60:1094–7.
13. Renton AE, Majounie E, Waite A, et al. A hexanucleotide repeat expansion in C9ORF72 is the cause of chromosome 9p21-linked ALS-FTD. Neuron. 2011;72:257–68.
14. Dickson DW. Parkinson's disease and parkinsonism in. Cold Spring Med Harb Perspect. 2012;2:1–15.
15. Marshall K, Hale D. Lewy body dementia. Home Healthc Now. 2021;39:107–8.
16. Watanabe H, Riku Y, Hara K, Kawabata K, Nakamura T, Ito M, Hirayama M, Yoshida M, Katsuno M, Sobue G. Clinical and imaging features of multiple system atrophy: challenges for an early and clinically definitive diagnosis. J Mov Disord. 2018;11:107–20.

17. Shrivastava A. The hot cross bun sign. Radiology. 2007;245:606–7.
18. Way C, Pettersson D, Hiller A. The 'hot cross bun' sign is not always multiple system atrophy: etiologies of 11 cases. J Mov Disord. 2019;12:27–30.
19. Hegde AN, Mohan S, Lath N, Lim CCT. Differential diagnosis for bilateral abnormalities of the basal ganglia and thalamus. Radiographics. 2011;31:5–30.
20. Aquino D, Bizzi A, Grisoli M, Garavaglia B, Bruzzone MG, Savoiardo M, Chiapparini L. Age-related iron deposition in the basal ganglia : quantitative methods: results: conclusion. Neuroradiology. 2009;252:165–72.
21. Kruer MC, Boddaert N, Schneider A, Houlden H, Bhatia KP, Gregory A, Anderson JC, Rooney WD, Hogarth P, Hayflick SJ. Neuroimaging features of neurodegeneration with brain iron accumulation. Am J Neuroradiol. 2012;33:407–14.
22. Mascalchi M, Lolli F, Della Nave R, Tessa C, Petralli R, Gavazzi C, Politi LS, Macucci M, Filippi M, Placentini S. Huntington disease: volumetric, diffusion-weighted, and magnetization transfer MR imaging of brain. Radiology. 2004;232:867–73.
23. Kassubek J, Juengling FD, Kioschies T, et al. Topography of cerebral atrophy in early Huntington's disease: a voxel based morphometric MRI study. J Neurol Neurosurg Psychiatry. 2004;75:213–20.
24. Wang S, Melhem ER, Poptani H, Woo JH. Neuroimaging in amyotrophic lateral sclerosis. Neurotherapeutics. 2011;8:63–71.
25. Mascalchi M. The cerebellum looks normal in Friedreich ataxia. Am J Neuroradiol. 2013;34:3480.
26. Meira AT, Arruda WO, Ono SE, de Carvalho Neto A, Raskin S, CHF C, HAG T. Neuroradiological findings in the spinocerebellar ataxias. Tremor Other Hyperkinet Mov. 2019;9:1–8.
27. Yoon HJ, Kim JH, Jeon T, Yoo SY, Eo H. Devastating metabolic brain disorders of newborns and young infants. Radiographics. 2014;34:1257–73.
28. Kartikasalwah AL, Ngu LH. Leigh syndrome: MRI findings in two children. Biomed Imaging Interv J. 2010;6:1–4.

Hydrocephalus and CSF Disorders

Afshin Ameri and Neel Madan

INTRODUCTION

- Cerebrospinal fluid (CSF) surrounds the brain and spinal cord and moves around with each heartbeat.
- Alterations in CSF production, movement, and absorption can affect neurologic health.
- With increased CSF fluid, hydrocephalus or increased water results.
- A number of surgical techniques can be used to intervene when hydrocephalus occurs.
- Alterations in CSF fluid volume or pressure can also result, with both increased pressure/volume (idiopathic intracranial hypertension) as well as decreased pressure/volume (CSF leak).

OVERVIEW OF THE CEREBROSPINAL FLUID (CSF)

- Choroid plexus: CSF is mainly produced by the epithelial cells of the choroid plexus located in the temporal horns and body of the lateral ventricles, foramen of Monro, roof of the third ventricle, and medullary part of the fourth ventricle extending into the lateral apertures.
- Brain interstitial fluid and ventricular ependyma can also contribute to CSF fluid via aquaporin channels.
- In the adult brain, there is approximately 150 mL of CSF fluid (the majority of which is in the subarachnoid space), with three to four times that volume produced and reabsorbed every day.
- CSF bulk flow: Lateral ventricles→Foramen of Monro→Third ventricle→Aqueduct of Sylvius→Fourth ventricles→Foramina of Luschka to the cerebellopontine angle cistern and foramen of Magendie to the cisterna magna.
- Pulsatile flow: CSF moves with each cardiac cycle, with intracranial blood volume expanding in systole, propelling CSF to move to the spine, and return during diastole (Monro-Kelly doctrine).
- CSF flow in the subarachnoid space is multidirectional.
- Most of CSF is absorbed by arachnoid villi found along the venous sinuses.
- However, the importance of alternative drainage mechanisms is increasingly being recognized, with fluid homeostatsis related to the glymphatic system; fluid drainage occurs via perivascular spaces and leptomeningeal arteries (with a role for aquaporin channels), with drainage through the cribriform plate into the head and neck [1].
- Basal cistern patency is crucial to CSF flow.

OVERVIEW OF CSF IMAGING TECHNIQUE

- The two components of CSF circulation are bulk flow (the mechanism by which CSF moves from choroid plexus to arachnoid granulation) and pulsatile flow (back and forth movement of CSF due to cardiac pulsation). Typical CSF flow sequences assess pulsatile flow, with bulk flow harder to assess by routine imaging techniques.
- A typical CSF flow sequence utilizes a phase-contrast technique and can be both qualitative and quantitative (Fig. 18.1).

A. Ameri · N. Madan (✉)
Tufts University School of Medicine, Boston, MA, USA
e-mail: aameri@tuftsmedicine.org

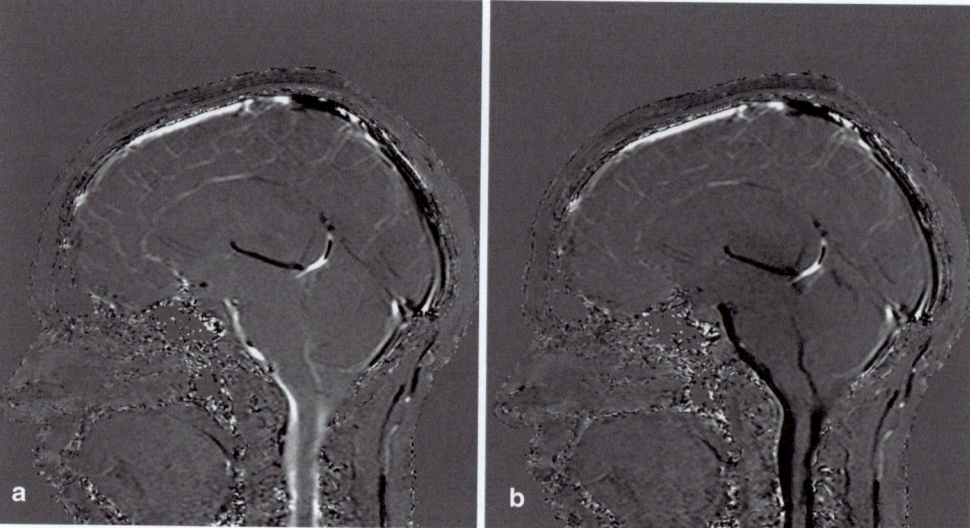

Fig. 18.1 Normal CSF flow phase contrast imaging. CSF flow phase images demonstrate (**a**) caudal flow during systole, which is white, and (**b**) cranial flow during diastole, which is black. The foramen of Monro, cerebral aqueduct, and basilar cisterns demonstrate brisk asynchronous biphasic flow

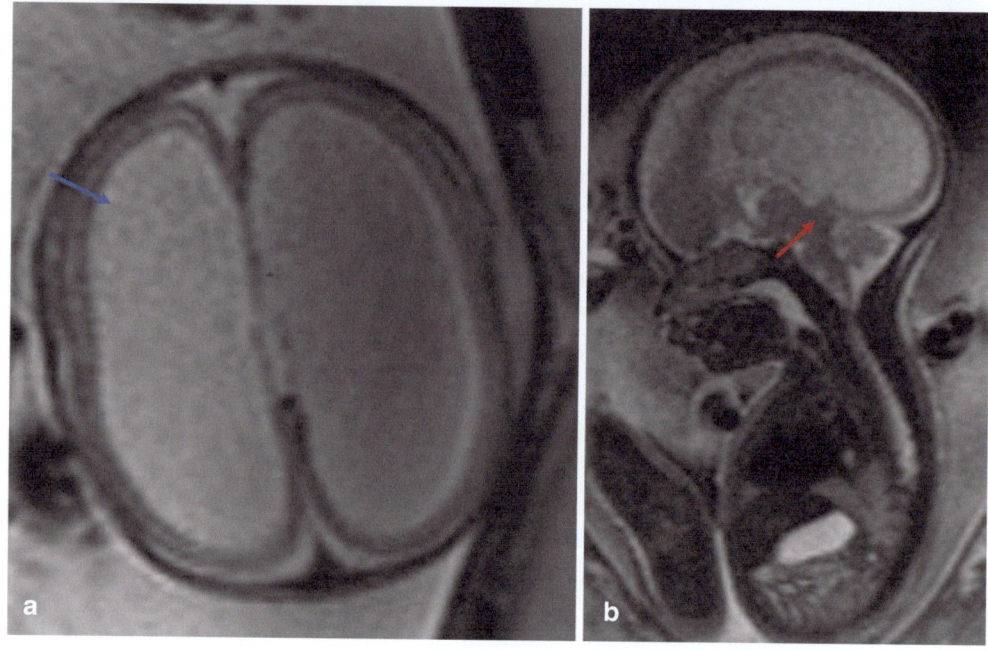

Fig. 18.2 Congenital aqueductal stenosis. Single-shot T2 axial (**a**) and sagittal (**b**) fetal MRI in a 27-week gestational fetus demonstrates marked dilatation of the lateral ventricles (blue arrow) with the absence of the cerebral aqueduct (red arrow), consistent with congenital aqueductal stenosis

- CSF flow can also result in a number of artifacts in the brain and spine, with signal nulling due to the movement on routine anatomic images.

HYDROCEPHALUS

- Alterations in the amount or movement of CSF fluid can result in accumulation of CSF fluid, resulting in increased intracranial pressure.
- Commonly subdivided by the point of obstruction.

Intraventricular (Obstructive) Hydrocephalus

- Hydrocephalus caused by obstruction in the ventricular system [2, 3].
- Multiple etiologies can lead to this entity including congenital and acquired disorders.
  - Congenital etiologies include arachnoid webs at the level of the cerebral aqueduct (Fig. 18.2) as well as a range of malformations, including those affecting the posterior fossa such as Dandy-Walker malformation, Chiari 2 malformations, and so on.
  - Acquired disorders most commonly include hemorrhage or mass such as a neoplasm (Fig. 18.3) or cyst also resulting in obstruction.
- Can be acute or chronic.

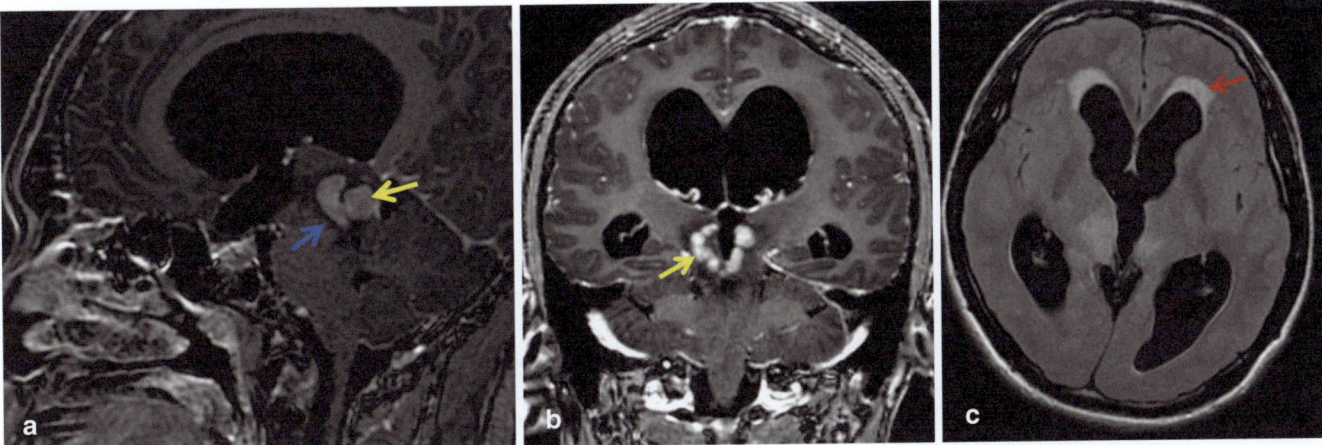

Fig. 18.3 Obstructive pineal germinoma. A 20-year-old presented with progressive blurry vision with sagittal (**a**) and coronal (**b**) T1 post-contrast MRI images showing a lobulated, enhancing mass (yellow arrows) centered in the region of the pineal gland/tectum and extending into the thalamus, with compression of the cerebral aqueduct (blue arrow). Axial FLAIR image (**c**) demonstrates an enlargement of the lateral and third ventricles, with periventricular FLAIR hyperintensity reflecting transependymal edema (red arrow)

- Obstruction results in the accumulation of CSF in the ventricles, with subsequent ventricular expansion, and increased pressure, which can reduce cerebral perfusion.
- Imaging features include ventriculomegaly above the level of obstruction with indistinct margins of the ventricles most pronounced around the horns of the lateral ventricles. The latter entity is not seen with chronic obstruction.

Extraventricular (Communicating) Hydrocephalus

- Previously referred to as communicating hydrocephalus [2].
- Obstruction is outside the ventricular system.
- Can occur from the foramina at the base of the brain to the level of absorption at the arachnoid granulations.
- Most commonly due to subarachnoid hemorrhage but can be due to a host of other etiologies, including infection (Fig. 18.4), inflammation, or leptomeningeal tumor.
- MRI can show signal changes in the subarachnoid space.
- A heavily weighted thin slice T2 sequences steady-state free precession sequence (also known as *Fast Imaging Employing Steady-state Acquisition*, FIESTA, constructive interference in steady state CISS, or balanced fast field echo, BFFE) is best able to show membranes or other reasons for obstruction.
- The cause may not be identified.

Overproduction Hydrocephalus

- Uncommon, with an increase in the ventricles due to overproduction of CSF fluid.
- Most commonly seen with choroid plexus papilloma (Fig. 18.5) (or carcinoma), an unusual neoplasm. Typically seen in young children.

Normal Pressure Hydrocephalus (NPH)

- Form of extra-ventricular hydrocephalus.
- Presents with the classic triad of dementia, urinary incontinence, and gate apraxia (though frequently not all of these symptoms will be present).
- Ventriculomegaly with normal CSF pressure, but diagnosis depends on clinical findings, imaging studies, and response to high-volume lumbar tap.
- Imaging findings that raise the possibility of NPH (Fig. 18.6):
  - The lateral and third ventricles are dilated while the fourth ventricle is normal, with ventriculomegaly disproportionate to sulci.
  - The callosal angle is acute.
  - Tight high convexity with effacement of parafalcine sulci.
- Treatment is placement of a VP shunt, although not all patients respond, and long-term outcome is variable.

CSF Shunts and Complications

- Placement of a shunt is most common treatment for obstructive hydrocephalus [2, 3].
- However, they can frequently fail, requiring shunt adjustment.

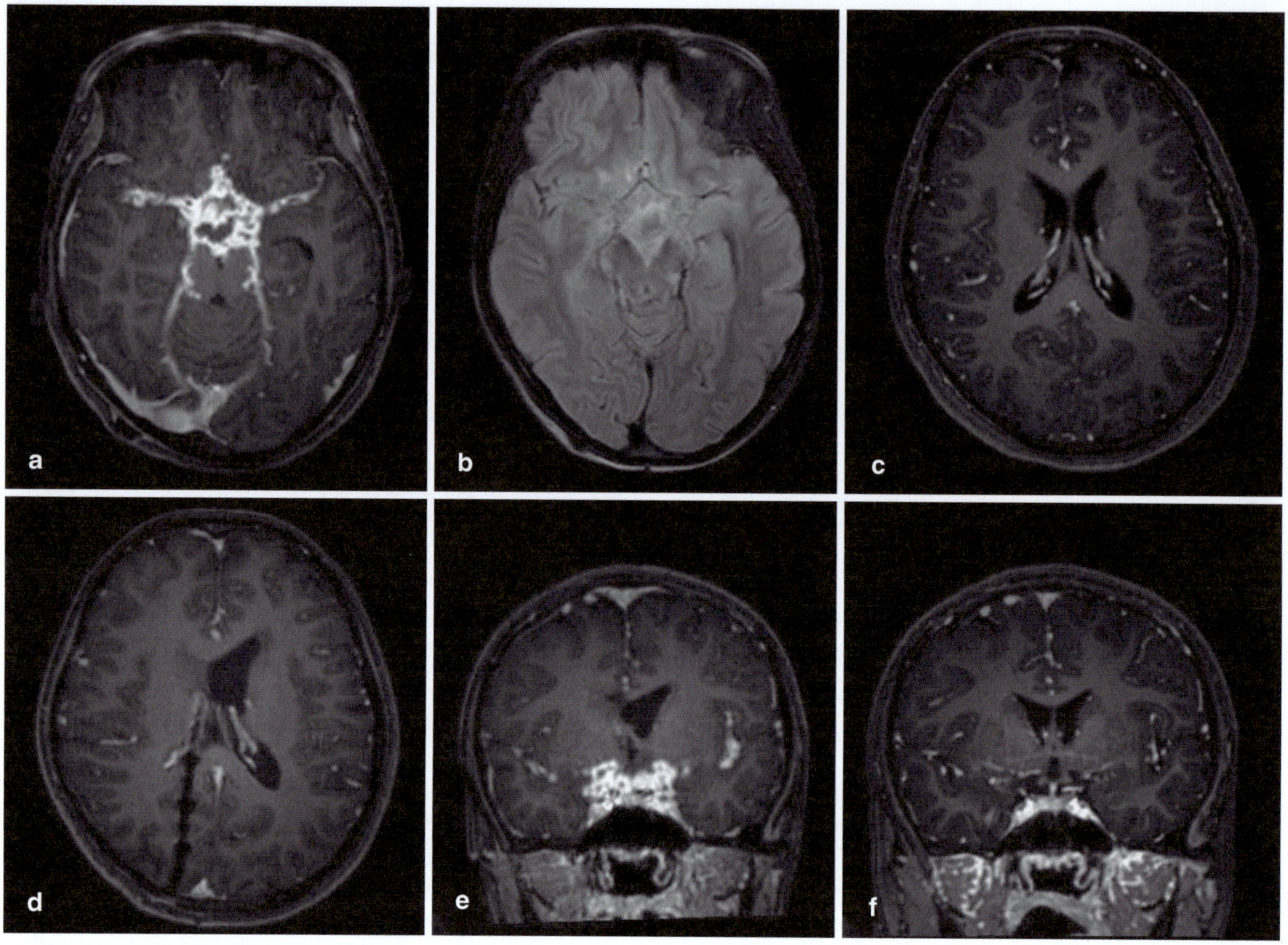

Fig. 18.4 Leptomeningeal tuberculosis. Axial T1 post-contrast image (**a**) demonstrates marked enhancement in the basal cisterns, with associated FLAIR hyperintensity (**b**). T1 post-contrast axial (**d**) and coronal (**e**) images demonstrate ventriculomegaly on the left s/p decompression with a ventriculostomy catheter on the right, from extraventricular hydrocephalus. Compare to T1 post-contrast axial (**c**) and coronal (**f**) from 4 months earlier where there is leptomeningeal enhancement with no evidence of hydrocephalus

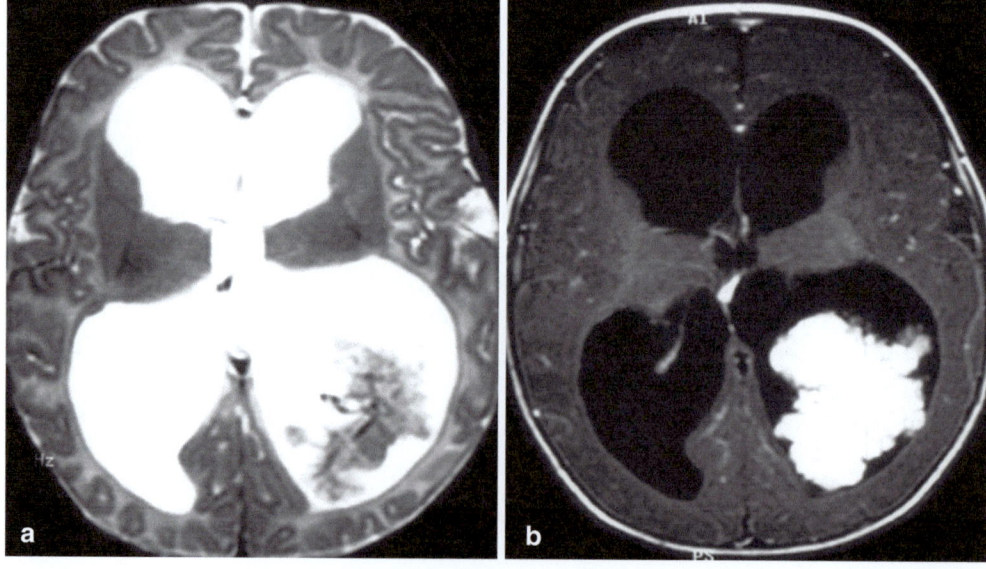

Fig. 18.5 Choroid plexus papilloma. Axial T2 (**a**) and axial T1 post-contrast (**b**) images demonstrate a large frond-like enhancing mass in the left lateral ventricle trigone, with marked enlargement of the lateral ventricles secondary to overproduction of CSF fluid

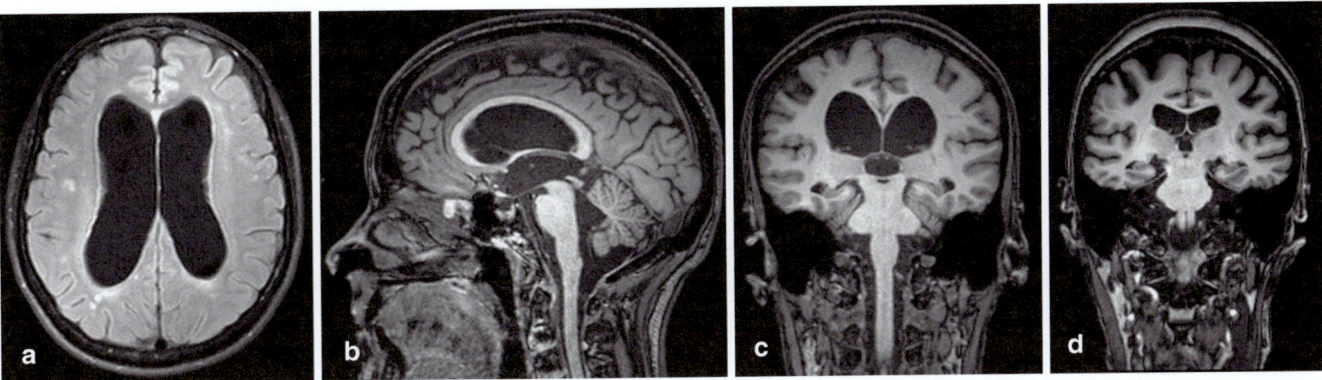

Fig. 18.6 Normal pressure hydrocephalus. Axial FLAIR (**a**) and sagittal T1 (**b**) images demonstrate enlargement of the lateral and third ventricles with relatively normal sulcal spaces and fourth ventricle. Coronal T1 image (**c**) demonstrates an acute callosal angle with effacement of the parafalcine sulci. Compare to coronal T1 (**d**) in a patient with diffuse cerebral volume loss

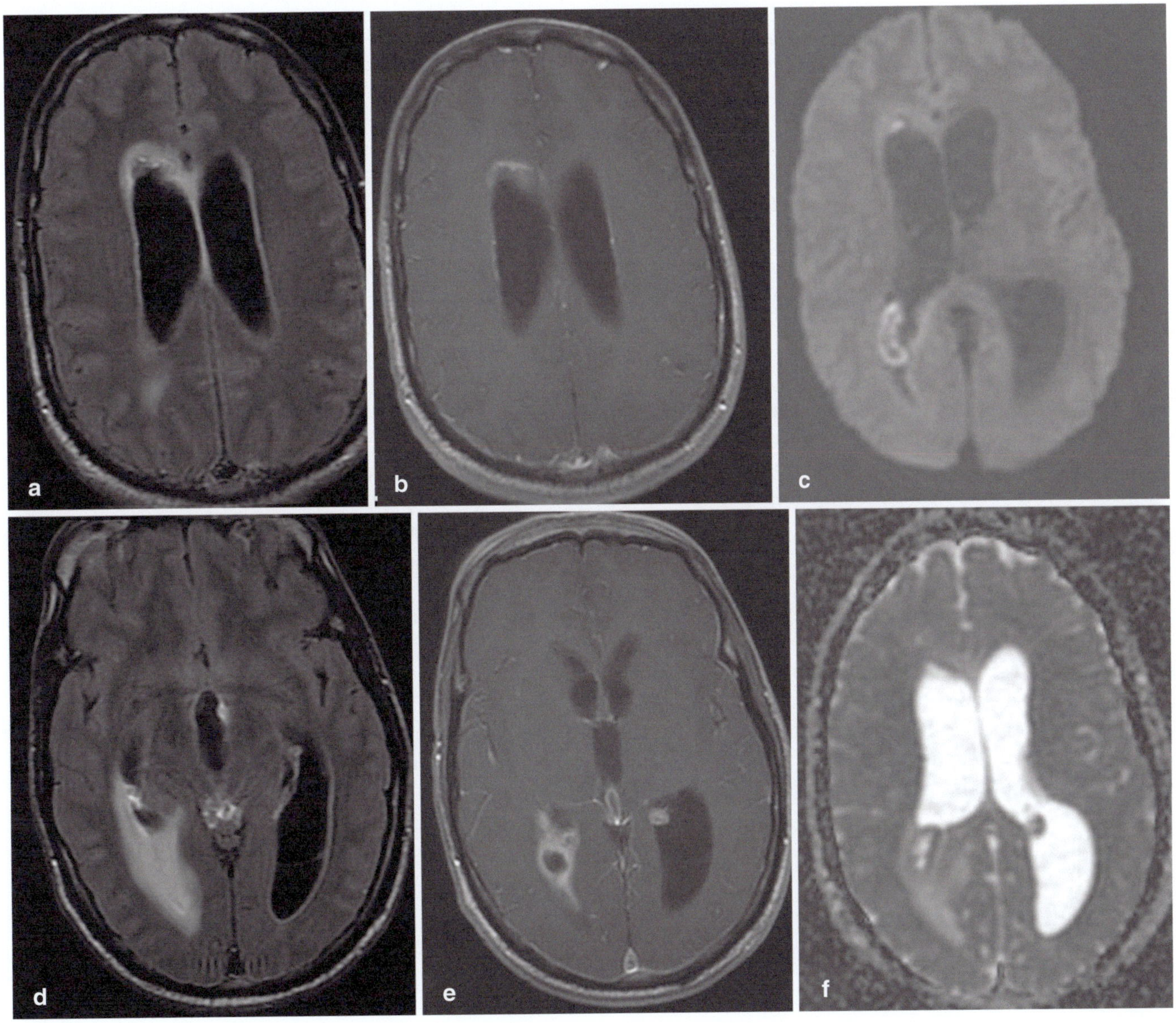

Fig. 18.7 Aspergillus ventriculitis secondary to infected shunt catheter. MRI demonstrates FLAIR hyperintensity (**a** and **d**) of the ependyma extending into the periventricular white matter with corresponding enhancement on post-contrast T1 images (**b** and **e**) as well as a combination of restricted and facilitated diffusion on diffusion trace image (**c**) and corresponding ADC map (**f**), reflecting an aspergillus ventriculitis secondary to an infected shunt catheter

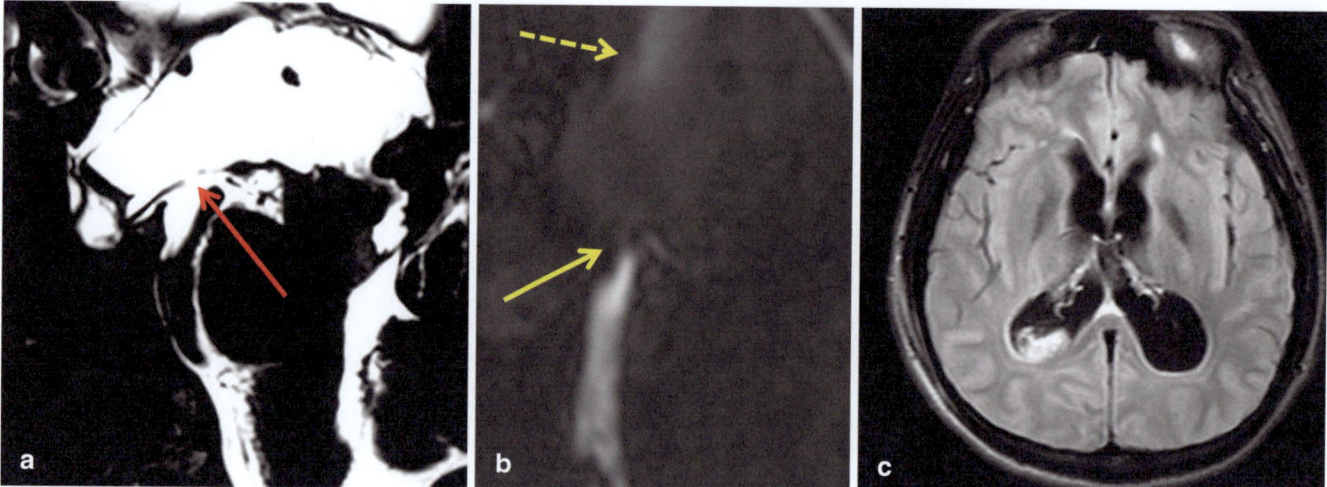

Fig. 18.8 Successful ETV. Patient with obstructive pineal germinoma from Fig. 18.3, status post-endoscopic third ventriculostomy. Sagittal steady-state free precession (SSFP, FIESTA/CISS/BFFE) MRI (**a**) shows a defect in the floor of the third ventricle (red arrow). Sagittal phase contrast image (**b**) shows CSF flow through the stoma (*solid arrow*) and foramen of Monro (*dotted arrow*). Axial FLAIR (**c**) demonstrates decreased transependymal edema (compared to Fig. 18.3c)

- Imaging is needed, in comparison with prior studies to assess for enlarging or shrinking the size of the ventricles.
- Shunts can fail for a number of reasons:
  o Mechanical failure due to shunt disruption.
  o Programmable valve failure.
  o Infection (Fig. 18.7).
  o Slit-like ventricle: Scarred ventricular walls result in coaptation of the ventricular walls, preventing expansion when pressure changes result; thus, the ventricles will remain small even if the shunt malfunctions.

Endoscopic Third Ventriculostomy (ETV)

- Increasingly used as a first attempt to regain communication between the third ventricle and the suprasellar cistern via a neurosurgical endoscopic approach through the floor of the third ventricle (Fig. 18.8).
- Potentially prevents the necessity for lifetime use of a shunt catheter.

ALTERATIONS IN CSF PRESSURE/VOLUME

- The complex nature of CSF fluid dynamics is increasingly being recognized.
- Opening pressure reflects only one measure of the overall system, and alterations in CSF volume likely play an important role in neurologic health.

Idiopathic Intracranial Hypotension (IIH)

- Elevated intracranial pressure (ICP) not secondary to an intracranial mass, cerebral venous thrombosis, or a leptomeningeal process [4].
- Formerly referred to as Pseudotumor cerebrii.
- Predilection for obese patients as well as females.
- Clinical symptoms include headache, tinnitus, and visual disturbances.
- Papilledema most common finding on examination.
- Diagnosis confirmed with elevated opening pressure, >25 cm CSF.
- Venous stenosis has been implicated, though unclear if this causes IIH due to venous outflow obstruction or is an effect of IIH with increased ICP resulting in venous compression.

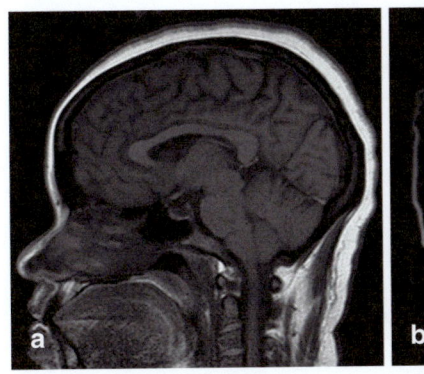 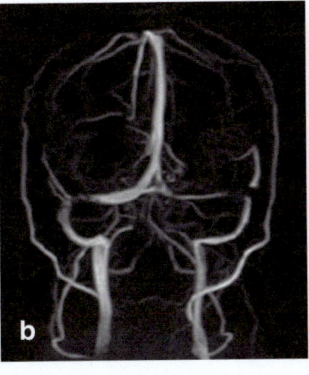 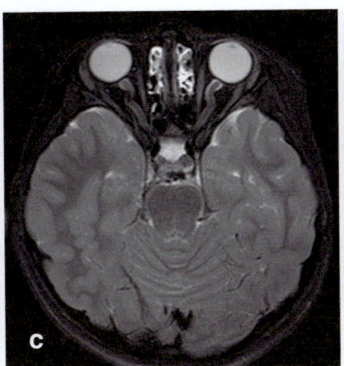 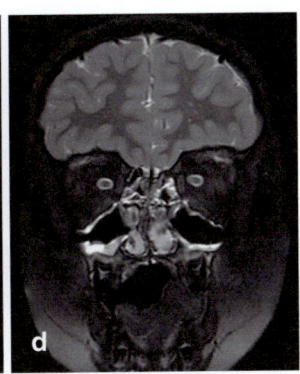

Fig. 18.9 Idiopathic intracranial hypertension. Sagittal T1 (**a**) demonstrates a partially empty Sella. 3D MPR from an MRV (**b**) demonstrates stenotic distal transverse sinuses bilaterally. Coronal T2 (**c**) and axial T2 images (**d**) show tortuosity and dilatation of the optic nerve sheath, in addition to posterior scleral flattening and papilledema

- Mechanism unclear; potentially related to alterations in the glymphatic pathway.
- Imaging (Fig. 18.9):
  - Most importantly used to exclude alternative diagnoses.
  - Imaging can be normal.
  - Imaging findings associated with IIH:
    - Flattening of the posterior globes.
    - Dilated optic nerve sheath with or without increased tortuosity.
    - Partially empty sella.
    - Bilateral transverse venous stenosis.
- Treatment includes weight loss, acetazolamide (Diamox), and serial CSF removal.

CSF Leaks/Spontaneous Intracranial Hypotension

- When there is a violation of the dura, CSF leaks outside the subarachnoid space.
- Can be congenital or acquired; acquired CSF leaks can be iatrogenic (e.g., lumbar puncture and surgery), post-traumatic (e.g., fracture and dural tear), or spontaneous.

Cranial Leaks

- Typically occur in the paranasal sinuses and result in rhinorrhea or in the temporal bones and result in otorrhea.
- Present with complaints of fluid discharge, and are at risk of intracranial infection.
- Imaging:
  - CT modality of choice for detecting a bone defect with fluid in the nasal cavity, paranasal sinuses, or mastoid air cells.
  - CT or nuclear medicine cisternography can also be helpful in localizing a CSF leak site.
  - MRI helpful when concerned for a cephalocele, to evaluate for herniation of CSF and/or brain into the defect.

Spinal Leaks

- CSF leaks in the spine cause a range of symptoms, but most commonly patients present with positional headaches, commonly with an occipital predominance; other symptoms include tinnitus, visual disturbances, neck pain, and brain fog, though in severe cases, patients can present with encephalopathy or coma [5].
- Diagnosis is made by a combination of symptoms and one of the following:
  - Cranial imaging findings of CSF leak.
  - Spinal imaging showing evidence of a CSF leak.
  - Low opening pressure (<6 cm CSF, though very uncommon).
  - Response to a blood patch.
- Cranial imaging findings of a CSF leak (seen in 70–80% of patients) include:
  - Diffuse dural thickening and enhancement.
  - Distension of the dural sinuses.
  - Downward displacement of brain/brain sag.
  - Spontaneous subdural hematomas and hygromas.

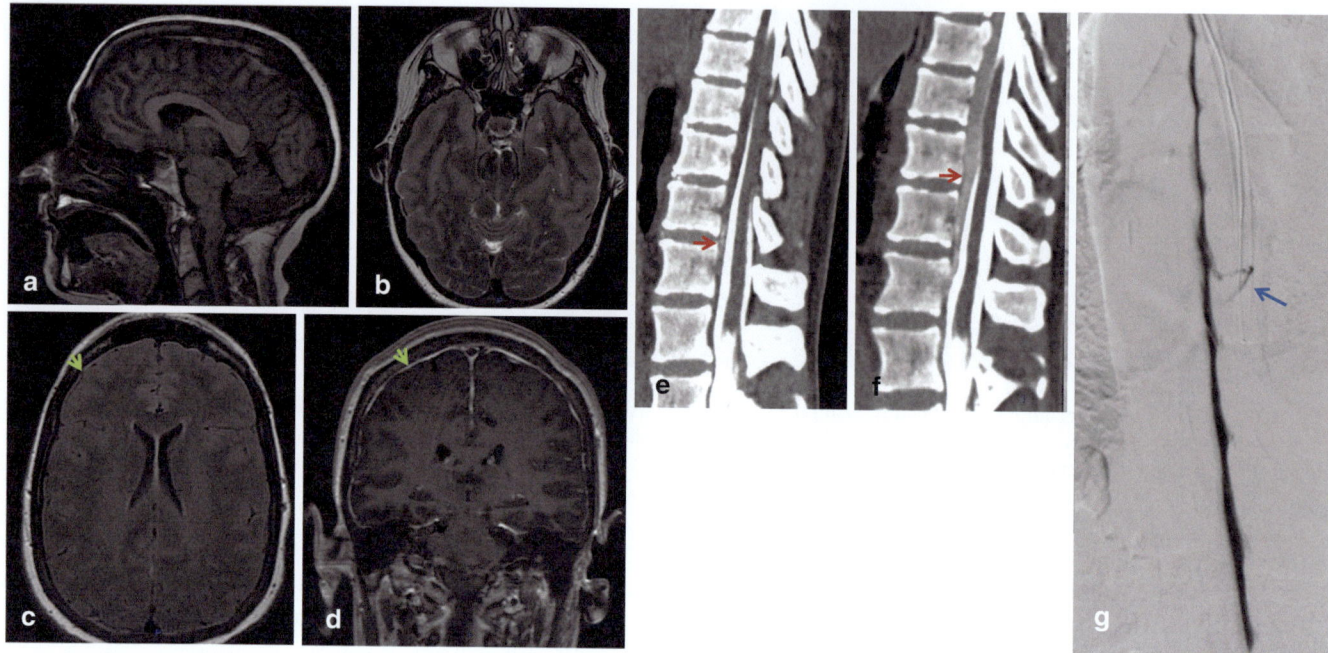

Fig. 18.10 Spontaneous intracranial hypotension. Brain MRI shows typical stigmata of a CSF leak including sagittal T1 (**a**) and axial T2 (**b**) images showing significant brain sag, with cerebellar tonsillar descent, downward movement of the brain, narrowing of the basilar cisterns, and reduction of the mamillopontine distance. Axial FLAIR (**c**) and coronal T1 post-contrast images (**d**) demonstrate thickening and enhancement of the dura (green arrows). Spinal imaging including sagittal reformat demonstrated an extradural fluid collection, which filled with contrast on dynamic CT myelogram (**e** and **f**, red arrows). A digital subtraction myelogram in another patient shows a CSF-venous fistula (**g**, blue arrow)

- Spinal imaging findings of a CSF leak include (Fig. 18.10):
  - Extradural fluid collection.
  - CSF Venous fistula (detected by digital subtraction myelography or dynamic CT myelography).
  - Venous plexus engorgement.
- Treatment:
  - Conservative measures include bed rest, fluid replenishment, and caffeine.
  - Non-targeted high-volume epidural blood patch.
  - For those not responding to non-targeted blood patches, further imaging workup to diagnose the location of the CSF leak with targeted blood or fibrin glue patch, venous embolization (for CSF-venous fistulas), or surgery may be options.

References

1. Carlstrom LP, Eltanahy A, Perry A, et al. A clinical primer for the glymphatic system. Brain. 2022;145(3):843–57. https://doi.org/10.1093/brain/awab428.
2. Kartal MG, Algin O. Evaluation of hydrocephalus and other cerebrospinal fluid disorders with MRI: an update. Insights Imaging. 2014;5(4):531–41. https://doi.org/10.1007/s13244-014-0333-5.
3. Khalatbari H, Parisi MT. Management of hydrocephalus in children: anatomic imaging appearances of CSF shunts and their complications. AJR Am J Roentgenol. 2021;216(1):187–99. https://doi.org/10.2214/AJR.20.22888.
4. Juhász J, Hensler J, Jansen O. MRI-findings in idiopathic intracranial hypertension (Pseudotumor cerebri). Rofo. 2021;193(11):1269–76. https://doi.org/10.1055/a-1447-0264.
5. Schievink WI. Spontaneous intracranial hypotension. N Engl J Med. 2021;385(23):2173–8. https://doi.org/10.1056/NEJMra2101561.

Intracranial Cysts

Angela L. Kanna, Salar Hakham, and Neel Madan

INTRODUCTION

- Cysts are a very common finding in the brain.
- Important to recognize the common imaging features of simple and complex cysts.
- Cysts can be separated into intra-axial and extra-axial lesions.

IMAGING CHARACTERISTICS OF CYSTS

- Simple, Fluid-Filled Cysts.
  - On CT, will be isodense to CSF fluid, measuring 0–20 Hounsfield units, with a thin wall that may enhance.
  - On MRI, will follow CSF signal on all sequences, being dark on T1 and FLAIR, bright on T2, dark on diffusion imaging, and bright on the ADC map, with a thin wall that may enhance.
- Complex Cysts.
  - On CT, may have higher density due to proteinaceous fluid, hemorrhage, or calcium, and may have a thicker wall or septation(s).
  - On MRI, will have similar complex features that lead to increased signal on T1 or FLAIR, darker signal on T2, and may also appear brighter on diffusion imaging and darker on the ADC map.
  - If cysts have thicker or nodular areas of enhancement, neoplasm needs to be considered.

Supplementary Information The online version contains supplementary material available at https://doi.org/10.1007/978-3-031-55124-6_19.

A. L. Kanna · N. Madan (✉)
Tufts University School of Medicine, Boston, MA, USA
e-mail: akanna@tuftsmedicine.org

S. Hakham
Beverly Hospital, Montebello, CA, USA

LOCATION

- The initial step in correctly diagnosing an intracranial cyst is determining its location, as the differential for intra-axial (within the brain parenchyma) and extra-axial (outside the brain parenchyma) cystic masses is different.
- Additionally, some locations such as the sellar and suprasellar region or the pineal region have specific differential diagnoses.

EXTRA-AXIAL LESIONS

Arachnoid Cyst

- Benign, congenital intracranial, extra-axial CSF-filled sac which does not communicate with the ventricular system [1].
- May occur at any age, but more common in adults.
- Often asymptomatic and discovered incidentally. Symptoms vary based on cyst size and location (headache, dizziness, and sensorineural hearing loss). Giant arachnoid cysts may cause obstructive hydrocephalus (especially when associated with the foramen of Monro, or mass effect on the midbrain tectum with obstruction at the cerebral aqueduct).
- The majority (50–60%) are located in the middle cranial fossa, 10–20% along the cerebellopontine angle, and 10% are suprasellar/intrasellar.
- Size is highly variable, from a few millimeters to giant.
- Imaging characteristics are those of a simple cyst (Fig. 19.1).
- Often no intervention is necessary. If symptomatic, endoscopic resection, fenestration, and cystoperitoneal shunt are common treatment options.

Cavum Velum Interpositum Cyst

- Rare, benign, simple cyst located in the potential space of the velum interpositum (Fig. e19.1).

© The Author(s), under exclusive license to Springer Nature Switzerland AG 2024
B. A. Vachha et al. (eds.), *What Radiology Residents Need to Know: Neuroradiology*, What Radiology Residents Need to Know,
https://doi.org/10.1007/978-3-031-55124-6_19

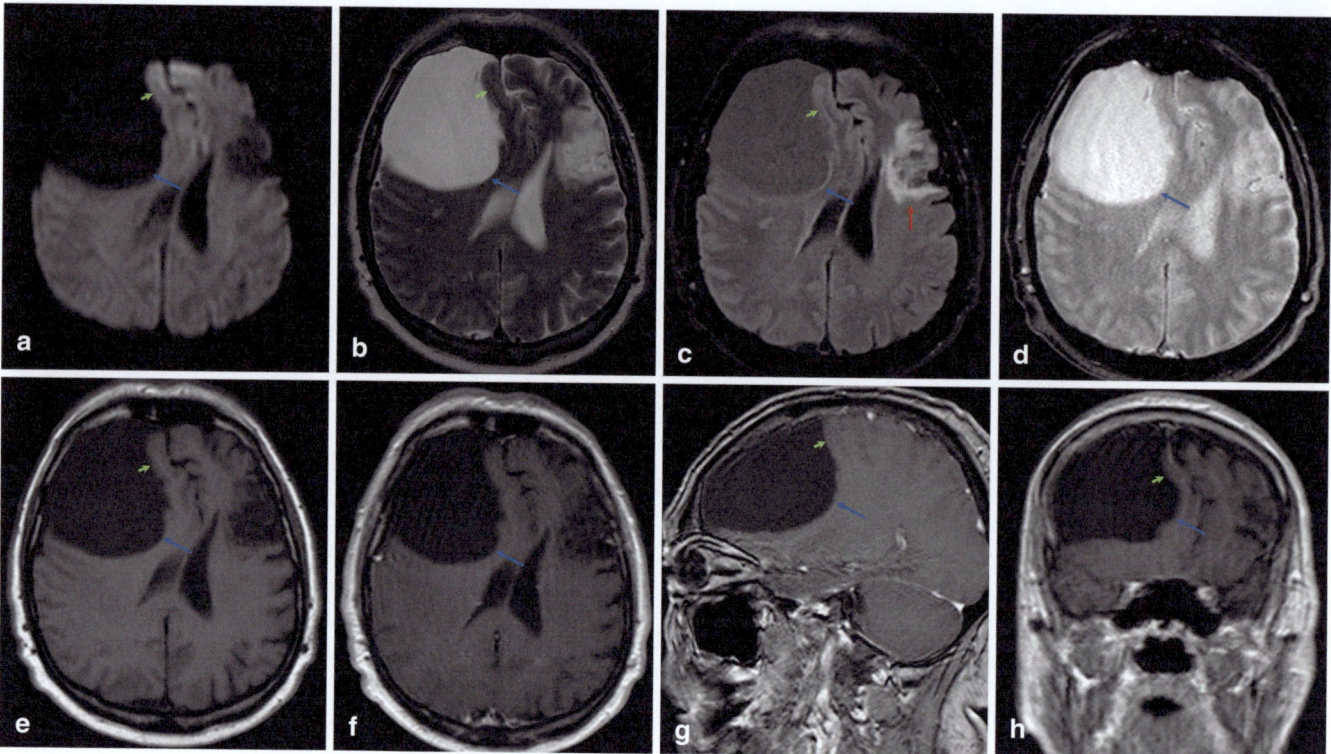

Fig. 19.1 Arachnoid cyst. Right frontal extra-axial cystic lesion (blue arrow) displaces the underlying brain and follows CSF on nearly all sequences (axial diffusion-weighted imaging (DWI) (**a**), T2 (**b**), FLAIR (**c**), GRE (**d**), T1 (**e**), and axial (**f**), sagittal (**g**), and coronal (**h**) T1 post-contrast images), with incomplete suppression on FLAIR. Note a thin rim of gray matter can be seen in the brain parenchyma (green arrow), displaced by the cyst, identifying this as extra-axial in location and not intra-axial. Incidentally, an area of encephalomalacia is also noted in the left frontal lobe (red arrow)

- (All electronic images (Figs. e19.1–e19.15) can be found on this chapter's website on SpringerLink: https://doi.org/10.1007/978-3-031-55124-6_19)
- Velum interpositum is located between two layers of the tela choroidea of the third ventricle, in between the internal cerebral veins and the posterior medial choroidal artery.
- Triangular shape with wide base posteriorly and anterior apex.
- When enlarged, located behind the foramen of Monro, beneath the columns of the fornices and abutting the pineal gland.
- Usually small in size (less than 1–2 cm).
- Majority are clinically silent and discovered incidentally. Larger cysts (greater than 1 cm) may cause headaches from aqueduct compression and hydrocephalus and are associated with brain anomalies [2].
- Usually, no intervention is required. If symptomatic, surgical (endoscopic) fenestration may be performed.

Epidermoid Cyst

- Congenital inclusion of ectodermal epithelial elements, which typically presents in adult life (20–60 years old) [3].
- May remain clinically silent for many years; the most common symptom is headache. Additional symptoms depend on location and mass effect on adjacent structures:
  - Neuropathy of cranial nerves V, VII, and VIII are commonly seen with a cerebellopontine angle mass.
  - Seizures may occur if the tumor is located in the sylvian fissure.
- The vast majority (90%) are intradural in location (basal cisterns, cerebellopontine angle, fourth ventricle), and 10% are extradural in the skull or spine.
- Slow-growing and variable in size.
- Complex cysts, which can be differentiated from arachnoid cysts with increased DWI, decreased ADC, and/or heterogeneously increased FLAIR signal (Figs. 19.2 and e19.2).

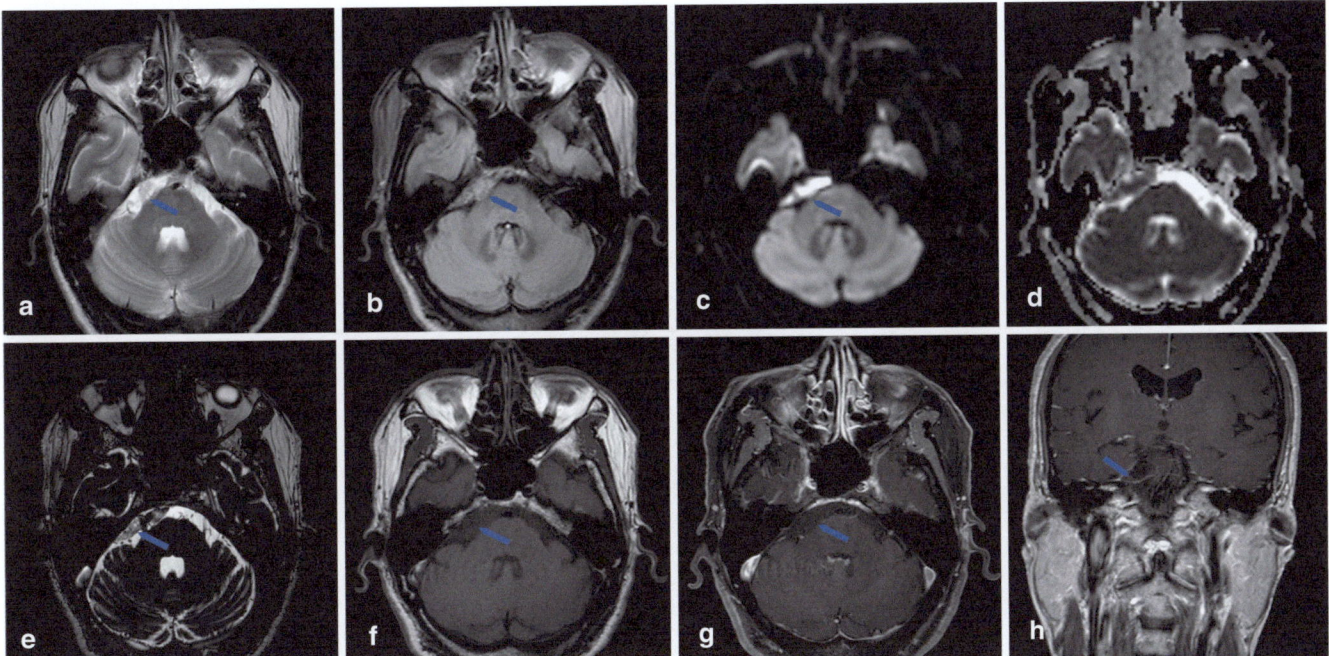

Fig. 19.2 Epidermoid cyst. Axial T2 (**a**), FLAIR (**b**), DWI (**c**), ADC (**d**), BFFE (**e**), T1 (**f**), T1 post-contrast (**g**), and coronal T1 post-contrast (**h**) images show a cystic structure (blue arrows) which is difficult to perceive on some sequences (T1, **f**), but does not follow CSF signal on FLAIR (**b**) and DWI/ADC (**c**, **d**) maps in the right cerebellopontine angle where it is most apparent. The imaging characteristics are thus consistent with an epidermoid cyst

- Complete microsurgical resection is the goal of treatment.
  - Aggressive total removal may cause significant cranial neuropathy, but recurrence is common if incompletely removed.
  - Subarachnoid dissemination of contents during surgery can cause chemical meningitis.

Dermoid Cyst

- Benign, epithelial inclusion cyst containing dermal elements (hair follicles and sebaceous and sweat glands), which commonly occurs in the second to the third decades of life [4].
- May be asymptomatic. When symptomatic, most commonly headaches and seizures.
- Midline, most commonly suprasellar or in the posterior fossa, with variable size.
- Unilocular, cystic lesion with fat (Fig. 19.3).
  - CT will have negative Hounsfield Units from fat; can have capsular calcification.
  - On MRI, T1 hyperintense related to fat, T2 heterogeneous with chemical shift artifact, and may have thin rim of enhancement.
- Complications include obstructive hydrocephalus, hypopituitarism, diabetes insipidus, and visual symptoms (if suprasellar in location).

- Cyst rupture causes chemical meningitis (subarachnoid/intraventricular spread of contents), with fat droplets in subarachnoid space on CT and MRI, as well as possible leptomeningeal enhancement.
- Management is complete surgical excision, and the cyst may recur.
- Subarachnoid dissemination may also occur intraoperatively, which may or may not cause symptoms (justifies "wait-and-see" approach).

Neurenteric Cyst

- Rare, endodermal derived developmental lesion arising from the persistence of the embryonic neurenteric canal [1].
- More common in spine, than intracranially; when intracranial, most commonly seen in the ventral posterior fossa.
- Variable size, but most commonly small.
- Incidental, or when large, can present with headaches, neck pain, or seizures.
- Smoothly marginated cysts which are frequently iso to hyperintense to CSF on T1 and hyperintense to CSF on T2 images; however, may have complex features (Fig. 19.4).
- Differentiated from epidermoids which are usually more lateral with restricted diffusion.

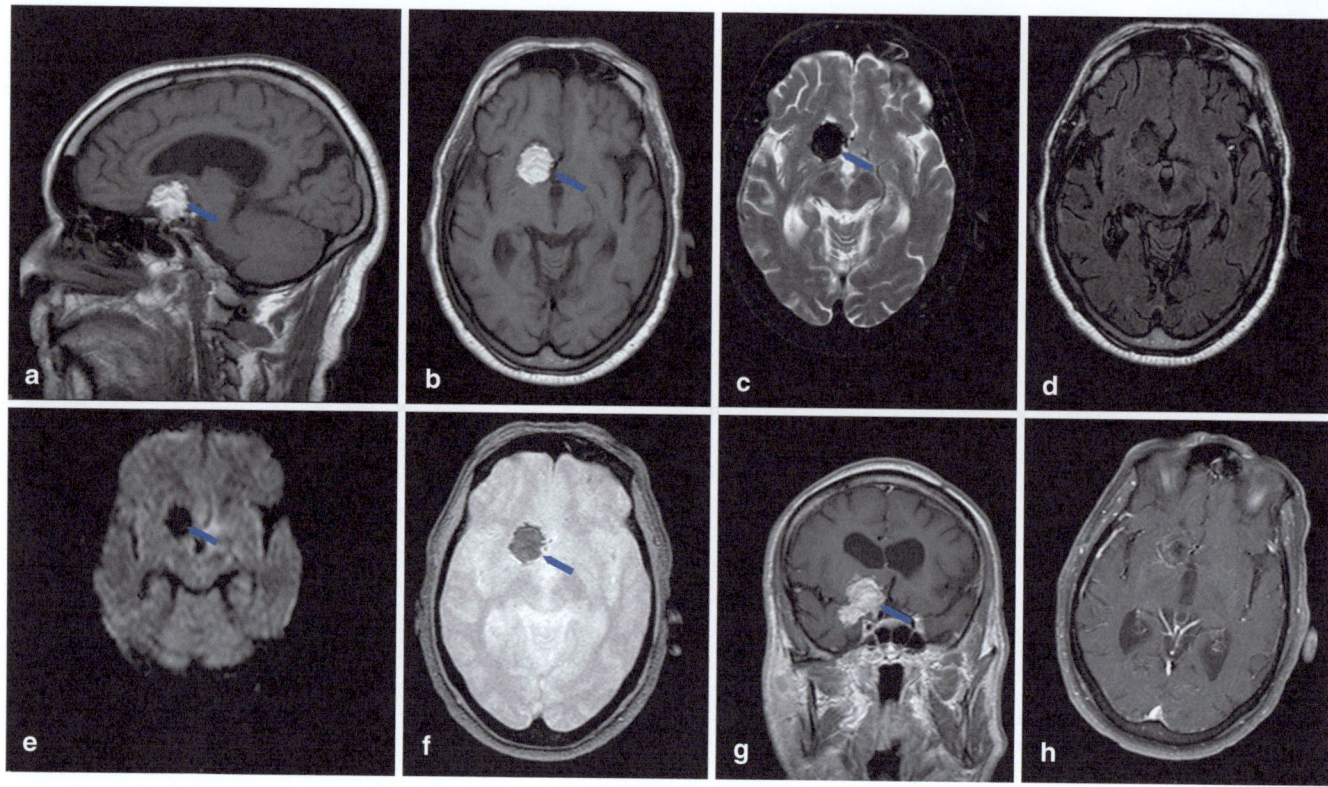

Fig. 19.3 Dermoid cyst. Sagittal T1 (**a**), axial T1 (**b**), T2 (**c**), FLAIR (**d**), DWI (**e**), and T2* (**f**) as well as post-contrast coronal T1 (**g**) and axial T1 with fat suppression (**h**) images demonstrate a lesion (blue arrow) in the right suprasellar region with intrinsic T1 hyperintensity (**b**) reflecting fat, which is hypointense on the remainder of the sequences with minimal enhancement, consistent with a dermoid cyst

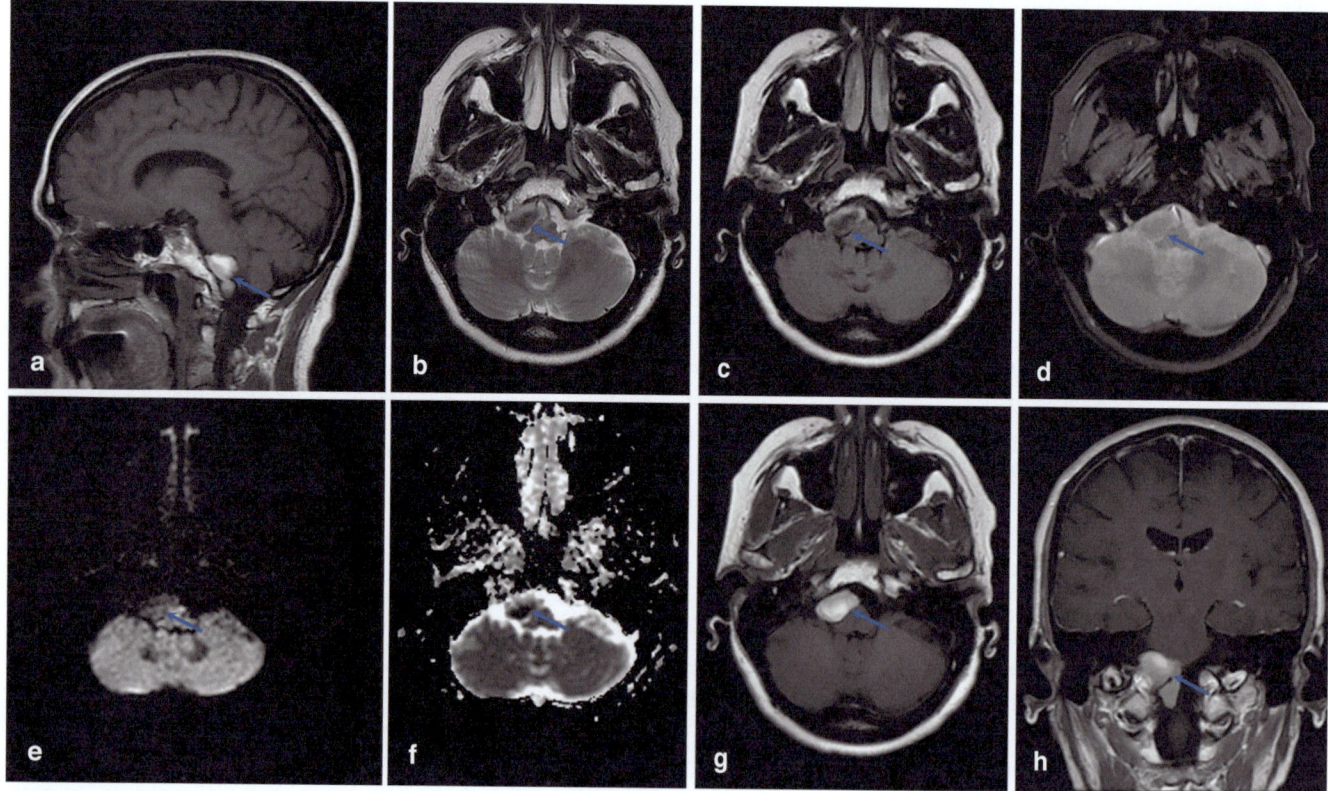

Fig. 19.4 Neurenteric cyst. Sagittal T1 (**a**), axial T2 (**b**), FLAIR (**c**), T2* (**d**), DWI (**e**), ADC (**f**), and axial (**g**) and coronal T1 post-contrast (**h**) images demonstrate a mass in the cerebellomedullary angle (blue arrows) which is intrinsically T1 hyperintense with variable signal intensity on T2 (**b**) and DWI/ADC (**e**, **f**), which on pathology was found to represent a neurenteric cyst. Dermoid is also in the differential diagnosis given the T1 hyperintensity, but the location is typical of a neurenteric cyst

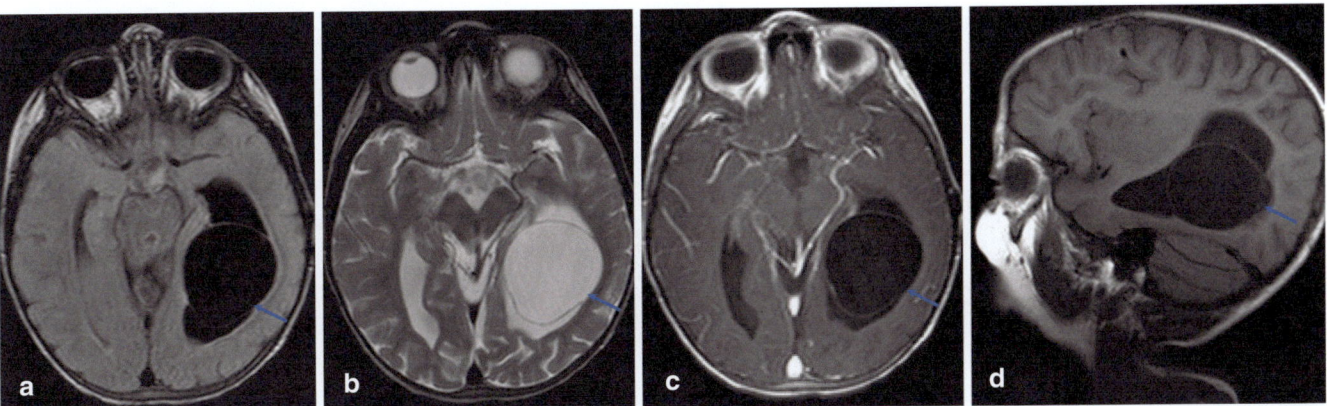

Fig. 19.5 Intraventricular cyst. Large simple, cystic lesion (blue arrows) within the left lateral ventricle of a 5-year-old patient which follows CSF signal on axial FLAIR (**a**), T2 (**b**), T1 post-contrast (**c**), and sagittal T1 without contrast (**d**), consistent with a simple intraventricular cyst

Choroid Plexus Cyst

- Benign cyst of the choroid plexus, typically seen in neonates (and typically regress) and older adults, though can be seen at any age [1].
- Typically asymptomatic and discovered incidentally. Rarely present with obstructive hydrocephalus due to ventricular obstruction.
- Most commonly located in the atria of the lateral ventricles, less commonly the third ventricle. May be unilateral or bilateral.
- Usually small in size (2–20 mm). Large cysts (greater than 20 mm) are rare.
- May be simple or complex cysts, without solid/enhancing components (Fig. 19.5).
- Xanthogranulomas are another name for complex cysts of the choroid plexus (Fig. e19.3). If the cystic lesion exhibits a thick and nodular enhancing rim, consider intraventricular cystic metastasis (Fig. e19.4).
- Management depends on risk factors and location:
  o Fetal choroid plexus cysts have been associated with increased risk of trisomy 21 or 18; although trisomy screening is now typically performed with blood tests.
  o Isolated choroid plexus cysts with no additional risk factors are considered clinically insignificant. Only a concern if large and in a location where obstructive hydrocephalus is a risk.

Ependymal Cyst

- Benign, congenital ependymal-lined cyst, typically seen in adults younger than 40 years old [1].

- Location is intraventricular (lateral ventricle more commonly than the third and fourth ventricles). Additional less common sites include cerebral parenchyma, temporoparietal and frontal lobe white matter, and rarely the subarachnoid space (Fig. e19.5).
- Usually small (2–3 mm), but sizes up to 8–9 cm have been reported.
- Typically asymptomatic, but may cause headache, seizure, gait disturbance, and dementia from CSF flow obstruction or increased intracranial pressure.
- Conservative management is indicated if asymptomatic. Surgical excision or decompression results in rapid resolution of symptoms.

Colloid Cyst

- Epithelial-lined cyst containing mucin. Peak age at diagnosis third to fourth decades of life (rare in children) [1].
- Vast majority (greater than 99%) are wedged into the foramen of Monro. The location is virtually pathognomonic (Fig. 19.6).
- Typically very small in size (1–2 mm), although up to 3 cm has been reported.
- Approximately half are asymptomatic and discovered incidentally. May present with headache (50–60%), nausea, vomiting, memory loss, altered personality, gait disturbance, and visual changes.
- Acute foramen of Monro obstruction leads to rapid onset hydrocephalus, herniation, and possibly, death.
- Treatment is surgical resection through an image-guided endoscopic approach. Less-favored options include stereotactic aspiration and ventricular shunting.

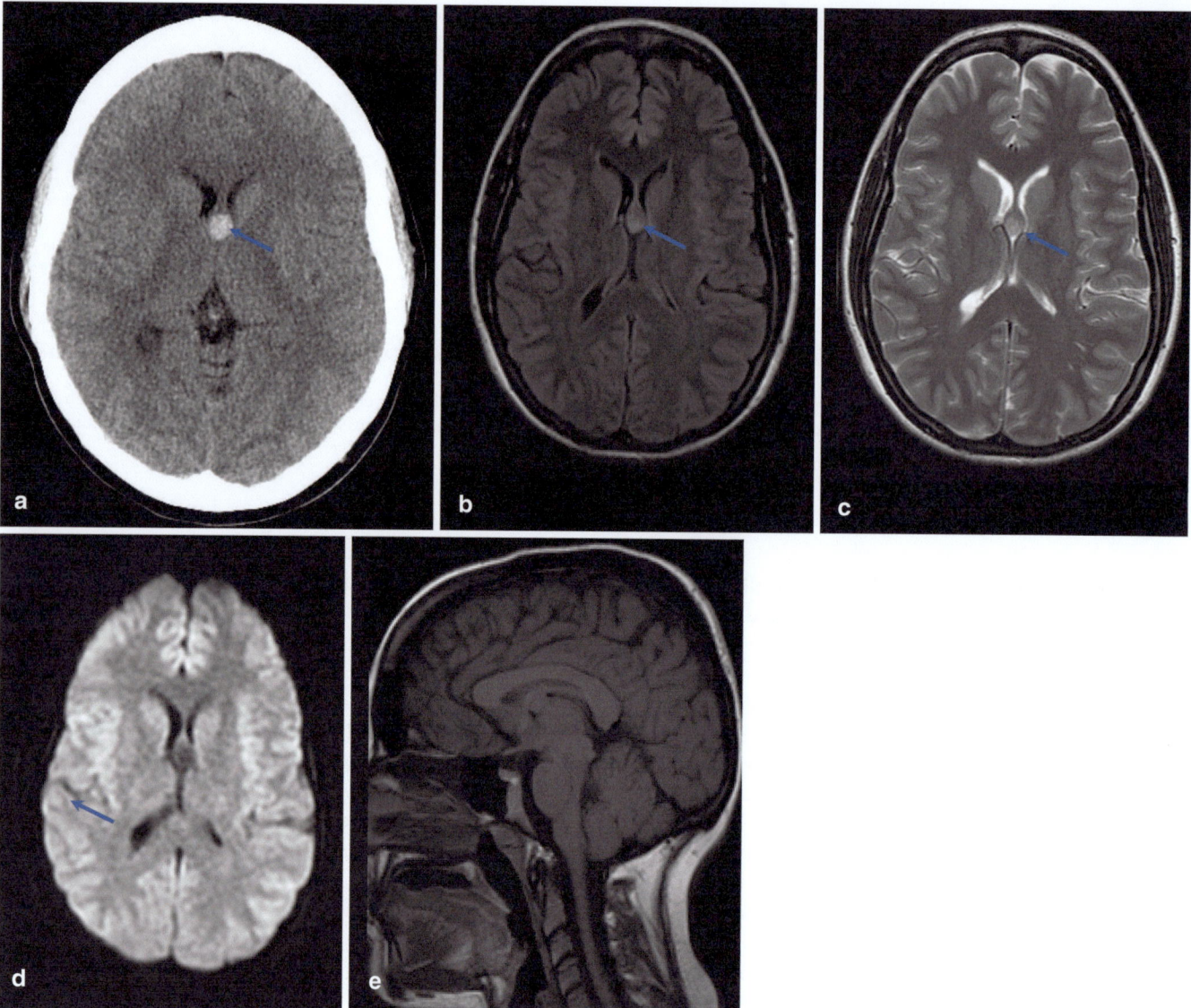

Fig. 19.6 Colloid cyst. Classic CT (**a**) appearance of a colloid cyst (blue arrows), with a hyperdense rounded lesion centered in the anterior third ventricle at the level of the foramen of Monro. Corresponding MRI shows variable signal intensity on axial FLAIR (**b**), axial T2 (**c**), axial DWI (**d**), and sagittal T1 (**e**)

Pineal Cyst

- Benign intrapineal glial-lined cyst [5].
- May occur at all ages, with an incidence of approximately 25% in healthy adults.
- Most are located above and clearly distinct from the tectum (Fig. e19.6).
- Usually small in size, majority are less than 1 cm, but can be large.
- Majority are clinically silent and discovered incidentally.
  - Larger cysts (greater than 1 cm) may cause headaches from compression of the cerebral aqueduct resulting in hydrocephalus.
  - "Pineal apoplexy" may rarely occur (severe headache, cyst hemorrhage, rarely with acute hydrocephalus, and sudden death).
- Usually, no intervention is needed. If symptomatic, stereotactic aspiration or resection/biopsy is performed to exclude malignancy.
- Imaging characteristic is that of simple cysts, though there can be multiple septations, rim enhancement, or regions of enhancement.
- When complex features exist, cannot be distinguished from neoplasm (pineocytoma) on the basis of imaging studies alone (Fig. e19.7).

Rathke Cleft Cyst

- Non-neoplastic cyst from persistence of embryonic Rathke's pouch, with mean age at diagnosis 45 years [6].
- Also known as Pars Intermedia Cyst.
- Most are asymptomatic and found incidentally. Symptomatic cysts present with pituitary dysfunction, visual disturbances, headache, and rarely apoplexy.
- Most are completely intrasellar in location (40%), but 60% of the time have a suprasellar extension, characteristically arising between the adeno- and neurohypophysis (Fig. 19.7).
- Size is usually between 5 and 15 mm in diameter when symptomatic, and occasionally, they may become very large.
- Typically simple cyst which is best seen on post-contrast imaging as a region of non-enhancement relative to the normal pituitary tissue; can have complex cystic features.
- If asymptomatic, conservative management is indicated. If symptomatic, aspiration or partial excision may be performed, but recurrence occurs in approximately 30%.
- Differential diagnosis includes a pituitary adenoma with hemorrhage (pituitary apoplexy, Fig. e19.8), a craniopharyngioma (Fig. e19.9), a cystic pituitary adenoma (Fig. e19.10), as well as infundibular cyst (Fig. e19.11).

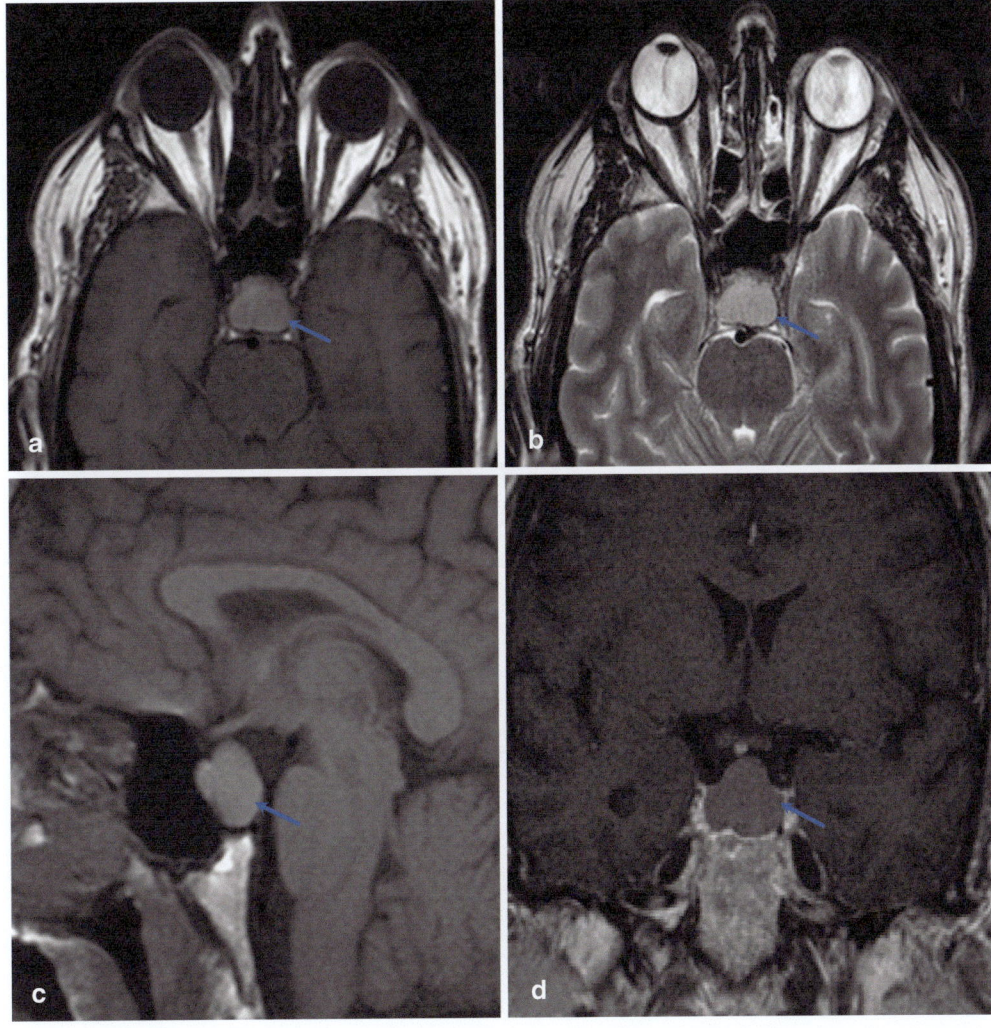

Fig. 19.7 Rathke cleft cyst. Axial T1 (**a**) and T2 (**b**), sagittal T1 (**c**), and coronal T1 post-contrast (**d**) images show an intermediate intensity sellar mass with suprasellar extension (blue arrows), without definite enhancement and without a solid component pathologically proven to be a Rathke cleft cyst

INTRA-AXIAL CYSTS

Neuroglial Cyst

- Also known as a neuroepithelial cyst or glioependymal cyst [1].
- Benign, congenital glial-lined cyst which may be seen at any age.
- Can be seen anywhere along the neural axis, but most commonly seen in the frontal lobe (Figs. 19.8 and e19.12).
- When intracranial, the cysts are most often asymptomatic (most common) or cause headaches. If intraspinal, they may cause cord compression and myelopathy.
- Simple cyst; if complex features, especially a solid/enhancing component, must consider a cystic neoplasm.
- Management options include observation or total surgical excision, based on symptoms.
- Differential diagnoses include infectious cysts such as an intracranial abscess/cerebritis (Fig. e19.13) and neurocysticercosis (Fig. e19.14).

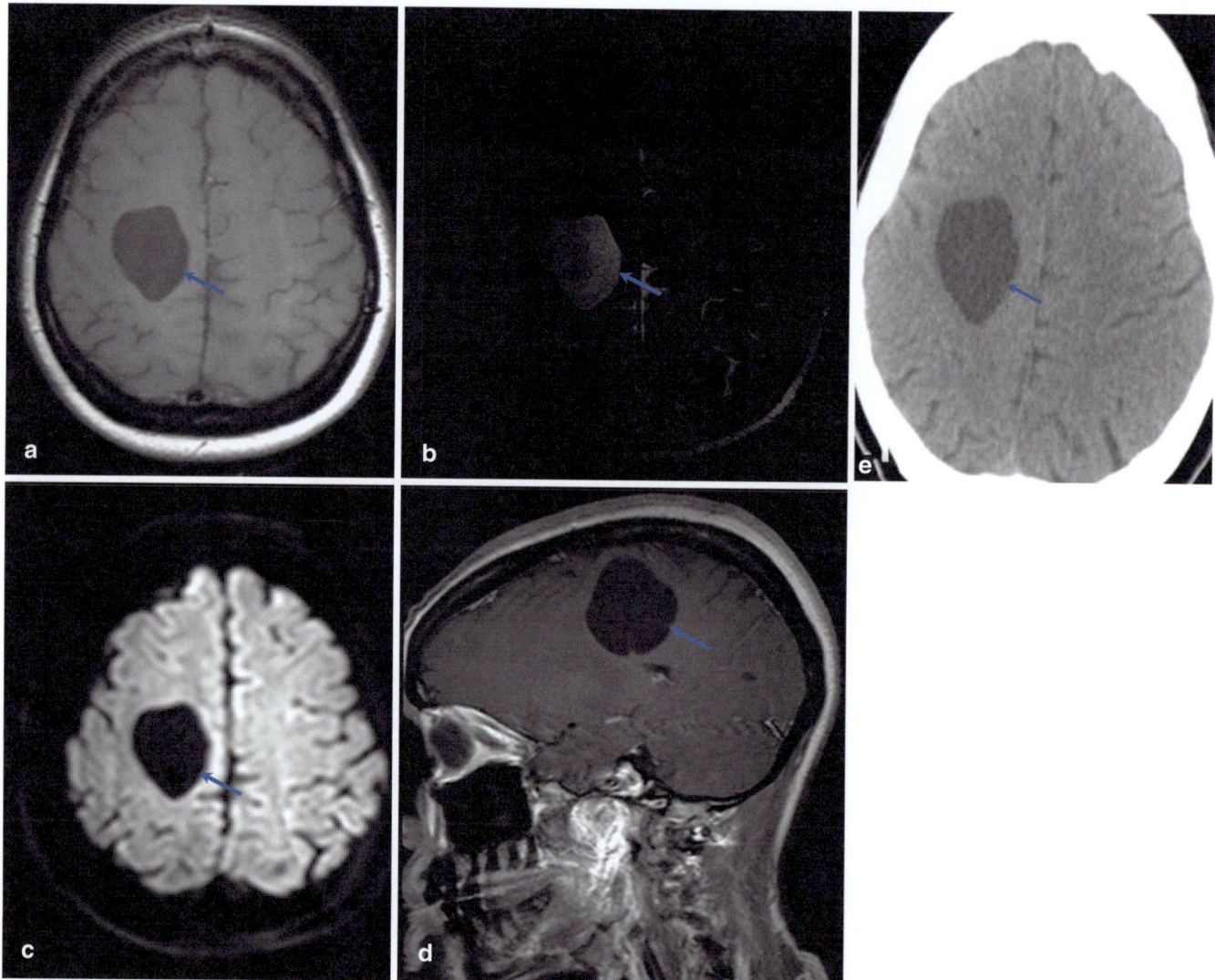

Fig. 19.8 Neuroglial cyst. Axial T2 (**a**), axial FLAIR (**b**), DWI (**c**), and sagittal T1 post-contrast (**d**) images demonstrate an intra-axial cystic centered in the right frontal lobe (blue arrow), which follows CSF on all sequences, demonstrates minimal complexity and shows incomplete suppression on FLAIR images. (**e**) CT images show a cystic mass (blue arrow)

Porencephalic Cyst

- Parenchymal CSF-filled cavity lined by reactive gliosis (Fig. 19.9) [1, 7].
  - Congenital cysts result from a destructive process in-utero (typically venous infarct or arterial infarct, though hemorrhage or infection also possible).
  - Acquired cysts result from an injury later in life (head trauma, surgery, infarct, or infection).
- Usually communicates with the ventricular system, usually unilateral although can be bilateral.
- Size varies from small to enormous (with communication with subarachnoid space).
- Symptoms depend on the location and size of the injury and can be asymptomatic or present with mild developmental delay, or spastic hemiplegia. Other associations include severe neurological deficits, mental and psychomotor developmental delay, and intractable epilepsy.

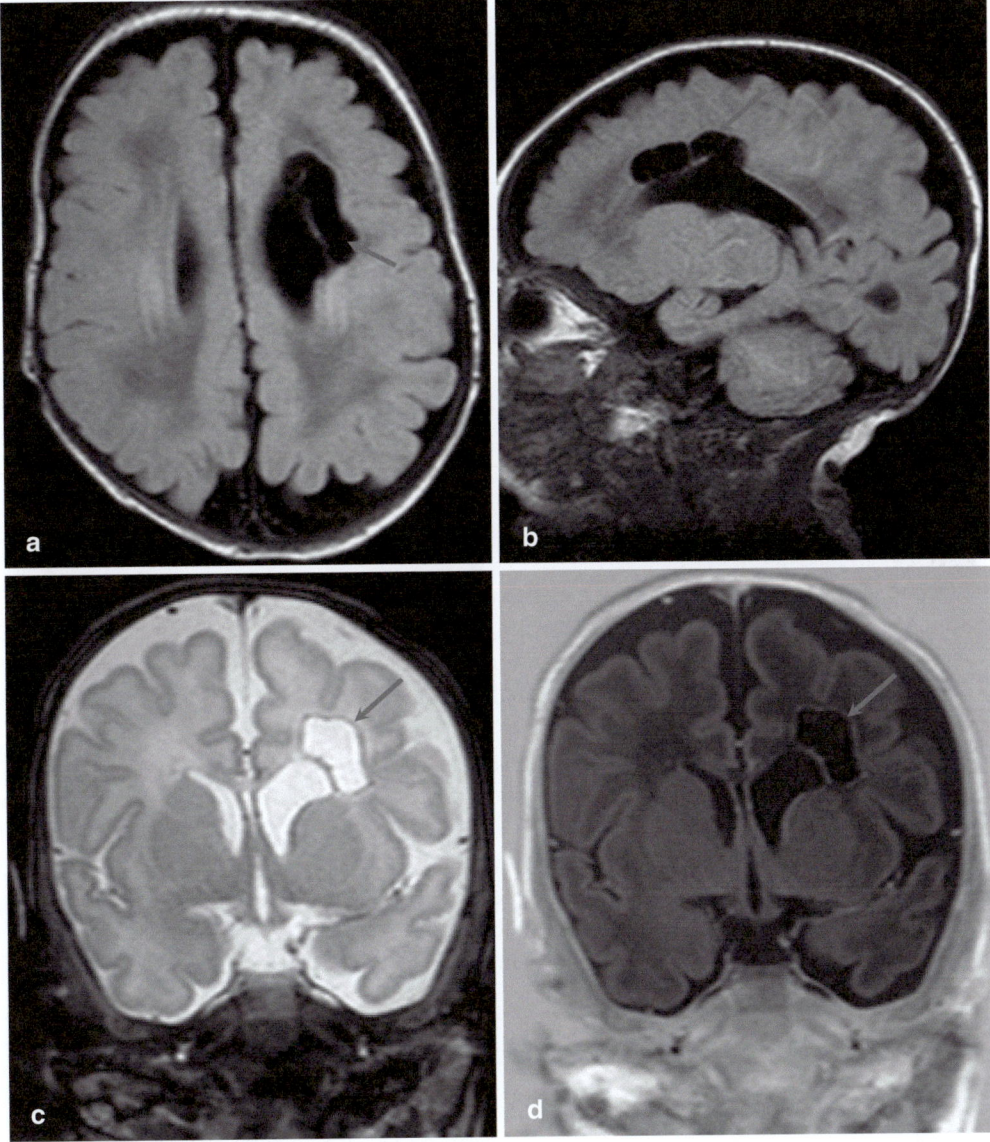

Fig. 19.9 Porencephalic cyst. Axial FLAIR (**a**), sagittal FLAIR (**b**), coronal T2 (**c**), and coronal T1 double inversion recovery (**d**) images demonstrate a cystic lesion (blue arrows) located at the frontal horn of the left lateral ventricle with volume loss in the brain parenchyma and ex vacuo dilatation of the ventricle reflecting sequela of prior vascular insult

Fig. 19.10 Giant tumefactive perivascular spaces. Axial T2 (**a**) and sagittal T1 post-contrast (**b**) images demonstrate multiple, large cystic spaces (blue arrows) in the brain parenchyma which were stable over time, consistent with perivascular spaces

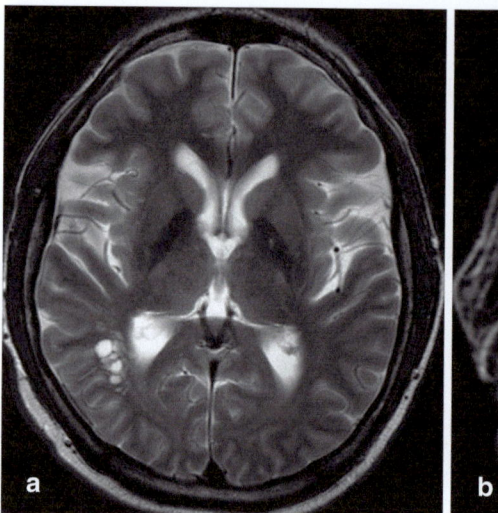
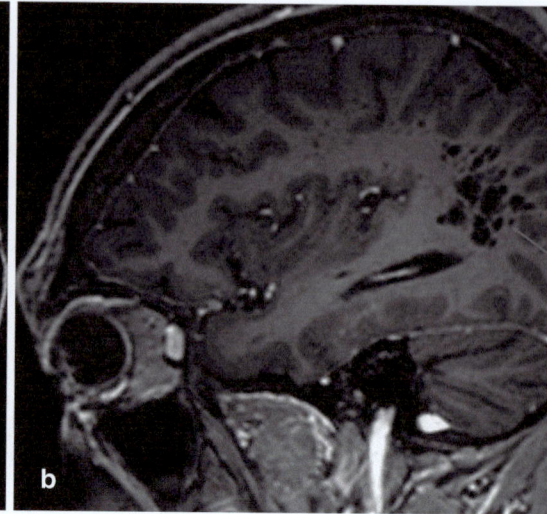

- No treatment is usually warranted, but if acute or refractory symptoms are present, options include placement of a cystoperitoneal shunt, or fenestration to the lateral ventricles (if the cyst does not communicate with the ventricular system). For intractable epilepsy, surgical resection may be warranted.

Enlarged Perivascular Spaces

- Fluid-filled spaces that follow CSF signals that may be seen at all ages [8, 9].
- Occur in any location, but mostly in the basal ganglia. Other common sites include the midbrain, thalami, and deep white matter. Rarely involve the cortex.
- Usually 5 mm in size or less, but occasionally attain large size where sometimes referred to as "Giant" or "tumefactive" perivascular spaces (Fig. 19.10). If these occur in the midbrain, may cause mass effect and obstructive hydrocephalus.
- Typically asymptomatic and discovered incidentally.
- "Leave me alone" lesion that should not be mistaken for ominous disease; cystic neoplasm. If midbrain lesions cause obstructive hydrocephalus, a shunt may be placed.

Connatal Cyst

- Also known as coarctation of the lateral ventricles or frontal horn cysts [10].
- Mostly located adjacent to the superolateral margins of the frontal horns of the lateral ventricles; occasionally seen along the body of the lateral ventricles (Fig. e19.15).
- No intervention is indicated, though needs to be differentiated from other cystic lesions.

References

1. Osborn AG, Preece MT. Intracranial cysts: radiologic-pathologic correlation and imaging approach. Radiology. 2006;239(3):650–64. https://doi.org/10.1148/radiol.2393050823.
2. Moradi B, Rahmani M, Kia K, Kazemi MA, Tahmasebpour AR. Cavum velum interpositum cysts in normal and anomalous fetuses in second trimester of pregnancy: comparison of its size and prevalence. Taiwan J Obstet Gynecol. 2019;58(6):814–9. https://doi.org/10.1016/j.tjog.2019.09.016.
3. Ren X, Lin S, Wang Z, et al. Clinical, radiological, and pathological features of 24 atypical intracranial epidermoid cysts. J Neurosurg. 2012;116(3):611–21. https://doi.org/10.3171/2011.10.JNS111462.
4. Liu JK, Gottfried ON, Salzman KL, Schmidt RH, Couldwell WT. Ruptured intracranial dermoid cysts: clinical, radiographic, and surgical features. Neurosurgery. 2008;62(2):377–84; discussion 384. https://doi.org/10.1227/01.neu.0000316004.88517.29.
5. Pu Y, Mahankali S, Hou J, et al. High prevalence of pineal cysts in healthy adults demonstrated by high-resolution, noncontrast brain MR imaging. AJNR Am J Neuroradiol. 2007;28(9):1706–9. https://doi.org/10.3174/ajnr.A0656.
6. Binning MJ, Liu JK, Gannon J, Osborn AG, Couldwell WT. Hemorrhagic and nonhemorrhagic Rathke cleft cysts mimicking pituitary apoplexy. J Neurosurg. 2008;108(1):3–8. https://doi.org/10.3171/JNS/2008/108/01/0003.
7. Epelman M, Daneman A, Blaser SI, et al. Differential diagnosis of intracranial cystic lesions at head US: correlation with CT and MR imaging. Radiographics. 2006;26(1):173–96. https://doi.org/10.1148/rg.261055033.
8. Caner B, Bekar A, Hakyemez B, Taskapilioglu O, Aksoy K. Dilatation of Virchow-Robin perivascular spaces: report of 3 cases with different localizations. Minim Invasive Neurosurg. 2008;51(1):11–4. https://doi.org/10.1055/s-2007-1022538.
9. Salzman KL, Osborn AG, House P, et al. Giant tumefactive perivascular spaces. AJNR Am J Neuroradiol. 2005;26(2):298–305.
10. Tan ZYJ, Naidoo P, Kenning N. Ultrasound and MRI features of connatal cysts: clinicoradiological differentiation from other supratentorial periventricular cystic lesions. Br J Radiol. 2010;83(986):180–3. https://doi.org/10.1259/bjr/10458905.

Normal Spine Anatomy and Imaging

20

Peter Liaw, Charissa Kim, Mike Bao, Elisa Flower, and Yu-Ming Chang

Vertebral Anatomy

BONES [1, 2]

- Typically composed of 24 vertebrae separated by intervertebral discs along with variably fused sacral and coccygeal segments:
  - Cervical (seven vertebrae).
  - Thoracic (twelve vertebrae).
  - Lumbar (five vertebrae).
  - Sacrum and coccyx (five sacral and four rudimentary coccygeal segments).
- Each vertebra can be grossly divided into two parts (Figs. 20.1 and 20.2):
  - Body—located anteriorly, responsible for weight-bearing, and progressively increases in height caudally.
  - Neural arch—located posteriorly.
- Neural arch structures (Figs. 20.1, 20.2, 20.3, and 20.4):
  - Spinal canal (aka vertebral foramen)—osseous ring containing the spinal cord.
  - Pedicle—bilateral posterior protrusions from the posterolateral vertebral body that form lateral walls of the spinal canal.
  - Lamina—bilateral posteromedial protrusions from the posterior pedicles, forming posterior walls of the spinal canal.
  - Neuroforamen (aka neural foramen or intervertebral foramen)—lateral passage out of the spinal canal bound by pedicles superiorly and inferiorly, containing spinal nerve roots, dorsal root ganglion, fat, and blood vessels.
- Structures arising from the neural arch (Figs. 20.1, 20.2, 20.3, and 20.4) include:
  - Transverse process—bilateral, project posterolaterally from where the pedicle and lamina fuse.
  - Spinous process—project posteriorly midline.
  - Superior and inferior articular processes—project posterosuperiorly and posteroinferiorly, respectively, from where the pedicle and lamina fuse. Together, they form the facet joint.
  - Superimposition of the transverse process, pedicle, inferior facet, superior facet, portion of the lamina between the facets, known as the pars articularis, and spinous process on oblique plain radiographs creates the famous "Scottie Dog Sign" (Fig. 20.5b).
    - Transverse process forms the nose.
    - Pedicle forms the eye.
    - Inferior facet forms the front leg.
    - Superior facet forms the ear.
    - Pars articularis forms the neck.
    - Lamina and spinous process forms the body.
    - Superior facet of the opposite side forms the tail.
    - Inferior facet of the opposite side forms the hindleg.
- The vertebral bodies contain prominent torturous veins called basivertebral veins which drain to the external vertebral veins along the outer surfaces of the vertebral bodies or internal vertebral veins in the epidural space (Figs. 20.2 and e20.1).

  (All electronic images (Figs. e20.1–e20.2) can be found on this chapter's website on SpringerLink: https://doi.org/10.1007/978-3-031-55124-6_20)

Supplementary Information The online version contains supplementary material available at https://doi.org/10.1007/978-3-031-55124-6_20.

P. Liaw · C. Kim · M. Bao · E. Flower · Y.-M. Chang (✉)
Radiology Department, Beth Israel Deaconess Medical Center, Boston, MA, USA
e-mail: pliaw@bidmc.harvard.edu; ckim16@bidmc.harvard.edu; mbao@bidmc.harvard.edu; eflower@bidneedham.org; ychang2@bidmc.harvard.edu

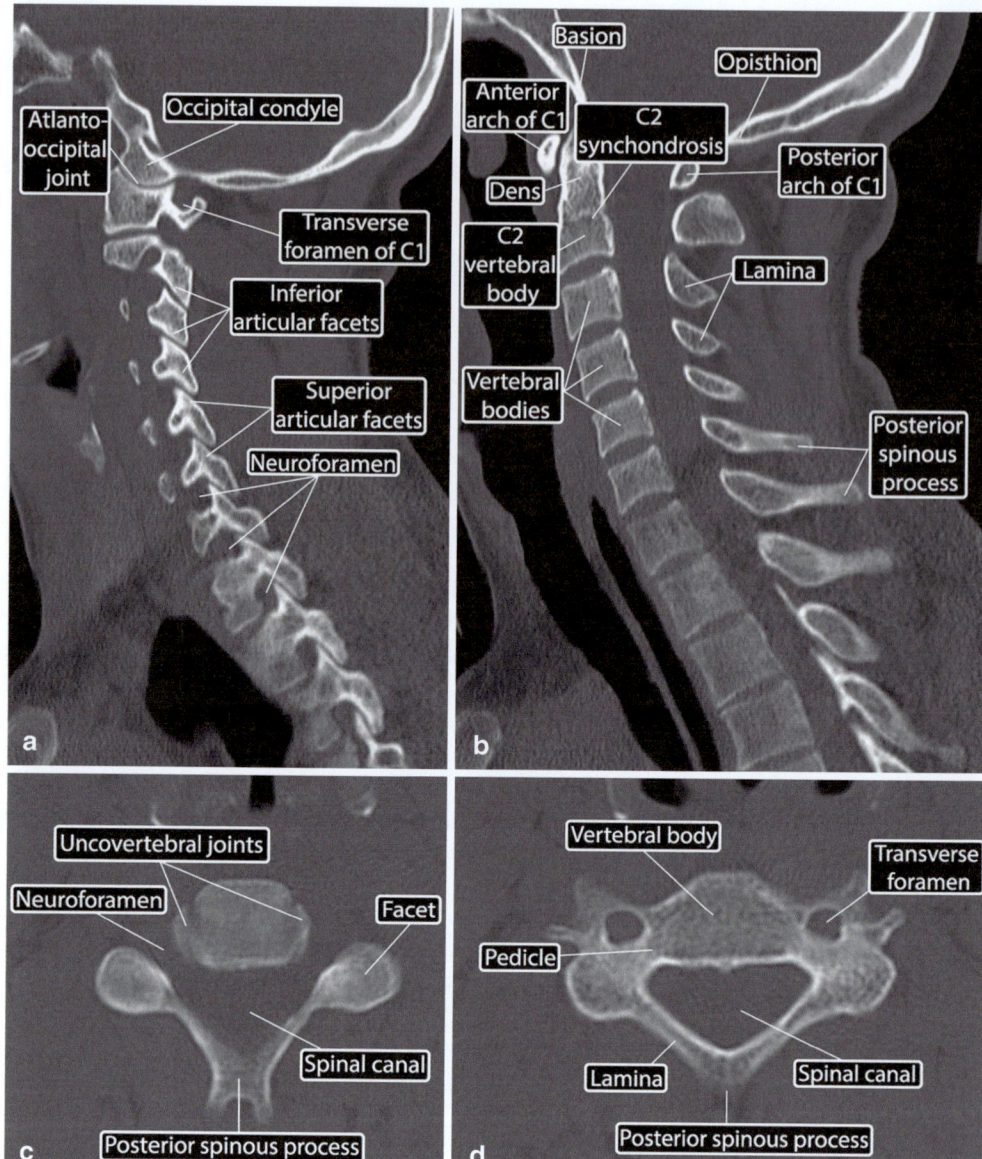

Fig. 20.1 (**a**) **Right parasagittal CT image of the cervical spine demonstrating the atlanto-occipital and atlantoaxial joints and articulating facets**. The neuroforamina of the visualized upper thoracic spine is also noted. Cervical neuroforamina are best evaluated on axial images given their oblique relationship to the vertebral body and spinal canal (see below on panel **c**). (**b**) Midline sagittal CT image of the cervical spine demonstrating the normal relationship of the foramen magnum, C1 and C2, as well as the vertebral bodies and posterior elements. The anterior midline margin of the foramen magnum is called the basion, an important landmark for anatomic measurements. The posterior midline margin of the foramen magnum is called the opisthion, also an important landmark for anatomic measurements. (**c**) Axial CT image of C5 at the level of the neuroforamen. Notice the oblique relationship of the neuroforamen relative to the vertebral body and spinal canal as well as the presence of uncovertebral joints which exist only in the cervical spine. (**d**) Axial CT image of C5 at the level of the transverse foramen which contains the vertebral arteries

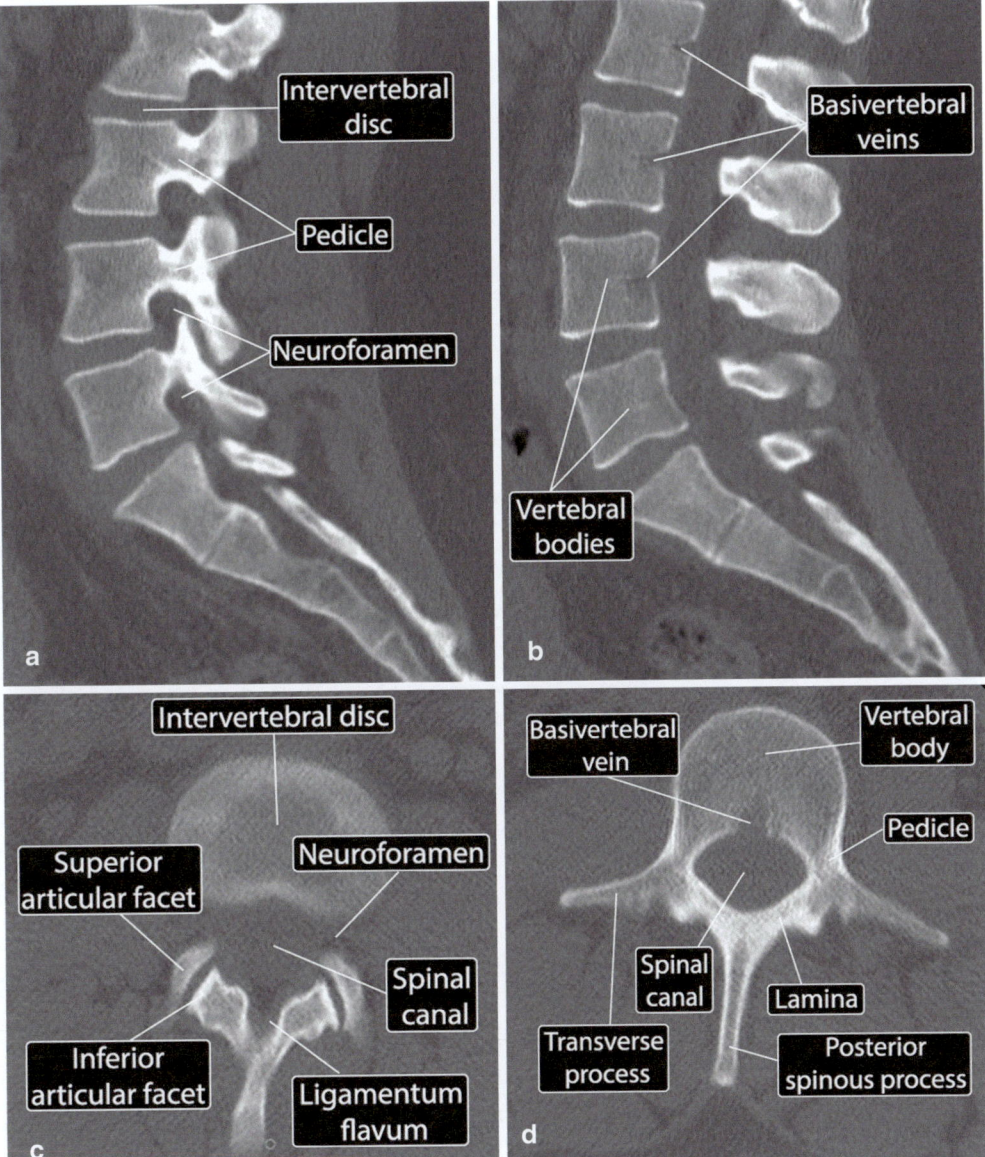

Fig. 20.2 (a) Right parasagittal CT image of the lumbar spine (spanning L2-sacrum) demonstrating the articulating facets and neuroforamen. (b) Midline sagittal CT image of the lumbar spine (spanning L2-sacrum). Midline triangular hypodensity of the posterior vertebral bodies represents the basivertebral veins. (c) Axial CT image of L3 at the level of the neuroforamen. Unlike the cervical spine, the neuroforamen of the lumbar spine (and thoracic spine) is oriented perpendicular to the axis of the vertebral bodies and spinal canal. (d) Axial CT image of L3 at the level of the transverse processes

Fig. 20.3 (**a and b**) **Midline sagittal T2-weighted image of the cervical spine demonstrating the normal anatomic relationship of the skull-base, C1 and C2, vertebral bodies, and posterior elements**. MRI allows for the evaluation of the contents of the spinal canal and neuroforamen as well as ligaments, paraspinal muscles, and other soft tissues. MRI also allows for evaluation of the intervertebral discs and marrow of the vertebrae. (**c**) Representative axial T2-weighted image of the cervical spine. Note the normal artifactual T2 hypointense signal in the CSF caused by CSF pulsation

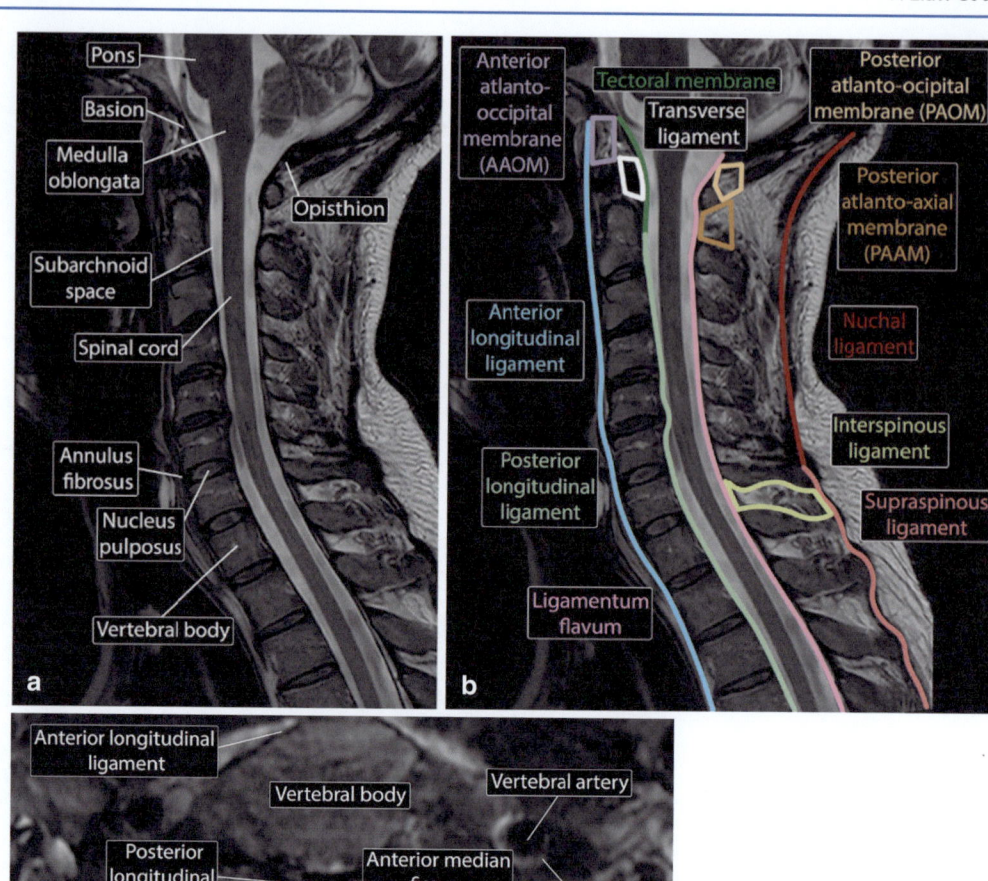

20 Normal Spine Anatomy and Imaging

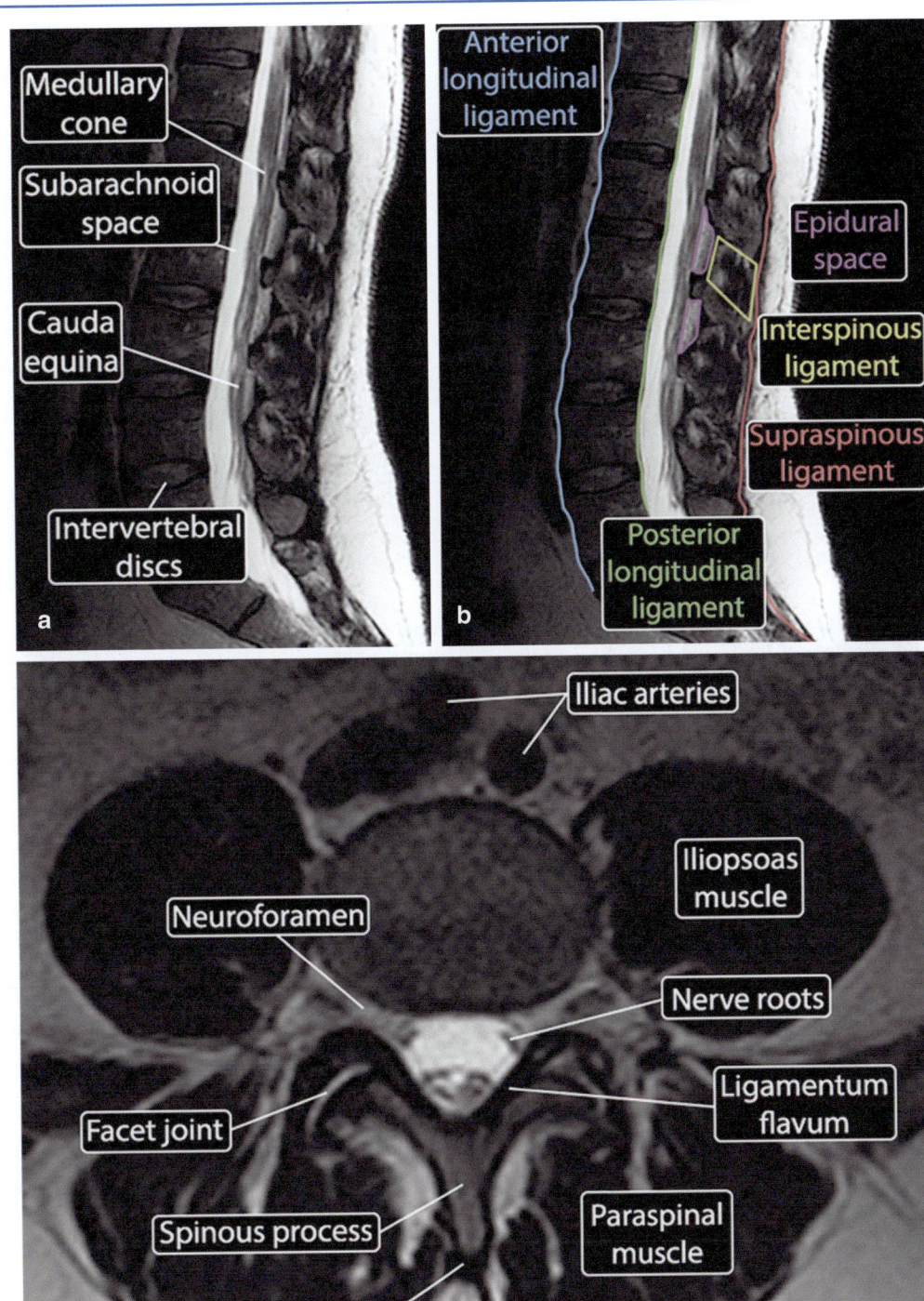

Fig. 20.4 (a and b) Midline sagittal T2-weighted image of the lumbar spine demonstrating normal appearance and position of the conus medullaris (aka medullary cone), cauda equina, vertebral bodies, and posterior elements. The conus medullaris has been reported to terminate from T11 to the mid-L3 level but is typically found between T12–L1 and L1–L2. (c) Representative axial T2-weighted image of the lumbar spine at the level of the neuroforamen

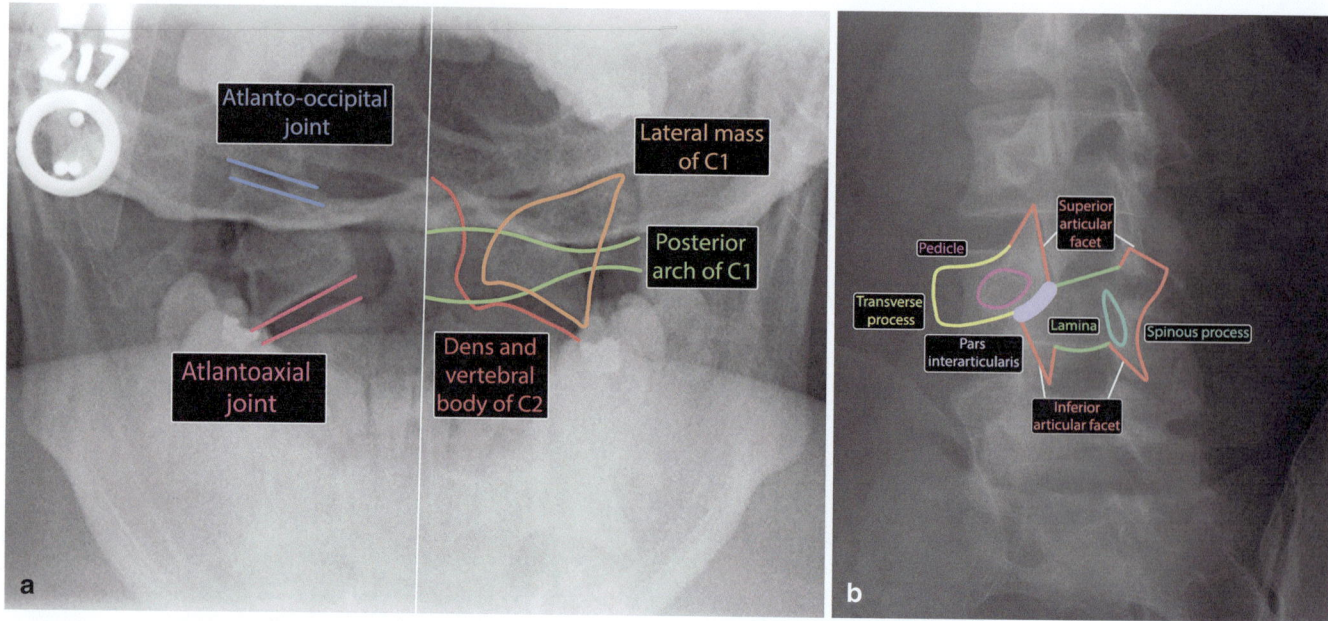

Fig. 20.5 (a) Odontoid view showing the normal atlanto-occipital and atlantoaxial joints and C1 and C2 relationship on plain film radiograph (X-ray). (b) Oblique radiograph of the lumbar spine demonstrating the "Scottie dog sign," comprised of superimposed posterior elements. The transverse process represents the nose of the dog. The pedicle forms the eye, inferior articular facet forms the front leg, superior articulating facet forms the ear, the pars interarticular (the portion of the lamina between the facets) forms the neck, the opposite side inferior articulating facet forms the hind leg, and the opposite side superior articulating facet forms the tail

Ligaments [1, 2] (Figs. 20.3 and 20.4)

- Anterior longitudinal ligament.
  - Band of fibers that extend along the ventral surface of the spine, attaching to the atlas and axis cranially and blending into the presacral fibers caudally.
  - The deepest fibers span one intervertebral level, the intermediate layer spans two or three vertebrae, and the superficial layer connects four or five vertebrae.
  - It most firmly attaches to the articular lip of each vertebral body and loosely attaches to the connective tissue encircling the annulus.
- Posterior longitudinal ligament.
  - Band of fibers located within the vertebral canal and extends from the dens (tectorial membrane) cranially to the sacrum caudally.
  - The posterior longitudinal ligament is separated from the spinal cord dura by the epidural space. This space can be effaced in the setting of trauma (epidural hematoma), infection (epidural abscess), or masses.
- Ligamentum flavum (aka yellow ligament).
  - Paired ligament that connects the spinal laminae and forms the posterior wall of the spinal canal.
  - Laterally, the ligamentum flavum is fused with the capsule of the facet joints, forming the boundaries of the intervertebral neural foramina.
  - Similar to the posterior longitudinal ligament, the ligamentum flavum is separated from the adjacent dura by the epidural space and can become effaced in the setting of trauma, infection, or masses.
- Interspinous ligament.
  - Attachments: ventrally continuous with the ligamentum flavum. Connects the anterior margin of the caudal spinous process and the inferior margin of the cranial spinous process.
  - Consists of a ventral, middle, and dorsal part. The middle is thickest and often oriented in an "s" configuration.
- Supraspinous ligament.
  - Attachment: spinous process apices from C7 to L3 or L4.
  - Absent at the L5/S1 level and is replaced by the medial tendons of the erector spinae muscle.
  - Continuous with the dorsal part of the interspinous ligament.

20 Normal Spine Anatomy and Imaging

Intervertebral Discs and Facet Joints [1–3] (Figs. 20.1, 20.2, 20.3, and 20.4)

INTERVERTEBRAL DISCS

- Articulate with vertebral endplates of adjacent vertebral bodies from C2 to S1 forming fibrocartilaginous joints to provide cushioning for the spine.
- The nucleus pulposus is located centrally, whereas the annulus fibrosus is located peripherally (Fig. 20.3a).
- Cartilaginous endplates, made from hyaline cartilage, produce flat central depression on the vertebral endplate.
- When discs herniate into the epidural space (Fig. 20.6), they are localized to the:
  o Central zone (if eccentric, the herniation can be categorized as right central or left central).
    - Because the posterior longitudinal ligament is strongest and thickest at the midline, a central protrusion will typically deflect to one side or another.
  o Lateral recess (which is also used interchangeably with the term subarticular zone, although some authors specifically apply lateral zone only at the level of the pedicles).
- Discs can also herniate into the:
  o Foraminal zones (within the neuroforamina).
  o Extraforaminal zones (outside the neuroforamina along the lateral aspects of the vertebral body).
  o Anterior zone (along the anterior body of the vertebra).
- The above disc herniation nomenclature is typically applied to the lumbar spine and not to the cervical or thoracic vertebrae.

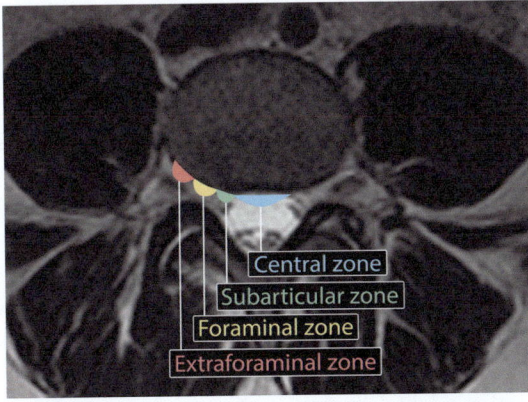

Fig. 20.6 Representative schematic of nomenclature localizing disc herniations. Disc herniations in the central zone typically deviate slightly off midline to the right or left given the thickness of the posterior longitudinal ligament at midline. Not shown is the lateral recess as this is found at the level of the pedicles

FACET (Aka Zygapophyseal) JOINTS

- Synovial-lined articular joint within a fibrous capsule.
- Joins the pedicle-lamina junction between the inferior articular process of one vertebral level and the superior articular process of the subjacent vertebral level (Figs. 20.1 and 20.2).
- Stabilized by the posterior ligamentous complex which contains the ligamentum flavum, interspinous ligament, and supraspinous ligament (Figs. 20.3 and 20.4).
- Facet joints at the cervical and thoracic levels are oriented in the coronal plane and hence are better evaluated in the axial or sagittal plane, whereas at the lumbar spine are oriented in the sagittal plane and hence are better viewed in the axial plane.
- Facet joint tropism refers to asymmetric variations in paired facet joints.

Distinctive Bony and Ligamentous Anatomy [1, 2, 4, 5]

CERVICAL SPINE

- Generally shared characteristics include:
  o Uncinate process (Figs. 20.1c, 20.7b, and 20.8c) at the lateral aspect of superior vertebral bodies that form uncovertebral (aka Luschka) joints (between C3 and C7).
  o The uncinate processes are unique to the cervical spine.
  o Bifid spinous processes (except C7).
  o Bilateral transverse foramina transmitting vertebral arteries (except C7).
- Unique cervical vertebrae (Figs. 20.7 and 20.8).
  o C1 (aka atlas) is a ring consisting of anterior and posterior arches and paired lateral masses instead of a vertebral body. CI articulates with the dens and occipital condyles through the atlantoaxial and atlanto-occipital joints, respectively.
  o C2 (aka axis) has a superiorly oriented odontoid process or dens, which lies just posterior to the C1 anterior arch and provides functional head rotation at the atlantoaxial joint.
  o C7 has small transverse foramina that does not contain vertebral arteries. It also has a rounded (not bifid) and prominent palpable spinous process (called vertebra prominens).
- Nuchal ligament (Fig. 20.3b).

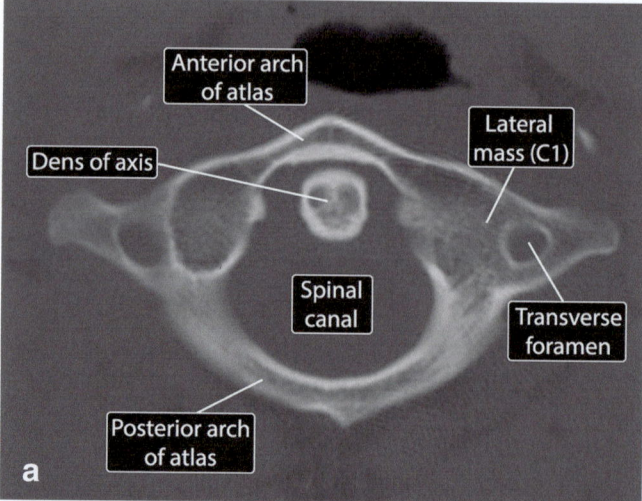

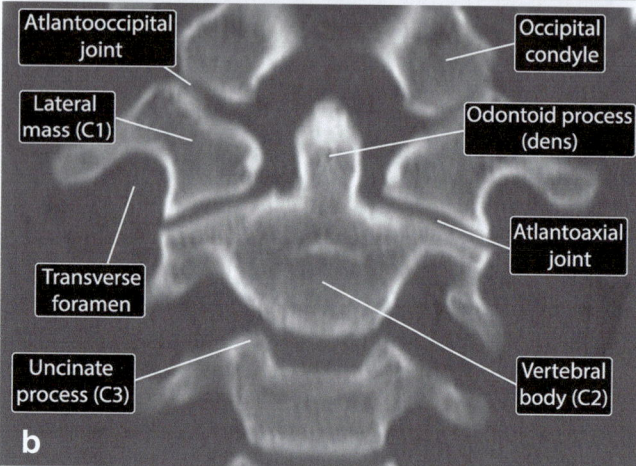

Fig. 20.7 (a) Axial CT image of C1 demonstrating its unique ring-shaped morphology without a vertebral body and its relationship with the dens (aka odontoid process) of C2. (b) Coronal CT image centered on C2 showing the unique presence of the dens (aka odontoid process) as well as the normal relationship of C1 with the occipital condyles and C1 with C2. Again, note the uncinate process that only exists in the cervical spine

- Composed of two parts [6]:
  - Lamellar: anterior double-layered portion containing fatty areolar tissue.
  - Funicular: posterior fibrous component composed of fused layers of the lamellar portion.
- Attachment: The funicular portion connects the external occipital protuberance cranially to the C7 spinous process caudally.
- Continues below C7 as the interspinous ligament in the thoracic spine.
- Covered by multiple layers of cervical fascia and aponeurosis of the trapezius muscle.
- The lamellar portion also extends from the external occipital protuberance to the C7 spinous process. Anteriorly, the paired layers are attached to the spinous process of the cervical spine and are inseparable from the interspinous ligaments.

CRANIOCERVICAL JUNCTION (Figs. 20.3b, 20.9, and e20.2)

- The craniocervical junction features unique anatomy and biomechanics which allows for a range of motion not seen in other parts of the spine.
- Comprised the occipital condyles, C1, C2, and their articulations.
- Important ligaments crucial for maintaining the stability of the craniocervical junction include:
  - Cruciate ligaments (aka cruciform; Fig. 20.9a).
    - Composed of three separate ligaments:
      - Superior longitudinal fibers.
      - Transverse ligaments.
      - Inferior longitudinal fibers.
    - Provides stability during motion (flexion, extension, and lateral movement) of C1 on C2.
    - Avulsion of the transverse ligament requires internal fixation as healing with external immobilization alone is slim [7].
  - Alar ligament (Fig. 20.9a).
    - Paired ligaments from the foramen magnum adjacent to the occipital condyles to the dens of the axis (C2).
    - Injury to the alar ligaments can result in upper cervical hypermobility and, most severely, occipitocervical dislocation.
  - Apical ligament.
    - Attachments: the tip of the odontoid process of C2 to midline anterior rim of the foramen magnum (basion).
    - Often seen as a vestigial structure without significant contribution to craniocervical stability.
- Craniocervical junction injuries can result in severe morbidity. The following craniocervical intervals are key measurements, especially in the setting of trauma, to rule out suspected injuries (Fig. e20.2):
  - Atlantodental interval = distance between C1 anterior arch and dens:
    - >3 mm in men or >2.5 mm in females is abnormal on radiographs.
    - > 2 mm is abnormal in adults on CT.

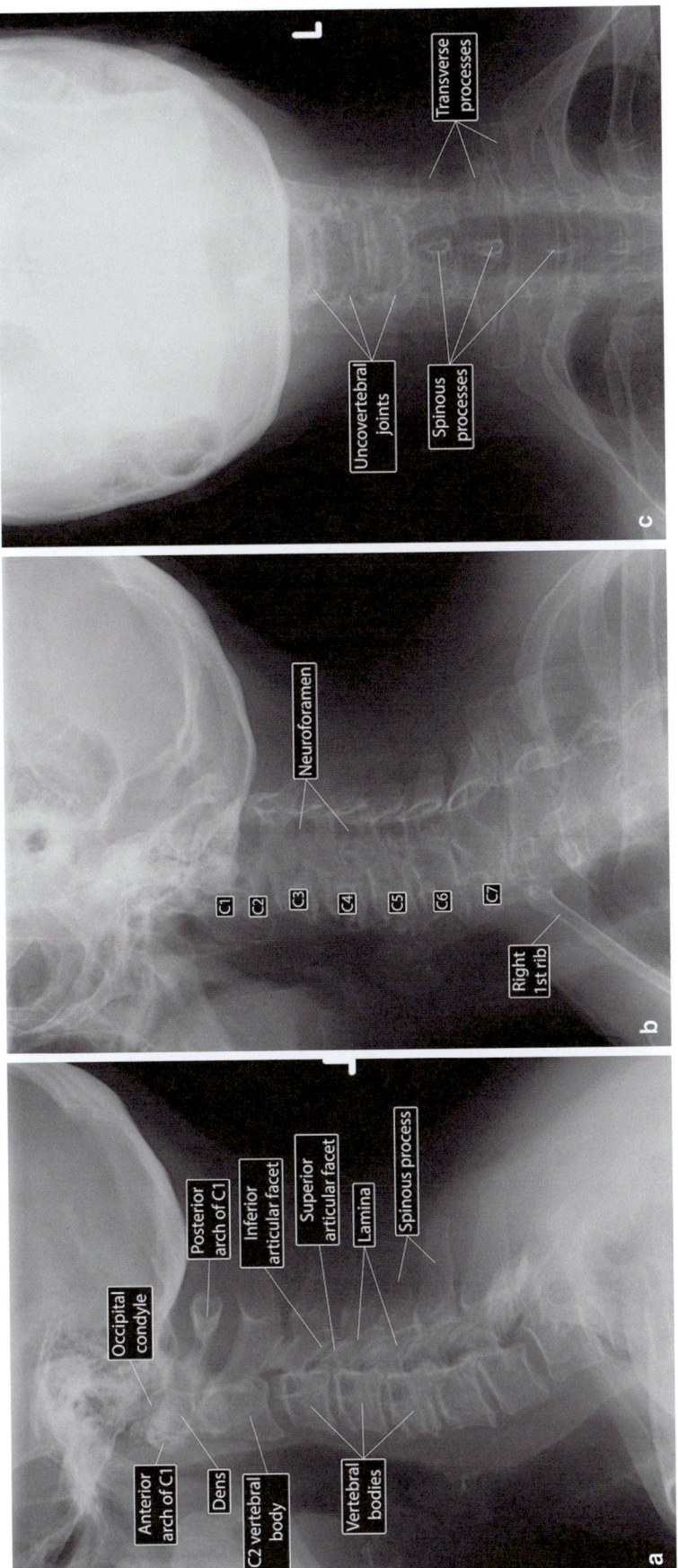

Fig. 20.8 Allowing for degenerative changes in this older patient, representative plain film radiographs of the cervical spine on (a) left lateral view, (b) left anterior oblique view, and (c) anterior–posterior view. The oblique radiographic views of the cervical spine allow for evaluation of the neuroforamen. The neuroforamen being evaluated is opposite to the patient's positioning. In a left anterior oblique view, the right neuroforamina would be assessed

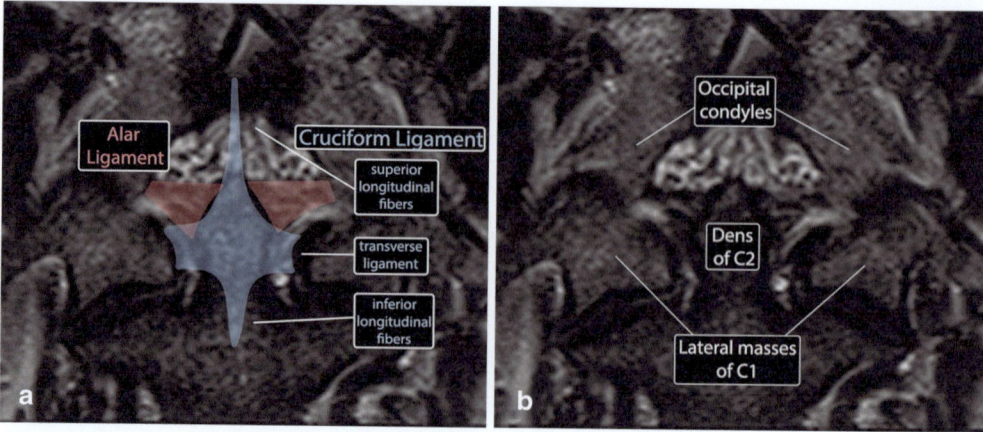

Fig. 20.9 (a) Coronal schematic representation of the cruciform (aka cruciate) ligament and alar ligaments overlayed on a coronal T2-weighted image of the craniocervical junction. The ligament is posterior to the dens and comprises the superior longitudinal fibers, the transverse ligaments, and inferior longitudinal fibers. (b) Coronal T2-weighted image of the craniocervical junction

- >5 mm is abnormal in children on radiographs.
- >3 mm is abnormal in children on CT.
  o Basion-dens interval = distance between basion and tip of the dens:
  - >12 mm is abnormal in adults on radiographs.
  - >10 mm is abnormal in adults on CT.
  o Powers ratio = basion to posterior arch of C1/opisthion to anterior arch of C1:
  - On CT, a power ratio > 0.9 is abnormal.
  - On radiographs, a power ratio > 1.0 is abnormal.

THORACIC SPINE

- At T2–T8, the thoracic vertebra articulates with each rib at three points:
  o Superior demifacet articulates with its corresponding rib at the costovertebral joint.
  o Costal facet along the transverse process again articulates with the rib at the costotransverse joint.
  o Inferior demifacet articulates with the inferior rib.
- T9 may have the variable presence of a demifacet. T10 may have a complete facet if T9 does not have demifacets, whereas if T9 has demifacets so will T10.
- T1, T11, and T12 vertebrae have additional minor differences in anatomy:
  o T1 more resembles the lower cervical vertebrae in morphology and contains a complete facet for the first rib and a demifacet for the second rib.
  o T11 and T12 contain a costal facet for the atypical 11th rib without facets on the transverse processes.
  o T12 resembles a lumbar vertebrae.

LUMBAR SPINE

- Pars interarticularis of the lumbar spine are located between the superior and inferior articular processes bilaterally and seen at the junction of the pedicle and lamina on the axial plane (Fig. 20.5b).
- L5 transverse processes are thick, short, and pyramidal in shape.
- Iliolumbar ligaments.
  o Paired ligaments (anterior/posterior and bilaterally) of the last lumbar vertebra. However, this landmark cannot be reliably used to identify the L5 vertebrae in cases of lumbosacral transitional vertebrae.
  o Laterally, the anterior and posterior iliolumbar ligaments insert at the iliac tuberosity.
  o Functions to provide stability of the lower lumbar spine and pelvis.

SACRUM AND COCCYX

- Fused five sacral and four rudimentary coccygeal segments that are not separated by intervertebral discs.
- Sacrum.
  o Formed by the sacral body centrally and paired sacral ala, which articulates with the ilium at the sacroiliac joint.
  o Sacral promontory is the anterior edge of the superior sacral facet.
  o Posteriorly, the median sacral crest represents fused spinous processes.
  o Sacral canal is the inferior continuation of the spinal canal and contains the caudal equina, which terminates inferiorly at the sacral hiatus.

20 Normal Spine Anatomy and Imaging

- Coccyx.
  - Formed by modified small vertebral bodies, without spinal canal or large processes.
  - Labeled as "Co#," as "C#" is used to denote cervical spine levels.

VARIANT ANATOMY [8–11]

- C1 posterior arch incomplete fusion anomalies are common.
- C2.
  - Os odontoideum is congenital failure of fusion between dens and C2 vertebral body and can lead to atlantoaxial instability.
  - Persistent ossiculum terminale appears similar to os odontoideum but is located at the tip of the dens and is considered stable.
- Arcuate foramen represents unilateral or bilateral calcification of the C1 posterior atlanto-occipital membrane that transmits the vertebral artery.
- Limbus vertebra is a well-corticated triangular vertebral body corner, usually at the anterosuperior corner.
- Transitional vertebrae, which may be unilateral or bilateral.
  - Cervical ribs are accessory ribs at C7. They can cause thoracic outlet syndrome by compressing the brachial plexus or subclavian vessels.
  - Lumbar rib at L1.
  - Lumbosacral transitional vertebra, including lumbarization of S1 and sacralization of L5.

Spinal Canal and Spinal Cord [2, 12–14]

EPIDURAL SPACE (Figs. 20.4b and 20.10)

- The space between the ligamentum flavum and the dura.
- Extends from the foramen magnum to the sacral hiatus where it terminates at the sacrococcygeal ligament.
- Communicates with the paravertebral spaces bilaterally.
- Contains fat, veins (including the anterior and posterior internal vertebral plexuses (Supplementary Fig. e20.1), and arteries.
- It is a common site for analgesia as well as a possible site of infection.

SPINAL MENINGES (Fig. 20.10)

- The connective layers that wrap concentrically around the spinal cord, spinal nerve roots, and the spinal vasculature.
- The three layers of the spinal meninges are:
  - Dura Mater.
    - Extends from the foramen magnum caudally, terminating as the filum between the S1 and S2 vertebral bodies.
    - Only has one dural layer, unlike the cranial meninges.
    - Attaches laterally to the periosteum of the margin of the neuroforamen.
    - Attaches ventrally via anterior epidural ligaments (aka ligaments of Hoffman).

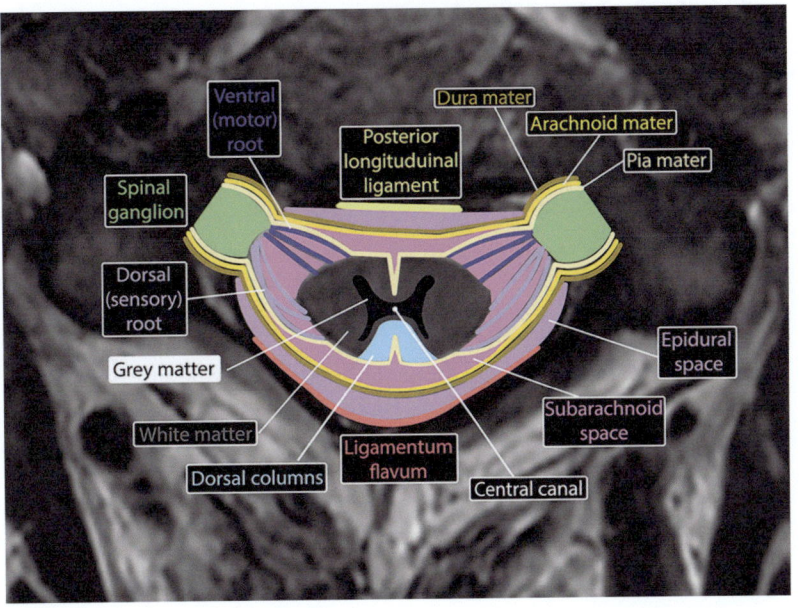

Fig. 20.10 Axial schematic representation of the spinal canal, spinal cord, nerve roots, meninges, posterior longitudinal ligament, ligamentum flavum, and epidural space at the cervical level. Not pictured are arachnoid trabeculations/septa or dentate ligaments

- Anterior midline epidural ligament that attaches to the posterior longitudinal ligament is also called the ligament of Trolard.
  ○ Arachnoid Mater.
    - Thin membrane deep to the dura mater enveloping the spinal cord, spinal nerve roots, cauda equina, spinal vessels, and intradural segment of the radicular vessels.
    - Attachments between the arachnoid and dura mater are fragile thin strands of collagen.
    - Attachments between the arachnoid and pia mater are web-like trabeculations.
  ○ Pia Mater.
    - Deepest layer and attaches directly to the glia limitans of the spinal cord, fusing into the filum terminale inferiorly.
    - Forms 20 pairs of dentate ligaments.
      ■ Bilateral extensions which pierce the arachnoid and attach to the inner dura which helps to stabilize the cord.
    - As stated above, the arachnoid and pia mater fuse laterally. Subpial collagen separates the spinal pia mater from the glia limitans of the spinal cord. Vessels coursing in the subarachnoid space have a leptomeningeal layer continuous with the pia mater.

SUBDURAL SPACE

- A potential space between the dura and arachnoid mater that does not exist under physiological conditions.
- Emerges under conditions where neurothelial cells break up along the dura-arachnoid surface.

SUBARACHNOID SPACE

- Subarachnoid space is located between the arachnoid mater and pia mater.
  ○ Filled with CSF.
  ○ Continuous with the subarachnoid space at the foramen magnum.
  ○ Terminates between S1 and S2.
  ○ Inferior to the conus medullaris, the spinal subarachnoid space forms the lumbar cistern.
  ○ The dentate ligaments (described above in Pia Mater) divide the spinal subarachnoid space into the ventral and dorsal chambers.
  ○ Arachnoid trabeculations form a dorsal septum that separates the dorsal chamber into right and left compartments.
  ○ Laterally, the subarachnoid space encompasses the spinal nerve roots and nerves, merging with the pia mater.
  ○ Vessels and nerve roots traverse the subarachnoid space.

Spinal Cord (Figs. 20.3 and 20.10)

GENERAL ANATOMY

- The spinal cord extends from the foramen magnum to approximately L2.
- Larger in the cervical (C5–T1) and lumbar (T11–Conus) regions (known as cervical and lumbar enlargements).
- Caudally, the conus medullaris is anchored to the coccygeus via the filum terminale.
- Separated into 31 segments (8 cervical, 12 thoracic, 5 lumbar, 5 sacral, and 1 coccygeal) with each segment giving rise to a pair of spinal nerves that exit via the neuroforamina.
- Spinal nerve naming convention:
  ○ Spinal nerves C1–C7 exit above their respective vertebrae.
  ○ The eighth cervical nerve exits between C7 and T1.
  ○ Spinal nerves T1–Co1 exit below their respective vertebrae (i.e. at the L4–L5 level, the exiting nerve is L4 and the traversing nerve is L5).
- Each spinal nerve attaches to the spinal cord via a ventral and dorsal root, which are composed of several rootlets.
  ○ Axons of motor neurons make up the ventral rootlets.
  ○ Axons of sensory neurons make up the dorsal rootlets.
- Dorsal roots.
  ○ Arises from the spinal cord at the dorsolateral sulcus.
  ○ Composed of sensory fibers from skin, subcutaneous tissue, deep tissue, and viscera.
  ○ Each dorsal nerve root has a corresponding dorsal root ganglion or spinal ganglion which is located in the neuroforamen.
    - Dorsal root ganglion is susceptible to compression and is an important consideration in low back pain and radiculopathy.
- Ventral roots.
  ○ Arises from the spinal cord at the ventrolateral sulcus.
  ○ Composed mostly of efferent somatic motor nerve fibers.
- The spinal cord is hemisected anteriorly by the anterior median fissure (sulcus) and posteriorly by the posterior median fissure (sulcus).
- White matter.
  ○ Myelinated axons that are located on the outer portion of the spinal cord.

- White matter axon bundles are broadly subdivided into columns:
  - Dorsal (posterior) columns contain fasciculi cuneatus and gracilis. They carry sensory information from mechanoreceptors such as vibration, conscious proprioception, and fine touch.
    - Fasciculus gracilis carries information from T7 and below and is thus present in the entire spinal cord.
    - Fasciculus cuneatus carries information from C1 to C6 and is found lateral to the fasciculus gracilis at these levels.
  - Lateral columns contain the corticospinal tract, which is the principal motor pathway.
  - Ventral (anterior) columns contain the spinothalamic tracts, which carry sensory information involving pain, pressure, and temperature as well as coarse touch.
- Gray matter.
  - Located in the interior of the spinal cord in a "butterfly" or H-shaped pattern and is divided into dorsal (posterior), ventral (anterior), and lateral horns.
  - Dorsal horn contains neurons that carry sensory information.
  - Ventral horn contains the bodies of motor neurons.
  - Laterals horns are found from T1–L2 and contain the bodies of the sympathetic nervous system
- Central Canal.
  - CSF-filled space lined with ependyma located centrally within the cord in the gray matter.
  - Typically 1–2 mm in width.

BLOOD SUPPLY

- The spinal cord is supplied by 3 longitudinal arteries.
  - A single anterior spinal artery supplies the anterior two-third of the spinal cord.
    - Arises from the V4 segments of the vertebral artery.
    - Travels caudally along the anterior median fissure.
    - Reinforced by branches arising from the vertebral, ascending cervical, deep cervical, posterior intercostal, subcostal, lumbar, and lateral sacral arteries.
    - The Artery of Adamkiewicz is an important supplier to the T8 cord and caudally.
      - This forms the dominant supply of the lower spinal cord.
      - Injury to this vessel can result in anterior cord infarct.
      - Famously makes a "hair-pin" turn as it anastomoses with the anterior spinal artery.
      - Arises from either the posterior intercostal, subcostal, or lumbar arteries which arise from the aorta.
  - Paired posterior spinal arteries.
    - Arises from the posterior inferior cerebellar artery or potentially the distal vertebral artery.
    - Travels caudally along the posterolateral aspects of the cord.
    - Also receives vascular supply from sources to the anterior spinal artery.

Brachial Plexus [15, 16]

- Formed from the ventral rami of C5–T1 (with some contribution from C4 and T2).
  - Provides sensory and motor innervation of the upper extremity.
  - Five components (from proximal to distal):
    - Roots (ventral rami from spinal nerves):
      - Innervation of the scalene and longus colli muscles (C5–C8).
      - Long thoracic nerve innervates the serratus anterior muscle (C5–C7).
      - Phrenic nerve innervates the diaphragm (C5).
      - Dorsal scapular nerve innervates the rhomboid and levator scapulae muscles (C5).
    - Trunks (as the nerves exit the posterior triangle of the neck between the anterior and middle scalene muscles):
      - Upper trunk = C5 and C6 ventral rami:
        - Suprascapular nerve supplies the supraspinatus and infraspinatus muscles and sensation to the acromioclavicular and glenohumeral joints.
        - Subclavian nerve innervates the subclavius muscle.
      - Middle trunk = continuation of C7 nerve.
      - Inferior trunk = C8 and T1.
    - Divisions (between the clavicle and first rib):
      - Anterior.
      - Posterior.
    - Cords (named based on relation to the axillary artery):
      - Posterior.
        - Upper subscapular nerve (C5–C6) innervates the subscapularis muscle.
        - Middle subscapular nerve (C6–C8), also known as the thoracodorsal nerve, innervates the latissimus dorsi muscle.
        - Lower subscapular nerve (C5–C6) innervates the subscapularis and teres major muscles.

- Medial.
  - Medial pectoral nerve (C8–T1) innervates the pectoralis major and minor.
  - Medial brachial cutaneous nerve (C8–T1) provides sensory innervation from the medial aspect of the arm.
  - Medial antebrachial cutaneous nerve (C5–C6) provides sensory innervation from the lateral aspect of the arm.
- Lateral.
  - Lateral pectoral nerve (C5–C7) innervates the pectoralis major muscle.
- Terminal nerves.
  - Musculocutaneous nerve (C5–C7) innervates the biceps brachii, coracobrachialis, and brachialis muscles. Also becomes the lateral antebrachial cutaneous nerve providing sensory innervation from the lateral upper forearm.
  - Median nerve (C6–T1 from the medial and lateral cords) innervates the pronator teres, flexor carpi radialis, palmaris longus, and flexor digitorum superficialis muscles. This nerve also provides sensory innervation to the lateral 3 ½ fingers of the palm.
  - Ulnar nerve (C8–T1 from the medial cord) innervates the flexor digitorum profundus and flexor carpi ulnaris muscle, as well as muscles in the hand and fingers. This nerve also provides sensory innervation to the small finger and half of the ring finger.
  - Axillary nerve (C5–C6 from the posterior cord) innervates the deltoid and teres minor muscles.
  - Radial nerve (C5–T1 from the posterior cord) innervates triceps brachii, anconeus, extensor carpi radialis longus, brachioradialis, supinator, and extensor carpi radialis brevis muscles. This nerve also provides sensory innervation to the dorsal aspect of the thumb, index, and middle fingers.

Imaging of the Spine

Many of the fine anatomic structures detailed above are beyond the resolution of standard commonly used imaging techniques, even MRI. However, knowledge of their existence, even structures we cannot routinely visualize, plays a vital role in localizing pathology, inferring injuries that require urgent intervention and understanding the imaging appearance of pathology and normal artifacts that may appear (especially with MRI).

Plain Radiograph [17]

CERVICAL SPINE (Fig. 20.8)

- Anterior posterior (AP).
- Lateral (Lat).
- Oblique.
  - Assesses the neuroforamina.
  - In an AP Oblique, the patient will be positioned in either a right posterior oblique (RPO) or left posterior oblique (LPO) position. The neuroforamina examined is opposite the patient's positioning.
    - In other words, an RPO will assess the LEFT foramina.
- Flexion and extension.
  - Assesses dynamic instability.
- "Swimmer's View."
  - Lateral view taken with one of the arms up (as in a crawl stroke) to better assess the cervicothoracic junction.
- PEG view (aka open mouth view; Fig. 20.5a).
  - AP projection of the C1 and C2 with the patient's mouth open.
  - The "peg" refers to the odontoid (dens) of C2.
  - Primarily used to detect odontoid or Jefferson fractures.

THORACIC SPINE

- AP.
- Lat (with arms raised forward to uncover the thoracic spine).

LUMBOSACRAL SPINE

- AP.
- Lat.
- Flexion and extension.
  - Assesses dynamic instability.
- Oblique.
  - Assesses the articulating facets.

20 Normal Spine Anatomy and Imaging

CT [2]

CERVICAL, THORACIC, AND LUMBAR SPINE

- Axial soft tissue and bone algorithm.
- Sagittal and coronal bone algorithm.

MRI (Standard Noncontrast) [1, 2]

CERVICAL, THORACIC, AND LUMBAR SPINE

- Sagittal T1-weighted.
  - Vertebral cortical bone is hypointense.
  - Bone marrow is hyperintense to disc or muscle due to fatty marrow in adults.
  - Disc.
    - Annulus fibrosis is hypointense.
    - Nucleus pulposus is slightly hypointense to bone marrow.
  - Ligaments are hypointense.
  - Fat is hyperintense (e.g., epidural fat).
  - CSF is hypointense.
  - Cord and nerve roots are isointense and similar to disc signal.
  - Large blood vessels demonstrate signal voids.
- Sagittal and axial T2-weighted.
  - Vertebral cortical bone is hypointense.
  - Bone marrow is hyperintense due to fatty marrow in adults.
  - Disc (Fig. 20.3a).
    - Annulus fibrosis is hypointense.
    - Nucleus pulposus is slightly hyperintense.
  - Ligaments are hypointense.
  - Fat is hyperintense (e.g., epidural fat).
  - CSF is hyperintense.
  - Cord and nerve roots are isointense.
    - On axial sequences, gray and white matter differentiation can be better visualized with gray matter slightly hyperintense relative to white matter.
  - Large blood vessels demonstrate signal voids.
  - Venous structures such as basivertebral veins will be hyperintense due to flow phenomenon (Fig. e20.1).
- Sagittal STIR (or other fat-suppressed techniques).
  - Vertebral cortical bone is hypointense.
  - Bone marrow is mildly hypointense due to the suppression of fatty marrow.
  - Disc.
    - Annulus fibrosis is hypointense.
    - Nucleus pulposus is slightly hyperintense.
  - Ligaments are hypointense.
  - Fat is suppressed (e.g., epidural fat).
  - CSF is hyperintense.
  - Cord and nerve roots are isointense.
  - Large blood vessels demonstrate signal voids.
  - Venous structures such as basivertebral veins or venous plexus will be hyperintense due to the slow flow phenomenon.
- Axial GRE (typically applied in the cervical spine).
  - Accentuates disc, cartilage, and venous hyperintense signal to help separate ligaments and disc material from bone and differentiate between osteophyte and herniated disc.
  - Differentiates gray and white matter, with gray matter hyperintense relative to the white matter.
  - Venous structures such as basivertebral veins or venous plexus are hyperintense.

COMMON MRI ARTIFACTS [2, 18] (Figs. 20.3 and 20.11)

- Gibbs (Fig. 20.11a).
  - Also known as truncation or ringing artifact is characterized by parallel lines formed through an image next to a high-contrast interface such as the CSF and spinal cord.
  - This can result in the false appearance of a syrinx.
- CSF pulsation (Figs. 20.3 and 20.11a, b).
  - CSF pulsates with the cardiac cycle. Systole increases intracranial pressure which is transmitted throughout the CSF caudally.
  - This results in time of flight and turbulent flow artifact which appears hypointense on T2-weighted sequences.
  - Arachnoid trabeculations form septa in the subarachnoid space, which along with the dentate ligaments form separate chambers. This results in the often segmented appearance of CSF pulsation artifact on axial T2-weighted images (Fig. 20.11b).
- Entry slice phenomenon (Fig. 20.11c).
  - Occurs when unsaturated spins in blood first enter into a slice or slices. It is characterized by the bright signal CSF on T1-weighted images.

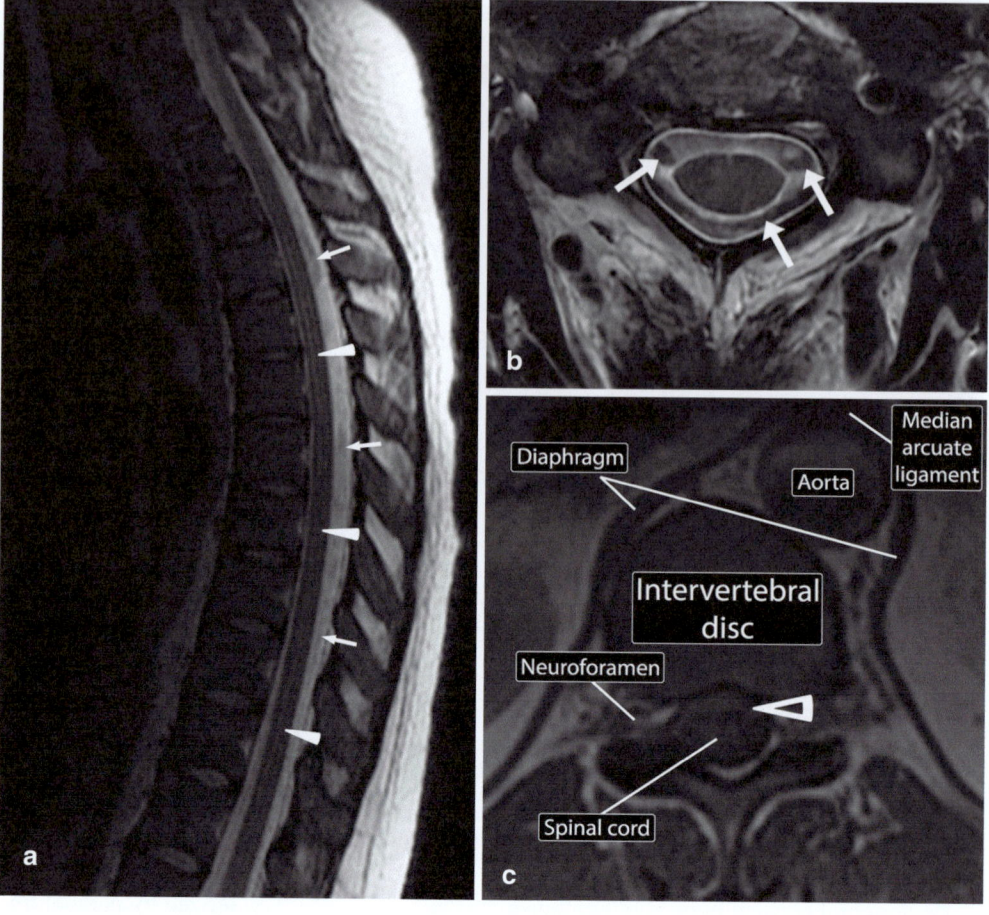

Fig. 20.11 (a) Sagittal T2-weighted image through the thoracic spine. Arrowheads point to Gibbs artifact (aka truncation or ringing artifact), which is a series of parallel lines adjacent to high-contrast interfaces. In the cord, this could be mistaken for syringohydromyelia. Small arrows point to regions of CSF pulsation artifact. (b) Axial T2-weighted image through the cervical spine. Arrows indicate regions of CSF pulsation artifact. (c) Axial T1-weighted image through the T12–L1 level. The arrowhead indicates a T1 hyperintense signal in the ventral CSF space compatible with the "entry slice" phenomenon. (Not shown: corresponding sagittal T1-weighted imaging through this level demonstrates no signal abnormality)

References

1. Bogduk N. Functional anatomy of the spine. Handb Clin Neurol. 2016;136:675–88.
2. Shanechi AM, Kiczek M, Khan M, Jindal G. Spine anatomy imaging: an update. Neuroimaging Clin N Am. 2019;29(4):461–80.
3. Fardon DF, Williams AL, Dohring EJ, Murtagh FR, Gabriel Rothman SL, Sze GK. Lumbar disc nomenclature: version 2.0: recommendations of the combined task forces of the North American Spine Society, the American Society of Spine Radiology and the American Society of Neuroradiology. Spine J. 2014;14(11):2525–45.
4. Diel J, Ortiz O, Losada RA, Price DB, Hayt MW, Katz DS. The sacrum: pathologic spectrum, multimodality imaging, and subspecialty approach. Radiographics. 2001;21(1):83–104.
5. Lirette LS, Chaiban G, Tolba R, Eissa H. Coccydynia: an overview of the anatomy, etiology, and treatment of coccyx pain. Ochsner J. 2014;14(1):84–7.
6. Kadri PA, Al-Mefty O. Anatomy of the nuchal ligament and its surgical applications. Neurosurgery. 2007;61(5 Suppl 2):301–4; discussion 4
7. Yashar MKS, Feiz-Erfan I, Dickman CA. Chapter 12: C1-C2 Trauma Injuries and Stabilization Techniques. In: Kim D, Vaccaro A, Dickman C, Cho D, Lee S, Kim I, editors. Surgical anatomy and techniques to the spine. 2nd ed. Saunders/Elsevier; 2013.
8. Carr RB, Fink KR, Gross JA. Imaging of trauma: Part 1, Pseudotrauma of the spine—osseous variants that may simulate injury. AJR Am J Roentgenol. 2012;199(6):1200–6.
9. Chang KZ, Likes K, Davis K, Demos J, Freischlag JA. The significance of cervical ribs in thoracic outlet syndrome. J Vasc Surg. 2013;57(3):771–5.
10. Konin GP, Walz DM. Lumbosacral transitional vertebrae: classification, imaging findings, and clinical relevance. AJNR Am J Neuroradiol. 2010;31(10):1778–86.
11. Smoker WR, Khanna G. Imaging the craniocervical junction. Childs Nerv Syst. 2008;24(10):1123–45.
12. Bican O, Minagar A, Pruitt AA. The spinal cord: a review of functional neuroanatomy. Neurol Clin. 2013;31(1):1–18.
13. Gailloud P. Spinal vascular anatomy. Neuroimaging Clin N Am. 2019;29(4):615–33.
14. Sakka L, Gabrillargues J, Coll G. Anatomy of the spinal meninges. Oper Neurosurg (Hagerstown). 2016;12(2):168–88.
15. Bayot ML, Nassereddin A, Varacallo M. Anatomy, shoulder and upper limb. Treasure Island, FL: Brachial Plexus. StatPearls; 2022.
16. Gilcrease-Garcia BM, Deshmukh SD, Parsons MS. Anatomy, imaging, and pathologic conditions of the brachial plexus. Radiographics. 2020;40(6):1686–714.
17. Lampignano JKL. Bontrager's textbook of radiographic positioning and related anatomy. 9th ed; 2017.
18. Lisanti C, Carlin C, Banks KP, Wang D. Normal MRI appearance and motion-related phenomena of CSF. AJR Am J Roentgenol. 2007;188(3):716–25.

Congenital and Developmental Malformations of the Spine

21

Anna Y. Li, Tarik F. Massoud, and Hisham Dahmoush

Terminology

Several terms that may be confusing and that are used extensively throughout the rest of the chapter are defined below.

- Neural placode—a segment of flat, non-neurulated embryonic neural tissue [1].
- Tethered cord syndrome—a clinical syndrome of progressive neurologic deterioration that results from chronic traction on the usually low-lying conus medullaris [1–3].
  o May be accompanied by a low-lying conus (see discussion on the development of the conus medullaris below), tight filum terminale, or related to developmental anomalies such as an intraspinal lipoma, lipomyelomeningocele (LMMC), or diastematomyelia [1].
  o May also result post-operatively following repair of a myelomeningocele (MMC), tight filum terminale, intraspinal lipoma, caudal agenesis, and so on [1, 3].
  o Cannot be excluded based on imaging findings as this is a clinical diagnosis.
  o Clinical manifestations: Abnormal reflexes, incontinence, spastic gait, motor and sensory dysfunction, and lower extremity deformities [1, 3].

- Spina bifida—incomplete/defective fusion of the osseous posterior elements of the vertebrae [4, 5].
- Spina bifida occulta—a more specific term than spina bifida which assumes that the spinal cord is normal and covered with skin despite the defective or incomplete fusion of the osseous vertebral posterior elements [5].
- Open spinal dysraphism (OSD)—neural tube defect whereby neural tissue is externally exposed through a spina bifida and skin defect [1].
- Closed spinal dysraphism (CSD)—neural tube defect whereby neural tissue is covered by skin.
  o Cutaneous stigmata are seen in up to 50% of patients [1].
- Syringomyelia—a fluid-filled cavity formed by cerebrospinal fluid (CSF) dissection of the spinal cord [6, 7].
  o Greater than 3 mm in diameter.
    - The term "prominent central canal" is preferred for the dilation of the central canal to the upper limit of normal (2–3 mm).
  o Extends lateral to, or is independent of, the central canal of the cord.
  o Typically involves the lower cervical or upper thoracic cord.
- Hydromyelia—ependymal-lined dilation of the central canal of the spinal cord [6, 7].
- Syringohydromyelia—syrinx involves the central canal and the spinal cord parenchyma; a term used when the distinction between syringomyelia and hydromyelia is not possible on imaging [6, 7].

Supplementary Information The online version contains supplementary material available at https://doi.org/10.1007/978-3-031-55124-6_21.

A. Y. Li
Department of Radiology, Stanford University School of Medicine, Palo Alto, CA, USA
e-mail: annayli@stanford.edu

T. F. Massoud
Department of Radiology, School of Medicine, Stanford University, Stanford, CA, USA
e-mail: tmassoud@stanford.edu

H. Dahmoush (✉)
Department of Radiology, Lucile Packard Children's Hospital at Stanford, Palo Alto, CA, USA
e-mail: dahmoush@stanford.edu

Brief Overview of Normal Development

An understanding of the embryologic development of the spine provides the foundation for comprehension of congenital spinal malformations. The development of the spine and spinal canal along with the spinal cord is a highly coordinated series of consecutive events that begins

Table 21.1 Congenital spinal malformation by stage of embryogenesis [4, 8]

Embryologic stage	Weeks of gestation	Anomaly
Gastrulation (notochord development)	Weeks 2–3	• Split notochord syndromes (i.e., diastematomyelia) • Neurenteric cyst/fistula • Caudal regression syndrome (CRS) • Segmental spinal dysgenesis
Primary neurulation (development of the brain and upper 90% of the spinal cord)	Weeks 3–4	• Open spinal dysraphism (e.g., myelocele and myelomeningocele) • Closed spinal dysraphism (e.g., lipomyelocele and lipomyelomeningocele) • Dermal sinus tract • Spinal inclusion cysts
Secondary neurulation (development of the lower 10% of the spinal cord and filum terminale)	Weeks 5–6	• Filar fibrolipoma • Tight filum terminale • Persistent terminal ventricle • Terminal myelocystocele • Sacrococcygeal teratoma • CRS
Segmentation	Weeks 4–6	• Spinal segmentation and formation anomalies

early in gestation. The four main sequential and partially overlapping processes are described below. Table 21.1 summarizes the types of spinal dysraphism by the embryologic stage during which the developmental error occurs [4, 8].

GASTRULATION (Weeks 2–3 of Gestation)

- Gastrulation begins on day 14 of gestation when the primitive streak, a stripe of thickened epiblast with totipotent cells, appears along the midline of the embryo's dorsal surface [4, 5, 9]. The epiblast contains the cells that will become the ectoderm. A focal thickening at the cephalad end of the primitive streak becomes the Hensen node [5, 9].
- Cells then invaginate between the epiblast and the endoderm at the primitive pit, a central depression that forms in the primitive streak [5, 9]. These cells form the mesoderm.
- The bilaminar embryonic disk is converted to a trilaminar disk composed of ectoderm, mesoderm, and endoderm [5, 9].
- The notochordal process is formed by a portion of the invaginating cells in the midline which migrate along the craniocaudal axis [5, 9].
- The notochord itself forms after the resorption of the floor of the notochordal process around day 20 [5, 9].

PRIMARY NEURULATION (Weeks 3–4 of Gestation)

- Responsible for the development of the brain and the upper 90% of the spinal cord [4, 9].
- On day 18, the notochord and the overlying ectoderm interact resulting in the formation of the neural plate, which rapidly elongates along with the underlying notochord [4, 5].
- The neural plate transforms into a neural groove on days 18–20, with thickened lateral margins of the groove that will eventually become neural crest cells [4].
- The neural plate then folds on itself to form a neural tube that closes bidirectionally around day 21 [5].
- The subsequent process of disjunction involves the detachment of the neural tube from the overlying ectoderm [4].
- Cells at the border of the neuroectoderm and ectoderm detach to form neural crests; neural crests subsequently fragment and become the primordia of the ganglia, giving rise to sensory innervations [5].
- The closure of the posterior neuropore defines the end of primary neurulation [9].

SECONDARY NEURULATION (Weeks 5–6 of Gestation)

- Responsible for development of the lower 10% of the spinal cord and the filum terminale [9].
- The distalmost portions of the notochord and the neural tube merge inferiorly at the caudal cell mass [4]. Infolding of the neural plate forms the secondary neural tube, which gives rise to the sacrum, coccyx, and L5 vertebral body [4, 9].
- The secondary neural tube subsequently undergoes cavitation until it contains a central canal, via a process termed canalization [9].
- Around day 38, the caudal cell mass decreases in size via apoptosis leading to the formation of the filum terminale

as well as the tip of the conus medullaris in a process called retrogressive differentiation [8, 9].
- The terminal ventricle is an expansion of the ependymal canal at the conus that represents a remnant of the lumen of the secondary neural tube [9].

SEGMENTATION (Weeks 4–6 of Gestation)

- Development of the vertebral column progresses simultaneously with that of the neural tube [5].
- A somite plate develops on each side of the neural tube, which then segments into somites. By the end of the fifth week, 42 pairs of somites are seen [5].
- Somites develop central cavitation with the internal side giving rise to the sclerotome [5]. The sclerotome migrates toward the notochord and gives rise to the vertebral primordial.

DEVELOPMENT AND ASCENT OF THE CONUS MEDULLARIS

- Early on in embryogenesis, each neural segment corresponds to the same segment of the spinal canal, and the spinal cord extends to the caudal end of the canal with each nerve root coursing laterally toward its neural foramen [7].
- However, as the embryo matures, vertebral bodies grow faster than the spinal cord, and the distal aspect of the cord undergoes retrogressive differentiation, leading to a relative ascent of the spinal cord within the canal and nerve roots traveling more caudal within the thecal sac to reach their respective exiting neural foramina [7].
- At 24 weeks of gestation, the conus should be no lower than the L3 level [7].
- At 33–40 weeks of gestation, the conus reaches its adult level at or cranial to the L1–L2 disc space and is usually located above the mid-L2 vertebral level by 2–3 months of age.
- After 2–3 months of age, if the conus terminates below the L2 inferior endplate, it is considered abnormal, and evaluation for a tethering mass should be considered [7].

Approach to Classification and the Role of Imaging

A systematic approach to classification of spinal dysraphism, based on the method described by Tortori-Donati and Rossi, is dependent on the initial clinical assessment of whether the spinal dysraphism is open or closed, as in if the neural tube defect is open to the air with exposure of the neural elements or covered by skin [3, 4, 9]. If the spinal dysraphism is closed, the malformation can be further classified by the presence or absence of an associated subcutaneous mass [2, 9]. Closed spinal dysraphic states without a subcutaneous mass may be subdivided further into simple and complex states (see Fig. 21.1). Table 21.2 highlights key differences between open and closed spinal dysraphism [2, 3, 8].

ULTRASOUND (US)

- Useful screening tool in neonates or small infants with suspected cord tethering, especially when a dimple is seen in the skin above the gluteal cleft is complex or large (greater than 5 mm) [1]. Evaluation of the location of the conus medullaris is an important aspect of screening.
- Specific indications for ultrasound of the neonatal spine in the setting of dysraphism include lumbosacral stigmata of spinal dysraphism, further evaluation of clinically suspected neural tube defects, spectrum of caudal regression syndrome, and post-operative assessment of cord re-tethering [2].
- A detection rate of 80–90% of OSDs has been reported with the use of high-frequency US transducer and three-dimensional (3D) US [2].
- In addition to operator dependence, US evaluation is limited by ossification of the neural arches and is generally not possible after 6 months of age [2].

COMPUTED TOMOGRAPHY (CT)

- Given the concerns regarding radiation dose exposure in children, CT is reserved for the evaluation of specific osseous features such as bony spurs, skeletal dysplasias, and vertebral anomalies [2].
- Tailoring the field of view (FOV) in addition to other techniques to reduce radiation dose is crucial to minimize radiation exposure in the pediatric population.

MAGNETIC RESONANCE IMAGING (MRI)

- Prenatal/fetal MRI is a crucial aspect in the selection of operative candidates for fetal surgical repair of open dysraphism and helps guide the prenatal counseling and management process [10].
- In OSD, the goals of pre-operative evaluation include defining the size and level of the open defect, identifying the presence of hindbrain herniation, and defining the

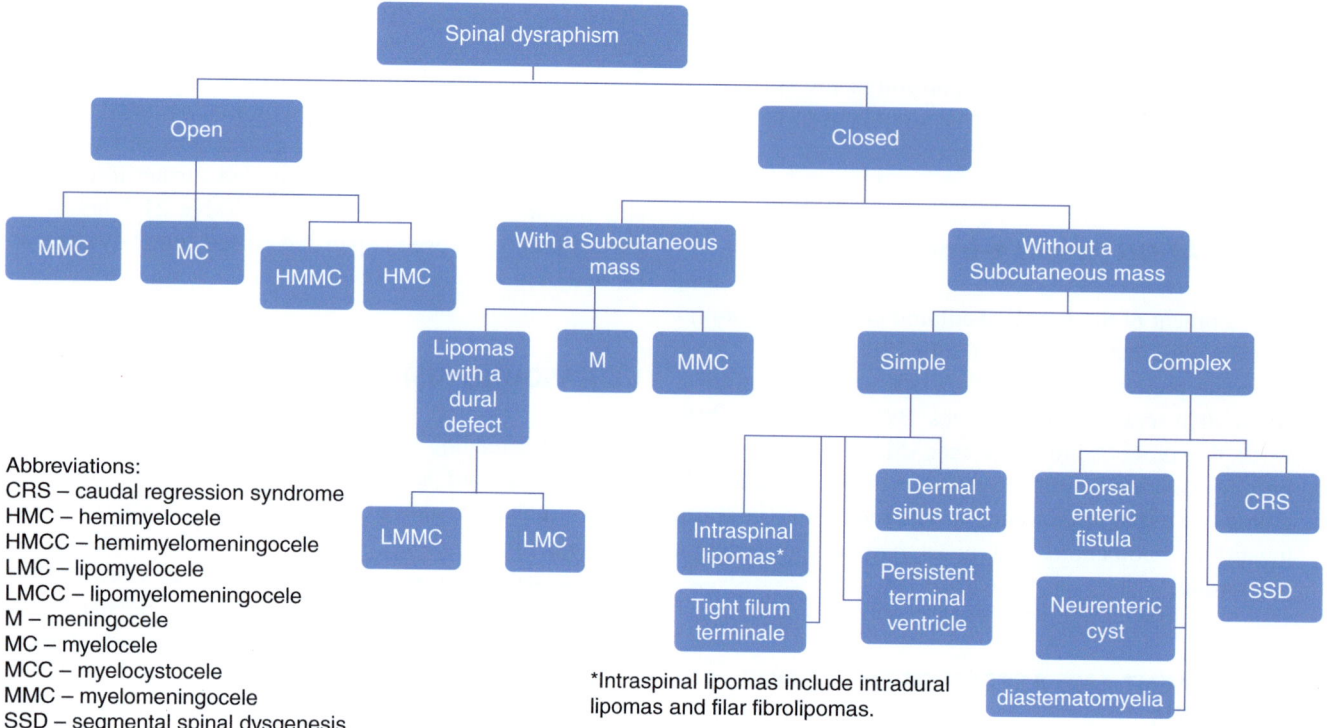

Fig. 21.1 Classification of spinal dysraphism, based on Tortori-Donati and Rossi method. *Intraspinal lipomas include intradural lipomas and filar fibrolipomas. Abbreviations: *CRS* caudal regression syndrome, *HMC* hemimyelocele, *HMMC* hemimyelomeningocele, *LMC* lipomyelocele, *LMMC* lipomyelomeningocele, *M* meningocele, *MC* myelocele, *MCC* myelocystocele, *MMC* myelomeningocele, *SSD* segmental spinal dysgenesis

Table 21.2 Comparison of open and closed spinal dysraphism [2, 3, 8]

Characteristic	Open spinal dysraphism	Closed spinal dysraphism
Etiology	• Incomplete or segmental defective closure of the neural tube results in a neural placode that fails to detach from the adjacent surface ectoderm	• Premature disjunction of the neural tube from the adjacent surface ectoderm before the neural tube is completely closed
Clinical presentation	• Midline, skin-deficient swelling over the back • CSF leakage • Complications such as meningitis or hydrocephalus may be the presenting symptoms	• A skin-covered mass over the back or neurocutaneous stigmata (e.g., sacral dimple and patch of hair)
Imaging	• Sac over the neural tube defect with the extension of the subarachnoid space through bony defect and the presence of neural tissue within the sac	• Low-lying or blunted conus medullaris, thickened and fatty filum, intradural or subcutaneous lipoma, fixed dorsal position of the cord on US, among specific entities
Treatment	• Prenatal surgery OR • C-section delivery with the closure of the spinal defect within the first 48 h after birth • May require ventricular shunting	• Post-natal surgery to address spinal cord tethering and possible resection of an associated lesion
Prognosis	• Worse prognosis (injury to the neural placode from deranged neuroarchitecture and chronic exposure to amniotic fluid)	• Better clinical and neurologic prognosis (lower risk of scoliosis, may be able to walk)
Associated anomalies	• Chiari 2 malformation	• Omphalocele-extrophy-imperforate anus-spinal defects (OEIS) complex

anatomic relationship between the neural placode and nerve roots [10].
- In CSD, the goals of pre-operative evaluation include delineating the type, location, and extent of dysraphism; specifically, the location of the lipoma–placode interface, level of the cord termination, status of the conus and filum, and presence of tethering are crucial to report [2].
- MRI also allows the identification of associated intraspinal lesions with the malformation, such as dermoid and epidermoid cysts [4].
- Intracranial evaluation for hydrocephalus is often performed concurrently, as shunting of CSF may be achieved at the time of repair of the spinal malformation [2, 4].
- In the post-operative setting, MRI is important in the detection of complications including infection, CSF leak, adhesions, re-tethering, and dermoid/epidermoid cyst formation [2].

Open Spinal Dysraphism

- OSD is one of the most common congenital abnormalities of the central nervous system (CNS) and is nearly always detected prenatally.
- Maternal serum screening with alpha-fetoprotein (AFP) can detect up to 90% of OSDs [10]. Elevated acetylcholinesterase also confirms the presence of an OSD, and amniocentesis can be performed to identify fetal karyotype prior to fetal surgery [10].
- OSD results from defective closure of the primary neural tube, which results in a neural placode that fails to detach from the adjacent surface ectoderm [5].
- Imaging findings:
    - There is a deficiency of the soft tissues and bones overlying the neural tube defect with absent vertebral posterior elements at the level of the defect [2].
    - The neural placode is flattened and either at the same level with the cutaneous surface, i.e., myelocele (MC), or pushed dorsal to the adjacent skin within a CSF-filled sac formed by extension of the subarachnoid space through the spina bifida, i.e., MMC [2, 3].
    - The conus medullaris is usually not formed, and the cord is low-lying and dysplastic.
    - Syringohydromyelia may be seen as superior to the OSD [5].
- The clinical presentation of patients with OSD includes a skin and soft tissue deficient area of swelling over the midline back, and patients may present with CSF leakage, meningitis, or hydrocephalus [2].

- Clinical features common to both OSD and CSD include neurogenic bladder and bowel, progressive scoliosis, and lower extremity abnormalities including leg-length discrepancy and spasticity [1, 2].
- Diagnostic concerns:
    - Type 2 CM.
    - Hydrocephalus.
    - Post-operative complications.
- > 90% of children with an OSD have an associated type 2 CM [2, 6, 9]. (See complete discussion on the Chiari malformations later in this chapter.)
    - Chronic leakage of CSF at the level of the neural placode leads to incomplete/defective expansion of the rhomboencephalic vesicle, limiting normal growth of the skull base and posterior fossa [5].
- Goals of pre-operative imaging:
    - Determine the type of OSD and level of defect.
    - Need to image the entire spine to exclude the presence of syringohydromyelia or other associated anomalies, e.g., diastematomyelia [4].
- Goals of post-operative imaging:
    - Evaluate the status of the neural placode.
    - Evaluate for complications such as hydromyelia, epidermoid/dermoid cysts, and cord re-tethering [4].

MYELOMENINGOCELE (Fig. 21.2)

- >98% of OSDs [8].
- Neural placode protrudes beyond the spinal canal and through an osseous and cutaneous defect via expansion of the subarachnoid space [1, 7].
- Nerve roots may appear stretched as they traverse the dilated subarachnoid space toward the neural foramina [4, 5].

MYELOCELE (Fig. 21.3)

- Much less common than MMC.
- Neural placode is either deep to or at the level of the skin surface, without expansion of the subarachnoid space [3, 8].

ENTITIES RELATED TO DIASTEMATOMYELIA

- Hemimyelomeningocele—one of the hemicords of the split spinal cord fails to neurulate and results in an MMC. Extremely rare.
- Hemimyelocele—one of the hemicords of the split spinal cord fails to neurulate and forms an MC. Extremely rare.

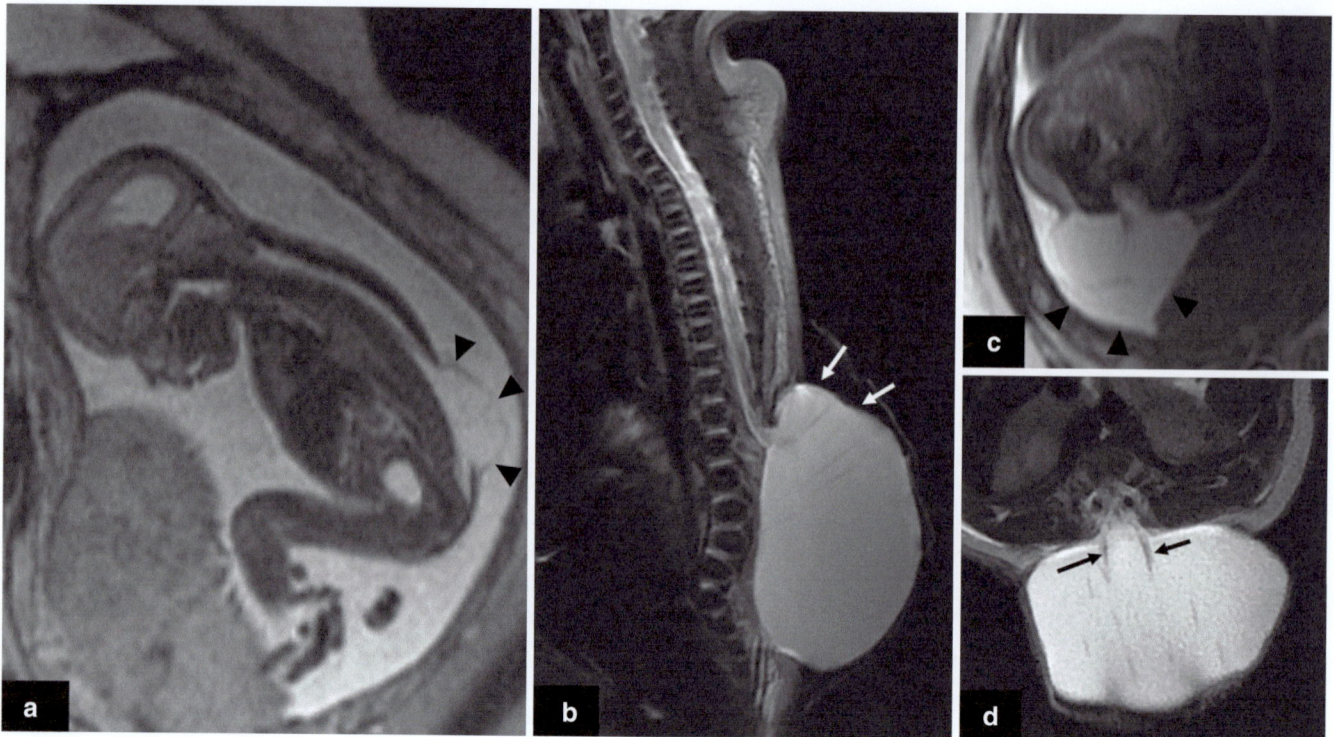

Fig. 21.2 Myelomeningocele. Prenatal MRI sagittal and axial T2-weighted images show an open neural tube defect involving the lower thoracic to the lower sacral levels, with a CSF-filled sac protruding beyond the level of the adjacent skin superior and inferior to the sac (**a, c**; black arrowheads), consistent with a myelomeningocele. Postnatal MRI sagittal and axial T2-weighed images of a different patient on the first day of life show a myelomeningocele with a CSF-filled sac protruding beyond the level of the skin with traversing nerve roots (**b**, white arrows; **d**, black arrows)

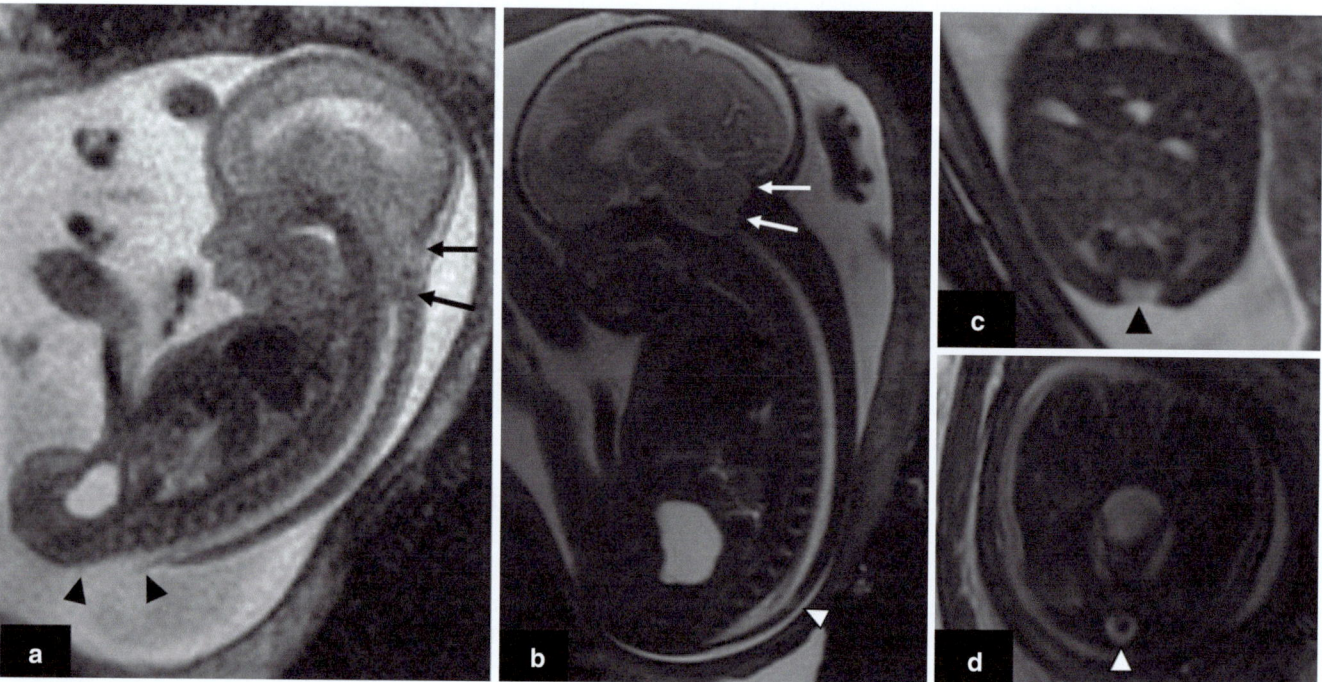

Fig. 21.3 Myelocele. Prenatal MRI sagittal and axial T2-weighted images show an open neural tube defect involving the lumbosacral spine, whereby the neural placode is at the level of the skin (**a, c**; black arrowheads), consistent with a myelocele. There is hindbrain herniation into the cervical spinal canal and effacement of the fourth ventricle in a Chiari 2 malformation configuration (**a**, black arrows). The neural tube defect was surgically repaired in utero at 24 weeks. Sagittal and axial T2-weighted images of the post-surgical prenatal MRI at 31 weeks show closure of the previously seen neural tube defect (**b, d**; white arrowheads) along with near-complete reversal of hindbrain herniation (**b**, white arrows)

Closed Spinal Dysraphism

- CSDs result from premature disjunction of the neural tube from the adjacent surface ectoderm before the neural tube is completely closed [5].
  - Interaction of mesenchymal tissue with the inner lining of the neural tube induces excess fat production [5].
  - *Not* associated with Chiari 2 malformation because no CSF leakage occurs when the overlying skin is closed.
- Clinical presentation:
  - Skin-covered mass at the midline back.
  - Cutaneous stigmata: Midline dimple, focal patch of hair, hemangioma, dermal sinus, skin tag, and tail-like appendages [2].
  - Lower extremity deformities.
  - Anal and genitourinary (GU) anomalies, e.g., imperforate anus.
    - Omphalocele-extrophy-imperforate anus-spinal defects (OEIS) complex—associated with CSDs rather than OSDs [2].
- Prognosis: Better clinical and neurologic prognosis than with OSDs.
  - The neural placode is less injured than in OSDs where the placode is damaged by chronic exposure to the amniotic fluid.
  - Patients may still be able to walk but suffer from bowel and bladder dysfunction.
  - Lower risk of scoliosis than seen with OSDs.

CLOSED SPINAL DYSRAPHISM *WITH* A SUBCUTANEOUS MASS

- Lipomas with a dural defect.
  - Characterized by a subcutaneous fatty mass above the intergluteal crease.
  - Results from a defect in primary neurulation where mesenchymal tissue enters the neural tube and differentiates into lipomatous tissue.
  - The lipomatous tissue traverses a spina bifida and is contiguous with the epidural space and subcutaneous fat.
  - The size of the lipoma may vary and pose a cosmetic issue with surgical reduction often performed later in life [5].
  - Goals of pre-operative imaging:
    - Identification of the placode–lipoma interface.
    - The presence of mass effect exerted by the lipoma on the placode may result in partial rotation of the placode with asymmetric protrusion of the meninges posterior to the spinal canal.
  - LMMC (Fig. 21.4).
    - The placode–lipoma interface is external to the spinal canal, specifically, posterior to the posterior margin of the spinal canal owing to the expansion of the subarachnoid space.
  - Lipomyelocele (LMC) (Fig. 21.5).
    - The placode–lipoma interface is within the spinal canal; there is no posterior expansion of the subarachnoid space.
- Meningocele (Fig. 21.6).
  - A meningocele is a herniation of a CSF-filled sac lined by the dura and arachnoid mater, which may extend laterally through a neural foramen versus anteriorly or posteriorly through a sacral defect/spina bifida.
    - Posterior meningocele—more common in the lumbosacral region than occipital or cervical and least common in the thoracic region.
    - Anterior meningocele—most common in a presacral location.
  - Although the spinal cord is not within a meningocele, the cord may be tethered to the neck of the meningocele [1, 2, 8].
  - Elongated nerve roots and filum terminale can traverse the sac of the meningocele.
  - Associations [4]:
    - Neurofibromatosis type 1.
    - Marfan syndrome.
    - Currarino triad—sacral agenesis abnormalities, anorectal malformation, and presacral mass consisting of a teratoma, anterior sacral meningocele, or both (see later).
- Myelocystocele.
  - Myelocystoceles are extremely rare anomalies that involve herniation of spinal cord containing an expanded central canal/terminal syrinx within a meningocele [1].
  - The dilated central canal herniates through a posterior spina bifida [8].
  - The syrinx and meningocele components do not communicate [4].
  - Results when neurulation is nearly complete except for a small placode that connects to the inner cutaneous surface [1].
  - A terminal myelocystocele (versus non-terminal or cervical myelocystocele) involves the herniation of a large terminal syrinx into a posterior meningocele through a spina bifida [4].
  - Non-terminal myelocystoceles are most common at the cervical or cervicothoracic levels [3].
  - Associations: OEIS complex [2, 4].

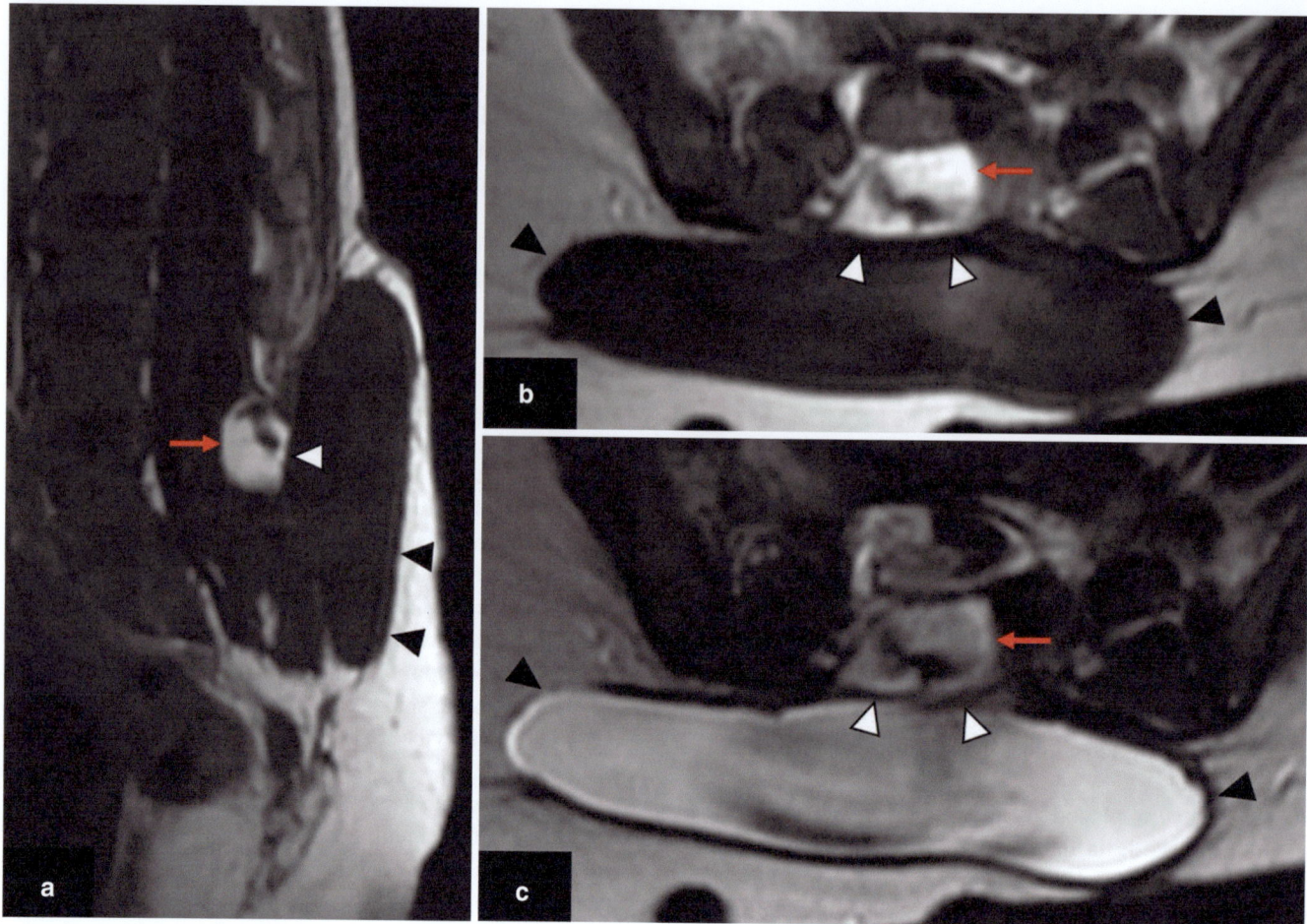

Fig. 21.4 Lipomyelomeningocele. Sagittal T1-weighted (**a**), axial T1-weighted (**b**), and axial T2-weighted (**c**) images of a 4-month-old show a lumbosacral spina bifida with a CSF-filled sac extending posteriorly to the spinal canal (black arrowheads) associated with an intraspinal lipoma (red arrows). The neural placode–lipoma interface is just outside of the spinal canal (white arrowheads)

CLOSED SPINAL DYSRAPHISM *WITHOUT* A SUBCUTANEOUS MASS

CSDs without an associated subcutaneous mass can be divided into two main categories of simple or complex anomalies.

- Simple.
  - Intraspinal lipoma—includes intradural, intramedullary, and filar lipomas.
    - Intradural lipoma (Fig. e21.1).
      - Consist of a dorsal midline lipoma within a completely formed dural sac.
      - The lumbosacral location is the most common and is associated with tethered cord syndrome [3].
      - Cervicothoracic lipomas are more likely to present later with symptoms of spinal cord compression.
    - (All electronic images (Figs. e21.1–e21.13) can be found on this chapter's website on SpringerLink: https://doi.org/10.1007/978-3-031-55124-6_21)
  - Filar fibrolipoma (Fig. 21.7).
    - Consist of fibrolipomatous thickening of the filum terminale.
    - Caused by an anomaly of secondary neurulation whereby persistence of mesodermal elements within the filum terminale which differentiate later into adipose tissue [2].
    - Can be considered a normal variant if there is no tethered cord syndrome or cord compression.
      - Incidental filar fibrolipomas are seen in 1.5–5% of normal adults in 4–5% of autopsies [2].
    - On MRI, T1 hyperintense signal intensity with thickening of the filum terminale is seen. Axial T1-weighted images without fat saturation are the most sensitive series.

21 Congenital and Developmental Malformations of the Spine

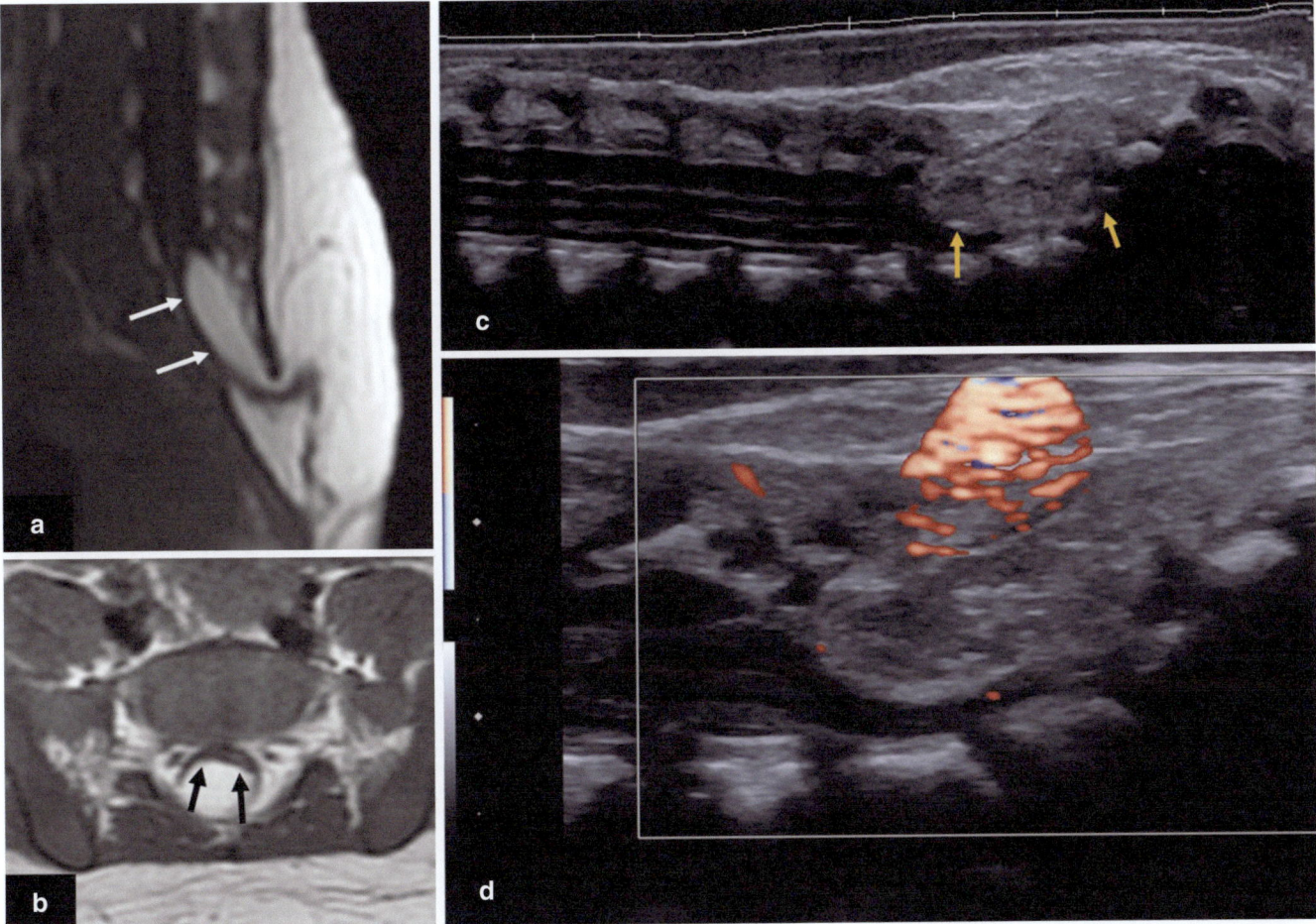

Fig. 21.5 Lipomyelocele. Sagittal (**a**) and axial (**b**) T1-weighted images in a 3-month-old show a neural tube defect at the lower sacral levels with intraspinal lipoma in contiguity with a prominent subcutaneous lipomatous mass (**a**, white arrows). The placode–lipoma interface remains within the spinal canal (**b**, black arrows), consistent with a lipomyelocele. Sagittal grayscale ultrasound images demonstrate a lumbosacral hyperechoic mass within the spinal canal (**c**, yellow arrows) without substantial internal vascularity on Doppler ultrasound images (**d**), which corresponds to the lipomatous mass seen on MRI

- Tight filum terminale (Fig. e21.2).
  - Characterized by a shortened and thickened (>2 mm in diameter) filum.
  - May result in a low-lying (below L2–L3), tethered conus medullaris, caused by an impaired ascent of the conus.
  - May be associated with a lipoma or less frequently with a cyst [5].
  - Caused by abnormal differentiation of the secondary neural tube [4].
- Persistent terminal ventricle (Fig. e21.3).
  - Characterized by a persistent small ependymal-lined intramedullary cavity within the conus medullaris directly above the filum terminale.
  - Caused by incomplete closure of the central canal in the conus.
  - Enlargement of the persistent ventricle in a more cyst-like appearance may reflect an anatomic variation or obstruction.

- On MRI, no contrast enhancement should be seen, and the lesion should be stable or decrease in size over time.
- Dermal sinus tract (Figs. 21.8 and e21.4).
  - A dermal sinus tract (DST) consists of an epithelial-lined fistulous communication that extends from the skin surface to the dura, subarachnoid space, or spinal cord and causes tethering [2].
    - Tracts may contain dermal or neuroglial components.
  - Caused by focal incomplete disjunction of the neuroectoderm from the surface ectoderm which closes dorsal to the neural tube [5].
  - Most common in the lumbosacral location.
  - Associated with spinal dermoid cysts at the level of the cauda equina or conus. (See the section on dermoid cysts later in this chapter.)
  - Clinical manifestations:

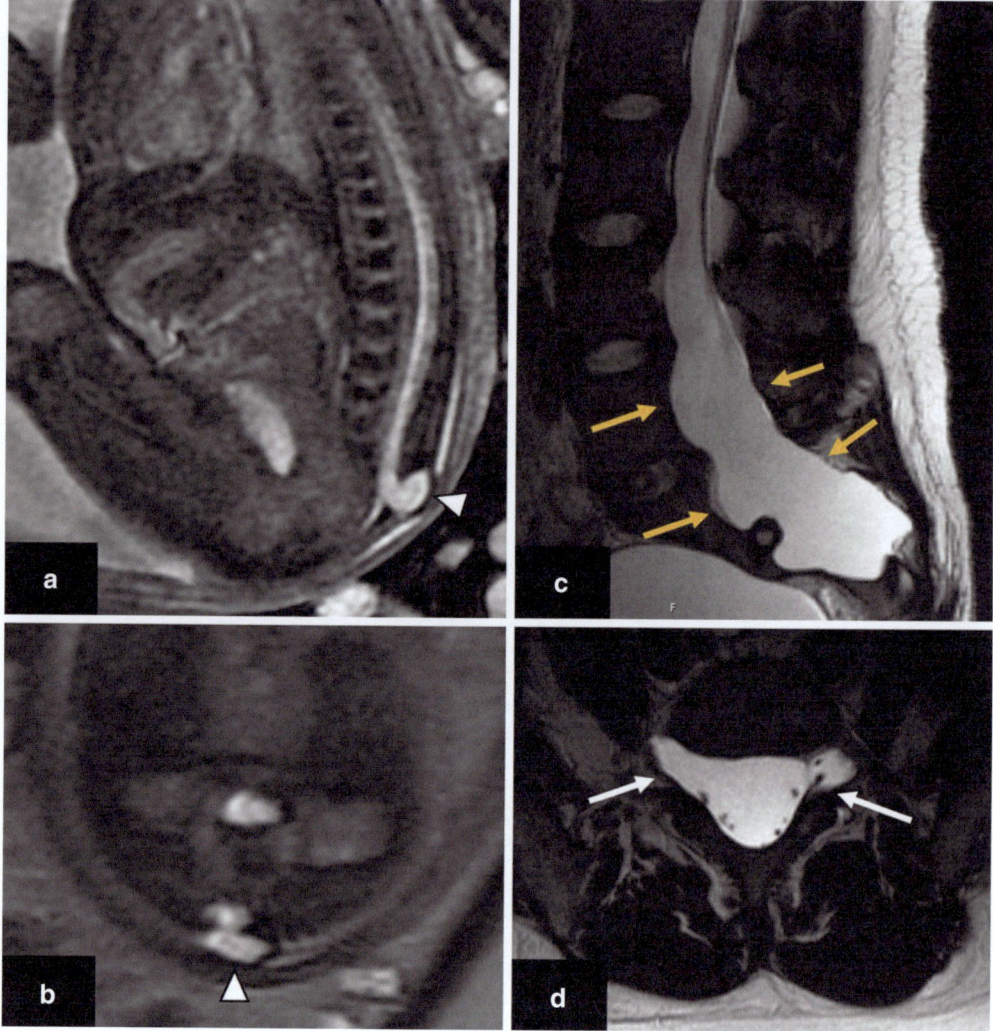

Fig. 21.6 Meningoceles. Prenatal MR sagittal (**a**) and axial (**b**) T2-weighted images show a CSF-intensity outpouching arising from the spinal canal through a sacral spina bifida without neural tissue within the outpouching (**a, b**; white arrowheads). Sagittal (**c**) and axial (**d**) T2-weighted images in a 23-year-old male with neurofibromatosis 1 (different patient) demonstrate lumbosacral dural ectasia (**c**, yellow arrows) with prominent lateral meningoceles at the L5 level (**d**, white arrows)

- A midline skin dimple/cutaneous pit or pinpoint ostium at the back from which CSF leaks intermittently, especially when the neonate is crying.
- Cutaneous stigmata such as hairy nevus, hyperpigmented patch, or hemangioma.
- All fistulous openings above the gluteal crease are clinically presumed to communicate with the subarachnoid space until proven otherwise [9].
- Complications:
    - Infection—may manifest as a local bacterial infection, meningitis, or abscess formation.
- Imaging findings:
    - On MRI, a T1- and T2-hypointense tract extending from the cutaneous dimple to the spinal canal can be seen, especially well-seen on non-fat saturated images.
    - The tract may end in an intradural lipoma in up to 50% of cases, with associated cord tethering [5].
- Surgical repair is important to prevent infection of the tract.
    - Complete resection of an associated intradural lipoma is important to prevent complications and tethering [5].
- Associations: Tethered cord syndrome, lipo(myelomeningocele), dermoid cysts, and vertebral segmentation anomalies.
- Complex.

Complex CSDs without an associated subcutaneous mass can be divided into disorders of midline notochordal integration or notochordal formation.

 ○ Disorders of midline notochordal integration.
- Dorsal enteric fistula—a fistulous communication forms between the skin surface and bowel. Extremely rare.
- Neurenteric cyst (Fig. e21.5).
    - A localized form of the dorsal enteric fistula which consists of a cyst lined with mucin-secreting epithelium in the spinal canal with

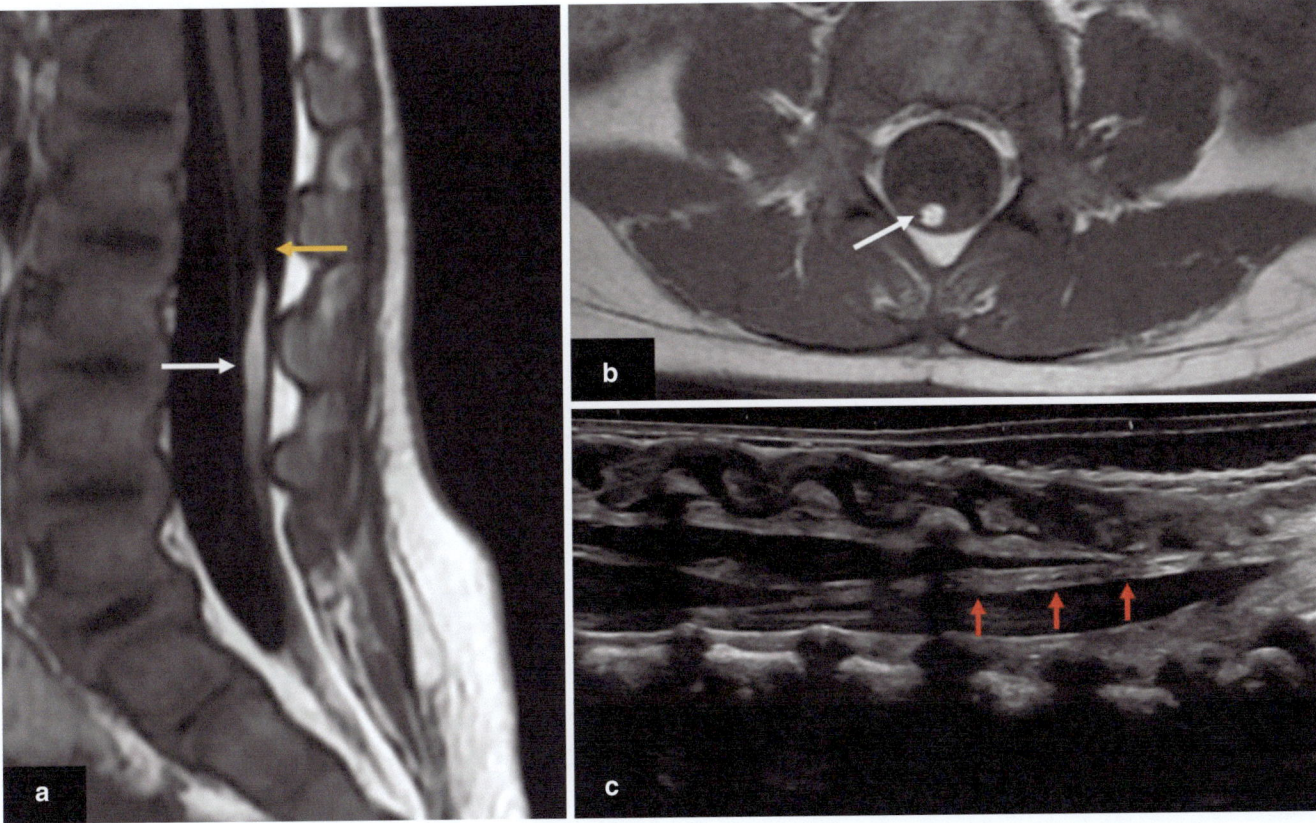

Fig. 21.7 Filar fibrolipoma. Sagittal (**a**) and axial (**b**) T1-weighted images in a 15-month-old male demonstrate lipomatous thickening of the filum terminale (**a** and **b**, white arrows) with a slightly low-lying conus medullaris that terminates just inferior to the L2 vertebral body (**a**, yellow arrow). Sagittal ultrasound image demonstrates an echogenic structure extending from the conus caudally (**c**, red arrows), consistent with a filar fibrolipoma

- has a connection to the spinal cord and/or vertebra [2].
  - The cyst may communicate with extraspinal components in the mediastinum or mesentery through a vertebral defect or attach to the vertebra or the GI tract by a fibrous stalk [2].
  - Most common location is anterior to the cord at the cervicothoracic level where the lesion presents as a posterior mediastinal mass, passing through an osseous dysraphic opening called a Kovalesky canal [3].
    - Mass effect may cause airway or esophageal compression.
  - The intraspinal component of the cyst may cause neurologic deficits.
  - Imaging findings:
    - A cystic structure that is isointense to hyperintense to CSF on T1- and T2-weighed images (high protein content).
    - No contrast enhancement.

- Split cord malformation/diastematomyelia (DMM) (Fig. 21.9).
  - Characterized by the separation of the spinal cord into two hemicords with each hemicord containing one ventral and one dorsal nerve root as well as one central canal.
  - Usually symmetric but can vary in length of involvement.
  - Most common at the lumbar or thoracic levels.
  - Generally diagnosed on prenatal US or fetal MRI.
  - Caused by an abnormally widened primitive streak which leads ectoderm cells to form two more laterally positioned (rather than midline) hemi-notochords in parallel, divided by intervening primitive streak cells [5].
    - Primitive streak cells that differentiate into cartilage and bone result in type 1 diastematomyelia.

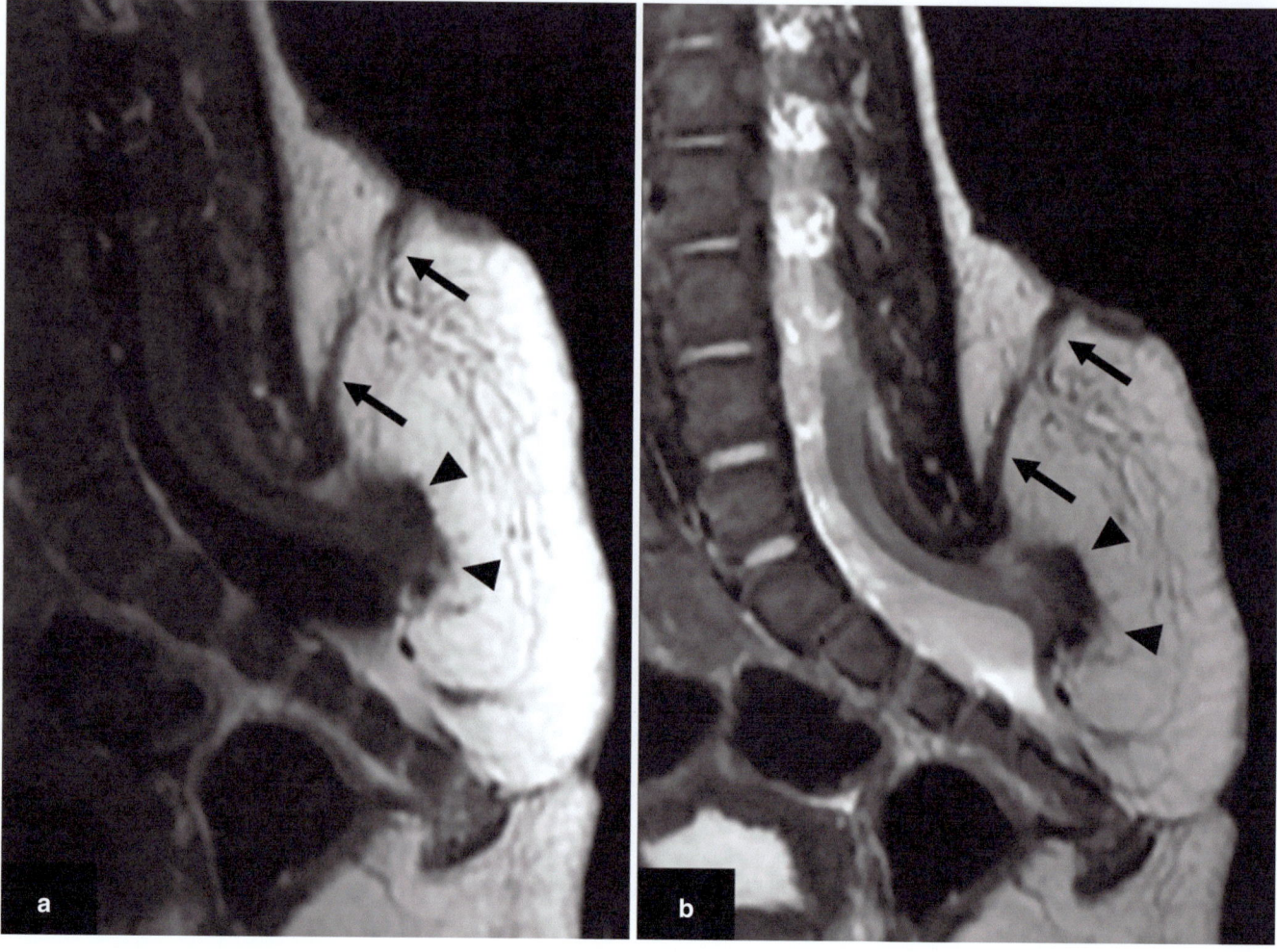

Fig. 21.8 Dermal sinus tract. Sagittal T1-weighted (**a**) and sagittal T2-weighted (**b**) images in a 4-month-old female demonstrate a T1 and T2 hypointense tract (black arrows) extending from the spinal canal/ dura at the upper sacral level and communicating with the overlying skin surface. A lipomyelomeningocele is also seen (black arrowheads)

- ♦ Primitive streak cells that are resorbed result in type 2 diastematomyelia.
- ▪ Type 1:
  - ♦ Each hemicord is contained within its own dural sac, with the two dural sacs separated by an extradural osseous or cartilaginous septum/spur.
  - ♦ Tethering of the cord by the spur and syringomyelia are common causes of symptoms [1, 4].
- ▪ Type 2:
  - ♦ Two hemicords are contained within a single dural sac.
  - ♦ An intervening fibrous septum may separate the hemicords but is uncommon.
  - ♦ More likely to be asymptomatic if no septum is present.
  - ♦ The presence of syringohydromeylia may cause symptoms.

- ▪ Imaging findings:
  - ♦ Prenatal US or MRI shows cord splitting. Orthogonal planes (axial and coronal images) are more helpful than sagittal images.
  - ♦ Plain radiography may show a spindle-shaped, area of focal widening of the spinal cord on frontal views.
  - ♦ CT may demonstrate osseous bone spurs better than MRI although MRI is ideal for evaluation of the spinal cord and canal anatomy.
  - ♦ Imaging of the entire spinal canal needs to be performed as DMM can be multifocal, and the additional associated findings such as cord tethering, vertebral segmentation anomalies, and syringohydromyelia need to be evaluated.

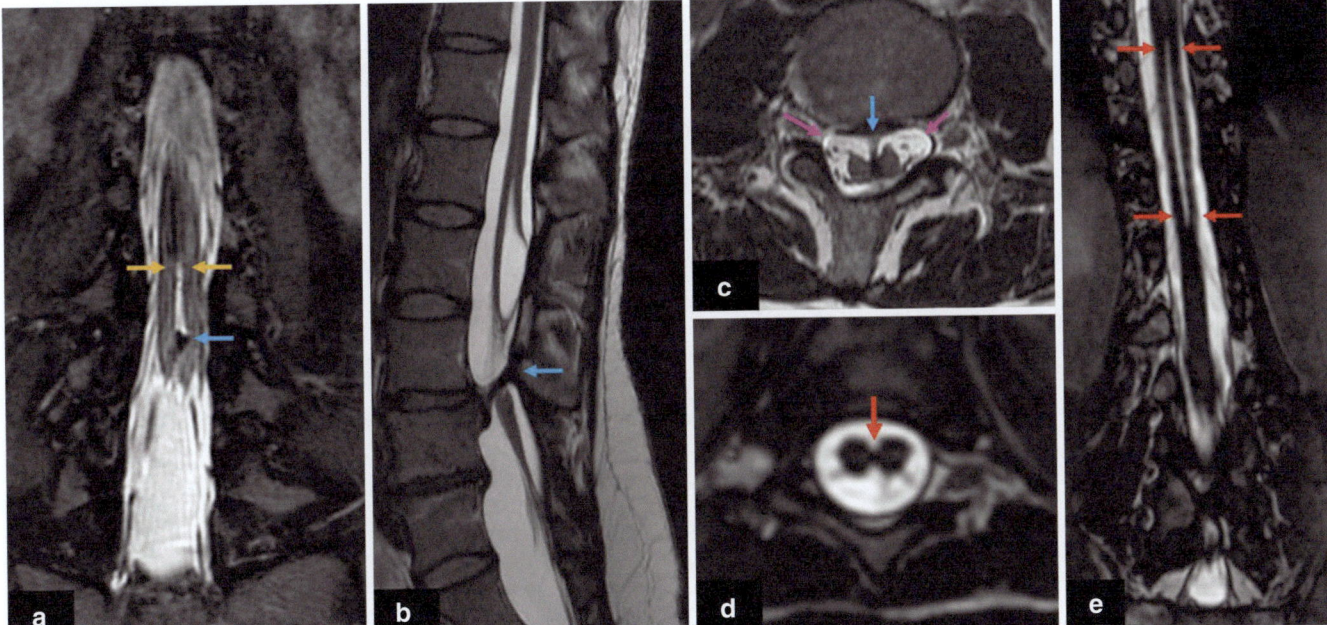

Fig. 21.9 Diastematomyelia. Coronal (**a**), sagittal (**b**), and axial (**c**) T2-weighted images in a 39-year-old female show splitting of the upper lumbar spinal cord (yellow arrows). Each hemicord is contained within its own dural sac (**c**, pink arrows) which is separated by a bony bar (**a–c**, blue arrows), consistent with type 1 diastematomyelia. Axial (**d**) and coronal (**e**) FIESTA images in a 5-year-old female (different patient) demonstrate a split spinal cord from the mid-thoracic to the upper lumbar levels (red arrows). Both hemicords are contained within a single dural sac, consistent with type 2 diastematomyelia

- ■ Associations:
  - ♦ Scoliosis.
  - ♦ Vertebral segmentation anomalies—more common in type 1.
  - ♦ Low-lying conus, filar fibrolipomas, and tight filum terminale—more common in type 2.
  - ♦ Tethered cord syndrome—seen in up to 90% of cases [5].
  - ♦ Cutaneous stigmata—seen in 50–70% of cases [5].
    - ❖ Focal patch of hair is common in the upper thoracic spine.
- o Disorders of notochordal formation—an absent notochordal segment results in the absence of the corresponding spinal cord and spine elements.
  - • Caudal regression syndrome (CRS) (Fig. 21.10).
    - ■ Total or partial agenesis of the distal spinal column, which includes the spinal cord and vertebrae.
    - ■ Vertebral anomalies range from the absence of coccygeal segments to the agenesis of inferior thoracic vertebrae, although the sacrum and coccyx are the most commonly affected.
    - ■ The two types of CRS depend on the level of the cord terminus and the morphology of the conus.
      - ♦ Type 1 [1, 9]:
        - ❖ High position of the cord terminus and thecal sac (above S2).
        - ❖ The conus medullaris terminates abruptly, demonstrating a "hatchet" or wedge shape.
        - ❖ The most inferior intact vertebra is usually between L5 and S2.
        - ❖ More severe type.
      - ♦ Type 2 [1, 9]:
        - ❖ Low position of the cord terminus, e.g., may terminate as low as the S2 level if tethering is present.
        - ❖ Only the tip of the conus medullaris may be absent with tethering as a common association.
        - ❖ Less severe vertebral dysgenesis with only the lowest sacral or coccygeal segments absent.
        - ❖ A tight filum terminale or associated mass such as a lipoma, LMMC, or anterior sacral meningocele may be present.
    - ■ Associations:
      - ♦ Maternal diabetes.
      - ♦ Syndromes/complexes:
        - ❖ OEIS complex.
        - ❖ Currarino syndrome.
        - ❖ Vertebral defects, anal atresia, cardiac defects, tracheoesophageal fistula, renal anomalies, limb abnormalities syndrome (VACTERL).

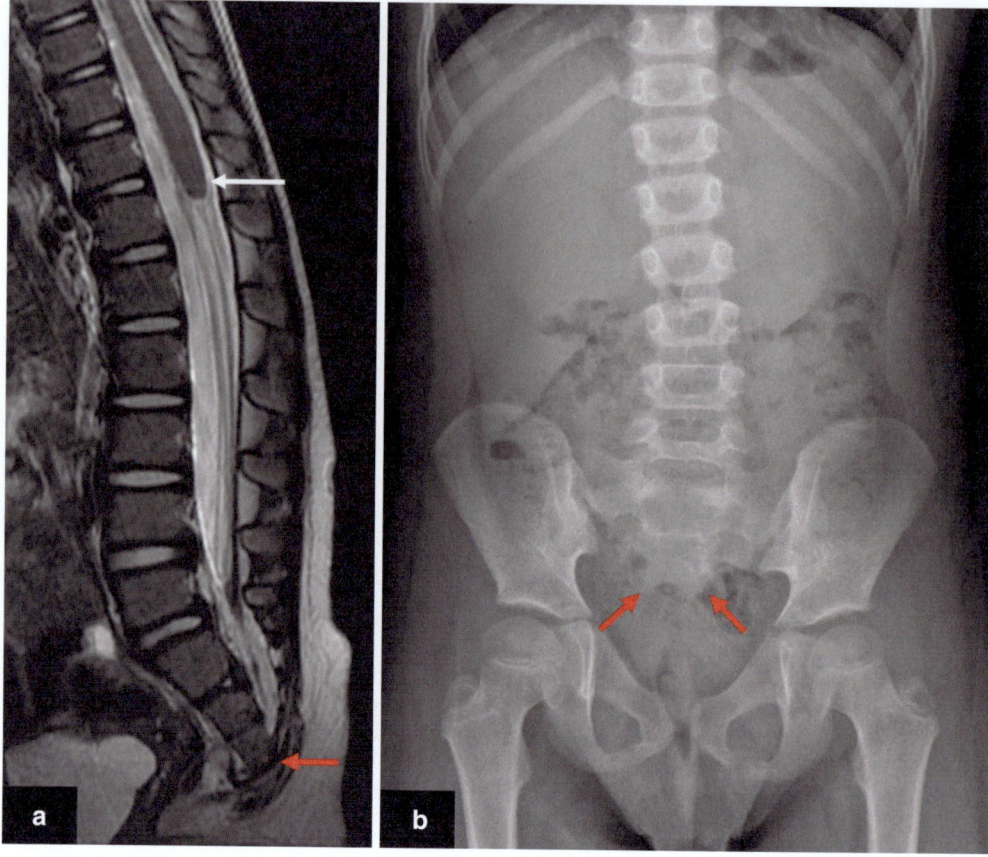

Fig. 21.10 Caudal regression. The sagittal T2-weighted image shows transitional lumbosacral lumbarized S1 and the characteristic blunted appearance of the conus medullaris ("hatchet" or wedge-shaped conus) which terminates at the L1 level (**a**, white arrow). There is associated hypoplasia of the lower sacrum and coccyx (red arrows), seen on MRI (**a**) as well as the frontal radiograph (**b**)

- Segmental spinal dysgenesis (SSD).
    - Extremely rare anomaly characterized by abnormal development of a segment of the lumbar or thoracolumbar spine along with the respective spinal cord and/or nerve roots at the level.
    - Vertebrae are generally intact above and below the abnormal segment.
    - Congenital paraparesis or paraplegia and congenital lower limb deformities. The paraplegia results from the spinal cord being separated into two unconnected cranial and caudal portions.
    - Imaging findings:
        - Thin or indiscernible spinal cord with an absent vertebral segment and kyphosis at the affected level.
        - A bulky and low-lying cord segment can be seen in the caudal spinal canal.
    - Associations:
        - Vertebral segmentation anomalies.
        - Severe scoliosis or kyphoscoliosis.

Spinal Inclusion Cysts

- The spinal inclusion cysts or congenital spinal cysts make up 1–2% of pediatric intraspinal tumors but may constitute up to 17% of spinal tumors in the first year of life and up to 10% of spinal tumors in patients under 15 years of age [7, 11].
- Seen commonly in relation to spinal dysraphism and are most frequently seen with a dermal sinus tract [12].
- May be congenital or acquired [12]:
    o Congenital:
        - Result from cutaneous ectodermal inclusions during neural tube formation between the third and fifth weeks of gestation [11, 13].
        - More likely to present with infection [11].
    o Acquired:
        - Result from implanted dermal elements from prior instrumentation (e.g., surgery and lumbar punctures) [11, 12].
- Location:
    o Most commonly within the intradural extramedullary compartment.
    o The lumbosacral location is more common than the thoracic and cervical locations.
    o Dermoid cysts are more common in the spine than epidermoid cysts.
- Symptoms are related to mass effect, infection, or cord tethering [11].
    o Slowly progressive myelopathy and chemical meningitis can also be seen [7].
- Dermoid and epidermoid cysts may be difficult to distinguish on imaging but are of low practical relevance to the

Table 21.3 Spinal inclusion cysts [11–13]

Characteristic	Dermoid cyst	Epidermoid cyst
Etiology	Ectodermal origin with skin structures from the dermal layer	Ectodermal origin tissue with keratin-containing desquamated epidermal cells and lined by squamous epithelium
Demographics	M = F, typical presentation at <20 years of age	M > F, typical presentation at 30–50 years of age
Location	Mostly lumbosacral and cauda equina	Uniformly distributed along the spine
Imaging findings	May have a fat signal within the lesion, non-enhancing, may show restricted diffusion	T1 hypointense, T2 hyperintense, non-enhancing, more commonly restricts diffusion
Presentation	Spinal pain, slowly progressive myelopathy, chemical meningitis	
Complications	Infection (local infection, meningitis, abscess), cord compression, tethered cord syndrome	
Associations	Dermal sinus tracts (up to 20%), myelomeningocele, spina bifida and vertebral anomalies, Currarino syndrome, split cord malformation, intraspinal lipomas	
Treatment	Surgical resection	

surgeon or prognostic relevance to the patient as the clinical presentation, surgical management, and prognosis are similar [11]. Table 21.3 details important differentiating points between dermoid and epidermoid cysts [11–13].

- Complications:
  - Local mass effect—may result in pain and cord compression.
  - Infection—may lead to abscess or subdural empyema formation if severe [11].
- Associations:
  - DST:
    - Most common association (20% of spinal inclusion cysts develop in association with DST).
    - Squamous cells from the epithelial-lined tract may become a nidus for inclusion cyst formation.
  - Spina bifida and vertebral segmentation anomalies.
  - Currarino triad—a dermoid or epidermoid cyst may constitute the presacral lesion.
  - Diastematomyelia.
  - Intraspinal lipomas.

DERMOID CYSTS (Fig. e21.4)

- Round/ovoid or multilobulated mass that is lined by squamous epithelium and contains skin appendages (e.g., hair follicles, sweat glands, and sebaceous glands) [7].
- Can form within or along a DST and may be subcutaneous, epidural, intradural extramedullary, or intramedullary [11].
- Lumbosacral and caudal equina location is more common than at the cervical or thoracic levels.
- Symptoms usually manifest before age 20 years.
- Imaging findings:
  - Hypointense to hyperintense with macroscopic fat on T1 and hyperintense on T2.
  - Signal dropout on fat-saturated MR images in lipid-rich lesions.
  - No enhancement.
  - May show restricted diffusion.

EPIDERMOID CYSTS (Fig. e21.6)

- Consists of keratin-containing desquamated epidermal cells and stratified squamous epithelial cells lined by epidermal elements of the skin [7].
- Symptoms manifest in early adulthood (third to fifth decade).
- Epidermoid cysts are uniformly distributed along the spine, rather than more commonly in the lumbosacral region as are dermoid cysts.
- Imaging findings:
  - T1 hypointense, T2 hyperintense (due to water and protein contents).
  - More commonly shows restricted diffusion than dermoid cysts.
  - No enhancement is seen.

Sacrococcygeal Teratomas (Fig. e21.7)

- SCTs are large, complex solid and cystic masses that are caudal to the coccyx and contain tissues derived from all three germ layers.
- They arise from the totipotent cells of the caudal cell mass.
- They are the most common tumors of the fetus and neonate.
- Most are benign.
- Occur in a 3:1 ratio of females to males.
- Classified as types 1–4 [2]:
  - Type 1—external to the pelvis.
  - Type 2—equally external and internal to the pelvis.
  - Type 3—primarily internal to the pelvis.
  - Type 4—internal to the pelvis.
- Fetal hydrops is an important clinical concern as it may result from the tumor's large size.

- Imaging findings:
  - Lesion may appear as a combination of cystic, solid, or mixed components.
    - Greater than 50% of lesions contain calcium [2].
  - Plain radiography may show a soft tissue mass in the sacrococcygeal region with foci of calcification.
  - On MRI, heterogeneous enhancement with variable signal on T1- and T2-weighted images is seen, depending on the internal contents.
  - Post-natal MR can delineate the extent of displacement/mass effect and infiltration of the pelvic organs.
  - Intraspinal extension is rare.
- Definitive treatment involves complete resection of the SCT along with the coccyx to decrease the risk of recurrence.
- Associations:
  - Polyhydramnios (in utero).
  - Anorectal and genital anomalies.
  - Cardiac anomalies such as ventriculoseptal defect.
  - Hip dislocation.
  - Vertebral anomalies (e.g., spina bifida and sacral agenesis).

Chiari Malformations

- CM types 1–3 are associated with caudal descent of various portions of the hindbrain into the upper cervical spinal canal. The differences between different types of Chiari malformations are summarized in Table 21.4 [6, 10, 14, 15].
- Osseous abnormalities commonly associated with CM in general include:
  - Vertebral segmentation and fusion abnormalities.
  - Klippel-Feil syndrome.
  - Atlanto-occipital assimilation.
  - Retroflexed odontoid process.
  - Scoliosis.

TYPE 1 (Chiari 1 Deformity) (Fig. e21.8)

- Chiari 1 deformity is the current preferred terminology since malformation implies that there is an inherent developmental abnormality, which is not the case in this disorder.
- It is defined by caudal migration of the cerebellar tonsils >5 mm inferior to the foramen magnum [6].
- Incidentally seen in 1–4% of patients who receive imaging evaluation of the CNS [6].
- Causes:
  - Congenital—inadequacy of the paraxial mesoderm after the neural tube is closed, which leads to insufficient development of the occipital somites [6].
  - Acquired—cerebellar tonsillar descent secondary to intracranial hyper- or hypotension [14].
- Signs and symptoms are related to compression of the posterior fossa and spinal canal.

Table 21.4 Chiari malformations (CM) [6, 10, 14, 15]

	Type 1	Type 2	Type 3
Definition	• Caudal migration of cerebellar tonsils ≥5 mm below the foramen magnum • Chiari 1 deformity is the current preferred terminology	• Caudal migration of brainstem, cerebellum, and fourth ventricle through foramen magnum with inferior displacement of cervical spinal cord	• CM 2 with low occipital or high cervical encephalocele
Key imaging features	• Caudal tonsillar ectopia with peg-like configuration • Angled cerebellar folia • Anterior flattening of the midbrain, pons, and medulla • Effaced CSF at foramen magnum • Hydrocephalus rare	• Small posterior fossa • Caudal herniation of the hindbrain • Tectal beaking • Towering cerebellum • Prominent Massa intermedia • Hydrocephalus in up to 90%	• Cerebellar or low occipital encephalocele • Other findings in CM 2
Associated anomalies	• Syringohydromyelia (50–75%) • Retroflexed dens • Platybasia and basilar invagination • Klippel-Feil syndrome.	• Callosal dysgenesis • Falx defects (interdigitating gyri) • OSD present in ≥90% (lumbar myelomeningocele) • Syringohydromyelia (25–45%) • Gray matter anomalies (e.g., polymicrogyria and heterotopias) • Luckenschadel (lacunar skull)	• Corpus callosum dysgenesis • Hydrocephalus • Syringohydromyelia
Clinical issues	• Most common • Up to 50% asymptomatic • Valsava-induced suboccipital headache, neck pain	• Maternal folate deficiency • Myelomeningocele and hydrocephalus at birth	• Encephalocele • Microcephaly
Developmental error	• Inadequacy of paraxial mesoderm after neural tube closure, leading to insufficient development of occipital somites	• Non-closure of the caudal end of the neuropore, leading to inadequate distension of ventricles and disorganized CNS development	• Non-closure of the rostral end of the neuropore

- Children—oropharyngeal dysfunction, headaches, scoliosis, as well as altered pain, temperature, and vibratory sensation (related to a holocord syringohydromyelia).
- Adults—headache (exacerbated by activities that increase intrathoracic pressure), neck pain, and syncope.
- Additional symptoms include lower cranial nerve dysfunction, symptoms related to cerebellar and brainstem compression (e.g., nystagmus, opthalmoplegia, and tongue atrophy), and upper and lower extremity neurologic deficits related to syringomyelia.
- Imaging findings [6, 16]:
  - Caudal descent of the cerebellar tonsils which have a pointed "peg-like" morphology and obliquely/inferiorly angled cerebellar folia.
  - Caudal descent of the cervicomedullary junction may be present in severe cases.
  - Effaced CSF spaces and crowding at the foramen magnum.
  - Anterior flattening of the midbrain, pons, and medulla.
  - Altered CSF flow dynamics on phase-contrast CSF flow studies [16].
  - Hydrocephalus is rare.
  - Abnormalities of the posterior fossa/skull-base and craniovertebral (CVJ) junction—up to 50% of Chiari 1 deformity patients.
    - Retroflexed dens.
    - Platybasia and basilar invagination.
    - CVJ fusion anomalies.
    - Scoliosis.
    - Klippel-Feil syndrome.

TYPE 2 (CM 2) (Fig. e21.9)

- CM 2 is defined by caudal descent of the brainstem, cerebellum, and fourth ventricle through the foramen magnum with inferior displacement of the cervical cord [6].
- Caused by a defect in primary neurulation which leads to open spinal dysraphism and continuous CSF leak in the amniotic cavity [4].
  - Lack of adequate fourth ventricular distension from low CSF pressure results in a persistently small posterior fossa as well as disorganized CNS development, which may result in callosal dysgenesis, anomalous neural migration, and defects of the falx [2].
- Symptoms include [6, 16]:
  - Neonatal—central apnea, inspiratory stridor, vocal cord palsy, dysphagia, and bradycardia.
  - Older children—motor dysfunction, e.g., hypotonia, hypertonia, and deterioration of sphincter function [15].

- Imaging findings [6, 16]:
  - Caudal descent of the hindbrain and towering of the cerebellum (superior displacement of the cerebellum through the tentorial incisura).
    - Banana sign—appearance of the cerebellum wrapping around the brainstem with effacement of the fourth ventricle and usually the cisterna magna, often first seen on ultrasound.
  - Tectal beaking.
  - Enlarged massa intermedia (connection between the medial thalami).
  - Elongated brainstem with fusion of the colliculi.
  - Low-lying and hypoplastic tentorium.
  - Elongation and stenosis of the cerebral aqueduct.
  - Hypoplasia/aplasia of cranial nerves.
  - Osseous abnormalities:
    - Luckenschadel—lacunar skull.
    - Lemon sign—bony scalloping of the frontal calvarium.
    - Scalloping of the clivus.
  - Ancillary findings:
    - Hydrocephalus—in 90% of CM 2 patients [6].
    - Syringohydromyelia—up to 24-45% of CM 2 patients [6].
    - Falcine insufficiency (e.g., fenestrations and hypoplasia), seen as interdigitating gyri.
    - Hypogenesis/agenesis of the corpus callosum.
    - Stenogyria (multiple small gyri usually after CSF diversion).
    - Subependymal gray matter heterotopias.
    - An OSD is associated with CM 2 in >90% of cases, and thus MMCs are commonly seen in conjunction.

TYPE 3 (CM 3) (Fig. e21.10)

- Most rare of the CM.
- Defined by findings seen in CM 2 along with a low occipital or high cervical encephalocele.
- Caused by non-closure of the rostral end of the neuropore.
- Neonates present with a cystic mass in the cervical or occipital region.
- Older children may exhibit ataxia, hypotonia, and developmental delay.
- Imaging findings:
  - CM 2 findings (see previous section).
  - Cerebellar or low occipital encephalocele with a possible extension of the dural venous sinuses and brain tissue into the encephalocele.
  - Associations: Partial or complete agenesis of the corpus callosum.

Syndromes and Anomalies Associated with Congenital Spinal Malformations

Table 21.5 lists some of the syndromes associated with congenital spinal malformations [1, 2, 4, 5].

CURRARINO SYNDROME (Fig. e21.11)

- The Currarino triad includes:
  - Partial sacral agenesis (Scimitar sacrum).
  - Anorectal malformations.
  - Presacral mass—meningoceles (most common), teratomas, epidermoid, or dermoid cysts (least common) [1].

KLIPPEL-FEIL SYNDROME AND VERTEBRAL SEGMENTATION ANOMALIES

- Klippel-Feil syndrome is defined by cervical spine segmentation anomalies (Fig. e21.12).
  - Most common at the C2–C3 level, with C5–C6 as the second most common level of involvement.
  - Associations:
    - Congenital scoliosis.
    - Sprengel's deformity—congenital asymmetric elevation of the scapula (see Fig. e21.12).
    - Cervical ribs and rib abnormalities.
    - Deafness.
    - Cardiac anomalies.
    - Genitourinary tract abnormalities.

NEUROFIBROMATOSIS TYPE I (NF 1) (Fig. e21.13)

- Congenital malformations of the spine in the setting of NF1 are only a small subset of the myriad multi-organ clinical manifestations.

Table 21.5 Syndromic associations of congenital spinal malformations [1, 2, 4, 5]

Anomaly	Associated syndrome(s)
Chiari I	• Klippel-Feil
Meningocele	• NF1 • Marfan
Myelocystocele	• OEIS complex
Caudal regression syndrome	• OEIS complex • Currarino triad • VACTERL
Segmental spinal dysgenesis	• VACTERL • Klippel-Feil
Vertebral segmentation anomalies	• Alagille

- Notable osseous findings include:
  - Scoliosis.
  - Vertebral body scalloping.
- Non-osseous findings include:
  - Dural ectasia.
  - Meningoceles.
  - Neurofibromas may involve the nerve roots at any level along the entire spine.
    - Degeneration into malignant peripheral nerve sheath tumors may occur (MPNST).

References

1. Schwartz ES, Rossi A. Congenital spine anomalies: the closed spinal dysraphisms. Pediatr Radiol. 2015;45:413–9.
2. Reghunath A, Ghasi RG, Aggarwal A. Unveiling the tale of the tail: an illustration of spinal dysraphisms. Neurosurg Rev. 2021;44:97–114.
3. Rufener SL, Ibrahim M, Raybaud CA, Parmar HA. Congenital spine and spinal cord malformations—pictorial review. Am J Roentgenol. 2010;194:26–37.
4. Grimme JD, Castillo M. Congenital anomalies of the spine. Neuroimaging Clin N Am. 2007;17:1–16.
5. Huisman TAGM, Rossi A, Tortori-Donati P. MR imaging of neonatal spinal dysraphia: what to consider? Magn Reson Imaging Clin N Am. 2012;20:45–61.
6. Hiremath SB, Fitsiori A, Boto J, Torres C, Zakhari N, Dietemann JL, Meling TR, Vargas MI. The perplexity surrounding chiari malformations—are we any wiser now? Am J Neuroradiol. 2020;41:1975–81.
7. Schwartz ES, Barkovich AJ. Congenital anomalies of the spine. In: Barkovich AJ, Raybaud CA, editors. Pediatric neuroimaging. 6th ed. Philadelphia, PA: Wolters Kluwer; 2019. p. 973–1042.
8. Rufener S, Ibrahim M, Parmar HA. Imaging of congenital spine and spinal cord malformations. Neuroimaging Clin N Am. 2011;21:659–76.
9. Rossi A, Martinetti C, Morana G, Severino M, Tortora D. Diagnostic approach to pediatric spine disorders. Magn Reson Imaging Clin N Am. 2016;24:621–44.
10. Nagaraj UD, Kline-Fath BM. Imaging of open spinal dysraphisms in the era of prenatal surgery. Pediatr Radiol. 2020;50:1988–98.
11. Thompson DNP. Spinal inclusion cysts. Childs Nerv Syst. 2013;29:1647–55.
12. Karthigeyan M, Singh K, Salunke P, Gupta K. Co-existent epidermoid and dermoid in a child with spinal dysraphism. Childs Nerv Syst. 2021;37:2087–90.
13. McNutt SE, Mrowczynski OD, Lane J, Jafrani R, Rohatgi P, Specht C, Tubbs RS, Zacharia TT, Rizk EB. Congenital spinal cysts: an update and review of the literature. World Neurosurg. 2021;145:480–491.e9.
14. Cotes C, Bonfante E, Lazor J, Jadhav S, Caldas M, Swischuk L, Riascos R. Congenital basis of posterior fossa anomalies. Neuroradiol J. 2015;28:238–53.
15. Spazzapan P, Bosnjak R, Prestor B, Velnar T. Chiari malformations in children: an overview. World J Clin Cases. 2021;9:764–73.
16. Osborn AG, Hedfund GL, Salzman KL. Posterior fossa malformations. In: Osborn's brain imaging, pathology anatomy. 2nd ed. Salt Lake City, UT: Elsevier Inc.; 2018. p. 1169–94.

Spine Trauma

Alexander M. Khalaf, Tarik F. Massoud, and Syed S. Hashmi

Introduction

The diagnosis of spinal trauma is an essential skill for radiologists to develop given the potential for devastating clinical outcomes. The most common causes of spinal injuries are motor vehicle accidents, falls, sports, and violence (e.g., gunshots). After blunt trauma, the thoracolumbar spine is the most common site of spinal injury, followed by the cervical spine and the sacrum [1, 2]. Spine trauma has a myriad of manifestations that radiologists should recognize, and a thorough understanding of anatomy, mechanisms of injury, and imaging findings is necessary for accurate diagnosis.

Modalities

- Cervical spine imaging is indicated when acute cervical spine injury is suspected and one of the following *Nexus* (National Emergency X-Radiography Utilization Study) criteria are present:
  - Posterior midline cervical spine tenderness.
  - Intoxicated or altered mental status.
  - Focal neurologic deficit.
  - Painful injury outside the spine that distracts away from a possible coexisting spine injury.
- Multiple competing criteria exist for determining when imaging is indicated in the setting of suspected thoracolumbar spine injury, but they are generally similar to the *Nexus* criteria for cervical spine trauma.
- Computed tomography (CT) is the gold standard in the setting of suspected acute spinal trauma.
  - Approximately two-thirds of fractures visualized on CT will be occult on radiography.
  - While CT is primarily indicated to identify fractures and assess for spinal malalignment, it can also demonstrate findings suggestive of pathology that would be better characterized on MRI, for which a follow-up trauma protocol MRI can be obtained.
  - Dual-energy CT is also becoming more readily available and has demonstrated value in the identification of:
    - Marrow edema—which can suggest that a fracture is more acute as opposed to chronic, and help identify subtle fractures that may have otherwise been missed on standard CT.
    - Disc edema—suggestive of disc injury [3].
- MRI is often considered the next step, and its superior tissue contrast makes it the ideal modality for the following indications:
  - Ligamentous injury.
  - Intervertebral disc injury.
  - Cord injury.
  - Hemorrhage and large vessel injury, e.g., vertebral arteries.
  - Differentiating acute from chronic fractures (assessing for marrow edema).
  - Differentiating benign osteoporotic and malignant pathologic vertebral fractures.

Three-Column Concept

- The most widely used classification system for thoracolumbar fractures and often for cervical fractures.
- Spinal columns are defined from anterior to posterior:
  - Anterior column—anterior longitudinal ligament (ALL), anterior two-thirds of the vertebral body.

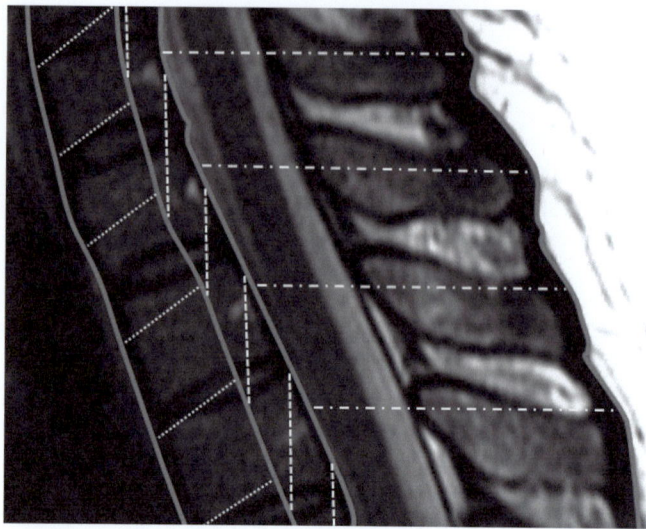

Fig. 22.1 Three-column concept. Oblique lines = anterior column; vertical lines = middle column; horizontal lines = posterior column

- Middle column—posterior one-third of the vertebral body, posterior longitudinal ligament (PLL).
- Posterior column—pedicles, lamina, spinous process, ligamentum flavum, interspinous ligament, and supraspinous ligament (Fig. 22.1) [4].
- The pattern of column involvement is used to predict the risk of spinal instability and thus potential cord injury.
- Disruption of structures in ≥2 contiguous columns is considered an unstable injury.
- Stable fractures can usually be treated with bracing and rest, whereas unstable ones require surgical intervention.

Types Of Spinal Fractures

- Compression and burst fractures.
  - Mechanism—axial loading.
  - Vertebral compression fractures involve loss of vertebral body height without involvement of the posterior margin of the vertebral body. These include anterior wedge collapse, superior endplate collapse, and biconcave endplate collapse.
  - Burst-type compression fractures are similar but involve the posterior margin.
  - Burst fractures often result in bony retropulsion, which increases the risk of cord injury, and are thus considered potentially unstable (Fig. 22.2) [5].
- Vertebra plana.
  - Defined as near-complete vertebral body height loss.
  - May be associated with trauma or osteoporosis, and often occurs with pathologic fractures in the setting of Langerhans cell histiocytosis, osteomyelitis, and malignancy.
- Spondylolysis/pars interarticularis defect.
  - Defect in lumbar vertebrae pars interarticularis, which is the portion of bone connecting the superior and inferior articular facets (Fig. e22.1).
  - (All electronic images (Figs. e22.1–e22.15) can be found on this chapter's website on SpringerLink: https://doi.org/10.1007/978-3-031-55124-6_22)
  - Developmental or acquired secondary to trauma.
  - Not to be confused with spondylosis, which broadly refers to degenerative changes of the spine, or spondylolisthesis, which refers to anterior (anterolisthesis) or posterior (posterolisthesis) subluxation of a vertebra relative to the one below it.
  - Often develop secondary spondylolisthesis, usually an anterolisthesis of the affected vertebral body.
- Jefferson fracture.
  - Mechanism—axial loading.
  - Analogous to a compression fracture of C1 with involvement and distraction of both the anterior and posterior elements (Fig. e22.2).
- Hangman's fracture.
  - Mechanism—hyperextension.
  - Bilateral traumatic pars interarticularis fractures of C2 (Fig. 22.3).
  - Commonly associated with anterolisthesis of C2 on C3 with widening of the spinal canal.
  - Considered unstable if disc space widening, angulation of fragments, or C2 on C3 anterolisthesis ≥2 mm is present.
- Dens Fractures.
  - Type 1.
    - Fracture to superior tip of dens.
    - Stable injury.
  - Type 2.
    - Fracture at the base of the dens.
    - Unstable injury.
  - Type 3.
    - Dens fracture which extends into the body of C2.
    - Considered to be potentially unstable (Fig. 22.4) [6].
- Flexion teardrop fracture.
  - Mechanism—high impact flexion.
  - Anterior inferior endplate fracture with a fragment in the shape of a "teardrop," and both anterior and posterior longitudinal ligament disruption with retrolisthesis of the affected vertebra.
  - Considered unstable injury with a high propensity for cord injury and resulting neurological deficits [7].
- Extension teardrop fracture.
  - Mechanism—extension.
  - Cervical fracture with anterior inferior endplate fracture with teardrop morphology, and ALL injury only.

22 Spine Trauma

Fig. 22.2 Burst fracture. (**a**) Lateral radiograph depicting L1 vertebral body fracture with vertebral body height loss. (**b**) Sagittal T2 MRI which better depicts disruption of the vertebral body posterior margin with bony fragment retropulsion resulting in a mass effect on the cauda equina

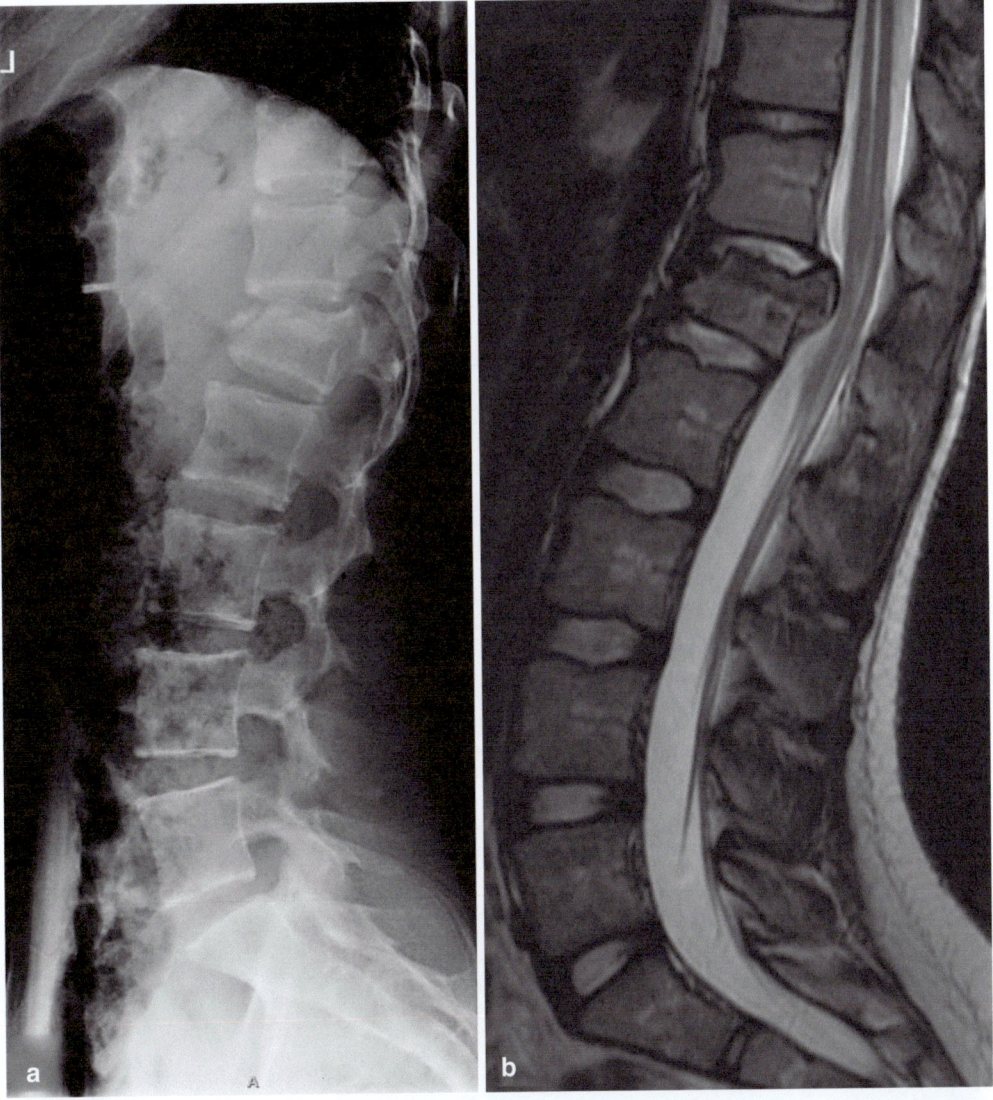

Fig. 22.3 Hangman's fracture. (**a**) Axial CT with fracture lines through the bilateral C2 pars interarticularis. (**b**) Sagittal CT view of right-sided pars interarticularis fracture

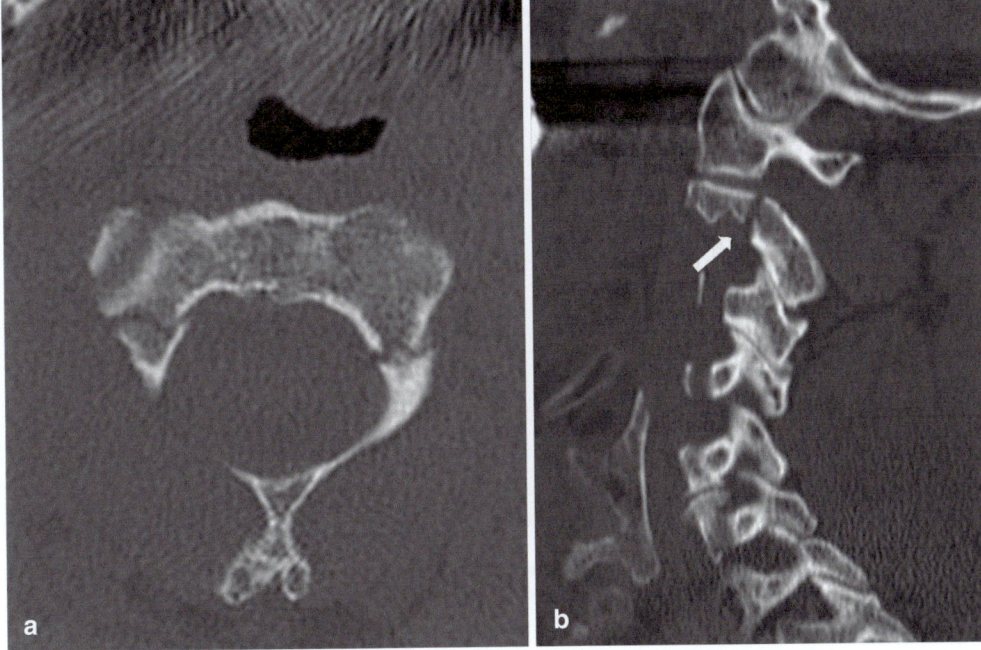

- Stable spinal injury if the patient's neck is in extension, and unstable if in flexion. This is related to the latter resulting in ligamentum flavum buckling with cord impingement in the setting of ALL injury (Fig. 22.5) [7].
- Clay-shoveler fracture.
  - Oblique spinous process fracture historically ascribed to upward thrusting motion during shoveling, more commonly seen in the setting of posterior blunt trauma to a flexed cervicothoracic spine.
    - Most often occurs from C6 to T3 (Fig. e22.3) [8].
- Chance fracture.
  - Mechanism—high-impact motor vehicle collisions with the seatbelt acting as a fulcrum with distraction injury through all three spinal columns.

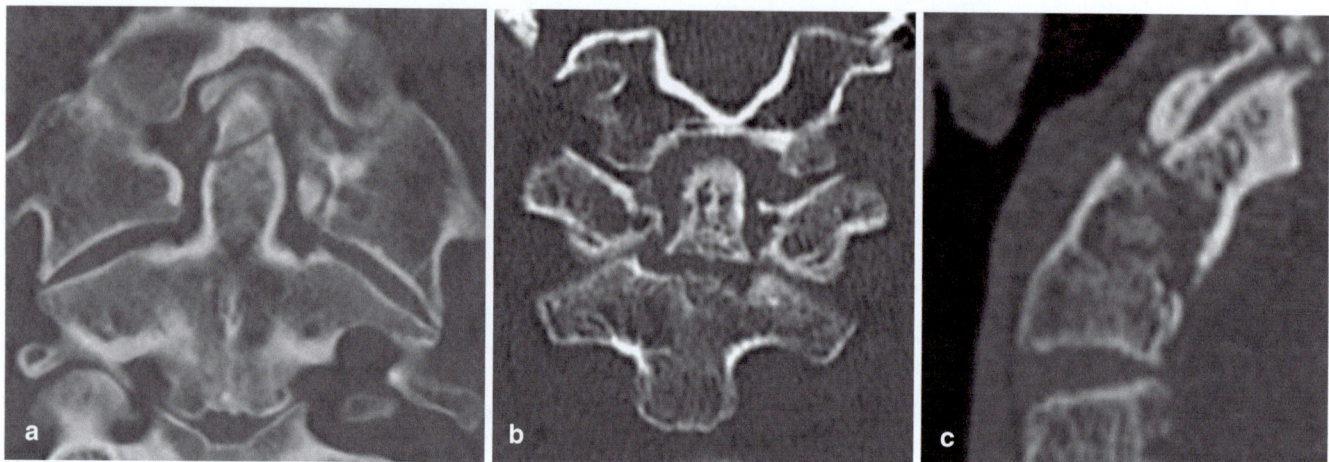

Fig. 22.4 Dens fractures. (**a**) Type 1 dens fracture which is isolated to the cranial tip of the dens. (**b**) Type 2 dens fracture at the base of the dens. (**c**) Type 3 dens fracture involving the base of the dens, and with extension into the anterior C2 body

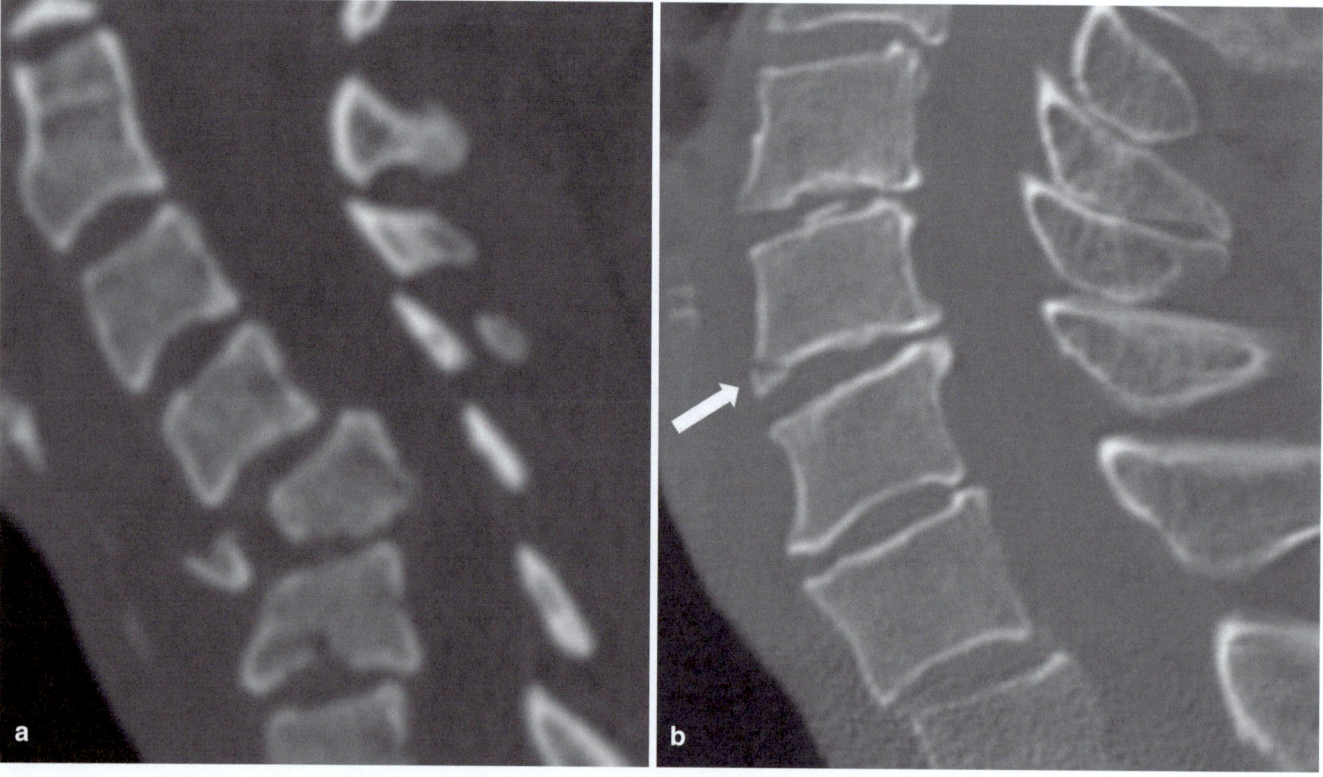

Fig. 22.5 Flexion and extension teardrop fractures. (**a**) C5 and C6 flexion teardrop fractures with marked displacement and rotation of C5 anteroinferior endplate fragment, and posterior subluxation of C5. (**b**) Minimally displaced extension teardrop fracture

- Occurs in the thoracolumbar spine with anterior wedge-shaped vertebral body fracture and horizontally oriented distracted fracture line through the more posterior vertebrae. Ligamentous injury involving the ligamentum flavum, interspinous, and supraspinous ligaments is also common (Fig. e22.4).
- It is also possible to have an entirely soft tissue Chance injury which extends through the intervertebral disc and ligamentous structures, as well as a combined osseous and soft tissue injury.
- Considered to be an unstable injury, with a strong association with intra-abdominal trauma, especially aortic injury [9].
• Chalk (or carrot) stick fractures.
- Spinal fractures that occur in the setting of fused spines secondary to conditions such as:
  • Ankylosing spondylitis.
  • Ossification of the posterior longitudinal ligament (OPLL).
  • Diffuse idiopathic skeletal hyperostosis (DISH).
  • Surgical spinal fusion.
- The fused column of vertebral segments acts as a fulcrum that can fracture with relatively low-impact trauma related to poor dissipation of the force of impact.
- Fractures typically occur in the cervicothoracic spine along a disco-vertebral junction and demonstrate a broken chalk stick-like morphology.
- These are highly unstable fractures relating to all three columns behaving as a single unit secondary to multi-level fusion (Fig. e22.5) [10].
• Limbus fracture/posterior ring apophyseal fracture.
- Mechanism—chronic repetitive microtrauma.
- Fracture occurring only in pediatric patients along the posterior apophyseal ring, which is a secondary ossification center where the vertebral endplate attaches to the intervertebral disc.
- Most commonly localized to the lumbar spine.
- Characterized by a small osseous fragment along the posterior vertebral endplate (Fig. e22.6) [11].
• Transverse process fracture.
- It occurs most commonly within the lumbar spine.
- In isolation, transverse fractures are stable, but they are associated with other clinically significant injuries.
- Approximately 50% of patients with a transverse process fracture in the lumbar spine will have concurrent intra-abdominal injury [12].
- Cervical spine transverse process fractures should be closely inspected for the involvement of the transverse foramina, and if present, a CTA should be performed to exclude vertebral artery injury.
• Sacral fractures.
- Traumatic fractures result from either transmitted forces through the pelvic ring or direct impact, such as falling from a height onto the buttocks.
- The most commonly used classification system for traumatic sacral fractures is the Denis Classification system, which broadly is defined as follows:
  • Zone 1 Fracture—Involving the sacral ala lateral to the neuroforamina.
  • Zone 2 Fracture—Involving the neuroforamina, but not extending to the spinal canal.
  • Zone 3 Fracture—Involving the spinal canal.
- Zone 2 and 3 fractures are associated with an increasing probability of radiculopathies and neurological deficits.
- Traumatic sacral fractures can additionally be associated with diastasis of the sacroiliac joint, which is generally identified by the presence of joint space widening.
- Insufficiency fractures of the sacrum occur secondary to normal biomechanical stress in the setting of abnormal bone, which most commonly includes osteoporosis in the elderly.
  • Given marked osseous demineralization in these patients, fracture lines can be difficult to appreciate. If the radiograph and CT are negative, but an insufficiency fracture is still highly suspected, an MRI or Tc99m-MDP bone scan can be performed [13].
• Coccygeal fractures.
- Fractures of the coccyx are frequently missed on imaging which may relate to:
  • Significant normal variation in coccygeal contour, shape, and degree of osseous fusion between segments among patients.
  • Imaging inadvertently not including the entire coccyx in the FOV.
  • Perceived lack of clinical importance.
- Although most coccygeal fractures will heal with conservative management, some patients will present weeks to months after the trauma with chronic refractory pain at the site, which may be related to nonunion, malunion, or subluxation of the sacrococcygeal joint [14, 15].

Differentiating Benign Osteoporotic And Malignant Pathologic Vertebral Fractures

- Vertebral body compression/burst fractures secondary to osteoporosis and malignancy can have overlapping imaging findings but have vastly different management and prognostic implications.
- Therefore, identifying an underlying malignant/metastatic lesion in the setting of a vertebral fracture is essential.
- Benign vertebral body fracture Findings.
  - Fracture is often limited to the vertebral body.
  - CT—Well-demarcated sharp fracture lines resembling puzzle pieces on CT (i.e., *puzzle sign*).
  - FDG PET—Increased uptake at the site of fracture that normalizes by 3 months.
  - MRI findings.
    - Enhancement of vertebrae that should resolve by 3 months.
    - Hypointense linear horizontal lines on T1- and T2-weighted sequences.
    - *Fluid sign*—T2 hyperintense linear or triangular region within the vertebral body (Fig. e22.7).
- Malignant pathologic fractures findings.
  - Fractures often extend into posterior elements.
  - Convex margin of the posterior vertebral body.
  - Presence of adjacent soft tissue mass.
  - CT—Aggressive osteolytic changes (Fig. 22.6).
  - FDG PET—Increased uptake that persists beyond 3 months with possible worsening [16].

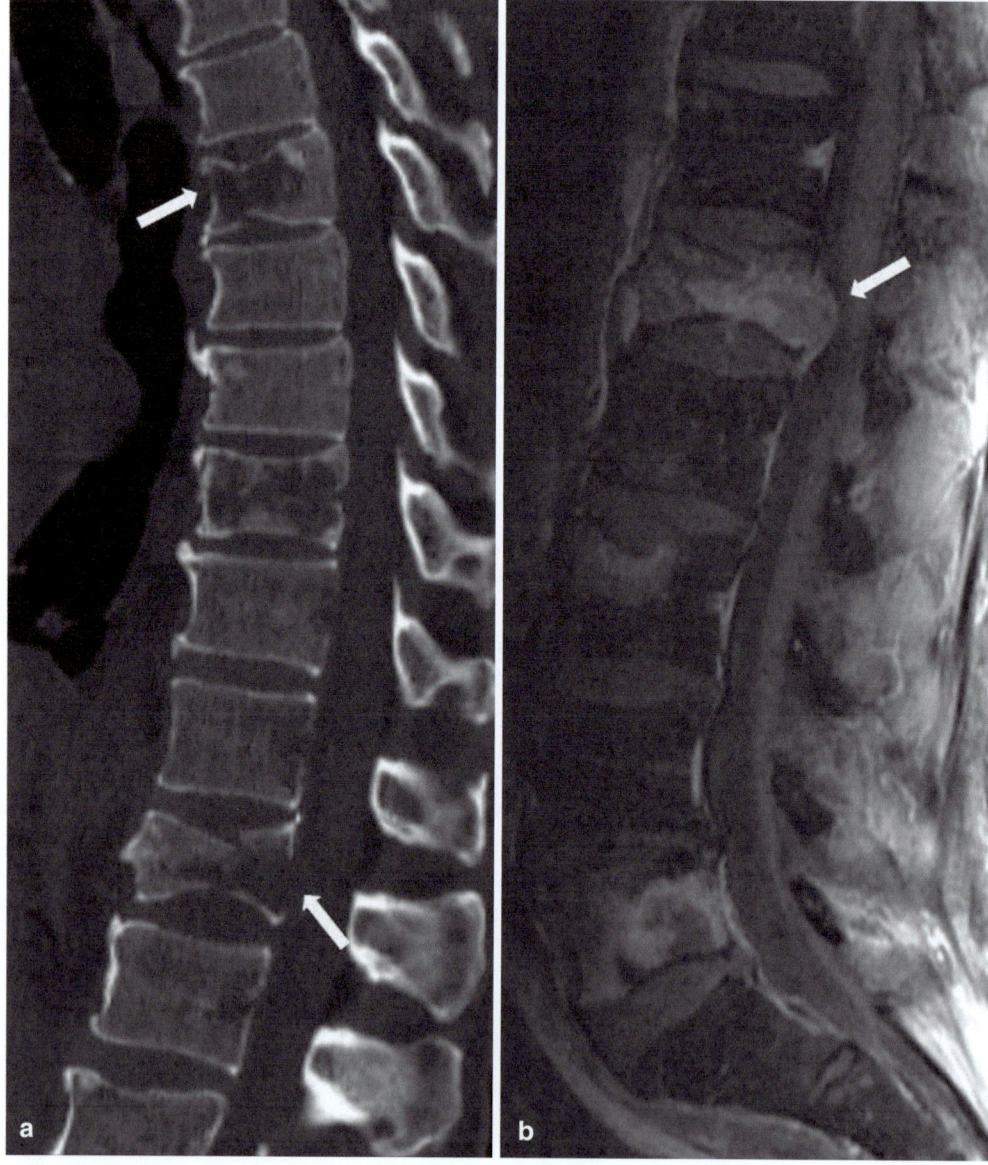

Fig. 22.6 Malignant vertebral body fractures. (**a**) Vertebral body fractures with underlying osteolytic lesions resulting in cortical breakthrough (arrows). (**b**) Sagittal T1 post-contrast sequence demonstrating vertebral body fracture with underlying heterogeneous enhancing lesion resulting in a convex margin of the dorsal margin (arrow)

- MRI.
  - Enhancement of vertebrae that increases over time or persists beyond 3 months.
  - Mass-like confluent T1 hypointensity which effaces normal T1 hyperintense fatty marrow.
  - Presence of diffusion restriction.

Spinal Fracture Mimics

- Odontoid/dens variants.
  - The dens fuse to the C2 body at the subdental synchondrosis, with the latter persisting into adulthood as a sclerotic line that can be confused for a fracture.
  - An os terminale is a small secondary ossification center cranial to the tip of the dens which may fail to fuse appropriately with the dens by adulthood.
  - An os odontoideum is a well-corticated osseous fragment adjacent to the dens that is larger than an os terminale and can be in a similar location as the os terminale (i.e., orthotopic os odontoideum) or more displaced (i.e., dystopic os odontoideum) (Fig. e22.8).
- Intercalary bone—triangular ossifications that occur along the anterior margin of intervertebral discs (Fig. e22.9).
- Limbus vertebra.
  - Originates from herniation of the intervertebral disc through the corner of a vertebral endplate.
  - Results in well-corticated triangular fragments most commonly seen along an antero-superior end-plate of the lumbar spine (Fig. e22.10) [17].

Subluxations And Dislocations

- Facet malalignment spectrum.
  - Most commonly occurs in the cervical spine.
  - Continuum of facet displacement:
    - Facet subluxation—mild partial facet malalignment.
    - Perched facet—near-complete subluxation verging on dislocation of the facet joint with the superior facet "perched" along the cranial margin of the inferior facet.
    - Locked (or jumped) facet—complete dislocation of the facet joint with the superior facet "locked" ventrally to the inferior, now "naked," facet (Fig. 22.7). On axial CT images, the normal facet joint is described as having a "hamburger bun" appearance. When the joint is dislocated, the naked facet appearance is also called the "reverse hamburger bun sign."
  - Bilateral facet dislocation.
    - Bilateral locked facets with injury to all spinal ligaments.
    - Unstable injury with a high incidence of cord injury.
  - Unilateral facet dislocation.
    - Unilateral locked facet.
    - Less severe than bilateral type, and with stability determined by the extent of other associated fractures and ligamentous injuries [18].
- Atlanto-occipital Dissociation.
  - Mechanism—high-impact trauma, most commonly motor vehicle accidents.
  - Identified by widening of the basion-dental interval, which is the distance between the basion (i.e., anterior

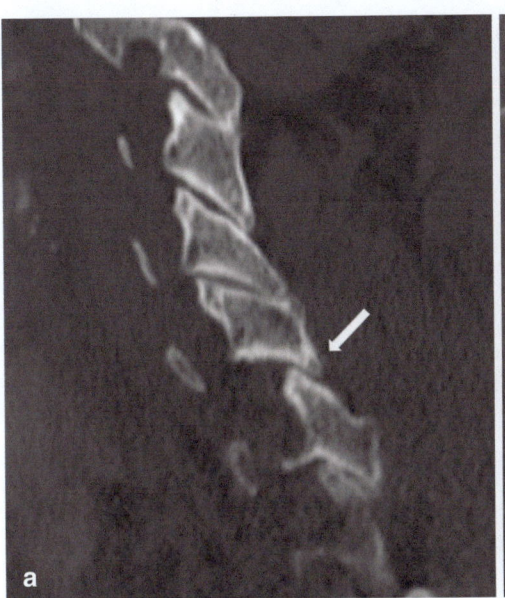 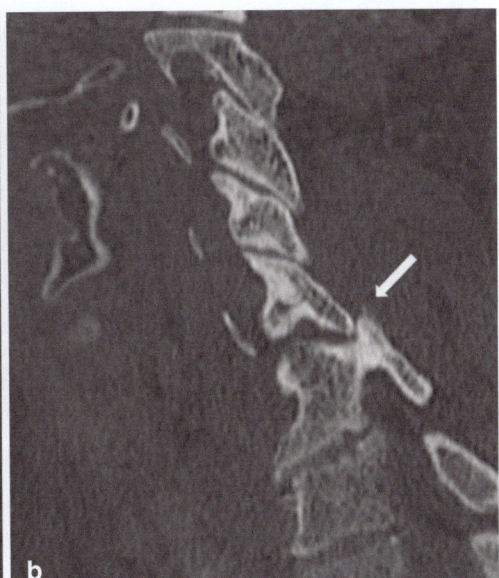

Fig. 22.7 Facet malalignment. (**a**) Perched facet with superior facet only minimally articulating with the inferior facet near the cranial margin. (**b**) Naked facet with complete disarticulation of the superior and inferior facets and with the superior facet "locked" anteriorly

midpoint of the occipital bone at the foramen magnum) and the dens in the sagittal plane. The normal value is ≤1.0 cm.
- MRI is often required to assess for craniocervical ligament, brain stem, and upper cervical cord injury.
- Unstable injury.
- Atlanto-axial subluxation.
  - Associated with numerous etiologies, including pediatric retropharyngeal abscesses causing craniocervical ligamentous laxity (i.e., Grisel syndrome), Down syndrome, inflammatory arthropathies (e.g., rheumatoid arthritis), and trauma.
  - Various directions of subluxation including anteroposterior, rotatory, vertical, and lateral subluxation.
  - Imaging findings include.
    - Widened atlanto-dental interval which is ≥3 mm in adults, and ≥10 mm in pediatrics in the flexed position (Fig. e22.11).
    - Dens projecting above the foramen magnum.
    - Asymmetry of the lateral atlantoaxial joints.
  - Stability varies with the type of subluxation and extent of other associated injuries [19–21].

Extramedullary Hematomas

- Epidural hematomas occur superficial to the dura and thecal sac, and subdural hematomas occupy the potential space between the dura and arachnoid membrane, with the latter commonly manifesting as the *inverted Mercedes-Benz sign* on axial MRI.
- These entities are most commonly spontaneous in the setting of anticoagulation or coagulopathy but can also be seen in the setting of trauma.
- MRI is the modality of choice for diagnosis.
- Unfortunately, the temporal progression of MRI signal characteristics for intracranial intra-axial hemorrhages cannot be applied to those in the extramedullary compartments of the spine owing to the absence of a blood–brain barrier.
- Therefore, diagnosis of spinal epidural and subdural hematomas is best accomplished using clinical context and by analyzing both T1- and T2-weighted sequences for loculated collections in these separate compartments that are distinct from CSF (Fig. 22.8) [22].

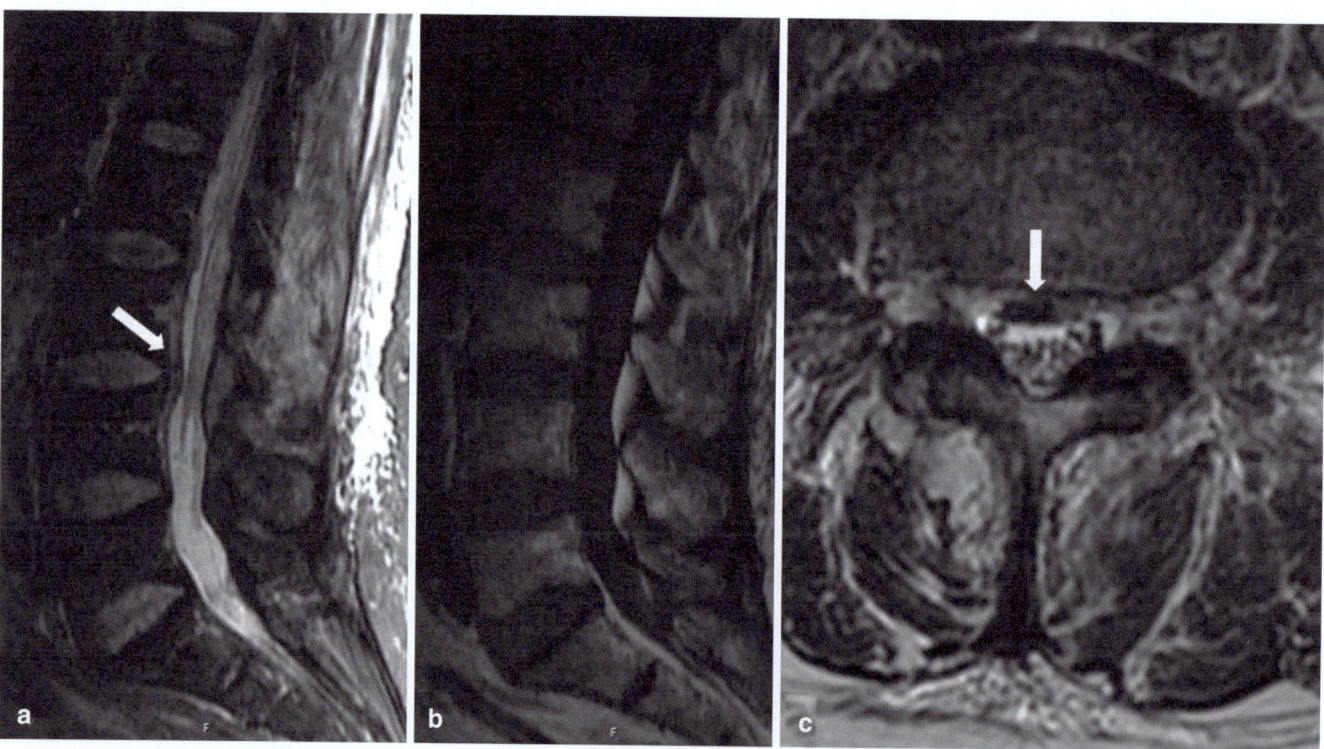

Fig. 22.8 Spinal epidural hematoma. (**a**) Sagittal T2 fat-suppressed sequence demonstrating isointense collection in the L3–L4 ventral epidural compartment (arrow). (**b**) This collection is notably occult on sagittal T1 imaging. (**c**) Axial view of this ventral epidural collection (arrow) which appears more hypointense on this T2-weighted non-fat-suppressed sequence

22 Spine Trauma

Intervertebral Disc Injury

- Intervertebral disc injuries are best demonstrated on MRI, and manifest as follows:
  o Edema—hyperintense T2 signal which is greater than adjacent unaffected levels.
  o Hemorrhage—focal hypointense T2 signal which is less than adjacent unaffected levels, and cannot be accounted for by intradisc gas or calcifications.
  o Annular tear and/or disc rupture—focal or multifocal T2 hyperintensity with or without herniation of disc material into adjacent vertebral endplate or spinal canal [23].

Soft Tissue And Ligamentous Injury

- Injuries of the paravertebral soft tissues are common in the setting of spinal trauma and primarily include edema and hemorrhage.
- In the cervical spine, the anterior prevertebral soft tissue is a classic site for trauma-related edema and/or hematoma.
  o This is best assessed in the midline sagittal plane on CT or radiograph where the soft tissue thickness anterior to the vertebral body can be quickly assessed for thickening. This is best assessed qualitatively, as there is significant variability between patients as to the normal degree of thickness.
  o Pseudothickening can occur if the patient has an excessively flexed neck during imaging and would resolve upon reimaging in a more neutral position.
  o On MRI, edema and/or hematoma can be visualized as thin linear or focal signal abnormalities that are distinct from adjacent normal-appearing soft tissue.
  o Notably STIR sequences, which are T2-weighted inversion recovery sequences that suppress surrounding fat signal, will highlight edema the best.
- Throughout the remainder of the spinal perivertebral space, trauma can result in edema and hemorrhage within the adjacent subcutaneous fat and paraspinal musculature.
  o Edema—Manifests as fat stranding and hypoattenuation on CT, as well as T2 hyperintensity on STIR sequences.
  o Hemorrhage—Focal collection in the setting of trauma with variable CT and MRI appearance depending on acuity.
- Spinal ligamentous injury is best evaluated on MRI, and its primary manifestations include:
  o Strain—Increased T2 signal without evidence of discontinuity.
  o Tear—Increased T2 signal with partial or complete discontinuity, and potential malalignment of associated osseous structures (Fig. e22.12).

Spinal Cord Injury

- Cord trauma manifestations.
  o Swelling—Increased cord caliber with or without cord signal abnormality.
  o Edema—Increased T2 signal within the cord.
  o Contusion—Central focus of T2 isointensity and peripheral hyperintensity which persists for days following trauma.
  o Hemorrhage—Best identified greater than 24 h after trauma on GRE sequences as the focus of increased susceptibility.
  o Compression—Trauma-related (i.e., fracture fragment, hematoma, etc.) thecal sac CSF effacement with mass effect on the cord.
  o Transection (partial or complete)—Discontinuity of normal cord contour (Fig. 22.9) [24, 25].
- Incomplete spinal cord syndromes—Cord injury/insult patterns secondary to trauma, syringohydromyelia, neoplasm, and other processes.
  o Central cord syndrome.
    - Etiology—Hyperextension injury in the setting of spondylosis.
    - Small lesion—Affects decussating bilateral spinothalamic tracts (STT) with resulting loss of bilateral pain and temperature sensation in a band of two to three spinal segments below the spinal injury.
    - Large lesion—Affects bilateral STTs and corticospinal tracts (CSTs) with resulting bilateral motor, pain, and sensory deficits preferentially affecting the upper extremities, and to a lesser degree the lower extremities.
  o Brown-Sequard syndrome.
    - Etiology—Penetrating trauma (e.g., gunshot wound) resulting in hemicord lesion.
    - Affects ipsilateral STT, CST, and posterior columns with resulting ipsilateral motor, light touch, and proprioception deficits at and below the lesion, and contralateral pain and temperature sensation deficits in two to three spinal segments below the lesion.
  o Anterior cord syndrome.
    - Etiology—Anterior spinal artery-related ischemia is the most common cause, but in the setting of trauma can be related to anterior cord impingement by fracture fragments or disc displacement.
    - Affects the bilateral STTs and CSTs with resulting motor deficits at and below the lesion, and pain and

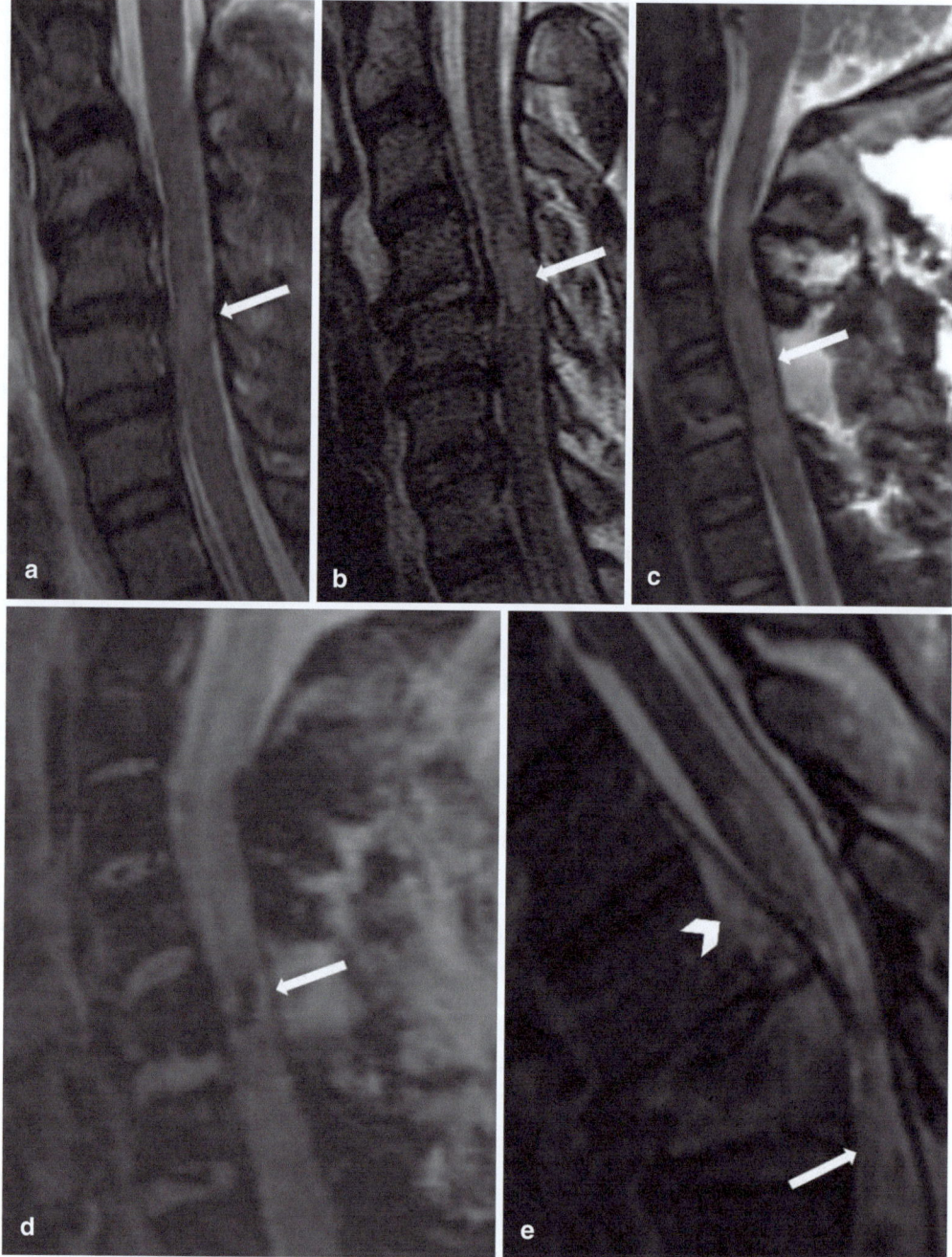

Fig. 22.9 Cord injury. (**a**) Sagittal T2 sequence demonstrating isolated cord edema (arrow). (**b**) Sagittal T2 sequence with focal contusion manifesting as the focus of hyperintensity with a more central isointense signal (arrow). (**c**) Sagittal T2 sequence showing cord swelling with regional CSF effacement (arrow). (**d**) Sagittal GRE sequence with the focus on increased susceptibility within the cord compatible with hemorrhage (arrow). (**e**) Sagittal T2 sequence demonstrating severe traumatic injury with burst fracture and severe retropulsion, epidural hematoma (chevron), and focal non-visualization of the spinal cord suggestive of transection (arrow)

temperature sensation deficits in two to three spinal segments below the lesion.
- Posterior cord syndrome.
    - Etiology—Uncommonly caused by trauma, with multiple sclerosis, vitamin B12 deficiency, and metastases being more common causes.
    - Affects the bilateral posterior columns with resulting bilateral light touch and proprioception deficits at and below the lesion.
- Conus medullaris syndrome.
    - Etiology—Numerous etiologies that result in compression of the conus including trauma, degenerative changes, and tumors.
    - Physical exam findings include upper motor neuron (e.g., hyperreflexia and hypertonia) and lower motor neuron (e.g., hyporeflexia and hypotonia) signs, as well as saddle anesthesia, and bowel/bladder dysfunction.
- Cauda equina syndrome.
    - Etiology—Similar to conus medullaris syndrome, but with compression of the cauda equina nerve roots in the lumbosacral spine.
    - Physical exam findings are comparable with conus medullaris syndrome, but without upper motor neuron signs [26].

Brachial Plexus Injury

- Brachial plexus anatomy.
  - The brachial plexus is supplied by the C5–T1 nerve roots, although 50% of patients will have some degree of variant anatomy.
  - Each spinal nerve is formed from the convergence of the dorsal (afferent) and ventral (efferent) rootlets, which then distally branch into dorsal and ventral rami (Fig. e22.13).
  - The ventral rami of C5–T1 are what form the brachial plexus, with the proximal to distal architecture labeled as roots, trunks, divisions, cords, and branches.
  - A common mnemonic used to remember this framework is "Rad Techs Drink Cold Beer" (Fig. e22.14).
  - The most important anatomical detail related to brachial plexus injury (BPI) is the distinction between pre- and post-ganglionic structures.
    - The pre-ganglionic structures include the dorsal/ventral nerve rootlets within the thecal sac extending into the neuroforamen, at the approximate location of the dorsal root ganglion (DRG), with the post-ganglionic structures distal to the DRG.
    - Pre-ganglionic injuries can be managed with nerve transfers.
    - In contrast, post-ganglionic injuries can be managed conservatively or with nerve grafts depending on the severity.
- Etiology.
  - Mechanistically occurs with traction-related injuries of the upper extremities.
  - The most common causes include motor vehicle collisions and birth-related trauma (e.g., Duchenne and Erb palsies).
  - Less commonly sport, occupational, and gun-shot-related trauma can result in BPI.
  - BPI results in variable upper extremity musculature weakness, depending on the specific site of involvement.
- Imaging.
  - BPI is best evaluated with high-resolution MRI, and additional CT myelogram may be useful.
  - Compression and traction injuries to the nerves are more common than complete transections.
  - Direct signs of preganglionic injury.
    - Anatomic discontinuity of nerve roots extending up to neuroforamen.
    - Asymmetric enhancement and/or T2 signal of nerve root.
  - Direct signs of postganglionic injury—similar to preganglionic injury, but findings are distal to the neuroforamen (Fig. e22.15).
  - Indirect signs of pre- and post-ganglionic injury—abnormal enhancement and/or T2 signal within ipsilateral paraspinal musculature innervated by the brachial plexus, reflective of denervation.
  - Indirect signs of preganglionic injury.
    - Contralateral deviation of the cord owing to loss of traction by the injured side.
    - Pseudomeningocele extending into the ipsilateral neural foramina (Fig. 22.10) [27, 28].

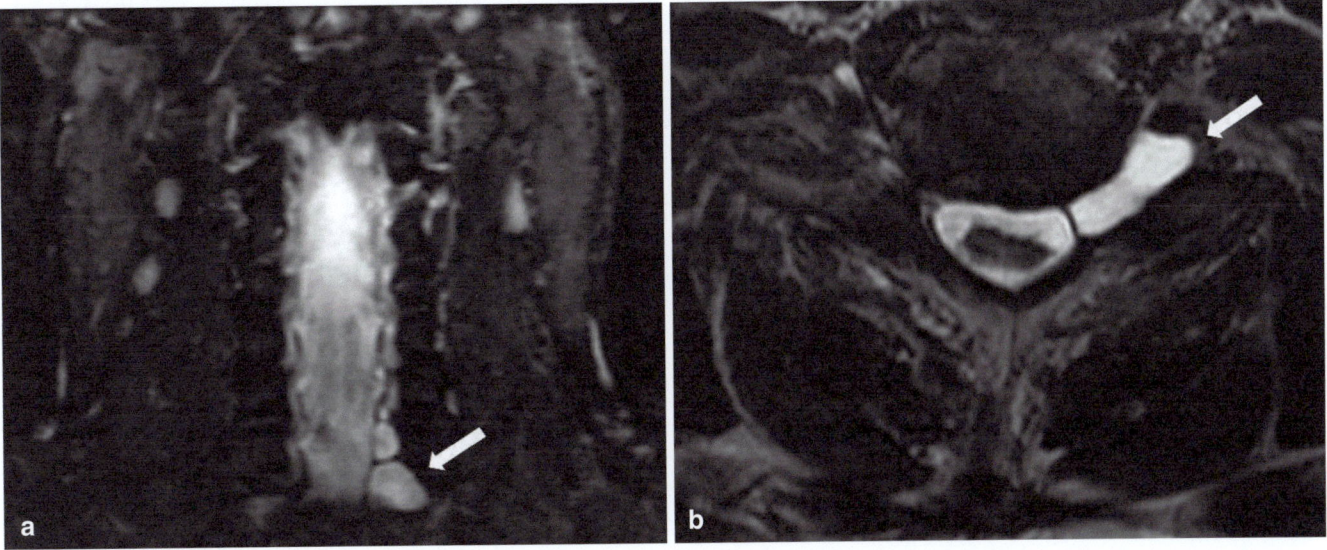

Fig. 22.10 Pre-ganglionic brachial plexus injury. (**a**) Coronal T2 sequences demonstrating two pseudomeningoceles within left C6–C7 and C7–T1 neural foramina (arrow). (**b**) Axial view of the larger C7–T1 neural foraminal pseudomeningocele

References

1. Beckmann N, West OC, Nunez D, et al. ACR appropriateness criteria—suspected spine trauma. American College of Radiology. 2018. https://www.acr.org/Clinical-Resources/ACR-Appropriateness-Criteria. Accessed 3 March 2022.
2. Parizel PM, Van Der Zijden T, Gaudino S, et al. Trauma of the spine and spinal cord: imaging strategies. Eur Spine J. 2010;19(SUPPL. 1):8–17. https://doi.org/10.1007/s00586-009-1123-5.
3. Bäcker HC, Wu CH, Perka C, Panics G. Dual-energy computed tomography in spine fractures: a systematic review and meta-analysis. Int J Spine Surg. 2021;15(3):525–35. https://doi.org/10.14444/8074.
4. Denis F. The three column spine and its significance in the classification of acute thoracolumbar spinal injuries. Spine (Phila Pa 1976). 1983;8(8):817–31. https://doi.org/10.1097/00007632-198311000-00003.
5. Vaccaro AR, Lehman RA, Hurlbert RJ, et al. A new classification of thoracolumbar injuries: the importance of injury morphology, the integrity of the posterior ligamentous complex, and neurologic status. Spine (Phila Pa 1976). 2005;30(20):2325–33. https://doi.org/10.1097/01.brs.0000182986.43345.cb.
6. Hsu WK, Anderson PA. Odontoid fractures: Update on management. J Am Acad Orthop Surg. 2010;18(7):383–94. https://doi.org/10.5435/00124635-201007000-00001.
7. Dreizin D, Letzing M, Sliker CW, et al. Multidetector CT of blunt cervical spine trauma in adults. Radiographics. 2014;34(7):1842–65. https://doi.org/10.1148/rg.347130094.
8. Cancelmo JJ. Clay shoveler's fracture. A helpful diagnostic sign. Am J Roentgenol Radium Therapy, Nucl Med. 1972;115(3):540–3. https://doi.org/10.2214/ajr.115.3.540.
9. Groves CJ, Cassar-Pullicino VN, Tins BJ, Tyrrell PNM, McCall IW. Chance-type flexion-distraction injuries in the thoracolumbar spine: MR imaging characteristics. Radiology. 2005;236(2):601–8. https://doi.org/10.1148/radiol.2362040281.
10. Tomar SS. Chalkstick fracture: a catastrophic injury. Asian J Neurosurg. 2021;13(2):383–5. https://doi.org/10.4103/ajns.AJNS_167_13.
11. Yen CH, Chan SK, Ho YF, Mak KH. Posterior lumbar apophyseal ring fractures in adolescents: a report of four cases. J Orthop Surg (Hong Kong). 2009;17(1):85–9. https://doi.org/10.1177/230949900901700119.
12. Patten RM, Gunberg SR, Brandenburger DK. Frequency and importance of transverse process fractures in the lumbar vertebrae at helical abdominal CT in patients with trauma. Radiology. 2000;215(3):831–4. https://doi.org/10.1148/radiology.215.3.r00jn27831.
13. White JH, Hague C, Nicolaou S, Gee R, Marchinkow LO, Munk PL. Imaging of sacral fractures. Clin Radiol. 2003;58(12):914–21. https://doi.org/10.1016/S0009-9260(03)00270-8.
14. Skalski MR, Matcuk GR, Patel DB, Tomasian A, White EA, Gross JS. Imaging coccygeal trauma and coccydynia. Radiographics. 2020;40(4):1090–106. https://doi.org/10.1148/rg.2020190132.
15. Maigne JY, Doursounian L, Jacquot F. Classification of fractures of the coccyx from a series of 104 patients. Eur Spine J. 2020;29(10):2534–42. https://doi.org/10.1007/s00586-019-06188-7.
16. Mauch JT, Carr CM, Cloft H, Diehn FE. Review of the imaging features of benign osteoporotic and malignant vertebral compression fractures. Am J Neuroradiol. 2018;39(9):1584–92. https://doi.org/10.3174/ajnr.A5528.
17. Carr RB, Tozer Fink KR, Gross JA. Imaging of trauma: part 1, pseudotrauma of the spine—osseous variants that may simulate injury. Am J Roentgenol. 2012;199(6):1200–6. https://doi.org/10.2214/AJR.12.9083.
18. Anaya JEC, Coelho SRN, Taneja AK, Cardoso FN, Skaf AY, Aihara AY. Differential diagnosis of facet joint disorders. Radiographics. 2021;41(2):543–58. https://doi.org/10.1148/rg.2021200079.
19. Rojas CA, Hayes A, Bertozzi JC, Guidi C, Martinez CR. Evaluation of the C1-C2 articulation on MDCT in healthy children and young adults. Am J Roentgenol. 2009;193(5):1388–92. https://doi.org/10.2214/AJR.09.2688.
20. Riascos R, Bonfante E, Cotes C, Guirgui M, Hakimelahi R, West C. Imaging of atlanto-occipital and atlantoaxial traumatic injuries: what the radiologist needs to know. Radiographics. 2015;35(7):2121–34.
21. Joaquim AF, Ghizoni E, Tedeschi H, Appenzeller S, Riew KD. Radiological evaluation of cervical spine involvement in rheumatoid arthritis. Neurosurg Focus. 2015;38(4):E4. https://doi.org/10.3171/2015.1.FOCUS14664.
22. Braun P, Kazmi K, Nogués-Meléndez P, Mas-Estellés F, Aparici-Robles F. MRI findings in spinal subdural and epidural hematomas. Eur J Radiol. 2007;64(1):119–25. https://doi.org/10.1016/j.ejrad.2007.02.014.
23. Sander AL, Laurer H, Lehnert T, et al. A clinically useful classification of traumatic intervertebral disk lesions. Am J Roentgenol. 2013;200(3):618–23. https://doi.org/10.2214/AJR.12.8748.
24. Mahmood NS, Kadavigere R, Ramesh AK, Rao VR. Magnetic resonance imaging in acute cervical spinal cord injury: a correlative study on spinal cord changes and 1 month motor recovery. Spinal Cord. 2008;46(12):791–7.
25. Kulkarni MV, McArdle CB, Kopanicky D, et al. Acute spinal cord injury: MR imaging at 1.5 T. Radiology. 1987;164(3):837–43. https://doi.org/10.1148/radiology.164.3.3615885.
26. Kunam VK, Velayudhan V, Chaudhry ZA, Bobinski M, Smoker WRK, Reede DL. Incomplete cord syndromes: clinical and imaging review. Radiographics. 2018;38(4):1201–22. https://doi.org/10.1148/rg.2018170178.
27. Yoshikawa T, Hayashi N, Yamamoto S, et al. Brachial plexus injury: clinical manifestations, conventional imaging findings, and the latest imaging techniques. Radiographics. 2006;26(suppl_1):133–44. https://doi.org/10.1148/rg.26si065511.
28. Vijayasarathi A, Chokshi FH. MRI of the brachial plexus: a practical review. Appl Radiol. 2016;45(4):9–18.

Degenerative Disease of the Spine and Spinal Arthritides

Brian Rigney, Shivam Kaushik, and Amish Doshi

- **Degenerative disease** of the spine and **spinal arthritides** are extraordinarily common and pose a significant health care burden.
- Degenerative changes and arthritides can involve the **intervertebral disc**, facets, and ligamentum flavum.
- Symptoms most commonly occur due to nerve root compression which can result in radicular pain or localized inflammatory changes which can result in axial back pain.
- Symptoms occur due to nerve root compression which can result in radicular pain or localized inflammatory changes which can result in axial back pain [1].
- Nerve roots can be compressed within the spinal canal, the subarticular zone, or neural foramen.
- Consistent and detailed characterization with appropriate grading of associated findings is important to patient management.
- A variety of multidisciplinary groups have proposed consensus nomenclature guidelines including Spine 2.0 which should be adhered to whenever possible.

Disc Degeneration

- Normal **intervertebral disc** is composed of central gelatinous nucleus pulposus and fibrous peripheral annulus fibrosis.
- With age, the nucleus pulposus can become dehydrated which is known as disc desiccation.
- Disc desiccation is manifested as a loss of normal T2 hyperintense signal within the annulus fibrosis (Fig. 23.1).
- Loss of disc height is common and can occur at multiple levels (Fig. 23.1).
- An annular fissure is usually a degenerative defect in one or more layers of the annulus fibrosis. An annular fissure appears as a linear T2 or STIR hyperintense signal in the annulus fibrosis (Fig. 23.1) and is often best seen on the sagittal plane.

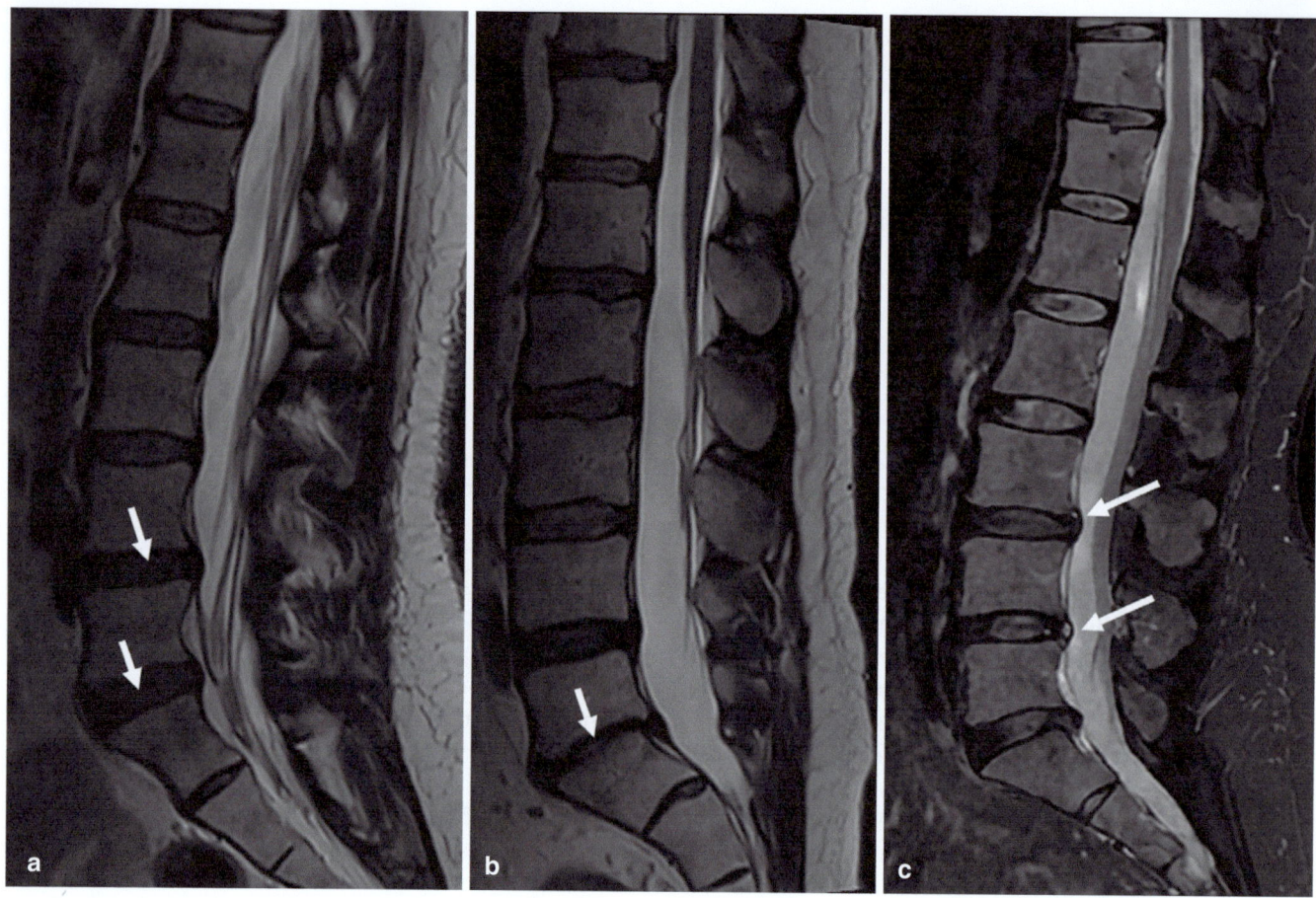

Fig. 23.1 Disc degeneration. (**a**) A sagittal T2 image demonstrates disc desiccation with loss of normal T2 hyperintense signal within annulus fibrosis at L4–L5 and L5–S1 (arrows). (**b**) A sagittal T2 image demonstrated loss of normal disc height at L5–S1 (arrow). (**c**) A sagittal T2 image demonstrates annual fissures at L3–L4 and L4–L5 (arrows)

Vertebral Body Endplate Degeneration

- The vertebral body endplate comprises f a thin layer of hyaline cartilage.
- Functions in conjunction with **intervertebral disc** as an axial load-bearing unit.
- Degeneration results in a pattern of subchondral marrow signals that were described and classified by **Modic** [2].
- **Modic** type 1 changes: represent bone marrow edema. Can be associated with active back pain.
  - Characterized by low T1 signal, high T2 signal, and high STIR signal (Fig. 23.2).
- **Modic** type 2 changes: represent fatty metaplasia. Less likely to be associated with active back pain.
  - Characterized by high T1 signal, high T2 signal, and low STIR signal (Fig. 23.2).
- **Modic** type 3 changes: represent subchondral fibrosis/sclerosis. Chronic in nature with an unclear clinical significance.
  - Characterized by low T1 signal, low T2 signal, and low STIR signal (Fig. 23.2).

Fig. 23.2 Upper Panel (Modic type 1 changes) (**a**) **Low T1 signal subchondral marrow signal (white arrows)**. (**b**) High T2 subchondral marrow signal (white arrows). (**c**) High subchondral STIR signal (white arrows). Middle Panel (Modic type 2 changes) (**a**) High T1 signal subchondral marrow signal (white arrows). (**b**) High T2 subchondral marrow signal (white arrows). (**c**) Low subchondral STIR signal (white arrows). Lower Panel (Modic type 3 changes) (**a**) Low T1 signal subchondral marrow signal (white arrows). (**b**) Low T2 subchondral marrow signal (white arrows). (**c**) Low subchondral STIR signal (white arrows)

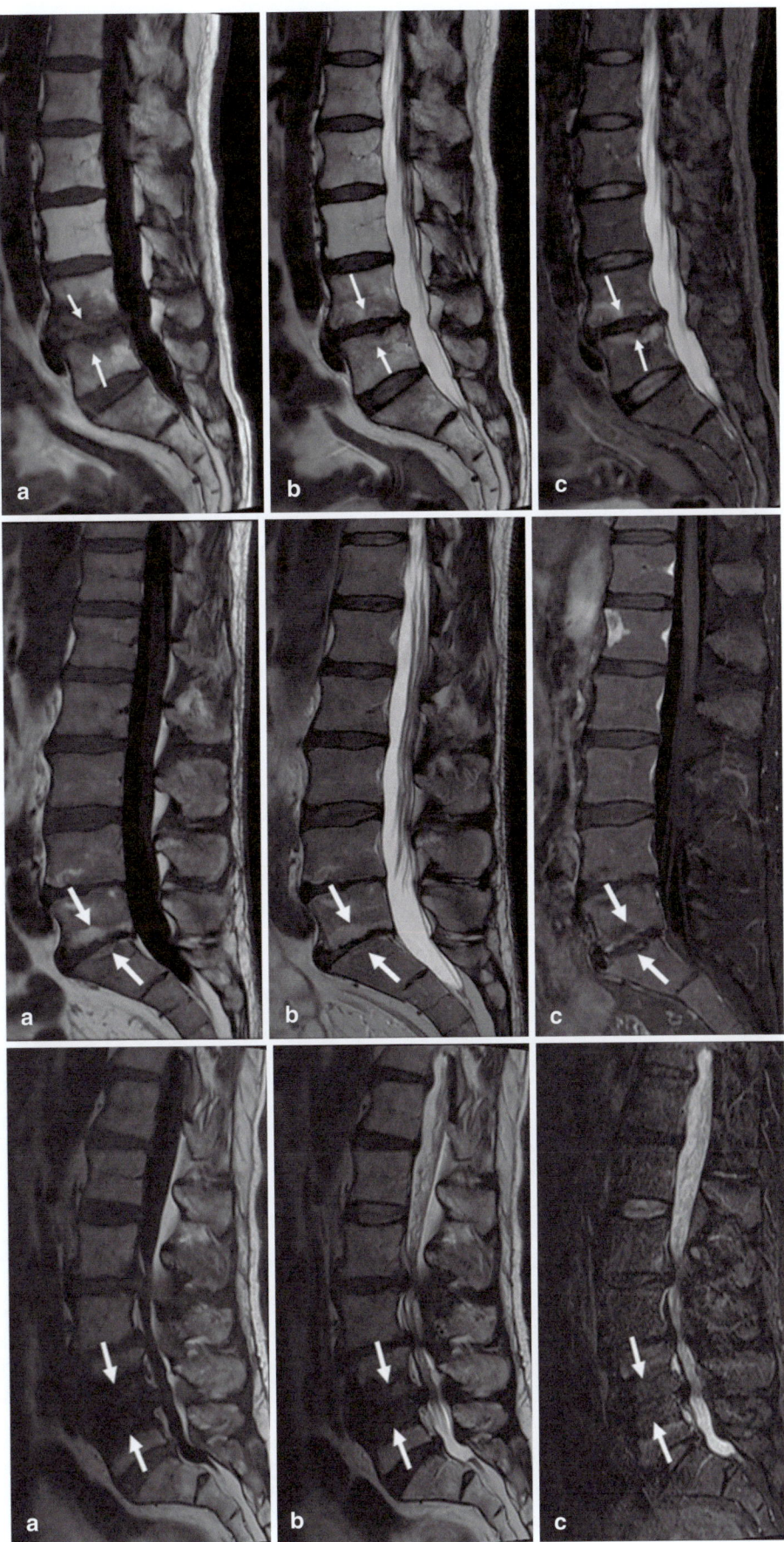

Disc Bulges and Herniations

- A **disc bulge** or **herniation** is the displacement of disc material beyond the normal limits of the disc margin.
- A **disc herniation** may involve nucleus pulposus or annulus fibrosis.
- A **disc herniation** should encompass less than 90 ° of the disc circumference and can be classified as either a protrusion or extrusion (Fig. 23.3).
- A **disc protrusion** is defined as a **herniation** with a neck that is wider than the distance from the base to the dome (Fig. 23.3) [3].
- A **disc extrusion** is defined as a **herniation** with a distance from the base to the dome that is wider than the neck (Fig. 23.3).
- An extruded disc fragment may be discontinuous from the parent disc and may become sequestered.
- A sequestered disc can migrate superiorly or inferiorly.
- A **disc bulge** is defined as the displacement of disc material by greater than 90 ° of the disc circumference (Fig. 23.3) [3].
- A **disc bulge** can be circumferential or asymmetric.
- The location of a **herniation** determines which nerve root is affected and is classified into zones: central, subarticular, foraminal, or extra-foraminal (Figs. 23.4 and e23.1).
- (All electronic images (Figs. e23.1–e23.7) can be found on this chapter's website on SpringerLink: https://doi.org/10.1007/978-3-031-55124-6_23)
- Central and subarticular **disc herniations** may compress the descending/traversing nerve roots.
- Foraminal or extra-foraminal **disc herniations** may compress the exiting or far lateral nerve roots.
- A **disc herniation** may extend through a gap in the endplate into the vertebral body and is commonly referred to as a Schmorl's node (Fig. e23.2).

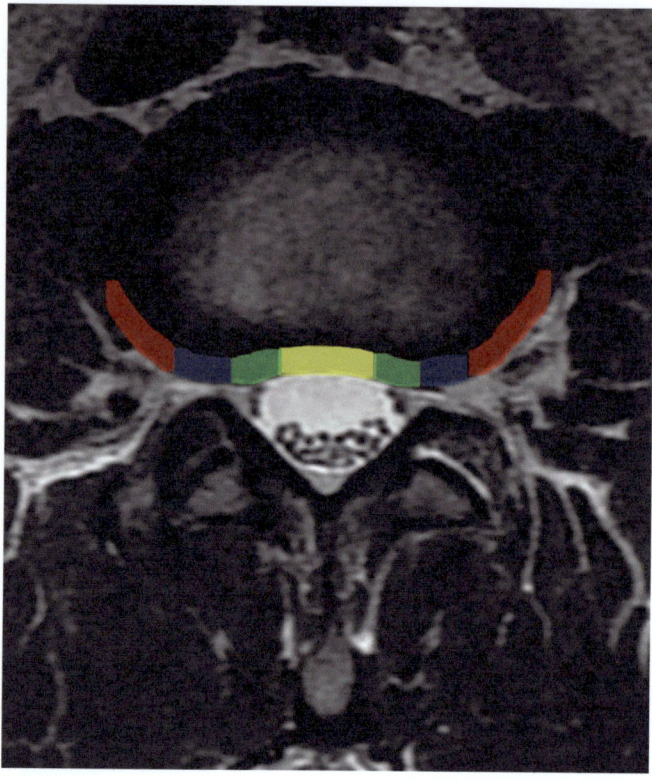

Fig. 23.4 Disc herniation locations. Central zone (yellow). Subarticular zone (green). Neural foramina (blue). Extra-foraminal zone (red)

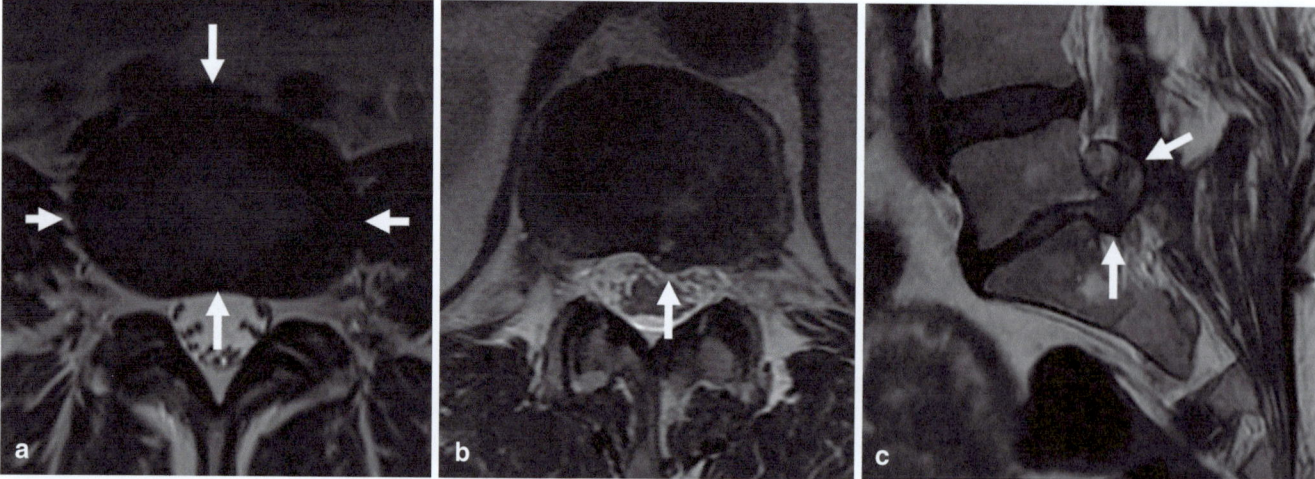

Fig. 23.3 Disc bulges and herniation. (a) Circumferential **disc bulge** extending beyond the margin of the normal disc (white arrows). (b) **Disc protrusion** with a neck that is wider than the distance from the base to the dome (white arrows). (c) **Disc extrusion** with a distance from the base to the dome that is wider than the neck (white arrows)

Arthrosis

- Synovial joints in the spine can undergo the same degenerative process as other synovial joints in the body including cartilage loss, osteophyte formation, sclerosis, and subchondral cystic changes.
- Uncovertebral joints are found in the cervical spine between C3 and C7. This joint involves an articulation between the paired superiorly projecting uncinate processes and the lateral aspect of the vertebral body above forming the ventral margin of the vertebral body.
- Uncovertebral arthrosis can contribute to **neural foraminal stenosis** in the cervical spine.
- Facet joint arthrosis can contribute to neural foraminal and spinal canal narrowing anywhere in the spine.
- Facet joint arthrosis is often accompanied by ligamentum flavum thickening/hypertrophy which can contribute to **spinal canal stenosis** (Fig. 23.5).
- Facet joint effusions can be associated with spinal instability (Fig. 23.5).
- Reactive bone marrow or soft tissue signal changes can occur in the setting of active degeneration.

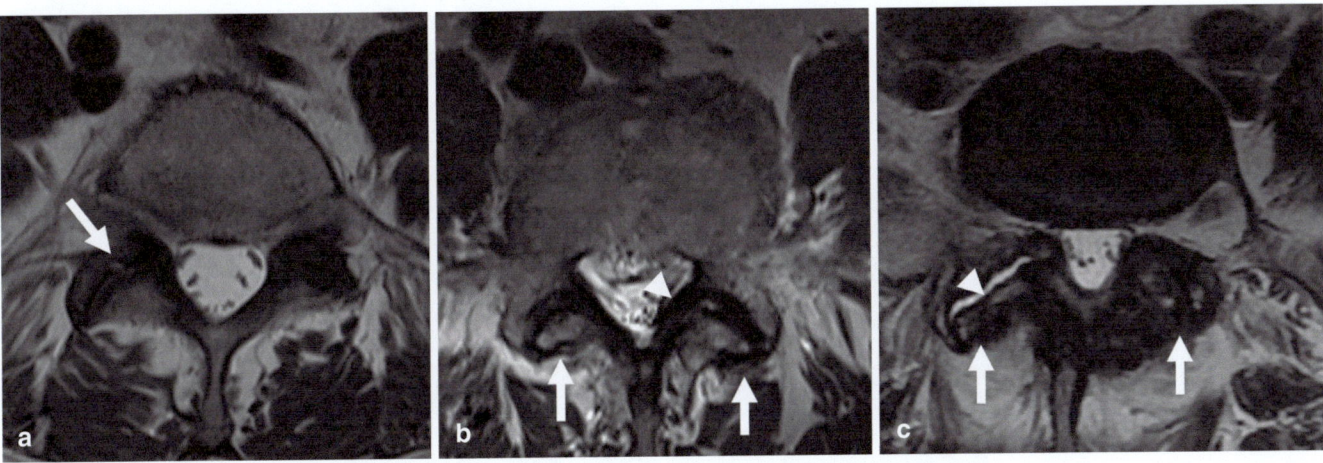

Fig. 23.5 Facet joint degenerative arthrosis. (**a**) An axial T2 image demonstrates mild facet arthrosis with a small subchondral cyst (arrows). (**b**) Moderate facet arthrosis with osteophyte formation (arrows) and ligamentum flavum thickening (arrowhead). (**c**) Severe facet arthrosis with more prominent osteophyte formation (arrows) and a facet joint effusion (arrowhead)

Synovial Cysts

- Spinal **synovial cysts** contain synovial fluid and communicate with the facet joint (Fig. 23.6).
- Associated with a degenerated facet joint (Fig. 23.6).
- Can project into the spinal canal and cause spinal canal or **subarticular stenosis** (Fig. 23.6) and result in nerve root impingement or compression causing radicular symptoms.
- Cyst contents are typically T2 and STIR hyperintense with peripheral T2 hypointensity of the cyst wall [4].
- Fluid with the cyst may be complex and include debris or hemorrhage (Fig. 23.6) and result in heterogeneous T2 and STIR signals.
- The cyst wall can calcify (Fig. 23.6).

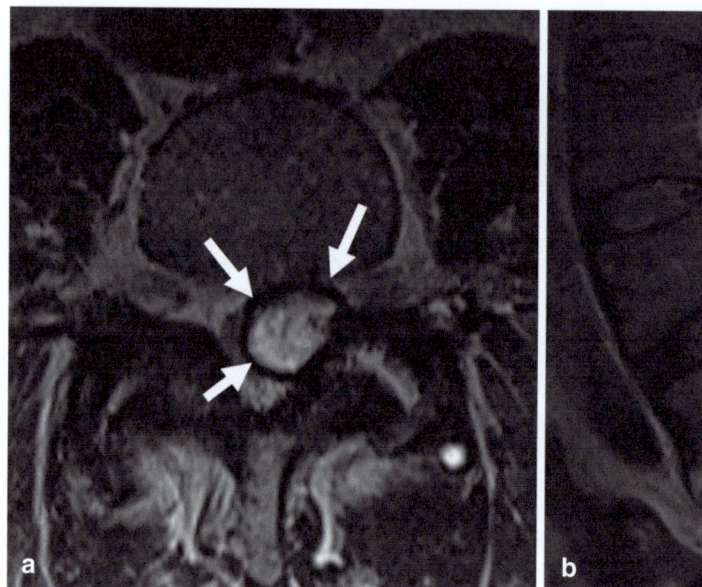

Fig. 23.6 Synovial cysts. (**a**) An axial and sagittal (**b**) T2 image demonstrates underlying degenerative facet arthrosis with a T2 hyperintense **synovial cyst** arising from the left ventral facet joint. There is inhomogeneity of signal centrally within the cyst which may reflect debris or mineralization and peripheral low T2 signal which is compatible with mineralization (arrows). There is a resultant severe spinal canal and left **subarticular stenosis**

Spondylolisthesis

- Involves the translation of one vertebral body relative to another.
- Anterolisthesis involves the anterior displacement of a vertebral body relative to the vertebra below.
- Retrolisthesis involves the posterior displacement of a vertebral body relative to the vertebra below.
- Can occur because of a variety of underlying etiologies including congenital abnormalities, a lesion involving the pars interarticularis, degenerative changes, and trauma.
- Most common in the lumbar spine but can occur anywhere in the vertebral column.
- Lumbar spondylolisthesis can be graded based on the position of the posterior inferior corner of the vertebral body above relative to the superior endplate of the vertebral body below. The vertebral body can be divided into four quadrants with corresponding Grades I–V (Fig. 23.7).
    o Grade I: 0–25%, Grade II: 26–60%, Grade III: 51–75%, Grade IV: 76–100%, Grade V: >100%.

Spondylolysis

- Defined as a defect in the pars interarticularis.
- The pars interarticularis is the part of the lamina interposed between the superior and inferior articular facet joints.
- A pars defect can be traumatic or degenerative in nature (Fig. 23.8).
- Pars interarticularis defects can be bilateral or unilateral (Fig. 23.8).
- Often associated with spondylolisthesis (Fig. 23.8).
- The spinal canal is typically widened, and the neural foramina can be narrowed (Fig. 23.8).

Spinal Stenosis

- Reliable characterization of spinal stenosis is important in the communication of findings between referrers and directing management.

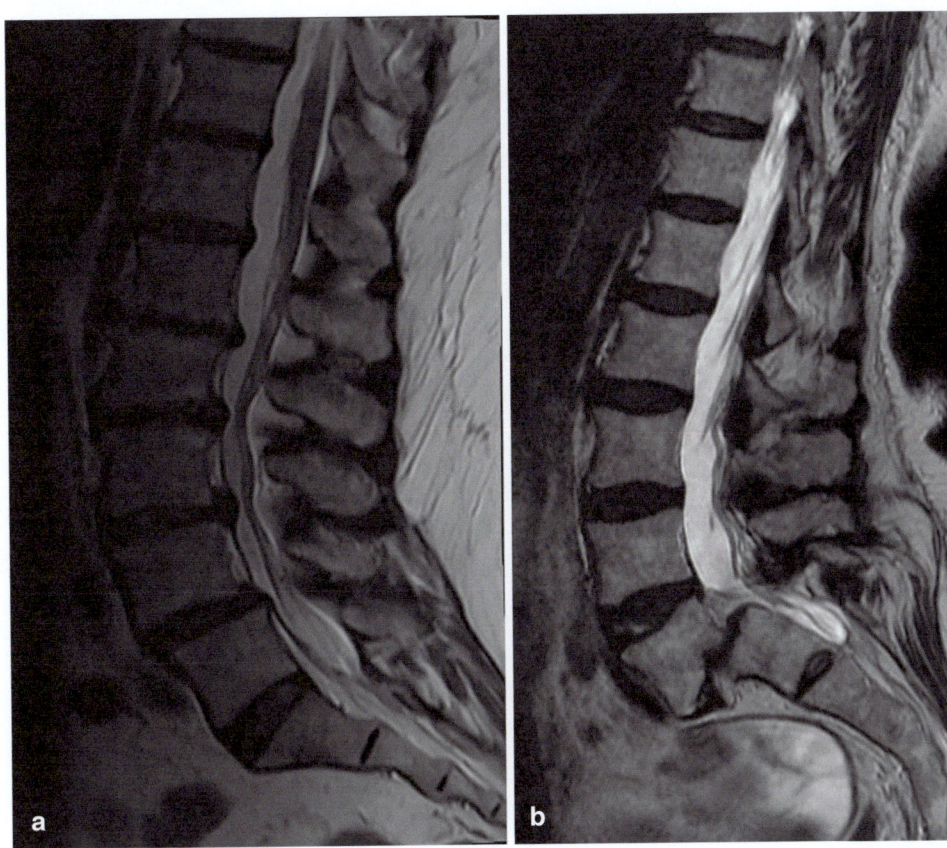

Fig. 23.7 Spondylolisthesis. (**a**) The sagittal T2 image of the lumbar spine demonstrates Grade I anterolisthesis at L3–L4 and L4–L5. (**b**) The sagittal T2 image of the lumbar spine demonstrates Grade II anterolisthesis at L5–S1

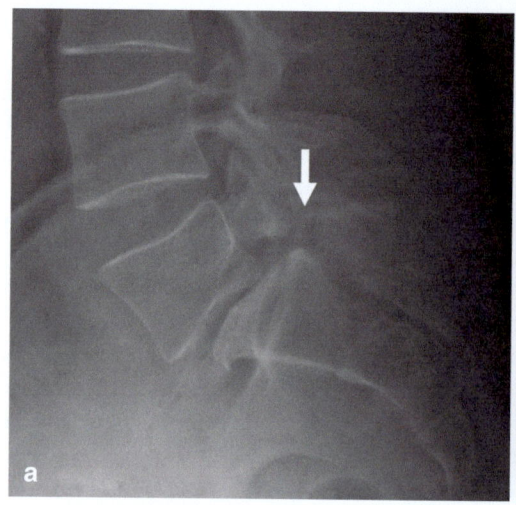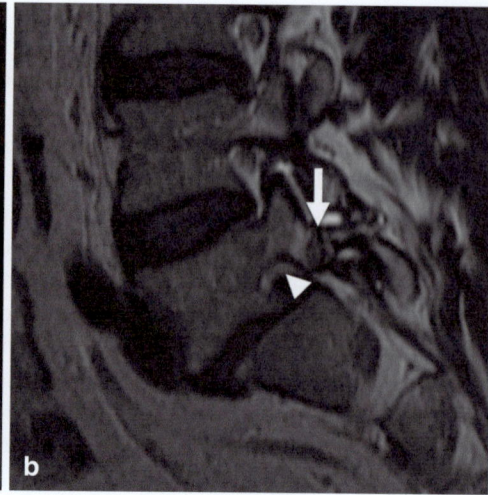

Fig. 23.8 Spondylolysis. (**a**) A lateral radiograph of the lumbar spine demonstrates anterolisthesis at L5-S1 and a L5 pars interarticularis defect (arrow). (**b**) A sagittal T2 image of the lumbar spine demonstrates anterolisthesis, the L5 pars interarticularis defect (arrow) and resultant severe neural foraminal narrowing (arrowhead)

- There are a variety of classification systems that have been developed.
- **Spinal canal stenosis** [5]:
    - Spinal cord compression can occur when **spinal canal stenosis** occurs above the level of the conus medullaris.
    - **Spinal canal stenosis** can cause radicular symptoms or neurogenic claudication.
    - The extent of **spinal canal stenosis** is best determined on the axial T2 sequence.
    - Below the level of the conus medullaris the descending nerve roots should be freely distributed within CSF.
    - When the spinal canal is mildly narrowed, the anterior margin of the thecal sac is flat or concave and there may be slight crowding of the descending nerve roots in the subarticular zone (Fig. 23.9).
    - When the spinal canal is moderately narrowed, there is a concave margin of the thecal sac ventrally and crowding of the nerve roots in the thecal sac which may be somewhat indistinct (Fig. 23.9).
    - When the spinal canal is severely narrowed there is complete effacement of CSF in the thecal sac and the nerve roots are indistinct (Fig. 23.9).
- **Neural foraminal stenosis:**
    - Paired opening at the lateral margin of the spinal canal that allows for the passage of exiting nerve roots.
    - Bound by disc and endplate ventrally, facet joint dorsally, and pedicles superiorly and inferiorly.
    - The exiting nerve is normally surrounded by fat with a "keyhole" like morphological appearance (Fig. e23.3).
    - The extent of **neural foraminal stenosis** in the cervical spine is best assessed on the axial T2 and axial GRE sequences.
    - The extent of **neural foraminal stenosis** in the lumbar spine is best assessed on the sagittal T1 and sagittal T2 sequences. The axial T2 can also be complimentary.
    - When the neural foramen is mildly narrowed, there is a loss of epidural fat on two or three sides of the exiting nerve (Fig. e23.3) [6].
    - When the neural foramen is moderately narrowed, there is a loss of epidural fat on three or four sides of the exiting nerve root (Fig. e23.3) [6].
    - When the neural foramen is severely narrowed, there is complete loss of epidural fat throughout the foramen or compression of the exiting nerve root (Fig. e23.3) [6].
- **Subarticular stenosis:**
    - The lateral aspect of the thecal sac where the descending nerve roots course just before entering the neural foramina.
    - The extent of lateral recess stenosis is best accessed on the axial T2 sequence.
    - Characterized by the effect on the descending nerve roots.

Nerve roots can be contacted, displaced, or compressed (Fig. e23.4) [7].

Fig. 23.9 Spinal stenosis.
(**a**) Normal caliber of the spinal canal. (**b**) Mild **spinal canal stenosis** with flattening of the thecal sac and slight crowding of the descending nerve roots in the subarticular zone. (**c**) Moderate spinal canal narrowing with a concave margin of the thecal sac ventrally and crowding of the nerve roots in the thecal sac. (**d**) Severe spinal canal narrowing complete effacement of CSF in the thecal sac and indistinct nerve roots [5]

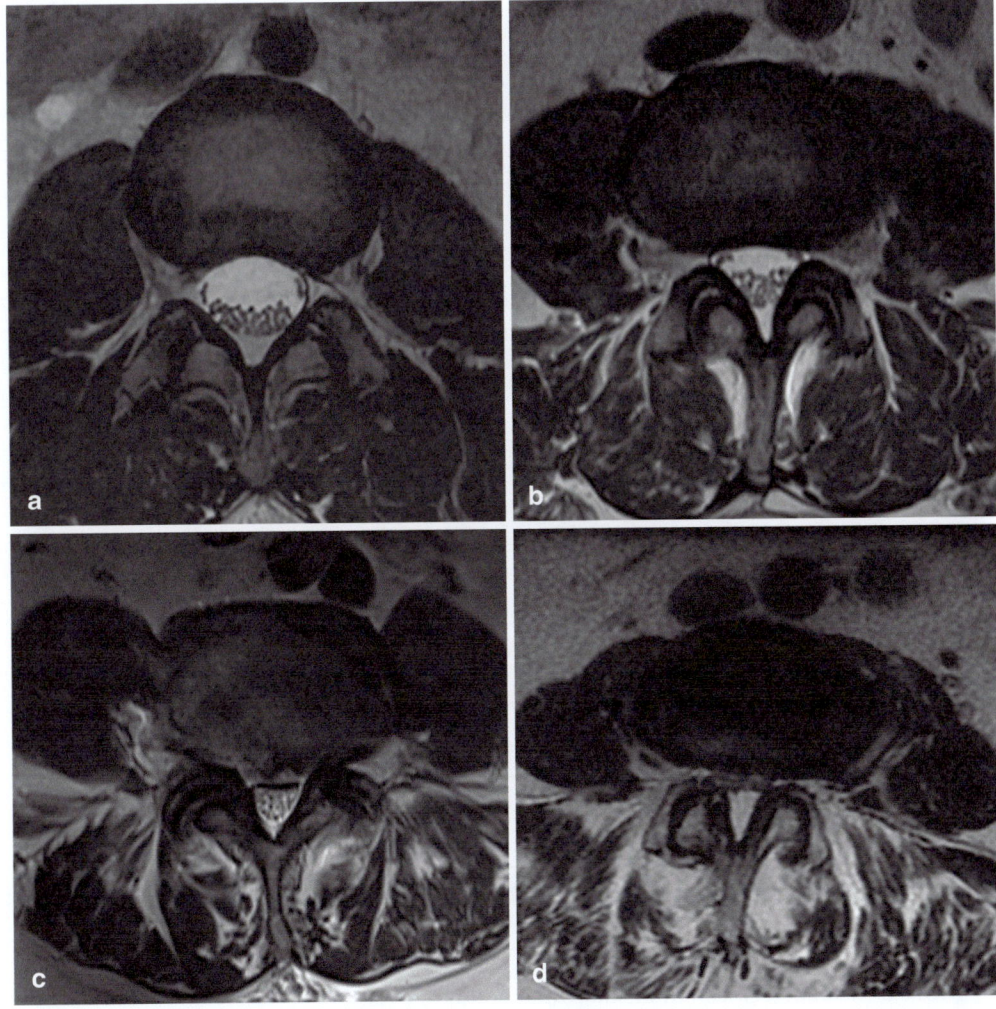

Ossification of the Posterior Longitudinal Ligament (OPLL)

- OPLL involves the formation of calcification/bone along the posterior longitudinal ligament (Fig. 23.10).
- Most frequently involves the cervical spine (Fig. 23.10).

OPLL can contribute to **spinal canal stenosis** (Fig. 23.10) [8].

Fig. 23.10 Ossification of the posterior longitudinal ligament. (**a**) Sagittal and axial (**b**) CT images of the cervical spine demonstrate ossification of the posterior longitudinal ligament (arrows). There is resultant severe **spinal canal stenosis**

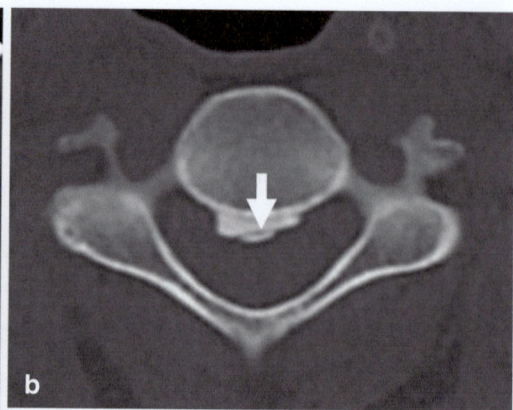
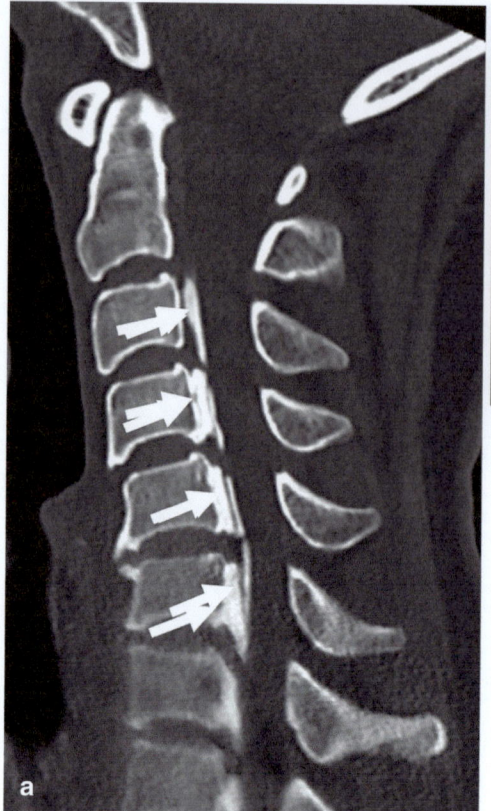

Diffuse Idiopathic Skeletal Hyperostosis (DISH)

- DISH is a relatively common idiopathic condition that involves bony proliferation at sites of tendinous and ligamentous insertion of the spine [9, 10].
- Most commonly affects older individuals with a male predominance.
- Characterized by "flowing" ossification along the anterolateral margins of at least four contiguous vertebral bodies (Fig. 23.11).
- DISH most commonly involves the thoracic spine but can occur anywhere along the neuroaxis (Fig. 23.11).
- Patients are susceptible to fractures due to altered biomechanics.

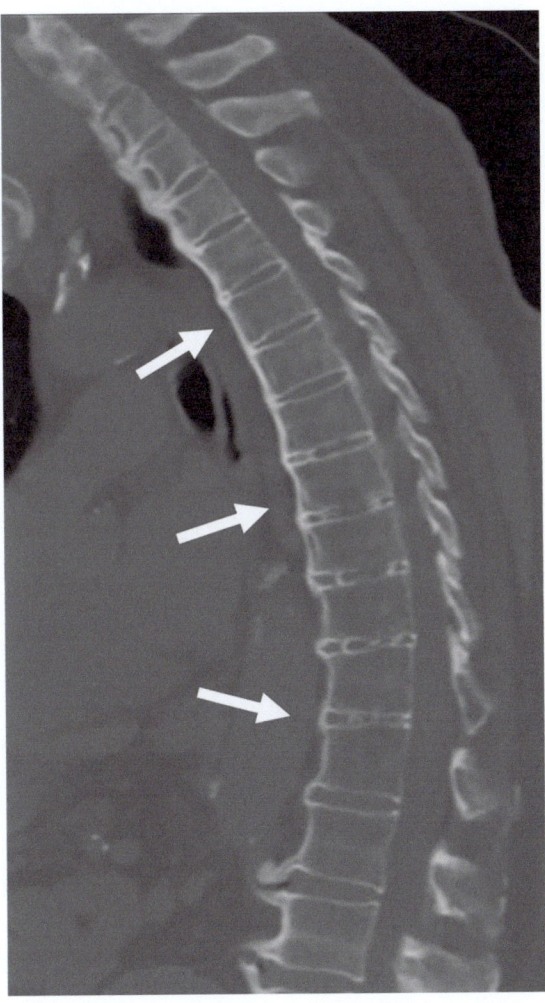

Fig. 23.11 Diffuse idiopathic skeletal hyperostosis (DISH). Sagittal CT image of the thoracic spine demonstrates "flowing" ossification along the anterolateral margins of at least four contiguous vertebral bodies (arrows)

Scheuermann Disease

- Scheuermann disease is a relatively common idiopathic condition that affects adolescent individuals.
- A proposed mechanism is avascular necrosis which leads to Schmorl's nodes and wedge compression deformities.
- Scheuermann disease most commonly involves the thoracic spine and leads to a kyphotic deformity.
- To meet the classical definition of Scheuermann disease, the Sorensen criteria must be met (Fig. e23.5) [11]:
  o Thoracic spine kyphosis >40 ° or thoracolumbar spine kyphosis >30 °.
  o At least three adjacent vertebral bodies demonstrate wedging of >5 °.

Seronegative Spondyloarthropathies

- **Seronegative spondyloarthropathies** are a group of four inflammatory arthropathies [12, 13].
- This group of disorders by definition have negative rheumatoid factors and are usually HLA-B27 positive.
- The four **seronegative spondyloarthropathies** are ankylosing spondylitis (AS), psoriatic arthritis, reactive arthritis, and inflammatory bowel disease (IBD) associated arthropathy.
- Sacroiliitis is a hallmark of these conditions which involves the inferior synovial portion of the joint.
- Symmetric sacroiliitis is seen with AS- and IBD-associated arthropathy.
- Asymmetric sacroiliitis is seen with psoriatic arthritis and reactive arthropathy.
- AS is more common in men and patients commonly present with back pain and stiffness.
- AS is associated with a variety of other conditions, including pulmonary fibrosis, aortitis, and cardiac conduction defects [14].
- The earliest radiologic findings in AS involve the sacroiliac joints followed by invariable involvement and ankylosis of the spine.
- Patients with a fully ankylosed spine are susceptible to fractures due to altered biomechanics even with minor trauma.
- The earliest radiologic findings in AS are symmetric erosive changes and sclerosis of both sacroiliac joints.
- Spine involvement in AS follows a sequence that ascends from the lumbar to the cervical spine.
  o Romanus lesions are erosive changes that involve the anterior superior or anterior inferior aspect of the vertebral bodies at the attachment of annulus fibrosis due to enthesitis.
  o Shiny corners are sclerotic changes that form at the location of former Romanus lesions (Fig. e23.6).
  o Squaring of the vertebral body at the margins of the disc occurs due to erosive changes (Fig. e23.6).
  o Delicate syndesmophytes form which connect adjacent vertebral body margins.
  o The classic bamboo spine is seen with advanced disease where there are confluent bridging delicate syndesmophytes (Fig. 23.12).
  o The classic dagger sign can be seen with advanced disease where there is confluent ankylosis of the spinous processes (Fig. 23.12).
- IBD-associated arthropathy has variable spine involvement which can be identical to AS.

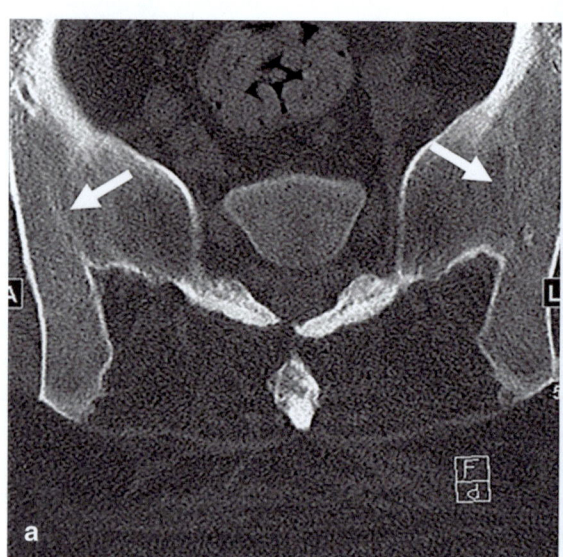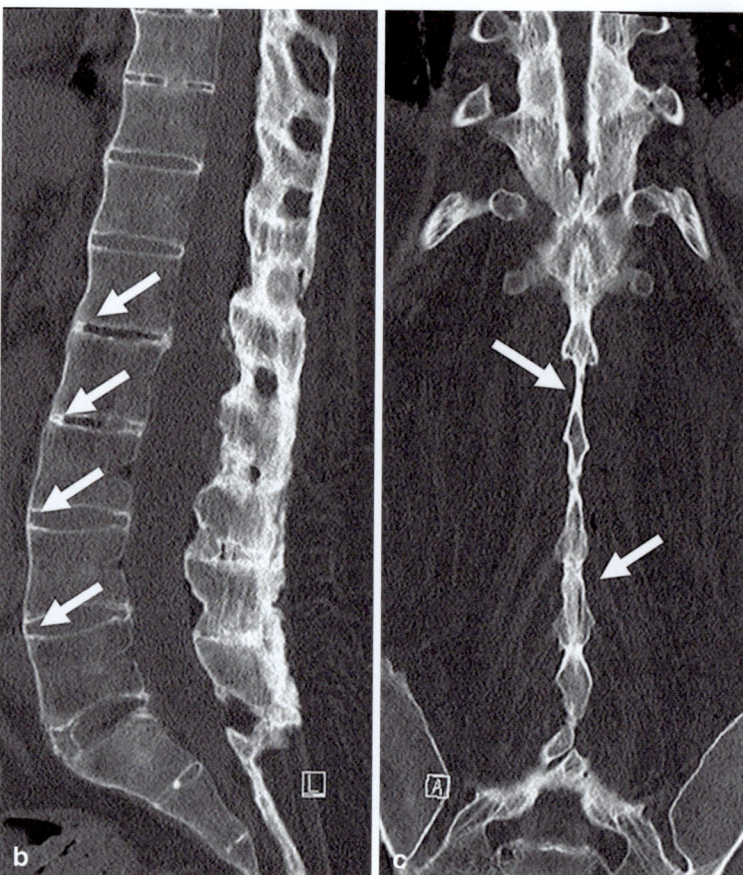

Fig. 23.12 Ankylosing spondylitis. (**a**) An axial CT image demonstrates diffuse ankylosis of both sacroiliac joints (arrows). (**b**) A sagittal CT image of the lumbar spine demonstrates the classic "bamboo spine" with confluent bridging delicate syndesmophytes (arrows). (**c**) A coronal CT image of the lumbar spine demonstrates the "dagger" sign with diffuse ankylosis of the spinous processes (arrows)

- Psoriatic arthritis and reactive arthritis can variably lead to bulky bridging osteophytes and are often indistinguishable from each other [12, 13].

Rheumatoid Arthritis

- **Rheumatoid arthritis** (RA) is an autoimmune disorder that attacks synovial joints.
- Associated with a positive rheumatoid factor (RF).
- Patients typically present with symmetric joint pain, swelling, and morning stiffness.
- Erosive changes are the radiographic hallmark.
- Small joints of the hands and feet are most affected early in the disease.
- Larger joints and the cervical spine can be affected with advanced disease.
- Characteristic findings of RA in the cervical spine are erosions of the dens and atlantoaxial subluxation (Fig. e23.7).
- Ligamentous laxity can develop in the setting of chronic inflammation (Fig. e23.7).
- Inflammatory granulation tissue can be seen behind the dens and is commonly referred to as Pannus. This can lead to stenosis of the spinal canal (Fig. e23.7) [15].
- The dens can protrude through the foramen magnum and impress on the cervical medullary junction or brain stem which is referred to as basilar invagination (Fig. e23.7).

References

1. Meucci RD, Fassa AG, Faria NM. Prevalence of chronic low back pain: systematic review. Rev Saude Publica. 2015;49:1. https://doi.org/10.1590/S0034-8910.2015049005874. Epub 2015 Oct 20. PMID: 26487293; PMCID: PMC4603263
2. Modic MT, Steinberg PM, Ross JS, Masaryk TJ, Carter JR. Degenerative disk disease: assessment of changes in vertebral body marrow with MR imaging. Radiology. 1988;166(1 Pt 1):193–9. https://doi.org/10.1148/radiology.166.1.3336678.
3. Fardon DF, Williams AL, Dohring EJ, Murtagh FR, Gabriel Rothman SL, Sze GK. Lumbar disc nomenclature: version 2.0: recommendations of the combined task forces of the North American Spine Society, the American Society of Spine Radiology and the American Society of Neuroradiology. Spine J. 2014;14(11):2525–45. https://doi.org/10.1016/j.spinee.2014.04.022. Epub 2014 Apr 24

4. Liu SS, Williams KD, Drayer BP, Spetzler RF, Sonntag VK. Synovial cysts of the lumbosacral spine: diagnosis by MR imaging. AJR Am J Roentgenol. 1990 Jan;154(1):163–6. https://doi.org/10.2214/ajr.154.1.2104702.
5. Lee GY, Lee JW, Choi HS, Oh KJ, Kang HS. A new grading system of lumbar central canal stenosis on MRI: an easy and reliable method. Skeletal Radiol. 2011;40(8):1033–9. https://doi.org/10.1007/s00256-011-1102-x. Epub 2011 Feb 1. Erratum in: Skeletal Radiol. 2011 Aug;40(8):1127. Guen, Young Lee [corrected to Lee, Guen Young]; Joon, Woo Lee [corrected to Lee, Joon Woo]; Hee, Seok Choi [corrected to Choi, Hee Seok]; Kyoung-Jin, Oh [corrected to Oh, Kyoung-Jin]; Heung, Sik Kang [corrected to Kang, Heung Sik]
6. Lee S, Lee JW, Yeom JS, Kim KJ, Kim HJ, Chung SK, Kang HS. A practical MRI grading system for lumbar foraminal stenosis. AJR Am J Roentgenol. 2010;194(4):1095–8. https://doi.org/10.2214/AJR.09.2772.
7. Sartoretti E, Wyss M, Alfieri A, Binkert CA, Erne C, Sartoretti-Schefer S, Sartoretti T. Introduction and reproducibility of an updated practical grading system for lumbar foraminal stenosis based on high-resolution MR imaging. Sci Rep. 2021;11(1):12000. https://doi.org/10.1038/s41598-021-91462-2. Erratum in: Sci Rep 2021 Sep 15;11(1):18732. PMID: 34099833; PMCID: PMC8184791
8. Yamashita Y, Takahashi M, Matsuno Y, Sakamoto Y, Yoshizumi K, Oguni T, Kojima R. Spinal cord compression due to ossification of ligaments: MR imaging. Radiology. 1990;175(3):843–8. https://doi.org/10.1148/radiology.175.3.2111569.
9. Tsukamoto Y, Onitsuka H, Lee K. Radiologic aspects of diffuse idiopathic skeletal hyperostosis in the spine. AJR Am J Roentgenol. 1977;129(5):913–8. https://doi.org/10.2214/ajr.129.5.913.
10. Cammisa M, De Serio A, Guglielmi G. Diffuse idiopathic skeletal hyperostosis. Eur J Radiol. 1998;27(Suppl 1):S7–11. https://doi.org/10.1016/s0720-048x(98)00036-9.
11. Summers BN, Singh JP, Manns RA. The radiological reporting of lumbar Scheuermann's disease: an unnecessary source of confusion amongst clinicians and patients. Br J Radiol. 2008;81(965):383–5. https://doi.org/10.1259/bjr/69495299.
12. Jacobson JA, Girish G, Jiang Y, Resnick D. Radiographic evaluation of arthritis: inflammatory conditions. Radiology. 2008;248(2):378–89. https://doi.org/10.1148/radiol.2482062110.
13. Hermann KG, Althoff CE, Schneider U, Zühlsdorf S, Lembcke A, Hamm B, Bollow M. Spinal changes in patients with spondyloarthritis: comparison of MR imaging and radiographic appearances. Radiographics. 2005;25(3):559–69; discussion 569–70. https://doi.org/10.1148/rg.253045117.
14. Schueller-Weidekamm C, Mascarenhas VV, Sudol-Szopinska I, Boutry N, Plagou A, Klauser A, Wick M, Platzgummer H, Jans L, Mester A, Kainberger F, Aström G, Guglielmi G, Eshed I. Imaging and interpretation of axial spondylarthritis: the radiologist's perspective—consensus of the Arthritis Subcommittee of the ESSR. Semin Musculoskelet Radiol. 2014;18(3):265–79. https://doi.org/10.1055/s-0034-1375569. Epub 2014 Jun 4. Erratum in: Semin Musculoskelet Radiol. 2014 Nov;18(5):523
15. Sommer OJ, Kladosek A, Weiler V, Czembirek H, Boeck M, Stiskal M. Rheumatoid arthritis: a practical guide to state-of-the-art imaging, image interpretation, and clinical implications. Radiographics. 2005;25(2):381–98. https://doi.org/10.1148/rg.252045111. PMID: 15798057

Tumors and Tumor-Like Lesions of the Spine and Spinal Cord

Kimberly Seifert, Tarik F. Massoud, and Austin Trinh

Spine

BONE-FORMING TUMORS:

- **Pearl:** Generally, better evaluated on **X-ray and/or CT**.
- Enostosis (Bone island):
  - Benign, probably congenital or developmental.
  - Dense compact bone.
  - Imaging appearance:
    - X-ray/CT: Round dense/sclerotic focus.
    - MRI: T1 and T2 hypointense, no enhancement.
    - Scintigraphy: <10% show activity.
- Osteoid osteoma (Fig. 24.1):
  - Most common benign vertebral tumor in the pediatric population.
  - Osteoblastic lesion.
  - Nidus of osteoid tissue surrounded by sclerotic/reactive bone.
  - Less than 2 cm in size (larger lesions are referred to as osteoblastoma – see below).
  - Second to third decade of life.
  - Male predilection 3:1.
  - Located in the posterior elements, most commonly in the lumbar spine.
  - The classic presentation is night pain relieved by aspirin:
    - Can cause painful scoliosis with convexity pointing away from the lesion.
  - Treatment: surgical resection or radiofrequency ablation.
  - Imaging appearance:
    - X-ray/CT: radiolucent nidus with surrounding reactive sclerosis:
      - May have a central sclerotic dot.
      - CT is the modality of choice for evaluation.
    - MRI: nonspecific appearance with low to intermediate on T1 and heterogeneous T2 with surrounding edema.
    - Scintigraphy:
      - Focal increased uptake.
      - Double density sign is fairly specific and is a central focus of increased uptake within the lower surrounding activity.

Pearl: Posterior elements differential (GO TAPE):

- Giant cell tumor.
- Osteoid osteoma/osteoblastoma.
- Tuberculosis.
- Aneurysmal bone cyst.
- Paget's disease.
- Eosinophilic granuloma.

- Osteoblastoma:
  - Histologically similar to osteoid osteoma.
  - >2 cm in size.
  - Second to third decade of life.
  - Male predilection 2:1.
  - Clinical presentation: insidious, dull, achy pain, worse at night, and minimal relief with aspirin.
  - Can be locally aggressive, rapidly increases in size, and causes cortical destruction.
  - Treatment: surgical excision with possible preoperative embolization, or percutaneous ablation/curettage with bone grafting:
    - Recurrence rate = 10–15%.
  - Imaging appearance: overall similar to osteoid osteoma, however larger than 2 cm:

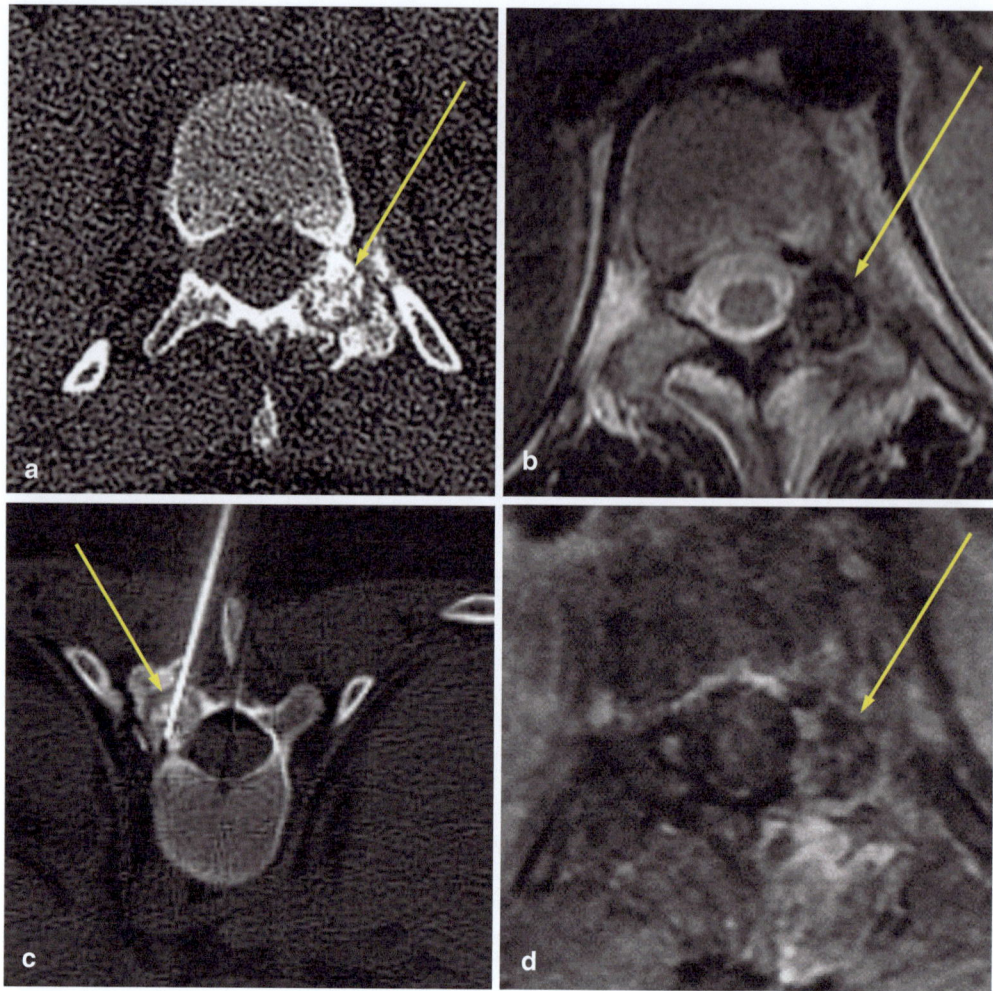

Fig. 24.1 Osteoid osteoma. (**a**) CT demonstrating nidus with surrounding sclerotic bone and central calcification. (**b**) T2 low signal compatible with sclerosis. (**c**) CT-guided ablation. (**d**) Post-contrast T1 with surrounding enhancement secondary to inflammatory changes

- X-ray/CT: expansile lytic lesion with rim of reactive sclerosis:
    - May have internal calcification.
    - Approximately 20% with associated aneurysmal bone cysts.
- MRI: nonspecific low to intermediate signal on T1, and low to intermediate signal on T2, enhances post-contrast (highly vascular).
- Scintigraphy: nonspecific increased uptake.
- Osteosarcoma (Fig. e24.1).
  (All electronic images (Figs. e24.1–e24.15) can be found on this chapter's website on SpringerLink: https://doi.org/10.1007/978-3-031-55124-6_24):
    - High-grade malignant osteoblastic lesion.
    - More commonly found outside the spine.
    - Primary lesions typically occur before the age of 20 years.
    - Slight male predominance.
    - Predilection for the thoracic and lumbar spine posterior elements.
    - Patient presentation: pain, compression, or palpable mass.
    - Multiple subtypes:
        - Conventional most common: osteoid matrix.
        - Sclerosing osteoblastic osteosarcoma: marked mineralization of the vertebral body with an ivory vertebra.
        - Telangiectatic osteosarcoma: cystic architecture that mimics an aneurysmal bone cyst with fluid/fluid levels on MR:
            - In comparison with ABCs, thick, enhancing, nodular soft tissue surrounds the cystic components.
    - Can occur secondary to radiation therapy, Paget's disease, bone infarcts, and osteoblastoma and will present in the elderly.
    - Treatment: chemotherapy and surgical excision with possible radiation.
    - Imaging will demonstrate a permeative, aggressive lesion with enhancement.

CARTILAGE-FORMING TUMORS:

- Osteochondroma (Fig. e24.2):
  - Developmental lesion, NOT **a neoplasm:**
    - Separation of a fragment of the growth plate cartilage, leading to a projection from the bone with a cartilage cap.
    - Enlarges with normal growth, usually with no further growth after skeletal maturity.
  - Typically solitary and sporadic:
    - Multiple lesions—consider hereditary multiple exostoses.
  - Most common in the cervical spine, with a predilection for the atlantoaxial region.
  - More common near the tip of the spinous process or transverse process.
  - Secondary lesions can occur at the periphery of the radiation field.
  - Imaging appearance:
    - X-ray/CT: demonstrates marrow and cortical continuity and does not evaluate cartilage components.
  - MRI: used to evaluate the cartilage cap, which normally thins with age:
    - In adults, a cartilage cap >1 cm thick is concerning for chondrosarcoma (see additional information below).
- Chondroblastoma:
  - Benign tumor that involves the vertebral body and posterior elements.
  - Third decade of life.
  - Classical presentation: back pain with possible neurological symptoms.
  - Treatment: local curettage or resection (complete vertebrectomy):
    - High rate of recurrence.
  - Imaging appearance:
    - X-ray/CT: geographic lucent lesion with sclerotic borders.
    - MRI: T1 isointense, T2 heterogeneous, with heterogeneous enhancement of lesion and surrounding bone and soft tissue.
- Chondrosarcoma (Fig. 24.2):

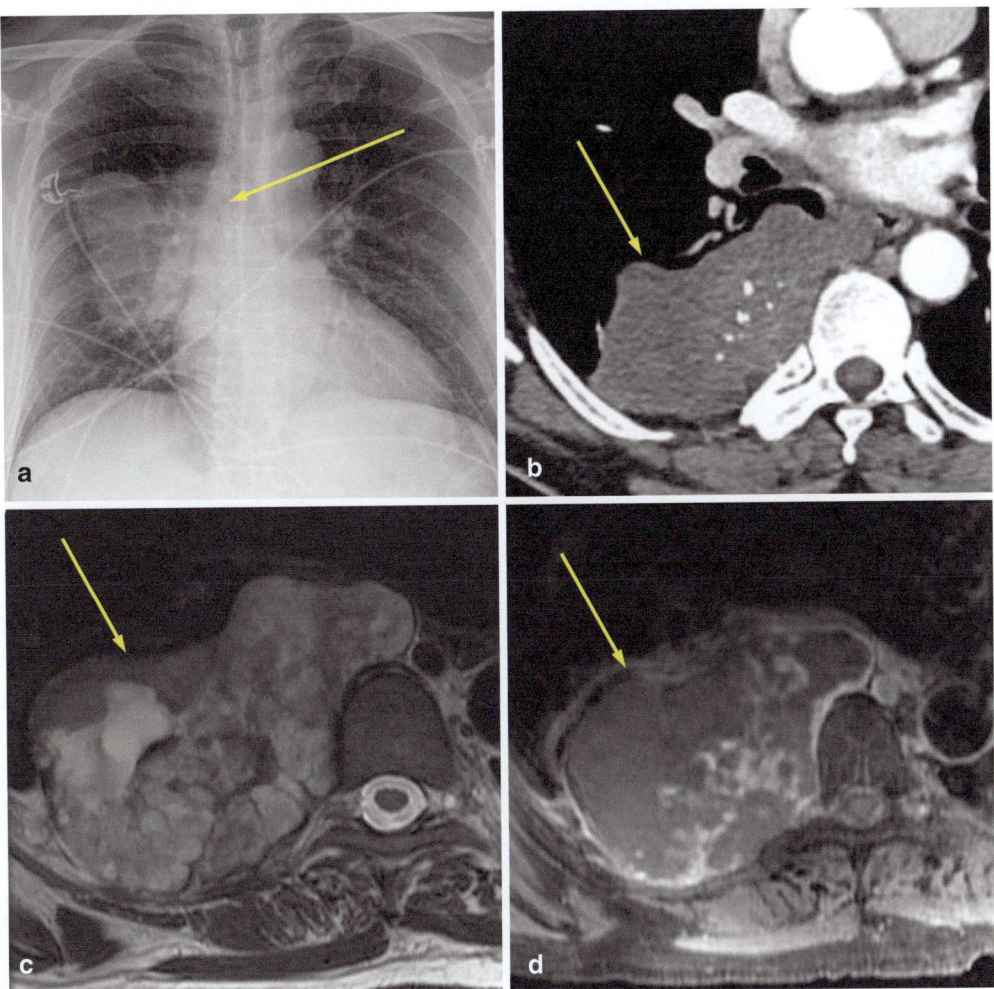

Fig. 24.2 Chondrosarcoma. (**a**) Radiograph and (**b**) CT with chondroid matrix. (**c**) T2 heterogeneous hyperintense signal, with (**d**) heterogeneous enhancement

- Second most common primary malignant tumor of the spine.
- Occurs between 30 and 70 years of age.
- Men more common (4:1).
- Occurs in the posterior elements with possible extension to the vertebral body.
- Large, calcified mass with osseous destruction and can extend through intervertebral discs.
- Treatment: en bloc resection:
  - High risk of recurrence.
- Imaging appearance:
  - X-ray/CT: chondroid matrix.
  - MRI: calcified portions with signal void, nonmineralized portions hyperintense on T2 owing to hyaline cartilage and water content, heterogeneous enhancement reflects growth.

MISCELLANEOUS BONE TUMORS

- Eosinophilic granuloma (Fig. e24.3):
  - Histology demonstrates Langerhans cell histiocytosis.
  - Classified as a tumor of undefined neoplastic nature.
  - Peak occurrence between 5 and 10 years with male predominance.
  - Presentation: pain that improves with bed rest:
    - Lab analysis may include mild elevation of ESR, eosinophilia, and leukocytosis.
  - Typical spine lesion with vertebral body collapse (vertebra plana).
  - Imaging appearance:
    - X-ray/CT: vertebral body collapse, preservation of posterior elements.
    - MRI: hypointense on T1 and heterogeneous hyperintense on T2.
    - Scintigraphy: increased uptake.
- Plasmacytoma (Fig. 24.3a–c):
  - Focal proliferation of malignant plasma cells.
  - Thought to represent an early stage of multiple myeloma.
  - >60 years of age.
  - Vertebral body is the most common site with possible extension to pedicles.
  - Presents with a single collapsed vertebra:

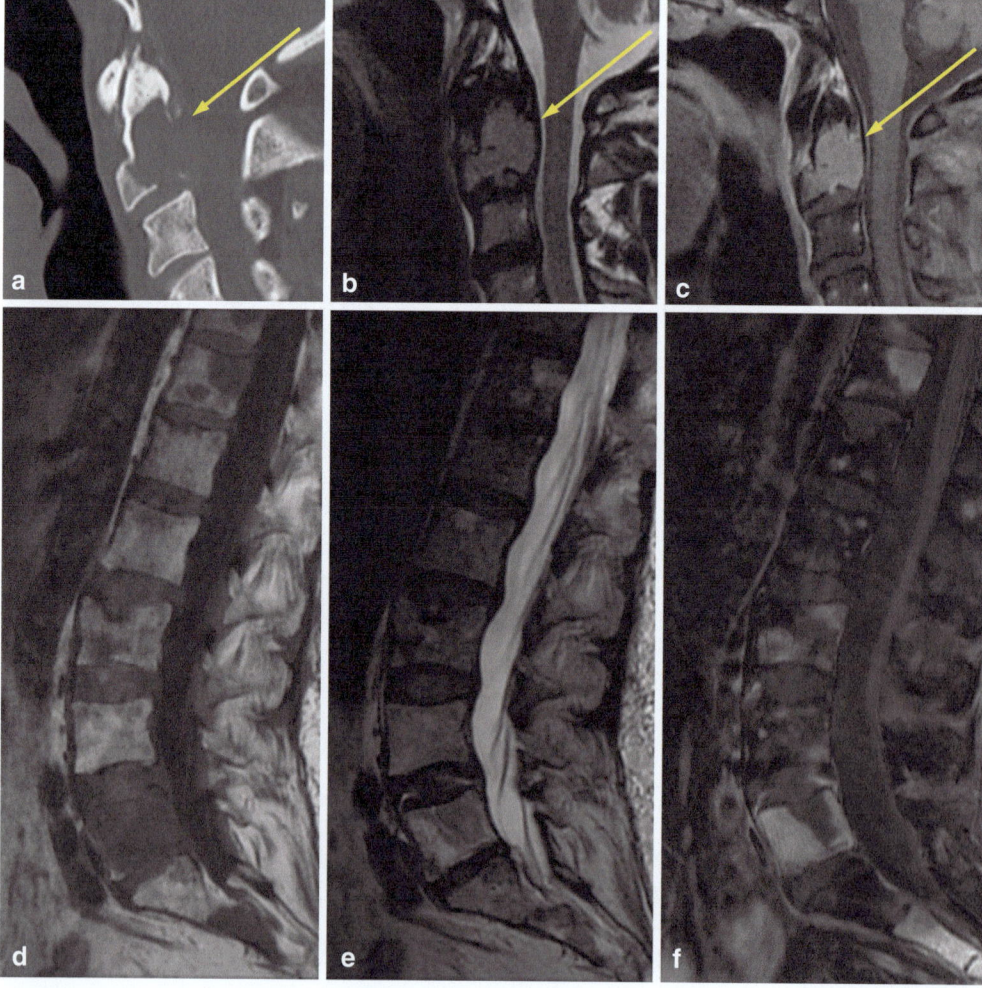

Fig. 24.3 Spectrum of plasmacytoma (a–c) and multiple myeloma (d–f). (a) CT with lytic lesion, (b) T2 mildly hyperintense, and (c) enhancement of a solitary plasmacytoma. Heterogeneous hypointense signal on both (d) T1 and (e) T2, with (f) heterogeneous enhancement

- Focal endplate fractures can be seen, as well as the involvement of the intervertebral disc.
  o Imaging appearance:
    - X-ray/CT: mixed pattern, predominantly lytic:
      ▪ Hollow vertebral body or pedicle.
      ▪ Cortical thickening can create a minibrain appearance.
    - MRI: hypointense on T1, hyperintense on T2, and marked enhancement.
- Multiple myeloma (Fig. 24.3d–f):
  o Most common primary malignant tumor of the spine (with chordoma).
  o Plasma cell proliferation.
  o Clinical presentation: bone pain with anemia.
  o Imaging appearance:
    - X-ray/CT: multiple well-circumscribed lytic lesions:
      ▪ General osteopenia less common presentation.
    - MRI: hypointense T1, hyperintense T2, enhances, restricted diffusion.
    - Scintigraphy: typically negative.
    - PET/CT: increased uptake.
- Lymphoma (Fig. e24.4):
  o Primary osseous lymphoma is rare (1–3%):
    - Diffuse large B-cell is the most common.
    - Fifth to seventh decades.
    - Male predilection (8:1).
  o Secondary lymphoma is more common:
    - Vertebral metastasis occurs from hematogenous spread.
  o Treatment: chemotherapy and radiation.
  o Imaging appearance:
    - Unifocal or multifocal.
    - X-ray/CT: can have sclerotic, lytic, or mixed appearance:
      ▪ *Ivory vertebra* more common in Hodgkin lymphoma.
    - MRI: heterogeneous low T1 and T2 signal with homogenous enhancement.
    - Scintigraphy: increased uptake.
- Ewing sarcoma (Fig. e24.5):
  o Primary tumor in the spine is less common; however, metastatic disease often affects the spine, including local invasion from paraspinal masses.
  o Second decade of life, slight male predilection.
  o Small round cell tumor.
  o Necrosis is common.
  o Imaging appearance:
    - Imaging appearance can vary depending on whether the lesion is primary versus secondary and can be unifocal versus multifocal.
    - X-ray/CT: lytic appearance which may cause pathologic compression of the vertebral body, with possible large extraosseous soft tissue component.
    - MRI: heterogeneous hypointense on T1, hyperintense on T2, with enhancement.
- Vertebral venous malformation (formerly hemangioma) (Fig. 24.4):
  o **Most common benign neoplasm:**
    - Can be locally aggressive.
  o Pathology: vascular spaces displacing bone.
  o Presentation: typically asymptomatic; however, can cause pain usually when bone expansion is present.
  o More common in the thoracic spine.
  o Imaging appearance:
    - X-ray/CT: corduroy cloth, jail bar, polka dot, salt and pepper signs.
    - MRI: the presence of variable fat and water in typical hemangiomas results in T1 and/or T2 hyperintensity, that saturates on fat saturation, and enhances owing to vascular component:
      ▪ Atypical lipid-poor will appear hypointense on T1.
    - Scintigraphy: varies from photopenic to moderate increased uptake.
- Chordoma (Fig. 24.5):
  o **Most common primary malignant tumor of the spine (with multiple myeloma).**
  o Arises from the remnants of the notochord:
    - Hysaliphorous cells are the hallmark of chordoma.
  o Tumor can have a heterogeneous makeup, including fluid, gelatinous material, acute and chronic blood products, necrosis, and calcifications or sequestered bone.
  o Fifth and sixth decades.
  o Male predominant (2:1).
  o The most common location is a sacrococcygeal region, midline.
  o Presentation: insidious subtle symptoms owing to slow growth.
  o Treatment: en bloc resection with possible radiation:
    - High rate of recurrence and high rate of metastasis.
  o Imaging appearance:
    - X-ray/CT: soft tissue lobulated mass spanning several segments and sparing discs with possible amorphous calcifications.
    - MRI: iso- or hypointense on T1, hyperintense on T2, with possible scattered areas of blood products and calcifications, moderate heterogeneous enhancement.
- Aneurysmal bone cyst (ABC) (Fig. 24.6a–c):
  o Reclassified as a tumor of undefined neoplastic nature.

Fig. 24.4 Vertebral venous malformation (hemangioma). (**a**) T1 and (**b**) T2 hyperintense that saturates with (**c**) fat saturation technique

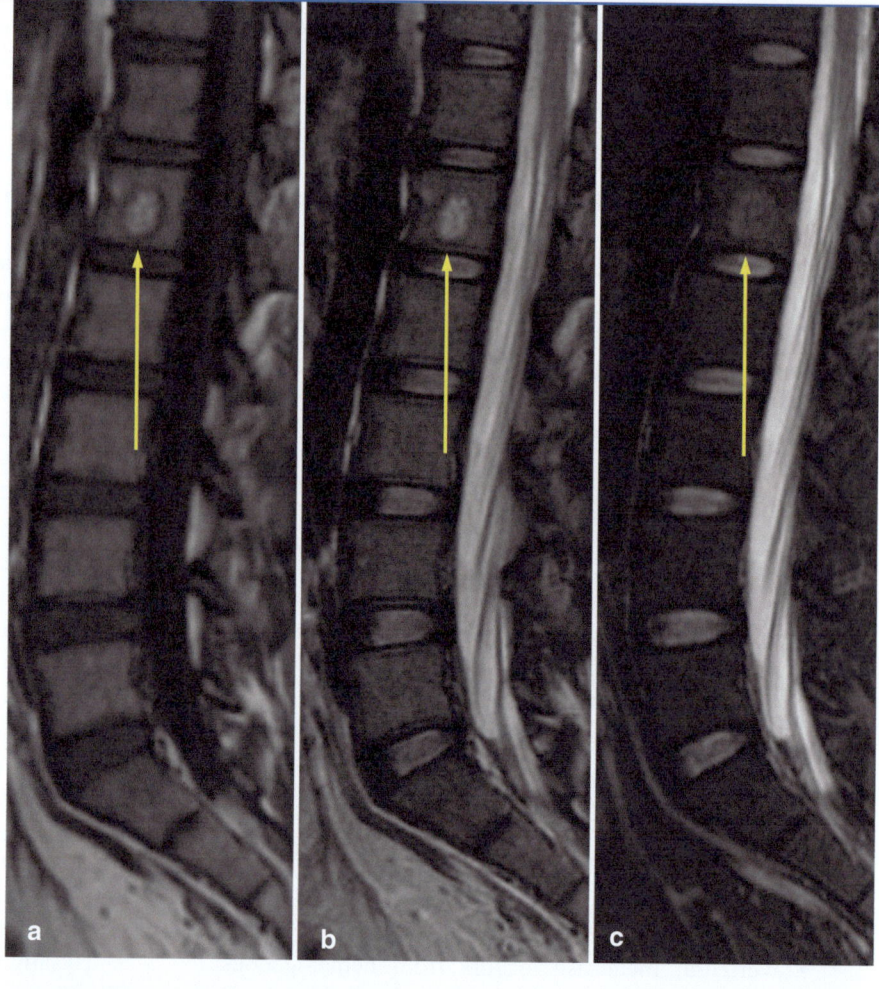

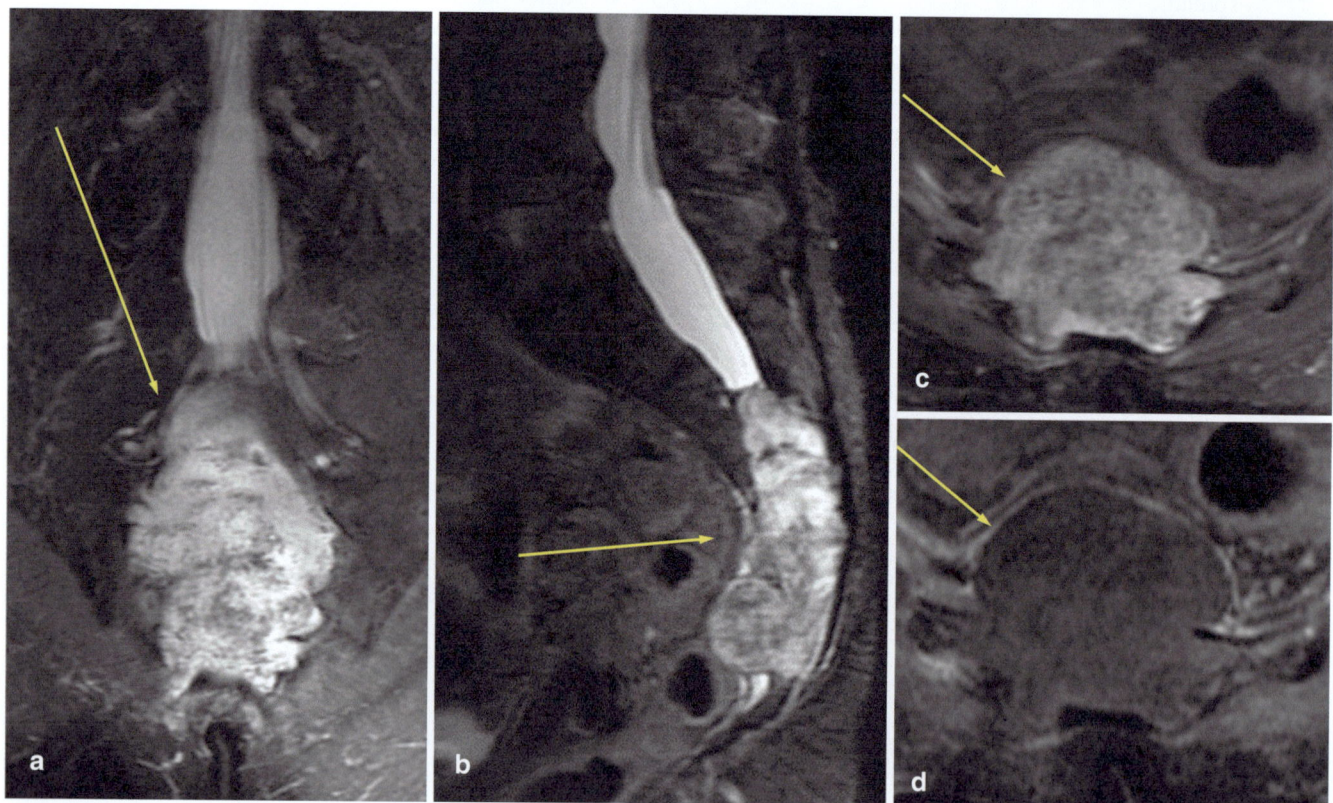

Fig. 24.5 Chordoma. Coronal (**a**), sagittal (**b**), and axial T2 (**c**) with a heterogeneous sacrococcygeal mass, without enhancement (**d**)

- Blood-filled cystic spaces separated by osteoclast-like giant cells.
- Often originating from a pre-existing lesion, which creates a diagnostic dilemma:
  - Giant cell tumor, osteoblastoma, angioma, chondroblastoma, fibrous lesions, osteosarcoma, and metastatic carcinoma.
- First to third decade.
- Slight female predilection.
- Thoracic and lumbar spine most common, and typically in posterior elements.
- Presentation: pain and swelling.
- Imaging appearance: appearance overlaps with giant cell tumor:
  - X-ray/CT: well-circumscribed lucency. Internal septations and fluid–fluid levels may be seen.
  - MRI: Fluid–fluid levels with signal characteristics of blood products, smooth enhancement of septa:
    - Nodular enhancement is suspicious of ABC arising from malignant lesions.
  - Scintigraphy: Moderate to intense uptake along the periphery *doughnut sign*.
- Giant cell tumor (GCT) (Fig. 24.6d–f):
  - Made up of ovoid mononuclear cells and osteoblastic giant cells.
  - Small percentage occurs in spine:
    - Usually in sacrum, lateralized to wing.
  - Second to fourth decade.
  - Female predilection.
  - Treatment: resection:
    - Risk of sarcomatous transformation with radiation.
  - Imaging appearance: often with a concurrent ABC:
    - X-ray/CT: lytic lesion with cortical expansion:
      - **NO sclerotic rim.**
    - MRI: hypo- to intermediate signal on T1, heterogeneous on T2, may have scattered blood products, nodular enhancement if seen may help differentiate from ABC.
    - Scintigraphy: Increased uptake.
- Fibrous dysplasia:
  - Benign fibro-osseous lesion.
  - In general, fibrous dysplasia can be monostotic (only occurring in one bone) or polyostotic.
  - Vertebral involvement is rare:
    - More common in patients with extraspinal polyostotic disease, with spinal polyostotic disease being extremely rare.
  - Presentation: typically asymptomatic; however, can cause pain and fracture.
  - Imaging appearance:
    - X-ray/CT: mild expansile lesion with a sclerotic rim with a characteristic ground-glass matrix.
    - MRI: hypo- to intermediate signal on T1, variable on T2, may have scattered blood products, enhances.
    - Scintigraphy: Mild to marked increased uptake.
- Metastatic disease:
  - **Most common malignant tumor of the spine.**
  - The third most common site for metastatic disease is the spine.
  - Osteolytic metastases (lung, breast, thyroid, kidney, colon, and neuroblastoma) slightly more common than osteoblastic (prostate, breast, lymphoma, carcinoid, GI mucinous adenocarcinoma, neuroblastoma, and medulloblastoma).
  - Typically multiple and variable in size.

MIMICS OF BONE TUMORS

- Schmorl's node (Fig. e24.6a–c):
  - Herniation of disc material through the vertebral body endplate into the marrow:
    - Typically with edema in the acute phase (high T2 signal).
    - Chronic Schmorl's node will have a sclerotic rim.
  - Can have an atypical appearance that mimics a lytic lesion:
    - Identifying endplate defects helps with the diagnosis.
- Infection (Fig. e24.6d–f):
  - Infection can present as a tumor-like lesion, more common in certain infections:
    - Spinal tuberculosis.
    - Echinococcus.
  - Pearl: Vertebral body infection typically spares the disc, look for other signs of infection in the paraspinal tissues.
  - Chronic infection can predispose patients to the development of bone tumors and is considered a precancerous condition.
- Paget disease (Fig. e24.6g):
  - Chronic metabolic disorder with abnormal bone remodeling.
  - >40 years of age.
  - Sarcomatous transformation is rare.
  - Imaging appearance:
    - X-ray/CT: expanded sclerotic vertebra with picture frame or ivory vertebra appearance:
      - Progresses from lytic to mixed to sclerotic.
    - MRI: heterogeneous appearance.
    - Scintigraphy: Increased uptake on all phases.
- SAPHO syndrome:
  - Synovitis, acne, pustulosis, hyperostosis, and osteitis.
  - When seen in the spine, it presents as multiple corner lesions.

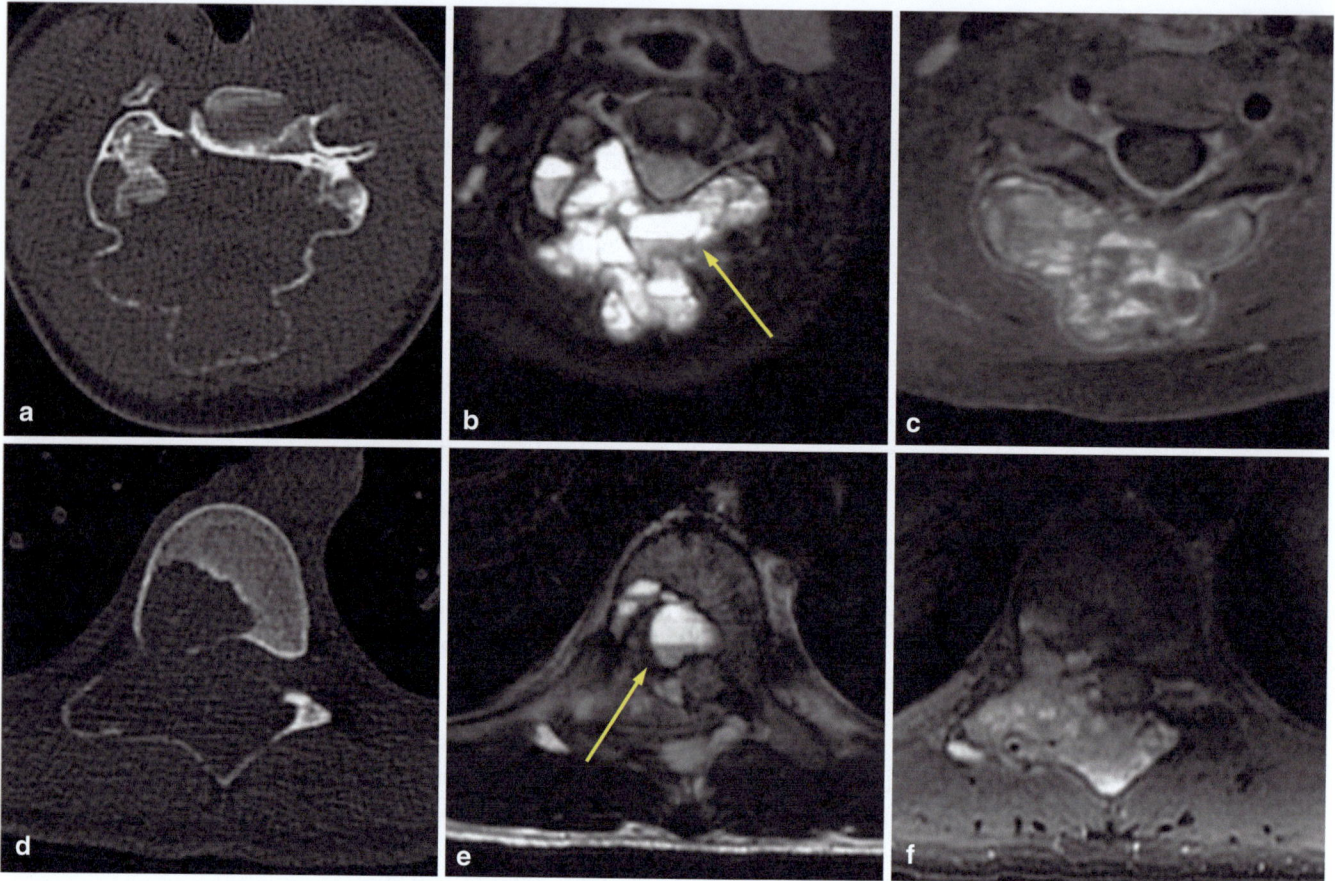

Fig. 24.6 Aneurysmal bone cyst (top row a–c) and giant cell tumor (bottom row d–f) share imaging features with an expansile lytic lesion on CT (a and d), fluid–fluid levels seen well on T2 (b and e), with enhancement (c and f)

- Imaging appearance:
  - X-ray/CT: sclerosis, osteolysis, and periostitis.
  - MRI: heterogeneous appearance.
  - Scintigraphy: most sensitive to identifying lesions.
- Brown tumor (Fig. e24.6h):
  - Sequela of hyperparathyroidism.
  - Imaging appearance: Well-defined lytic lesion, MRI may appear cystic or solid and demonstrate enhancement.
  - Histologically undifferentiated from giant cell tumor.
  - Re-mineralizes after parathyroidectomy.
- Renal osteodystrophy (Fig. e24.6i):
  - Secondary to chronic renal failure.
  - Imaging appearance:
    - Rugger Jersey Spine with sclerotic bands at the top and bottom of vertebral bodies.
    - Dense on X-ray/CT, low signal on MRI.
  - Can cause secondary hyperparathyroidism and associated Brown tumors (see above).
- Osteopetrosis (Fig. e24.6j):
  - Impaired osteoclastic resorption.
  - Diffuse involvement is common.
  - Presentation: fracture secondary to weakened bones.
  - Dense cortical bone on X-ray/CT, MRI with low signal.

Spinal Canal And/Or Cord Tumors

Pearl: Differential is based on location.

INTRAMEDULLARY

- Astrocytoma (Fig. 24.7):
  - Most common intramedullary mass in pediatric patients.
  - Located eccentrically, although often too large to accurately localize.
  - Associated with neurofibromatosis 1 (NF1).
  - The most common histology is pilocytic astrocytoma (WHO I):
    - Higher grades (diffuse and anaplastic WHO II/III) are typically found in the older population.
    - Enhancement correlates to a higher grade.
  - Imaging appearance:
    - MRI: T1 isointense, T2 hyperintense, patchy enhancement.
- Spinal cord glioblastoma (Fig. e24.7):
  - Rare high-grade (WHO IV) glial tumor:
    - May be primary or metastatic from a brain glioblastoma.

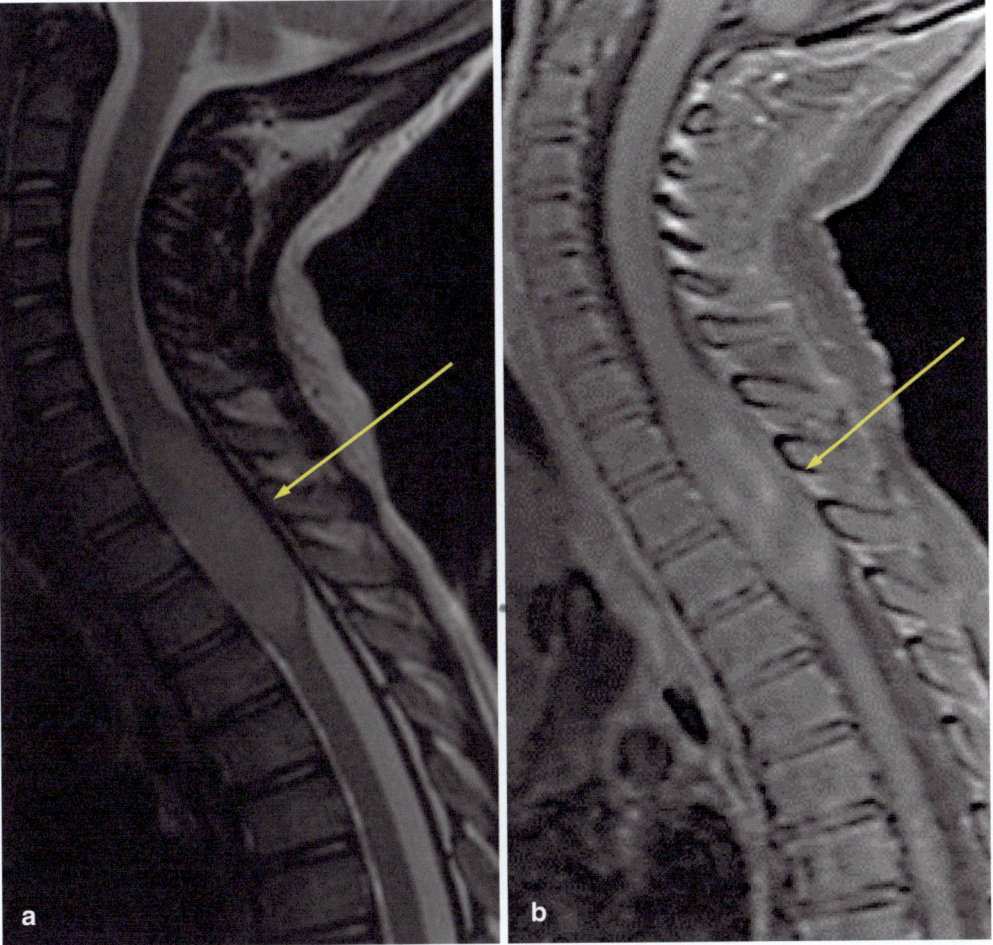

Fig. 24.7 Pilocytic astrocytoma. Expansile T2 hyperintense mass (**a**) with patchy enhancement (**b**) suggestive of a higher grade

- Can occur in both intramedullary and extramedullary spaces.
- Imaging appearance:
  - Demonstrates heterogeneously enhancement, angiogenesis, and necrosis.
- Overall poor prognosis.
- Ependymoma (Fig. 24.8):
  - **Most common intramedullary mass in adults**.
  - Arise from the ependymal lining of the central canal, and thus will **be located in the canal and central cord**.
  - Patients with neurofibromatosis 2 (NF2) will typically have multiple tumors that present at a younger age.
  - WHO grade II:
    - Anaplastic variant is high-grade (WHO III) with increased cellularity, mitotic activity, and aggressive imaging features.
  - Treatment: Gross total resection with radiation therapy for anaplastic variant.
  - Imaging appearance:
    - T1 hypo- to isointense.
    - T2 iso- to hyperintense.
    - **Pearl: cystic components and hemosiderin cap with surrounding cord edema and/or syrinx.**
    - Enhancement of the soft tissue component.
- Subependymoma (Fig. e24.8):
  - Rare.
  - WHO I.
  - Arise from subependymal glial progenitor cells, thus located paramedian.
  - Treatment: resection although typically not easy to dissect resulting in subtotal resection.
  - Imaging appearance:
    - Paramedian location.
    - Expansile, lobulated T2 hyperintense nonenhancing mass, bamboo leaf sign.
- Hemangioblastoma (Fig. 24.9):
  - **Third most common intramedullary tumor**.
  - Arises from mesenchymal hemangioblast cells, which are located in the leptomeninges:
    - Can manifest in both intra and extramedullary spaces.
  - Nonaggressive (WHO I).
  - **Pearl:** Multiple lesions – think von Hippel-Lindau syndrome.
  - Imaging characteristics:
    - Hypervascular enhancing tumor centered at the pial surface.
    - "Leaky vessels" cause a cyst-with-nodule appearance.

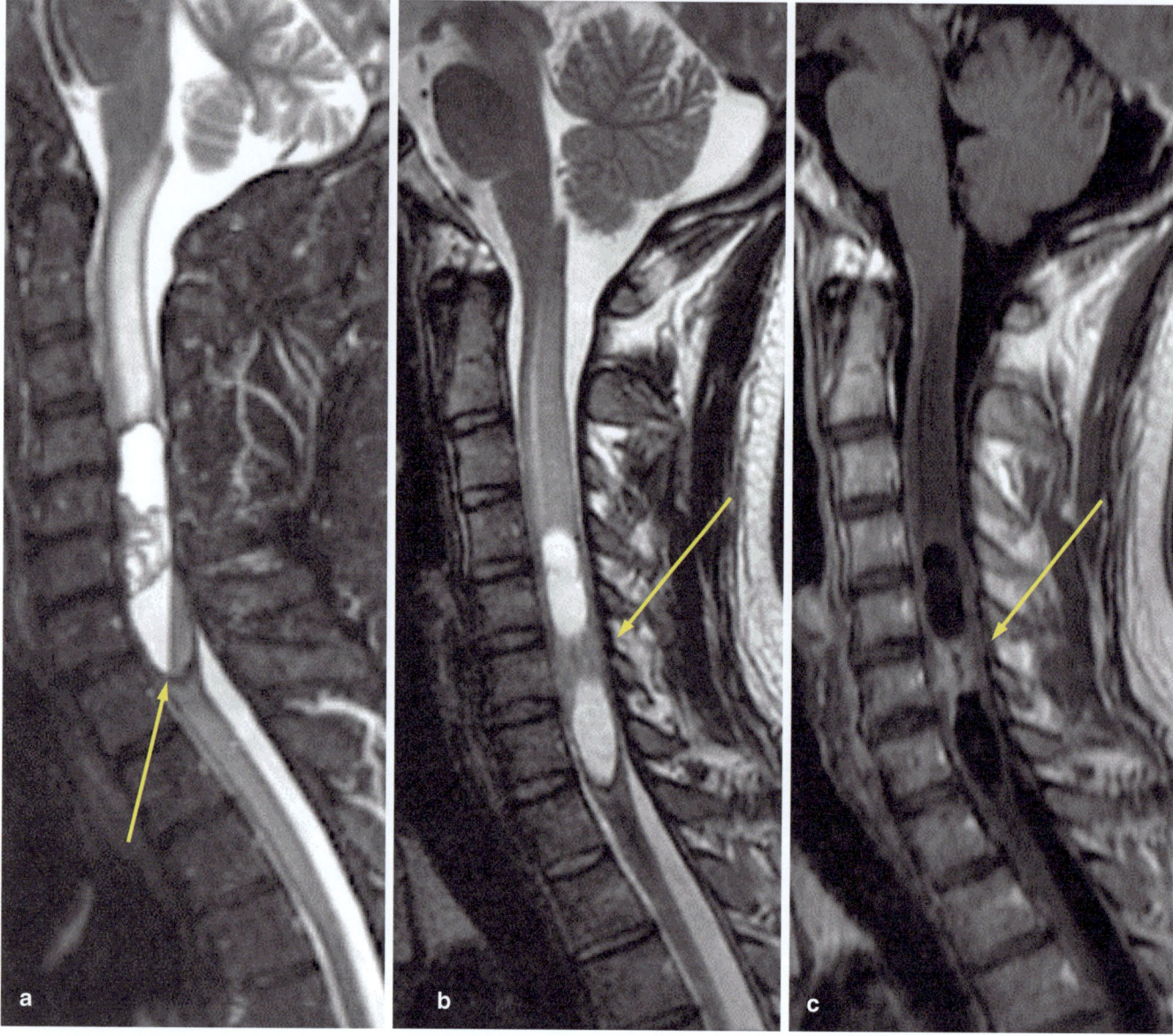

Fig. 24.8 Ependymoma. Heterogeneous mass on T2 with cystic component, syrinx, fluid–fluid layer of hemorrhage, and hemosiderin cap (**a**). T2 (**b**) and post-contrast (**c**) with mass, cystic component, and cord edema

CAUDA EQUINA/FILUM TERMINALE

- Myxopapillary ependymoma (Fig. 24.10):
  - Low grade (WHO II).
  - Arises from the ependymal cells of the filum terminale and therefore will be located at or just below the conus.
  - Presents in young adults, female predilection.
  - Presentation: low back pain.
  - Imaging appearance:
    - Well-circumscribed enhancing solid mass with possible cystic and hemorrhagic changes.
    - Large masses may remodel the spinal canal.
- Nerve sheath tumors:
  - See below in the intradural/extramedullary section.
- Paraganglioma (Fig. e24.9):
  - Arise from neuroendocrine cells.
  - Presentation: lower back pain with possible sciatica.
  - More common in middle-aged adults.
  - Slight male predilection.
  - Imaging appearance:
    - Well-circumscribed mass, isointense T1, iso- to hyperintense T2, may have blood products with a hemosiderin cap, can see salt-and-pepper sign secondary to flow voids, and intensely enhancing.
    - Vessels along the surface are common.
    - May show some adjacent bony erosion – best seen on CT.
- Metastases:
  - Drop metastases:
    - The most common primary CNS tumor is medulloblastoma.
    - The most common systemic tumor is breast.

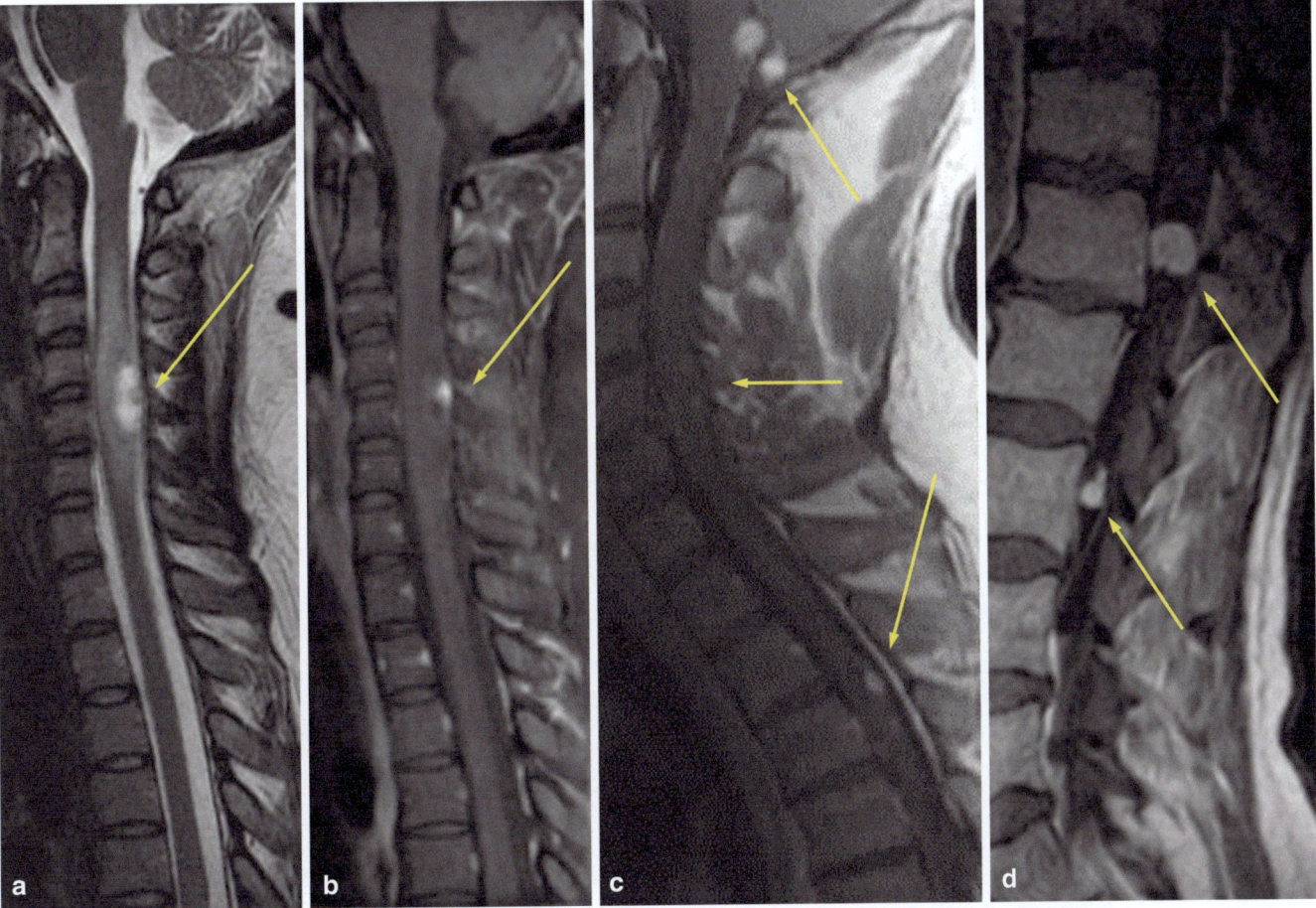

Fig. 24.9 Hemangioblastoma. Sporadic appearance with cyst and nodule (**a**), with nodule demonstrating avid enhancement (**b**). Multiple avidly enhancing lesions in a patient with confirmed VHL (**c** and **d**)

INTRADURAL/EXTRAMEDULLARY

- Meningioma (Fig. 24.11):
  - **Most common intradural/extramedullary tumor.**
  - Low-grade WHO I most common:
    - Higher grades may have rapid growth or local aggressive features.
  - Thoracic spine most common.
  - Female predilection (9:1).
  - Associated with NF2.
  - Previous radiation is a risk factor.
  - Presentation: results from compression of the spinal cord.
  - Treatment: surgical resection:
    - Recurrence rates are variable, higher with increasing grades, young patients, males, ventrally located, and presence of a dural tail.
  - Imaging appearance:
    - Well-circumscribed mass, T1 hypo- to isointense, T2 iso- to mild hyperintense, homogenously enhances.
  - Pearl: The presence of a dural tail helps with diagnosis; however, not always present in the spine.
  - Calcifications may be present on CT; however, less common than intracranial meningiomas.
- Solitary fibrous tumor (previously hemangiopericytoma) (Fig. e24.10):
  - Rare, WHO II/III.
  - Fourth to sixth decade.
  - Thoracic spine most common site for primary location, however is rare.
  - Local invasion from paraspinal tumor is more common and can be intradural or extradural.
  - Associated with NAB2 and STAT6 genetic mutations.
  - Imaging appearance:
    - T1 iso to hypointense, T2 hyperintense with avid enhancement.
    - Bone destruction is a common feature.
    - Angiography may show an intense vascular blush and feeding vessels similar to paragangliomas.
- Peripheral Nerve Sheath Tumor:
  - Schwannoma (Fig. 24.12a, b):

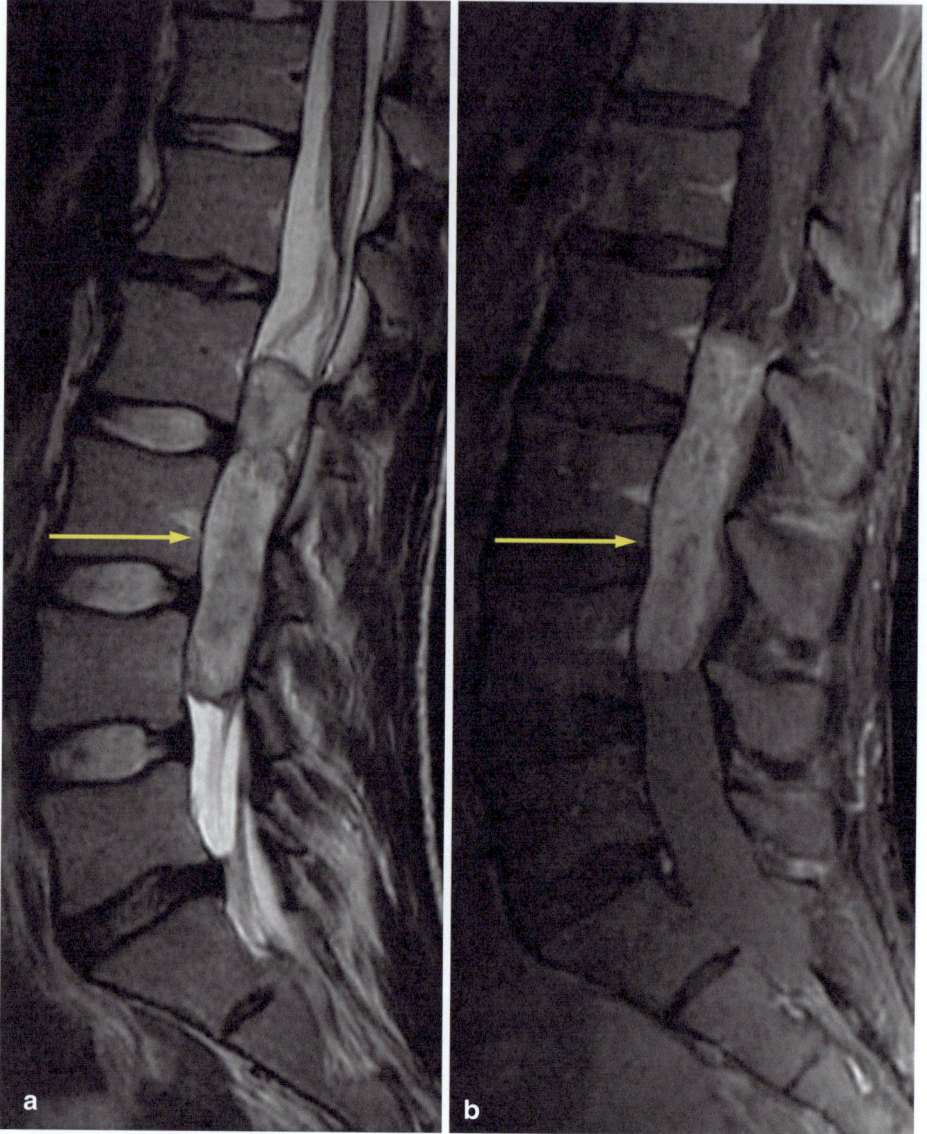

Fig. 24.10 Myxopapillary ependymoma. Well-circumscribed heterogeneous mass associated with the filum terminale with cystic and hemorrhagic areas (**a**), which demonstrates enhancement (**b**)

- Second most common intradural/extramedullary tumor.
- WHO I.
- Associated with NF2.
- Arises from Schwann cells, especially in the dorsal root.
- Foraminal involvement is common.
- Surgical resection for symptomatic lesions.
- Imaging appearance:
  - Well-circumscribed T1 hypointense, T2 hyperintense enhancing mass.
  - Expands the neural foramen without destruction.
  - Cystic degeneration can occur in larger masses and can mimic a malignant peripheral nerve sheath tumor.
  - Schwannomatosis can appear as multiple small enhancing nodules, similar to metastatic disease.
- Neurofibroma (NF) (Fig. 24.12c, d):
  - Associated with NF1:
    - Less commonly associated with Noonan syndrome with multiple lentigines (NSML).
  - Cervical spine is the most common location.
  - Arises from connective tissue of peripheral nerve sheaths, especially the endoneurium.

24 Tumors and Tumor-Like Lesions of the Spine and Spinal Cord

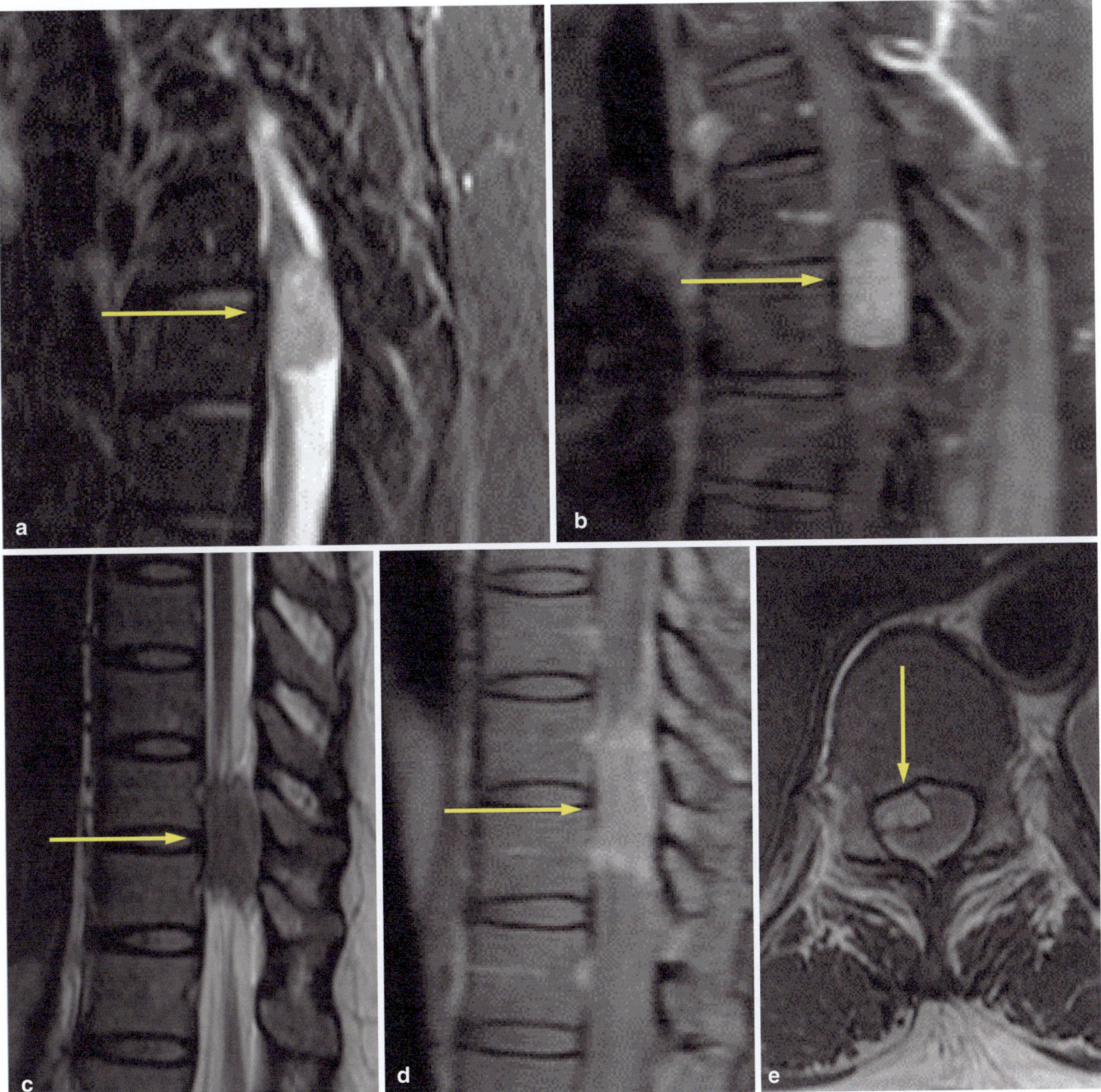

Fig. 24.11 Meningioma. Homogeneous extramedullary mass which displaces the cord without significant edema (**a** and **c**), with homogenous enhancement (**b–e**)

- Tumor encases rather than displaces the nerve roots.
- Imaging appearance similar to Schwannomas:
  - A *target sign* with hyperintense rim and central low signal is more common with neurofibromas than schwannomas.
- Plexiform tumors with a *bag of worms* appearance.
- Malignant peripheral nerve sheath tumor (MPNST) (Fig. 24.12e, f):
  - Rare.

- Associated with NF1.
- Prior radiation is a risk factor.
- Imaging appearance is similar to schwannomas and neurofibromas, especially in smaller tumors:
  - Enlarging painful peripheral nerve sheath tumors is suspicious for transformation.
  - Typically larger than 5 cm.
  - Can have areas of necrosis and hemorrhage related to rapid growth.

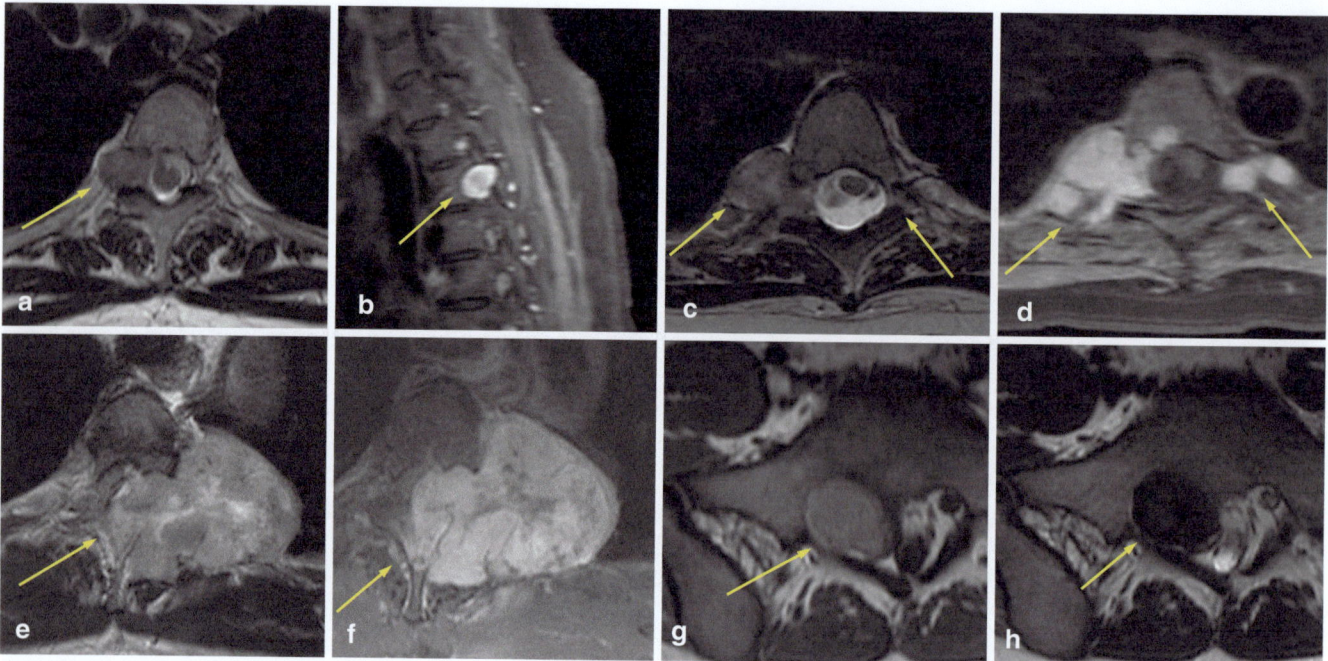

Fig. 24.12 Peripheral nerve sheath tumor spectrum. Typical Schwannoma—T2 hyperintense (**a**), homogeneously enhancing (**b**), and expanding the neural foramen. Typical neurofibromas in a patient with NF1—multiple T2 hyperintense (**c**) and homogeneously enhancing (**d**) masses extended from the neural foramina. Features of a malignant peripheral nerve sheath tumor included heterogeneous T2 signal (**e**) and heterogeneous enhancement (**f**) with the suggestion of areas of necrosis and hemorrhage and destruction of the adjacent osseous structures. Malignant melanotic peripheral nerve sheath tumors—well-circumscribed T1 hyperintense (**g**) and T2 hypointense (**h**) mass secondary to the presence of melanin

- Can arise sporadically, or from a conventional schwannoma, neurofibroma, ganglioneuroblastoma/ganglioneuroma, or pheochromocytoma.
  ○ Malignant melanotic nerve sheath tumor (Fig. 24.12g, h):
    - Extremely rare pigmented mass.
    - Can be sporadic or genetic (Carney complex).
    - High rate of metastases.
    - Treatment: surgical resection with possible radiation.
    - Imaging appearance:
      ▪ Well-circumscribed mass, **T1 hyperintense,** and very low on T2 dependent on the concentration of **melanin**, with enhancement.
- Leptomeningeal metastases:
  ○ Imaging will present with leptomeningeal nodular and/or thick linear enhancement:
    - Can occur in patients with known malignancy or be the initial presentation.
    - Most common with melanoma, breast, small cell lung carcinoma, leukemia, and lymphoma.
  ○ CSF analysis can confirm.

EXTRADURAL

- Bone tumors:
  ○ Extending from vertebrae into the epidural spaces.
  ○ See tumors of the spine in the previous section.
- Metastases:
  ○ Some malignancies metastasize directly to the epidural space and will present as an enhancing epidural mass.
  ○ Breast.
  ○ Melanoma.
  ○ Lymphoma:
    - Can localize to the epidural space, or paravertebral space with extension through the neural foramen.
- Meningioma:
  ○ A small portion of meningiomas are completely extradural.
  ○ See imaging details in the previous section.
- Peripheral nerve sheath tumors:
  ○ Typically extend from the intradural space.
  ○ See imaging details in the previous section.

EXTREMELY RARE SPINAL CANAL/CORD TUMORS

- Melanocytic tumors (Fig. e24.11):
  o Melanocytes arise from the neural crest cells.
  o Wide range of benign and malignant variants—meningeal melanocytoma, melanoma, melanocytosis, and melanomatosis:
    • Metastatic melanoma more common than primary tumors.
  o Can manifest in both intra- and extramedullary spaces.
  o Imaging appearance: MR iso- to hyperintense on T1 and hypo- to isointense on T2 related to melanin content, with enhancement. Metastatic disease will typically present with multiple lesions.

  Pearl: Intrinsic T1 high signal differential—hemorrhage, melanin, proteinaceous material, and fat (can do a fat saturation technique or CT to rule this out).

- Oligodendroglioma (Fig. e24.12):
  o Rare glial cell tumor (WHO II):
    • Anaplastic oligodendroglioma (WHO III).
  o Drop metastases more common than primary tumor.
  o Imaging appearance: heterogeneous T1 and T2 with enhancement.
- Ganglioglioma (Fig. e24.13):
  o Glioneuronal tumor (WHO I/II).
  o More common in pediatrics.
  o Imaging features: expansile mass:
    • Requires pathologic evaluation as imaging features can overlap with astrocytoma (which is more common in this age group).
    • Calcifications and remodeling/bony expansion of the spinal canal are more common with gangliogliomas.
    • High-grade features (cystic changes and enhancement) suggest anaplastic variant (WHO III).
- Lymphoma:
  o Primary lymphoma in the cord is rare and typically presents as diffuse large B-cell in middle-aged adults with symptoms similar to demyelinating diseases.
  o Metastatic disease (Fig. e24.14) is more common:
    • Can present as both intramedullary and extramedullary.
    • Can also present as a local invasion of the cord from adjacent structures.
    • Imaging appearance is nonspecific, similar to other metastatic lesions.
- Metastases:
  o Intramedullary metastases are uncommon.
  o Enhancing lesions with surrounding edema:
    • **A more intense rim of peripheral or flame-shaped enhancement is highly specific**.
  o Lung and breast most common.

MIMICS OF SPINAL CANAL/CORD TUMORS

- Degenerative disc disease (Fig. e24.15a, b):
  o Most common extradural "mass":
    • Typically extends from the intervertebral disc, but may also present after migration and sequestration.
  o Can rarely present as an intradural mass.
  o Synovial cysts can arise from the facet joints.
- Inclusion cysts:
  o Abnormal inclusion of ectoderm, mesoderm, or endoderm during embryogenesis:
    • Typically associated with spinal dysraphism.
  o Can manifest in both intra- and extramedullary spaces.
  o Treatment is surgical resection if symptomatic.
  o Can be acquired secondary to trauma or surgery.
  o Epidermoid cysts (Fig. e24.15c):
    • Contains keratinizing squamous epithelium.
    • More frequently in thoracic location.
    • Cystic appearance on imaging:
      ▪ More likely to restrict diffusion.
  o Dermoid cyst:
    • Includes additional tissues, such as hair follicles and sweat and sebaceous glands.
    • More common in the lumbosacral spine.
    • Cystic appearance on imaging:
      ▪ Less likely to restrict diffusion.
      ▪ Presence of fat density/signal.
  o Spinal lipoma (Fig. e24.15d):
    • Abnormal inclusion of mesoderm during embryogenesis.
    • Can manifest in both intra and extramedullary spaces.
    • **Will follow fat density and signal on imaging, no enhancement**:
      ▪ MR should be performed with fat saturation technique or additional CT showing fat density to differentiate from late subacute hematoma as this will also appear T1 and T2 hyperintense.
  o Neuroenteric cyst:
    • Abnormal inclusion of endoderm during embryogenesis:
      ▪ Respiratory and intestinal cells.
    • More commonly located ventral to the spinal cord.
    • Cystic appearing on imaging with varying signal secondary to mucin content, no enhancement.
- Hematoma (Fig. e24.15e, f):
  o Can occur from multiple causes:
    • Trauma/surgery/procedural:
      ▪ Epidural space will localize to the outside of the thecal sac.
      ▪ Subdural space hemorrhage may cause an *inverted Mercedes-Benz* sign.

- Blood patch in the epidural space or unexpected intrathecal blood patch injection in the subarachnoid space.
  - Aneurysm rupture will involve the subarachnoid space.
- Compressive myelopathy (Fig. e24.15g, h):
  - Can appear as an expansile lesion with enhancement.
  - Pancake enhancement that typically spares the gray matter is specific.
- Post-surgical changes:
  - Fibrosis/scar will enhance homogeneously.
- Cord infarction (Fig. e24.15i, j):
  - Classical imaging feature of *owl's or snake eyes* sign with an anterior spinal cord infarct.
  - Will enhance in the subacute phase.
- Inflammatory conditions:
  - MS (Fig. e24.15k, l), NMO, ADEM, or transverse myelitis:
    - Less common subacute combined degeneration, sarcoidosis, and HIV myelopathy.
  - Causes focal inflammation of the cord.
  - Can enhance in an active phase.
- Vascular:
  - Arteriovenous fistulas/arteriovenous malformations (Fig. e24.15m, n):
    - Type 1:
      - Most common (85%).
      - Dural AVF.
      - Causes venous congestion with multiple enlarged extramedullary veins and cord edema.
      - Presentation: middle-aged male with progressive lower extremity weakness and sensory deficits.
        - Foix-Alajouanine syndrome.
    - Type 2:
      - Intramedullary nidus.
    - Type 3:
      - Juvenile.
    - Type 4:
      - Perimedullary near the conus.
      - Associated with hereditary hemorrhagic telangiectasia.
  - Cavernous malformation (Fig. e24.15o, p):
    - Low flow capillary malformation.
    - Mulberry or popcorn appearance with varying ages of blood products and peripheral rim of hemosiderin.
    - No enhancement and little to no surrounding edema.

Further Reading

1. Rodallec MH, Feydy A, Larousserie F, et al. Diagnostic imaging of solitary tumors of the spine: what to do and say. Radiographics. 2008;28(4):1019–41.
2. Shih RY, Koeller KK. Intramedullary masses of the spinal cord: radiologic-pathologic correlation. Radiographics. 2020;40(4):1125–45.
3. Wang X, Gao J, Wang T, Li Z, Li Y. Intraspinal dermoid and epidermoid cysts: long-term outcome and risk factors. J Spinal Cord Med. 2020;43(4):512–7.
4. Koeller KK, Shih RY. Intradural extramedullary spinal neoplasms: radiologic-pathologic correlation. Radiographics. 2019;39(2):468–90.
5. Solomou G, et al. Extramedullary malignant melanotic schwannoma of the spine: case report and an up to date systemic review of the literature. Ann Med Surg (Long). 2020;59:217–23.
6. Mohajeri Moghaddam S, Bhatt AA. 1. Insights Imaging. 2018;9:511–26.
7. Brinjikji W, Nasr DM, Cloft HJ, Iyer VN, Lanzino G. Spinal arteriovenous fistulae in patients with hereditary hemorrhagic telangiectasia: a case report and systematic review of the literature. Interv Neuroradiol. 2016;

Spine Infection

Nicole Levy and Michael J. Hoch

By Organism

DISCITIS AND OSTEOMYELITIS

BACTERIAL DISCITIS/OSTEOMYELITIS
- Infection of the disc space and the surrounding vertebral endplates.
- Usually the result of hematogenous spread of infection, or less likely from the direct contiguous spread.
- Most frequently seen in the lumbar spine, and at only one level.
- *Staphylococcus aureus* is the most common causative organism, though *Streptococcus*, *Escherichia coli*, and *Proteus* are other common causes.
- Vertebral osteomyelitis may be seen without discitis, usually related to hematogenous spread.
- Bacterial discitis has some imaging features differentiating it from Tuberculous discitis and mimics such as neoplasm and dialysis-related spondyloarthropathy (Table 25.1).
- Imaging Findings:
  - Acute (Fig. 25.1):
    - MRI is the most specific method for diagnosis.
    - Discitis with associated edema and fluid in the disc will manifest as T1 hypointensity, T2 hyperintensity, and enhancement [1].
    - Vertebral osteomyelitis similarly has T1 hypointensity, T2 hyperintensity, and enhancement, particularly in the endplates, though this can also be seen in endplate degenerative changes.
    - Diffusion-weighted imaging, if performed, can show restricted diffusion. This can help differentiate from non-infectious changes [2].
    - Endplate erosive changes, sclerosis, and fragmentation are better visualized on CT compared with MRI and can help differentiate from degenerative changes.
    - Loss of disc space height and hypodensity in the disc space are also important CT findings.
    - Nuclear medicine bone scan will be hot on all three phases.
  - Late discitis and associated findings (i.e., epidural abscess and kyphosis; Fig. e25.1).
    - (All electronic images (Figs. e25.1–e25.3) can be found on this chapter's website on SpringerLink: https://doi.org/10.1007/978-3-031-55124-6_25):
    - As discitis progresses, there may be a loss of intervertebral disc height.
    - Infection can spread into the epidural space and result in an associated epidural abscess or phlegmon.
    - Paraspinal abscess and surrounding soft tissue infection can also be present.
    - Infection of the facet joint (facetitis) can also occur, especially when there is surrounding infection in the surrounding paraspinal soft tissues.
    - Significant erosive changes can cause a focal kyphosis, possibly worsening mass effect on the spinal canal.
    - Resolving infection may show reactive bone formation and sclerosis (best seen on CT) and normalization of marrow signal on MRI.

Table 25.1 Imaging features of bacterial discitis, tuberculosis, and possible mimics (neoplasm and dialysis spondyloarthropathy)

Condition	Disc space	Paraspinal involvement	Posterior element involvement	Spread
Bacterial	• Always involved early • T2 bright	Sometimes	Uncommon	Contiguous
Tuberculosis	Spared early	Usually large fluid collection	Common	Skip areas anteriorly
Neoplasm	Very rarely involved	Extraosseous mass	Common	Noncontiguous
Dialysis	• Focal erosions • Can be T2 dark	Rare	Uncommon	Cervical (most common)

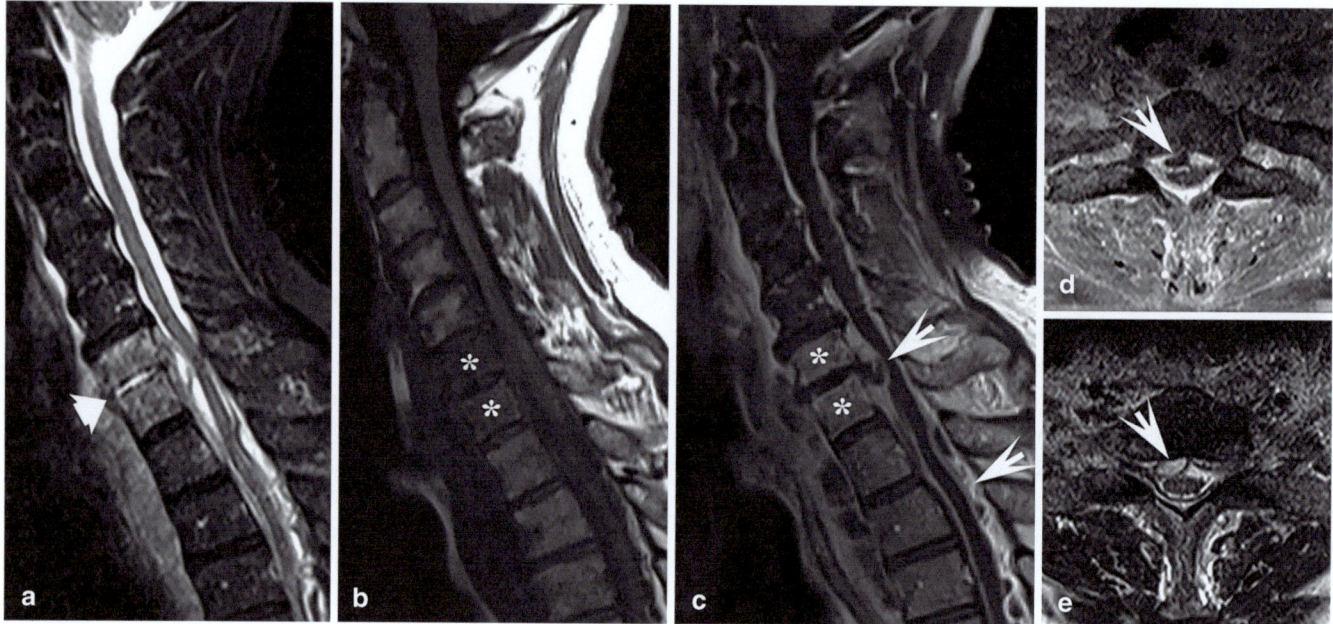

Fig. 25.1 Bacterial discitis/osteomyelitis. (**a**) Sagittal STIR image of the cervical spine showing edema within the infected C6–C7 disc (arrow head) and adjacent vertebral bodies. (**b, c**) Sagittal T1 pre- and post-contrast images demonstrating enhancement of the C6 and C7 vertebral bodies (asterisks). There is a large peripheral enhancing multi-loculated circumferential epidural abscess (arrows) originating from the C6–C7 disc. (**d, e**) Axial T1 post-contrast and T2 images show the peripheral enhancing and T2 hyperintense epidural abscess (arrows) expanding the epidural space with mass effect on the dura and thecal sac

TUBERCULOUS (TB) DISCITIS

- The most common granulomatous infection of the spine, *Mycobacterium tuberculosis* is also known as Pott's disease.
- Has a more indolent and insidious onset and progression of symptoms compared with bacterial infection.
- Many patients also have pulmonary tuberculosis (~50%).
- Typically involves the thoracic spine and progresses anterior to posterior.
- Commonly involves the posterior elements.
- Lack of proteolytic enzymes in Mycobacterial infections has been proposed as the reason why there is relative sparing of the disc space with a subligamentous spread of infection.
- More likely to involve multiple levels and have entire vertebral body involvement compared with bacterial infection.
- Imaging Findings (Fig. 25.2):
  - Typically has destructive changes in the vertebral bodies, with progression of untreated disease leading to vertebral collapse and anterior wedging causing the classic "gibbus" deformity with focal kyphosis [3].
  - MR imaging findings of vertebral osteomyelitis including T1 hypointensity, T2 hyperintensity, and enhancement and CT findings of cortical erosions and sclerosis are often indistinguishable from bacterial osteomyelitis.
  - Signal in the disc may be normal on unenhanced imaging, though post-contrast imaging usually shows enhancement.
  - Frequently also has epidural and paraspinal extension, including psoas abscess:
    - Paraspinal abscesses usually have a well-defined, smooth enhancing rim, and can be large.
    - Paraspinal calcified masses are highly specific for TB.

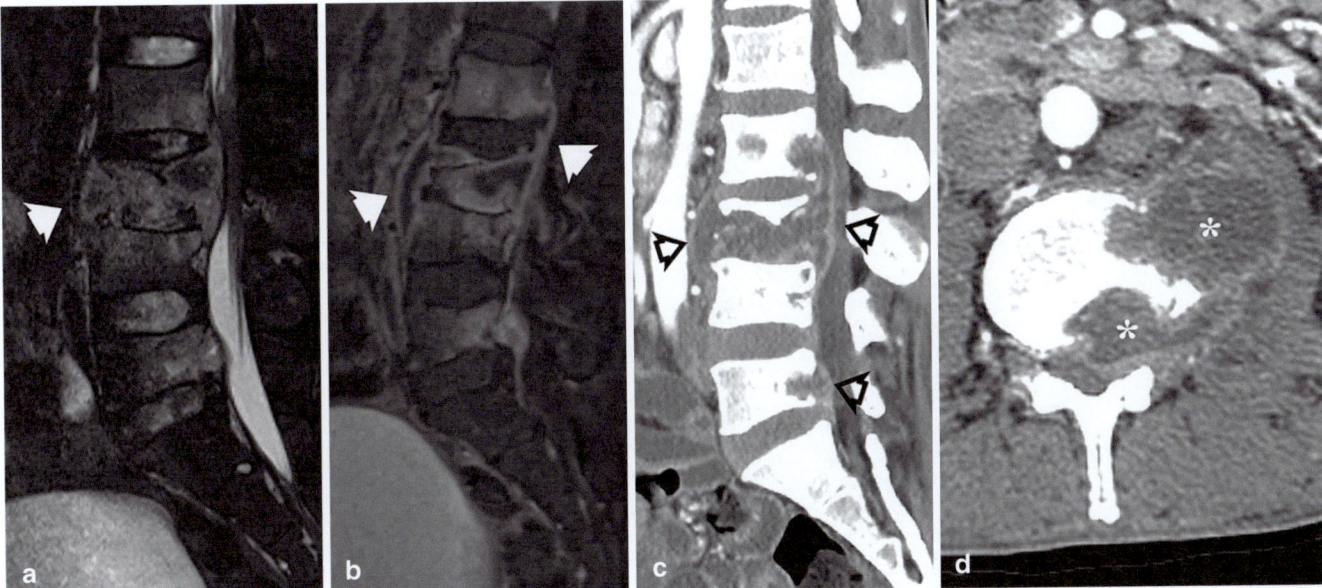

Fig. 25.2 Tuberculosis osteomyelitis. (**a**) Sagittal STIR image of the lumbar spine demonstrating edema and destruction of the L3 vertebral body (arrow head). (**b**) Sagittal fat saturated T1 post-contrast image with subligamentous spread of disease to the L2 and L4 vertebrae along the anterior and posterior longitudinal ligaments (arrow heads). (**c**) Sagittal CT with IV contrast showing peripheral enhancing collections spreading along the ligaments (black outlined arrow heads) with relative sparing of the disc spaces. (**d**) Peripheral enhancing epidural abscess with contiguous large left psoas muscle abscess (asterisks) on axial CT with IV contrast

ATYPICAL INFECTION

FUNGAL

- Usually has a slower, more indolent presentation than bacterial infection.
- More commonly seen in immunocompromised patients or in patients in certain endemic regions.
- Common fungal infectious species that may affect immunocompromised patients include *Aspergillus*, *Candida*, and *Mucor*.
- Common fungal infectious species that may affect immune-competent patients include *Coccidioides*, *Histoplasma*, and *Blastomyces*. These have certain regional predilections.
- Fungal discitis/osteomyelitis usually involves the anterior vertebral body and is associated with paraspinal involvement.
- Imaging Findings:
  o Findings on MRI are usually less striking than those seen with bacterial infection, and the T1 hypointensity, T2 hyperintensity, and enhancement may all be milder.
  o Aspergillus spondylodiscitis may appear almost identical to that of pyogenic infection, with the exception that the disc will not be T2 hyperintense on MRI and the normal nuclear cleft in the disc may be preserved (uncommon with bacterial infection).
  o Aspergillus and Blastomyces infections often span multiple levels and may skip levels, traveling via subligamentous spread.
  o Coccidiomycosis spinal infection more frequently presents as leptomeningeal disease with leptomeningeal nodularity and enhancement though may also present as spondylodiscitis [4].
  o Candidiasis often presents with microabscesses (similar to its presentation in the abdominal organs), with an imaging appearance of multiple tiny T2 hyperintense foci, and can have subdural and even intramedullary extension (Fig. 25.3).

PARASITIC

- Very uncommon source of spinal infections.
- May be associated with certain regions [5].
- While there are many parasitic infections that can involve the CNS, the most common diseases are neurocysticercosis and schistosomiasis.
- Toxoplasmosis also commonly involves the CNS, particularly in AIDS patients, though it very rarely involves the spine.
- Neurocysticercosis CNS infection is caused by ingestion of the egg of the parasitic tapeworm *Taenia solium* and hematogenous distribution into the CNS compartments:

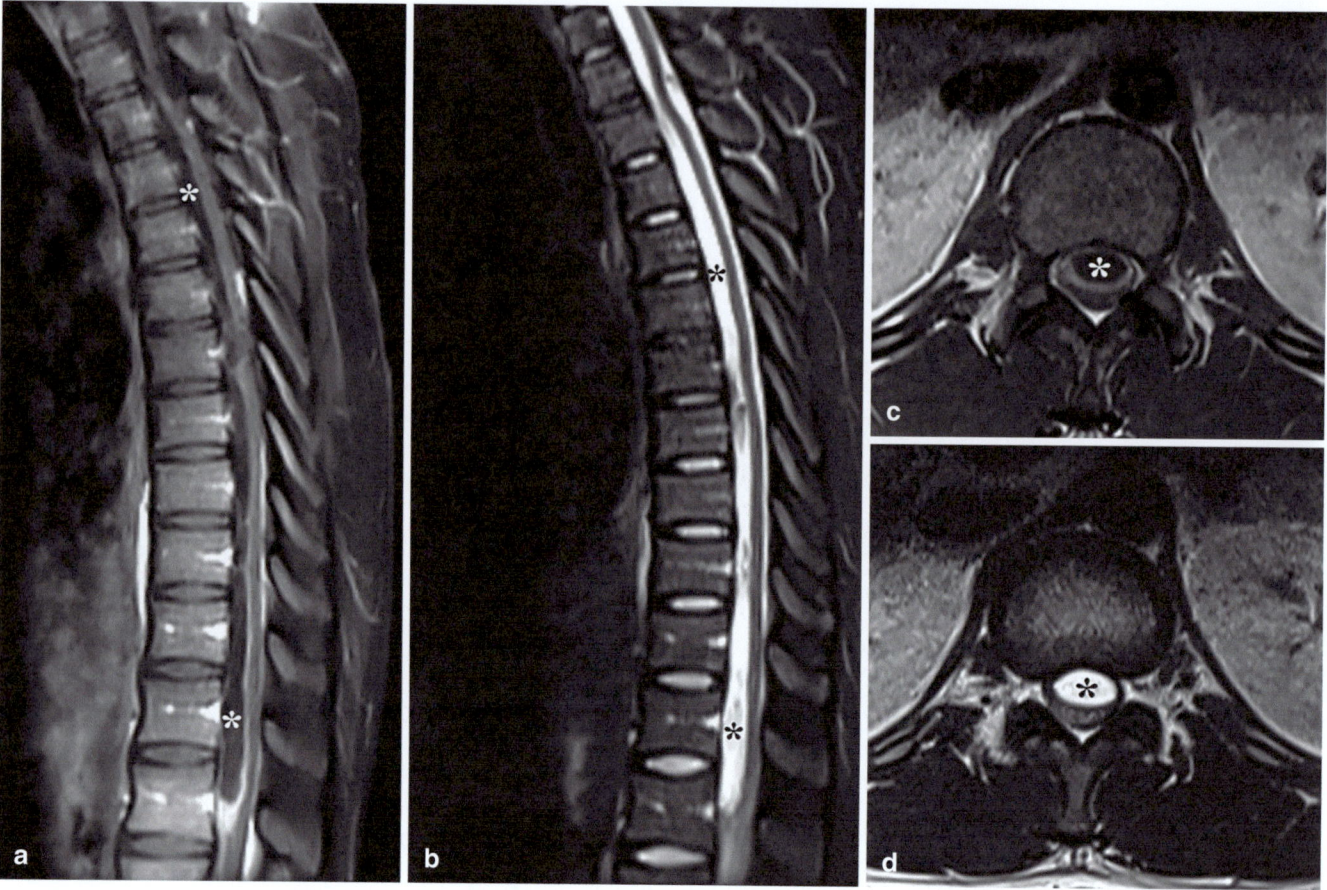

Fig. 25.3 Candida subdural empyema. (**a**, **b**) Sagittal fat saturated T1 post-contrast and STIR images of the thoracic spine showing a large multilevel peripheral enhancing and STIR hyperintense ventral subdural collection (asterisks). (**c**, **d**) Axial T1 post-contrast and T2 images demonstrate the collection (asterisks) compresses the thoracic cord but does not displace the dura (in contrast to Fig. 25.1d and e where the epidural abscess displaces the dura)

- Spinal involvement is much less common than intracranial involvement.
- While intramedullary infection is more common intracranially, spinal infection most often presents in the intradural extramedullary space (Fig. 25.4).
- MRI findings include cystic intradural lesions with signal intensity similar to CSF on all sequences and variable cyst wall enhancement.
- MR findings can be subtle, with mass effect on the cord being a clue to the presence of cystic lesions, and as such, CT myelography may be helpful in visualizing the cysts.
- Spinal intramedullary infection may be similar to intracranial infection, with a classic central scolex and surrounding cyst, or may be nonspecific and very challenging to distinguish from other infectious and noninfectious conditions.

- Schistosomiasis infections are caused by ingestion of the *Schistosoma* parasitic worm:
  - Infection is very rare in the United States though it is endemic in other parts of the world.
  - Can result in an acute onset intramedullary infection, more often in the lower cord, with imaging findings related to the granulomatous reaction to the parasitic egg with nodular, T2 hyperintense lesions with heterogeneous enhancement of the eggs and granulomas. This imaging appearance can mimic neoplasm or vascular lesions.
  - Radiculitis tends to have more indolent development of symptoms and can occur independently or along with myelitis, and often has imaging findings of thickening of the cauda equina nerve roots with associated leptomeningeal enhancement.

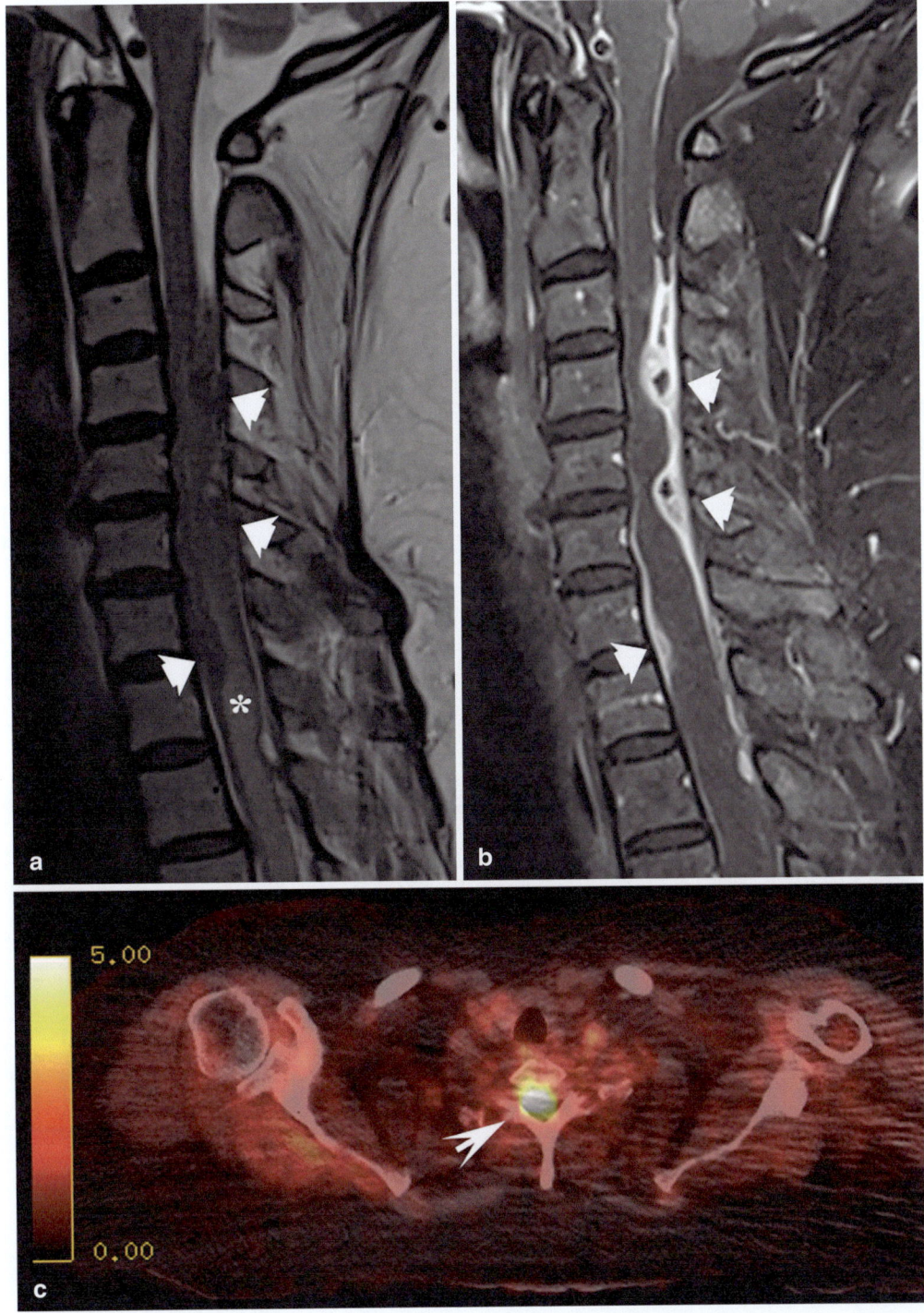

Fig. 25.4 Neurocysticercosis. (**a**) Sagittal T2 image of the cervical spine shows a multilevel hypointense infectious process along the dorsal and ventral surfaces of the cord (arrow heads). There is cord edema (asterisk). (**b**) Sagittal fat saturated T1 post-contrast image shows a corresponding multiloculated enhancing process in the CSF space coating the surfaces of the cord (arrow heads). (**c**) FDG-PET scan reveals increased metabolic activity (arrow)

IMMUNOCOMPROMISED CONDITIONS

- Immunocompromised conditions can both directly cause infection and can put these patients at risk for infection by typical opportunistic organisms.

HIV MYELITIS AND MYELOPATHY

- Typically presents with progressive spastic paresis, loss of sensation, and ataxia.
- Occurs in late-stage HIV/AIDS.

- HIV myelitis is caused by direct infection of the cord by the virus and is usually seen alongside severe cerebral disease involvement.
  - Imaging Findings:
    - MRI findings are similar to other cases of myelitis and typically show T2 hyperintense signal and patchy enhancement with no specific pattern (Fig. 25.5).
    - More common in the thoracic spine.
    - Increasing cranial spread as disease progresses.
- HIV vacuolar myelopathy is caused by spongy degeneration within the white matter of the cord and is the most common myelopathy in HIV patients.
  - Imaging Findings:
    - The most common imaging finding of HIV vacuolar myelopathy is cord atrophy with volume loss [6].
    - Classic MR imaging appearance of high T2 signal in the posterior columns (very similar to subacute combined degeneration; Fig. 25.7c).
  - Imaging appearance can be variable and may look like anything from a normal cord signal to central cord T2 hyperintensity.
  - Usually does not enhance.
- These patients are also more likely to have infectious myelitis from certain opportunistic viral (HSV, VZV, CMV), parasitic (toxoplasmosis), and bacterial (TB, syphilis) organisms [7].

CYTOMEGALOVIRUS (CMV) POLYRADICULOMYELITIS

- CMV is fairly mild or asymptomatic in the immune-competent host.
- It is never fully cleared from the body, so reactivation of the latent virus can occur at any time.
- More severe illness can be seen in those with some form of immunosuppression, including AIDS, prior transplantation, and chemotherapy or other immune-suppressing medications:

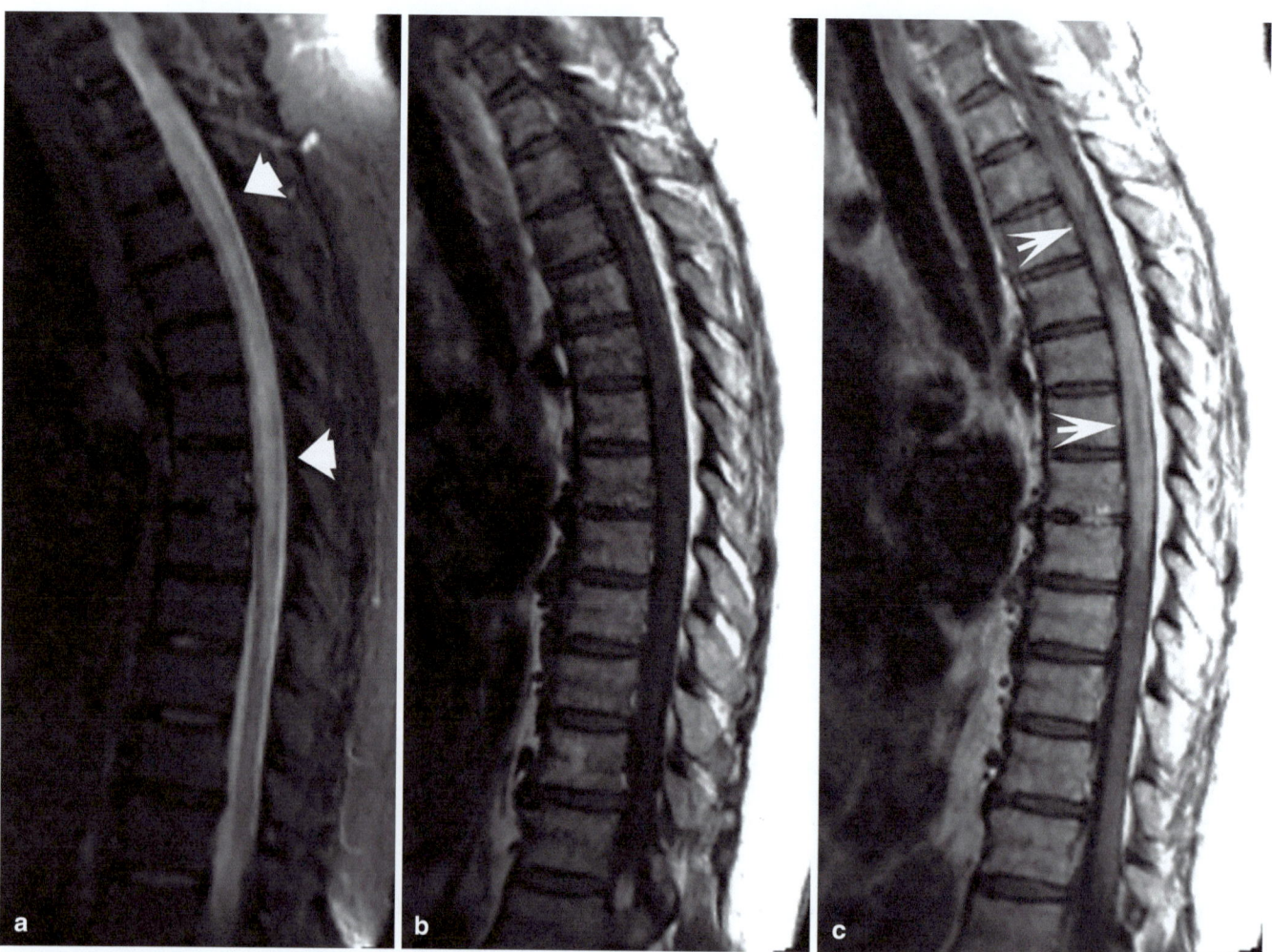

Fig. 25.5 HIV myelitis. (a) Sagittal T2 image of the thoracic spine showing diffuse longitudinal T2 hyperintensity of the cord (arrow heads). (b, c) Sagittal T1 pre- and post-contrast images showing corresponding widespread patchy enhancement of the cord in no specific pattern (arrows)

- o Lumbosacral polyradiculopathy can be seen in HIV patients with CD4 levels <40/μL.
- Spinal manifestation presents as myelitis or polyradiculomyelitis.
- Similar to other myelitis cases, it presents with radicular pain, progressive ascending paralysis, and autonomic dysfunction.
- Strongly associated with Guillain–Barre syndrome.
- Imaging Findings:
  - o Most common MRI finding is lumbosacral radiculitis or arachnoiditis with diffuse thickening of the cauda equina nerve roots best visualized on axial T2 images and hyperenhancement on post-contrast imaging (Fig. 25.6).
  - o Has a tendency to involve the ventral nerve roots.
  - o Severe cases of CMV polyradiculomyelitis may have central intramedullary T2 hyperintensity.

IMMUNE RECONSTITUTION INFLAMMATORY SYNDROME (IRIS)

- After starting antiretroviral therapy, patients with AIDS are at an increased risk for developing CNS-IRIS:
  - o Can be associated with herpes infections (CMV, herpes zoster), mycoses, or mycobacterial infections.
  - o Recurrent myelopathy due to TB.
- Imaging Findings:
  - o Increased pial enhancement and edema surrounding tuberculomas (TB-IRIS).
  - o Increased size and enhancement of ring or nodular tuberculomas.

By Location

INTRAMEDULLARY

MYELITIS

- Broad term for inflammation of the spinal cord, from a wide variety of causes [8].
- May be due to direct viral infection of the cord or post viral immunologic attack.
- Infectious myelitis is most commonly viral in origin, though can also be bacterial or fungal.
- Symptoms present over hours to days and can be variable, though are typically bilateral and generally include paresis, sensory dysfunction, and autonomic abnormalities.
- Appearance on imaging has a large overlap with demyelinating disease, and infectious etiologies may also have overlapping imaging features with each other, making clinical history, lab tests, and CSF testing very important in establishing a diagnosis (and in many cases, the cause is idiopathic) [9, 10].

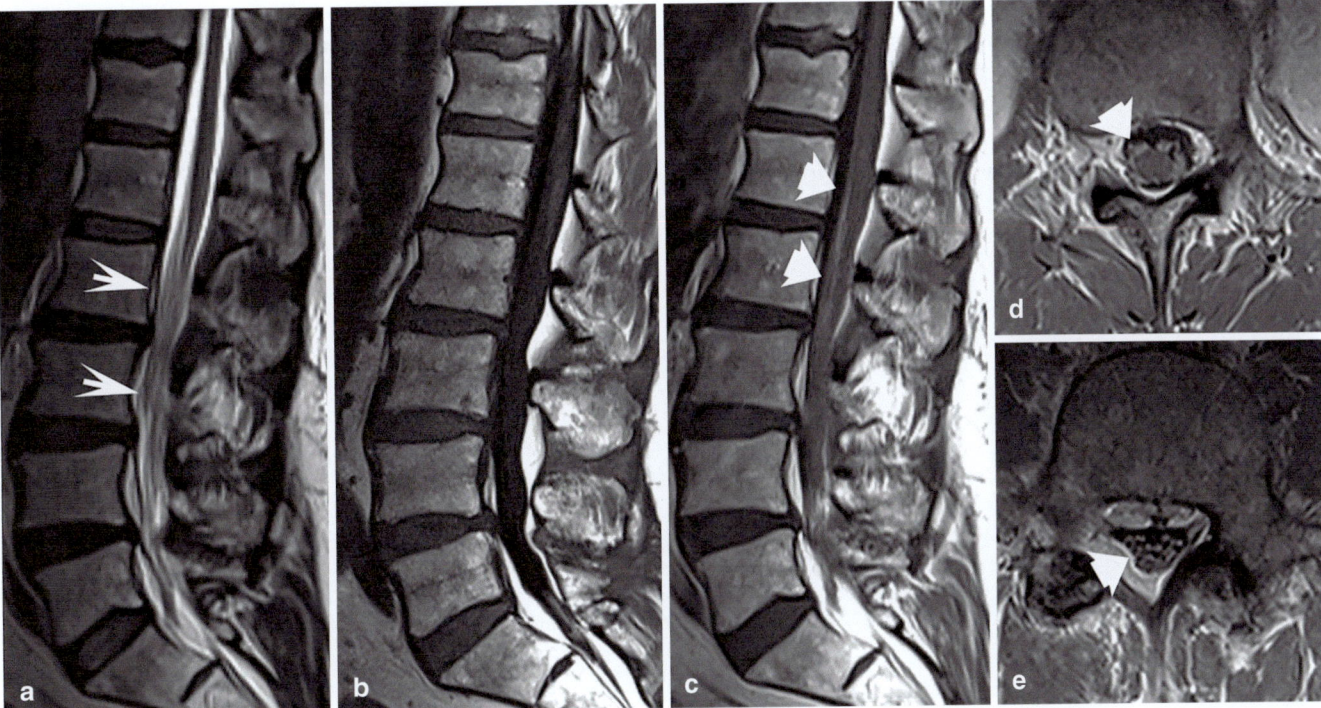

Fig. 25.6 Cytomegalovirus polyradiculopathy. (**a**) Sagittal T2 image of the lumbar spine with thickened nerves of the cauda equina (arrows). (**b, c**) Sagittal T1 pre- and post-contrast images demonstrating cauda equina diffuse smooth enhancement (arrow heads). (**d, e**) Axial T1 post-contrast images showing diffuse enhancement of both the ventral and dorsal cauda equina nerves (arrow heads)

- Certain patterns of involvement of the cord have been associated with different infectious sources, helping to narrow a differential diagnosis [11] (Table 25.2).
- Imaging Findings:
  - MRI is the ideal modality for evaluation.
  - In general, MRI demonstrates T2 hyperintense signal within the cord, with cord expansion sometimes seen.
  - Enhancement is variable and may be nonexistent, patchy, or extensive.
  - Craniocaudal extent of signal abnormality is variable, though usually spans multiple levels.
  - Centromedullary involvement is the least specific appearance and is usually central, symmetric, and round or ovoid in the axial plane, possibly involving the whole transverse dimension of the cord:
    - Some examples include CMV, EBV, Enterovirus, Lyme disease, viral hepatitis, *Campylobacter jejuni*, and *Mycoplasma*.
  - Anterior predominant involvement usually manifests as fairly symmetric involvement of the anterior horns due to the propensity of certain viruses to affect the motor neuron pools:
    - Can result in acute flaccid paralysis (AFP) or a poliomyelitis-like syndrome.
    - Patients present with flaccid paralysis and areflexia of involved limbs usually without sensory deficits.
    - Tends to affect the pediatric population.
    - Severe cases can involve the lower brainstem.
    - AFP can also be seen with a centromedullary pattern if the lesion is large enough to affect the anterior horn cells.
    - Some AFP agents include West Nile virus (Fig. 25.7a), Poliovirus, Enterovirus-71, and Enterovirus-D68 (Fig. 25.8).
  - Lateral involvement usually indicates involvement of certain tracts preferentially and is commonly associated with HSV and can be seen with retrovirus HTLV I and II.
  - Posterior involvement is usually related to involvement of the dorsal columns, and is commonly seen in VZV (unilateral; Fig. 25.7b), HIV vacuolar myelopathy (Fig. 25.7c), and syphilis.

INTRAMEDULLARY ABSCESS

- Very rare complication of a spinal cord infection, and usually evolves from infectious myelitis of the cord.
- Spread can be hematogenous, via direct spread of adjacent infection, direct implantation (from trauma or iatrogenic), or from a congenital sinus tract.
- Usually develops approximately 1 week after the onset of infection.
- Most often caused by *Staphylococcus aureus* and *Streptococcus* organisms.
- *Baceteroides, Haemophilus,* and *Listeria monocytogenes* are other causative organisms.
- Imaging Findings (Fig. 25.9):
  - Again best visualized with MRI.
  - As with other abscesses elsewhere, will appear as a rim enhancing fluid collection on MRI post-contrast sequences.
  - Cord expansion is usually present.
  - If diffusion imaging is obtained, will have central diffusion restriction.
  - Typically, there is extensive surrounding T2 hyperintense signal abnormality.
  - Abscess capsule can have low T2 signal giving a double-rim appearance of bright T2 edema surrounding a low T2 capsule.

Table 25.2 Myelitis by characteristic location

Location	Central	Anterior	Lateral	Posterior
Diagram				
Conditions	CMV EBV Enterovirus Viral hepatitis	Coxsackie Enterovirus Polio West Nile	HSV HTLV	HIV Syphilis VZV

CMV Cytomegalovirus, *EBV* Epstein–Barr virus, *HSV* Herpes simplex virus, *HTLV* Human T-lymphotrophic virus, *HIV* Human immunodeficiency virus, *VZV* Varicella-zoster virus

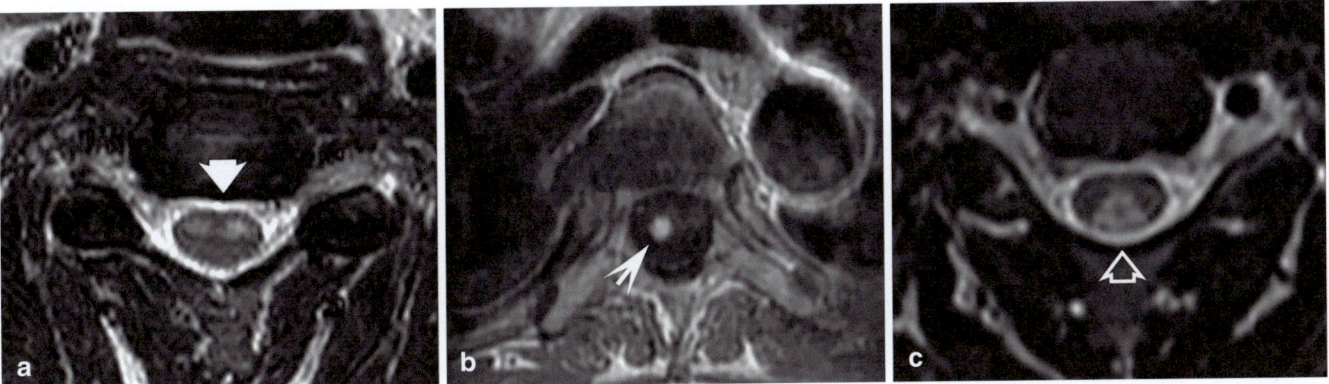

Fig. 25.7 Viral myelitis by location. (**a**) Axial T2 image of the cervical spine in a case of West Nile myelitis affecting the anterior horn cells (arrow head). (**b**) Axial T1 post-contrast image of the thoracic spine showing unilateral cord enhancement in a case of Varicella-Zoster myelitis (arrow). (**c**) Axial T2 image of the cervical spine in a case of HIV vacuolar myelopathy with hyperintensity affecting the posterior columns (white outlined arrow head)

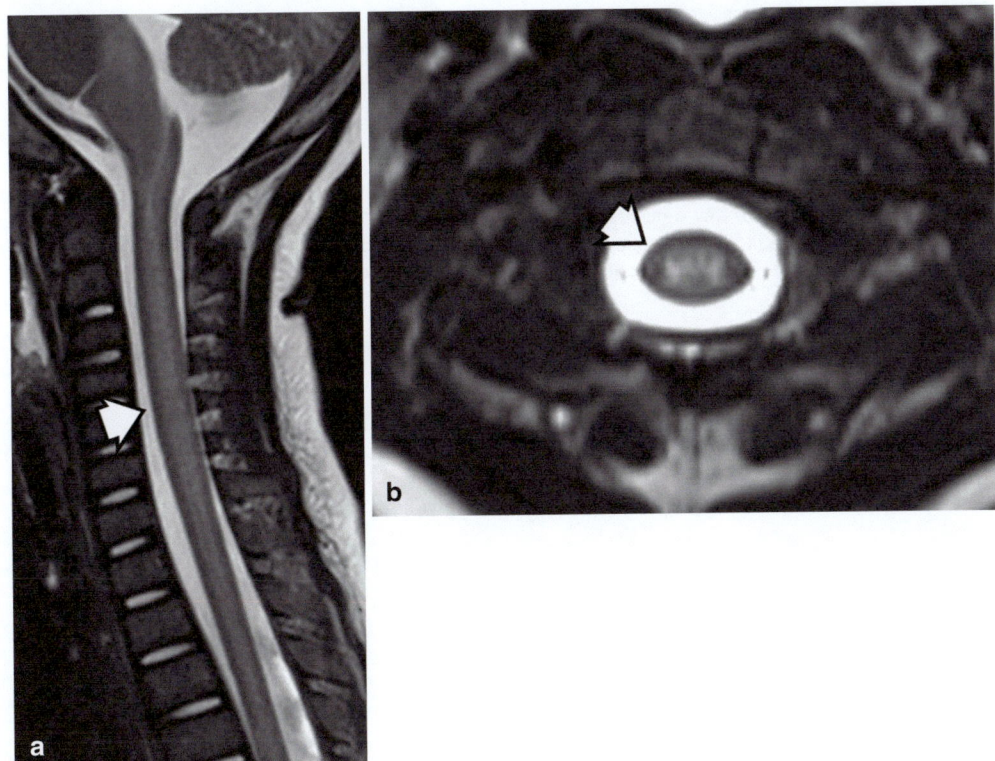

Fig. 25.8 Acute flaccid myelitis. (**a**) Sagittal T2 image of the cervical cord in a pediatric patient with enterovirus reveals a longitudinal hyperintensity with cord expansion (arrow head). (**b**) Axial T2 image shows a gray matter pattern of cord edema (arrow head). There was no enhancement

EXTRAMEDULLARY

LEPTOMENINGEAL DISEASE/NEURITIS

- Infection is isolated to the leptomeningeal spaces in the spine and is often related to spread of CNS infection from another location, most commonly from epidural or intracranial infection.
- Pyogenic meningitis can involve the spinal meninges, though imaging findings may not often be apparent.
- Tuberculous meningitis is more likely to involve the spine than other etiologies may, and can occur from direct extension of bony spinal infection, hematogenous dissemination, or extension from intracranial infection.
- Lyme neuritis caused by *Borrelia burgdorferi* and transmitted by tick bite can cause CNS involvement with white

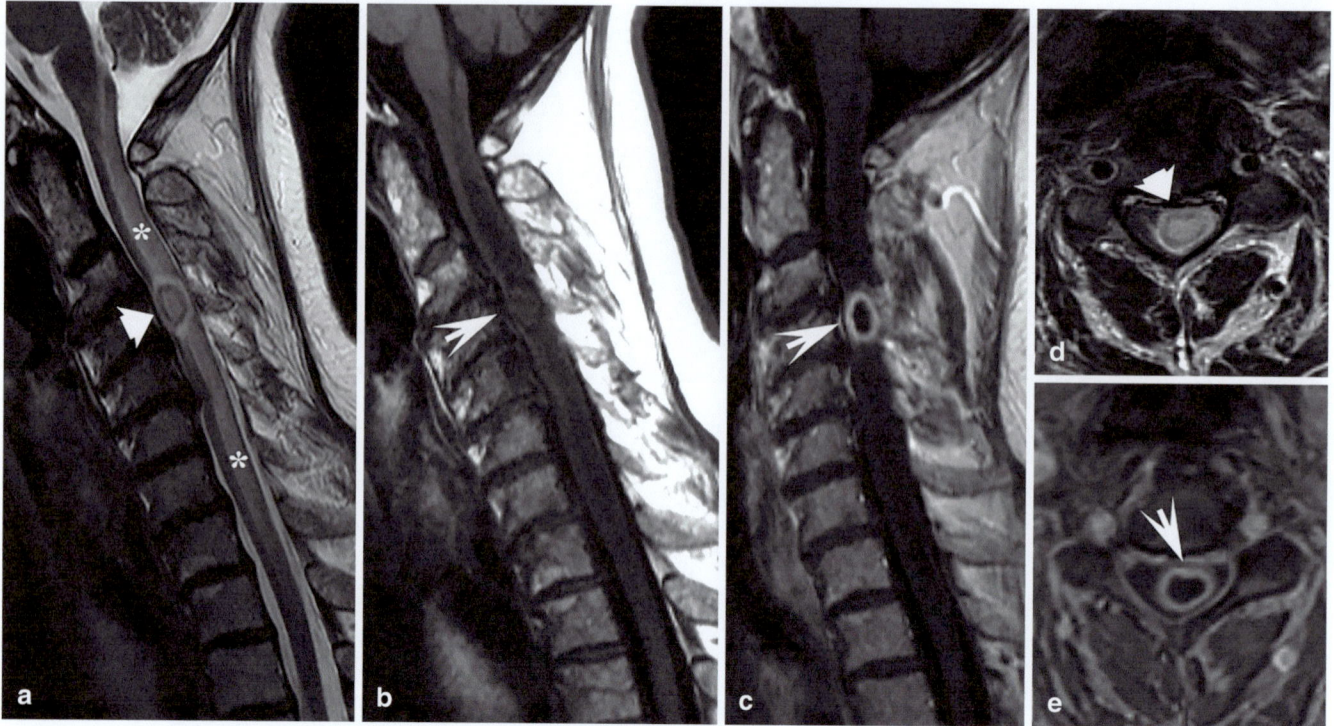

Fig. 25.9 Listeria cord abscess. (**a**) Sagittal T2 image shows an ovoid lesion of the cervical cord with a double rim of low signal capsule surrounded by high signal edema (arrow head). There is extensive cord edema (asterisks) disproportionate to the size of the lesion. (**b, c**) Sagittal T1 pre- and post-contrast images demonstrate peripheral enhancement of the lesion. (**d, e**) Axial T2 and T1 post-contrast images show the double rim (arrow head) and peripheral enhancement (arrow) of the intramedullary abscess

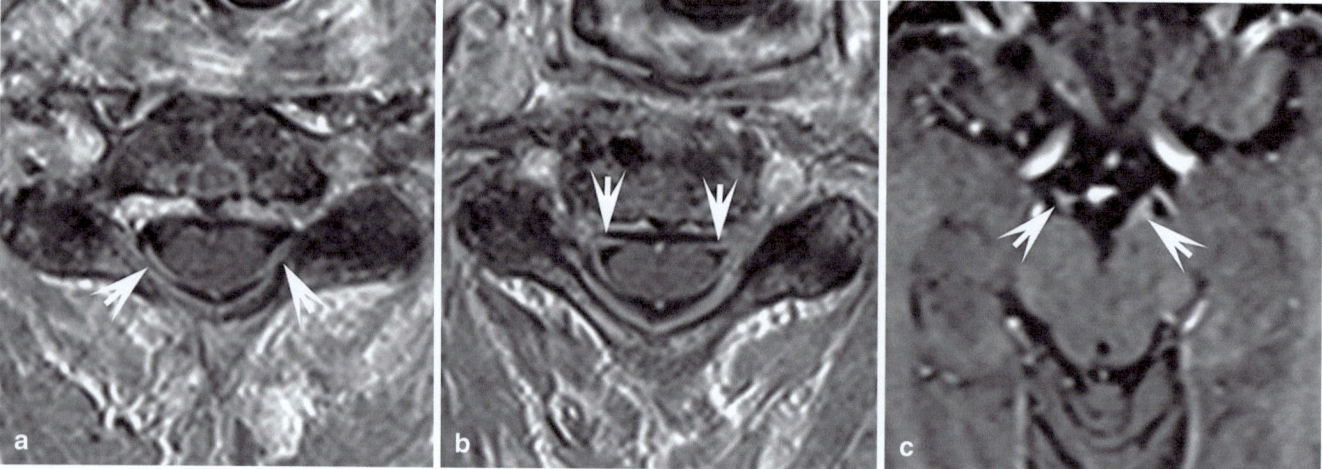

Fig. 25.10 Lyme neuritis. (**a, b**) Axial T1 post-contrast images demonstrate enhancement of the dorsal and ventral nerves (arrows) at different levels of the cervical cord. (**c**) Axial T1 post-contrast image of the brain shows enhancement of the oculomotor nerves, CN3 (arrows)

matter lesions in the brain, leptomeningeal, cranial nerve, and cauda equina enhancement (Fig. 25.10).
- Imaging Findings:
  - MRI is the main imaging modality for diagnosis.
  - Post-contrast sequences will likely be the most useful and may show nodular and linear enhancing foci along the pial surfaces in the spine, involving both the surface of the cord and the nerve roots.
  - Dural thickening may be present, along with loculated collections in the intradural or subdural compartments.
  - TB meningitis is more likely to have imaging findings compared with many bacterial cases, with the presence of associated abscess, granulomatous phlegmon, and linear and nodular enhancing foci being highly concerning.

ARACHNOIDITIS

- A broad term meaning inflammatory disorder of the spinal leptomeninges and arachnoid spaces, most notably involving the nerve roots.
- Can be caused by infectious sources or inflammatory sources (based on exposure to certain irritants such as blood or some contrast agents).
- Look for a patient history include prior surgery, trauma, or infectious meningitis.
- Intradural adhesions begin to form as a result of infection/inflammation with varying degrees of severity.
- Imaging Findings (Fig. e25.2):
  o Axial T2-weighted MR images are best for visualizing the nerve root morphology.
  o Enhancement may or may not be present.
  o Has a variable appearance in the lumbar spine, with thickening and clumping of the nerve roots and loss of the ability to see individual nerve roots.
  o Empty thecal sac appearance occurs when all the nerve roots are clumped peripherally along the dural margin, giving the illusion of the cauda equina nerve roots being missing.
  o Pseudofilum appearance occurs when all the nerve roots clump centrally into one large conglomerate.
  o Tuberculous arachnoiditis is somewhat unique in appearance, and concern should be raised if there is leptomeningeal thickening, nodular enhancement along the spinal cord and nerve roots, and cord involvement.

EXTRADURAL

EPIDURAL ABSCESS

- Loculated infected collection in the epidural space.
- A result of either direct or hematogenous extension of infection. Direct extension is more common, and is typically due to adjacent vertebral osteomyelitis/discitis or less likely direct inoculation.
- Most common organism is *Staphylococcus aureus*, with Gram-negative bacteria, anaerobes, mycobacteria, and fungal sources being less common.
- Look for a history of IV drug use, weakened immune system, urinary tract infection, and prior surgery to the area.
- Symptoms are usually related to mass effect but can result in cord edema from cord compression from an adjacent collection.
- Subdural infected collections are very similar to epidural abscesses though much less common, and can be seen with a history of instrumentation (i.e., lumbar puncture, anesthesia, etc.).
- Imaging Findings (Fig. e25.3):
- Best evaluated by MRI.
  o Primary epidural abscesses are usually located in the dorsal epidural space, while abscesses associated with vertebral infection are in the anterior/ventral epidural space.
  o T1 hypointense, T2 hyperintense, peripherally enhancing collection with central necrosis.
  o Often has associated phlegmon (infected material not yet organized into a collection) characterized as more homogeneous soft tissue enhancement.
  o Infection can span multiple vertebral levels or can affect non-contiguous levels ("skip lesions").
  o Subdural empyema can have a similar appearance but is located within the dark dural margins, compared with the epidural abscess which is outside of the dura. This distinction is best visualized on T2-weighted sequences.

Suggestions For Further Reading

References 12–15 are suggested for further reading.

Acknowledgements The authors would like to thank Dr. Ben Cohen and Dr. Ryan Peterson for their case contributions to this chapter.

References

1. Sundaram VK, Doshi A. Infections of the spine: a review of clinical and imaging findings. Appl Radiol. 2016:10–20. https://doi.org/10.37549/AR2301. Published online.
2. Hoch MJ, Rispoli J, Bruno M, Wauchope M, Lui YW, Shepherd TM. Clinical utility for diffusion MRI sequence in emergency and inpatient spine protocols. Clin Imaging. 2017;45:37–50. https://doi.org/10.1016/j.clinimag.2017.05.021.
3. Burrill J, Williams CJ, Bain G, Conder G, Hine AL, Misra RR. Tuberculosis: a radiologic review. RadioGraphics. 2007;27(5):1255–73. https://doi.org/10.1148/rg.275065176.
4. Crete RN, Gallmann W, Karis JP, Ross J. Spinal coccidioidomycosis: MR imaging findings in 41 patients. Am J Neuroradiol. 2018;39(11):2148–53. https://doi.org/10.3174/ajnr.A5818.
5. Faria do Amaral LL, Nunes RH, da Rocha AJ. Parasitic and Rare Spinal Infections. Neuroimaging Clin N Am. 2015;25(2):259–79. https://doi.org/10.1016/j.nic.2015.01.006.
6. Chong J, Rocco AD, Tagliati M, Danisi F, Simpson DM, Atlas SW. MR findings in AIDS-associated myelopathy. Published online 1999.
7. Richie MB, Pruitt AA. Spinal cord infections. Neurol Clin. 2013;31(1):19–53. https://doi.org/10.1016/j.ncl.2012.09.006.
8. Beh SC, Greenberg BM, Frohman T, Frohman EM. Transverse myelitis. Neurol Clin. 2013;31(1):79–138. https://doi.org/10.1016/j.ncl.2012.09.008.
9. Lee MJ, Aronberg R, Manganaro MS, Ibrahim M, Parmar HA. Diagnostic approach to intrinsic abnormality of spinal cord signal intensity. RadioGraphics. 2019;39(6):1824–39. https://doi.org/10.1148/rg.2019190021.

10. West T, Hess C, Cree B. Acute transverse myelitis: demyelinating, inflammatory, and infectious myelopathies. Semin Neurol. 2012;32(02):097–113. https://doi.org/10.1055/s-0032-1322586.
11. Yokota H, Yamada K. Viral infection of the spinal cord and roots. Neuroimaging Clin N Am. 2015;25(2):247–58. https://doi.org/10.1016/j.nic.2015.01.005.
12. Talbott JF, Narvid J, Chazen JL, Chin CT, Shah V. An imaging-based approach to spinal cord infection. Semin Ultrasound CT MRI. 2016;37(5):411–30. https://doi.org/10.1053/j.sult.2016.05.006.
13. Grill MF, Price RW. Central nervous system HIV-1 infection. In: Handbook of clinical neurology. Vol 123. Elsevier; 2014, pp 487–505. doi:https://doi.org/10.1016/B978-0-444-53488-0.00023-7
14. Hong SH, Choi JY, Lee JW, Kim NR, Choi JA, Kang HS. MR imaging assessment of the spine: infection or an imitation? RadioGraphics. 2009;29(2):599–612. https://doi.org/10.1148/rg.292085137.
15. DeSanto J, Ross JS. Spine infection/inflammation. Radiol Clin North Am. 2011;49(1):105–27. https://doi.org/10.1016/j.rcl.2010.07.018.

Spinal Cord Inflammation and Demyelination

Jason R. Lauer and William A. Mehan Jr.

Introduction

- Group of non-compressive, non-neoplastic myelopathic disorders affecting the spine.
- These include demyelinating disorders, cord manifestations of systemic inflammatory disorders, infection, infarction, and idiopathic.
- Besides imaging appearance, the patient's history, the timing of disease onset, and risk factor identification can be helpful in narrowing the differential diagnosis.

MULTIPLE SCLEROSIS (MS)

- Prototypical disorder, classically affecting younger patients (age 20–40 years) with a female predilection.
- Etiology remains unknown.
- 80–90% have spinal cord lesions [1, 2] (can satisfy one of the "dissemination in space" findings described by the McDonald criteria [3]).
- Brain MRI to evaluate for intracranial lesions and lumbar puncture to assess for CSF-specific oligoclonal bands may be helpful to further satisfy diagnostic criteria.

Imaging

- Lesions are characteristically T2 hyperintense and most conspicuous on STIR sequences.
- Lesion enhancement indicates active demyelination. Large lesions can show a specific pattern of "incomplete ring" enhancement, while smaller enhancing lesions solidly enhance [4].
- Lesions are typically longitudinally short (<2 vertebral bodies) and axially small (<50% cord surface area). Lesions are commonly peripherally distributed within the white matter tracts [4] (Fig. 26.1).
- The cervical cord is affected more frequently than the thoracic cord [5].

NEUROMYELITIS OPTICA SPECTRUM DISORDER (NMOSD)

- Inflammatory demyelinating disease affecting spinal cord, optic nerves, and to a lesser extent the brain parenchyma.
- Pathophysiology—autoantibody to the aquaporin-4 water channel, the most abundant water channel in the brain [6, 7].
- Compared with MS, NMOSD is significantly less common, affects a slightly older patient demographic (although a much stronger female predilection), and shows more severe clinical manifestations with an overall worse prognosis for the patient [8].

Imaging (Fig. 26.2)

- Spinal cord lesions are T2/STIR hyperintense, with signal intensity similar to CSF ("bright spotty lesion") quite specific for NMOSD [9] (Fig. 26.2c).
- Enhancement can be seen in the acute setting and can appear ill-defined and patchy.
- In contradistinction with MS, NMOSD lesions are longitudinally extensive (>3 vertebral bodies), axially larger (greater than two-thirds of the cord surface area), can appear expansile, and involve the central gray matter [10].

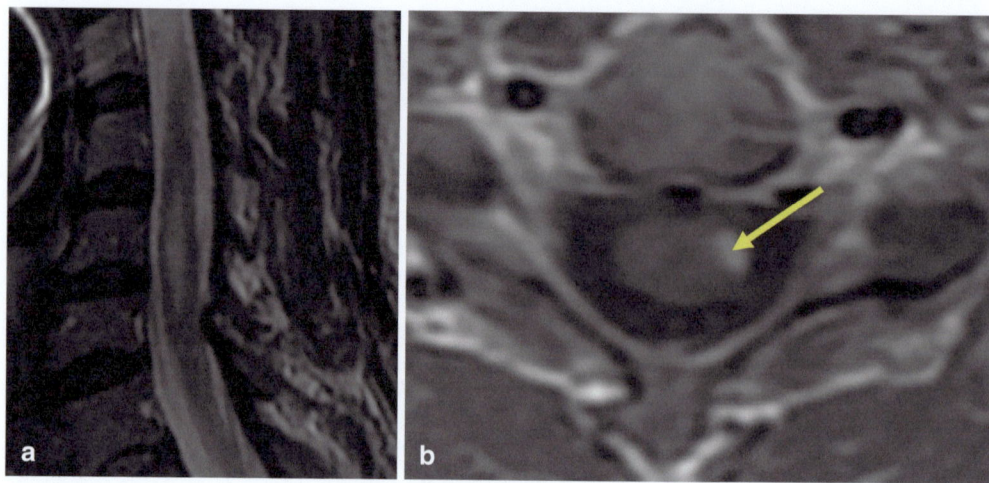

Fig. 26.1 Multiple sclerosis. (**a**) Sagittal T2-weighted image demonstrating an intramedullary T2 hyperintense lesion spanning less than three vertebral bodies in the cervical spine. (**b**) Note the enhancement and peripheral location on the axial T1 post-contrast image (arrow)

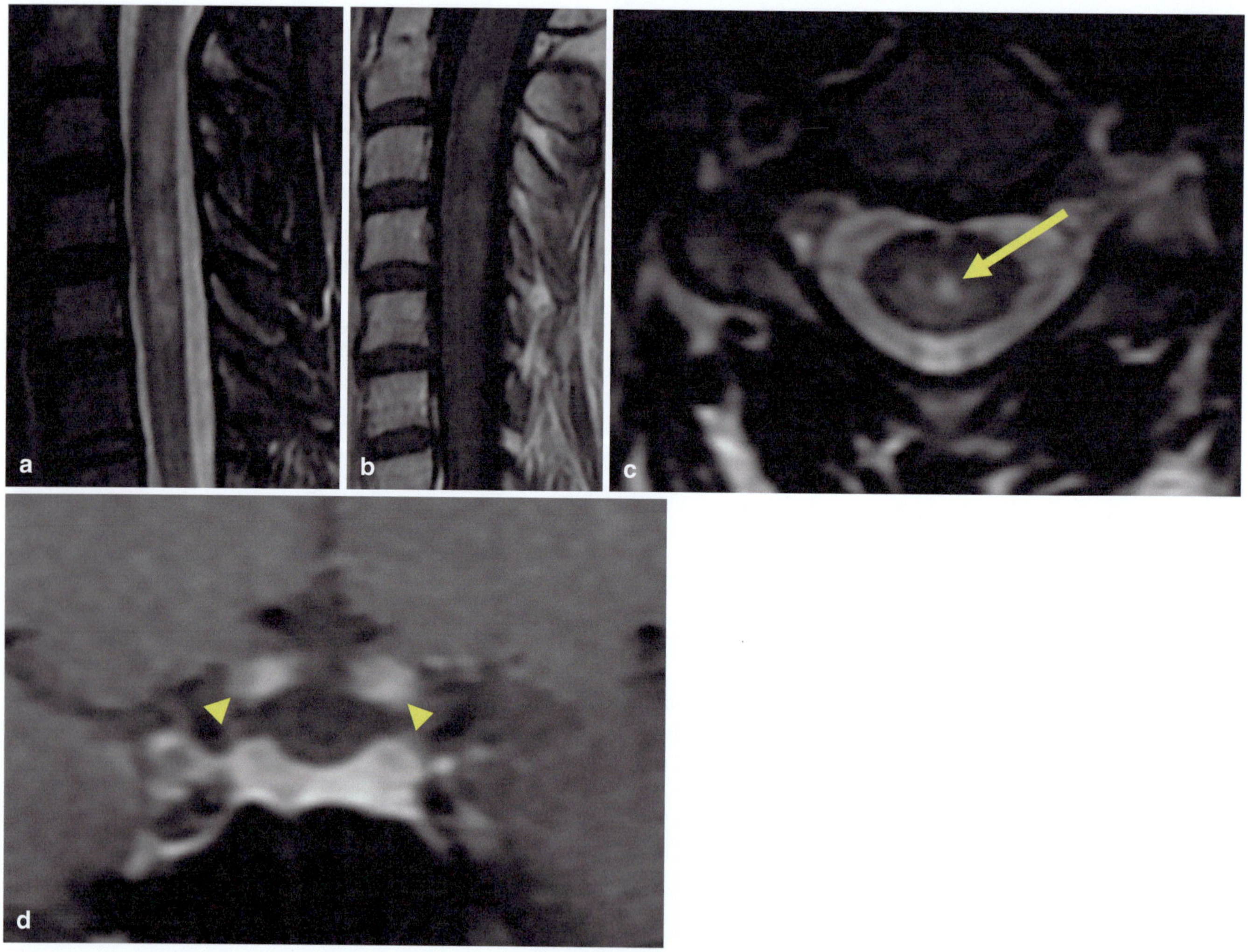

Fig. 26.2 Neuromyelitis optica spectrum disorder. (**a**) Sagittal T2-weighted and (**b**) sagittal T1-weighted post-contrast images demonstrate a T2 hyperintense intramedullary lesion with patchy enhancement spanning slightly greater than three vertebral levels. (**c**) Axial T2-weighted images through the lesion show a central CSF isointense focus within the lesion (arrow). Post-contrast fat-saturated images of the optic nerves in the same patient show avid optic nerve enhancement (arrowheads) (**d**)

ACUTE DISSEMINATED ENCEPHALOMYELITIS (ADEM)

- Inflammatory and demyelinating disorder affecting the spinal cord in 25% of cases [11].
- Usually affects children and young adults.
- Pathophysiology—immune-mediated response within 1 month of an antigenic exposure (post-viral or vaccine). Usually monophasic with complete recovery, although up to 10% of patients relapse within 3 months [11]. Further relapses suggest the presence of a chronic disease such as MS or NMOSD [12]. Other long-term sequelae include seizure disorder and optic neuritis [13, 14].

Imaging

- Spinal cord lesions are T2/STIR hyperintense and variable in size, although typically larger axially and longer longitudinally compared to MS lesions [15] (Fig. 26.3). Enhancement is variable. The thoracic cord is more commonly involved.
- Intracranial lesions can likewise be larger than typical MS plaques and can even involve deep gray nuclei [16].

MYELOPATHIES ASSOCIATED WITH SYSTEMIC INFLAMMATORY AND IMMUNE-MEDIATED DISEASES

- Spinal cord involvement, while uncommon, can occur in systemic diseases such as sarcoidosis ("neurosarcoid"), Behçet's ("neurobehçet's"), systemic lupus erythematosus, and Sjögren syndrome.
- Spinal cord manifestations are commonly nonspecific among the entities, with lesions appearing as non-expansile longitudinally extensive T2/STIR hyperintensity showing variable enhancement [17].
- Neurosarcoid sometimes features more specific findings including dorsal cord predominance, peripheral pial surface enhancement, and enhancement of the central canal [18] (Fig. 26.4).
- In the absence of specific spinal imaging findings, imaging findings in other body parts (such as the joints in SLE and the chest in sarcoid) along with clinical and laboratory data may be necessary to narrow down the diagnosis.

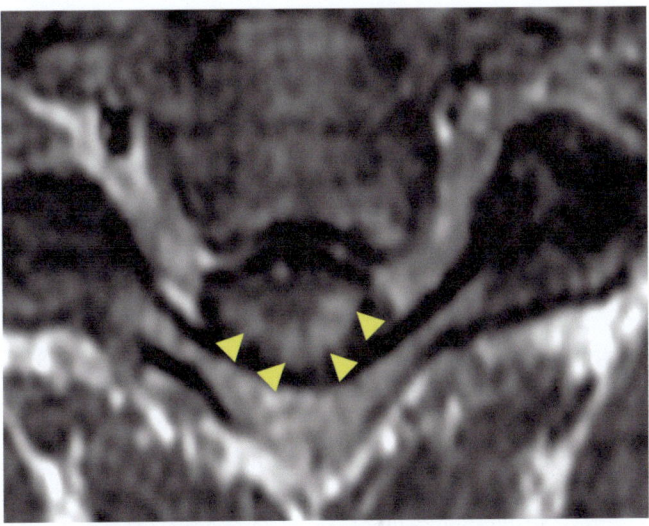

Fig. 26.4 Neurosarcoid. Axial T1 post-contrast image demonstrates a peripherally enhancing dorsal cord lesion (arrowheads)

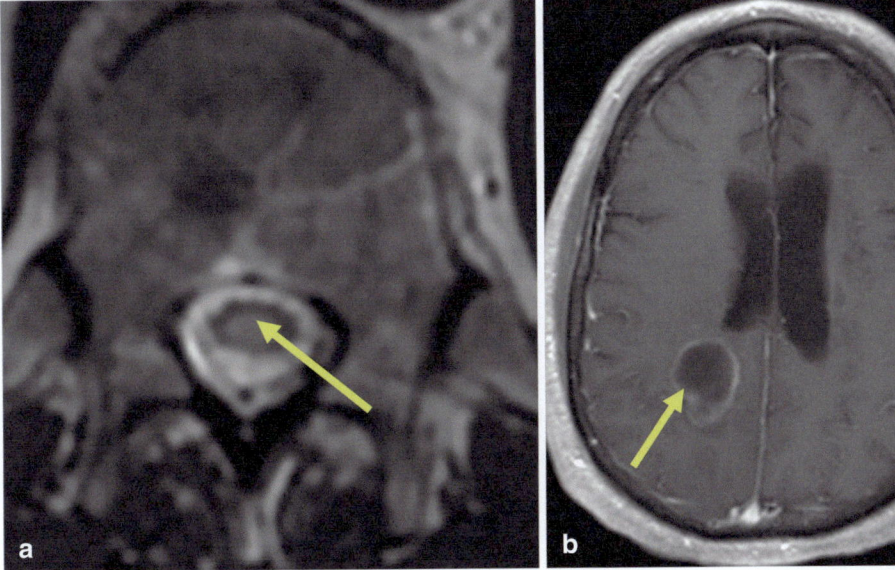

Fig. 26.3 Acute disseminated encephalomyelitis (ADEM): (a) axial T2-weighted images demonstrate a T2 hyperintense intramedullary lesion involving greater than two-thirds of cord surface area. (b) T1 post-contrast images of the brain in the same patient demonstrate a large dominant peripherally enhancing white matter lesion (arrow)

INFECTIOUS MYELITIS

- Uncommon cause for acute myelopathy.
- Typically viral with culprits including Enteroviruses (e.g., Polio and EV-71), Herpesviruses (e.g., HSV, VZV, and CMV), and Arboviruses (e.g., West Nile) [19]. Bacterial, fungal, and parasitic are rare pathogens in the absence of risk factors.
- Imaging overlap requires CSF culture and serology/PCR for a diagnosis.

Imaging (Fig. 26.5)

- Variable and nonspecific spinal cord T2/STIR hyperintensity, commonly longitudinally extensive, with variable enhancement.
- Specific patterns have been identified with enterovirus, which can involve the central gray/anterior horn, and VZV, which can involve the dorsolateral cord [20].
- Spinal cord abscess is a rare complication of pyogenic microbes and will appear similar to abscesses elsewhere in the body, including rim enhancement and central diffusion restriction.

SPINAL CORD INFARCTION

- Arterial ischemia is typically acute presentation and secondary to atherosclerotic disease, aortic surgery, trauma, fibrocartilaginous embolism, or idiopathic [21].
- Anterior spinal artery perfuses the anterior two-thirds of the spinal cord including the ventral horns, and the posterior spinal artery perfuses the posterior one-third of the spinal cord, including the dorsal columns [22].
- Anterior cord or total cord infarct patterns predominate. Pure isolated posterior cord infarcts are rare. This may be due to the differential vascular anatomy and collateralization of the posterior cord relative to the anterior cord [21]. The anterior horns are particularly involved due to the unique vulnerability of grey matter (particularly motor neurons) to anoxia [21, 23].
- Consequently, infarct in the anterior spinal artery territory will cause paralysis and bladder/bowel dysfunction with preservation of the dorsal column functions (proprioception and vibration).
- Spinal cord infarcts most commonly involve the cervical cord and thoracolumbar level [21].
- Venous ischemia can occur in the setting of arteriovenous fistulas as a result of venous hypertension and can mimic subacute arterial ischemia [24].

Imaging (Fig. 26.6)

- Similar to brain infarcts, the spinal cord shows segmental T2/STIR hyperintensity, high signal on diffusion-weighted images, and corresponding signal drop on the ADC map.
- The gray matter of the involved territory is predominantly involved, resulting in an "owl's eye" or "butterfly" configuration on axial images for anterior spinal artery infarcts [19, 21].
- Enhancement in the subacute phase can be seen.

SUBACUTE COMBINED DEGENERATION OF THE CORD (SACD)

- Describes the spinal cord manifestations of various metabolic derangements, most often caused by vitamin B-12 deficiency, but can also occur due to copper deficiency, vitamin E deficiency, and nitrous oxide toxicity [19].
- Clinical history, risk factor assessment, and laboratory data can be helpful in narrowing the diagnosis.
- Imaging features include longitudinally T2/STIR hyperintensity predominantly involving the dorsal columns, appearing as an "inverted V" [25] (Fig. 26.7).

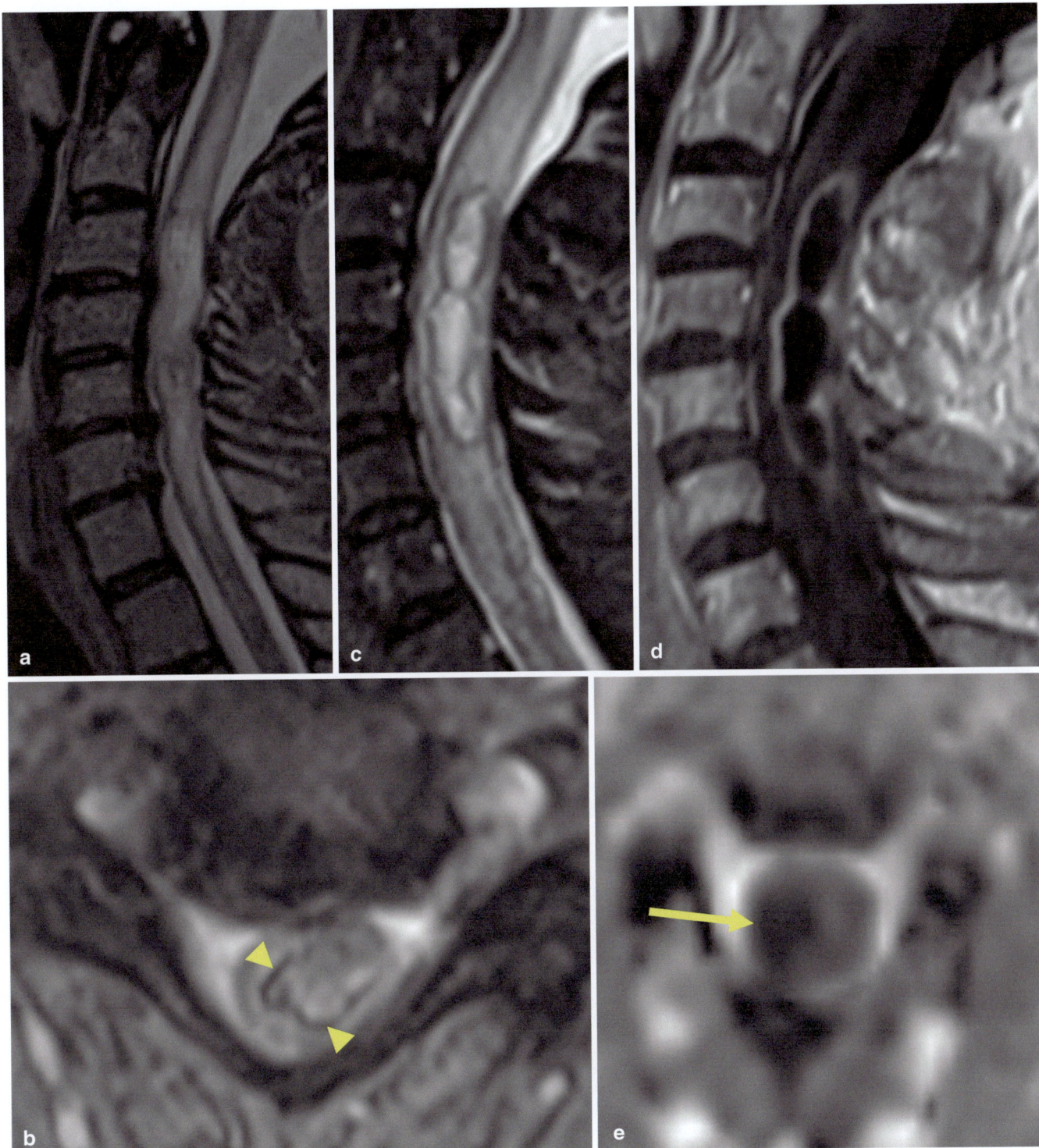

Fig. 26.5 Infectious myelitis. (**a**) Extensive T2/STIR hyperintensity with peripheral susceptibility (arrowheads) (**b**) within the cervical spinal cord in a patient with VZV encephalomyelitis. (**c**) Sagittal T2-weighted and (**d**) sagittal T1-weighted post-contrast images in a different patient with bacteremia demonstrating a T2 hyperintense, peripherally enhancing lesion in the spinal cord with surrounding vasogenic edema within the spinal cord. (**e**) ADC map confirming restricted diffusion consistent with abscess (arrow), a rare manifestation of pyogenic myelitis

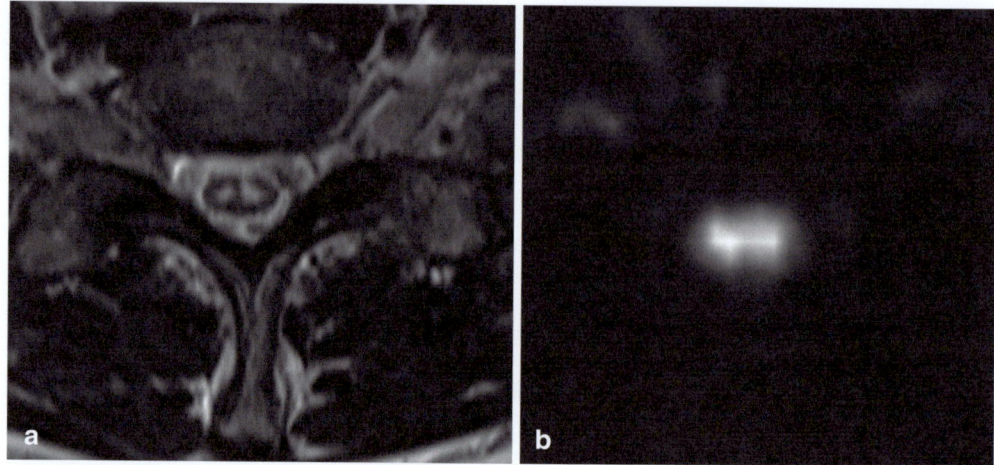

Fig. 26.6 Spinal cord infarction. (**a**) T2-weighted images demonstrating the "owl's eyes" pattern of signal abnormality due to the particular vulnerability of the grey matter to ischemia. (**b**) Diffusion-weighted images show restricted diffusion consistent with infarction

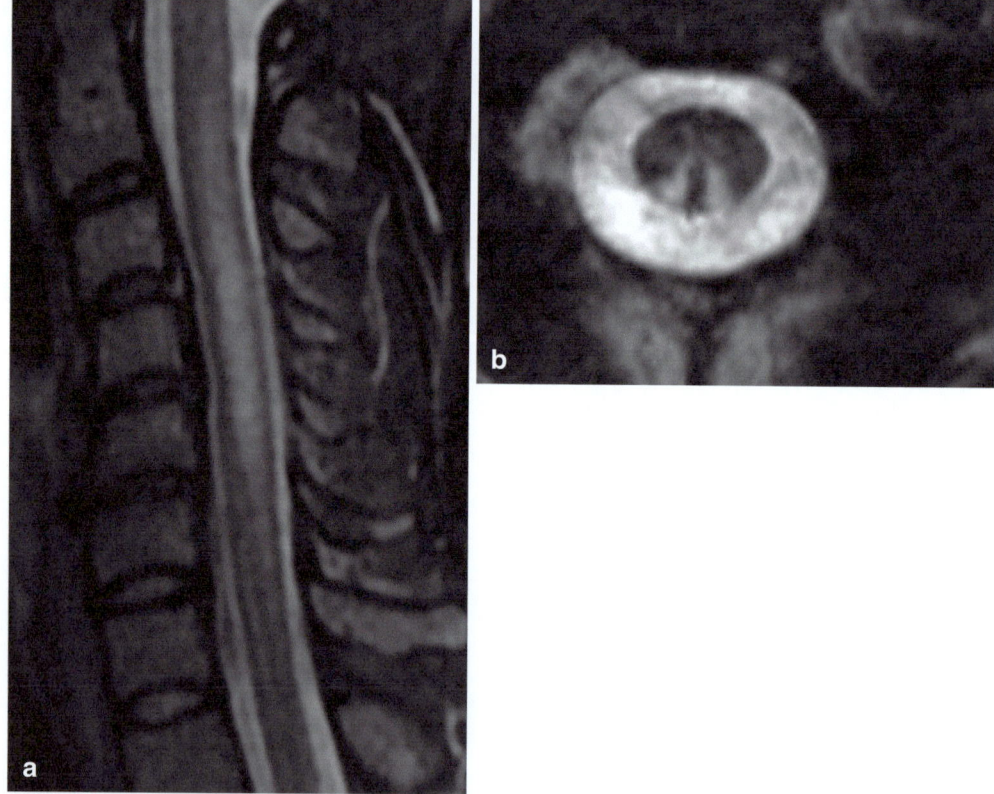

Fig. 26.7 Subacute combined degeneration of the spinal cord. (**a**) Longitudinally extensive intramedullary signal abnormality localizing to the dorsal columns on axial images (**b**) in a patient with nitrous oxide toxicity following 1 year of chronic recreational abuse

References

1. Bot JC, Barkhof F, Polman CH, et al. Spinal cord abnormalities in recently diagnosed MS patients: added value of spinal MRI examination. Neurology. 2004;62(2):226–33.
2. Gass A, Rocca MA, Agosta F, et al. MRI monitoring of pathological changes in the spinal cord in patients with multiple sclerosis. Lancet Neurol. 2015;14(4):443–54.
3. Thompson AJ, Banwell BL, Barkhof F, et al. Diagnosis of multiple sclerosis: 2017 revisions of the McDonald criteria. Lancet Neurol. 2018;17(2):162–73.
4. Grayev AM, Kissane J, Kanekar S. Imaging approach to the cord T2 hyperintensity (myelopathy). Radiol Clin North Am. 2014;52(2):427–46.
5. Kearney H, Miller DH, Ciccarelli O. Spinal cord MRI in multiple sclerosis—diagnostic, prognostic and clinical value. Nat Rev Neurol. 2015;11(6):327–38.

6. Lennon VA, Wingerchuk DM, Kryzer TJ, et al. A serum autoantibody marker of neuromyelitis optica: distinction from multiple sclerosis. Lancet. 2004;364(9451):2106–12.
7. Saadoun S, Papadopoulos MC. Aquaporin-4 in brain and spinal cord oedema. Neuroscience. 2010;168(4):1036–46.
8. Wingerchuk DM, Lennon VA, Lucchinetti CF, Pittock SJ, Weinshenker BG. The spectrum of neuromyelitis optica. Lancet Neurol. 2007;6(9):805–15.
9. Pekcevik Y, Mitchell CH, Mealy MA, et al. Differentiating neuromyelitis optica from other causes of longitudinally extensive transverse myelitis on spinal magnetic resonance imaging. Mult Scler. 2016;22(3):302–11.
10. Dutra BG, da Rocha AJ, Nunes RH, Maia ACMJ. Neuromyelitis optica spectrum disorders: spectrum of MR imaging findings and their differential diagnosis. Radiographics. 2018;38(1):169–93.
11. Tenembaum S, Chamoles N, Fejerman N. Acute disseminated encephalomyelitis: a long-term follow-up study of 84 pediatric patients. Neurology. 2002;59(8):1224–31.
12. Krupp LB, Tardieu M, Amato MP, et al. International Pediatric Multiple Sclerosis Study Group criteria for pediatric multiple sclerosis and immune-mediated central nervous system demyelinating disorders: revisions to the 2007 definitions. Mult Scler. 2013;19(10):1261–7.
13. Huppke P, Rostasy K, Karenfort M, et al. Acute disseminated encephalomyelitis followed by recurrent or monophasic optic neuritis in pediatric patients. Mult Scler. 2013;19(7):941–6.
14. Rossor T, Benetou C, Wright S, et al. Early predictors of epilepsy and subsequent relapse in children with acute disseminated encephalomyelitis. Mult Scler. 2020;26(3):333–42.
15. Thurnher MM, Cartes-Zumelzu F, Mueller-Mang C. Demyelinating and infectious diseases of the spinal cord. Neuroimaging Clin N Am. 2007;17(1):37–55.
16. Rossi A. Imaging of acute disseminated encephalomyelitis. Neuroimaging Clin N Am. 2008;18(1):149–61; ix.
17. Lee MJ, Aronberg R, Manganaro MS, Ibrahim M, Parmar HA. Diagnostic approach to intrinsic abnormality of spinal cord signal intensity. Radiographics. 2019;39(6):1824–39.
18. Zalewski NL, Krecke KN, Weinshenker BG, et al. Central canal enhancement and the trident sign in spinal cord sarcoidosis. Neurology. 2016;87(7):743–4.
19. Kranz PG, Amrhein TJ. Imaging approach to myelopathy: acute, subacute, and chronic. Radiol Clin North Am. 2019;57(2):257–79.
20. Yokota H, Yamada K. Viral infection of the spinal cord and roots. Neuroimaging Clin N Am. 2015;25(2):247–58.
21. Weidauer S, Nichtweiss M, Hattingen E, Berkefeld J. Spinal cord ischemia: aetiology, clinical syndromes and imaging features. Neuroradiology. 2015;57(3):241–57.
22. Santillan A, Nacarino V, Greenberg E, Riina HA, Gobin YP, Patsalides A. Vascular anatomy of the spinal cord. J Neurointerv Surg. 2012;4(1):67–74.
23. Gelfan S, Tarlov IM. Differential vulnerability of spinal cord structures to anoxia. J Neurophysiol. 1955;18(2):170–88.
24. Vargas MI, Gariani J, Sztajzel R, et al. Spinal cord ischemia: practical imaging tips, pearls, and pitfalls. AJNR Am J Neuroradiol. 2015;36(5):825–30.
25. Sun HY, Lee JW, Park KS, Wi JY, Kang HS. Spine MR imaging features of subacute combined degeneration patients. Eur Spine J. 2014;23(5):1052–8.

Spine: Vascular Pathologies

Victor Lam Shin Cheung and Sachin Kishore Pandey

Neurovascular Anatomy of the Spine

- The superficial arterial system of the spinal cord can be divided into the longitudinal arteries and the pial plexus [1].
  o Longitudinal arteries:
    - Single anterior spinal artery.
      ▪ Supplies the anterior two-thirds of the spinal cord.
      ▪ Originates from the intracranial (V4) segments of the vertebral arteries.
      ▪ Receives additional blood supply from the anterior radiculomedullary arteries.
    - Two posterior spinal arteries.
      ▪ Supplies the posterior one-third of the spinal cord.
      ▪ Originates from the intracranial vertebral arteries or posterior inferior cerebellar arteries.
      ▪ Receive additional blood supply from the posterior radiculomedullary arteries.
  o Pial plexus:
    - Represent an arterial network of anastomoses between the anterior and posterior spinal arteries on the surface of the spinal cord [1].
- Additional arterial supply is provided to the spine and spinal cord through segmental arteries.
  o Cervical spine:
    - Variable.
  o Thoracic spine:
    - Supreme intercostal artery.
    - Posterior intercostal arteries.
    - Subcostal arteries.
  o Lumbar spine:
    - Lumbar segmental arteries.
- The segmental arteries branch into radicular arteries that supply the spinal canal:
  o Radiculomeningeal/radiculoradial arteries: radicular arteries that supply the dura and nerve.
  o Radiculomedullary arteries: radicular arteries that supply the spinal cord.
    - Artery of cervical enlargement is the dominant anterior radiculomedullary artery in the cervical spine, usually located C4–C8 [1] (Fig. 27.1).
    - Artery of Adamkiewicz, also known as the radiculomedularris magna, is the dominant anterior radiculomedullary artery in the thoracolumbar spine, usually located between T8 and L1 (75–80%) and more commonly originating from the left [2] (Fig. 27.2).
- Venous system:
  o Variable, but mirrors vasculature of the arterial system.
  o Anterior and posterior spinal veins drain into radiculomedullary veins along the anterior or posterior spinal roots [3].
  o Intradural veins are valveless and thus rely on gravity, body position, and body cavity pressure changes in part for drainage pattern [1].

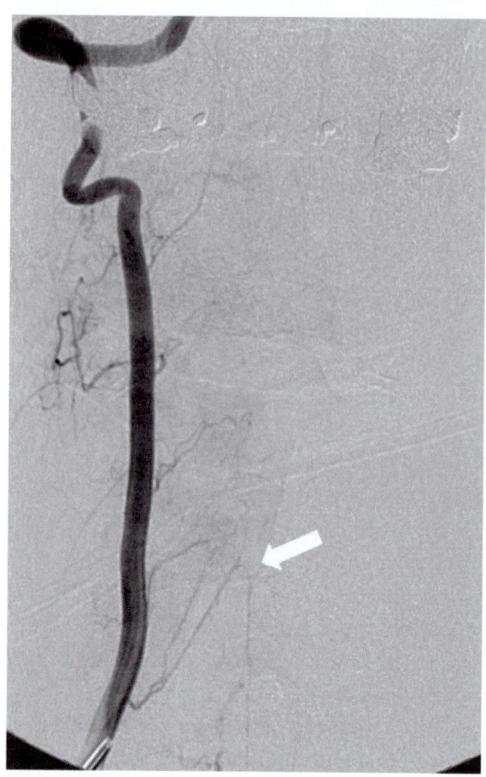

Fig. 27.1 Frontal subtraction angiographic projection of a right vertebral arterial injection demonstrating the artery of cervical enlargement (arrow) coursing medially and superiorly before making a characteristic hairpin turn

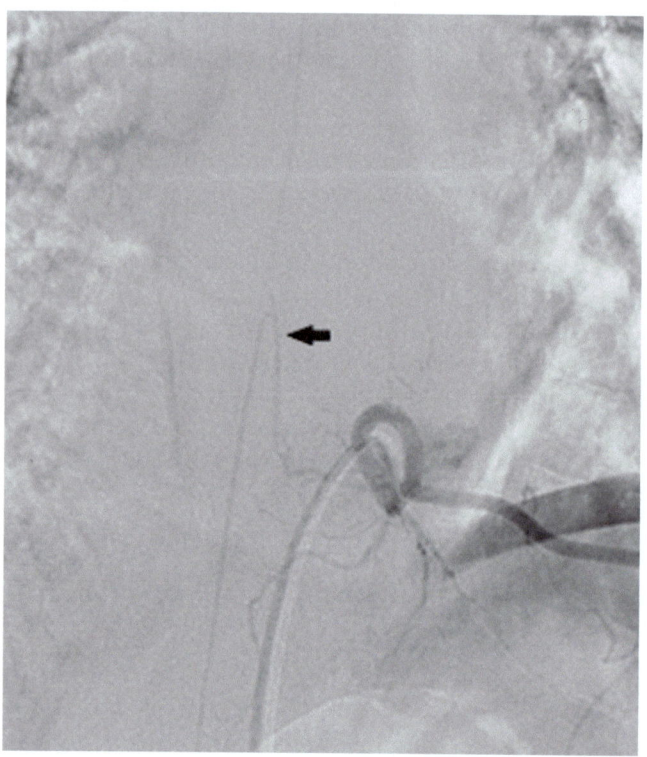

Fig. 27.2 Frontal subtraction angiographic projection of a spinal angiogram demonstrating the radiculomedullaris magna artery of Adamkiewicz arising from a T10 intercostal artery (arrow). The artery of Adamkiewicz ascends before making a characteristic hairpin turn

Vascular Pathologies of the Spine

- Arteriovenous shunting classifications:
  - Several different classification systems are used reflecting the contributions of authors from various medical specialties over several decades [4].
  - The most commonly used system is thus a composite of several contributions [5]:
    - Type I: Dural arteriovenous fistula (dAVF).
    - Type II: Intramedullary/glomus arteriovenous malformation.
    - Type III: Juvenile arteriovenous malformation.
    - Type IV: Intradural perimedullary arteriovenous fistula.

SPINAL DURAL ARTERIOVENOUS FISTULA (TYPE 1)

- Abnormal connection between a radiculomeningeal artery and a radicular vein typically located along the nerve root sleeve, causing venous hypertension and possible spinal cord edema.
- This is the most common spinal vascular arteriovenous shunt (~70% of all spinal arteriovenous shunts) [3].
- The majority (85%) of lesions are found below the T6 level [3].
- Most commonly affects middle-aged men (40–60 years), with a 5:1 predilection for males over females [3].
- Clinically, patients frequently present with paraparesis, back pain that may radiate to the lower legs, hypesthesia, paresthesias, impotence, and sphincter disturbances.
- The subacute myelopathic syndrome that can result from a dural arteriovenous fistula is also called Foix-Alajouanine syndrome (Fig. 27.3).

Imaging
- MRI will demonstrate spinal cord edema, with an enlarged cord, and hyperintense signal on T2W images extending across multiple segments.
- Numerous small, irregular vessel flow voids are found on the cord surface, which may enhance.
- Contrast-enhanced spinal angiography is less commonly useful in making the diagnosis but can be helpful to aid in targeting spinal angiography.
- Angiography is critical for the precise localization and characterization of vascular pathology.
- Selective angiography of the affected segmental artery demonstrates early venous filling and retrograde flow of the radiculomedullary veins into the spinal canal (Fig. 27.4).
- When a fistula is found, adjacent levels should be imaged to rule out additional radicular feeding arteries and identify possibly sensitive arteries (i.e., Artery of Adamkiewicz) which may alter treatment strategies.

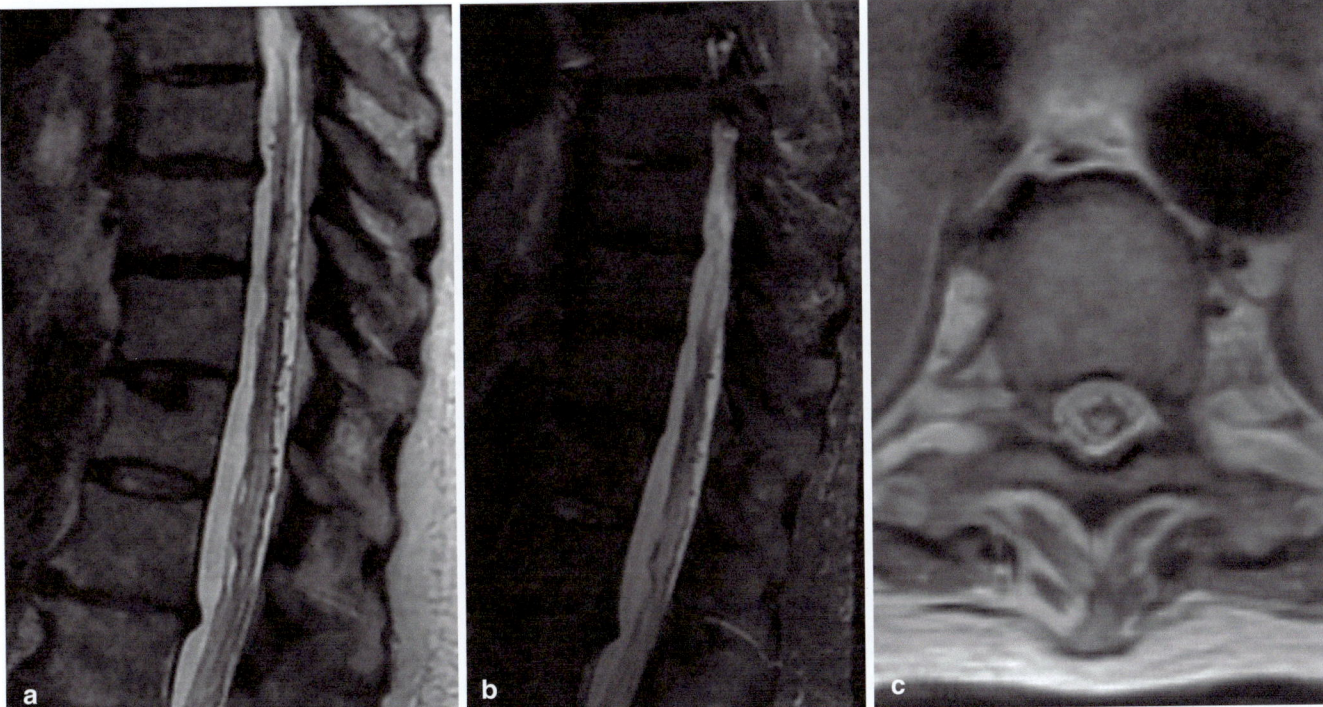

Fig. 27.3 A 61-year-old male with clinical Foix-Alajouanine syndrome. (**a**) Sagittal T2-weighted image and (**b**) sagittal STIR image demonstrating abnormal spinal cord signal hyperintensity in the lower cord and conus medullaris and abnormal perimedullary vascular flow voids. (**c**) Axial T2-weighted image confirms intramedullary signal abnormality

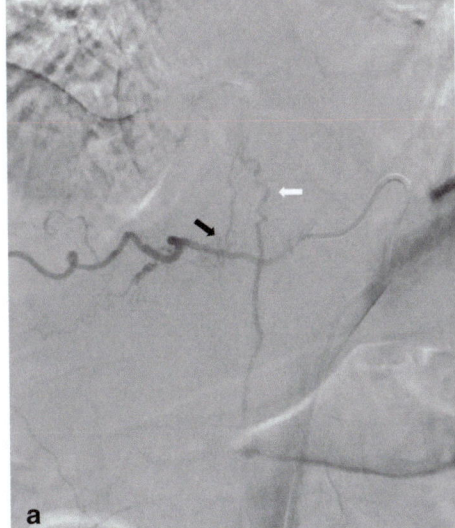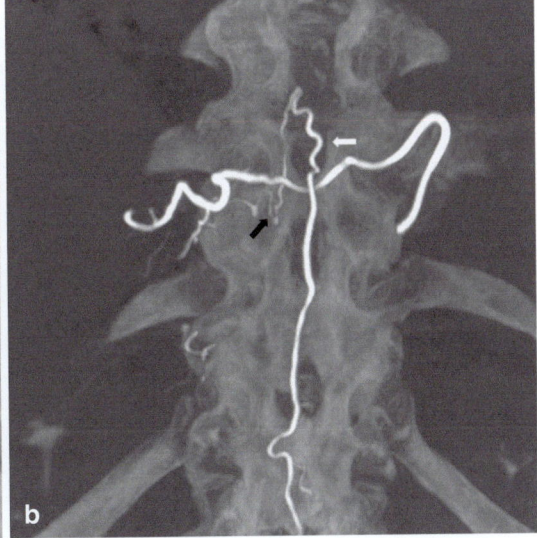

Fig. 27.4 Spinal dural arteriovenous fistula—Type I. (**a**) Frontal subtraction angiographic projection of a right T10 intercostal arteriogram demonstrating a prominent radiculomeningeal artery rapidly filling a vein at the nerve root sleeve (black arrow) which, in turn, drains into a distended, serpentine perimedullary vein (white arrow). (**b**) MIP reconstruction from a cone-beam CT angiogram acquired from the same vessel better delineates the fistula

Management

- Treatment is focused on the disconnection of the fistulous point.
- Surgical disconnection of the fistulae is the gold standard and most common form of treatment.
- Endovascular embolization using liquid embolic agents is also possible with successful treatment requiring embolic agent penetration across the site of the fistula.

SPINAL INTRAMEDULLARY ARTERIOVENOUS MALFORMATION (TYPE II)

- In distinction to an arteriovenous fistula, these lesions are true arteriovenous malformations and, as such, have a malformation nidus.
- The site of the nidus is intramedullary or within the spinal cord itself.

- Lesions are thus supplied by spinal cord arteries such as the radiculomedullary and radiculopial arteries and with drainage most commonly seen via pial veins.
    - After Type I lesions, these are the second most common spinal vascular shunting lesion (~20–45%) [3].
- Presentation is most common in the second to the fourth decade of life and, unlike Type I lesions, there is no clear sex predilection.
- The most common location is within the thoracic spine (51%) followed by the cervical (29%) [3].
- These malformations frequently present as spinal hemorrhage resulting in severe back pain.
- Spinal subarachnoid hemorrhage causing severe pain in these cases is also referred to as coup de poignard of Michon.
- Patients may also present with spinal cord symptoms including hypesthesia, paresthesia, weakness, bladder and bowel dysfunction, and impotence.

Imaging
- The malformation nidus will appear as a cluster of abnormal vascular flow voids within the spinal cord itself.
- Irregular, dilated perimedullary vascular flow voids are also commonly present.
- Cord edema due to venous congestion can also be present as hyperintensity on T2W imaging and focal dilatation of the spinal cord itself (Fig. 27.5).
- Hemosiderin deposits from nidal hemorrhage are also commonly present as hypointense T2W and T1W signals surrounding the nidus.
- Angiography is critical for precise localization and characterization of the vascular pathology (Fig. 27.6).
- Particular attention should be paid to the detection and localization of the artery of Adamkiewicz as well as to signs of angioarchitectural weakness such as feeding artery aneurysms and focal venous outflow stenosis.

Management
- The complexity of these lesions requires a multidisciplinary approach should be used as all treatment options are fraught with risk.
- Endovascular approaches with curative embolization from liquid embolic agents may be possible, but the risk of collateral ischemic damage to the spinal cord is high.
- Partial embolization strategies may be used to reduce risk by partial obliteration of specific areas of angioarchitectural weakness (i.e., focal aneurysms).
- Surgical resection can be possible for accessible lesions. Generally, dorsal lesions are more accessible.
- Radiosurgery is also possible but also carries the risk of collateral acute and chronic radiation-induced injury to the spinal cord.
- There is the promise of emerging genotype-guided targeted biological agents (i.e., trametinib) [6, 7].

SPINAL JUVENILE (METAMERIC) ARTERIOVENOUS MALFORMATION (TYPE III)

- These are the least common subtype of spinal arteriovenous shunting pathologies (~5–9%) [3].
- Generally, these involve the spinal cord as well as other tissues with a common metameric origin including the osseous spine, paraspinal soft tissue, and skin.

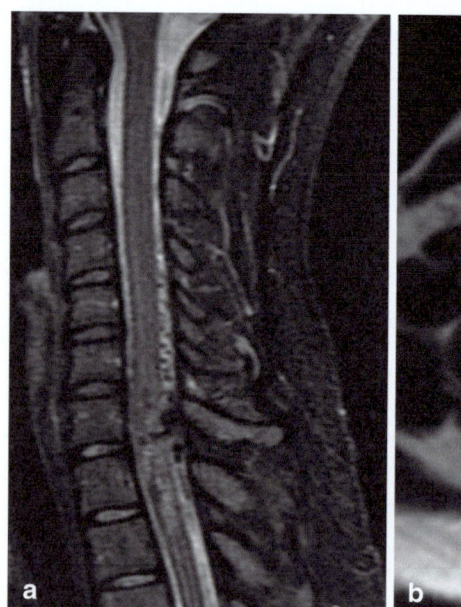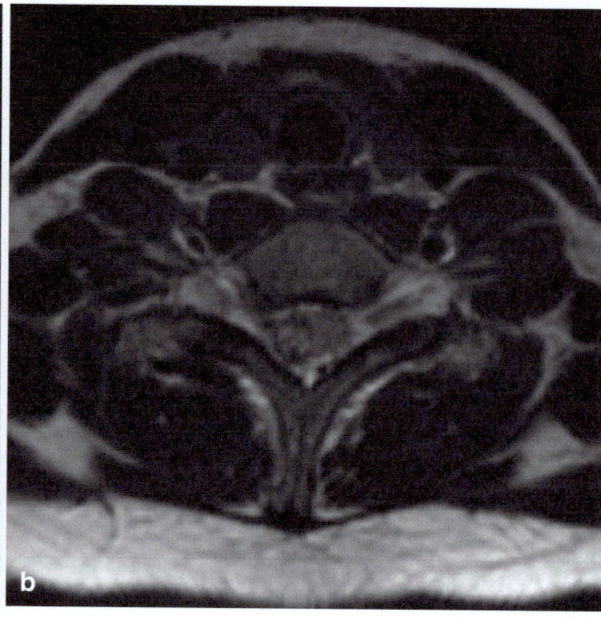

Fig. 27.5 Spinal intramedullary arteriovenous malformation—Type II. A 22-year-old female with acute onset numbness. (**a**) Sagittal and (**b**) axial T2-weighted images demonstrate abnormal expansion and hyperintense signal within the lower cervical cord. Abnormal vascular flow voids are also present within, and surrounding, the spinal cord

Fig. 27.6 Spinal intramedullary arteriovenous malformation—Type II. (**a**) Frontal subtraction angiographic projection of a superselective right feeding pedicle arteriogram in a late arterial phase demonstrating abnormal arteriovenous shunting into a vascular nidus with distended, ectatic perimedullary spinal veins (black arrow). (**b**) Frontal subtraction angiographic projection of a left subclavian arteriogram shown in an early arterial phase better delineates the nidal architecture (white arrows)

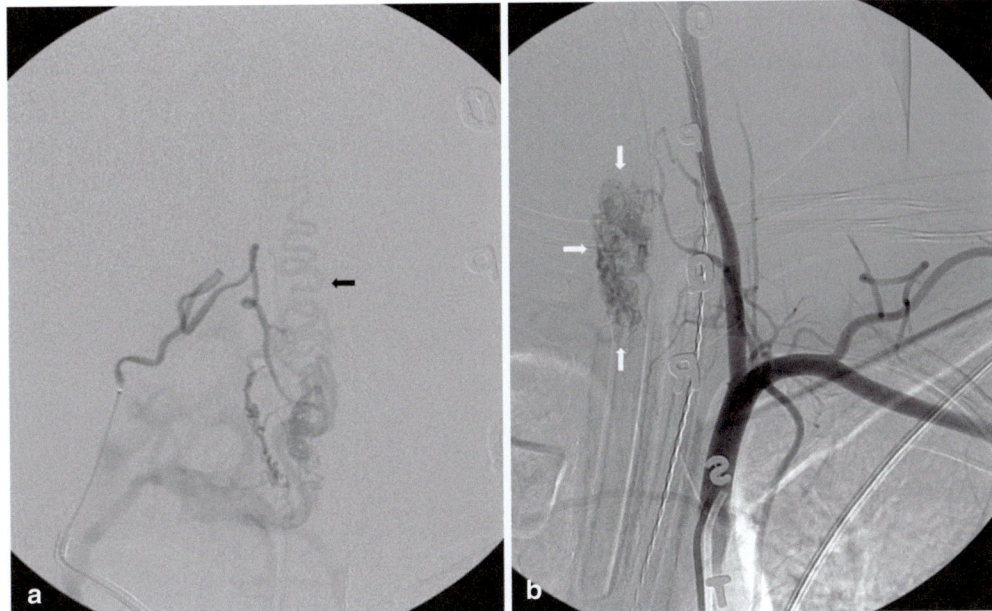

- There is no particular spinal zone predilection and there is a slight male predominance (2:1).
- The most common clinical presentation is in teenage patients with progressive neurologic deficits. Acute deficit without hemorrhage is slightly less common.
- Up to 12% of cases may also be detected incidentally.

Imaging
- Extensive, abnormal vascular flow voids can be found on T2W imaging within the spinal cord as well as variably within surrounding spinal and extraspinal tissues.
- Parenchymal spinal cord tissue can sometimes still be present within the interstices of the malformation.
- Spinal cord edema can also be found as a hyperintense signal on T2W images.
- Angiography allows for the characterization of feeding vessels, the extent of the nidus, venous drainage, and particular sites of angio-architectural weakness (Fig. 27.7).

Management
- The complexity of these lesions requires a multidisciplinary approach.
- Endovascular approaches generally focus on targeted, partial obliteration of specific areas of angio-architectural weakness (i.e., focal aneurysms) or symptomatic regions.
- There is the promise of emerging genotype-guided targeted biological agents (i.e., trametinib) [6, 7].

SPINAL INTRADURAL PERIMEDULLARY ARTERIOVENOUS FISTULA (TYPE IV)

- Arterio-venous fistula located on the pial surface of the spinal cord, rather than along the dura of the nerve root sleeve as with Type I lesions.
- These can encompass a variety of appearances ranging from single to multiple supplying vessels and some have even been described with small nidal components.
- Represent approximately 8–19% of spinal arteriovenous shunting pathologies [3].
- The large majority of patients will present with neurologic deficits with ~25–30% presenting with acute deficits.
- Presentation is most common between 18 and 50 years of age, and there may be a slight male predilection.
- Syndromic associations with Osler-Weber-Rendu, Proteus, Down, and Klippel-Trenaunay syndromes have been described [3].

Imaging
- Abnormal, perimedullary vascular flow voids are found on T2W images.
- In some cases, cord compression and even displacement can be found.
- Intrinsic signal abnormalities of the cord itself can also be found as a secondary effect.
- Angiography remains the gold standard for diagnostic confirmation and anatomic characterization including the

Fig. 27.7 Spinal juvenile arteriovenous malformation—Type III. A 10-year-old female with sudden onset of severe back pain. (**a**) Sagittal T2-weighted image demonstrates markedly distended vascular flow voids within the spinal canal as well as abnormal flow voids in the posterior half of the L1 vertebral body. (**b**) Frontal subtraction angiographic projection of a left L1 segmental arteriogram confirms the presence of a spinal cord arteriovenous malformation as well as abnormal arteriovenous malformation nidus within the L1 vertebral body itself

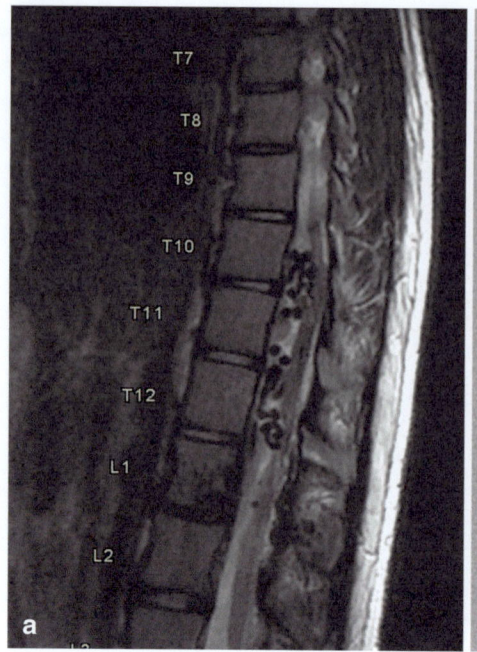 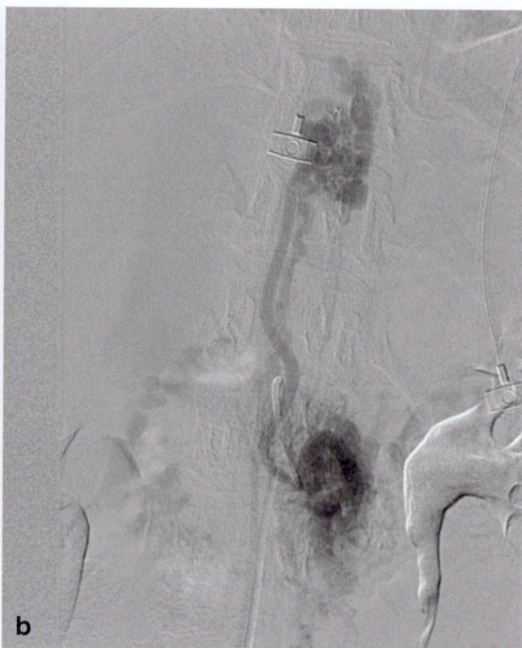

number of arterial feeding pedicles and the presence or absence of a nidal component.

Management

- Treatment is customized to the particular anatomy of a given shunt, but, generally, a combination of embolization and surgical resection is employed when necessary.

SPINAL CAVERNOUS MALFORMATION

- Intramedullary vascular malformations of dilated thin-walled capillary malformations with no intervening parenchymal tissue.
- There is no identifiable feeding artery, though up to one-third of cases may have an associated venous malformation.
- Though early reports suggested a female predominance, the largest series show no sex predilection.
- Lesional distribution closely follows spinal cord volume with most (>50%) being thoracic, followed by cervical and very few lumbar lesions.
- Approximately 9% of patients may have a family history of cavernous malformations [8].
- Annual hemorrhage rates vary between 0% and 4.5% with clinical presentations generally being either acute deficit, recurrent episodic deficits, or progressive neurologic decline [8].
- Motor weakness is the most common clinical symptom, followed by sensory deficit and pain.
- Management is generally observational, with surgical resection also being possible for some exophytic or severely symptomatic lesions.

Imaging

- Progressive deposition of hemosiderin leads to a hypointense rim on MR imaging surrounding a typically T2W hyperintense core. This can create a pathognomonic "popcorn"-type appearance.
- Less commonly, lesions may be more uniformly hyper- or hypo-intense.
- Lesions generally do not enhance with contrast administration (Fig. 27.8).

SPINAL CORD INFARCTION

- Fortunately, spinal infarction is rare. However, the prognosis remains poor.
- Etiologies are generally divided into pediatric causes such as trauma and cardiac malformations and adult causes such as atheromatous disease, aneurysms, aortic surgery, dissection, hypotension, drug use, and sickle cell disease among other causes.
- Clinical presentation is dependent on the anatomic location of infarction, though most infarctions share rapid symptom onset within 12 h [9].

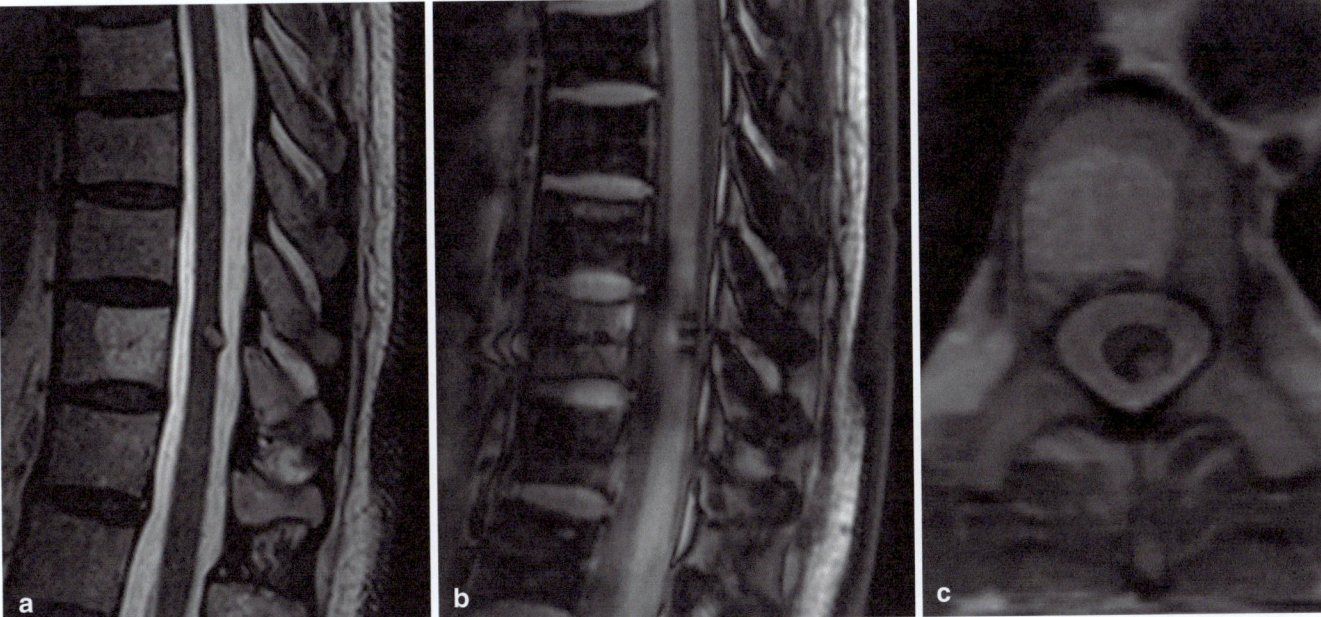

Fig. 27.8 Spinal cord cavernous malformation. A 32-year-old female with episodic lower extremity sensory abnormality. The sagittal T2-weighted image (**a**) demonstrates an exophytic lower thoracic spinal cord lesion with an intrinsic hyperintense signal and a thin hypointense rim. The sagittal gradient-echo image (**b**) confirms the susceptibility artifact associated with the rim of the lesion. The axial T2-weighted image (**c**) confirms the intramedullary location of the lesion

- Anterior spinal artery syndromes are most common and involve bilateral loss of motor function and pain/temperature sensation. Proprioception and vibration are relatively spared.
- Acutely, anterior spinal artery syndromes present with flaccidity and lost deep reflexes. Hyperreflexia and spasticity then occur over weeks.
- Anterior spinal artery syndromes involved in the rostral cervical cord can also compromise respiration.
- Posterior spinal artery syndrome is less common and involves loss of proprioception and vibratory sense below the injured level and total anesthesia at the injured level.
- Posterior spinal artery syndromes are generally unilateral.
- Sulco-commissural syndrome can occur from central sulcal artery occlusion and present with hemiparesis with the contralateral spinothalamic sensory deficit.
- Conus medullaris infarction can be clinically confused with cauda equina syndrome.
- Treatment is generally focused on treating the specific cause of ischemia if possible with the role of intravenous thrombolytics remaining unclear for most embolic etiologies.
- Radiologists may frequently be called upon to place lumbar drains in order to decrease intraspinal pressure and reduce the risk for cord infarction in cases of thoraco-abdominal aortic aneurysm surgery.

Imaging
- MRI is generally the mainstay of imaging evaluation with CT and angiography being much less useful.
- The spinal cord may be expanded in the acute phase.
- Hyperintense cord signal is typically seen on T2W images and both axial and sagittal planes of imaging can be helpful to localize the extent of injury and also help determine the possible arterial territory involved.
- Diffusion-weighted MR imaging can be helpful though has been more technically challenging than brain MRI due to flow artifacts, the length of the spinal cord, and the need for strong imaging gradients (Fig. 27.9).

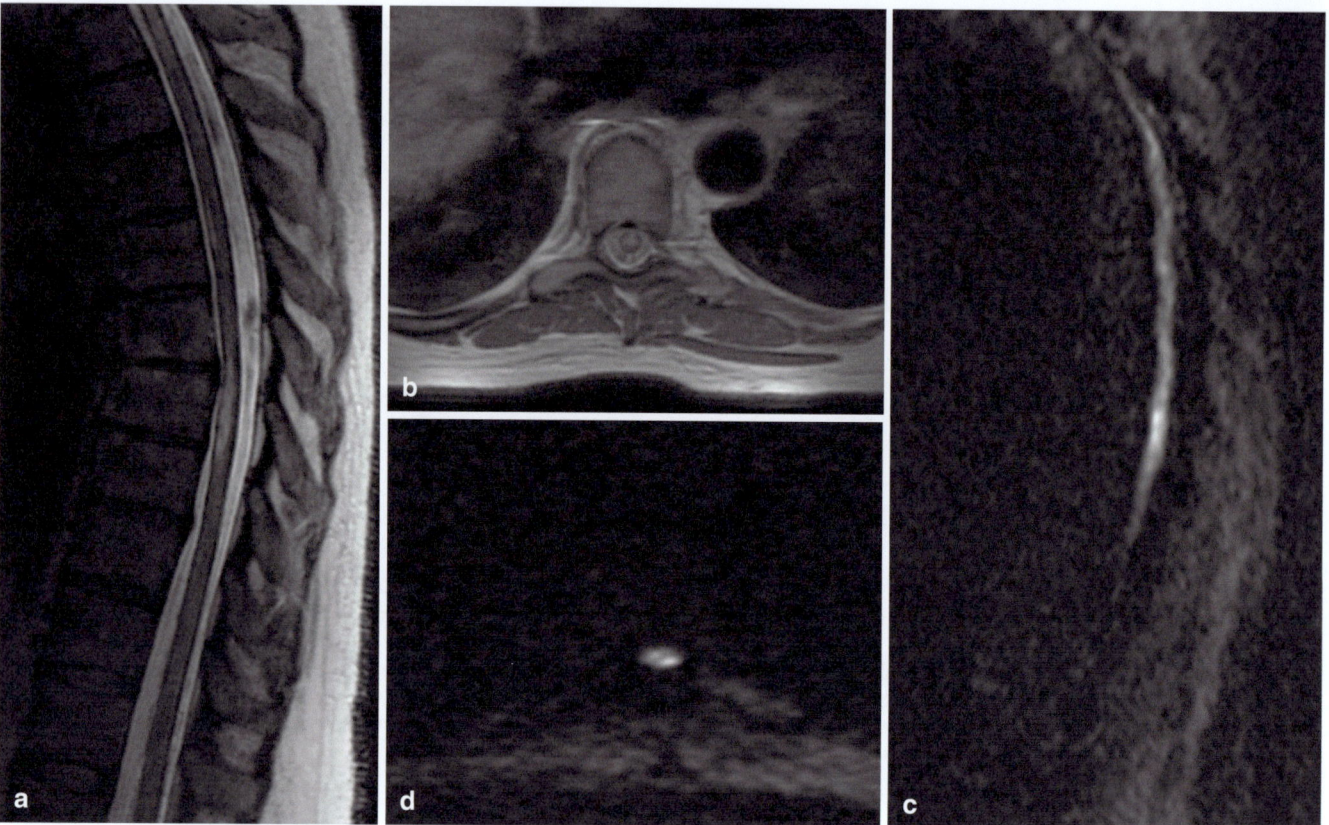

Fig. 27.9 A 68-year-old male with recent abdominal aortic aneurysm surgical repair. (**a**) Sagittal and (**b**) axial T2-weighted MRI demonstrating intramedullary abnormal hyperintense signal in the mid-thoracic spinal cord. (**c**) Sagittal and (**d**) axial diffusion-weighted images confirm abnormal prolongation of diffusivity in the same location, helping confirm the diagnosis of ischemic spinal cord infarction

References

1. Santillan A, Nacarino V, Greenberg E, et al. Vascular anatomy of the spinal cord. J Neurointerv Surg. 2012;4:67–74.
2. Taterra D, Skinningsrud B, Pękala PA, et al. Artery of Adamkiewicz: a meta-analysis of anatomical characteristics. Neuroradiology. 2019;61(8):869–80.
3. Saba L, Raz E. Neurovascular imaging: from basics to advanced concepts. Springer; 2016.
4. Rosenblum B, Oldfield EH, Doppman JL, et al. Spinal arteriovenous malformations: a comparison of dural arteriovenous fistulas and intradural AVM's in 81 patients. J Neurosurg. 1987;67(6):795–802.
5. Takai K. Spinal arteriovenous shunts: angioarchitecture and historical changes in classification. Neurol Med Chir (Tokyo). 2017;57(7):356–65.
6. Cooke DL, Frieden IJ, Shimano KA. Angiographic evidence of response to trametinib therapy for a spinal cord arteriovenous malformation. J Vasc Anom (Phila). 2021;2(3):e018.
7. Edwards EA, Phelps AS, Cooke D, et al. Monitoring arteriovenous malformation response to genotype-targeted therapy. Pediatrics. 2020;146(3):e20193206.
8. Gross BA, Du R, Popp AJ, et al. Intramedullary spinal cord cavernous malformations. Neurosurg Focus. 2010;29(3):E14.
9. Masson C, Pruvo JP, Meder JF, et al. Spinal cord infarction: clinical and magnetic resonance imaging findings and short term outcome. J Neurol Neurosurg Psychiatry. 2004;75:1431–5.

Imaging Anatomy of the Orbit, Sinus, and Mucosal Surfaces of the Neck

Nahil Matari and Akinrinola Famuyide

Orbit

BONY MARGINS

Anatomic relations of the structures surrounding the orbits are important clinically, particularly in the spread of infection and neoplasm [1].

The four borders of the orbits are formed by seven bones.

- The roof or superior wall is formed mostly by the frontal bone and to a lesser extent the lesser wing of the sphenoid bone. This separates the orbit from the intracranial compartment. See Fig. 28.1 [2].
- The floor or inferior wall is formed by the maxilla, palatine, and zygomatic bones. This separates the orbit from the maxillary sinus.
- The medial wall is formed by the lamina papyracea of the ethmoid bone, maxilla, lacrimal bone, and sphenoid bones. This separates the orbit from the ethmoid sinus.
- The lateral wall is formed by the zygomatic bone and the greater wing of the sphenoid bone. This separates the orbit from the overlying scalp soft tissues.

The orbit is cone-shaped where the apex is situated posteriorly and opens into the optic canal, superior orbital fissure, and inferior orbital fissure [3].

The connective tissue periosteum lining the orbit is known as the periorbita.

N. Matari
Diagnostic Radiology and Internal Medicine, Yale New Haven Health Greenwich Hospital, Greenwich, CT, USA

Columbia University Irving Medical Center, New York, NY, USA

A. Famuyide (✉)
Columbia University Irving Medical Center, New York, NY, USA

Department of Radiology, CUMC, New York, NY, USA

NewYork-Presbyterian, New York, NY, USA
e-mail: af3169@cumc.columbia.edu

GLOBE

The globe is made up of the anterior smaller segment and the posterior larger segment.

The eye is composed of three primary layers, the sclera, or the outer layer, of the uvea, or middle ear which is vascularized and contains pigmented tissue consisting of the choroid, ciliary body, and iris [4].

The inner layer is the retina which is the neural sensory portion of the eye.

The sclera is perforated 3 mm medial and 1 mm above the posterior pole by the optic nerve.

EXTRAOCULAR MUSCLES

There are six extraocular muscles that control eye movement. There are four rectus muscles—superior, inferior, medial, and lateral and two oblique muscles—superior and inferior. See Figs. 28.2 and 28.3.

- These are supplied by cranial nerves III, IV, and VI (pneumonic SO4, LR6, rest by CN3).

Retraction of the upper eyelid is performed by the levator muscle and the sympathetically innervated superior tarsal muscle also known as Mueller's muscle.

OPTIC NERVE

The optic nerve is a fiber tract of the central nervous system that originates in the ganglion cell layer of the retina. The optic nerve head insertion into the globe is at the optic disc [4].

The optic nerves pass posteriorly through the optic canal to join the optic chiasm.

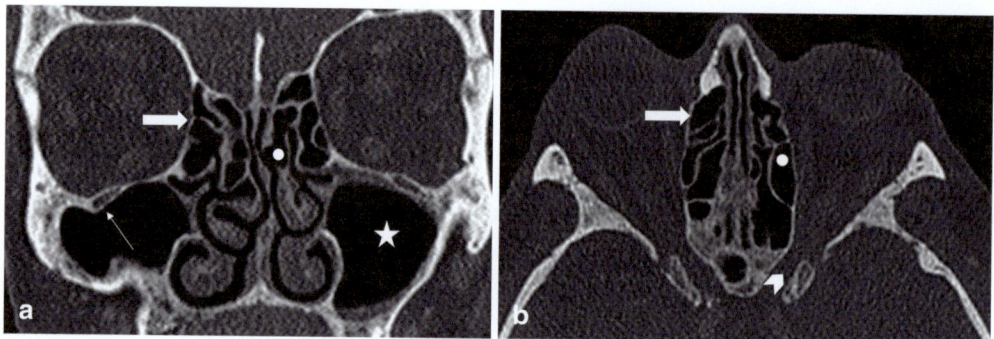

Fig. 28.1 Coronal (a) and axial (b) landmarks of the osseous orbit. The thick arrow shows the medial orbital wall formed primarily by the lamina papyracea. The ethmoid air cells (circle), maxillary sinus (star), infraorbital canal which transmits the V2 branch of the trigeminal nerve (thin arrow) and the optic canal (arrow head)

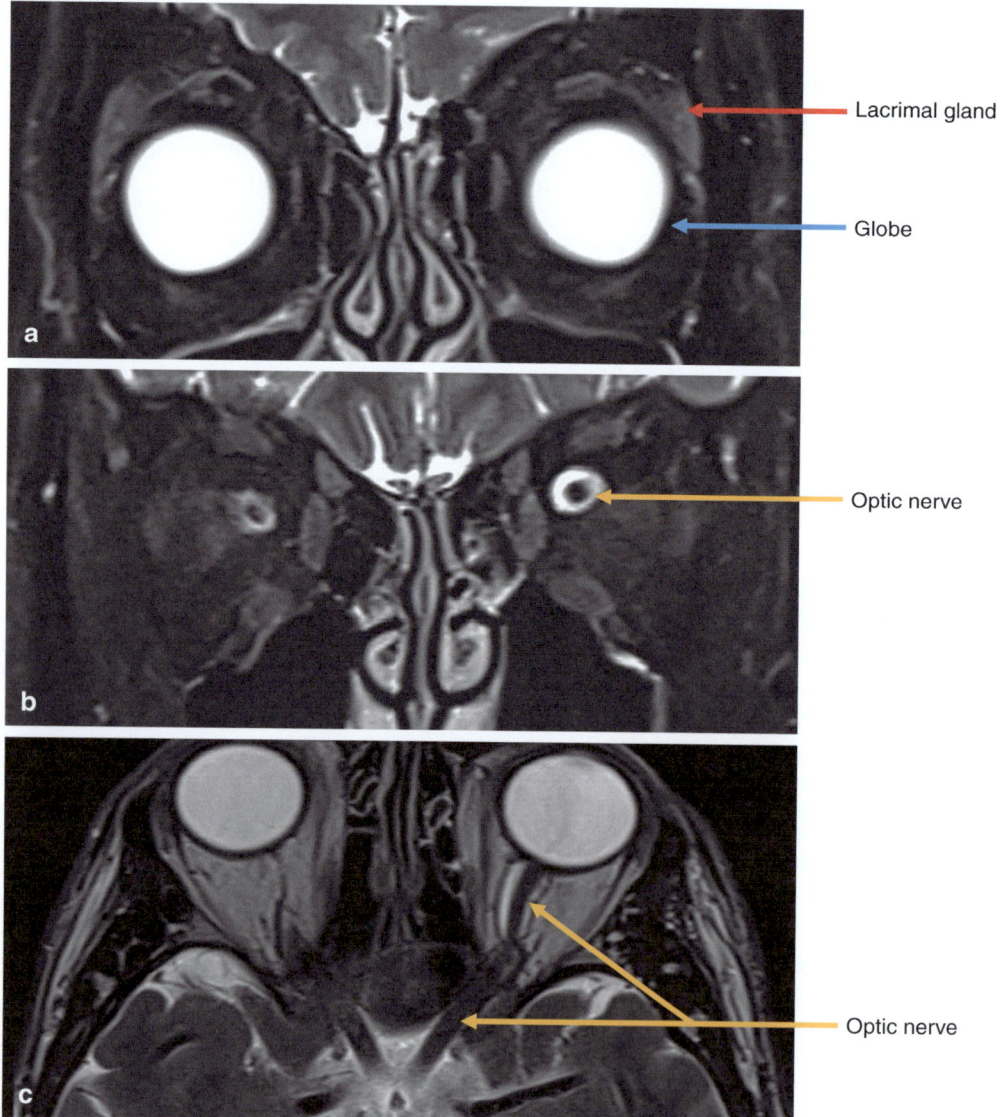

Fig. 28.2 Soft tissues of the orbit in coronal T2 fat-saturated (a and b) and axial T2 (c). This demonstrates the lacrimal gland, globe, and optic nerve. The left optic nerve (yellow) is normal and the right is atrophic

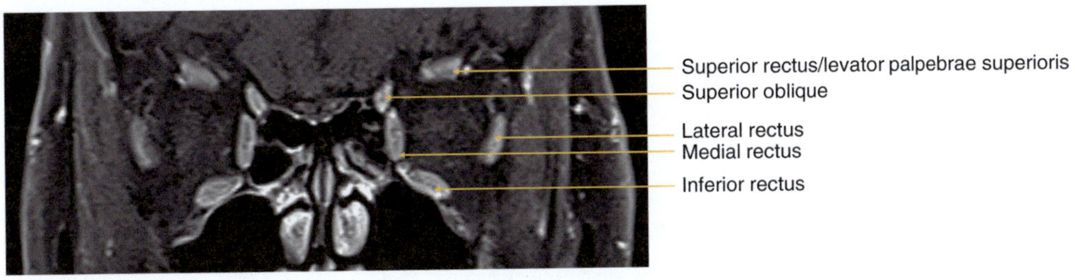

Fig. 28.3 Extraocular muscles are identified as the enhancing structures as above. The inferior oblique muscles are not well visualized in the image

LACRIMAL APPARATUS

The lacrimal gland is in the superolateral orbit behind the upper eyelid. It is situated in the extraconal orbit.

The lacrimal gland consists of the anterior palpebral and deeper orbital lobes. These lobes are demarcated by the lateral extension of the levator palpebrae superioris aponeurosis.

Tears produced by the gland pass medially across the surface of the cornea assisted by blinking. Tears drain medially to the lacrimal sac and then through the nasolacrimal duct into the nasal cavity, below the inferior turbinate [5].

Sinus

PARANASAL SINUSES

The paranasal sinuses originate as evaginations from the nasal fossa. They are lined by mucosa similar to that found in the nasal cavity and respiratory tract.

The sinuses comprise the ethmoid sinuses, frontal sinuses, sphenoid sinuses, and maxillary sinuses. See Figs. 28.4 and 28.5 [1].

- The frontal sinuses drain through the frontal recess and along with the anterior ethmoid air cells and ipsilateral maxillary sinus drain into the medial meatus.
- Drainage through the maxillary sinus into the middle meatus is through the ostiomeatal unit.
- The posterior ethmoid air cells and ipsilateral sphenoid sinus have a common drainage location to the sphenoethmoidal recess.

The nasal cavity contains bones extending from the lateral nasal wall known as turbinates. The nasal septum is in a midline structure with cartilaginous and osseous components [6].

Osseous components of the nasal septum have contributions from the ethmoid bone perpendicular plate, the vomer, the nasal crest of the palatine bone, the crus of the sphenoid bone, and the nasal crest of the maxillary bone [7].

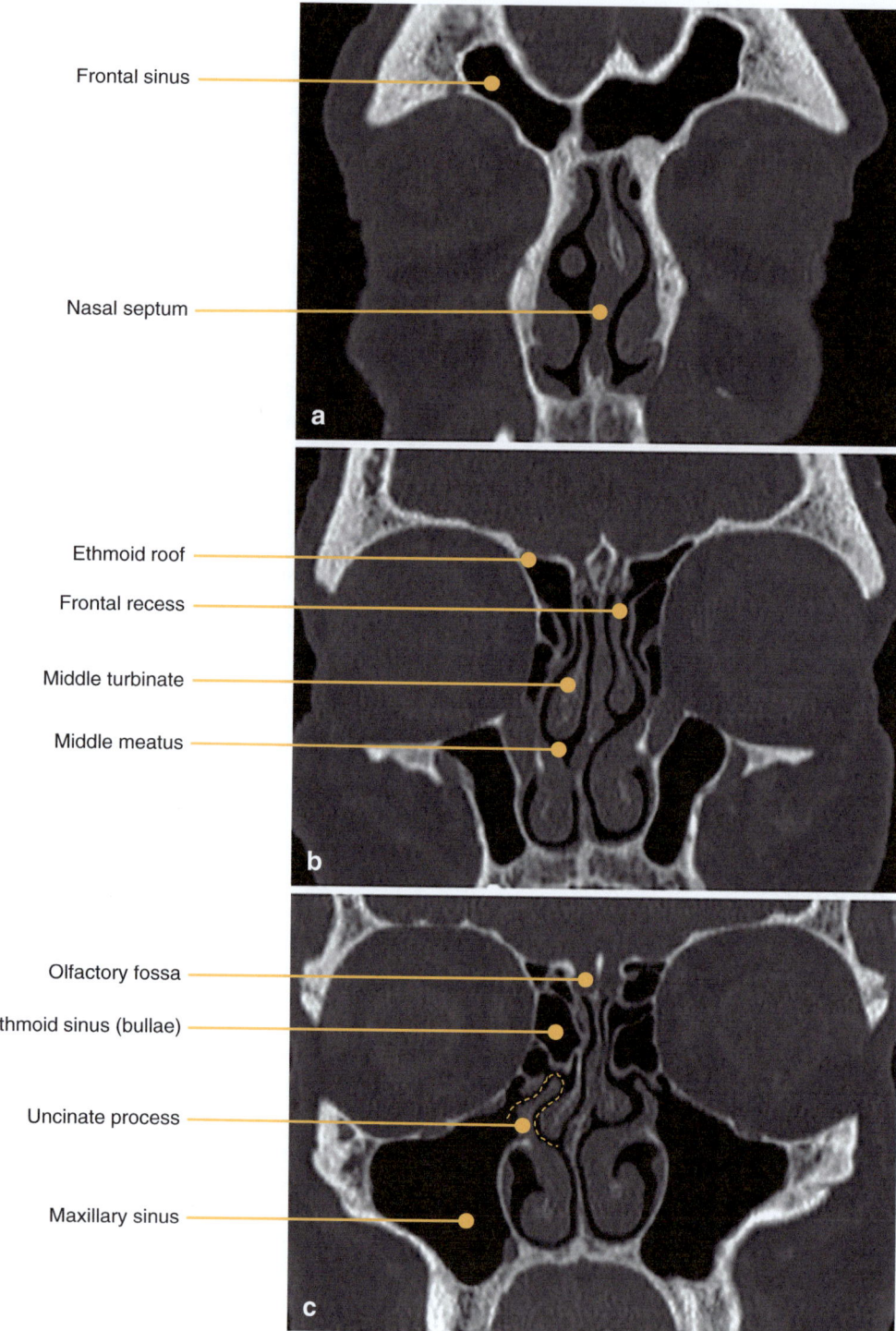

Fig. 28.4 Paranasal sinus anatomy as demonstrated on coronal CT of the sinus. Dashed line on image (**c**) is the drainage pathway of the ostiomeatal unit (OMU) coursing from the maxillary sinus to the middle meatus. It serves as the common drainage pathway for the frontal sinus, ipsilateral anterior ethmoid air cells, and ipsilateral maxillary sinus

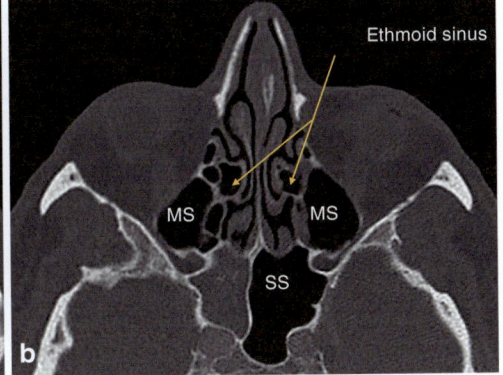

Fig. 28.5 Axial CT anatomy of the paranasal sinuses. Maxillary sinus, MS, sphenoid sinus, SS, with right sphenoid sinus opacified with intrasinus calcifications. The yellow dot represents the sphenoethmoidal recess which is the common drainage pathway for the posterior ethmoid air cells and ipsilateral sphenoid sinus

Mucosal Surfaces Of The Head And Neck

NASOPHARYNX

The nasopharynx forms the upper aspect of the aerodigestive tract.

The nasopharynx communicates with the middle ear via the eustachian tube.

- The opening of each eustachian tube is located along the upper and lateral walls of the nasopharynx with elevation of the overlying mucosa forming torus tubarius. The eustachian tube is prone to obstruction by nasopharyngeal masses.
- The fossa of Rosenmuller, a mucosa-lined recess, lies in the most superior part of the lateral nasopharyngeal recess. This is a common site of origin of nasopharyngeal cancer [8] (Fig. 28.6).

ORAL CAVITY

The oral cavity is separated into the oral cavity proper and vestibule. The oral cavity is divided into multiple subsites including the oral tongue, lips, floor of mouth, retromolar trigone, hard palate, buccal mucosa, and gingiva [9].

- It is a common site of infectious, neoplastic, and developmental processes.

Compartments of the oral cavity communicate with each other and additional spaces of the neck can transmit diseases such as infection, neoplastic processes, or developmental lesions (Fig. 28.7).

OROPHARYNX

The oropharynx is the area posterior to the oral cavity and includes the posterior one-third of the tongue known as the base of the tongue which contains the lingual tonsils, the palatine tonsils, posterior tonsillar pillars, soft palate, oropharyngeal mucosa, and associated constrictor muscles [10, 11].

The air-filled space posterior to the lingual tonsils is known as the vallecula. The valleculae are separated by the median glossoepiglottic fold.

The mucosa over the anterior aspect of the epiglottis is referred to as the lingual aspect of the epiglottis in contradistinction to the laryngeal aspect of the epiglottis (Fig. 28.8).

LARYNX

The larynx is responsible for maintaining the patent airway, protection from aspiration, and phonation. The larynx is composed of the vocal cords also known as vocal folds, the supraglottis, and the subglottis [12] (Fig. 28.9). The vocal folds fuse at the anterior commissure.

The false vocal folds also known as the ventricular vestibular folds are situated above the true vocal folds and comprise the supraglottis along with the epiglottis.

The subglottis traverses the region between the true vocal fold and the lower margin of the larynx.

HYPOPHARYNX

The hypopharynx extends from the level of the hyoid bone to the cricopharyngeus. On imaging, this caudal margin can be approximated by the lower level of the cricoid cartilage. Below this level, the cervical esophagus is formed.

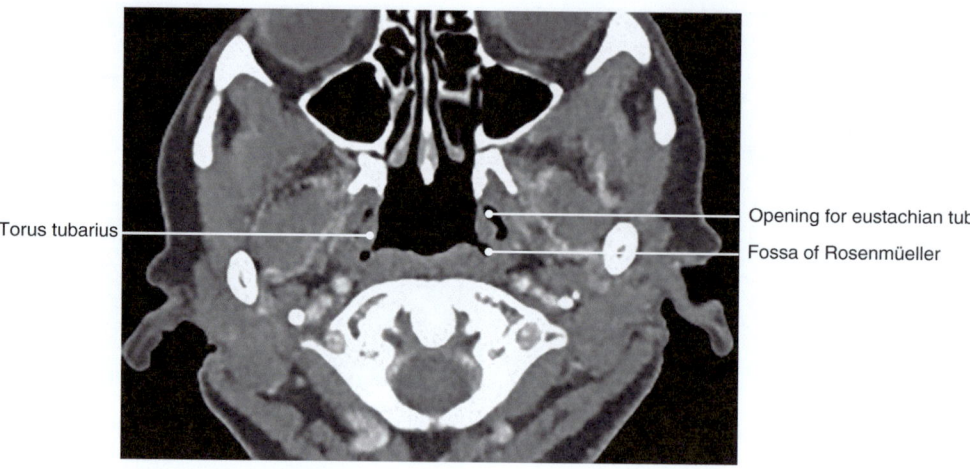

Fig. 28.6 Axial contrast-enhanced CT of the nasopharynx

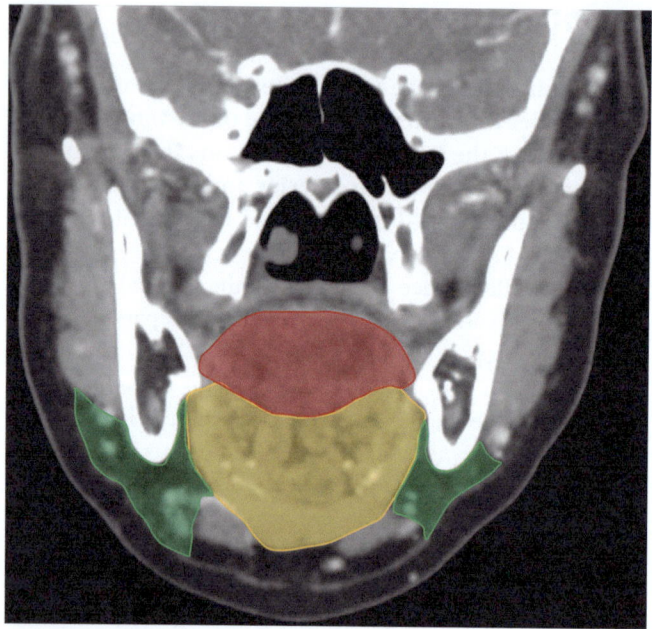

Fig. 28.7 Coronal CT showing the floor of mouth (yellow), tongue (red), and submandibular space (green)

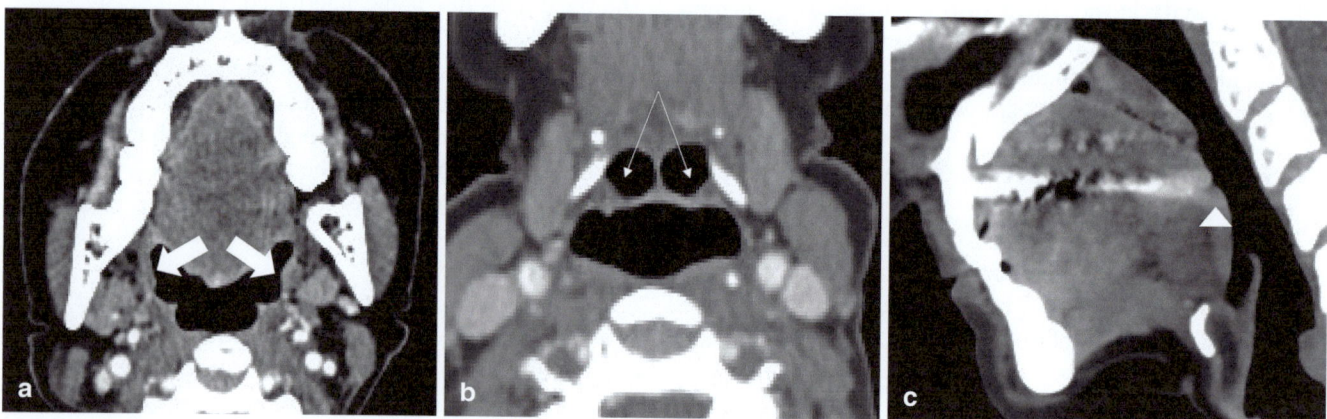

Fig. 28.8 Axial (a and b) and sagittal (c) contrast-enhanced CT demonstrating the palatine tonsils (thick arrows), vallecula (thin arrows), and the base of tongue where the lingual tonsils are situated (triangle)

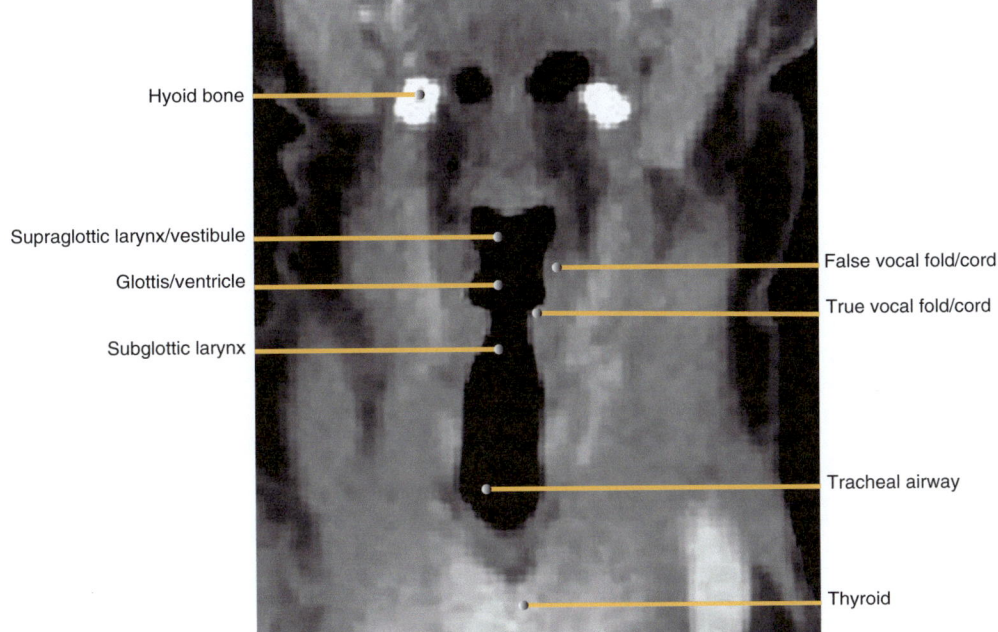

Fig. 28.9 Coronal contrast-enhanced CT of the larynx showing anatomic landmarks

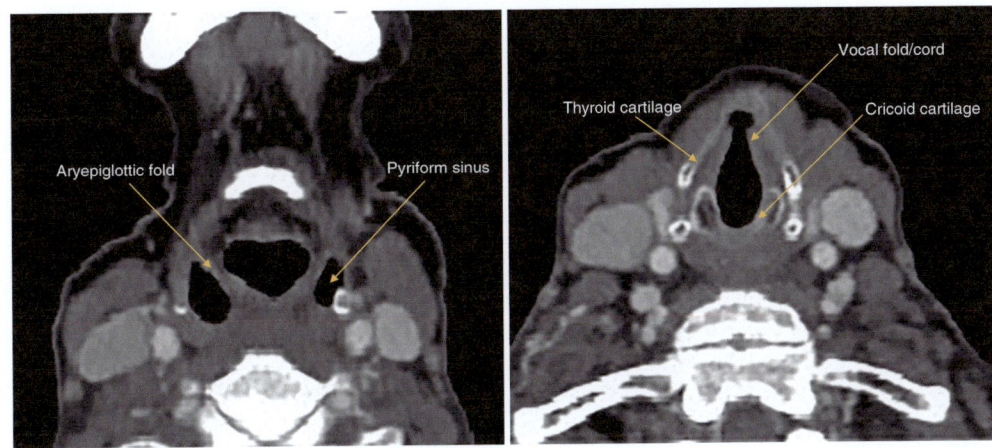

Fig. 28.10 Axial contrast-enhanced CT through the larynx demonstrating anatomic landmarks. The anterior aspect of the aryepiglottic fold is the laryngeal surface, and the posterior aspect is the hypopharyngeal surface

The hypopharynx is divided into the pyriform sinuses, the posterior hypopharyngeal wall, the hypopharyngeal (lateral) surface of the aryepiglottic, and the post-cricoid region [13] (see Fig. 28.10).

References

1. Som PM, Curtin HD. Head and neck imaging. Mosby; 1996.
2. Hande PC, Talwar I. Multimodality imaging of the orbit. Indian J Radiol Imaging. 2012;22:227–39.
3. Grech R, Cornish KS, Galvin PL, Grech S, Looby S, O'Hare A, Mizzi A, Thornton J, Brennan P. Imaging of adult ocular and orbital pathology—a pictorial review. J Radiol Case Rep. 2014; 8:1–29.
4. Gokharman D, Aydin S. Magnetic resonance imaging in orbital pathologies: a pictorial review. JBR-BTR. 2018;101:5.
5. Jung WS, Ahn KJ, Park MR, Kim JY, Choi JJ, Kim BS, Hahn ST. The radiological spectrum of orbital pathologies that involve the lacrimal gland and the lacrimal fossa. Korean J Radiol. 2007;8:336–42.
6. Hoang JK, Eastwood JD, Tebbit CL, Glastonbury CM. Multiplanar sinus CT: a systematic approach to imaging before functional endoscopic sinus surgery. AJR Am J Roentgenol. 2010;194:W527–36.
7. O'Brien WT Sr, Hamelin S, Weitzel EK. The preoperative sinus CT: avoiding a "CLOSE" call with surgical complications. Radiology. 2016;281:10–21.
8. Razek AAKA, King A. MRI and CT of nasopharyngeal carcinoma. Am J Roentgenol. 2012;198:11–8.
9. Law CP, Chandra RV, Hoang JK, Phal PM. Imaging the oral cavity: key concepts for the radiologist. Br J Radiol. 2011;84:944–57.
10. Som PM, Curtin HD. Head and neck imaging—2 volume set: expert consult—online and print. Mosby Elsevier; 2011.
11. Yousem DM, Chalian AA. Oral cavity and pharynx. Radiol Clin North Am. 1998;36:967–81, vii.
12. Silverman PM, Korobkin M. High-resolution computed tomography of the normal larynx. Am J Roentgenol. 1983;140:875–9.
13. Chen AY, Hudgins PA. Pitfalls in the staging squamous cell carcinoma of the hypopharynx. Neuroimaging Clin N Am. 2013;23:67–79.

Imaging of the Orbit (Infection, Inflammation, Benign, and Malignant Lesions)

Michael T. Starc and Azita Khorsandi

Orbital Imaging General Approach

- There are a limited number of pathologic orbital imaging patterns. Unfortunately, the same pattern of imaging may reflect a broad variety of etiologies, including infection, inflammation, and tumor. There are very few "pathognomonic" orbital imaging diagnoses.
- Accurate clinical history (including patient age, symptom duration, and presence of pain) is vital to localizing lesions prior to imaging and is key to shaping the differential diagnosis.
    - Exclusion of intracranial pathology should be the first step in any emergent situation. Recognition of clinical presentations that may benefit from both orbital and intracranial imaging is vital. These include bitemporal hemianopsia (suggesting suprasellar mass effect) or homonymous visual loss (as in occipital lobe infarction).
    - Unilateral eye symptoms suggest true orbital pathology that will benefit from dedicated imaging.
    - Clinical details including ophthalmoscopic examination will indicate if pathology is "ocular," i.e., involving the eye (globe) or "orbital," indicating pathology of the soft tissues and bony structures extrinsic to the eye.
- Imaging approach begins with the characterization of pathology as either localized or diffuse.
    - Localized lesions are centered in or isolated to a particular orbital structure i.e., globe, optic nerve, optic nerve sheath, extraocular muscle, lacrimal gland, and adjacent bone.
    - "Diffuse" or multicompartmental lesions have a separate differential but can be further subclassified by the involvement of preseptal or postseptal soft tissues, intraconal or extraconal fat, and infiltration of specific orbital structures.
    - The ultimate goal of orbital imaging of any lesion is to accurately define its anatomic boundaries and provide a useful, limited differential.
- CT represents the first line emergency imaging modality.
    - Best evaluates osseous structures and adjacent sinuses.
    - Essential for lesions arising from bone to define matrix and margins.
    - Best defines secondary bone findings in soft tissue lesions, i.e., smooth scalloping associated with long-standing masses versus aggressive erosive change in higher-grade tumors.
    - Calcification is readily identified which is helpful in certain diagnoses (i.e., retinoblastoma).
- MRI is the preferred diagnostic imaging modality for nearly all orbital pathologies [1].
    - Best soft tissue characterization, including of the optic nerve.
    - Best definition of tumor spread (perineural and intracranial).
    - Fat suppression is vital both for T2-weighted (STIR) and post-contrast T1 fat-saturated imaging.
    - Coronal imaging elucidates the majority of orbital anatomy most clearly and should be standard in addition to standard small field-of-view axial imaging.
    - DWI sequences are helpful for confirming abscess, tumor cellularity and optic nerve ischemia.

Orbital Infection

- Orbital infection is traditionally conceptualized as a spectrum from least severe to most severe as follows:
  - Preseptal cellulitis.
  - Orbital cellulitis (post-septal).
  - Subperiosteal abscess.
  - Intraorbital abscess (no longer confined by the periorbita).
  - Extraorbital complications (cavernous sinus thrombosis).
- The role of imaging is to define the extent of infection and therefore guide management, including potential surgical decompression, with the ultimate goal of vision preservation.
- By far the most common source of orbital infection is the adjacent paranasal sinuses.
- Contrast-enhanced CT is the modality of choice for initial evaluation, primarily due to ease of access, but also secondary to excellent definition of osseous structures including bony orbit, skull base, and paranasal sinuses.
- Contrast-enhanced MR provided better characterization of the soft tissues of the orbits. For complicated or aggressive infections, CT and MR are both indicated and complimentary.
- Preseptal cellulitis (Fig. e29.1a).
  (All electronic images (Figs. e29.1–e29.10) can be found on this chapter's website on SpringerLink: https://doi.org/10.1007/978-3-031-55124-6_29)
  - Most common presentation: erythema and superficial soft tissue swelling following regional trauma including from insect bites.
  - Infection is limited to the superficial tissues by the orbital septum, a plane of connective tissue dividing the orbit into superficial preseptal and deep post-septal spaces.
  - CT and MR will demonstrate infiltration of the superficial anterior periorbital soft tissues with preservation of retrobulbar fat signal.
- Postseptal cellulitis (Fig. e29.1b).
  - Also known as orbital cellulitis, intraorbital cellulitis.
  - Most common presentation: fever and pain in addition to superficial erythema in a patient with sinusitis.
  - Represents infection involving intraorbital soft tissues posterior to the orbital septum (retrobulbar). In sinusitis, there is transmission of pathogens either directly through foci of osseous dehiscence or through valveless veins. Morbidity is increased due to the potential involvement of vital adjacent structures including the optic nerve. Management often requires IV antibiotics. Invasive fungal infection should be considered in the immunocompromised.
  - Imaging with CT or MR will demonstrate heterogeneous stranding and infiltrative enhancement of the normally bland retrobulbar fat. MR may demonstrate posterior scleral thickening and enhancement as in scleritis. Myositis of extraocular muscles manifests as enlargement and enhancement.
- Subperiosteal abscess (Figs. 29.1 and Fig. e29.2).
  - Most common presentation: progressive proptosis, edema, pain, and double vision in a child with sinusitis.
  - Accumulation of purulent material within an avascular potential space between the bony orbit and the periosteum (periorbita) forming a space-occupying fluid collection.
  - Treatment is often based on the volume of abscess but always involves IV antibiotics.
  - Surgical drainage is required in greater than 50% of cases, more commonly in older patients and superior locations.
  - Imaging.
    - Rim enhancing extraconal lesion with broad contact with opacified paranasal sinus.
    - Most commonly medial (ethmoid, Fig. 29.1), less commonly superior or lateral (frontal sinus, Fig. e29.2).
    - Displace adjacent orbital soft tissues with bowing/enlargement of rectus musculature and resultant proptosis.
  - CT.
    - Stranding in intraconal fat reflecting cellulitis.
    - May see osseous thinning or dehiscence of orbital walls, although more commonly the bony orbit appears intact.
  - MRI.
    - As with any abscess, there will typically be T1 hypointense, T2 hyperintense fluid signal with diffusion restriction, and peripheral enhancement [2].
    - Often better demonstrates soft tissue infiltration and may be useful for subtle cases with high suspicion of orbital extension.
- Orbital abscess (Fig. e29.3a): collection of fluid no longer confined by the periosteum, typically in more severe infections. May reflect the hematogenous spread of infection in bacteremic or immunocompromised patients.
- Cavernous sinus thrombosis (Fig. e29.3b).
  - Sequelae of severe orbital infection with high morbidity. Should be considered in a patient with multiple cranial nerve palsies in addition to orbital pain.
  - Imaging demonstrates convex margins of cavernous sinuses with irregular enhancement and restricted diffusion. CT or MR angiography/venography demon-

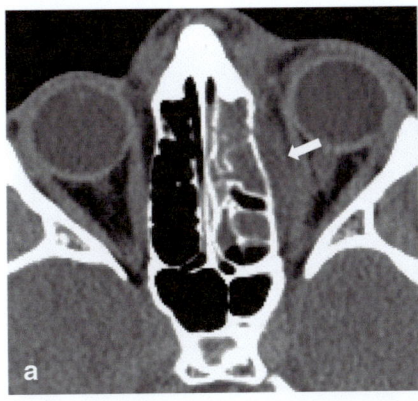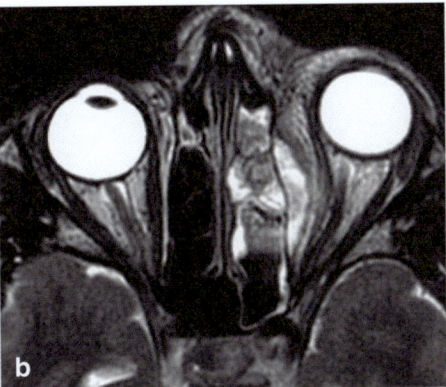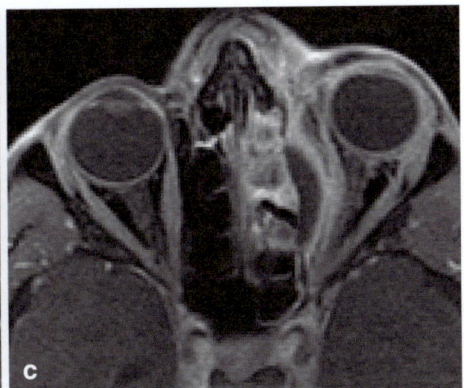

Fig. 29.1 Infection: subperiosteal abscess. (**a**) Axial noncontrast CT shows a thin low-density structure in the left extraconal fat between the lateral rectus muscle and opacified ethmoid air cells (arrow). (**b**) Axial T2 and (**c**) axial T1 contrast-enhanced MR images better define the T2 hyperintense fluid collection with peripheral enhancement and broad base along the left lamina papyracea

strates filling defects in cavernous sinuses and superior orbital veins.
- Top differential considerations.
  - Non-infectious inflammatory conditions (IOI and granulomatous disease) may mimic diffuse infiltration of cellulitis.
  - Trauma with fracture or foreign body and resultant retrobulbar hematoma/edema may coexist with infection.
  - Tumor (lymphoma, metastasis, and sarcoma in children) considered in atypical presentations or lack of clinical response.

Optic Neuritis (On)

- Most common presentation: acute vision loss and pain, most commonly in young adult females.
  - Spontaneous vision recovery is typical, although recurrence is also common.
  - ON often is the first presentation of multiple sclerosis (MS).
    - Over half of ON cases go on to develop MS, more commonly in females. The presence of brain lesions is also highly predictive of a subsequent MS diagnosis.
    - Conversely, ~70–90% of MS patients will have ON during their disease course.
  - In addition to MS, distinct clinical syndromes associated with ON are now recognized.
    - Neuromyelitis optica spectrum disorder (NMOSD, Devic syndrome). Typically aquaporin-4 (AQP4) antibody positive, classically with longitudinally extensive transverse myelitis.
    - MOG antibody-associated disease: myelin oligodendrocyte glycoprotein IgG positive. Younger patients (males) with optic disc edema, monophasic course, and better prognosis [3].
- Etiology is presumed to reflect an autoimmune response with autoreactive inflammation and likely reflects a combination of genetic risk factors and triggering stressors such as infection.
- Treatment: corticosteroid and IVIG help vision recovery in the short term, without proven long-term outcome alteration of underlying optic nerve disease course.
- Imaging: in general, contrast-enhanced MRI is the modality of choice; CT has little role in diagnosis.
- MR imaging of MS-associated acute optic neuritis (Fig. 29.2).
  - T1 contrast-enhanced images with fat saturation show central enhancement of the optic nerve itself in the active phase, most commonly within the intraorbital segment.
  - STIR or T2 fat-saturated images may show optic nerve mild enlargement and hyperintense signal acutely. Chronic sequela of optic neuritis manifests as atrophy of the optic nerve with persistent T2 hyperintense signal and nerve volume loss (increased fluid signal in adjacent nerve sheath).
  - DWI may reveal increased diffusivity (relatively hyperintense signal on DWI and ADC maps).
  - T2 FLAIR imaging of the brain is essential to evaluate for characteristic MS-defining T2 hyperintense lesions in periventricular, juxtacortical white matter, and posterior fossa.
  - Imaging of the spinal cord is also recommended to aid in diagnosis and clarify the extent of the disease.
- Findings suggesting NMOSD optic neuritis (Fig. e29.4a): bilateral or chiasm involvement, intracranial lesions following AQP4 distribution (midline periependymal lesions), and long segment spinal cord lesions.

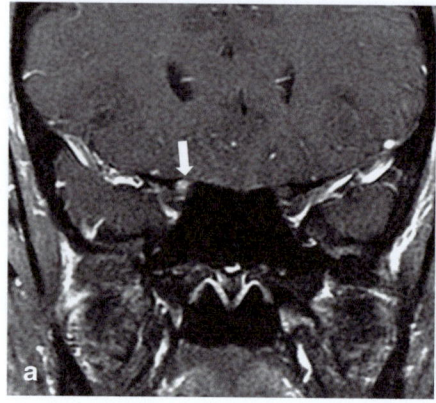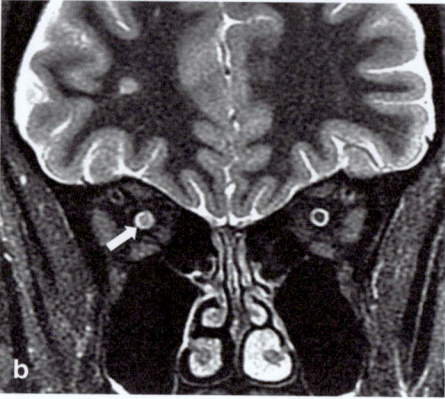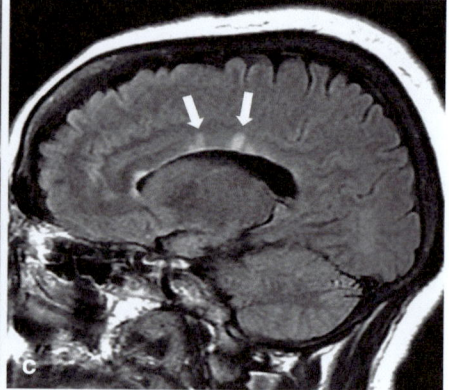

Fig. 29.2 Optic neuritis in multiple sclerosis. (a) Coronal T1 contrast-enhanced fat-saturated MR image shows asymmetric enhancement of the right optic nerve in the optic canal (arrow). (b) Coronal STIR MR image shows an asymmetric increased T2 signal in the right intraorbital segment of the optic nerve (arrow). (c) The sagittal T2 FLAIR image shows abnormal ovoid T2 hyperintense lesions radiating orthogonally from the ventricular margins characteristic of multiple sclerosis (arrows)

- Findings suggesting MOG antibody optic neuritis (Fig. e29.4b): anterior intraorbital optic nerve involvement, often bilateral with exuberant perineural enhancement.
- Top imaging differential considerations.
  - Ischemic optic neuropathy: different clinical presentation (elderly male with permanent visual defect), optic nerve restricted diffusion. May be seen in the setting of giant cell arteritis (GCA).
  - Infectious or inflammatory optic neuropathy (sarcoidosis): more often bilateral, evaluate for intracranial meningitis.
  - ADEM (acute disseminated encephalomyelitis): younger patient with large cerebral lesions, monophasic course.
  - Optic nerve sheath meningioma, optic nerve glioma, and idiopathic orbital inflammation: see discussion below.

Thyroid Eye Disease

- Also known as thyroid-associated orbitopathy, Graves ophthalmopathy.
- Most common presentation: indolent development of bilateral proptosis, lid lag/retraction leading to dry eyes, pain, and/or diplopia in middle-aged females with Graves' disease.
  - Less commonly seen in males and elderly, although often with more severe disease.
  - May progress to compressive optic neuropathy with vision loss.
  - >80% clinically hyperthyroid, although orbital symptoms may present prior to, during, or after hyperthyroid systemic findings.
  - Approximately one-third of cases are asymmetric.
- Pathology represents an autoimmune phenomenon related to the thyroid-stimulating hormone receptor found in orbital adipocytes and fibroblasts in addition to the thyroid.
  - Proliferative cytokine-mediated glycosaminoglycan (GAG) accumulation with muscle swelling.
  - Fibroblast proliferation with increased orbital fat formation.
  - Chronic stage with fibrosis and muscle atrophy.
- Treatment options include restoration of euthyroid state with supportive therapy for mild disease, corticosteroids for stabilization of acute progressive inflammation, and decompressive surgery.
- Imaging (Fig. 29.3).
- In general, there is a bilateral, relatively symmetric enlargement of extraocular muscles.
  - Characteristic distribution: "I'M SLOw" reflecting Inferior > Medial > Superior > Lateral > Oblique muscle involvement.
  - Typically spares tendinous insertions along the globe margins unless associated with acute inflammation.
  - Bilateral exophthalmos (proptosis) with increased orbital fat, fat stranding, and lacrimal gland anterior displacement [4].
- CT.
  - Muscle belly enlargement, often with internal low density due to GAG deposition, most commonly in the inferior rectus.
  - Essential for surgical planning or follow-up to characterize the bony orbit.
- MR.
  - All sequences may illustrate muscle belly enlargement and provide an excellent definition of soft tissue planes surrounding the optic nerve at the orbital apex.

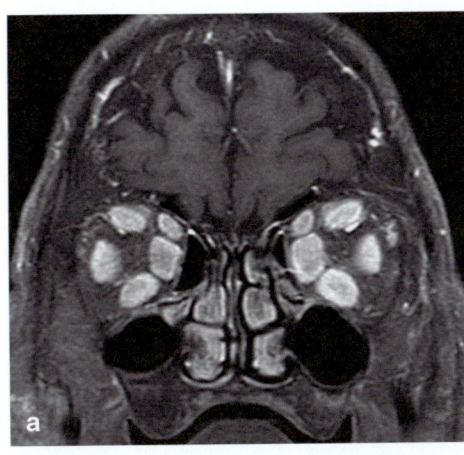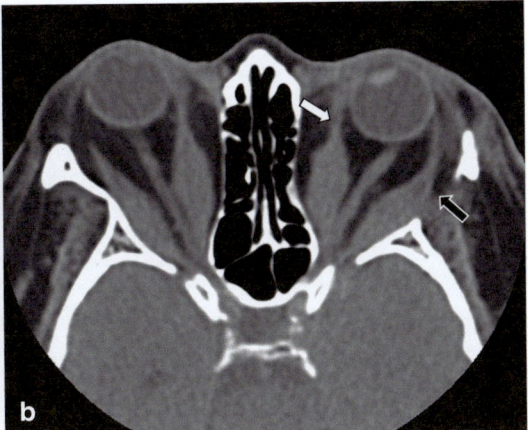

Fig. 29.3 Thyroid eye disease. (**a**) Coronal T1 contrast-enhanced fat-saturated MR shows diffuse symmetric enlargement of bilateral rectus musculature with inferior and medial rectus predominance. (**b**) Axial noncontrast CT shows rectus muscle belly enlargement with characteristic sparing of the tendinous insertions (white arrow). CT also demonstrates a left lateral osseous defect at prior decompressive surgery (black arrow)

- o T2 FS or STIR shows an increased signal in the active phase due to edema, with a relatively decreased signal chronically in fibrosis. Optic nerve edema or atrophy may be identified by increased nerve signal in severe cases.
- o T1 contrast-enhanced images may show relatively decreased muscle enhancement due to impaired circulation from mass effect. Ill-defined wispy enhancement of intraconal fat is seen in extramuscular involvement.
- Top imaging differential considerations: IOI, granulomatous disease, lymphoproliferative disease, and cellulitis.

Idiopathic Orbital Inflammation (Ioi)

- Also known as orbital pseudotumor.
- Most common presentation: subacute onset pain, proptosis, and diplopia in an adult of any age—slight predominance in females of older middle age.
- Disease variants include:
  - o Tolosa-Hunt: inflammation extending through the orbital apex to the cavernous sinus with painful ophthalmoplegia secondary to CN III, IV, and/or VI involvement.
  - o Sclerosing variant: progressive fibrosis, poorly responsive to typical therapy.
  - o IgG4-related orbital disease: fibrotic IgG4-positive plasma cell infiltrate on biopsy and elevated serum concentration of IgG4. May account for at least 5% of IOI.
- The pathophysiology of true "idiopathic" orbital inflammation is unknown but almost certainly reflects an autoimmune process.
- o IOI is therefore a diagnosis of exclusion following extensive workup, including the evaluation for IgG4-related disease.
- Treatment is with systemic corticosteroids with characteristic rapid response.
  - o Recurrence is not uncommon and may require repeat therapy or other systemic immunosuppression.
  - o Low-dose radiation therapy can be considered in poorly responding or aggressive cases.
- Imaging.
- In general, seen as "infiltrative," poorly defined enhancement of any portion of the orbit, more commonly unilateral.
- Specific sites of involvement (listed in order of prevalence with the most common first):
  - o Extraocular muscles, "myositic"—exhibit a pattern atypical for thyroid eye disease including isolated lateral rectus involvement, with less well-defined margins and extension to the tendinous insertions.
  - o Lacrimal gland.
  - o Globe (uveal-scleral) enhancement with extension to retrobulbar intraconal fat and perineural optic sheath, "anterior" pattern.
  - o Multifocal involvement, "diffuse" pattern.
  - o Orbital apex, intracranial, "apical" pattern as in Tolosa-Hunt.
- CT: Masslike irregular enhancement with the absence of bony remodeling or erosion.
- MR (Fig. 29.4):
  - o Typically T1 iso- to hypointense.
  - o T2 characteristics variable based on the amount of edema (hyperintense) versus cellularity/fibrosis (hypointense). Hypointense lesions in general suggest sclerotic or IgG4-related disease.

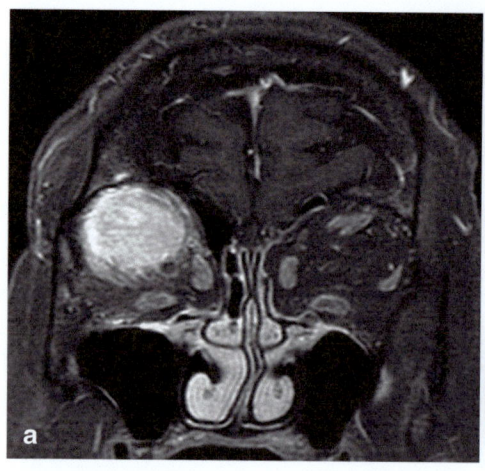 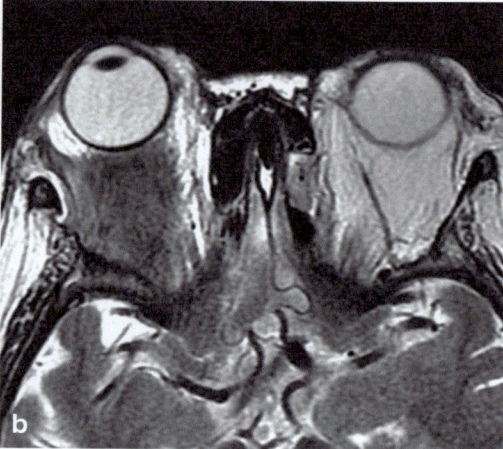

Fig. 29.4 **Idiopathic orbital inflammation.** (**a**) Coronal T1 contrast-enhanced fat-saturated MR shows right orbital masslike enhancement involving intraconal and extraconal fat with ill-defined margins. Enhancement is inseparable from the superior and lateral rectus muscu-lature. (**b**) Axial T2 MR image shows infiltrating mass abutting the posterior margin of the globe without deformation and marked T2 hypointense signal characteristic of sclerosing variant IOI

- T1 contrast-enhanced fat-saturated images ideally demonstrate the extent of infiltrative enhancement including potential perineural, intracranial, or cavernous sinus extension.
- Top differential considerations: As a diagnosis of exclusion, IOI deserves discussion in detail of the following differential etiologies:
  - Lymphoma and lymphoproliferative disorders are often indistinguishable on any imaging technique and may require biopsy for differentiation.
  - Thyroid eye disease shows a characteristic pattern of muscle involvement with better-defined smooth margins and sparing of tendinous insertions.
  - Granulomatous disease such as orbital sarcoidosis may also be indistinguishable on any modality. Characteristic intracranial manifestations of sarcoidosis may be evident including superficial/pial nodular enhancement. Sinonasal inflammatory erosive changes also support sarcoidosis or granulomatosis with polyangiitis. Imaging for systemic manifestations and clinical/laboratory correlation are essential.
  - Scirrhous orbital metastasis (Fig. e29.5) deserves special attention for its clinically and radiologically evident enophthalmos, which results from tumor infiltration and desmoplastic reaction. This has been most commonly described in breast carcinoma.
  - Cavernous carotid fistula typically presents more acutely with proptosis and edematous unilateral infiltration. Characteristic imaging findings include increased flow signal within the affected cavernous sinus and dilated superior ophthalmic vein on MRA.
  - Cellulitis also presents more acutely, ideally with an identifiable source on orbital imaging—i.e., sinusitis or superficial skin ulceration.

Dermoid/Epidermoid

- Most common presentation: young patient with slow-growing fixed mass along the superficial lateral margin of the orbit.
  - Adult presentation typically with larger, deeper masses.
  - Traumatic rupture results in regional inflammation and pain which may mimic infection.
- Etiology results from a congenital sequestration of ectodermal elements within deeper tissues, typically at a craniofacial suture site. Histopathology is required for differentiation.
  - Dermoid: contains adnexal remnants (sebaceous secretions, fat, and follicles).
  - Epidermoid: lacks the above and contains merely cholesterol/keratin debris.
- Treatment is surgical resection in its entirety including periosteal connection. Goals are often cosmetic in addition to prevention of potential rupture.
- Imaging.
- In general, well-defined superficial/anterior extraconal lesions centered along embryonic suture lines [5]:
  - Most commonly abutting frontozygomatic suture (superolateral).
  - Less commonly frontolacrimal suture (superomedial).
  - Internal cystic, fat, or mixed contents.
    - Dermoid: in general, more heterogeneous and may contain gross fat signal.
    - Epidermoid: homogenous.
- CT may demonstrate fat density with negative Hounsfield units in dermoid or fluid density in epidermoid (Fig. e29.6a).

- o Smooth osseous remodeling and thinning are not uncommon and do not suggest a more aggressive lesion.
- o Osseous cleft near a suture line may be seen.
- MR shows an encapsulated mass with:
  - o T1 range of signal characteristics: hyperintense if complex proteinaceous fluid with loss of signal on fat saturation if fatty elements, otherwise hypointense following simple fluid.
  - o T2 hyperintense if fluid or heterogeneous if mixed debris.
  - o DWI relative restricted diffusion is more common in epidermoid lesions although not pathognomonic (Fig. e29.6b).
  - o Post-contrast peripheral thin enhancement without nodularity.
- Top differential considerations:
  - o Dermolipoma: characteristic clinical fat containing lateral canthal mass.
  - o Subconjunctival fat prolapse: bilateral fat density continuous with orbital fat without encapsulation.
  - o Orbital vascular lesions.
  - o Lacrimal gland cyst/dacryocystocele: centered in lacrimal gland/apparatus.
  - o Orbital cellulitis: similar pattern of orbital inflammation, although usually with adjacent sinusitis.

Neurofibromatosis Type 1 (Nf1)

- Most common presentation: child with a distinct constellation of progressive developmental craniofacial asymmetry, cutaneous lesions, and visual impairment. (Please also refer to separate subsequent discussion of optic nerve glioma in NF1).
- Neurocutaenous syndrome with etiology due to the loss of NF1 tumor suppressor gene function on chromosome 17, with autosomal dominant inheritance and variable expression.
- Progressive orbital complications due to facial deformity with resultant proptosis, diplopia, glaucoma, and vision loss. Risk of degeneration into malignant peripheral nerve sheath tumors.
- Treatment of orbital manifestations is typically supportive and cosmetic with the goal of preserving functional vision.
- Imaging (Fig. e29.7):
  - o Optic nerve glioma: discussed in detail separately.
  - o Sphenoid wing dysplasia: CT ideally shows craniofacial osseous anomalies including changes in orbital volume and characteristic defects in the middle cranial fossa. MR best classifies the extent of associated extracranial herniation.
  - o Buphthalmos: unilateral asymmetric globe enlargement.
  - o Plexiform neurofibroma: infiltrative, multi-spatial, serpiginous, and sheetlike mass or masses with variable but often avid enhancement [6].
- Differential considerations: myriad given heterogeneous presentation.
  - o Rhabdomyosarcoma: most common pediatric primary orbital malignancy, infiltrative heterogeneous mass without a constellation of NF1 findings.
  - o Vascular lesions: multi-spatial enhancing lesions that may mimic plexiform neurofibroma.
  - o Sphenorbital cephalocele: isolated congenital middle cranial fossa defect containing meninges and or brain parenchyma.
  - o Primary congenital glaucoma: isolated enlarged globe with increased intraocular pressure.
  - o Coloboma (Fig. e29.8): defect along the posterior margin of the small globe with the retrobulbar cyst. May be sporadic or syndromic (i.e., CHARGE, Aicardi, and many others).

Retinoblastoma (Rb)

- Most common presentation: leukocoria, most commonly diagnosed before age 5 years although not apparent at birth.
  - o Most common pediatric intraocular tumor.
  - o Creamy white mass on ophthalmoscopy.
  - o Vision loss, strabismus, proptosis, neovascularization, and regional inflammation with more advanced disease.
- Sporadic (nongermline) accounts for a slight majority of all cases and most unilateral tumors.
- Inherited (autosomal dominant germline mutation RB1 gene, chromosome 13) accounts for bilateral tumors.
  - o Also possible are "trilateral" (pineal) and "quadrilateral" (suprasellar and pineal) diseases.
  - o Overall increased risk of other malignancies, most commonly osteogenic and soft tissue sarcomas.
- Classification based on size, location, subretinal/vitreous fluid seeding, multifocality, and additional clinical factors.
- Treatment: Vast majority of cases can be cured with modern techniques.
  - o Overall prognosis worsens with a degree of extraocular extension.
  - o Plaque radiotherapy, cryotherapy, and photocoagulation are all options for very small tumors.
  - o Ophthalmic artery chemosurgery (targeted intra-arterial chemotherapy) is the favored treatment for moderate to high-risk tumors.
  - o Enucleation is required if advanced and no chance of preserving vision.
- Imaging (Fig. 29.5).

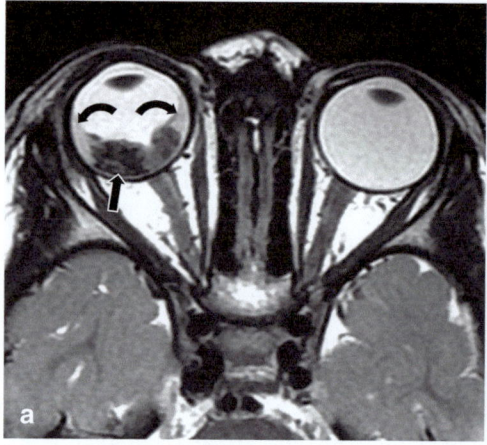 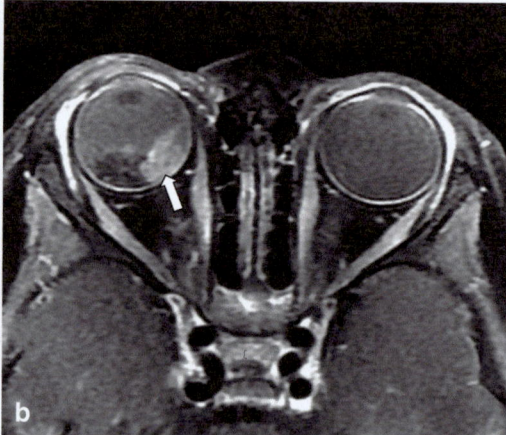 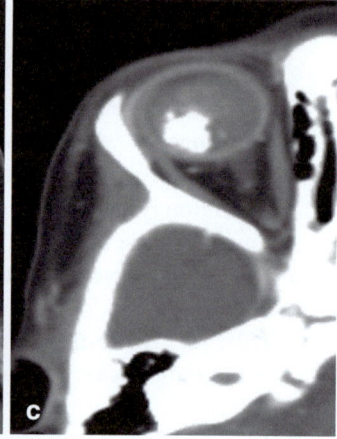

Fig. 29.5 Retinoblastoma. (**a**) Axial T2 MR shows a nodular mixed-intensity lesion in the posterior right globe with marked T2 hypointense calcification (black arrow) and subretinal fluid (curved arrows). (**b**) Axial T1 contrast-enhanced fat-saturated MR demonstrates solid enhancement of the tumor (white arrow) medially with adjacent low signal laterally representing a combination of exudate and calcification. (**c**) Axial CT shows coarse calcification within the right globe

- In general: globe mass with calcification in a child is RB until proven otherwise.
    - "Endophytic" pattern: growth into vitreous with vitreous seeding.
    - "Exophytic" pattern: growth into subretinal space with retinal detachment and exudate.
    - The goal is to evaluate for extraocular extension to the orbital soft tissues, optic nerve, and subarachnoid [7].
- CT readily shows calcifications in nearly all cases, punctate, coarse, or speckled.
- MR: essential for the classification of tumor extent.
    - T1 mildly hyperintense to vitreous, significantly T2 hypointense, with marked enhancement and diffusion restriction.
    - Characterize anterior chamber, choroidal thickening, scleral disruption, enhancement/enlargement of optic disc (prelaminar), or optic nerve (postlaminar).
    - Assess intracranial enhancement with attention to the suprasellar and pineal regions.
- Top differential considerations:
    - Coats disease: green-yellow mass, slightly older male child, normal-small globe without calcification, and hyperintense V-shaped retinal detachment/exudate on T1 and T2 without enhancement.
    - Persistent hyperplastic primary vitreous (PHPV): small globe without calcification, enhancing linear retrolental stalk hyaloid remnant Cloquet canal, and retinal detachment.
    - Retinopathy of prematurity: premature birth with vessels and fibroplasia, bilateral small hyperdense globes, may calcify.
    - Toxocariasis: parasitic uveal enhancement with calcification developing later.

Ocular Melanoma

- Most commonly arise from, and therefore referred to, as uveal melanoma or choroidal melanoma.
- Most common presentation: painless blurry vision, field loss, scotoma, retinal detachment, or asymptomatic in middle-aged to elderly patients.
- The most common intraocular (globe) tumor in adults.
- Arises from melanocytes in the uvea (choroid, ciliary body, or iris) in patients with genetic risk factors and sun exposure.
- Ophthalmoscopy shows an exophytic mass with adjacent exudate and retinal detachment.
- Significant risk of hematogenous metastatic systemic disease, most commonly to the liver.
- Management ranges from ultrasound observation and radiation therapy to enucleation based on size and symptoms. The prognosis depends on the size of the tumor and the invasion of local structures. Systemic disease may be managed with intrahepatic therapy or systemic immunotherapy.
- Imaging (Fig. 29.6).
- In general, solid enhancing mass arises from the posterior lateral globe.

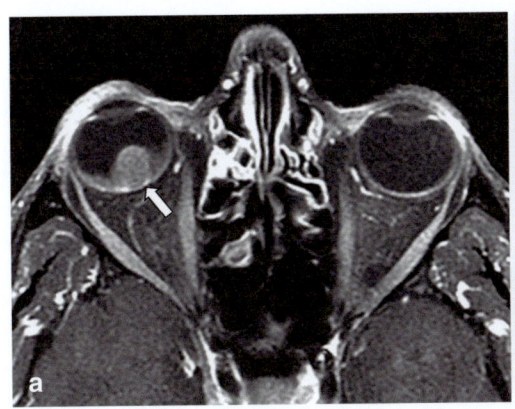
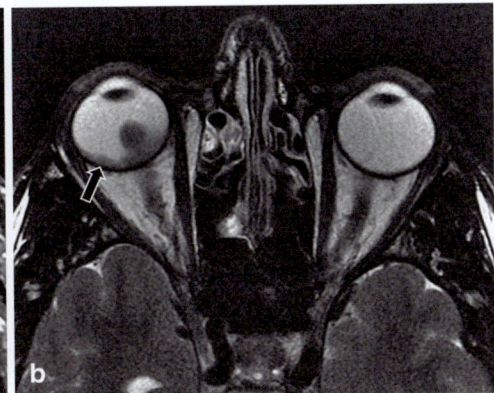

Fig. 29.6 Ocular melanoma. (**a**) Axial T1 contrast-enhanced fat-saturated MR shows a well-defined enhancing nodule (white arrow) arising from the enhancing choroid with adjacent shallow T1 intermediate subretinal detachment and exudate. There is no extraocular extension of enhancement. (**b**) Axial T2 MR shows corollary T2 hypointense nodule with intermediate mixed signal exudate (black arrow) extending medially and laterally

- o Broad choroidal base with smooth lobular, dome, or "mushroom" shaped, as seen with deeper penetration and retinal separation.
- o Less commonly, anterior mass arising from the ciliary body or iris.
- CT: enhancing mass which may show calcification following treatment.
- MR.
  - o T1 intrinsic signal of mass will vary based on melanotic pigment content, ranging from mildly to markedly hyperintense to vitreous.
  - o T2 hypointense to vitreous.
  - o Postcontrast T1 reveals homogeneous enhancement and allows differentiation from adjacent nonenhancing subretinal exudates, which demonstrate varying intermediate signals on precontrast sequences.
  - o Best modality for characterization of extraocular spread.
  - o MRI of the liver is useful to assess distant metastases at baseline, with additional body imaging with CT or PET for full systemic characterization as warranted.
- Top differential considerations: Choroidal metastasis, benign retinal detachment, retinoblastoma in pediatrics.

Optic Pathway Glioma (Opg)

- Presentation and course are highly variable based on clinical subtype and association with neurofibromatosis type 1 (NF1).
  - o Childhood syndromic (NF1): may be asymptomatic, with indolent progressive course followed by stability and potential regression in the second decade. Pathology is most often low-grade glioma (WHO grade 1–2).
  - o Childhood sporadic: vision loss with more rapid progression and relapse. These also represent almost entirely low-grade gliomas.
  - o Adult: rapid vision loss, rare with poor prognosis, representing high-grade gliomas.
- OPGs are also classified by anatomic location as either "anterior" (prechiasmatic optic nerve, considered here) or "posterior" (chiasmal/hypothalamic) [8].
- Treatment:
  - o With NF1 and anterior tumors, biopsy is generally not required, and observation is standard unless vision loss.
  - o Standard treatment begins with chemotherapy with radiation reserved for patients without NF1.
  - o Surgical debulking is associated with high morbidity but may be indicated for sporadic large or malignant tumors.
  - o Adults are generally managed as high-grade astrocytomas.
- Imaging.
- General: relatively long segment fusiform optic nerve enlargement with buckling of nerve.
- CT: calcification extremely rare, may show remodeled widened optic nerve canal.
- MR (Fig. 29.7).
  - o T1 similar and T2 hyperintense to brain parenchyma, with potential T2 focal hyperintense cystic spaces.
  - o Enhancement is variable and correlates with subtype.
- Subtype specific findings.
  - o Syndromic: often bilateral, smooth in contour without significant enhancement. Additional findings of NF1 may be present on imaging as discussed previously.
  - o Sporadic: unilateral with preferential involvement of the chiasm/prechiasmatic segments and enhancement with nodularity.

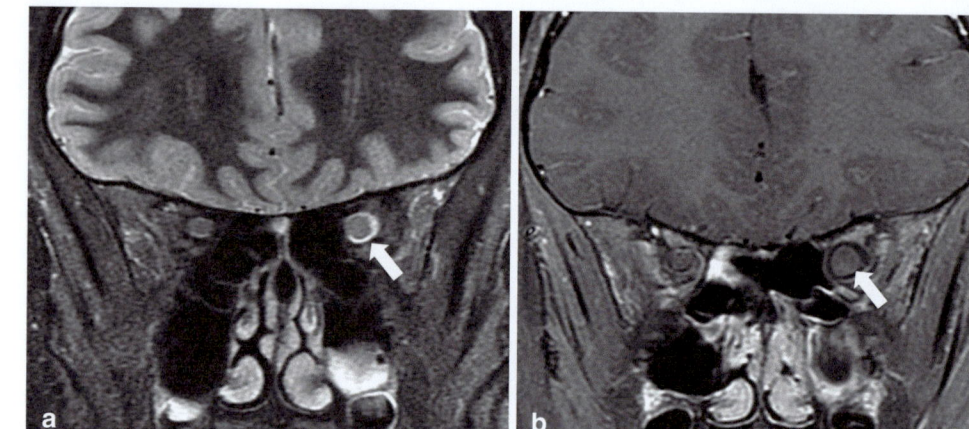
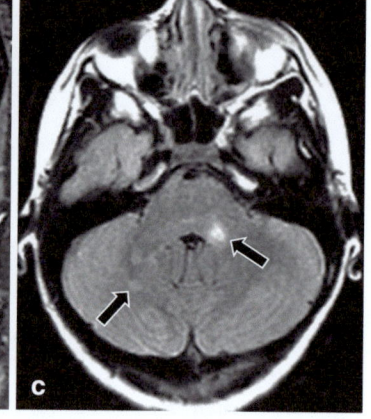

Fig. 29.7 Optic pathway glioma in NF1. (**a**) Coronal STIR and (**b**) T1 contrast-enhanced fat-saturated MR images show enlargement of the left optic nerve (white arrow) without significant enhancement in this syndromic case. (**c**) Axial T2 FLAIR MR image through the brain shows scattered foci of T2 hyperintensity (black arrows) compatible with intracranial vacuolization commonly seen in children with NF1

- - Adult: heterogeneous invasive enhancement.
- Top differential considerations: optic neuritis, optic nerve sheath meningioma, and IOI.

Optic Nerve Sheath Meningioma

- Most common presentation: indolent progressive painless unilateral vision loss with preserved central vision in a middle-aged female.
- Ophthalmoscopic examination: pallor and swelling of the optic disc with characteristic optociliary venous shunting.
- Etiology: tumor arising from arachnoid "cap" cells within the optic nerve sheath (dural sheath). There is an association with neurofibromatosis type 2, particularly in younger patients.
- Pathologic classification is identical to intracranial meningiomas with "meningothelial" the most common subtype. However, they are considered a distinct clinical entity from intracranial meningiomas with orbital extension.
- Management initially consists of careful surveillance on imaging and visual testing. Radiosurgery is the primary treatment modality to halt growth and preserve residual vision. Surgery is limited to aggressive cases with rapid growth or intracranial extension due to the high risk of postoperative vision loss.
- Imaging.
- General: MR is the modality of choice.
- CT: calcification may be seen in a minority of cases.
- MR (Fig. 29.8).
  - T1 with contrast and fat suppression best identifies markedly enhancing well-defined mass arising from the optic nerve sheath surrounding the non-enhancing optic nerve (*doughnut sign*).
    - Variable patterns of tubular/fusiform, en-plaque, or even eccentric masslike enhancement.
    - Characteristic "*Tram track*" appearance on axial images due to perioptic enhancement [9].
  - Noncontrast T1 and T2 signal characteristics are generally similar to soft tissue but variable due to cellularity and mineralization.
  - Increased T2 hyperintense CSF signal with the optic nerve sheath anterior to the tumor ("perioptic cysts") are sometimes seen and considered characteristic.
- Top differential considerations:
  - Optic neuritis and optic nerve glioma should demonstrate pathology centered in the nerve itself rather than the sheath, although this distinction may be difficult.
  - IOI, cellulitis, or lymphomatous disease with isolated perineural involvement are essentially indistinguishable.

29 Imaging of the Orbit (Infection, Inflammation, Benign, and Malignant Lesions)

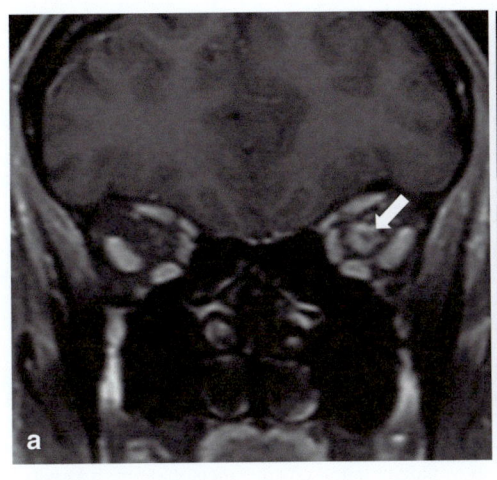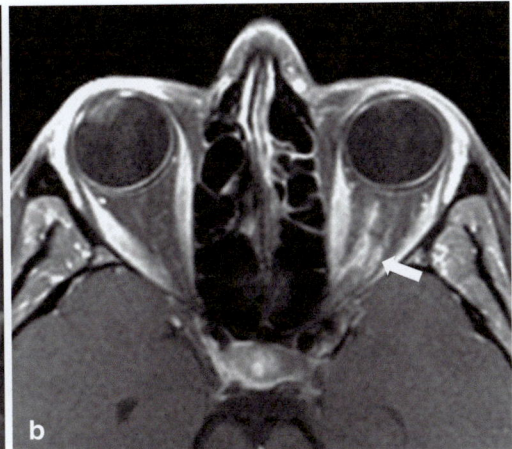

Fig. 29.8 Optic nerve sheath meningioma. (**a**) Coronal and (**b**) axial T1 contrast-enhanced fat-saturated MR images show enhancement of the intraorbital optic nerve sheath circumferentially surrounding the non-enhancing optic nerve (arrows). Axial images demonstrate a *tram-track* pattern of enhancement (arrow)

Orbital Cavernous Venous Malformation (Hemangioma)

- Most common presentation: incidentally discovered orbital intraconal mass in an adult.
  - Represents the most common adult orbital mass.
  - Larger lesions may present with diplopia or painless proptosis.
- Pathology: Slow flow venous vascular malformation with dilated "cavernous" vascular channels.
  - Commonly but incorrectly referred to as "hemangioma," as it is not a neoplasm.
  - Clinically and pathologically different from other facial hemangiomas.
- Imaging.
- General: well-defined, ovoid mass, usually intraconal.
- CT: Homogeneous non-contrast appearance with rare phleboliths. May smoothly remodel bone if large.
- MRI (Fig. 29.9):
  - T2 hyperintense with potential hypointense peripheral "pseudocapsule."
  - T1 progressive enhancement is nearly pathognomonic [10].
    - Early heterogeneous enhancement progresses to homogeneity.
    - The protocol can be designed to include a dedicated delayed phase or alternatively compare earlier acquired sequence to later sequence in the alternative plane.
- Top differential considerations:
  - Lymphatic malformation (Fig. e29.9):
    - Multi-spatial lobulated, multicystic lesion with thin peripheral or no enhancement.
    - Tendency to hemorrhage which results in symptoms from expansile mass effect.
    - Intralesional hemorrhage is evident as fluid-fluid levels of varying signal characteristics.
  - Venous varix:
    - Intermittent proptosis and pain with Valsalva.
    - Best diagnosed on dynamic contrast-enhanced CT obtained prior to and during Valsalva as a tubular enhancing lesion with expansion on provocative maneuvers.

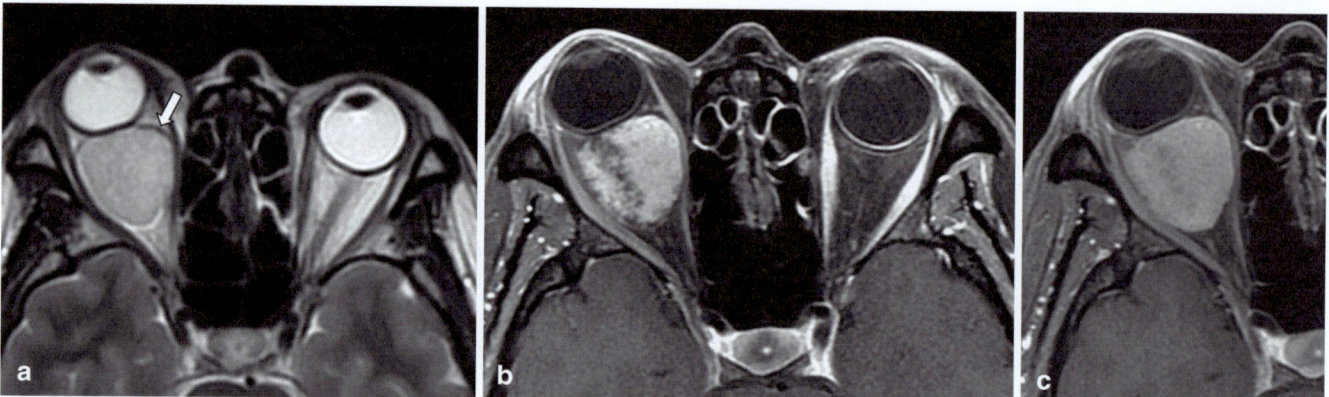

Fig. 29.9 Cavernous venous malformation (hemangioma). (a) Axial T2 MR shows a large intraconal well-defined strikingly hyperintense mass with a thin hypointense pseudocapsule with chemical shift artifact (arrow). Axial T1 fat-saturated contrast-enhanced images obtained (b) immediately following injection and (c) after a short delay show patchy initial enhancement that progressively becomes more uniform. Note is made of unusual mass effect on retrobulbar structures and globe in this case prompting surgical excision

Lymphoma And Lymphoproliferative Disorders

- Most common presentation: older patients with indolent painless proptosis, diplopia, and orbital mass.
- Pathologically, these represent a broad range of reactive and malignant lymphoproliferative lesions.
    - Benign: reactive, polyclonal, or atypical lymphoid hyperplasia, seen in younger patients and treated with steroids. Many cases of hyperplasia can be more accurately characterized as IgG4-related disease.
    - Malignant: lymphoma represents a monoclonal proliferation and overall is the most common adult orbital neoplasm.
        - Majority are low-grade B-cell origin and present without systemic symptoms, classified as extranodal marginal zone lymphoma (EZML) of mucosa-associated lymphoid tissue (MALT).
        - Rarely seen other types of lymphoma which carry worse prognoses including secondary orbital involvement of systemic disease.
        - Risk of systemic lymphoma increased, particularly if bilateral.
        - Treatment with radiotherapy with excellent local control and survival, with chemotherapy/immunotherapy reserved for aggressive lymphomas.
- Imaging (Fig. 29.10).
- Generally, solid uniformly enhancing mass anywhere in the orbit that engulfs and conforms to the shape of adjacent structures.
    - Isolated lacrimal, extraconal fat, extraocular muscle, and conjunctival lesions all possible.
    - Diffuse pattern of infiltration with intraconal and perineural extension.
    - Benign lymphoproliferative lesions are usually bilateral, and lymphoma is usually unilateral, but exceptions are common.
    - CT.
        - Noncontrast may be slightly hyperdense (due to increased cellularity) with diffuse homogenous enhancement.
        - Typically, there is no bone destruction unless aggressive histology.
    - MR.
        - High cellularity results in a T2 intermediate signal and restricted diffusion with decreased ADC values [11].
        - T1 homogeneous avid enhancement.
    - PET CT: FDG avid. Systemic imaging is recommended at diagnosis due to the elevated risk of systemic lymphoma.
- Top differential considerations: extremely broad differential due to the protean nature of lymphoma which may mimic IOI, sarcoidosis, thyroid eye disease, lacrimal gland epithelial tumor, orbital metastasis, and rarely cellulitis.

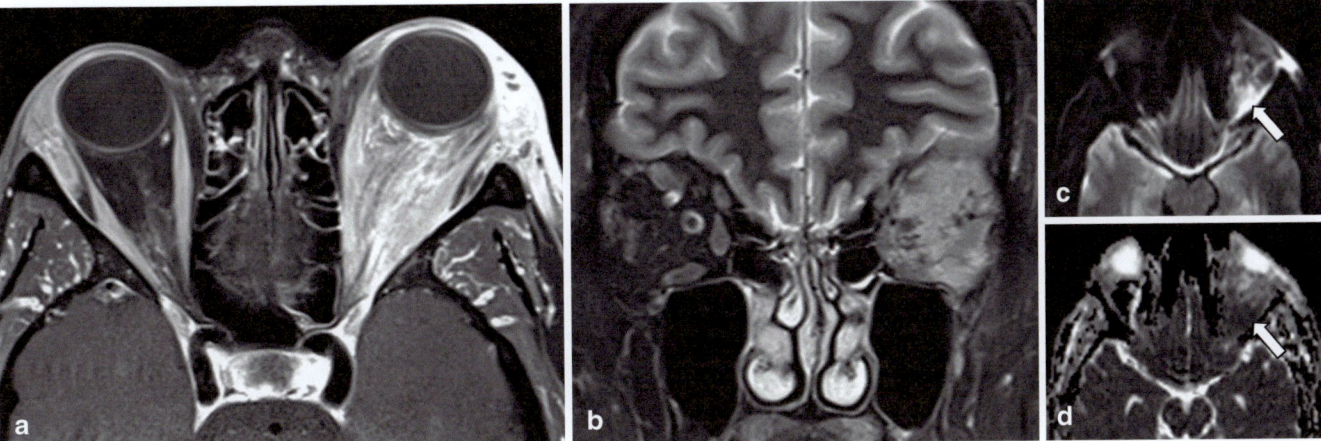

Fig. 29.10 Orbital lymphoma. (**a**) Axial T1 contrast-enhanced MR shows infiltrating enhancement of the left intraconal and extraconal retrobulbar fat with resultant proptosis, although no deformation of the globe. (**b**) Coronal STIR MR shows a T2 hyperintense signal throughout the intraconal and extraconal fat engulfing the optic nerve, rectus musculature, and vasculature. (**c**) Axial DWI and (**d**) ADC MR demonstrate relatively restricted diffusion (arrows)

Lacrimal Gland Mass

- Most common presentation: progressive proptosis and clinically evident mass; diplopia, pain, and sensory loss if higher grade epithelial malignancy (bone or perineural involvement).
- Lymphomas (discussed above) represent approximately 50% of lacrimal neoplasm.
- The remainder are masses of epithelial origin, of which approximately 50% represent benign Pleomorphic adenoma (a.k.a. benign mixed tumor). Often occur in middle age.
- Malignant epithelial lesions are overall rare, representing ~2% of orbital neoplasms, present in the elderly, and may represent malignant transformation.
  - Epithelial malignant pathologies include minor salivary origin (adenoid cystic carcinoma, carcinoma ex pleomorphic adenoma, and acinic cell carcinoma), squamous cell carcinoma, or adenocarcinoma.
  - Adenoid cystic carcinoma most common malignancy (~50%).
- Treatment:
  - Lymphoma: radiotherapy as above.
  - Benign pleomorphic adenoma: surgical excision without capsular disruption (seeding).
  - Epithelial malignancies are divided into low and high grades:
    - Low grade demonstrates a good prognosis following surgical resection.
    - High grade requires combined surgical resection and radiotherapy.
    - High incidence of local and regional/distant (perineural) recurrence, particularly with adenoid cystic carcinoma.
- Imaging (Fig. 29.11).
- In general, the first step is to confirm the presence of isolated unilateral mass. If there are bilateral findings, systemic etiologies should be considered as discussed below.
  - Lacrimal mass (superior lateral extraconal mass) more commonly arising from the orbital lobe of the gland with a regional mass effect.
    - Benign: smooth margins, oval, encapsulated.
    - Malignant: unilateral irregular lacrimal mass with extension to bone and nerves.
- CT.
  - Smooth osseous remodeling suggests benign, or lower-grade malignancy but may also be seen in higher-grade lesions.
  - Bone erosion and irregular destruction are the best predictors of malignancy on CT.
- MRI.
  - T2 hyperintense well-defined solidly enhancing mass with facilitated diffusion suggests pleomorphic adenoma.
  - Heterogeneous irregular mass with regions of significant T2 hypointensity worrisome for malignancy.
  - Perineural enhancement should be assessed with particular attention to the lacrimal nerve, frontal nerve, superior orbital fissure, cavernous sinus, and so on.
- Top differential considerations [12].
  - If unilateral:
    - Lymphoma: uniform signal mass or expansion conforming to adjacent structures.

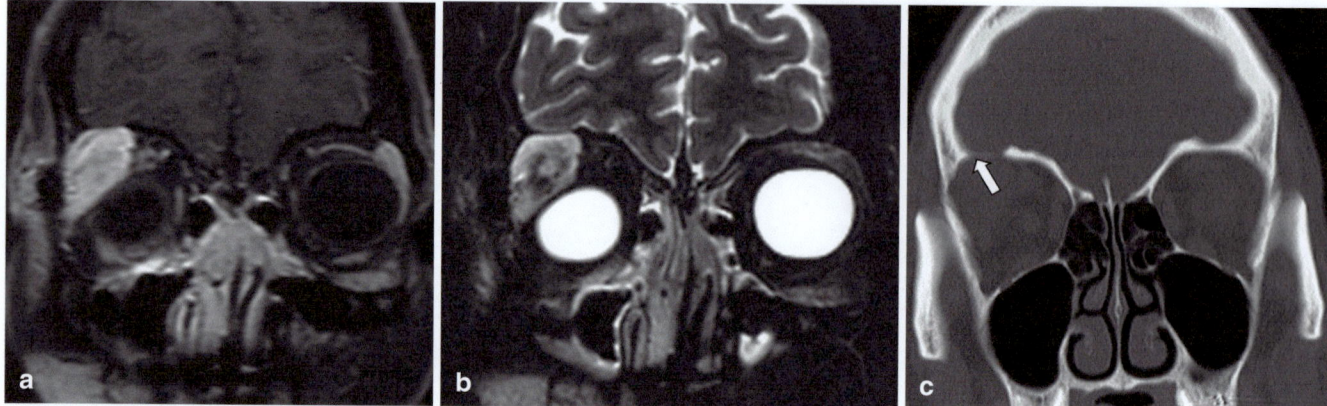

Fig. 29.11 Lacrimal gland epithelial neoplasm. (**a**) Coronal T1 post-contrast fat-saturated MR shows a solidly enhancing mass in the right superolateral orbit inseparable from the lacrimal gland. (**b**) Coronal STIR MR shows marked T2 heterogeneity as well as deformity of the adjacent globe. (**c**) Coronal noncontrast CT with bone algorithm best shows scalloped erosive remodeling of the orbital roof (arrow). Pathology proved to be adenoid cystic carcinoma

- Dacryoadenitis: painful tender enlargement with adjacent inflammatory changes on imaging.
- IOI: adjacent inflammatory change, involvement of additional orbital structures.
o If bilateral (Fig. e29.10):
  - Sjogren syndrome: enlargement and slightly heterogeneous enhancement early in the disease, atrophy in the late stage. No osseous changes. Parotid cystic change or calcifications at the margins of the study help confirm the imaging diagnosis.
  - Sarcoidosis (granulomatous disease): uniform enlargement and enhancement.
  - IgG4-related disease (Mikulicz syndrome).
  - Lymphoproliferative disorders.

References

1. Som PM, Curtin HD. Head and neck imaging. 5th ed. Elsevier; 2011.
2. Sepahdari AR, Aakalu VK, Kapur R, Michals EA, Saran N, French A, Mafee MF. MRI of orbital cellulitis and orbital abscess: the role of diffusion-weighted imaging. AJR Am J Roentgenol. 2009;193(3):W244–50. https://doi.org/10.2214/AJR.08.1838.
3. Dutra BG, da Rocha AJ, Nunes RH, Júnior MACM. Neuromyelitis optica spectrum disorders: spectrum of mr imaging findings and their differential diagnosis. Radiographics. 2018;38(1):169–93. https://doi.org/10.1148/rg.2018170141. Erratum in: Radiographics. 2018 Mar-Apr;38(2):662.
4. Debnam JM, Koka K, Esmaeli B. Extrathyroidal manifestations of thyroid disease: graves eye disease. Neuroimaging Clin N Am. 2021;31(3):367–78. https://doi.org/10.1016/j.nic.2021.04.006.
5. Gujar SK, Gandhi D. Congenital malformations of the orbit. Neuroimaging Clin N Am. 2011;21(3):585–602, viii. Epub 2011 Jun 25. https://doi.org/10.1016/j.nic.2011.05.004.
6. Jacquemin C, Bosley TM, Svedberg H. Orbit deformities in craniofacial neurofibromatosis type 1. AJNR Am J Neuroradiol. 2003;24(8):1678–82.
7. Sirin S, Schlamann M, Metz KA, Bornfeld N, Schweiger B, Holdt M, Schuendeln MM, Lohbeck S, Krasny A, Goericke SL. Diagnostic image quality of gadolinium-enhanced T1-weighted MRI with and without fat saturation in children with retinoblastoma. Pediatr Radiol. 2013;43(6):716–24. https://doi.org/10.1007/s00247-012-2576-y. Epub 2013 Jan 13.
8. Taylor T, Jaspan T, Milano G, Gregson R, Parker T, Ritzmann T, Benson C, Walker D, PLAN Study Group. Radiological classification of optic pathway gliomas: experience of a modified functional classification system. Br J Radiol. 2008;81(970):761–6. https://doi.org/10.1259/bjr/65246351.
9. Eddleman CS, Liu JK. Optic nerve sheath meningioma: current diagnosis and treatment. Neurosurg Focus. 2007;23(5):E4. https://doi.org/10.3171/FOC-07/11/E4.
10. Rootman DB, Heran MK, Rootman J, White VA, Luemsamran P, Yucel YH. Cavernous venous malformations of the orbit (so-called cavernous haemangioma): a comprehensive evaluation of their clinical, imaging and histologic nature. Br J Ophthalmol. 2014;98(7):880–8. https://doi.org/10.1136/bjophthalmol-2013-304460.
11. Haradome K, Haradome H, Usui Y, Ueda S, Kwee TC, Saito K, Tokuuye K, Matsubayashi J, Nagao T, Goto H. Orbital lymphoproliferative disorders (OLPDs): value of MR imaging for differentiating orbital lymphoma from benign OPLDs. AJNR Am J Neuroradiol. 2014;35(10):1976–82. https://doi.org/10.3174/ajnr.A3986. Epub 2014 May 29.
12. Gao Y, Moonis G, Cunnane ME, Eisenberg RL. Lacrimal gland masses. AJR Am J Roentgenol. 2013;201(3):W371–81. https://doi.org/10.2214/AJR.12.9553.

Imaging of Sinonasal Disease (Infection, Tumors)

Nathan Gruenhagen and Mohit Agarwal

Paranasal Sinus Anatomy Overview

- Paranasal sinuses are air-filled cavities around the nasal cavity. There are four pairs of paranasal sinuses—frontal, ethmoid, sphenoid, and maxillary. All paranasal sinuses are lined by respiratory epithelium.
- The superior, middle, and inferior turbinates are bony protuberances arising from the lateral wall of the nasal cavity. The superior, middle, and inferior meatuses are air passageways inferior and lateral to their respective turbinates.
- The anterior ethmoid air cells, frontal sinuses, and maxillary sinuses drain into the middle meatus via the hiatus semilunaris. The ostiomeatal unit includes the ethmoidal infundibulum, uncinate process, middle meatus, frontal recess, and hiatus semilunaris.
- The posterior ethmoid air cells and sphenoid sinuses drain into the superior meatus.
- Multiple named ethmoid air cells are important to recognize. The bulla ethmoidalis is located immediately posterior to the frontal recess and forms the roof of the middle meatus. An agger nasi cell is the anterior-most ethmoid air cell (Fig. e30.1) (All electronic images (Figs. e30.1–e30.15) can be found on this chapter's website on SpringerLink: https://doi.org/10.1007/978-3-031-55124-6_30), a Haller cell is located inferior to the orbit (Fig. e30.2), and an Onodi air cell is a posterosuperior ethmoidal air cell which extends superior to the sphenoid sinus.
- The drainage pathways and anatomic variations are important to identify on imaging, as blockages in the pathways are thought to contribute to inflammation of the sinuses, and variant anatomy can lead to risk of surgical complications if not appropriately identified.

Sinonasal Infections

ACUTE RHINOSINUSITIS

- Acute rhinosinusitis typically begins in the setting of an upper viral respiratory infection which gets complicated by bacterial superinfection.
- Complications include orbital and intracranial extension. Orbital complications are more frequently encountered and tend to occur in otherwise healthy young children less than 5 years of age [1].
- The key orbital complications to be aware of on imaging include orbital cellulitis, subperiosteal, and orbital abscess formation.
- Intracranial complications include subdural empyema, meningitis, cerebritis, and brain abscess. Intracranial complications most commonly occur secondary to frontal sinusitis.
- Infection may spread to the cavernous sinuses via the draining veins resulting in cavernous sinus thrombosis.

Imaging

- Imaging of acute bacterial rhinosinusitis is indicated when there are suspected complications.
- Air fluid levels within the paranasal sinuses could be indicative of acute rhinosinusitis in the appropriate clinical setting (Fig. e30.3). Peripheral mucosal thickening and gas bubbles can also be seen. However, air fluid levels can also be seen in intubated patients as a reactive phenomenon without infection.

Supplementary Information The online version contains supplementary material available at https://doi.org/10.1007/978-3-031-55124-6_30.

N. Gruenhagen · M. Agarwal (✉)
Medical College of Wisconsin, Milwaukee, WI, USA
e-mail: magarwal@mcw.edu

- Orbital cellulitis is seen as stranding of the orbital fat with inflammatory enhancing soft tissue adjacent to the involved sinus. Breech of the intervening bone is not necessary as the infection can spread to the orbit via the bridging veins [1].
- Rim-enhancing fluid collection, usually in the subperiosteal location, indicates the development of orbital abscess (Fig. 30.1).
- Subdural empyema is a collection of purulent material in the subdural space that develops most commonly as a complication of frontal sinusitis. The fluid collection shows rim enhancement and restricted diffusion on MRI (Fig. e30.4). The intervening bone may or may not be breeched [1].
- Smooth enhancement of adjacent pachymeninges and/or leptomeninges indicates the development of meningitis.
- Further complications may be seen in the form of cerebritis (Fig. 30.5) and intracranial abscess formation where focal edema/ abnormal long TR signal is seen in the brain parenchyma in the former, and rim-enhancing fluid collection with restricted diffusion is seen in the latter.
- Frontal bone osteomyelitis may develop with associated subperiosteal abscess formation, termed "Pott's puffy tumor," which presents as tender swelling on the forehead of a patient with frontal sinusitis (Fig. 30.2).
- Enlarged cavernous sinuses with convex margins and filling defects on post-contrast images should alert the radi-

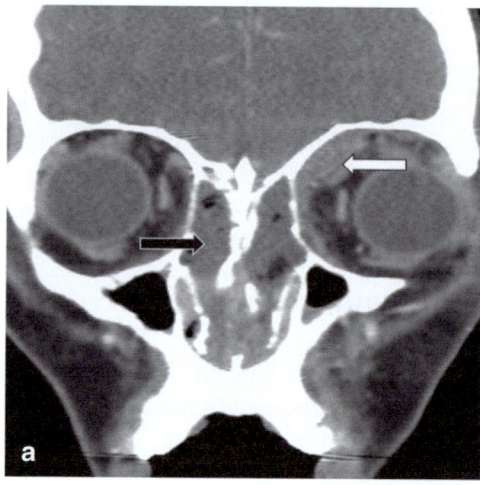
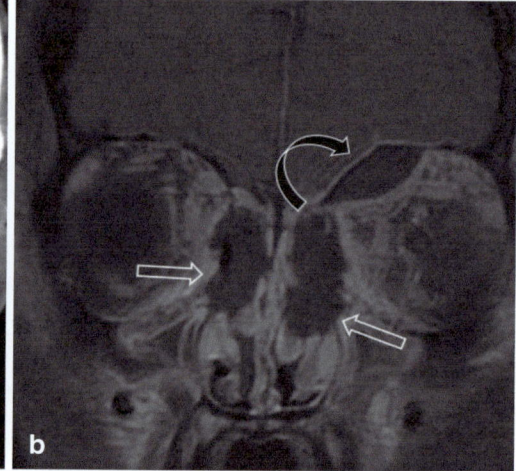

Fig. 30.1 Acute sinusitis complicated by orbital subperiosteal abscess. (a) Coronal soft tissue algorithm shows opacification of the nasal cavity (black arrow). Soft tissue attenuation is also seen along the medial aspect of the left orbit (white solid arrow). (b) Coronal postcontrast fat-suppressed T1W MRI demonstrates peripheral enhancement throughout the nasal cavity (white open arrows). Enhancement of the left medial orbit is also present with subperiosteal abscess formation seen along the superomedial left orbit (black curved arrow)

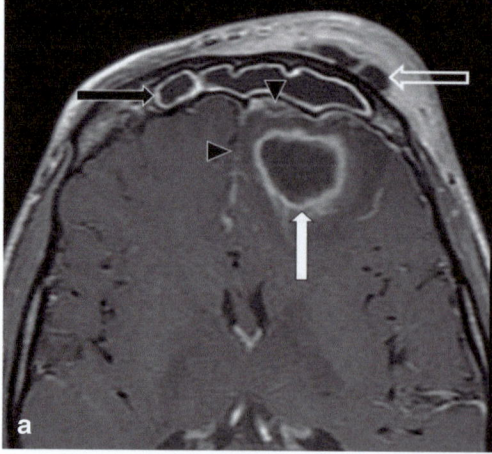
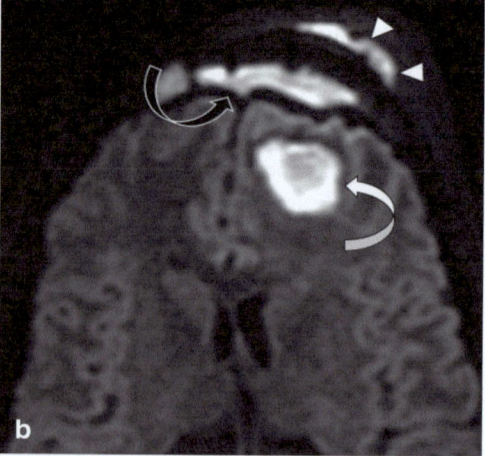

Fig. 30.2 Acute sinusitis complicated by Potts puffy tumor and intracranial abscess. (a) Axial postcontrast T1W MRI demonstrates opacification of the frontal sinuses with peripheral enhancement (black arrow). There is thickening and enhancement of the soft tissues overlying the left frontal sinus with fluid signal overlying the left frontal bone (open white arrow) representing Potts puffy tumor, which refers to a subperiosteal abscess as a complication of acute sinusitis. A ring-enhancing lesion is seen in the left frontal lobe compatible with abscess (white solid arrow). Meningeal thickening and enhancement are also seen overlying the left frontal lobe (black arrowheads). (b) The fluid collections within the frontal sinuses (curved black arrow), the forehead soft tissues (white arrowheads), and the brain (curved white arrow) demonstrate restricted diffusion on DWI MRI images suggestive of purulent material

ologist for the development of cavernous sinus thrombosis. The superior ophthalmic veins are dilated and there may be proptosis with enlargement of the extra-ocular muscles (Fig. 30.3).

ODONTOGENIC SINUSITIS

- Inflammatory dental disease can frequently be the cause of maxillary sinusitis.
- Periapical dental disease can result in bone dehiscence between the teeth and the alveolar recess of the maxillary sinus and can lead to dental infection spreading into the sinus.
- Important to check for this bone dehiscence in isolated maxillary sinus mucosal disease, especially that involving the alveolar recess (Fig. e30.5).

ACUTE INVASIVE FUNGAL SINUSITIS

- Aggressive infection typically occurs in diabetics and immunosuppressed patients.
- *Aspergillus* and *Mucormycetes* are the most frequently cultured organisms [2].

- Infection usually starts in the nasal cavity with ulceration of the nasal mucosa, with rapid progression within days to involve the paranasal sinuses, adjacent soft tissue, bone, and vascular structures.
- High mortality rate.

Imaging

- Imaging findings include mucosal thickening and opacification of the paranasal sinuses, commonly the ethmoid and sphenoid sinuses.
- Focal areas of bone erosion are seen with rapid progression of soft tissue thickening around the infected sinuses with the involvement of the premaxillary and retroantral soft tissues and the orbit (Fig. 30.4).
- Enhancing soft tissue within the sinuses and the soft tissues around the sinuses. Focal intervening areas of non-enhancement are an ominous sign and are indicative of necrotic/gangrenous tissue (black turbinate sign) [2].
- The process is angioinvasive, and arterial narrowing, occlusion, and pseudoaneurysm formation may be seen.

CHRONIC SINUSITIS

- Chronic sinusitis represents inflammation of the sinus mucosa for greater than 12 weeks.
- Disease processes with abnormal ciliary function such as cystic fibrosis and primary ciliary dyskinesis predispose to repeated sinus infections and chronic sinusitis.
- Imaging is indicated for presurgical planning, as chronic sinusitis is thought to be caused by obstruction of drainage pathways. Functional endoscopic sinus surgery is utilized to identify and remove any obstructing lesions.
- Delineation of variant anatomy is vital to avoid surgical complications.

Imaging

- Chronic sinusitis is demonstrated on imaging as a mucosal thickening and/or opacification of the affected paranasal sinuses. Thickening of the sinus walls can occur and is termed chronic osteitis (Fig. e30.6).
- There may be sinus atelectasis due to chronic obstruction and reduced volume of the sinus. Maxillary sinus atelectasis is associated with sagging of the orbital floor and enophthalmos [3].
- Areas of calcification/mineralization/inspissation may be seen.
- Fluid levels indicate an acute exacerbation of chronic sinusitis.

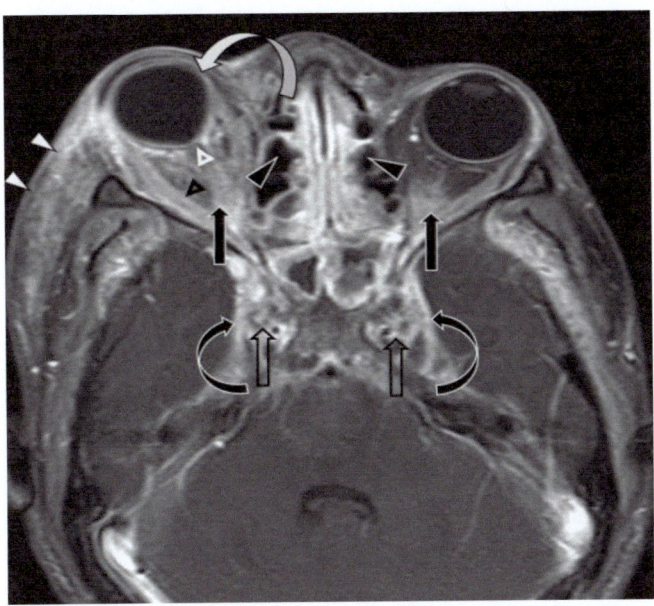

Fig. 30.3 Cavernous sinus thrombophlebitis. Axial postcontrast fat-suppressed T1W MRI shows enhancement throughout the ethmoid air cells (black arrowheads). Enlargement of the cavernous sinuses with regions of non-enhancement is compatible with thrombosis (black open arrows). Surrounding inflammatory changes result in enhancement surrounding the cavernous sinuses (black curved arrows). Additionally, right-sided proptosis is present (white curved arrow) with tenting of the globe (open white arrowhead). There is also thickening of the right-sided extra-ocular muscles (black open arrowhead), enhancement of right face soft tissues (white arrowheads), and infiltration of the right greater than left orbital soft tissues (black solid arrows)

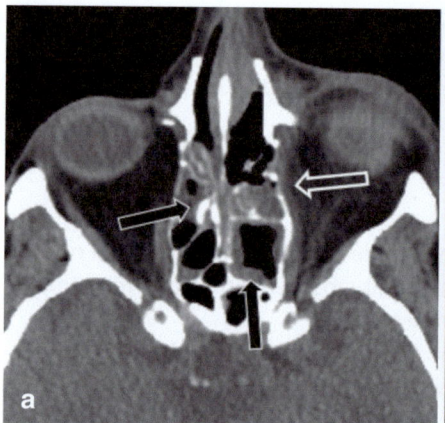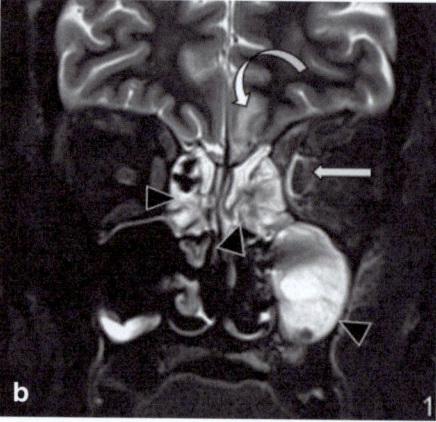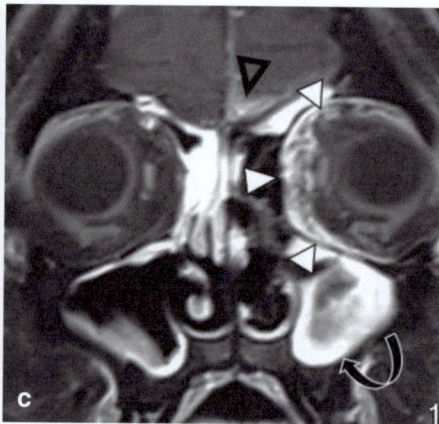

Fig. 30.4 Acute invasive fungal sinusitis. Acute onset left orbital pain in a patient on immunosuppressive therapy. (**a**) Axial soft tissue algorithm CT demonstrates mucosal thickening and opacification of multiple ethmoid air cells (black arrows). Soft tissue stranding is present within the medial left orbit (white open arrow). (**b**) Coronal STIR MRI shows a high T2 signal in the maxillary sinuses and ethmoid air cells (black arrowheads) with a high T2 signal also seen within the medial aspect of the orbit surrounding the medial rectus muscle indicating orbital invasion (white solid arrow). Increased T2 signal in the region of the left frontal lobe is compatible with intracranial extension (white curved arrow). (**c**) Coronal postcontrast fat-suppressed T1W MRI demonstrates diffuse enhancement throughout the paranasal sinuses (black curved arrow) with enhancement seen along the superior, medial, and inferior aspects of the left orbit (white arrowheads) compatible with the orbital spread of the infection. Enhancement overlying the left frontal lobe is compatible with intracranial extension (black open arrowhead)

ALLERGIC FUNGAL SINUSITIS

- Caused by a hypersensitivity reaction to fungi.
- Typically seen in immunocompetent patients as opposed to acute invasive fungal sinusitis which is seen in immunosuppressed patients.
- Patients typically have a history of atopy and asthma.

Imaging
- Allergic fungal sinusitis is characterized by the presence of thick eosinophilic fungal-laden mucin of "peanut-butter-like" consistency [3].
- Classic appearance includes opacification of multiple paranasal sinuses with hyper-attenuating components on CT and expansion of the affected sinuses.
- MR appearance can show variable T1 signal intensity. The profound central hypointense signal is seen on T2-weighted imaging, thought to be due to the deposition of heavy metals such as iron, manganese, and magnesium, which mimics air (Fig. 30.5). The mucosal lining that is pushed to the periphery of the sinus cavities enhances with contrast.
- This disease is noninvasive and does not demonstrate the aggressive features seen in acute invasive fungal sinusitis.

SINONASAL MYCETOMA

- Also known as "fungus balls", sinonasal mycetoma is a noninvasive infection associated with Aspergillus.
- This represents a chronic inflammatory response and is seen in immunocompetent patients.

Imaging
- Opacification of a paranasal sinus is seen with hyperattenuating components and dense calcifications seen on CT [2, 3].
- The maxillary sinus is most commonly involved and may demonstrate chronic osteitis.
- If extensive dense calcifications are present, may appear as T2 hypointense on MR imaging (Fig. e30.7).

ANTRONASAL/ANTROCHOANAL POLYP

- Polyps arise within the respiratory epithelium and are a result of hypertrophied respiratory epithelium consisting of edematous submucosa and mixed inflammatory infiltrate.
- When large, these polyps may cause obstruction of the nasal passages.

- One of the most common solitary polyps is the antronasal polyp.
- Treatment is surgical with complete removal of the intramaxillary component of the polyp to avoid recurrence.

Imaging

- Antronasal polyps arise in the maxillary sinus and extend into the nasal cavity via the maxillary infundibulum or via accessory maxillary ostia.
- Antronasal polyps can result in bony remodeling, typically enlarging the maxillary ostium as it passes through it resulting in a classic dumbbell-shaped low-density polypoid mass on CT. On MRI, they are usually of fluid intensity and show enhancement of the surrounding mucosa [4].
- Large lesions may extend into the pharynx via the posterior choana, thence termed antrochoanal polyps (Fig. 30.6).

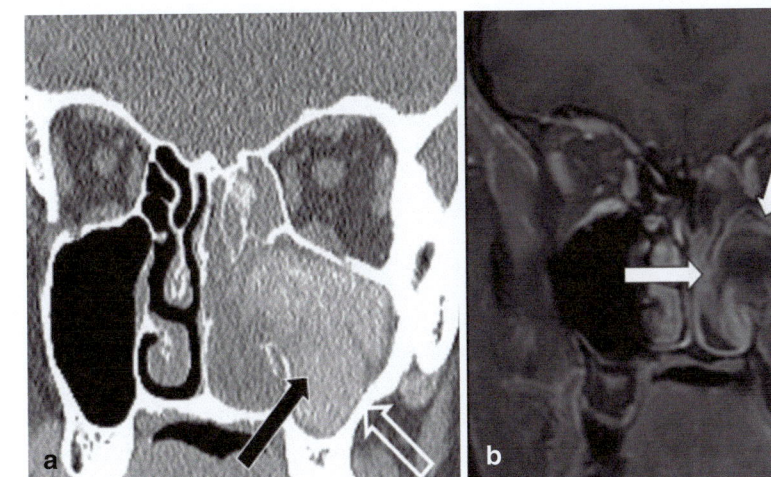
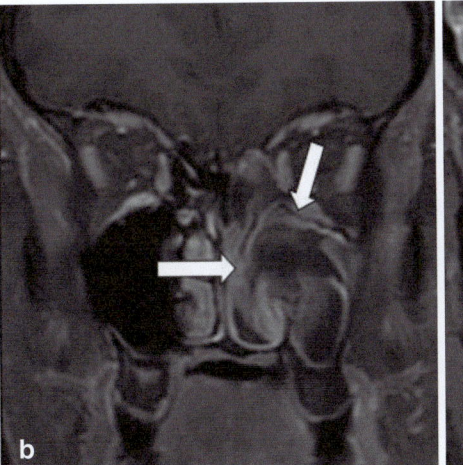
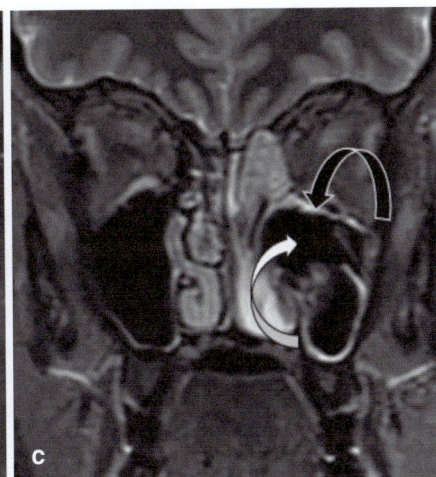

Fig. 30.5 Allergic fungal sinusitis. Left nasal obstruction in a patient with a history of asthma. (a) Coronal soft tissue algorithm CT shows opacification of the left maxillary sinus and nasal cavity with hyperattenuating components seen within the left maxillary sinus (black arrow). Chronic osteitis involving the left maxillary sinus walls is also seen (white open arrow). (b) Coronal postcontrast fat-suppressed T1W MRI demonstrates enhancing mucosa within the affected sinus (white arrows) with a lack of enhancement centrally within the sinus. (c) Coronal STIR MRI shows hyperintense mucosa (black curved arrow) and profound hypointense signal within the diseased sinus that mimics air (white curved arrow)

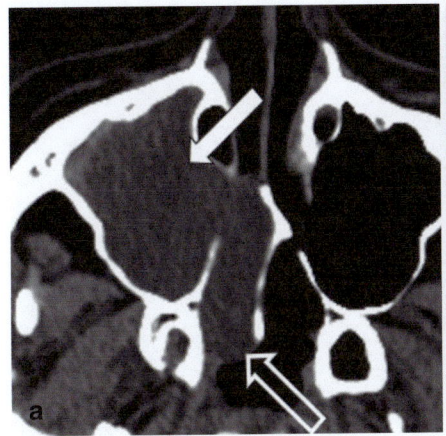
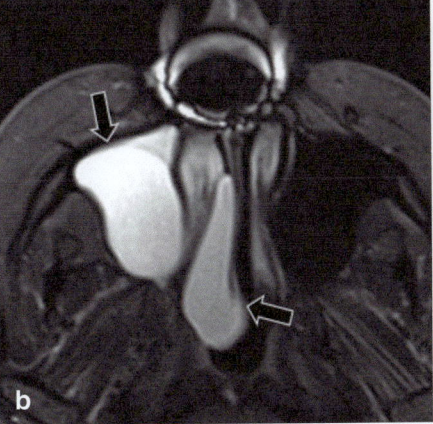
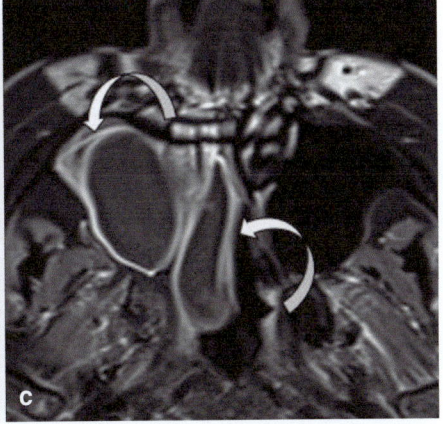

Fig. 30.6 Antrochoanal polyp. (a) Axial soft tissue algorithm CT shows complete opacification of the right maxillary sinus (white solid arrow) with extension of the lesion into the nasal cavity and right posterior choana (white open arrow). (b) Axial STIR MRI demonstrates a homogeneous high T2 fluid-like signal within the lesion (black arrows). (c) Axial postcontrast fat-suppressed T1W MRI demonstrates no enhancement of the lesion. The peripheral enhancement is due to the enhancing mucosa (white curved arrows)

SINONASAL POLYPOSIS

- The presence of multiple polyps is termed sinonasal polyposis.
- Pathogenesis is multifactorial with allergy, asthma, and other factors related to chronic sinus inflammation implicated in causation.

Imaging
- CT demonstrates multiple soft tissue masses arising within the nasal cavity and paranasal sinuses [5].
- Opacification of multiple sinuses with mucous secondary to obstruction is commonly seen (Fig. e30.8).
- Commonly associated with bone remodeling and demineralization.
- MR demonstrates diffuse T2 hyperintense lobular mucosal thickening.
- Contrast-enhanced MR demonstrates superficial enhancement of the mucosal tissue without central enhancement.

MUCOCELE

- Mucoceles result from chronic obstruction of the sinus drainage pathway with a collection of mucoid material in the sinus cavity and subsequent sinus expansion [6].
- Obstruction could be due to chronic inflammation, neoplasm, or post-surgical.
- Clinical symptoms depend on the location, with orbital symptoms being common due to encroachment by the expanded sinuses on the orbit.

Imaging
- The most common imaging appearance on CT is a low-density lesion with expansion of the affected sinus and remodeling of the sinus wall [6].
- Mucoceles containing proteinaceous material may demonstrate slightly higher density.
- Non-proteinaceous mucoceles demonstrate typical simple fluid characteristic on MR imaging, including hypointense signal on T1-weighted images and hyperintense signal on T2-weighted images (Fig. 30.7).
- The presence of proteinaceous material within a mucocele can increase the intrinsic T1 signal.
- Mucoceles typically do not demonstrate enhancement. If a thick peripheral enhancement is present, a superimposed infectious process could be present, termed "mucopyocele."

SARCOIDOSIS

- Sinonasal sarcoidosis is a granulomatous inflammatory condition, most common in African American females. It may occur as a part of multisystem sarcoidosis or more rarely as an isolated form [7, 8].
- Non-caseating granulomas are pathologic hallmarks of the disease.
- Nasal obstruction and sinusitis symptoms are the most common clinical features.
- Sinonasal sarcoidosis is typically diagnosed on biopsy.

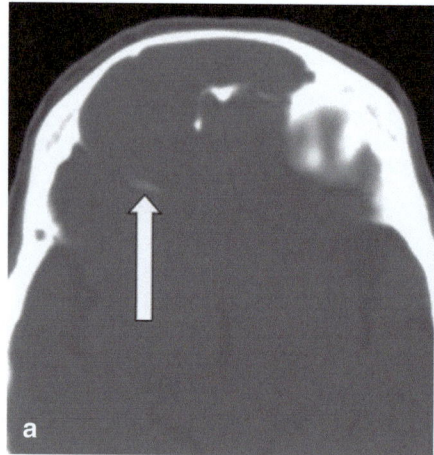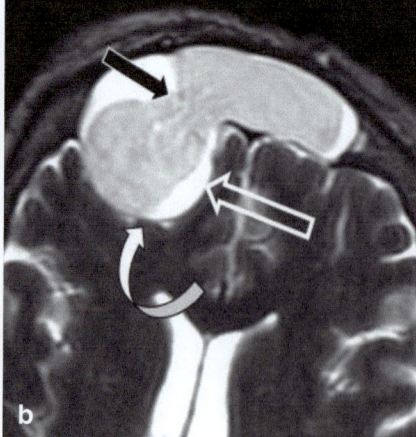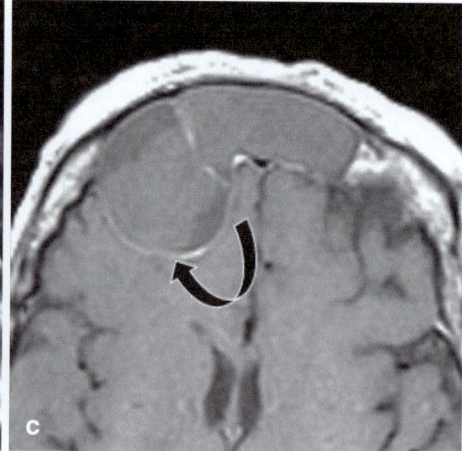

Fig. 30.7 Mucocele. (**a**) Axial soft tissue algorithm CT demonstrates opacification of the frontal sinuses with surrounding bony expansion (white arrow). (**b**) Axial T2W MRI shows a high T2 signal peripherally (open white arrow) and an intermediate T2 signal centrally within the sinuses (black solid arrow). (**c**) Axial postcontrast T1W MRI demonstrates no enhancement. Mild T1W hyperintensity is due to inspissated/proteinaceous contents (black curved arrow)

30 Imaging of Sinonasal Disease (Infection, Tumors)

Imaging

- Sinonasal sarcoidosis typically manifests as a paranasal soft tissue tumor with homogenous enhancement.
- Imaging findings can also include opacification of the sinuses similar to sinonasal polyposis.
- Cranial nerve involvement of systemic sarcoidosis may be seen concurrently, where retrograde extension along the nerves can be noted. Nerve involvement is best demonstrated on contrast-enhanced MRI [7, 8].

GRANULOMATOSIS WITH POLYANGIITIS

- Granulomatosis with polyanigiitis (GPA) is a granulomatous vasculitis involving small- to medium-sized arteries and is associated with antineutrphil cytoplasm antibodies (cANCA).
- GPA most commonly affects the kidneys, lungs, trachea, and nasal cavity.
- Common symptoms include nasal obstruction which can be mistaken for chronic sinusitis clinically.
- Diagnosis is usually made on biopsy.
- Systemic disease is usually treated with immunosuppressive agents.

Imaging

- Nasal cavity manifestations include soft tissue nodularity which can be associated with osseous erosions.
- Erosion of cartilage and bone can result in septal perforation and destruction of the turbinates. Collapse of the nasal cartilage may result in "saddle-nose" deformity [9].
- Bone erosion and chronic osteitis may be seen (Fig. e30.9).
- A rare complication is fistula formation between the oral and nasal cavities.

Overview of Sinonasal Neoplasm Imaging

- A wide variety of benign and malignant neoplastic processes can affect the paranasal sinuses.
- The main role of imaging in sinonasal tumors is tumor mapping, i.e., to describe the extent of the tumor and associated invasion. A determination of whether the tumor may be of a benign or malignant nature is also important [10–12].
- Tumor mapping aids in planning the surgical approach and radiation treatment field. Intracranial and orbital extension as well as perineural spread can alter the surgical course and radiation planning.
- MRI is the favored modality for tumor mapping and tumor surveillance following treatment.
- Tumors within a single sinus with well-circumscribed margins, homogeneous CT attenuation, and high T2 signal suggest a benign entity.
- Tumors extending beyond sinus walls with irregular margins, high CT attenuation, bone invasion, and low T2 signal suggest a possible malignant process.
- Pathology is required to determine the diagnosis in most cases.

Benign Tumors

OSTEOMA

- Benign tumor of fibro-osseous origin.
- Most common benign sinonasal tumor.
- Usually do not require treatment, unless they are large and obstruct sinus outflow tracts.
- Common in the frontal and ethmoid sinuses.
- The presence of multiple osteomas is associated with Gardner's syndrome, which is a form of familial adenomatous polyposis (FAP).

Imaging

- Ossification appears homogeneously dense on CT typically with round borders and no aggressive features (Fig. e30.10).
- Typically demonstrates a broad base along the bony sinus, although some may appear pedunculated.
- Ossified material appears dark on T2 imaging depending on the density of ossification.
- Fibrous components may occasionally be present and may result in enhancement and increased signal on T2-weighted images.

FIBROUS DYSPLASIA

- Fibrous dysplasia is another fibro-osseous lesion that can occur in medullary bone throughout the body including the paranasal sinuses, nasal cavity, and skull base.
- Occurs most commonly in the first decades of life and may continue until skeletal maturation.
- Polyostic fibrous dysplasia can be seen with McCune-Albright syndrome where endocrine abnormalities and classic café au lait skin lesions are also seen.

Imaging

- Classically appears as a "ground glass" matrix expanding osseous structures including the diploic space and thinning of the overlying cortex.
- Fibrous dysplasia does not respect suture lines and can affect multiple bones (Fig. 30.8).
- Diagnosis may be difficult on MR imaging where fibrous components can demonstrate hyperintense signal on T2-weighted images and enhancement on T1W + C images, resembling a neoplasm. CT imaging is characteristic, demonstrating the classic "ground glass" matrix and bone expansion.

OSSIFYING FIBROMA

- Benign fibro-osseous lesion occurs most commonly in females between ages 10 and 40 years of age.
- These are benign lesions but can demonstrate locally aggressive features.
- A high rate of recurrence is seen with incomplete resection.

Imaging

- Classic CT appearance is a round lesion with a peripheral sclerotic rim and soft tissue density centrally representing fibrous tissue.
- The lesions can be expansile and appear similar to fibrous dysplasia.
- MR appearance is variable and can demonstrate heterogeneous enhancement of the fibrous regions of the lesion.

SCHWANNOMA

- Schwannomas arise from the spindle cells of peripheral nerve sheaths and most commonly occur in the ethmoid sinuses when involving the sinonasal region [13].
- An increased incidence of sinonasal schwannomas is seen in neurofibromatosis type 2.
- Surgical excision is typically curative, and recurrence is rare.

Imaging

- Typically appear as expansile tumors resulting in bony remodeling.
- Sinonasal nerve sheath tumors demonstrate homogeneous CT attenuation and can have associated cysts.
- The typical MR appearance of nerve sheath tumors includes hypointensity on T1-weighted images and hyperintensity on T2-weighted images in a classic "target" pattern. The T2 signal intensity of sinonasal schwannomas is however lower than schwannomas in other parts of the body.
- Patchy enhancement pattern is seen on T1W + C.

PAPILLOMA

- Papillomas arise from the mucosal lining of the sinonasal tract, also known as the Schneiderian mucosa.
- The three subtypes of papilloma include exophytic (fungiform), inverted, and oncocytic papillomas in order of decreasing prevalence.

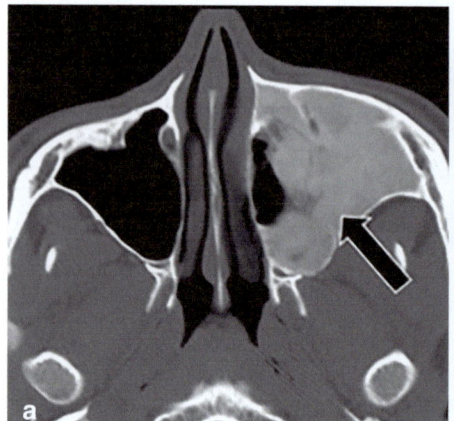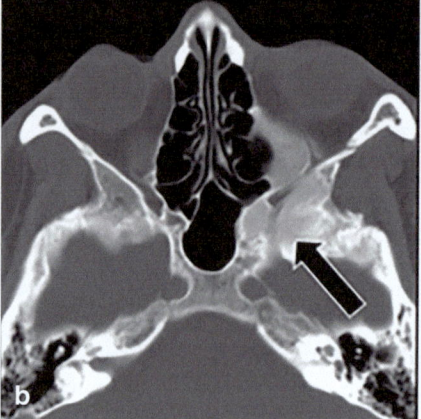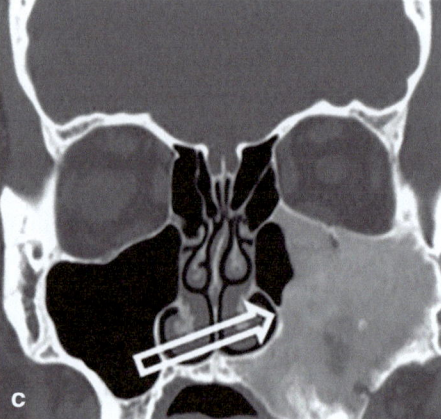

Fig. 30.8 Fibrous dysplasia. (**a**, **b**) Axial bone algorithm CT demonstrates characteristic bone expansion and "ground glass" appearance of the left maxilla (black arrows). The lesion also extends into the left sphenoid wing. Involvement of multiple bones is a feature of fibrous dysplasia. (**c**) Coronal bone algorithm CT shows the "ground glass" matrix, with bony overgrowth encroaching the left maxillary sinus lumen (white open arrow)

- Exophytic papillomas occur more commonly in males with malignant transformation being rare.
- Inverted papillomas also occur more commonly in males with 10% either coexisting with or degenerating into squamous cell carcinoma. HPV DNA has been isolated in approximately two-thirds of inverted papillomas with coexistent squamous cell carcinoma.
- Oncocytic papillomas demonstrate no gender predilection, and 10% of cases are estimated to undergo malignant transformation.
- Removal of the bony strut associated with inverted papillomas is important to prevent recurrence.

Imaging

- Inverted papillomas demonstrate classic imaging characteristics. These typically arise from the lateral wall of the nasal cavity and demonstrate a lobulated appearance and soft tissue attenuation on CT. Hyperostosis of the adjacent bone can be present, and a focal bony strut indicates the site of attachment of the lesion.
- On contrast-enhanced MRI, a classic convoluted "cerebriform" enhancement pattern is seen. The cerebriform enhancement is also apparent in T2-weighted imaging (Fig. e30.11).
- Loss of the cerebriform pattern can be indicative of malignant transformation.

JUVENILE NASOPHARYNGEAL ANGIOFIBROMA

- Most commonly occurs in young males presenting with epistaxis.
- Arises from the posterior choanal tissues in the sphenopalatine foramen.
- Angiography may be used to embolize the tumor prior to surgery to minimize blood loss. The most common feeding artery for this lesion is the internal maxillary branch of the internal carotid artery.

Imaging

- Highly vascular tumors, with intense contrast enhancement and multiple flow voids on MRI with heterogeneous T2 signal.
- The lesion occurs at the sphenopalatine foramen and commonly extends into the nasal cavity and pterygopalatine fossa (Fig. 30.9).
- These lesions are benign and cause bone modeling rather than destruction.

LOBULAR CAPILLARY HEMANGIOMA

- This is also known as pyogenic granuloma.
- Common clinical symptoms included epistaxis and facial pain.

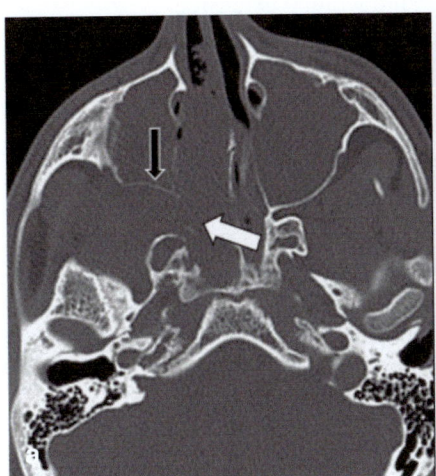
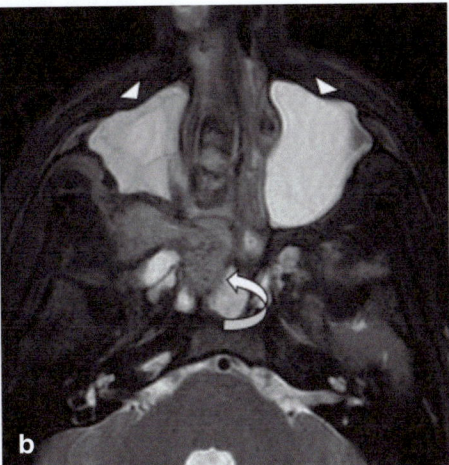
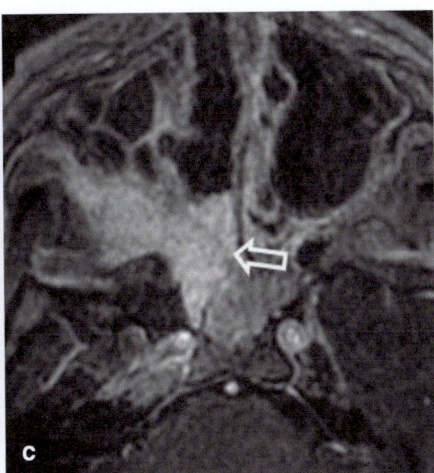

Fig. 30.9 Juvenile nasopharyngeal angiofibroma. (a) Axial bone algorithm CT shows a mass lesion centered at the right sphenopalatine foramen (white arrow) extending into the nasal cavity. There is bony remodeling with widening of the pterygopalatine fossa (black arrow). (b) Axial STIR MRI demonstrates T2 hyperintense signal throughout the mass (white curved arrow). Retained secretions are seen in the maxillary sinuses (white arrowheads). (c) Axial postcontrast fat-suppressed T1W MRI shows avid homogeneous enhancement of the mass (white open arrow)

- More commonly occurs in females. This can occur in all age groups with the most common incidence around age 40 years.
- Treatment is local surgical excision.

Imaging
- Noncontrast CT will demonstrate a slightly hypodense polypoid mass most commonly involving the nasal septum. The inferior turbinates are the second most frequent location [14].
- Contrast-enhanced CT and MR will typically demonstrate avid homogenous enhancement.
- MR imaging will demonstrate a T2 hyperintense mass. Flow voids may be present.
- Bone remodeling may be present.

VENOLYMPHATIC MALFORMATION

- Venolymphatic malformations are a subtype of vascular malformation composed of venous structures and dysplastic lymphatics. These are classified as low-flow mixed malformations.
- Venolymphatic malformations can occur in many places throughout the body and rarely can include the sinonasal region.
- If large enough, obstructive symptoms can develop.
- Sclerotherapy can be used to treat certain vascular malformations.

Imaging
- Imaging characteristics are similar to venolymphatic malformations elsewhere throughout the body.
- Manifest as lobulated fluid attenuation mass on CT. Intermediate to high signal intensity is seen on MRI with possible fluid–fluid levels [15].
- Adjacent remodeling of bone can be seen.
- If predominately venous, phleboliths within the soft tissues can be present.
- Typically demonstrate heterogeneous enhancement, although the lymphatic component of the lesion does not enhance.

Malignant Tumors

SQUAMOUS CELL CARCINOMA

- Most common sinonasal malignancy, typically occurring in males between the ages of 55 and 65 years.
- Multiple histologic subtypes exist including spindle cell, keratinizing, and non-keratinizing types.
- Exposure to nickel and wood dust is associated with the development of this cancer with a latency period of up to 30 years.
- HPV infection and pre-existing inverted papilloma are also risk factors [16].
- Distant and nodal metastatic diseases are uncommon.
- Diagnosis is usually delayed as symptoms can mimic chronic sinusitis.
- Treatment includes surgery and radiation.

Imaging (Fig. 30.10)
- Heterogeneously enhancing mass most commonly occurring in the maxillary sinus with aggressive features including frank osseous destruction and invasion into surrounding structures.
- MR signal characteristics include intermediate signal on T1-weighted images with interspersed regions of intrinsic T1 hyperintensity representing hemorrhage.
- Sinonasal squamous cell carcinoma demonstrates increased cellularity relative to other sinonasal malignancies and may thus demonstrate lower to intermediate T2 signal.
- Heterogeneous post-contrast enhancement.
- Orbital/intracranial extension may occur especially if the tumor involves ethmoid or frontal sinuses.
- Invasion of orbital fat and thickening of extraocular muscles are signs of orbital involvement.
- Nodular meningeal enhancement, brain parenchymal edema, and obvious enhancing mass in the brain parenchyma are signs of intracranial extension.
- Perineural tumor spread is not uncommon and usually involves the branches of CNV.

ADENOCARCINOMA

- Malignant tumor arising from surface epithelium or minor salivary rests with glandular differentiation.
- Divided histologically into intestinal type and non-intestinal type adenocarcinomas. Intestinal-type adenocarcinomas are associated with exposure to hardwood dust and leather processing chemicals [17].
- Intestinal type adenocarcinoma associated with occupational exposure occurs most commonly in the ethmoid sinuses.
- Non-intestinal type adenocarcinomas occur more commonly in the maxillary sinuses.
- Occur most commonly in males aged 55–60 years.

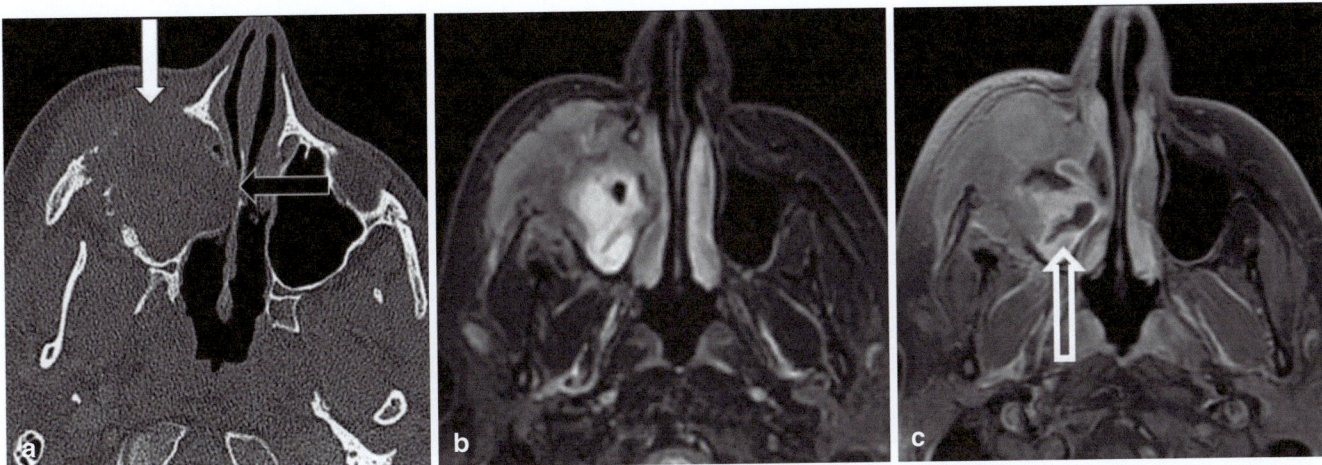

Fig. 30.10 Squamous cell carcinoma. (**a**) Axial bone algorithm CT demonstrates an invasive mass involving the right maxillary sinus with osseous erosion and invasion of the premaxillary soft tissues (white arrow) and extension into the nasal cavity (black arrow). (**b**) Axial STIR MRI demonstrates heterogeneous signals throughout the mass. (**c**) Axial postcontrast fat-suppressed T1W MRI demonstrates heterogeneous enhancement with areas of hypo-enhancement consistent with regions of necrosis (white open arrow)

Imaging (Fig. e30.12)

- CT imaging characteristics demonstrate poorly defined soft tissue mass that may result in bony destruction. Calcification can sometimes be present.
- Most commonly occurs in the nasal cavity and ethmoid sinuses.
- MR imaging characteristics include intermediate T1 signal and intermediate to high T2 signal with heterogeneous enhancement.
- Sinonasal adenocarcinoma tends to enhance less vividly than sinonasal squamous cell carcinoma.
- Tumors frequently involve the orbit and there may be intracranial extension.

ADENOID CYSTIC CARCINOMA

- Tumor arising from minor salivary glands with a high propensity for perineural spread [18].
- Most commonly occurs in the maxillary sinus followed by the nasal cavity.
- Presenting symptoms include facial pain relating to cranial nerve involvement, usually the maxillary division of the trigeminal nerve.
- More commonly results in distant metastatic spread compared with squamous cell carcinoma.

Imaging (Fig. e30.13)

- Imaging features are non-specific with the tumor resembling any other malignant lesion.
- Early and frequent perineural tumor spread is a feature.
- Infiltration of fat or soft tissue mass at the entry/exit sites of the branches of the CNV and widening/erosion of the osseous foramina/canals carrying the nerves are signs of perineural tumor.
- Abnormal/asymmetric enhancement of the nerves is also a useful clue to perineural tumor spread.
- Attention to the pterygopalatine fossa, foramen rotundum, and foramen ovale on imaging is important for the detection of perineural tumor spread.
- Skip lesions may occur along the course of the nerve, leading to falsely negative tumor margins and tumor recurrence following surgery.

ESTHESIONEUROBLASTOMA

- Tumor of neuroectodermal origin arising from olfactory mucosa in the superior nasal cavity.
- Bimodal age distribution, most commonly occurring in the second and sixth decades [19].
- Delayed recurrence may occur and has been seen with a latency of up to 20 years.
- Common presenting symptoms include nasal obstruction and epistaxis.
- Tumor resection and radiation therapy are the mainstays of treatment, with larger masses or disseminated disease also receiving chemotherapy.

Imaging (Fig. 30.11)

- CT appearance includes soft tissue mass with bony destruction, centered at the cribriform plate.
- MRI demonstrates intermediate T1 and T2 signals with avid homogeneous enhancement.

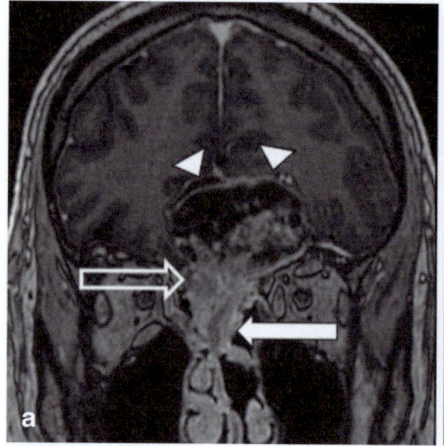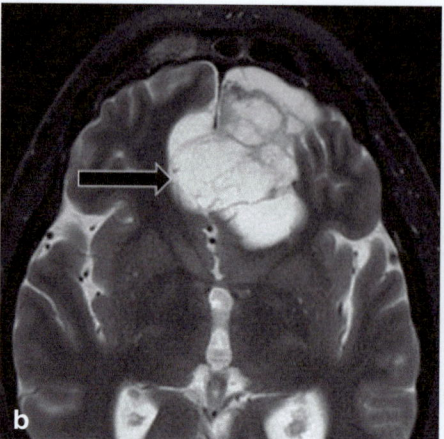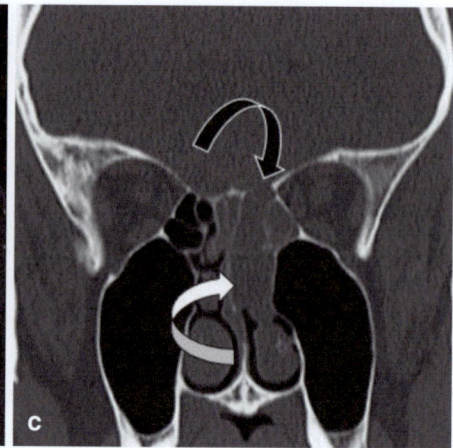

Fig. 30.11 Esthesioneuroblastoma. (**a**) Coronal T1 post-contrast MRI shows a mass centered in the superior nasal cavity within intracranial extension. The heterogeneously enhancing mass (solid white arrow) shows "waisting" at the skull base (open white arrow). Characteristic cysts are seen at the brain–tumor interface (white arrowheads). (**b**) Axial T2W MRI demonstrates the peritumoral cysts along the brain–tumor interface (black solid arrow). (**c**) Coronal bone algorithm CT demonstrates a soft tissue mass opacifying the nasal cavity (white curved arrow) with bony erosion at the skull base (black curved arrow)

- Associated with intracranial extension, which shows the characteristic dumbbell-shaped mass with slight narrowing or "waist" of the mass as it passes through the cribriform plate.
- When intracranial extension is present, characteristic peritumoral cysts at the brain–tumor interface are seen.
- The presence of somatostatin receptors on tumor cells allows it to be detected with DOTATATE, a radioisotope used to detect neuroendocrine tumors.
- Lymph node involvement is more commonly seen in esthesioneuroblastomas compared with other sinonasal malignancies.

SINONASAL UNDIFFERENTIATED CARCINOMA

- High-grade malignant epithelial tumor with aggressive features.
- Usually presents as a large (>4 cm) mass with osseous erosion and frequent intracranial or orbital invasion.
- More likely to result in distant metastasis than other sinonasal malignancies.
- The prognosis is poor even after complete resection and chemoradiation. Often, complete resection is difficult due to frequent orbit/intracranial involvement.

Imaging

- Predilection for the nasal cavity as opposed to the maxillary sinuses as seen in squamous cell carcinoma.
- On MRI, appears isointense to muscle on T1 with low to intermediate T2 signal.
- Heterogeneous enhancement and areas of necrosis are common.
- Highly aggressive features with osseous erosion and invasion of adjacent structures.

SINONASAL LYMPHOMA

- Highly cellular tumors derived from lymphoid tissues, divided into B-cell or T-cell subtypes.
- The B-cell subtype is more common in Western countries and more commonly affects the paranasal sinuses.
- The T-cell subtype is more common in Asian countries, affects a younger age group, more commonly involves the nasal cavity, and is associated with Epstein–Barr virus infection. The T-cell subtype also tends to demonstrate more aggressive features [20].

Imaging (Fig. e30.14)

- Typically hyperattenuating on CT, intermediate to low signal intensity on T2-weighted imaging, and demonstrate restricted diffusion due to their highly cellular nature.
- The mass typically demonstrates homogeneous avid enhancement.
- Orbital invasion and perineural tumor spread are common.
- Lymph node metastasis may be seen.

SINONASAL MELANOMA

- Malignant tumor arising from melanocytes migrated from the neural crest.

- Most commonly occurs in the nasal cavity but has also been seen to occur in the maxillary sinuses [21].
- Typically occurs in the sixth through eighth decades of life.
- Distant metastases are common and prognosis is poor. Wide local excision and radiation are the therapies of choice.

Imaging (Fig. e30.15)
- The paramagnetic nature of melanin gives this lesion characteristic intrinsic T1 hyperintensity, although lesions with low levels of melanin (non-melanotic melanomas) may demonstrate only intermediate or even low T1 signal.
- Despite the propensity for metastasis and poor prognosis, the lesion will typically demonstrate bony remodeling rather than destruction with non-invasive appearing margins on imaging.
- Homogeneous vivid contrast enhancement is seen owing to high tumor vascularity.
- Perineural tumor spread may be seen.

CHONDROSARCOMA

- Malignant tumors arise from mesenchymal cells and/or chondrocytes.
- Rarely occurs in the head and neck region, but can occur secondary to radiation or may be associated with genetic conditions such as Maffucci syndrome.
- Treatment is surgical resection with neoadjuvant chemoradiation. Late recurrences after many disease-free years have been known to occur, so long-term follow-up is advised.

Imaging
- Chondroid component on MRI appears bright on T2-weighted images with heterogeneous enhancement [22–24].
- Predilection for the nasal septum and maxillary sinuses.
- Characteristic appearance of chondroid matrix demonstrating an "arcs and rings" pattern, best seen on CT imaging.

OSTEOSARCOMA

- Malignant osteoid forming tumor arising from mesenchymal cells.
- The maxilla and mandible are the most common sites for craniofacial osteosarcoma [23].
- Peak incidence is seen in the third decade of life, later in life when compared with osteosarcomas in long bones.
- Predisposing factors include Paget's disease, fibrous dysplasia, and prior radiation therapy.
- Treatment includes surgical resection and chemotherapy.

Imaging (Fig. 30.12)
- CT imaging demonstrates a hyperdense mass with osteoid matrix. Poorly differentiated lesions may demonstrate predominately soft tissue attenuation with relatively little osteoid formation.
- Aggressive features such as local invasion and "sunburst" periosteal reaction are common.
- MR demonstrates low T1 and intermediate T2 signal intensity with moderate contrast enhancement.

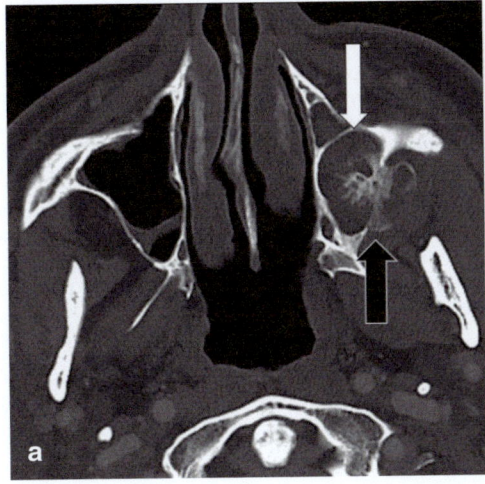
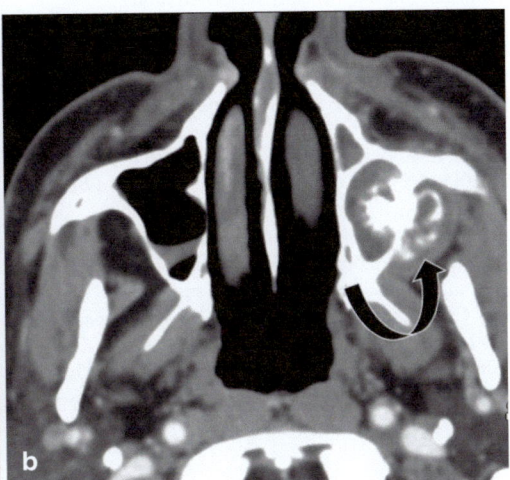

Fig. 30.12 Osteosarcoma. (a) Axial bone algorithm CT shows a mass involving the left maxillary sinus with osteoid matrix (black arrow) with opacification of the left maxillary sinus (white arrow). (b) Axial soft tissue algorithm CT demonstrates the mass with osteoid matrix and surrounding periosteal reaction (black curved arrow)

PLASMACYTOMA

- Soft tissue mass consisting of neoplastic monoclonal plasma cells in a patient with multiple myeloma or occurring as a solitary plasmacytoma.
- Can occur anywhere throughout the body, involving bone and extramedullary soft tissues. Solitary extramedullary non-osseous plasmacytoma most frequently occurs in the nasal cavity [25].
- If a lesion is diagnosed on biopsy as plasmacytoma, a work-up for multiple myeloma should be pursued if not previously performed which can include serum/urine protein electrophoresis and skeletal imaging via either CT or radiographs.

Imaging

- CT imaging typically demonstrates a soft tissue mass which can demonstrate osseous invasion of the skull base.
- MR signal characteristics include intermediate intensity on both T1- and T2-weighted images.
- The most common enhancement pattern is moderate homogeneous enhancement.

References

1. Dankbaar JW, van Bemmel AJ, Pameijer FA. Imaging findings of the orbital and intracranial complications of acute bacterial rhinosinusitis. Insights Imaging. 2015;6(5):509–18. https://doi.org/10.1007/s13244-015-0424-y.
2. DeShazo RD, O'Brien M, Chapin K, Soto-Aguilar M, Swain R, Lyons M, Bryars WC Jr, Alsip S. Criteria for the diagnosis of sinus mycetoma. J Allergy Clin Immunol. 1997;99(4):475–85. https://doi.org/10.1016/s0091-6749(97)70073-3.
3. Broderick D. The opacified paranasal sinus: approach and differential, Appl Radiol. https://appliedradiology.com/articles/the-opacified-paranasal-sinus-approach-and-differential
4. Meir W, Bourla R, Huszar M, Zloczower E. Antrochoanal polyp: updated clinical approach, histology characteristics, diagnosis and treatment, pathology—from classics to innovations, Ilze Strumfa and Guntis Bahs. IntechOpen; 2021. https://doi.org/10.5772/intechopen.96329.
5. Newton JR, Ah-See KW. A review of nasal polyposis. Ther Clin Risk Manag. 2008;4(2):507–12. https://doi.org/10.2147/tcrm.s2379.
6. Capra GG, et al. Paranasal Sinus Mucocele. Head Neck Pathol. 2012;6(3):369–72. https://doi.org/10.1007/s12105-012-0359-2.
7. DeShazo RD, et al. Diagnostic criteria for sarcoidosis of the sinuses. J Allergy Clin Immunol. 1999;103(5):789–95. https://doi.org/10.1016/s0091-6749(99)70421-5.
8. Joseph B, et al. Sinonasal sarcoidosis of the maxillary sinus and infraorbital nerve: a case report. J Korean Assoc Oral Maxillofac Surg. 2015;41(4):217. https://doi.org/10.5125/jkaoms.2015.41.4.217.
9. D'Anza B, Langford CA, Sindwani R. Sinonasal imaging findings in granulomatosis with polyangiitis (Wegener granulomatosis): a systematic review. Am J Rhinol Allergy. 2017;31(1):16–21. https://doi.org/10.2500/ajra.2017.31.4408.
10. Agarwal M, Policeni B. Sinonasal Neoplasms. Semin Roentgenol. 2019;54(3):244–57. https://doi.org/10.1053/j.ro.2019.03.001. Epub 2019 Mar 9.
11. Dean KE, et al. Imaging review of new and emerging sinonasal tumors and tumor-like entities from the fourth edition of the World Health Organization classification of head and neck tumors. Am J Neuroradiol. 2019;40:584. https://doi.org/10.3174/ajnr.a5978.
12. Kawaguchi M, Kato H, Tomita H, et al. Imaging characteristics of malignant sinonasal tumors. J Clin Med. 2017;6(12):116. Published 2017 Dec 6. https://doi.org/10.3390/jcm6120116.
13. Kumar S, Sayoo C. Sinonasal schwannoma: a rare sinonasal neoplasm. Indian J Otolaryngol Head Neck Surg. 2017;69(3):425–7. https://doi.org/10.1007/s12070-017-1125-2.
14. Baki A. Nasal cavity hemangiomas. In: Almasri M, Kummoona R, editors. Maxillofacial surgery and craniofacial deformity—practices and updates. IntechOpen; 2020. https://doi.org/10.5772/intechopen.90137.
15. Behravesh S, et al. Venous malformations: clinical diagnosis and treatment. Cardiovasc Diagn Ther. 2016;6(6):557–69. https://doi.org/10.21037/cdt.2016.11.10.
16. Lewis JS Jr. Sinonasal squamous cell carcinoma: a review with emphasis on emerging histologic subtypes and the role of human papillomavirus. Head Neck Pathol. 2016;10(1):60–7. https://doi.org/10.1007/s12105-016-0692-y.
17. Leivo I. Sinonasal adenocarcinoma: update on classification, Immunophenotype and molecular features. Head Neck Pathol. 2016;10(1):68–74. https://doi.org/10.1007/s12105-016-0694-9.
18. Michel G, et al. Adenoid cystic carcinoma of the paranasal sinuses: retrospective series and review of the literature. Eur Ann Otorhinolaryngol Head Neck Dis. 2013;130(5):257–62. https://doi.org/10.1016/j.anorl.2012.09.010.
19. Kumar R. Esthesioneuroblastoma: multimodal management and review of literature. World J Clin Cases. 2015;3(9):774. https://doi.org/10.12998/wjcc.v3.i9.774.
20. Shetty D, et al. Sinonasal T cell lymphoma: a case report. Indian J Otolaryngol Head Neck Surg. 2011;63(S1):16–8. https://doi.org/10.1007/s12070-011-0172-3.
21. Alves ISS, et al. Sinonasal melanoma: a case report and literature review. Case Rep Oncol Med. 2017;2017:8201301. https://doi.org/10.1155/2017/8201301.
22. Ferguson MS, et al. Management of sinonasal and skull base non-mesenchymal chondrosarcoma, a narrative review. Rhinology Online. 2018;1(1):94–103. https://doi.org/10.4193/rhinol/18.025.
23. Gore, Mitchell R. Treatment, outcomes, and demographics in sinonasal sarcoma: a systematic review of the literature. BMC Ear, Nose and Throat Disord vol. 18 4. 21 Mar. 2018, doi:https://doi.org/10.1186/s12901-018-0052-5.
24. Kharrat S, Sahtout S, Tababi S, Temimi S, Ben Miled M, Abid W, Zainine R, Nouira K, Menif E, Beltaief N, Besbes G. Chondrosarcoma of sinonasal cavity: a case report and brief literature review. Tunis Med. 2010;88(2):122–4.
25. Hazarika P, et al. Solitary extramedullary plasmacytoma of the sinonasal region. Indian J Otolaryngol Head Neck Surg. 2011;63(Suppl 1):33–5. https://doi.org/10.1007/s12070-011-0181-2.

Temporal Bone Imaging

Daniel Thomas Ginat

Anatomy

- CT is best for depicting the bony anatomy (Fig. 31.1), while MRI is best for depicting the labyrinthine and internal auditory canal contents.
- The external ear includes the auricle and external auditory canal, which extends medially to the tympanic membrane.
- The middle ear is an air-filled cavity within the petrous portion of the temporal bone that contains the ossicular chain and is bounded by the tympanic membrane laterally, the inner ear structures medially, the tegmen tympani superiorly, and the jugular wall (floor) inferiorly.
- The scutum is a sharp bony projection to which the tympanic membrane is attached superiorly.
- Prussak space is bordered by the pars flaccida and scutum laterally, the lateral malleal ligament superiorly, and the neck of the malleus medially.
- The tegmen is a thin plate of bone that separates the dura of the middle cranial fossa from the middle ear and the mastoid cavity.
- The posterior wall of the middle ear cavity is irregular and includes the facial recess, pyramidal eminence, sinus tympani, and round window niche.
- The ossicular chain is composed of three bones: malleus, incus, and stapes.
- The manubrium of the malleus is attached to the tympanic membrane, and the head of the malleus articulates with the body of the incus in the epitympanum, forming the incudomalleal joint, which has a characteristic "ice cream cone" configuration on axial images.
- The lenticular process of the incus extends from the long process of the incus to articulate with the head of the stapes, forming the incudostapedial joint.
- The footplate of the stapes attaches to the oval window of the vestibule.
- The inner ear is situated within the petrous portion and comprises the osseous labyrinth, which includes the cochlea, vestibule, and semicircular canals.
- The cochlea consists of 2 ½ to 2 ¾ turns formed by the basilar, middle, and apical turns, which are separated by the interscalar septa.
- Centrally within the cochlea is the cone-shaped spongy bone modiolus that houses the spiral ganglion.
- The vestibule is an ovoid space located superior and posterior to the cochlea that connects to the semicircular canals.
- There are three semicircular canals: lateral (horizontal), superior, and posterior. The posterior and superior semicircular canals share a common crus.
- The vestibular aqueduct normally measures up to 1 mm at the midpoint and 2 mm at the operculum.
- The internal auditory canal is a channel in the petrous bone that transmits the facial nerve, cochlear nerve, and superior and inferior vestibular nerves.
- The facial nerve is located superior to the cochlear nerve in the anterior portion of the internal auditory canal, for which there is the mnemonic "7 up, coke down" (Fig. 31.2).

Supplementary Information The online version contains supplementary material available at https://doi.org/10.1007/978-3-031-55124-6_31.

D. T. Ginat (✉)
Department of Radiology, University of Chicago, Chicago, IL, USA
e-mail: dtg1@uchicago.edu

Fig. 31.1 Temporal bone anatomy depicted on CT. (*SCC* Semicircular canal)

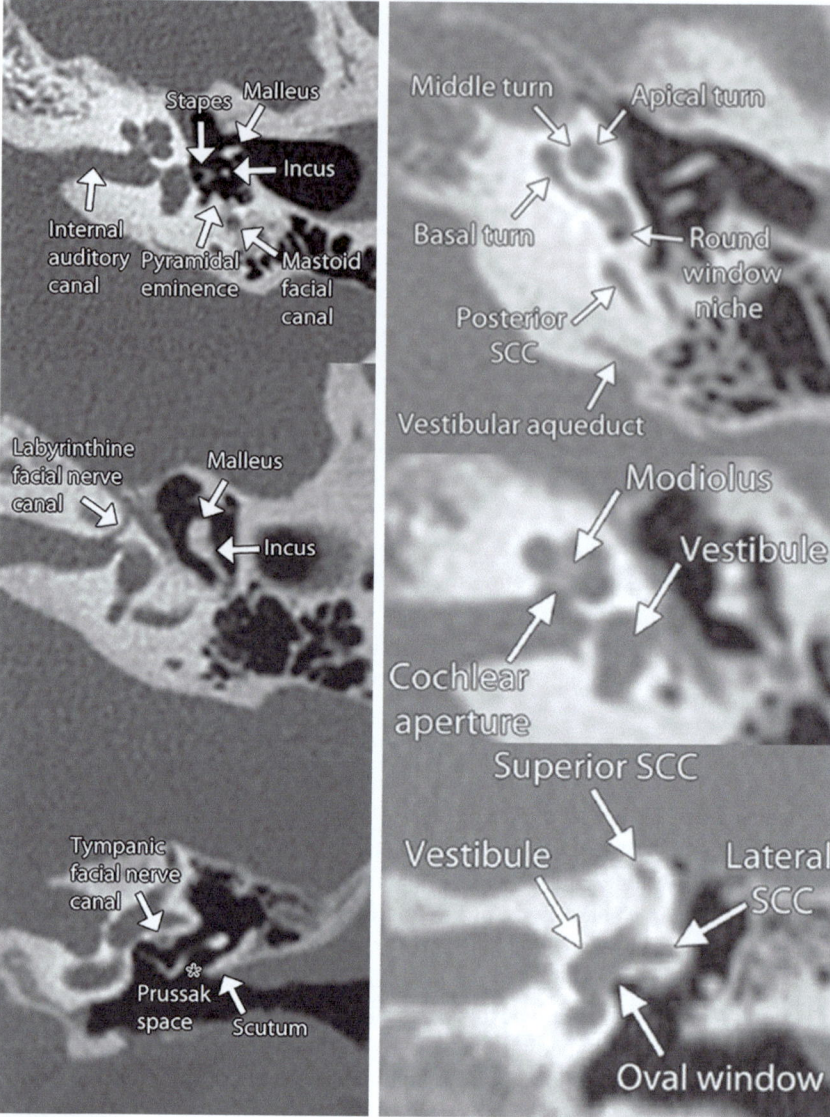

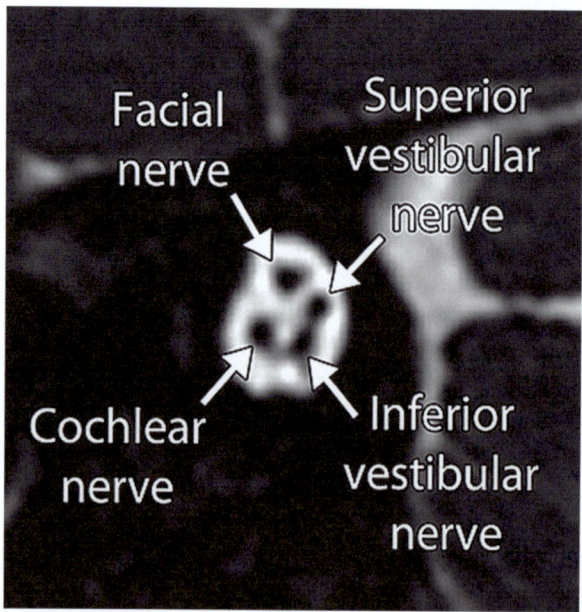

Fig. 31.2 Oblique sagittal T2-weighted MRI shows the contents of the internal auditory canal in cross-section

Incomplete Partition Type 2

- This is the most common inner ear anomaly, related to arrested development at the seventh week of gestation.
- The cochlea has deficient turns and modiolus, and the middle and apical turns coalesce to form a cystic apex (Fig. 31.3).
- The vestibular aqueduct is often enlarged.

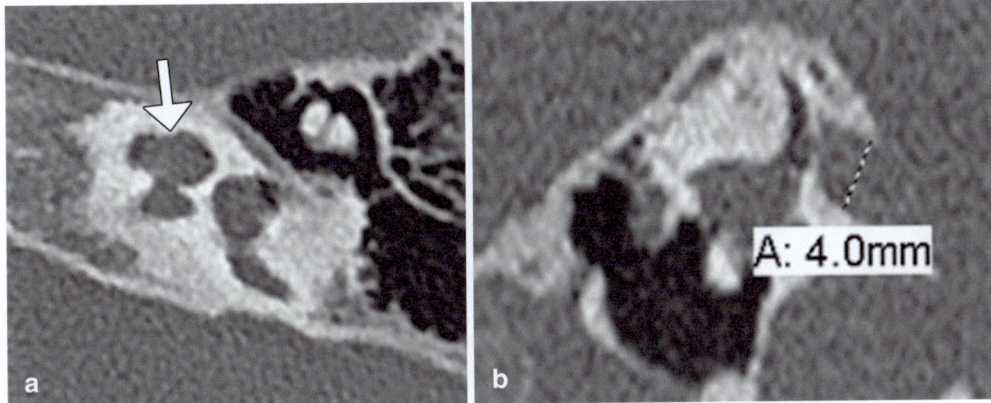

Fig. 31.3 Incomplete partition type 2. Axial CT image (**a**) shows deficient cochlear turns and modiolus (arrow). Sagittal CT image (**b**) shows an enlarged vestibular aqueduct (measuring 4 mm with the caliper)

Persistent Stapedial Artery

- Rare congenital vascular variant that arises from the hyoid artery.
- The vessel courses along the cochlear promontory and stapes, hence the name (Fig. 31.4).

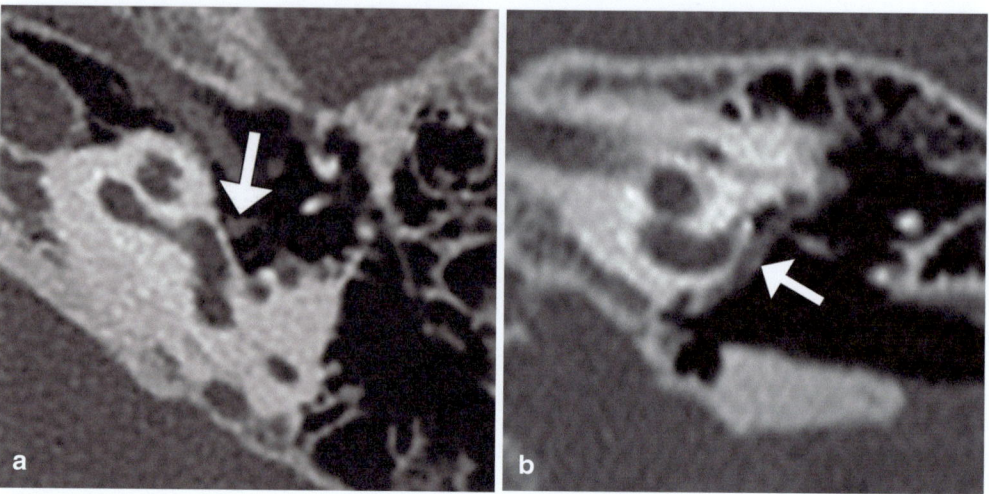

Fig. 31.4 Persistent stapedial artery. Axial (**a**) and coronal (**b**) CT images show the persistent stapedial artery (arrows) along the cochlear promontory and stapes

Aberrant Carotid Artery

- Aberrant internal carotid artery results from an anomalous connection between the inferior tympanic artery and caroticotympanic (hyoid) artery.
- Patients may present with a retrotympanic mass, hearing loss, and objective pulsatile tinnitus.
- Findings include a reduced-caliber ICA that enters the middle ear through the enlarged inferior tympanic canal within the caroticojugular spine.
- The aberrant ICA has a "figure of 7" configuration of 3D CTA or MRA MIP images (Fig. 31.5).
- Do not mistake it for a mass and biopsy!

Fig. 31.5 Aberrant carotid artery. Axial CTA image (**a**) shows the left internal carotid artery extending into the middle ear cavity (arrow). MRA MIP image (**b**) shows the abnormal left internal carotid artery with a figure of 7 configuration

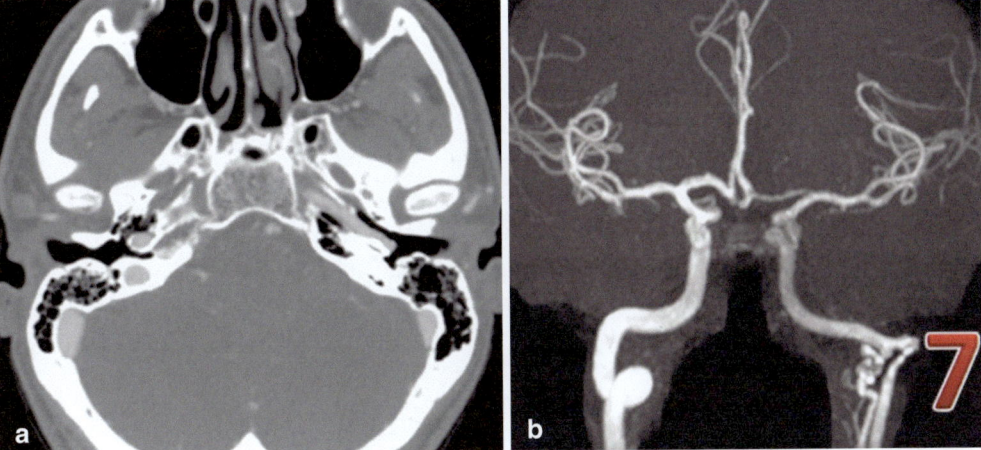

Cholesteatoma

- Cholesteatomas consist of a mass of desquamated keratin epithelium and can be acquired (98%) or congenital (2%).
- Acquired cholesteatoma is most often a complication of chronic otitis media with tympanic membrane perforation (pars flaccida).
- CT is the main modality used for imaging of temporal bone inflammation.
- Acquired pars flaccida cholesteatoma appears as an expansile lesion in Prussak space, often associated with erosion of the scutum and ossicles (Fig. 31.6).
- On MRI, cholesteatoma appears as a non-enhancing T2 hyperintense lesion with restricted diffusion on DWI (Fig. 31.7).
- Complications of cholesteatoma include erosion of the roof of the tegmen, meningoencephalocele, erosion of the facial canal, and perilymphatic fistula (communication between middle ear and inner ear).

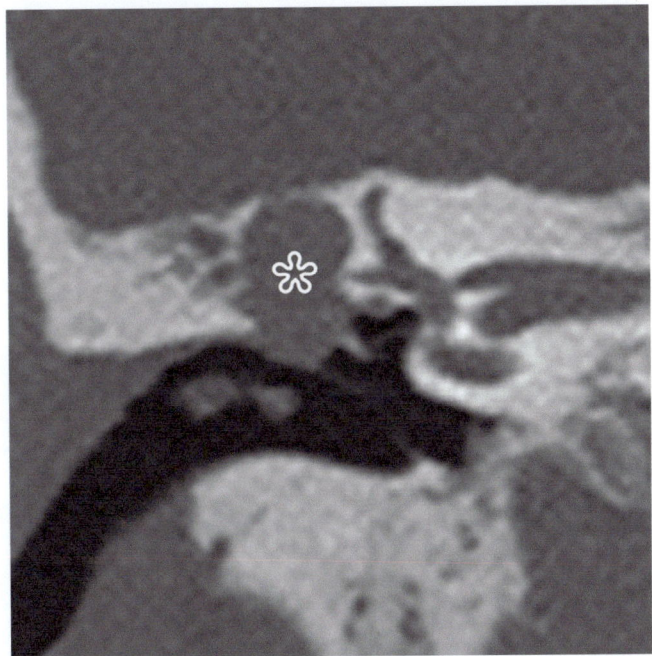

Fig. 31.6 Cholesteatoma. Coronal CT image shows an opacity (*) in Prussak space and attic with erosion of the ossicles and scutum

Cholesterol Granuloma

- Cholesterol granuloma (chocolate cyst) forms in the setting of eustachian tube dysfunction leading to ruptured blood vessels, which incites a foreign body giant cell reaction.
- Typical locations include the middle ear cavity and pneumatized petrous apex.
- On CT, there is typically a smooth expansile lucency.
- On MRI, the lesions typically appear as non-enhancing lesions with high signal intensity on T1 and T2 sequences, with a low signal rim peripherally (Fig. 31.8).

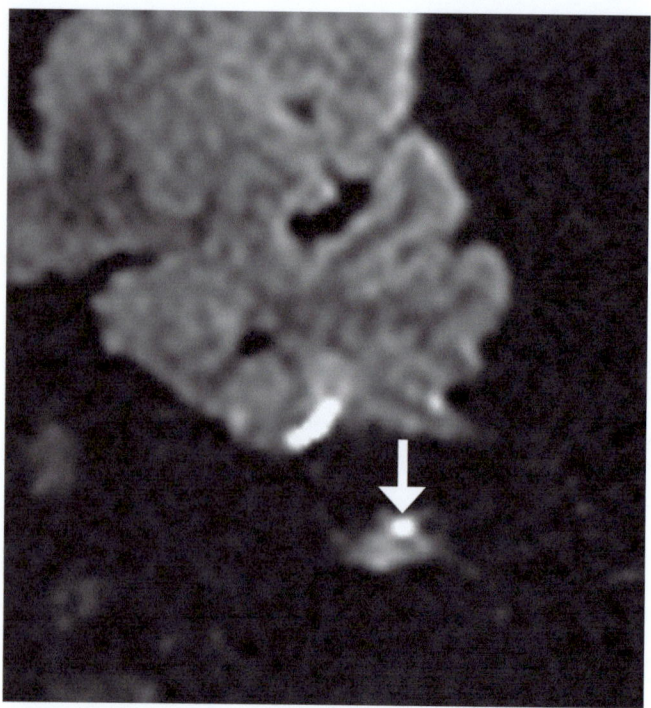

Fig. 31.7 Cholesteatoma. Coronal DWI shows a lesion (arrow) with restricted diffusion in the left temporal bone

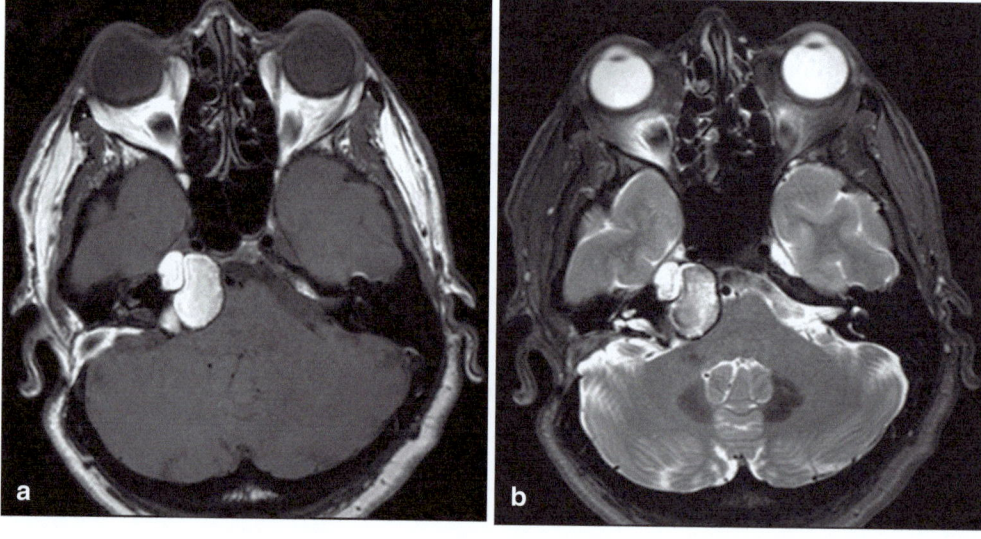

Fig. 31.8 Cholesterol granuloma. Axial T1-weighted (**a**) and T2-weighted (**b**) MR images show a hyperintense expansile lesion arising from the right petrous temporal bone

Superior Semicircular Canal Dehiscence

- Classically presents with vertigo, and nystagmus occurring in the setting of loud noises (Tullio phenomenon) due to a "third window phenomenon."
- CT shows deficient bone covering the semicircular canal (Fig. 31.9). Poschl (parallel to the plane of the SSC) and Stenver's (perpendicular to the plane of the SSC) views can be obtained to better visualize dehiscence.

Necrotizing Otitis Externa

- Necrotizing (malignant) external otitis tends to occur in elderly immunocompromised and diabetic patients.
- The infection is usually caused by *Pseudomonas aeruginosa*.
- Patients present with severe otalgia and otorrhea and there is a high mortality rate.
- Extensive bony erosions and soft tissue swelling along the external auditory canal can be demonstrated on CT (Fig. 31.10).
- Infection can then spread via fissures of Santorini into the soft tissues beneath the skull base, leading to skull base osteomyelitis.

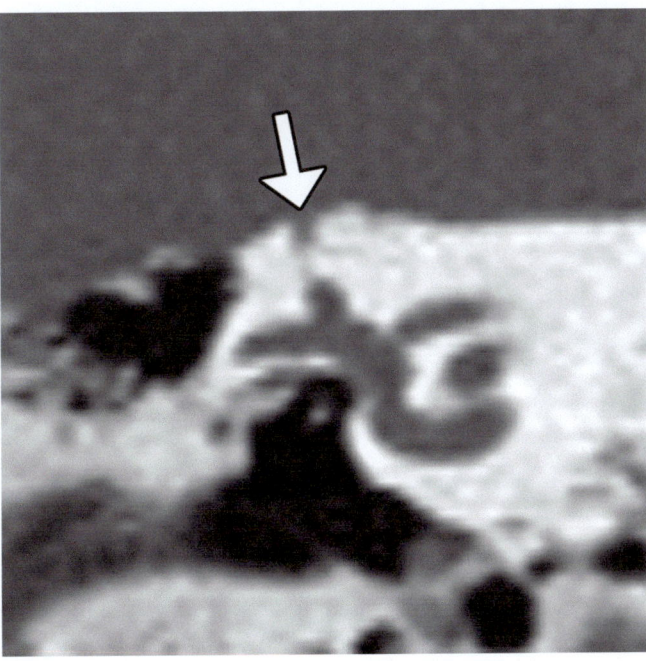

Fig. 31.9 Superior semicircular canal dehiscence. Oblique coronal CT image shows deficient bone covering the superior semicircular canal (arrow)

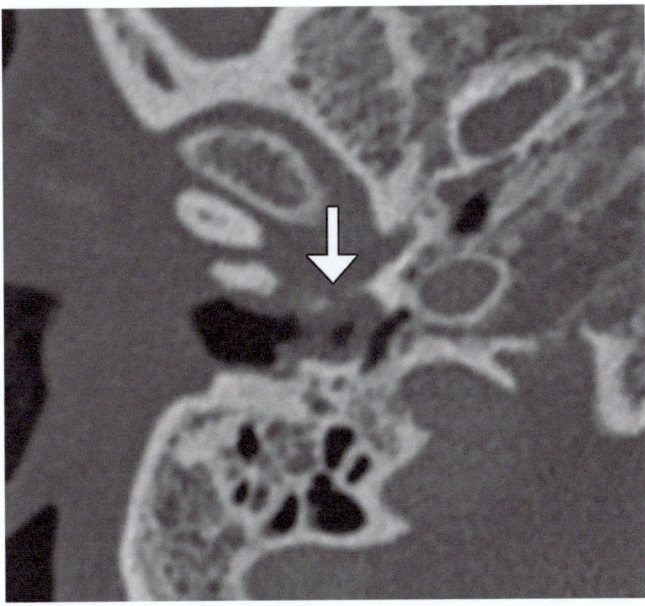

Fig. 31.10 Necrotizing otitis externa. Axial CT image shows soft tissue swelling in the right external auditory canal with bone erosions (arrow)

Otomastoiditis

- Acute otitis media is primarily a pediatric disease, usually caused by bacteria such as *Streptococcus* species or *Hemophilus influenza*.
- Imaging is usually not necessary in uncomplicated acute otitis media.
- Complicated mastoiditis is suggested clinically by the presence of postauricular erythema, tenderness, and edema. In this clinical situation, imaging is crucial to exclude complications, such as epidural empyema, abscess, and venous sinus thrombosis (Fig. 31.11).
- Coalescent mastoiditis represents the destruction of the mastoid trabeculae, which can extend to the inner or outer cortex (Fig. 31.12).

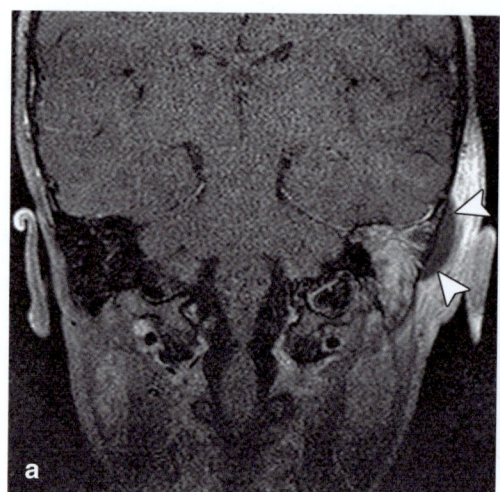 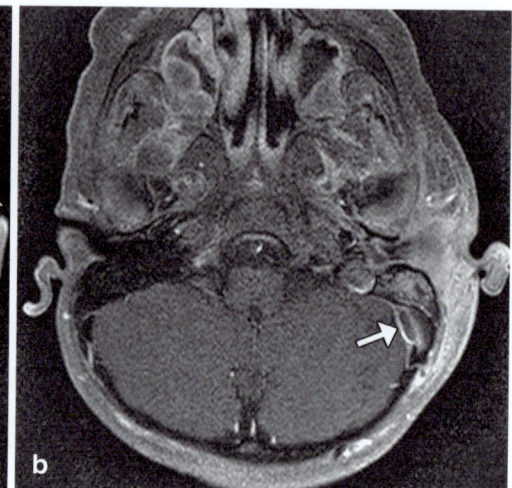

Fig. 31.11 Complicated acute mastoiditis. Coronal post-contrast T1-weighted MRI (**a**) shows enhancement of the left mastoid air cells and an overlying abscess (arrowheads) with regional cellulitis. Axial post-contrast T1-weighted MRI (**b**) shows associated venous thrombophlebitis (arrow)

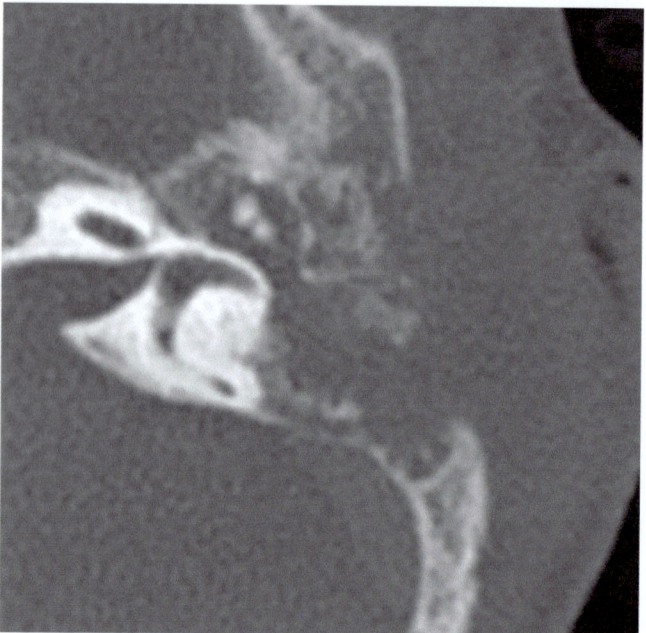

Fig. 31.12 Coalescent mastoiditis. Axial CT image shows extensive mastoid temporal bone erosions and tympanomastoid opacification

Petrous Apicitis

- Air cells and venous channels within the petrous apex that communicate with the middle ear can serve as a route for the spread of infection from the middle ear to the petrous apex leading to petrous apicitis.
- Gradenigo syndrome consists of otorrhea, abducens nerve paresis, and severe pain in the distribution of the trigeminal nerve due to local pachymeningitis.
- CT may demonstrate opacification of the air cells of the petrous apex with bone erosion and MRI findings include marrow T1 hypointensity, soft tissue abnormalities, and enhancement (Fig. e31.1).

  (All electronic images (Figs. e31.1–e31.13) can be found on this chapter's website on SpringerLink: https://doi.org/10.1007/978-3-031-55124-6_31).

Labyrinthitis

- Inflammation of the inner ear structures can be infectious or aseptic.
- In the acute setting, enhancement can be demonstrated within the inner ear structures on MRI (Fig. e31.2).
- In some cases, mineralization of the membranous labyrinth (labyrinthitis ossificans) ensues, whereby calcification is apparent on imaging (Fig. e31.3).

Herpes Zoster Oticus

- Herpes zoster oticus (Ramsay Hunt syndrome) results from varicella zoster viral infection.
- Patients typically present with peripheral facial nerve palsy associated with sensorineural hearing loss, tinnitus, vertigo with nystagmus, painful vesicular eruption within the external ear canal and of the auricle and the tympanic membrane, malaise, and fever.
- Diffuse enhancement of the facial nerve is a typical finding on MRI (Fig. e31.4).

Otospongiosis

- Otospongiosis is a primary osteodystrophy of the temporal bone with abnormal bone resorption and deposition. The disease usually appears in the fourth or fifth decades with a female predilection.
- Otoscopic examination may reveal a faint pink tinge reflecting the vascularity of the lesion, referred to as the Schwartze sign.
- Fenestral otospongiosis occurs just anterior to the oval window at a small cleft known as the fissula ante fenestram and results in conductive hearing loss.
- Cochlear otospongiosis is less common and can lead to sensorineural hearing loss.
- Imaging is mainly performed in cases of sensorineural or mixed hearing loss and the lesions appear as areas of demineralization on CT (Fig. e31.5).

Fractures

- Temporal bone fractures have been traditionally classified as transverse versus longitudinal versus oblique with respect to the long axis of the petrous bone and more recently as otic capsule violating versus otic capsule sparing.
- Regardless of the classification, the role of imaging is to evaluate for associated complications, including disruption of the ossicular chain (Fig. e31.6) and pneumolabyrinth (Fig. e31.7).
- Otic capsule-violating fractures are also more likely to be associated with facial nerve injury and cerebrospinal fluid leakage than otic capsule sparing fractures.

Encephalocele and Cerebrospinal Fluid Fistula

- Patients with temporal bone encephalocele and CSF fistula commonly present with persistent otorrhea and conductive hearing loss.
- Trauma is the most common cause, whether related to temporal bone fracture or surgery.
- Spontaneous leaks can occur from congenital anomalies in children and erosion by arachnoid granulations and intracranial hypertension in adults.
- Imaging studies are essential for determining the site of the CSF leak.
- High-resolution non-contrast CT is the initial diagnostic study of choice to identify a defect of the temporal bone, often in the tegmen, while MRI can help distinguish encephalocele from fluid (Fig. e31.8).

Schwannomas

- Schwannomas in the temporal bone region most commonly arise from the inferior vestibular nerve but can be intralabyrinthine or involve the facial nerve (Fig. e31.9).
- Schwannomas tend to display avid enhancement on MRI and can cause smooth bone remodeling.

Paragangliomas

- Paraganglioma is the second most common type of tumor involving the temporal bone and can arise from the jugulotympanic paraganglia along the nerves of Jacobson and Arnold.
- Glomus tympanicum refers to those confined to the tympanic cavity (arising from paraganglia cells along the nerve of Jacobson) and are found against the cochlear promontory (Fig. e31.10).
- Glomus jugulare refers to those tumors involving the jugular bulb and the base of the skull (arising from paraganglia cells along the nerve of Jacobson or Arnold).
- Paragangliomas are highly vascular and display avid enhancement and uptake on Dotatate scans.
- Lytic or permeative bone destruction is characteristic of glomus jugulare, which has "salt-and-pepper" appearance on MRI (Fig. e31.11).

Meningioma

- There are three subgroups of temporal bone meningiomas based on location: tegmen tympani, jugular foramen, and internal auditory canal meningiomas.
- Common to all temporal bone meningiomas is the presence of an intracranial enhancing dural-based component (Fig. e31.12).
- Tegmen tympani and jugular foramen meningiomas can extend into the middle ear cavity.
- In contrast, internal auditory canal meningiomas may demonstrate intralabyrinthine tumor spread.
- The tumors likely spread transosseously, although lack of frank bone destruction is characteristic for meningioma.

Endolymphatic Sac Tumor

- Endolymphatic sac tumor is a locally invasive papillary cystadenomatous tumor associated with von Hippel Lindau disease.
- On CT, the bone invaded by tumor has a moth-eaten, lytic appearance, often with intratumoral bone spicules.
- On MRI, areas of intrinsic T1 hyperintensity and T2 hyperintensity are common, reflecting blood products (Fig. e31.13).
- Enhancement is mild and usually heterogeneous.

Suggested Reading

Juliano AF, Ginat DT, Moonis G. Imaging review of the temporal bone: part I. Anatomy and inflammatory and neoplastic processes. Radiology. 2013;269(1):17–33.

Juliano AF, Ginat DT, Moonis G. Imaging review of the temporal bone: part II. Traumatic, postoperative, and noninflammatory nonneoplastic conditions. Radiology. 2015;276(3):655–72.

Anterior Skull Base

Gopi Nayak, Jesi Kim, and Mari Hagiwara

Anatomy (Figs. 32.1, 32.2, 32.3 and 32.4)

The anterior skull base (ASB) is formed by portions of the ethmoid, sphenoid, and paired frontal bones.

- Anterior border: posterior wall of the frontal sinuses.
- Posterior border: posterior edge of lesser sphenoid wing, anterior clinoid process, planum sphenoidale.
- Laterally, formed by the orbital plates of the frontal bone—forms roof of the orbits.
- Medially, formed by the ethmoid bone including the cribriform plate, crista galli, lateral lamella, and fovea ethmoidalis (ethmoid roof); and sphenoid bone—planum sphenoidale (anterior sphenoid roof).
- Cribriform plate, crista galli, and lateral lamella form the olfactory fossa which contain the olfactory bulbs (Cranial nerve I).
- Cribriform plate—thin bony interface between the olfactory fossa (intracranial compartment) and nasal cavity; multiple olfactory foramina in the cribriform plate convey olfactory nerves from the olfactory mucosa of the nasal cavity to the olfactory bulbs.
- Crista galli:
  o Superior bony projection from cribriform plate.
  o Attachment site for anterior falx cerebri.
- Foramen cecum:
  o Embryologic tract at the frontoethmoidal suture—anterior to crista galli (part of ethmoid bone).
  o During embryological development, it contains a dural diverticulum from the anterior cranial fossa to the superficial surface of the nose which then normally involutes [1].

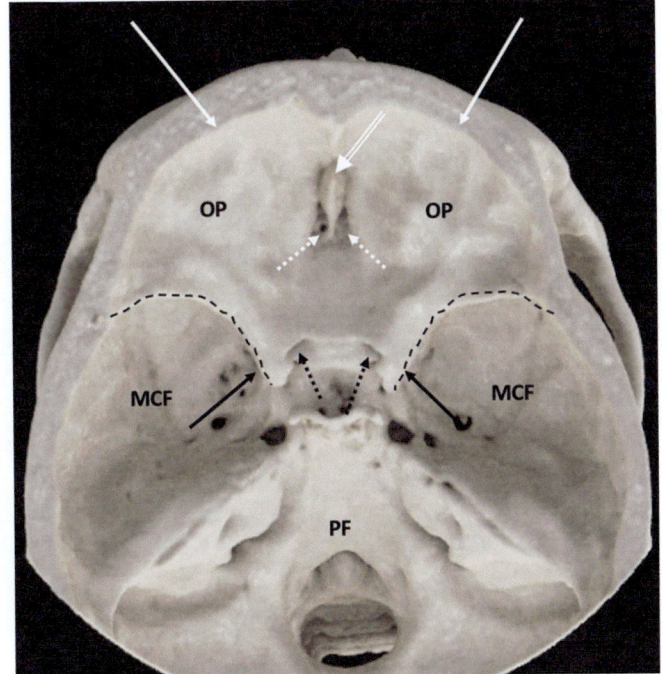

Fig. 32.1 Anatomy of the anterior skull base. Cinematic rendered image from noncontrast CT demonstrates the boundaries and anatomy of the anterior skull base. Anterior border—posterior wall of the frontal bone (solid white arrows). Posterior border—lesser wing of the sphenoid bone (dashed black line) including the anterior clinoid processes (solid black arrows). ASB is formed by the orbital plate (OP) of the frontal bones laterally, midline ethmoid bone centrally with the thin, perforated cribriform plate (dashed white arrows) and superiorly projecting crista galli (double lined arrow). Also seen are the planum sphenoidale (PS), optic canals (dashed black arrows), middle cranial fossa (MCF), and posterior fossa (PF). Image courtesy Dr. Matthew Young, NYU Langone Medical Center

G. Nayak (✉) · J. Kim · M. Hagiwara
Department of Radiology, NYU Langone Medical Center, New York, NY, USA
e-mail: gopi.nayak@nyulangone.org; Jesi.Kim@nyulangone.org; mari.hagiwara@nyulangone.org

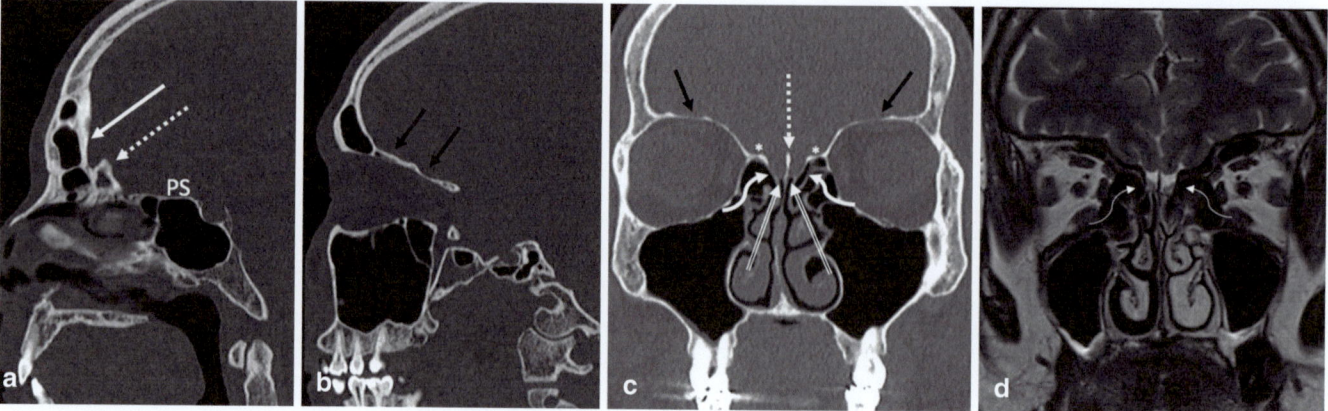

Fig. 32.2 Anatomy of the anterior skull base. Midline sagittal noncontrast CT image (**a**) demonstrates the ASB including the posterior wall of the frontal sinuses (solid white arrow), the crista galli (dashed white arrow), and planum sphenoidale (PS). Parasagittal noncontrast CT image at the level of the orbits (**b**) demonstrates the orbital plate of the frontal bone (solid black arrows) forming the roof of the orbit/lateral portion of the ASB. Coronal noncontrast CT image (**c**) through the ASB demonstrates the orbital plate of the frontal bone laterally (solid black arrows), fovea ethmoidalis (ethmoid roof) (*), lateral lamella (curved white arrows), cribriform plate (double lined white arrows), and crista galli (dashed white arrow). Coronal T2 weighted MRI image (**d**) demonstrates the olfactory bulbs (curved white arrows) sitting in the olfactory fossa (formed by the lateral lamella, cribriform plate, and crista galli)

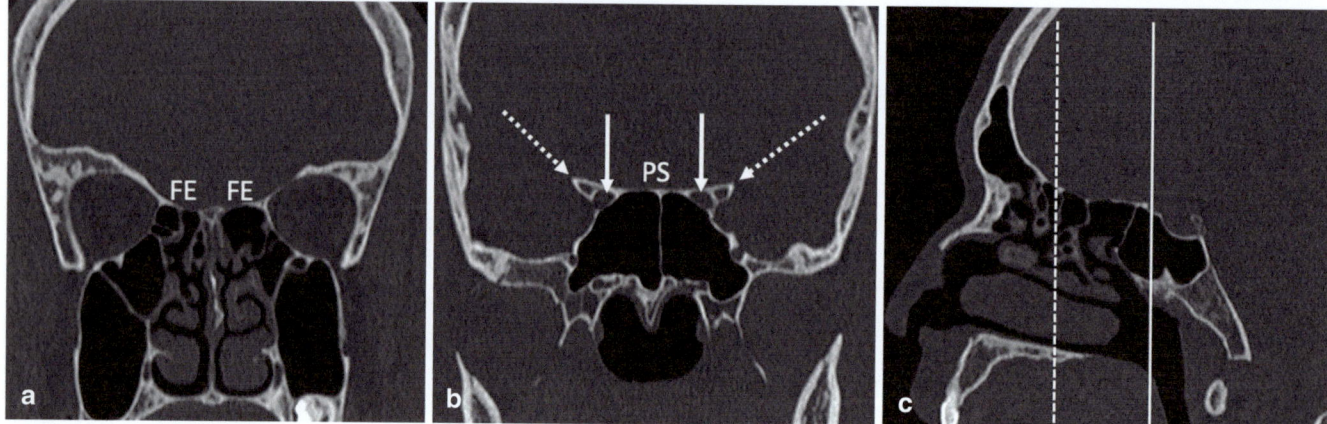

Fig. 32.3 Anatomy of the anterior skull base. Coronal CT images posterior to the cribriform plate at the level of the ethmoid roof/fovea ethmoidalis (FE) (**a**), and more posteriorly at the level of the sphenoid roof/planum sphenoidale (PS) (**b**). Sagittal CT image (**c**) demonstrates the corresponding area of anatomy with a dashed line corresponding to (**a**), and solid line corresponding to (**b**). Also seen in (**b**) are the anterior clinoid processes (dashed arrows) and optic canals (solid arrows)

- Incomplete regression of the tract can be associated with congenital midline abnormalities such as congenital nasal cephaloceles, nasal glial heterotopia, and epidermoid/dermoid cysts.
- Anterior clinoid process:
  - Medial portion of the lesser sphenoid wing.
  - Can be pneumatized by the sphenoid sinus or a variant ethmoid air cell ("Onodi" cell) extending superior or lateral to the sphenoid sinus.
  - Borders the superior orbital fissure and the optic canal—both open into the middle cranial fossa but can be involved by pathology affecting the anterior skull base.
- Optic canal:
  - Medial to the anterior clinoid process.
  - Transmits optic nerve, ophthalmic artery, and sympathetic nerve fibers.
- Superior orbital fissure:
  - Lateral to anterior clinoid process.
  - Transmits cranial nerves III, IV, V1, VI, and superior ophthalmic vein.
- Anterior ethmoid artery canals:
  - Variable positioning—at the skull base (relatively protected) or through the ethmoid air cells (at greater risk during endoscopic surgery).
  - Injury can result in lateral retraction with a rapidly expanding arterial intraorbital hematoma.

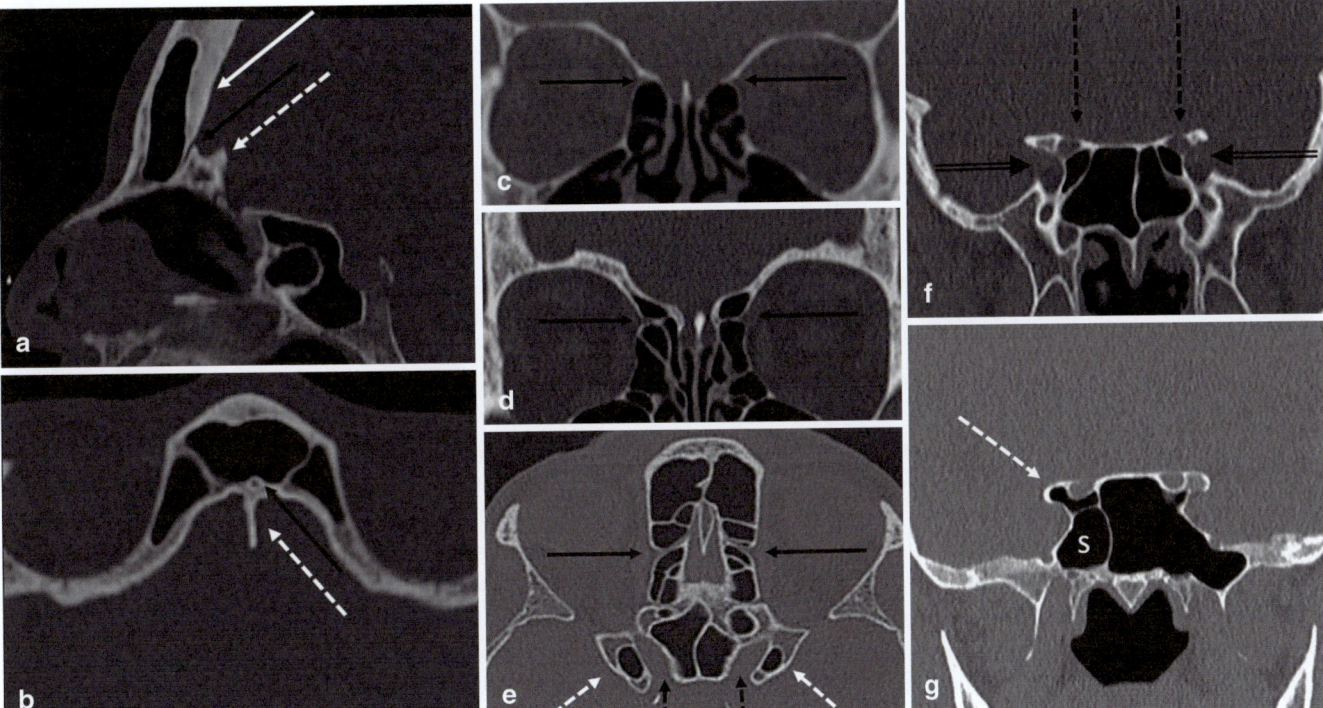

Fig. 32.4 Anatomy of the anterior skull base. Foramen cecum: Sagittal noncontrast CT (**a**) and corresponding axial CT image (**b**) demonstrate the residual tract of foramen cecum (solid black arrow) between the frontal bone anteriorly (solid white arrow) and the ethmoid bone/crista galli posteriorly (dashed white arrow). Anterior ethmoid artery canals: Coronal CT (**c**) demonstrates the anterior ethmoid artery canals (solid black arrows)—seen as a thin invagination along the superior aspect of the lamina papyracea in a relatively protected position traveling along the skull base. Coronal CT (**d**) demonstrates low-lying anterior ethmoid artery canals (solid black arrows) positioned inferior to the skull base traveling through the ethmoid air cells, placing them at high risk for injury during sinus surgery. Axial CT image (**e**) demonstrates the anterior ethmoid artery canals traversing the ethmoid air cells (solid black arrows). Also seen are pneumatized anterior clinoid processes (dashed white arrows), as well as the optic canals (dashed black arrows)—medial to the anterior clinoid process. Coronal CT (**f**) demonstrates the optic canals (dashed back arrows) medial to the anterior clinoid process. The superior orbital fissure (double black arrows) is inferolateral to the anterior clinoid process. Both transmit structures to the middle cranial fossa but are bordered by the anterior skull base. Coronal CT (**g**) demonstrates pneumatization of the right anterior clinoid process (dashed white arrow) by a variant ethmoid "Onodi" cell superior to the sphenoid sinus (S)

IMAGING CONSIDERATIONS

- CT:
  o Delineation of osseous changes.
    - Erosion or irregular, permeative changes margins suggest an aggressive lesion or pathologic process (can include infection/inflammation).
    - Smooth osseous changes, remodeling, and expansion suggest a benign or indolent process, however, can also be associated with some malignant processes [2].
  o Demonstrates characteristic bony changes of osseous lesions (can involve any part of the skull base; not limited to ASB).
    - Ground glass appearance suggests Fibrous Dysplasia.
    - Cortical and trabecular thickening suggests Paget's disease.

- MRI:
  o Evaluation for intracranial extension and orbital involvement—often confers a worse prognosis or higher tumor staging, and impacts surgical approach and treatment planning.
  o Dural or brain parenchymal invasion.
    - Nodular dural enhancement, or dural thickness >5 mm suggests dural invasion. Smooth thickening can reflect reactive or inflammatory changes [3].
    - Irregular parenchymal enhancement and vasogenic edema suggest parenchymal invasion [2].
  o Lesion characterization.
    - Diffusion restriction, low T2 signal suggest cellular lesion (e.g., lymphoma).
    - No diffusion restriction, high T2 signal suggests a relatively acellular lesion, or lesion with high mucin

content (e.g., low-grade minor salivary gland tumor).
  o Allows differentiation of masses from benign/inflammatory sinonasal mucosal disease [4].

Pathology

Pathology can originate from the bone itself, can be an intracranial process extending caudally, or a paranasal or orbital process extending cranially.

- Primary osseous pathology:
  o For example, fibrous dysplasia and Paget's disease—involvement not limited to the ASB.
  o Imaging findings are similar to those seen elsewhere in the body and skull base.
  o Attention should be paid to narrowing of involved.
- Congenital lesions associated with the ASB (Fig. 32.5) [1]:
  o Congenital nasal cephaloceles:
    • Persistent dural diverticulum extending through the ASB containing meninges and CSF (meningocele), or meninges, CSF, and parenchyma (meningoencephalocele).
    • Can be intranasal or extranasal.
    • Maintains direct connection to the intracranial compartment.
    • Risk of spread of infection to the intracranial compartment.
  o Nasal glial heterotopia:
    • A similar embryological mechanism to congenital nasal cephalocele, however, does not communicate with the intracranial compartment.
    • Contains meninges and neural tissue which has separated from the intracranial compartment. A thin non-communicating fibrous tract may be present.
  o Nasal dermoid/epidermoid cysts—midline epithelial lined cysts:
    • May present as a midline nasal cyst or skin pit along the glabella, nasal bridge, or columella.

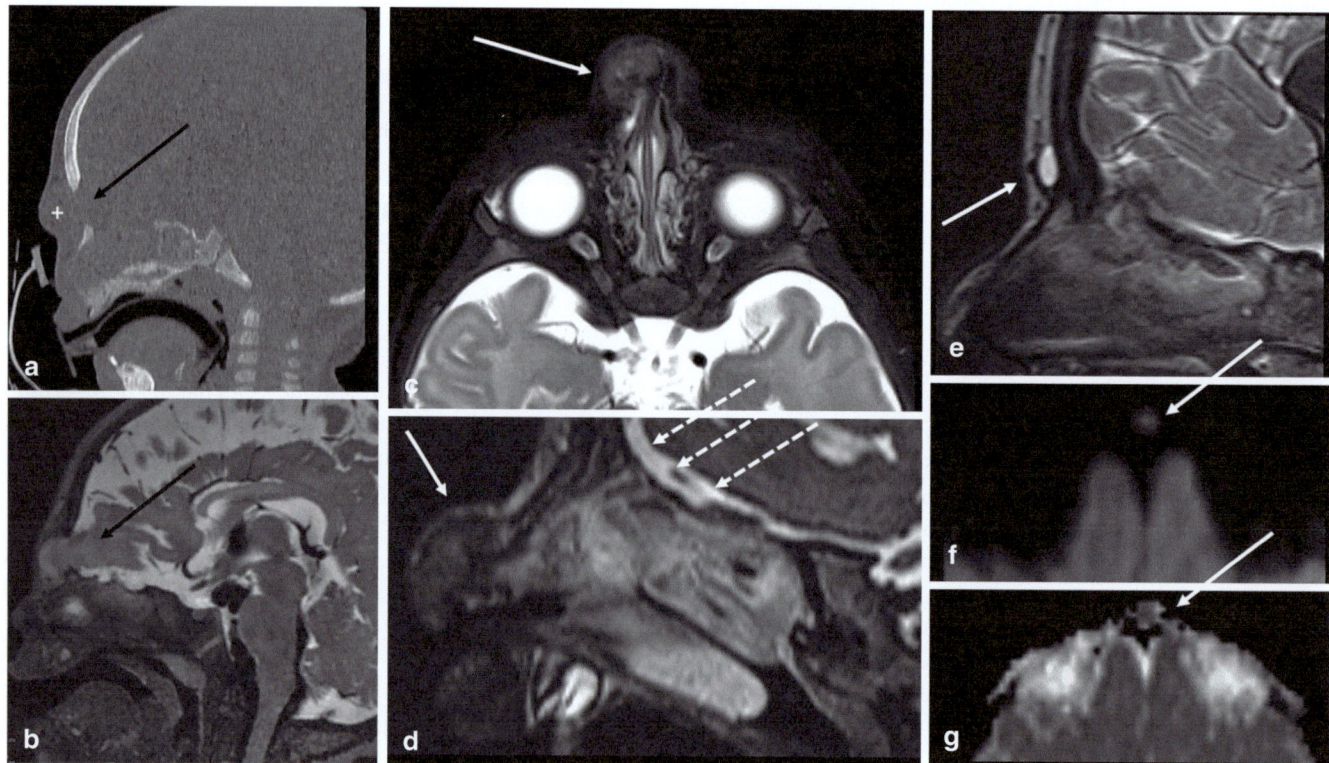

Fig. 32.5 Congenital midline lesions associated with the ASB. Sagittal noncontrast head CT in 6 month old (**a**) demonstrates an osseous defect at the nasofrontal junction (solid black arrow), with an overlying mass at the level of the glabella (+). Sagittal T2 MRI (**b**) demonstrates direct continuity of the brain parenchyma with the extranasal mass (solid black arrow) compatible with a nasal meningoencephalocele. Axial T2 MRI in a different patient (**c**) demonstrates a mass associated with the nasal dorsum and sidewall (solid white arrow). Sagittal T2 MRI (**d**) demonstrates no continuity of the mass (solid white arrow) with the intracranial compartment (dashed white arrows). Biopsy demonstrated gliotic neural tissue compatible with nasal glial heterotopia. Sagittal T2 MR image in a different patient (**e**) demonstrates a well-circumscribed T2 hyperintense lesion at the glabella (solid white arrow) without evidence of communication with the intracranial compartment. Axial DWI (**f**) and ADC maps (**g**) demonstrate diffusion restriction within the lesion (solid white arrows), compatible with a midline nasal epidermoid cyst

- Can be an isolated lesion or associated with a sinus tract extending to the intracranial compartment. Part of radiologic assessment is to exclude communication with anterior cranial fossa.
- Can become superinfected and cause meningitis if persistent communication exists.
- Imaging: (can have overlapping imaging features) [5, 6]:
  - Well-circumscribed, centrally nonenhancing lesion.
  - May have adjacent bony remodeling.
  - Epidermoids—fluid attenuation on CT and T2 hyperintense with possible diffusion restriction on MRI.
  - Dermoids may be fat density on CT with variable T1 signal on MRI.
  - May see enlarged foramen cecum or bifid crista galli.
- Intracranial pathology.
  - Meningiomas (Fig. 32.6):
    - Characteristic ASB locations—olfactory groove, planum sphenoidale.
    - Extra-axial, dural based lesion.
    - Relatively common, usually slow-growing tumor arising from arachnoid cap cells associated with the meninges.
    - Clues suggesting this diagnosis include adjacent hyperostosis and, along the ASB, pneumosinus dilatans (secondary expansion of an adjacent pneumatized sinus) [7].
    - MRI—usually homogenous enhancement. Can have internal mineralization inhomogeneous enhancement, low T1/T2 signal.
    - Due to the location, can encase and narrow olfactory bulbs or tracts, optic nerves and chiasm, and anterior circulation vessels.
- Cephalocele/CSF leak (Fig. 32.7):
  o Common areas include posterior table of the frontal sinus, fovea ethmoidalis, and cribriform plate.
  o CT is better for demonstrating the extent of osseous defect.
  o MRI helps confirm the presence of meninges and CSF alone (meningocele) versus the presence of brain parenchyma (meningoencephalocele).
  o CT cisternography with intrathecal contrast is useful to demonstrate site of active CSF leak.
  o Distortion and encephalomalacia/gliosis of the inferior frontal lobes can be an important clue to the diagnosis.
  o Can present as a nasal cavity mass—accurate diagnosis is important to avoid biopsy.
- Sinonasal pathology: goals of imaging are to distinguish benign from malignant processes and identify the extent of disease including skull base and intracranial involvement.
  o Benign/inflammatory—sinusitis and associated complications (Fig. 32.8):
    - Chronic sinus opacification—variable density on CT and signal intensity on MRI due to chronic inspissated sections with low water/high protein

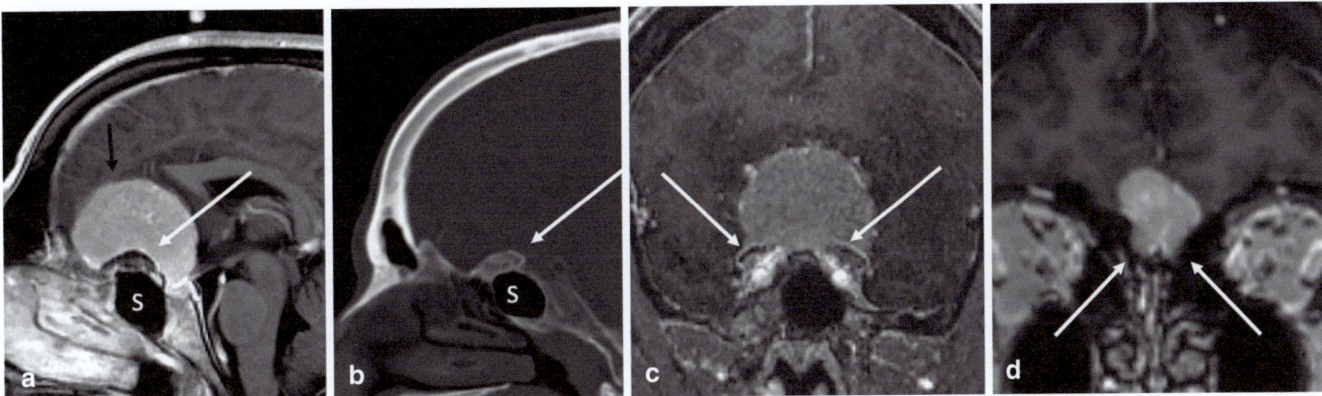

Fig. 32.6 Planum sphenoidale and olfactory groove meningiomas. Sagittal post-contrast T1 MRI image (**a**) demonstrates an avidly enhancing, extra-axial mass (solid black arrow) along the midline anterior skull base extending to the sella turcica. Adjacent hyperostosis of the planum sphenoidale (solid white arrow), also seen in sagittal CT image (**b**), and slight expansion of the sphenoid sinus (S), called "pneumosinus dilatans," are commonly associated with skull base meningiomas and are clues to the diagnosis. Coronal post-contrast T1 MRI image of the same lesion (**c**) demonstrates encasement of the optic nerves (indistinguishable from the mass) as they exit the optic canals adjacent to the anterior clinoid processes (solid white arrows). Coronal post-contrast T1 MRI image (**d**) demonstrates a different olfactory groove meningioma filling the olfactory fossa (solid white arrows) and encasing the olfactory bulbs (indistinguishable from the mass)

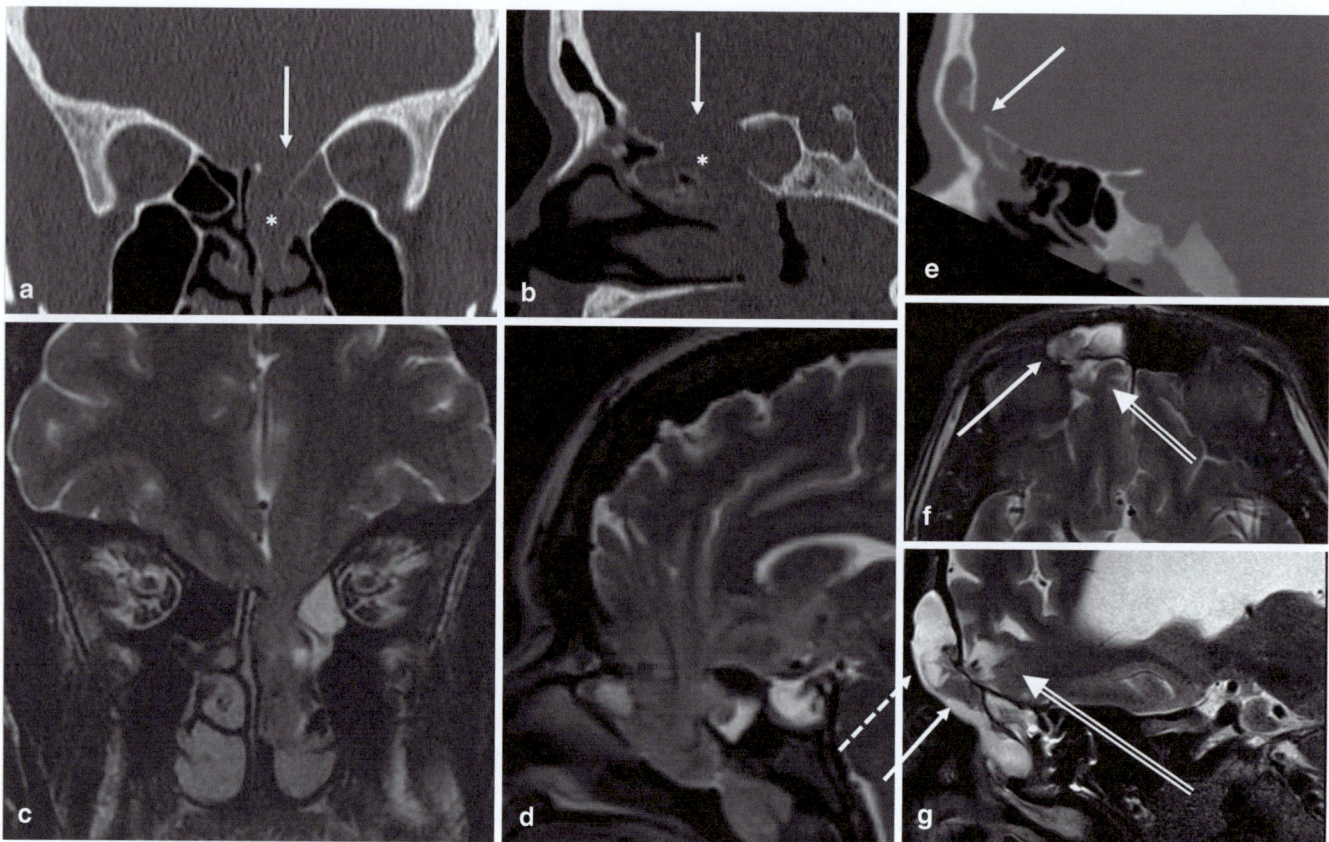

Fig. 32.7 Cephoceles. Coronal (**a**) and sagittal (**b**) images from noncontrast CT demonstrate a large defect in the left cribriform plate (solid white arrows) with nonspecific soft tissue in the adjacent nasal cavity (*). Corresponding coronal (**c**) and sagittal (**d**) T2-weighted MR images confirm the presence of herniated brain parenchyma through the ASB defect compatible with a meningoencephalocele. Sagittal noncontrast CT (**e**) demonstrates a defect in the posterior wall of the right frontal sinus (solid white arrow), and complete sinus opacification. Corresponding axial (**f**) and sagittal (**g**) T2-weighted MRI images demonstrate the presence of a small encephalocele (solid white arrows) surrounded by T2 hyperintense obstructed sinus secretions (dashed white arrows). Distortion and gliosis of the adjacent brain are a clue to the diagnosis (double white arrows)

content [2], or fungal colonization with associated mineral salt deposition [8]:
- Mixed areas of low and high density on CT.
- Areas of low T2 signal and high T1 signal on MRI.
- Mucocele formation:
  - Slow expansion of a sinus secondary to chronic outflow obstruction with continued mucin production.
  - Slow process results in smooth bony remodeling.
  - Can result in dehiscence of the sinus walls marginating the intracranial or intraorbital compartments.
  - Local mass effect can result in proptosis or obstruction of adjacent sinus cavities.
- Complicated bacterial or invasive fungal sinusitis—spread of infection beyond the sinus cavity:
  - Can result in intracranial infection through direct extension of infection through the anterior skull base.

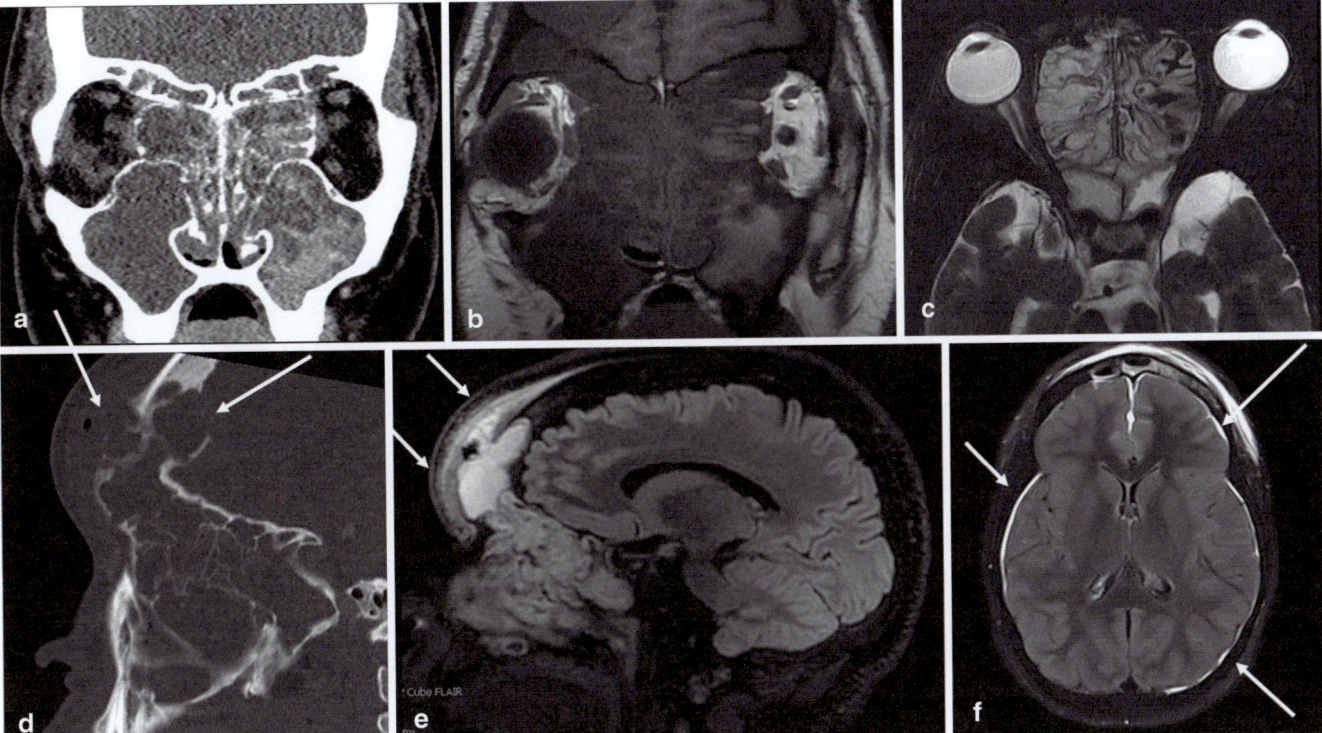

Fig. 32.8 Sinusitis and associated complications. Coronal noncontrast CT (**a**) in a patient with nasal polyposis and chronic allergic fungal pansinusitis presenting with acute bacterial superinfection. Mixed areas of high and low attenuation compatible with proteinaceous inspissated secretions and fungal mineralization. Note bilateral ethmoid and maxillary sinus expansion with bony remodeling (mucocele formation) and secondary mass effect on the orbital compartment. Corresponding coronal T1 (**b**) and axial T2 (**c**) demonstrate areas of heterogeneous signal intensity with intermixed areas of high T1 signal and markedly low T2 signal reflecting internal proteinaceous material and mineral deposition. Note again sinus expansion narrowing the orbital compartments. Sagittal noncontrast CT (**d**) demonstrates complete sinus opacification with frontal sinus mucocele formation with osseous remodeling, thinning, and areas of complete osseous dehiscence along the anterior and posterior frontal sinus walls (solid white arrows). Note abnormal soft tissue fullness and subcutaneous emphysema overlying the frontal bone compatible with a secondary subperiosteal abscess, sometimes referred to as "Pott's puffy tumor." Sagittal T2 FLAIR image (**e**) of the brain demonstrates dehiscence of sinus infection into the frontal soft tissues (solid white arrow) secondary to bacterial superinfection. Chronic thinning and demineralization of the posterior table of the frontal sinus/ASB allows easy access for the spread of infection to the intracranial compartment. Axial T2 FLAIR with fat saturation (**f**) in a different patient with Pott's puffy tumor demonstrates complex bilateral subdural fluid collections compatible with intracranial spread of infection (solid white arrows)

- ▪ "Pott's Puffy tumor": Frontal bone osteomyelitis with overlying subperiosteal abscess, usually secondary to sinusitis.
- o Malignant/aggressive (Figs. 32.9 and 32.10):
  - • CT and MRI are often complementary in the evaluation of malignant neoplasms.
  - • Esthesioneuroblastoma (olfactory neuroblastoma—neuroendocrine tumor):
    - ▪ Arises from olfactory mucosa of the superior nasal cavity.
    - ▪ Frequent intracranial extension through the cribriform plate—snowman or dumbbell configuration with a "waist" at the level of the cribriform plate.
    - ▪ Peritumoral cysts at the brain tumor interface are not specific, however, suggestive of the diagnosis [9, 10].
  - • Primary sinonasal cavity malignancies.
    - ▪ Varied histopathologies include squamous cell carcinoma (most common), adenocarcinoma,

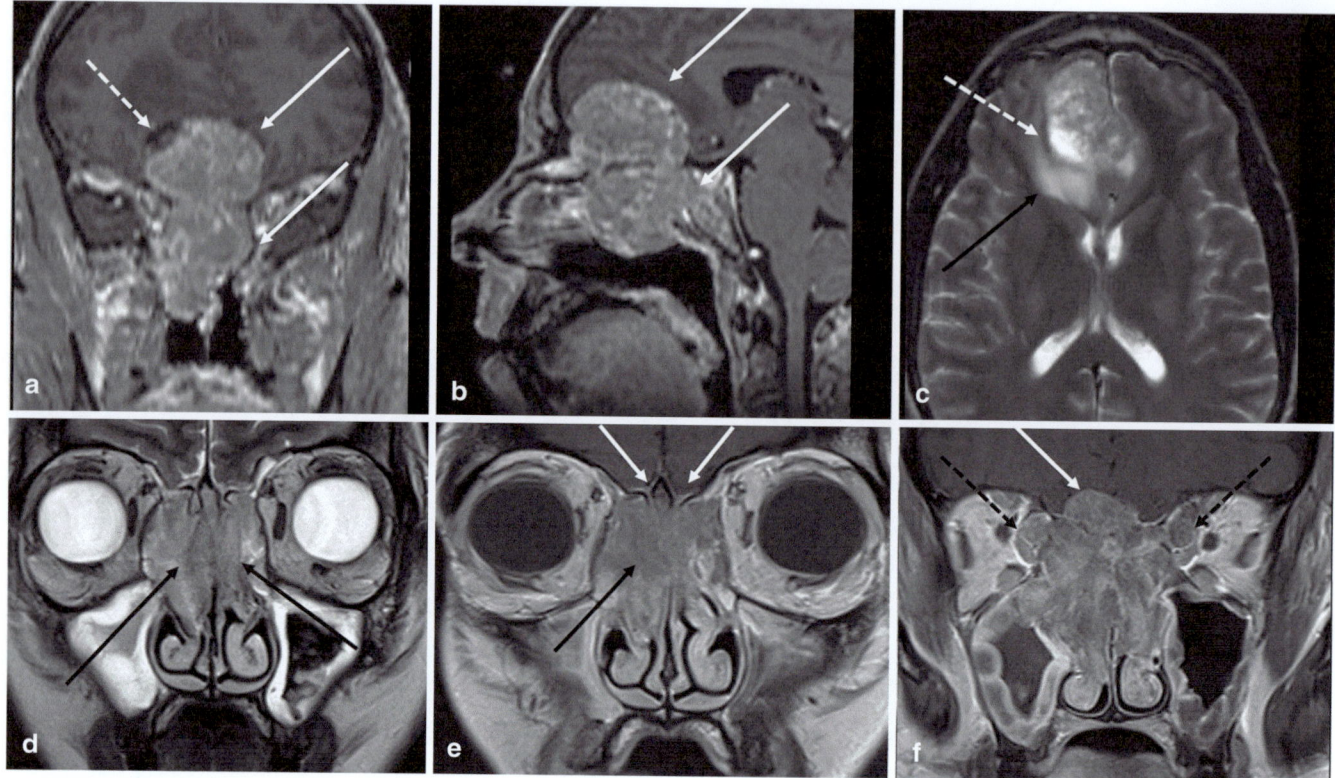

Fig. 32.9 Aggressive/malignant lesions of the sinonasal cavity. Upper row—Esthesioneuroblastoma. Coronal post-contrast T1 MR image (**a**) and sagittal post-contrast T1 image (**b**) demonstrate a dumbbell-shaped enhancing solid mass centered at the cribriform plate with superior intracranial and inferior nasal cavity/sinus extension (solid white arrows). Axial T2 MR image (**c**) in the same patient demonstrates a small cystic focus at the brain tumor interface (dashed white arrow), seen as the non-enhancing component in (dashed white arrow in a). Adjacent parenchymal edema (solid black arrow) suggests parenchymal invasion. Lower row—Sinonasal undifferentiated carcinoma (SNUC). Coronal T2-weighted (**d**) and post-contrast T1-weighted images (**e** and **f**) demonstrate a large heterogeneously enhancing mass centered in the superior sinonasal cavity (solid black arrows) with intracranial (solid white arrows) and intraorbital (dashed black arrows) invasion

sinonasal undifferentiated carcinoma, sinonasal melanoma, primary sinonasal lymphoma, among others.
- Imaging appearance can be similar with diagnosis requiring tissue sampling.
- Goal of imaging is to map extent of disease involvement including skull base/osseous destruction, intracranial and/or intra-orbital involvement.
  ♦ Signs of dural invasion—nodular dural enhancement, thickening >5 mm. Smooth dural thickening could reflect secondary reactive/inflammatory changes [3].
  ♦ Signs of parenchymal invasion—irregular enhancing margin at the brain tumor interface, adjacent parenchymal edema.
- Nonprimary or metastatic head and neck lesions:
  - Look for aggressive osseous erosion or invasion of adjacent structures.
  - Areas of lower T2 signal and diffusion restriction can help distinguish the mass from T2 bright inflammatory mucosal changes [4].

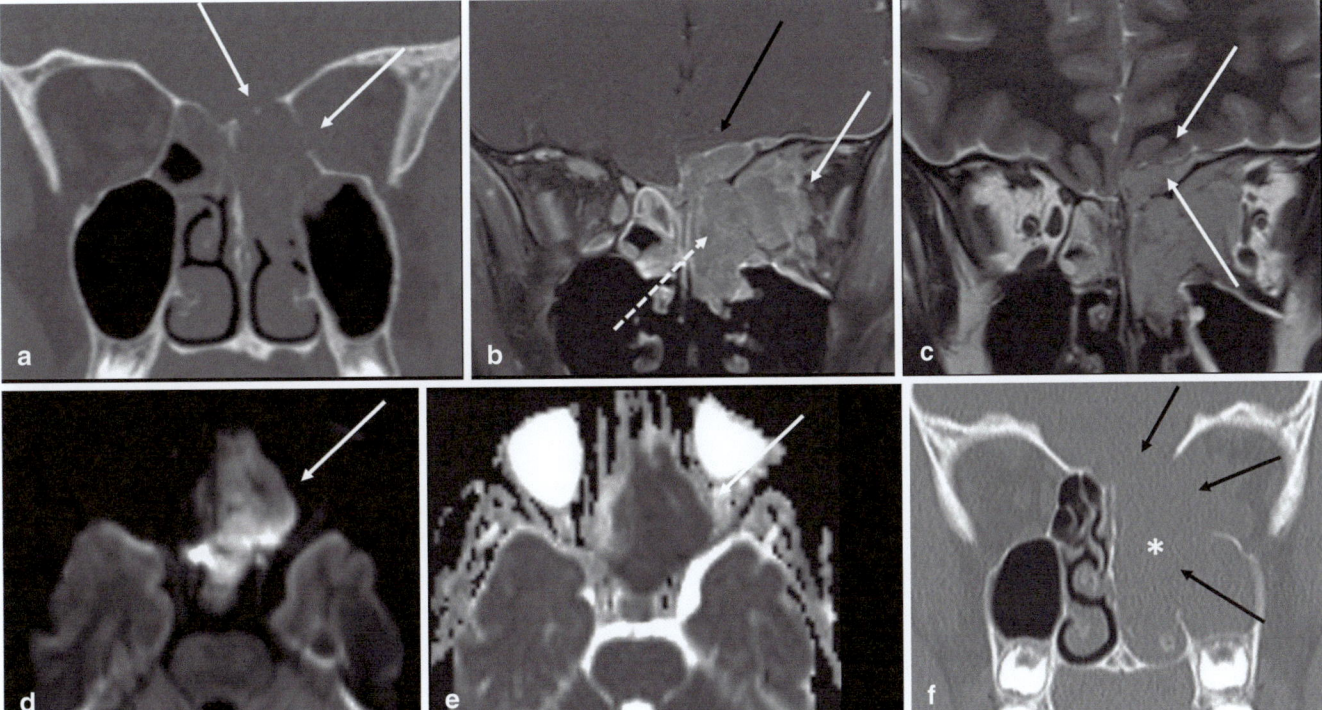

Fig. 32.10 Metastatic or systemic lesions involving the sinonasal cavity and ASB. Coronal noncontrast CT image (**a**) demonstrates partial soft tissue opacification of the sinonasal cavity in a 5-year-old patient. Erosion of the fovea ethmoidalis and left lamina papyracea (solid white arrows) are important clues suggesting an aggressive or malignant process rather than benign sinus disease. Coronal T1 postcontrast MR with fat saturation (**b**) demonstrates an enhancing solid lesion crossing the ASB with involvement of the intracranial (solid black arrow), orbital (solid white arrow), and sinonasal (dashed white arrow) compartments. Coronal T2 MR image (**c**) demonstrates a relatively smooth brain tumor interface (solid white arrow) with a partially visualized intervening CSF cleft and absence of parenchymal edema suggesting no brain parenchymal invasion. Axial DWI (**d**) and ADC maps (**e**) demonstrate marked lesion diffusion restriction (solid white arrows) compatible with high tumor cellularity, also reflected by relatively low lesion T2 signal in (**c**). Tumor pathology was consistent with rhabdomyosarcoma. Coronal noncontrast CT (**f**) in a different patient with rhabdomyosarcoma demonstrates complete opacification of the left nasal cavity and paranasal sinuses (*) with surrounding osseous erosion of the ASB, lamina papyracea, and sinus walls (solid black arrows)

References

1. Som PM, Curtin HD. Head and neck imaging. 5th ed. St. Louis: Mosby; 2011.
2. Raghavan P, Phillips CD. Magnetic resonance imaging of sinonasal malignancies. Top Magn Reson Imaging. 2007;18(4):259–67.
3. Eisen MD, Yousem DM, Montone KT, Kotapka MJ, Bigelow DC, Bilker WB, et al. Use of preoperative MR to predict dural, perineural, and venous sinus invasion of skull base tumors. AJNR Am J Neuroradiol. 1996;17(10):1937–45.
4. Som PM, Shapiro MD, Biller HF, Sasaki C, Lawson W. Sinonasal tumors and inflammatory tissues: differentiation with MR imaging. Radiology. 1988;167(3):803–8.
5. Lowe LH, Booth TN, Joglar JM, Rollins NK. Midface anomalies in children. Radiographics. 2000;20(4):907–22; quiz 1106–7, 12.
6. Rodriguez DP, Orscheln ES, Koch BL. Masses of the nose, nasal cavity, and nasopharynx in children. Radiographics. 2017;37(6):1704–30.
7. Parizel PM, Carpentier K, Van Marck V, Venstermans C, De Belder F, Van Goethem J, et al. Pneumosinus dilatans in anterior skull base meningiomas. Neuroradiology. 2013;55(3):307–11.
8. Zinreich SJ, Kennedy DW, Malat J, Curtin HD, Epstein JI, Huff LC, et al. Fungal sinusitis: diagnosis with CT and MR imaging. Radiology. 1988;169(2):439–44.
9. Schuster JJ, Phillips CD, Levine PA. MR of esthesioneuroblastoma (olfactory neuroblastoma) and appearance after craniofacial resection. AJNR Am J Neuroradiol. 1994;15(6):1169–77.
10. Som PM, Lidov M, Brandwein M, Catalano P, Biller HF. Sinonasal esthesioneuroblastoma with intracranial extension: marginal tumor cysts as a diagnostic MR finding. AJNR Am J Neuroradiol. 1994;15(7):1259–62.

Central Skull Base

Nikdokht Farid, Soudabeh Fazeli, Paul Manning, and Michael Shroads

Anatomy Overview [1]

- The central skull base represents a three-dimensional region that is roughly spherical in shape (Fig. e33.1).
- (All electronic images (Figs. e33.1–e33.10) can be found on this chapter's website on SpringerLink: https://doi.org/10.1007/978-3-031-55124-6_33).
- The superior pole is at the level of the optic chiasm and the inferior pole is at the level of the nasopharynx.
- The equator of the sphere encompasses the pterygopalatine fossa (PPF) anteriorly, the foramen ovale laterally, and the prepontine cistern posteriorly.
- The bones of the central skull base:
  - Sphenoid bone—clivus, pterygoid plates and processes, sella, and greater and lesser wings of sphenoid.
  - Temporal bone—petrous apex, petroclival fissure.
- Multiple canals, foramina, and fissures are present within the central skull base, which contain important neurovascular structures including cranial nerves II–VI (Fig. e33.2).
- CT and MR imaging are complementary in the evaluation of the complex anatomy and pathology of the central skull base.

Anatomical Variants [2]

- Arrested pneumatization of the sphenoid sinus (Fig. e33.3).
  - Occurs when developing respiratory epithelium does not extend into areas of the sphenoid body, which have already undergone fatty marrow conversion in preparation for sinus formation.
  - Imaging appearance on CT:
    - Bone window—lucent lesion with sclerotic margins and areas of curvilinear calcification.
    - Soft tissue window—fat attenuation.
  - Important to recognize this entity so as not to confuse it with true pathology.
- Asymmetric pneumatization of the petrous apex (Fig. e33.4).
  - Petrous apex can be pneumatized or non-pneumatized.
  - The non-pneumatized petrous apex can easily be identified on CT as an area of normal-appearing bone. However, on MRI it will appear as conspicuous T1 hyperintense marrow and could be mistaken for other entities such as cholesterol granuloma.
  - Normal bony contours and lack of bony expansion are key to recognizing this entity.
- Rare sphenoid and clival variants such as craniopharyngeal canal, canalis basilaris medianus, and fossa navicularis magna (Fig. e33.5).
  - Usually incidentally found but may facilitate the spread of infection to/from the central skull base.
  - Important to be familiar with these entities to avoid unnecessary work-up.

Supplementary Information The online version contains supplementary material available at https://doi.org/10.1007/978-3-031-55124-6_33.

N. Farid (✉) · S. Fazeli
University of California, San Diego, La Jolla, CA, USA
e-mail: nfarid@health.ucsd.edu; sfazelidehkordy@health.ucsd.edu

P. Manning
University of California, San Diego, La Jolla, CA, USA

VA Health System, San Diego, La Jolla, CA, USA
e-mail: pmanning@health.ucsd.edu

M. Shroads
Clinical Radiology & Imaging Sciences, Indiana University, Indianapolis, IN, USA
e-mail: mshroads@iuhealth.org

Developmental Lesions [2, 3]

- Ecchordosis physaliphora (Fig. 33.1).
  - Benign intradural hamartomatous lesion derived from residual notochord.
  - Asymptomatic, incidentally found on imaging, no growth.
  - Difficult to distinguish from chordoma based on histopathology, therefore imaging is key to diagnosis.
  - Characteristic location—retroclival, prepontine, intradural.
  - Imaging appearance on CT: well-defined lucent lesion along the dorsal aspect of the clivus.
  - Imaging appearance on MR: high signal on T2, low signal on T1, no enhancement, stalk-like connection to the clivus may be seen.
- Fibrous dysplasia (FD) (Fig. 33.2).
  - Mesenchymal disorder is characterized by benign expansion of bone.

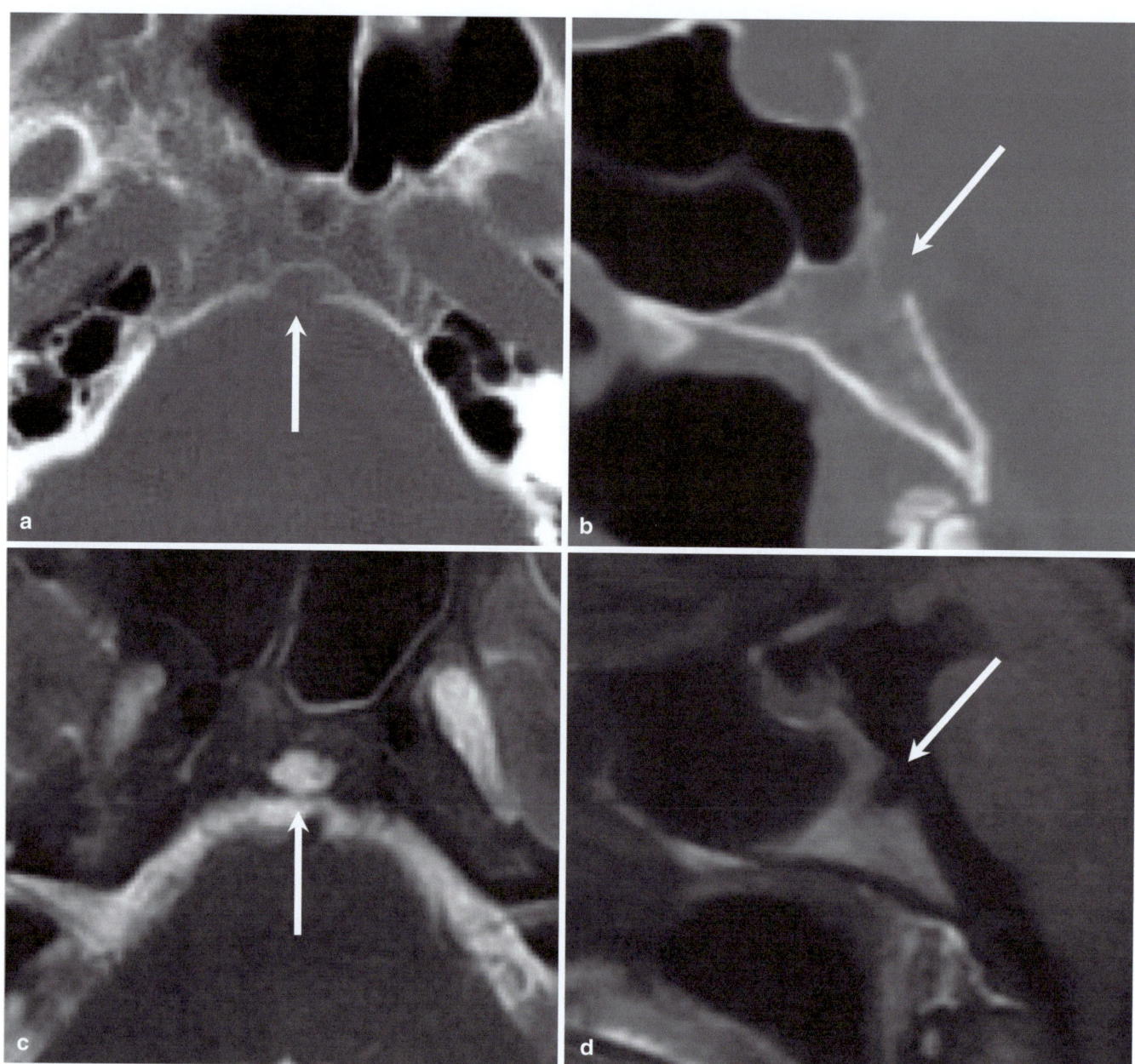

Fig. 33.1 Ecchordosis physaliphora. Axial (**a**) and sagittal (**b**) CT images demonstrate a well-defined lucent lesion on the dorsal aspect of the clivus. Axial T2-weighted (**c**) and sagittal T1-weighted (**d**) images demonstrate a well-defined lesion on the dorsal aspect of the clivus which is T2 hyperintense, T1 hypointense, and slightly lobulated

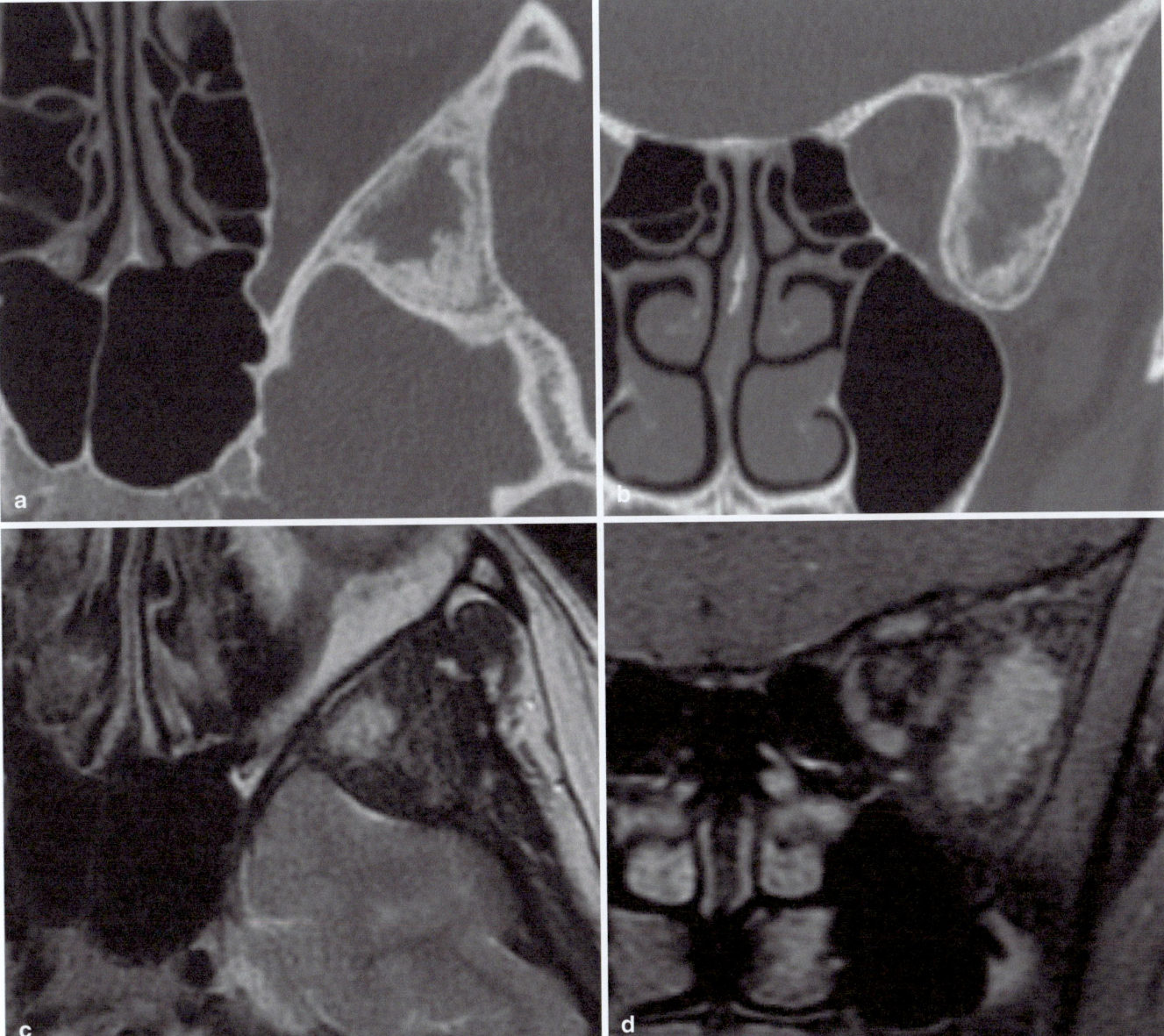

Fig. 33.2 Fibrous dysplasia. Axial (**a**) and coronal (**b**) CT images demonstrate a benign-appearing expansile lesion centered in the left greater wing of sphenoid with central lucency and peripheral sclerosis. Axial T2 (**c**) and coronal T1 post-contrast fat-suppressed (**d**) images demonstrates a predominantly T2 hypointense lesion with central T2 hyperintensity and associated enhancement

- o Skull and facial bones are involved in 10–25% of monostotic FD and in 50% of polyostotic FD.
- o Imaging appearance on CT: ground-glass pattern (56%), homogeneously dense pattern (23%), cystic pattern (21%).
- o Imaging appearance on MR: intermediate T1 signal, low T2 signal, enhances on post-contrast imaging.
- o Imaging appearance on PET: FDG avid.
- o CT is key for diagnosis as the MR and PET appearance may mimic tumor.

Osteodural Defects [4, 5]

- Osteodural defects can be acquired or congenital.
    - o Acquired are most common and can be due to iatrogenic causes (e.g., endoscopic sinus surgery), trauma, or elevated intracranial pressure.
    - o Close association between osteodural defects and idiopathic intracranial hypertension.

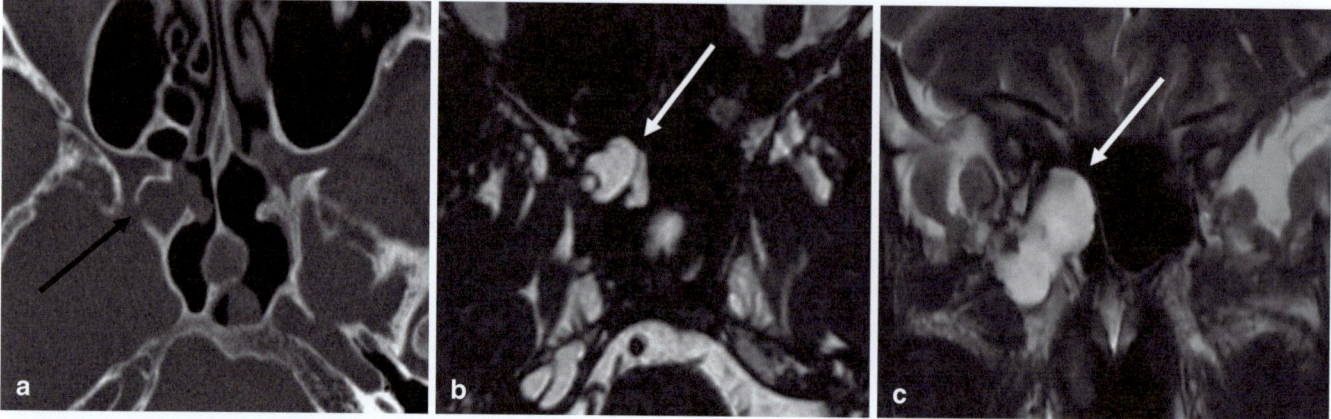

Fig. 33.3 Sphenoid sinus meningocele. Axial non-contrast CT image (**a**) demonstrates a focal osseous defect along the lateral wall of the right sphenoid sinus (black arrow) with associated opacification of the right lateral recess. Incidentally noted mucous retention cysts in the inter-sphenoid septum and in the left sphenoid sinus. Axial FIESTA (**b**) and coronal T2-weighted (**c**) images demonstrate a CSF outpouching (white arrow) extending medially through the defect into the right sphenoid sinus

- - Regardless of cause, the end result is communication between the subarachnoid space and the sinonasal or tympanomastoid cavity.
- Clinical manifestations include rhinorrhea, otorrhea, conductive or sensorineural hearing loss, meningitis, and seizures.
- Nomenclature is complex and depends on the contents of the defect.
  - Meningocele—only CSF and meninges herniating.
  - Meningoencephalocele/encephalocele—CSF, meninges, and brain parenchyma herniating.
  - Other associated terminologies include CSF leak, CSF fistula, and arachnoid diverticulum.
- Common locations include cribriform plate, sphenoid sinus (Fig. 33.3), petrous apex (Fig. e33.6), tegmen tympani (Fig. e33.7), and tegmen mastoideum.
- Imaging appearance on CT: osseous defect; air-fluid levels and opacification of the sinus, middle ear, or mastoid air cells; occasionally pneumocephalus.
- Imaging appearance on MR: CSF fluid signal, meninges, and/or brain parenchyma extending through the osseous defect; altered parenchymal signal intensity (due to edema or gliosis).

Petrous Apex-Specific Entities [6]

- The petrous apex is a pyramidal-shaped structure that is formed by the medial portions of the temporal bone and is bounded by the inner ear structures laterally, the petro-occipital fissure medially, the petro-sphenoidal fissure and ICA anteriorly, and the posterior cranial fossa posteriorly.

- Cholesterol granuloma (Fig. 33.4):
  - The most common lesion arises in the petrous apex.
  - Classically occurs in patients with a pneumatized petrous apex.
  - The pathogenesis is likely related to an initial obstruction of an air cell, which leads to the development of vacuum phenomenon, repeated cycles of hemorrhage and inflammatory response, and gradual expansion due to bone remodeling and resorption.
  - Imaging appearance on CT: expansile, well-defined, round, or ovoid lesion within the petrous apex with cortical thinning.
  - Imaging appearance on MR: typically hyperintense on both T1 and T2 (due to accumulation of blood breakdown products and proteinaceous debris), hypointense peripheral rim on T2 (due to hemosiderin deposition), possible subtle peripheral enhancement secondary to the inflammatory response.
  - Asymptomatic small cholesterol granulomas are managed conservatively, whereas large lesions and/or symptomatic lesions are treated with surgical drainage or cyst resection.
- Cholesteatoma:
  - Petrous apex cholesteatomas, also known as epidermoid cysts, are typically congenital, arising from aberrant ectoderm that is trapped during embryogenesis.
  - Classically seen in children and young adults.
  - They are slow growing and may be asymptomatic for years.
  - Progressive mass effect may cause hearing loss, cranial nerve palsies, or headache.
  - Imaging appearance on CT: non-enhancing expansile lesion in the petrous apex with variable degrees of bone destruction.

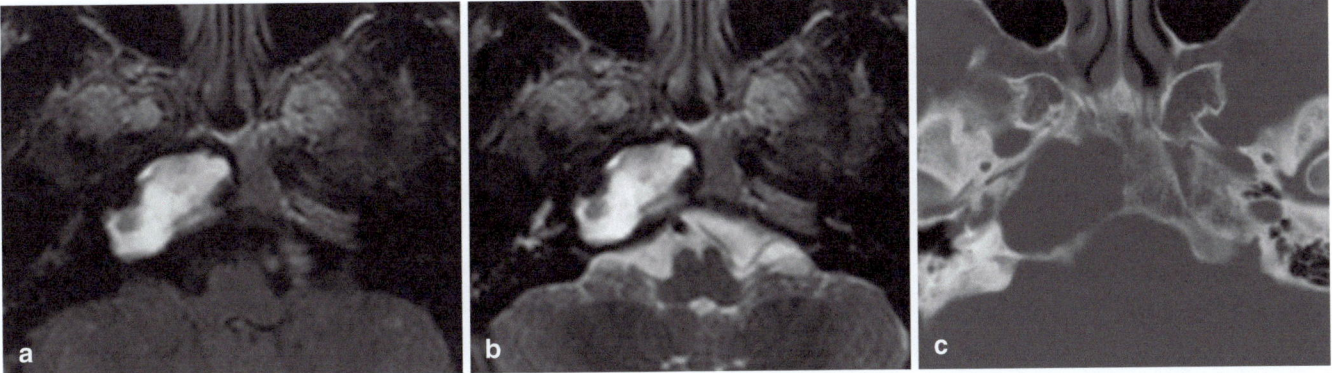

Fig. 33.4 Cholesterol granuloma. Axial T1-weighted (**a**) and T2-weighted (**b**) images demonstrate a well-defined T1 and T2 hyperintense lesion centered in the right petrous apex with a T1 and T2 hypointense peripheral rim. Axial non-contrast CT image (**c**) demonstrates a corresponding expansile and well-defined lesion with associated cortical thinning

- o Imaging appearance on MR: diffusion restriction on DWI/ADC is a characteristic feature that helps to differentiate cholesteatoma from other petrous apex entities, T1 hypointense and T2 hyperintense, typically with no enhancement.
- o Surgical excision or exteriorization is the treatment of choice.

- Petrous apex effusion (Fig. e33.8):
  - o Develops within a pneumatized petrous apex.
  - o Imaging appearance on CT: opacification and/or fluid level within the petrous apex, no bone remodeling, and preservation of bony septa.
  - o Imaging appearance on MR: high T2 signal intensity opacifying or layering in the petrous apex, no enhancement. May be high on T1 due to proteinaceous contents.

Infection/Inflammation [3, 7]

- Petrous apicitis (Fig. e33.9):
  - o Also known as apical petrositis.
  - o Refers to infection involving a pneumatized petrous apex; gram-positive cocci are the most commonly implicated organisms.
  - o Usually associated with severe otomastoiditis.
  - o Infection begins as an exudate limited to the petrous apex air cells, followed by bone involvement (osteomyelitis) and, in uncontrolled cases, spread to adjacent structures such as the meninges, extra-axial space, dural venous sinuses, and brain parenchyma.
  - o Gradenigo syndrome is the classic clinical presentation, though not seen in all cases, and consists of deep facial pain (due to trigeminal nerve involvement in Meckel's cave) and abducens nerve palsy (due to cranial nerve VI involvement in Dorello's canal).
  - o Imaging appearance on CT: opacification of the petrous apex air cells with varying degrees of osseous erosion.
  - o Imaging appearance on MR: fluid signal in a pneumatized petrous apex; heterogeneous, often peripheral enhancement; possible restricted diffusion.
  - o MRI is the preferred modality to evaluate for associated complications such as meningitis, epidural/subdural empyema, cerebritis, cerebral abscess, and thrombophlebitis.

- Skull base osteomyelitis (Fig. 33.5):
  - o Aggressive infection involving the central skull base +/− involvement of the temporal bone, external ear, and deep neck spaces.
  - o Most commonly occurs in elderly, diabetic, and immunocompromised patients.
  - o Pseudomonas aeruginosa is the most common causative organism.
  - o Clinical presentation is typically severe otalgia and otorrhea.
  - o Imaging appearance on CT: osseous erosions and destructive changes of the central skull base; soft tissue infiltration of the preclival soft tissues, external auditory canal, and infratemporal fossa with effacement of the normal fat planes.
  - o Imaging appearance on MR: replacement of the normal skull base marrow signal with T1 hypointensity, T2 hyperintensity, and enhancement.
  - o MRI is the preferred modality to evaluate for associated complications such as abscess formation, thrombophlebitis, cranial nerve involvement, and intracranial extension.
  - o Imaging findings can overlap with those of an aggressive malignancy; therefore, correlation with clinical data is of utmost importance.

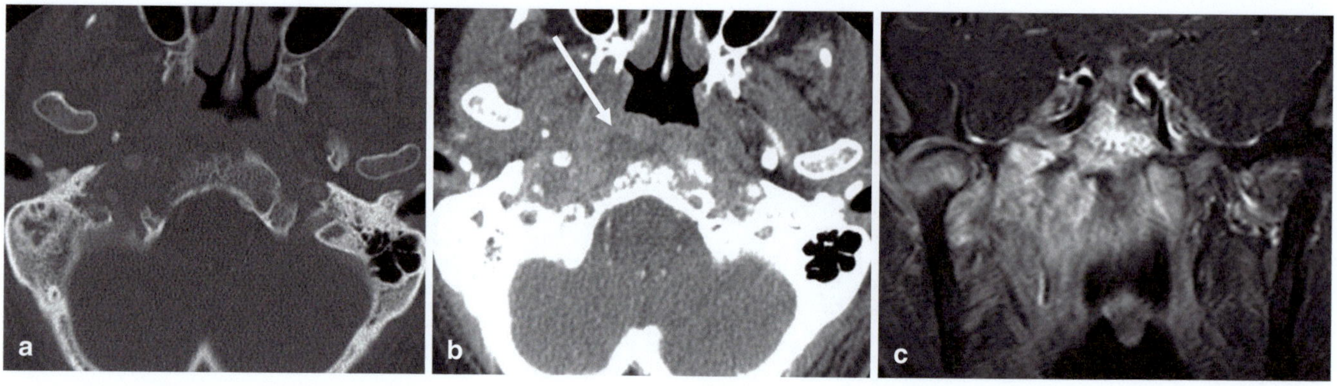

Fig. 33.5 Skull base osteomyelitis. Axial contrast-enhanced CT in bone algorithm (**a**) demonstrates destructive osseous changes involving the clivus and right petrous apex. Axial contrast-enhanced CT at the same level in soft tissue algorithm (**b**) demonstrates extensive inflammatory soft tissue in this region with encasement of the right internal carotid artery and effacement of the right parapharyngeal space. There is a region of low attenuation (arrow) concerning for phlegmon/early abscess formation. Coronal T1-weighted post-contrast fat-suppressed image (**c**) further demonstrates the extent of marrow and soft tissue enhancement with involvement of the right temporomandibular joint and infratemporal soft tissues

Neoplasms [7–10]

- Chordoma (Fig. 33.6):
    - Indolent, slow-growing, malignant neoplasm arising from notochordal remnants.
    - Most commonly occur at the sacrococcygeal region, clivus, and vertebral bodies.
    - In the clivus, they arise from the spheno-occipital synchondrosis in a midline location.
    - Three histologic subtypes: classical (conventional), chondroid, and dedifferentiated.
    - Imaging appearance on CT: well-circumscribed, expansile, midline soft tissue mass arising from the clivus with associated osseous erosions and internal cortical bone remnants; often hypoattenuating; mild-moderate enhancement.
    - Imaging appearance on MR: markedly T2 hyperintense mass with scattered foci of hypointensity (dirty cauliflower), iso- to hypointense on T1 with areas of hyperintensity representing hemorrhage or proteinaceous contents, variable enhancement (sometimes honeycomb-like).
    - Thumb sign: posterior extension of the mass into the prepontine cistern with indentation/compression of the pons.
- Chondrosarcoma (Fig. 33.7):
    - Malignant chondroid neoplasm arising from islands of cartilaginous rest cells at the skull base.
    - Arise off-midline, classically centered at the petro-occipital fissure.
    - May be associated with Ollier disease, Maffucci syndrome, or Paget disease.
    - Slow-growing, locally invasive tumor with several histopathologic variants and three histologic grades (grade 1/well differentiated is most common).
    - Imaging appearance can overlap with that of chordoma; therefore location is often key in differentiating with chordoma arising at the midline and chondrosarcoma arising off-midline.
    - Imaging appearance on CT: expansile, lytic soft tissue mass centered at the petro-occipital fissure, may have chondroid matrix (rings and arcs).
    - Imaging appearance on MR: T1 iso- to hypointense, T2 hyperintense, and variable heterogeneous enhancement.
- Meningioma (Fig. 33.8):
    - Arise from meningothelial arachnoid cells (i.e., arachnoid "cap" cells).
    - Most commonly occur along the convexities and falx, but approximately 20% involve the skull base including the parasellar region, cavernous sinus, and cerebellopontine angle cistern.
    - Central skull base meningiomas often cause visual symptoms, either by direct compression of the optic nerves or through the involvement of the cavernous sinus and its traversing nerve roots.
    - May encase and compress vascular structures such as the distal internal carotid artery and basilar artery.
    - Imaging appearance on CT: hyperdense extra-axial mass, associated calcification, adjacent bony sclerosis/hyperostosis.
    - Imaging appearance on MR: T1 iso-hypointense, T2 iso-hyperintense, avid homogenous enhancement, enhancing dural tail, elevated perfusion.

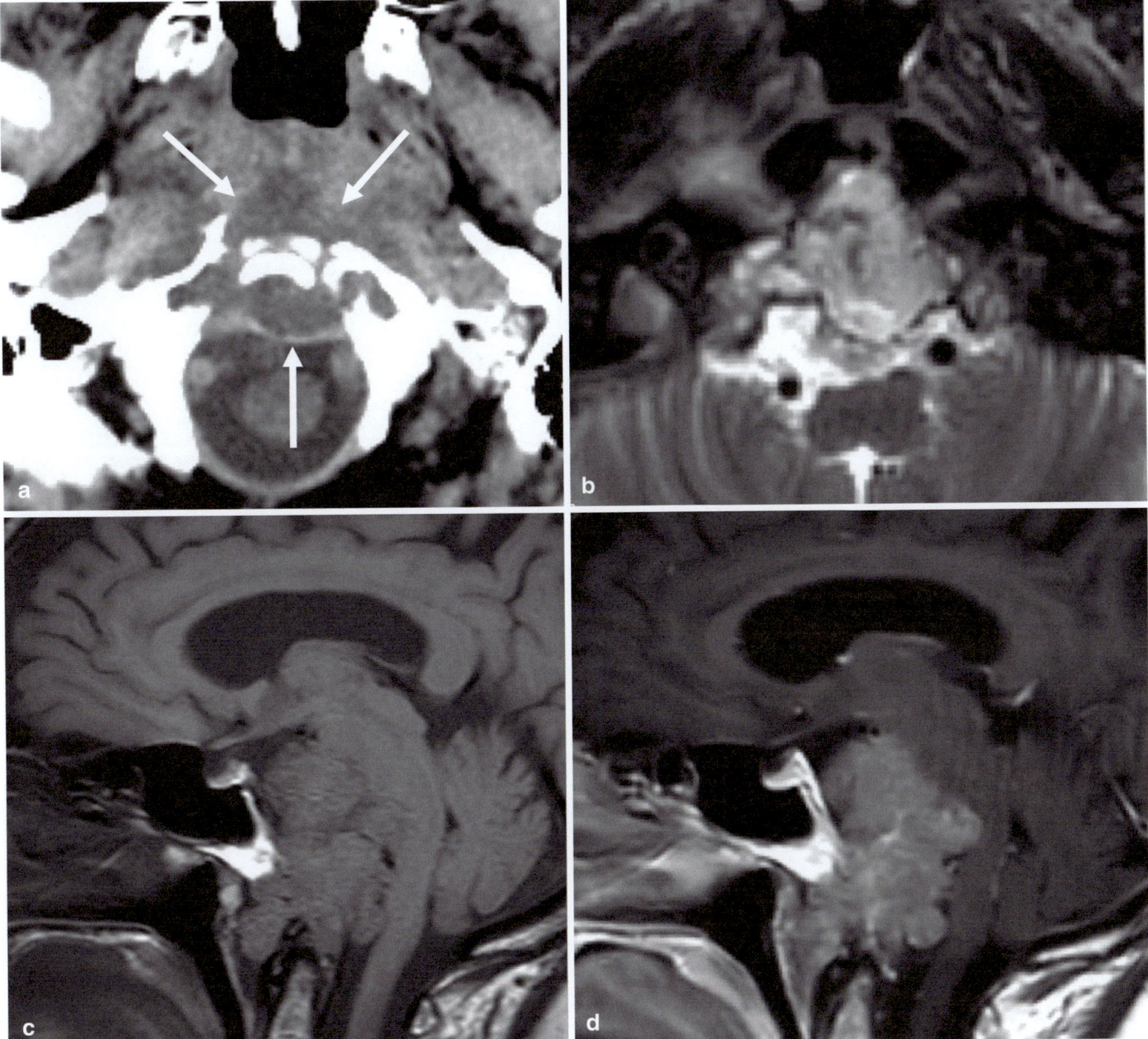

Fig. 33.6 Chordoma. Axial CT image (**a**) demonstrates a low attenuation, lobulated, midline clival mass (white arrows) with associated osseous erosions. Axial T2-weighted image (**b**) demonstrates that the mass is predominantly T2 hyperintense with a few areas of internal hypointensity and exerts mass effect upon the brainstem. Sagittal pre- (**c**) and post-contrast (**d**) T1-weighted images demonstrate mild diffuse enhancement of the lobulated mass

- ○ Associated with NF2, meningiomatosis, and prior radiotherapy.
- Schwannoma (Fig. 33.9):
  - ○ Benign tumor arising from nerve sheath Schwann cells.
  - ○ Can arise in any nerve, but vestibulocochlear nerve is most common (90%), followed by the trigeminal nerve (most common in the central skull base).
  - ○ Often demonstrate a dumbbell appearance if extending through multiple skull base compartments.
  - ○ Imaging appearance on CT: tubular extra-axial mass, smooth bony expansion/remodeling.
  - ○ Imaging appearance on MR: T1 iso-hypointense, heterogeneously T2 hyperintense, cystic components are common, enhancement may be homogeneous or heterogeneous.
  - ○ May be associated with downstream denervation changes such as edema and atrophy.
  - ○ Associated with NF2 and schwannomatosis.
- Metastasis (Fig. 33.10):

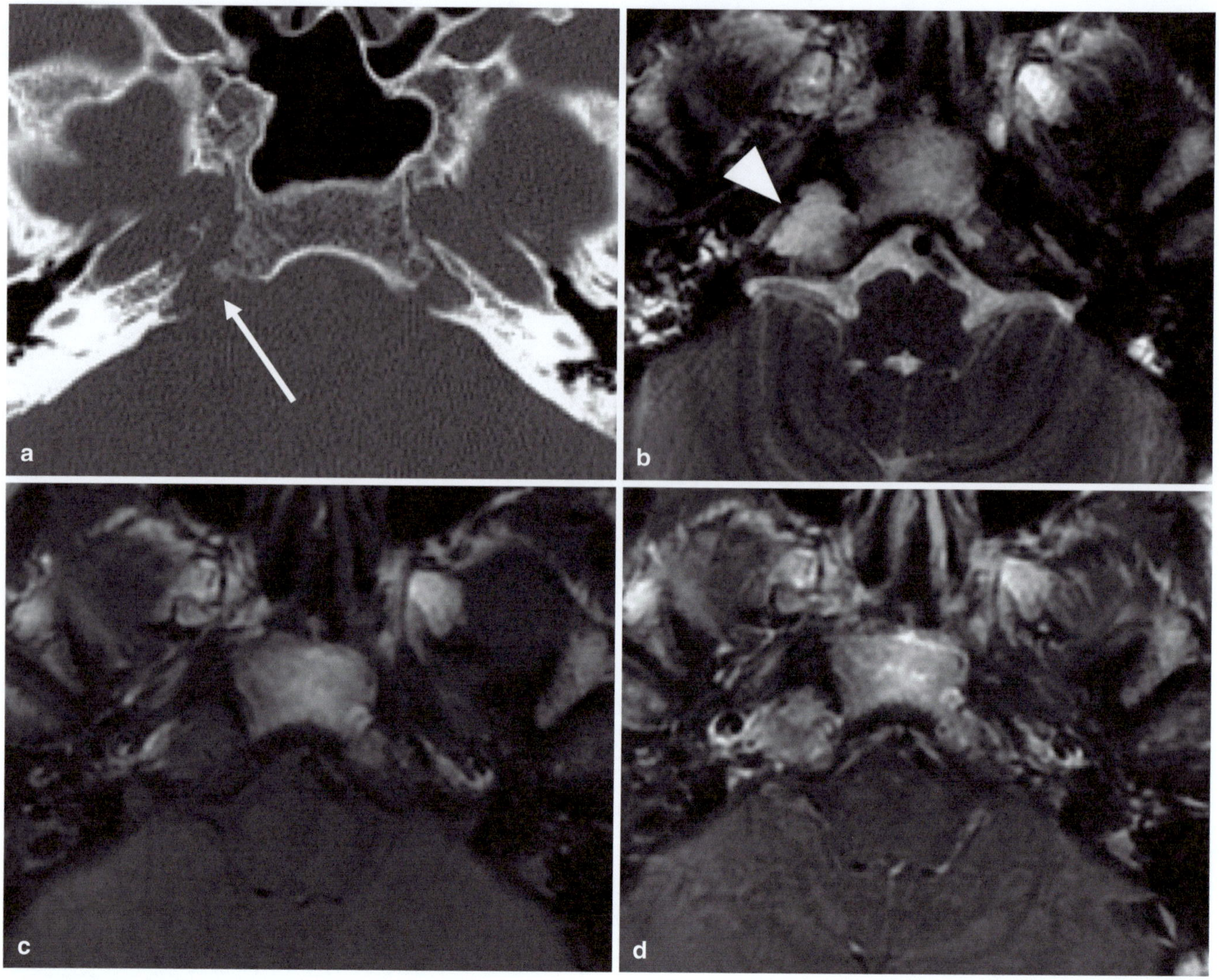

Fig. 33.7 Chondrosarcoma. Axial CT image (**a**) demonstrates a destructive mass centered at the right petro-occipital fissure (white arrow) with faint internal chondroid matrix. On T2-weighted imaging (**b**), the mass demonstrates T2 hyperintensity (white arrowhead). Pre-contrast (**c**) and post-contrast (**d**) T1-weighted imaging demonstrate mild heterogeneous enhancement of the mass

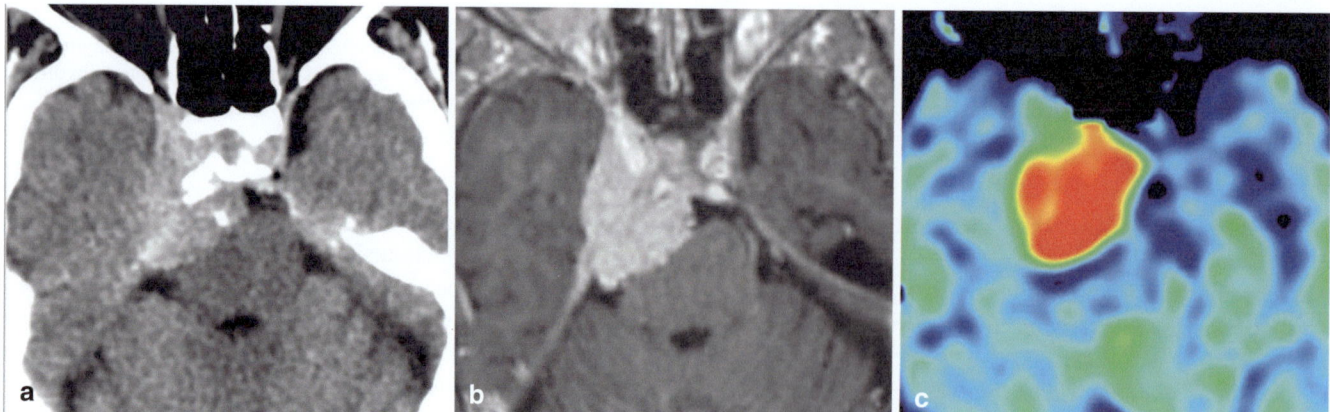

Fig. 33.8 Meningioma. Axial non-contrast head CT (**a**) demonstrates a hyperdense right parasellar mass centered in the right cavernous sinus and prepontine cistern with areas of internal calcification. Axial T1-weighted post-contrast image (**b**) demonstrates avid homogenous enhancement of the mass, and ASL perfusion image (**c**) demonstrates marked hyperperfusion of the mass

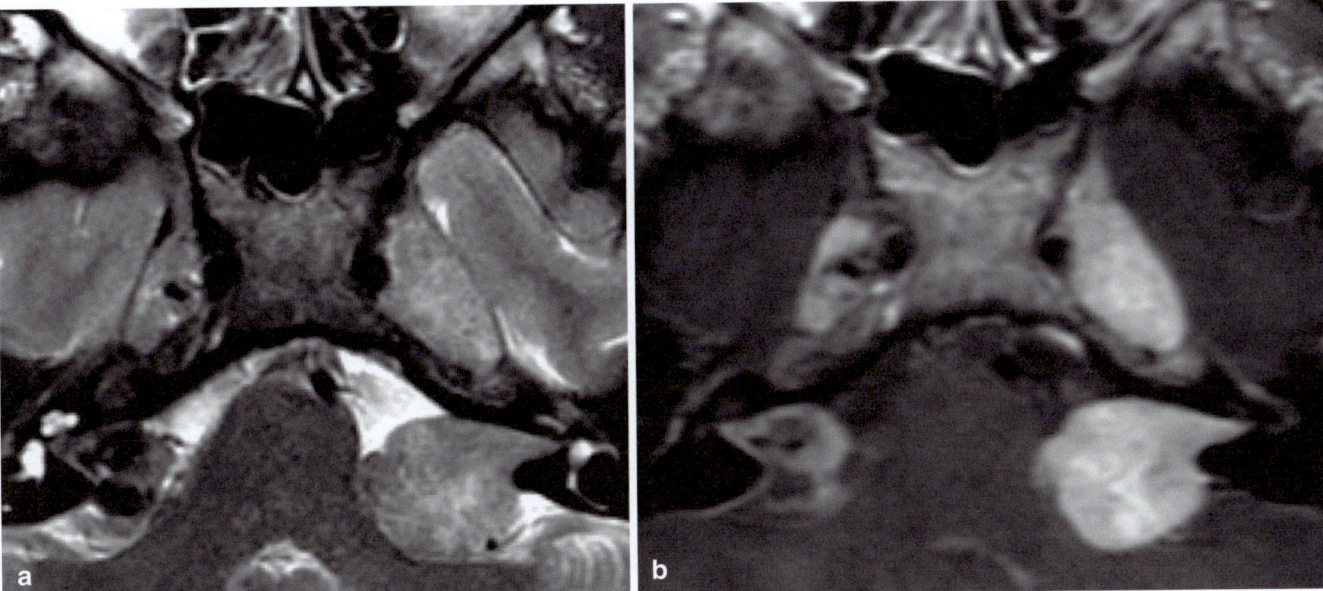

Fig. 33.9 Multiple schwannomas in NF2 patient. Axial T2-weighted image (**a**) and axial T1-weighted post-contrast image (**b**) demonstrate tubular, T2 heterogeneous, and enhancing masses extending along the course of the bilateral trigeminal nerves within Meckel's caves and along the course of the bilateral vestibular nerves within the cerebellopontine angle cisterns and internal auditory canals. Areas of T2 hypointense signal within the right vestibular schwannoma correspond to calcifications related to prior radiation therapy

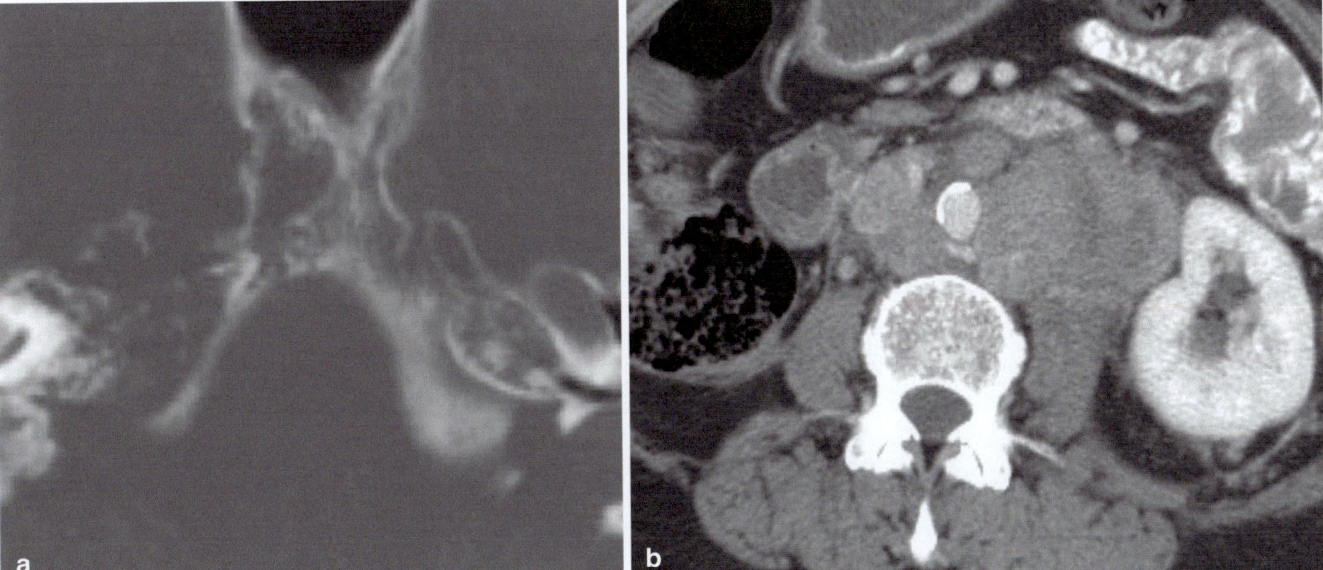

Fig. 33.10 Metastasis. Axial CT image of the head (**a**) demonstrates a destructive mass centered in the right petrous apex with extensive osseous erosions. Axial CT image of the abdomen (**b**) demonstrates extensive retroperitoneal lymphadenopathy in this patient with renal cell carcinoma status post prior right-sided nephrectomy

- ○ The clivus and petrous apex are frequent sites for osseous metastatic disease.
- ○ Osteolytic metastases are more common than osteoblastic metastases.
- ○ Multiplicity of lesions should increase suspicion of osseous metastatic disease.
- ○ Imaging appearance on CT:
  - • Osteolytic metastases—destructive lesion centered in the bone, often with erosive change and cortical breakthrough, no sclerotic rim.
  - • Osteoblastic metastases—ill-defined sclerotic lesion centered in the bone.
- ○ Imaging appearance on MR:

- Osteolytic metastases—T1 hypointense relative to normal bone marrow with enhancement on post-contrast fat-suppressed imaging.
- Osteoblastic metastases—T1 and T2 hypointense, often without enhancement.
- DWI may improve the detection of osseous metastases, particularly osteolytic metastases.
  o Involvement of adjacent vascular and neural structures must be carefully assessed.
  o Associated intracranial extension (pachymeningeal, leptomeningeal, and/or parenchymal) must also be carefully assessed.
- Multiple myeloma/plasmacytoma (Fig. 33.11):
  o Similar appearance to osteolytic metastatic disease.
  o Imaging appearance on CT:
    - Multiple myeloma—multiple, punched-out, lytic bone lesions.
    - Plasmacytoma—single lytic bone lesion without sclerotic borders, often with extraosseous extension into adjacent structures.
  o Imaging appearance on MR:
    - Background of marrow signal heterogeneity.
    - T1 hypointense relative to normal bone marrow with marked enhancement on post-contrast fat-suppressed imaging.
- Lymphoma (Fig. e33.10):
  o Primary skull base lymphoma is rare and can be a diagnostic challenge.
  o Secondary skull base lymphoma in the setting of extra-nodal disease is more common.
  o Clinical symptoms may include cranial nerve palsy such as diplopia, trigeminal neuropathy, or facial weakness.
  o Imaging appearance on CT: permeative bone destruction.
  o Imaging appearance on MR: typically iso- to hypo-intense on both T1 and T2, restricted diffusion on DWI/ADC.
- Perineural tumor spread (PNTS) (Fig. 33.12):
  o Extension of tumor along a nerve.

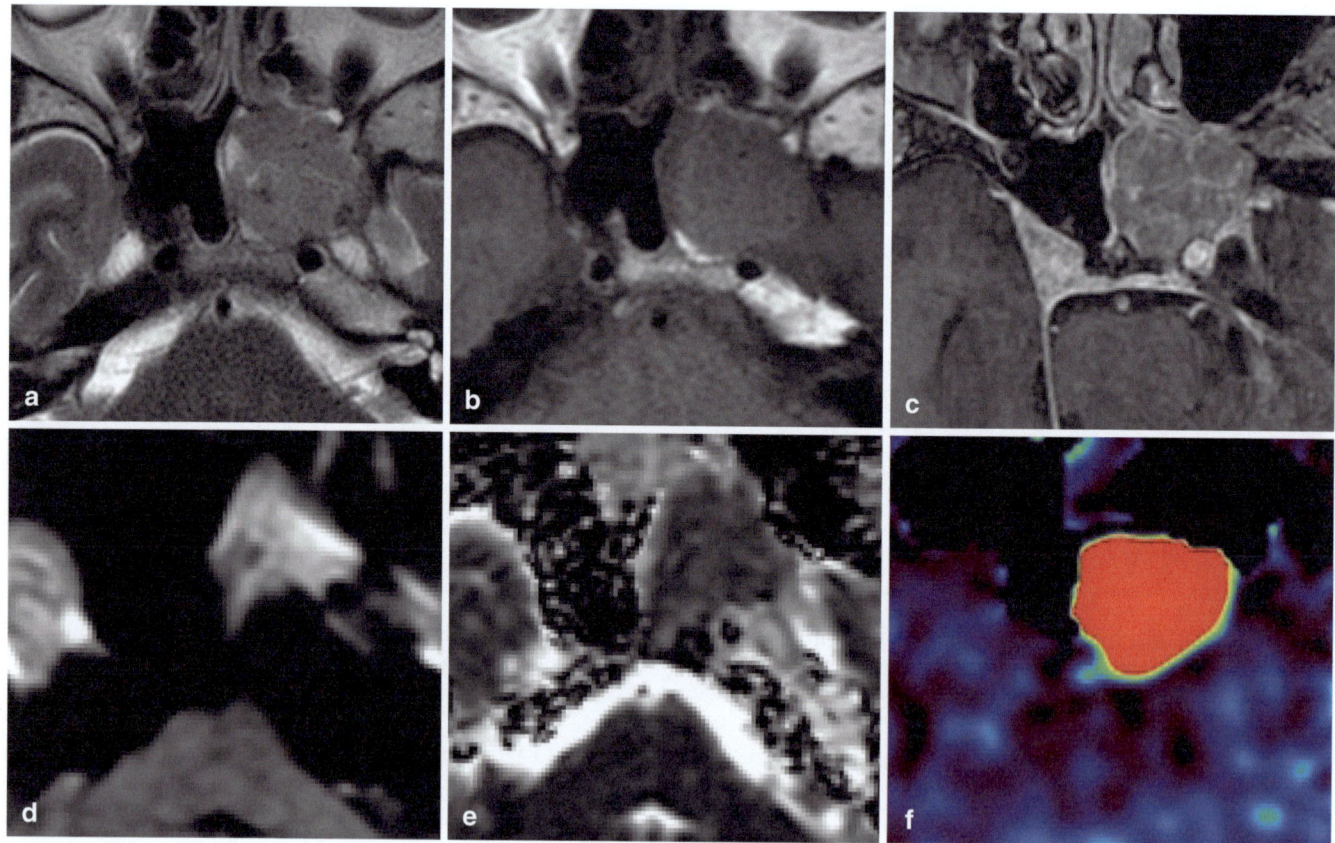

Fig. 33.11 Plasmacytoma/Multiple myeloma. Axial T2-weighted (**a**) and axial T1-weighted (**b**) images demonstrate a T2 and T1 iso-hypointense mass centered in the left sphenoid sinus with extension into the left cavernous sinus. Axial T1-weighted post-contrast image (**c**) demonstrates moderate, relatively homogeneous enhancement of the mass. Axial DWI and ADC images (**d**, **e**) demonstrate restricted diffusion within the mass compatible with a cellular tumor, and axial ASL perfusion image (**f**) demonstrates markedly elevated perfusion within the mass

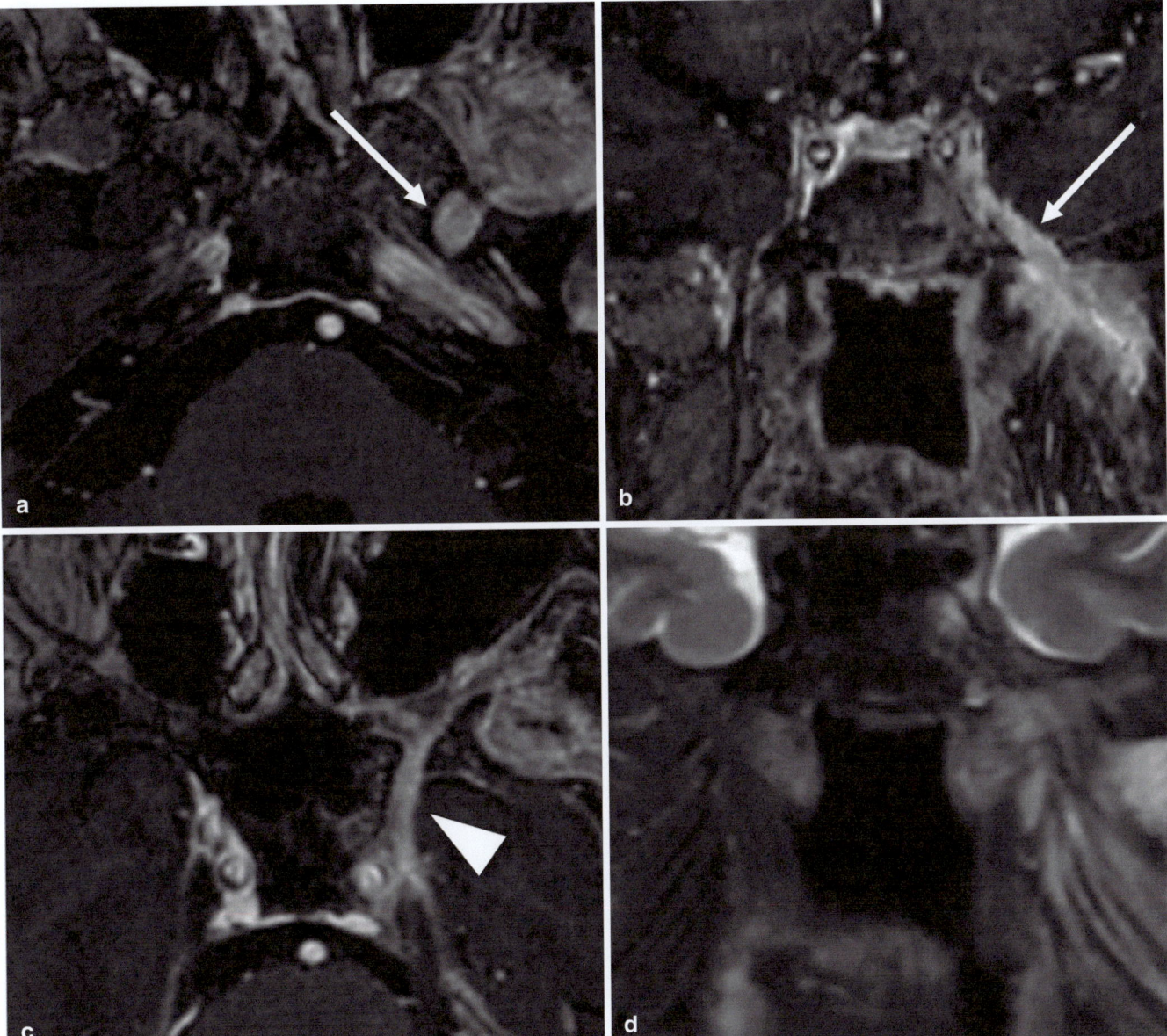

Fig. 33.12 Perineural tumor spread (in setting of basal cell carcinoma of the medial canthus). Axial (**a**) and coronal (**b**) T1-weighted post-contrast images demonstrate asymmetric thickening and enhancement of the left mandibular nerve (V3) within the left foramen ovale which is expanded (white arrows) and extending into the left masticator space. Axial T1-weighted post-contrast image (**c**) also demonstrates asymmetric thickening and enhancement of the left maxillary nerve (V2) within the left foramen rotundum (white arrowhead). Coronal T2-weighted image (**d**) demonstrates asymmetric T2 hyperintense signal within the left pterygoid muscles compatible with denervation edema due to perineural spread along the course of the left mandibular nerve

- Identification on imaging is critical as PNTS has significant implications for prognosis, staging, and treatment planning.
- Several malignancies have a propensity for PNTS including adenoid cystic carcinoma (most common malignancy associated with PNTS with a rate of up to 60%), squamous cell carcinoma, melanoma, and lymphoma.
- Maxillary (V2) and mandibular (V3) divisions of the trigeminal nerve and the facial nerve (VII) are most commonly involved.
- Important anastomotic pathways between the trigeminal and facial nerves including the auriculotemporal and the greater superficial petrosal nerves, where tumor can spread from one nerve to the other.
- Imaging appearance on CT: obliteration of the perineural fat within the skull base foramina, expansion and/or erosion of the skull base foramina.
- Imaging appearance on MR: asymmetric enhancement and thickening of the involved nerve, PNTS along a motor nerve may also manifest as denervation atrophy of the innervated muscles.

References

1. Chapman PR, Bag AK, Tubbs RS, Gohlke P. Practical anatomy of the central skull base region. Semin Ultrasound CT MR. 2013;34:381–92.
2. Dobre MC, Fischbein N. 'Do not touch' lesions of the skull base. J Med Imaging Radiat Oncol. 2014;58:458–63.
3. Conley LM, Phillips CD. Imaging of the central skull base. Radiol Clin North Am. 2017;55:53–67.
4. Alonso RC, de la Peña MJ, Caicoya AG, et al. Spontaneous skull base meningoencephaloceles and cerebrospinal fluid fistulas. Radiographics. 2013;33:553–70.
5. Schuknecht B, Simmen D, Briner HR, Holzmann D. Nontraumatic skull base defects with spontaneous CSF rhinorrhea and arachnoid herniation: imaging findings and correlation with endoscopic sinus surgery in 27 patients. AJNR. 2008;29:542–9.
6. Razek AA, Huang BY. Lesions of the petrous apex: classification and findings at CT and MR imaging. Radiographics. 2012 Jan;30(32):151–73.
7. Bag AK, Chapman PR. Neuroimaging: intrinsic lesions of the central skull base region. Semin Ultrasound CT MRI. 2013;34:412–35.
8. Kelly HR, Curtin HD. Imaging of skull base lesions. In: Giometto B, Pittock SJ, editors. Handbook of clinical neurology, vol. 135. Elsevier; 2016. p. 637–57.
9. Xing Z, Huang H, Xiao Z, Yang X, Lin Y, Cao D. CT, conventional, and functional MRI features of skull lymphoma: a series of eight cases in a single institution. Skeletal Radiol. 2019;48:897–905.
10. Abunimer A, Aiken A, Baugnon K, Wu X. Central skull base anatomy and pathology: a review. Semin Ultrasound CT MR. 2021;42:266–80.

Posterior Skull Base

Yuh-Shin Chang and Gul Moonis

Posterior Skull Base Lesions

ANATOMY

General Posterior Skull Base Anatomy (Fig. 34.1)

- The posterior skull base comprises five bones: the paired temporal and sphenoid bones and parts of the occipital bone (basilar, condylar, and squamous portion) [1, 2].
- **Boundaries:**
  o Anterior: dorsum sellae/posterior clinoid processes.
  o Anterolateral: petrous ridges of the petrous temporal bones = attachment site for tentorium cerebelli.
  o Posterior boundary: occipital bone.
- **Fissures, sutures and foramina:**
  o **Fissures:**
    - Petro-occipital fissure:
      ▪ Between the basiocciput medially and the petrous portion of the temporal bone laterally (Fig. 34.3b).
      ▪ Extends anteriorly into the foramen lacerum, posteriorly into the jugular foramen.
  o **Sutures:**
    - Occipitomastoid suture: between the mastoid portion of the temporal bone anteriorly and squamous occipital bone.
    - Occipitoparietal suture.
  o **Foramina:**
    - **Internal auditory meatus** (Fig. 34.1):
      ▪ Opening in the posterior wall of the petrous apex, superior to the jugular foramen.
      ▪ Leads through the porus acusticus (internal opening of internal auditory meatus) into the internal auditory canal (IAC).
      ▪ Contains: Cranial nerves (CN) VII–VIII (intracanalicular segment), labyrinthine artery.
    - **Stylomastoid foramen:**
      ▪ Vertically oriented foramen between the mastoid tip and styloid process.
      ▪ Contains: CN VII (mastoid segment) exits extracranially into the parotid space.
    - **Jugular foramen (JF):**
      ▪ Between the petrous temporal bone and occipital bone.
      ▪ Two parts: pars nervosa and pars vascularis.
    - **Hypoglossal canal:**
      ▪ Within the condylar part of the occipital bone.
      ▪ Contains: CN XII.
    - **Foramen magnum:** oval-shaped bony opening formed entirely by the occipital bone, anteriorly by the basilar part, laterally by the condylar part, and posteriorly by the squamous part of the occipital bone.
      ▪ Anterior margin is the basion, posterior margin is the ophistion.
      ▪ Contains: CN XI (spinal roots), medulla oblongata, vertebral arteries, anterior and posterior spinal arteries, bridging veins.

Supplementary Information The online version contains supplementary material available at https://doi.org/10.1007/978-3-031-55124-6_34.

Y.-S. Chang
Department of Radiology, Massachusetts Eye and Ear, Boston, MA, USA
e-mail: ychang3@mgb.org

G. Moonis (✉)
Department of Radiology, NYU Langone Medical Center, New York, NY, USA
e-mail: Gul.Moonis@nyulangone.org

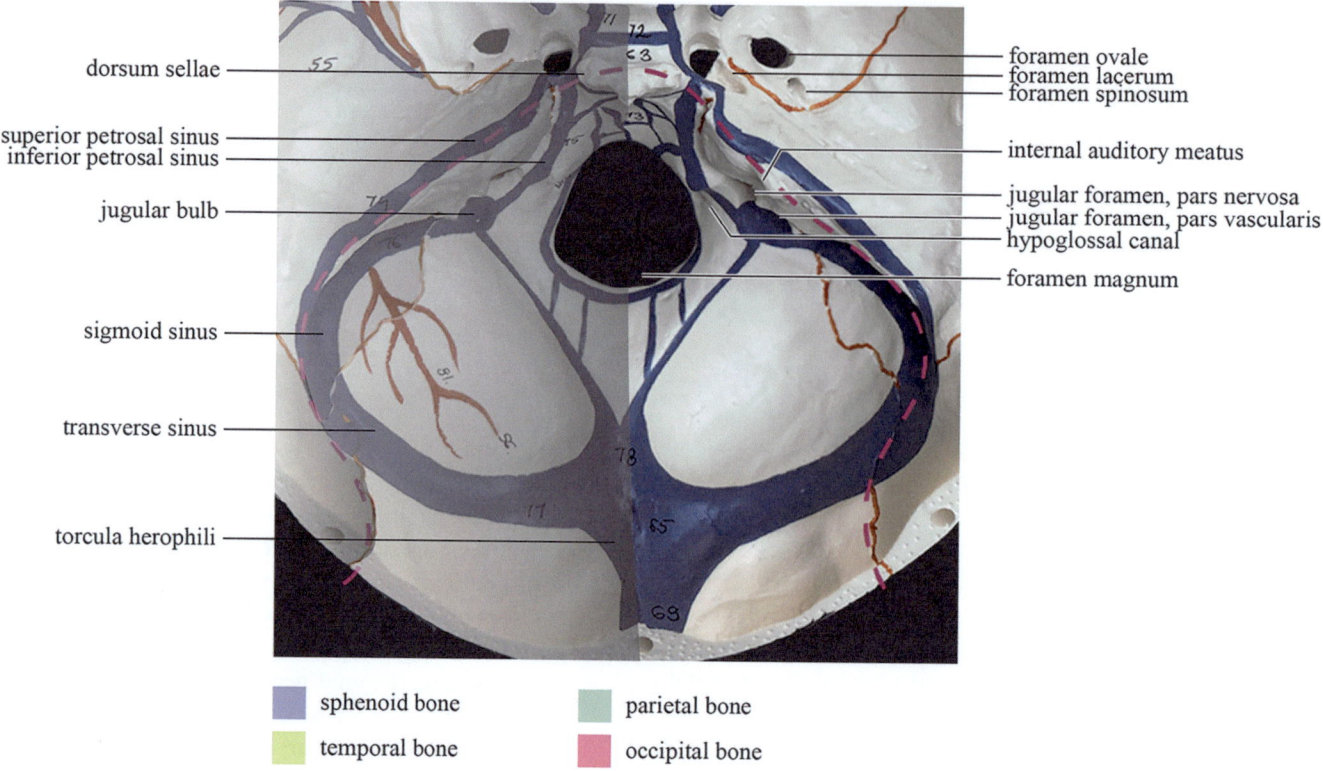

Fig. 34.1 Overview of posterior skull base anatomy. Overview of posterior skull base structures. Bones contributing to the posterior skull base are colored on the left: light blue, sphenoid bone; yellow: temporal bone; green: parietal bone; pink: occipital bone. The boundary of the posterior skull base is outlined by the pink line. The dorsum sellae and vascular structures are indicated on the left, foramina are shown on the right

Cerebellopontine Angle/Internal Auditory Canal Anatomy (Fig. 34.2)

- Cerebellopontine angle (CPA) cistern [1–4]: subarachnoid space in the anterior-posterior fossa centered around the IAC:
  - Boundaries (Fig. 34.2a, b):
    - Superior: variable definition, varies from tentorium cerebelli to CN V.
    - Inferior: CN IX–XI complex.
    - Anterior: posterior wall of the petrous temporal bone.
    - Posterior: Anterior pons, middle cerebellar peduncles, cerebellar hemispheres.
  - Contains: Facial nerve (CN VII), vestibulocochlear nerve (CN VIII), anterior inferior cerebellar artery loop, flocculus of the cerebellum, choroid plexus if extending from the fourth ventricle through the foramina of Luschka.
- IAC (Fig. 34.2c–h):
  - CSF-filled bony canal in the petrous portion of the temporal bone, connecting the CPA cistern to the auditory and vestibular organs.
  - Components (Fig. 34.2c–e):
    - Internal acoustic meatus/porus acusticus: medial/internal opening of the IAC adjacent to the CPA cistern.
    - IAC tapers distally toward the fundus.
    - Fundus: lateral end of the IAC. Several openings transmit nerves, including the cochlear nerve canal (also known as the cochlear fossette or cochlear aperture) for the cochlear nerve to the cochlea, facial nerve canal from the intracanalicular segment to the labyrinthine segment of the facial nerve and superior vestibular canal for the superior vestibular nerve (SVN).
      - Crista falciformis: horizontal bony crest in the fundus, separates CN VII and SVN in the superior compartment from the cochlear nerve and inferior vestibular nerve (IVN) in the inferior compartment.
      - Bill's bar: vertical bony crest in the fundus, further separates CN VII and SVN in the superior compartment.
  - Contains: CN VII anterosuperiorly, cochlear nerve anteroinferiorly, SVN posterosuperiorly, and IVN posteroinferiorly (Fig. 34.2c–e).

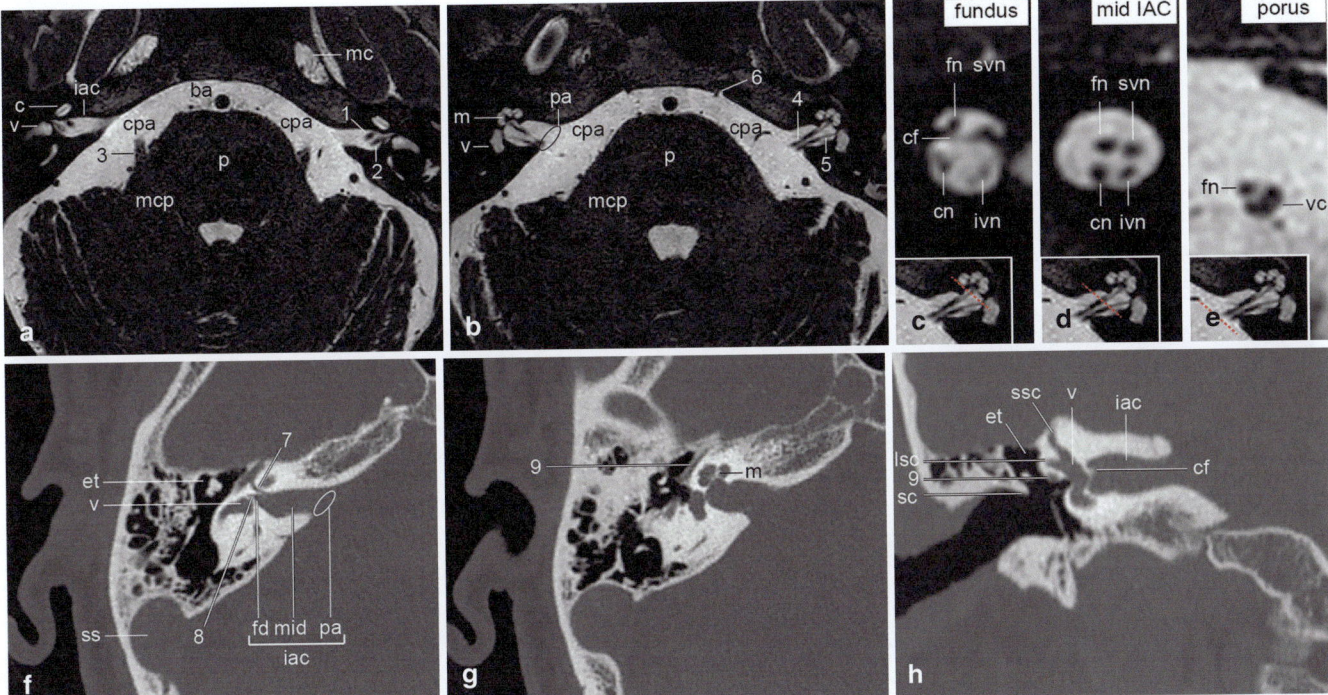

Fig. 34.2 Normal CT and MRI anatomy of the cerebellopontine angle/internal auditory canal region. (**a**, **b**) Axial T2-weighted CISS MR images at the level of the cerebellopontine angle (CPA)/internal auditory canal (IAC). Landmark structures are in letters, neural structures are numbered. 1: facial nerve, 2: superior vestibular nerve, 3: trigeminal nerve, 4: cochlear nerve, 5: inferior vestibular nerve, 6: abducens nerve (at Dorello's canal), 7: labyrinthine segment of the facial nerve, 8: superior vestibular nerve canal, 9: tympanic segment of the facial nerve. *ba* basilar artery, *c* cochlea, *cpa* cerebellopontine angle cistern, *mc* Meckel cave, *mcp* middle cerebellar peduncle, *p* pons, *pa* porus acusticus, *v* vestibule. (**c–e**) Oblique sagittal images through the left internal auditory canal. At the level of the fundus (**c**), a horizontally oriented crista falciformis (cf) separates the facial nerve (fn) and superior vestibular nerve (svn) superiorly from the cochlear nerve (cn) and inferior vestibular nerve (ivn). (**d**) In the mid-IAC, all 4 nerves are discretely seen. The facial nerve is anterosuperior, the cochlear nerve anteroinferior, the superior vestibular nerve posterosuperior, the inferior vestibular nerve posteroinferior. (**e**) Just anterior to the porus acusticus, the facial nerve is located anteriorly to and distinct from the vestibulocochlear nerve complex (vc), in a typical "ball (fn) in a catcher's mitt (vc)" appearance. (**f–h**) Axial CT images in bony reformat show landmark structures surrounding the IAC region. *Cf* crista falciformis, *et* epitympanum, *fd* fundus, *iac* internal auditory canal, *lsc* lateral semicircular canal, *m* modiolus of the cochlea, *sc* scutum, *ss* sigmoid sinus, *ssc* superior semicircular canal, *v* vestibule

- Mnemonic for the location of the nerves in the anterior compartment: "Seven (CN VII) up, Coke (cochlear nerve) down."
- Anterior inferior cerebellar artery loop:
  - Arises from the basilar artery and continues in the IAC as the internal auditory or labyrinthine artery.
  - Main arterial supply to the vestibular organs and cochlea.

Jugular Foramen Anatomy (Fig. 34.3)

- Located inferior to the internal acoustic meatus, between the petrous portion of the temporal bone superiorly and the basiocciput inferiorly (Fig. 34.1).
- Bordered anteromedially by the petrooccipital fissure, posteriorly by the groove for sigmoid sinus; posterolaterally by the occipitomastoid suture (Fig. 34.3b).
- 2 parts: the smaller anteromedial pars nervosa is partially divided from the larger posterolateral pars vascularis by a bony process termed the jugular spine or interjugular process.
  - Pars nervosa contains: CN IX, Jacobson nerve (tympanic branch of CN IX), inferior petrosal sinus (Fig. 34.3a, c).
  - Pars vascularis contains: CN X, CN XI, Arnold nerve (auricular branch of CN X), jugular bulb, meningeal branches of the ascending pharyngeal and occipital arteries (Fig. 34.3a, c).
- Inferiorly, the jugular foramen extends into the extracranial post-styloid parapharyngeal space, or carotid space. The adjacent carotid and hypoglossal canals also extend extra-cranially into the carotid space.
- Separated from the carotid canal by the caroticojugular spine and from the hypoglossal canal by the jugular tubercle (Fig. 34.4b).
- The right jugular foramen is asymmetrically enlarged compared to the left in 68% of cases.

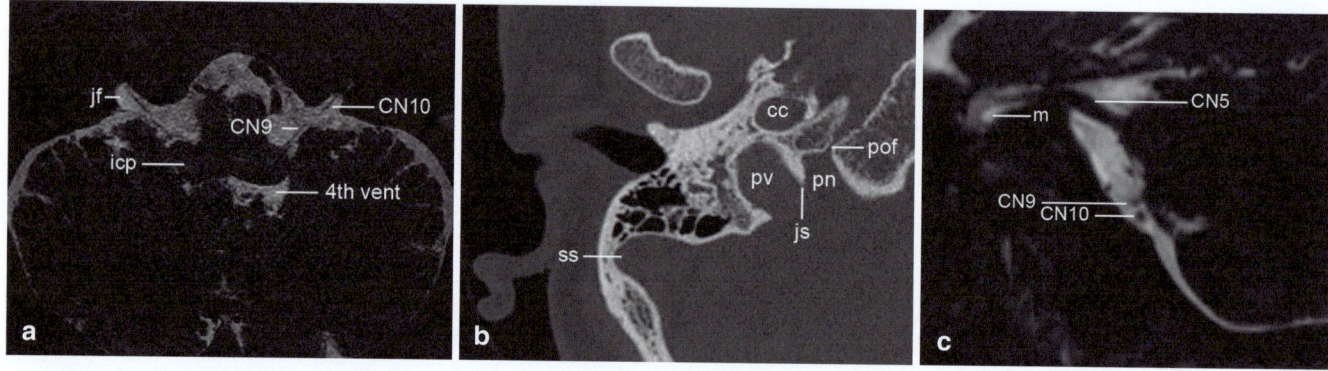

Fig. 34.3 Normal CT and MRI anatomy of the jugular foramen. (**a**) Axial and (**c**) sagittal heavily T2-weighted CISS MR image at the level of the jugular foramen (JF). (**b**) Axial CT image in bone algorithm of the JF. *Cc* carotid canal, *icp* inferior cerebellar peduncle, *jf* jugular foramen, *js* jugular spine, *m* Meckel's cave, *pn* pars nervosa, *pof* petro-occipital fissure, *pv* pars vascularis, *ss* sigmoid sinus, *fourth vent* fourth ventricle, *CN5* trigeminal nerve, *CN9* glossopharyngeal nerve, *CN10* vagus nerve

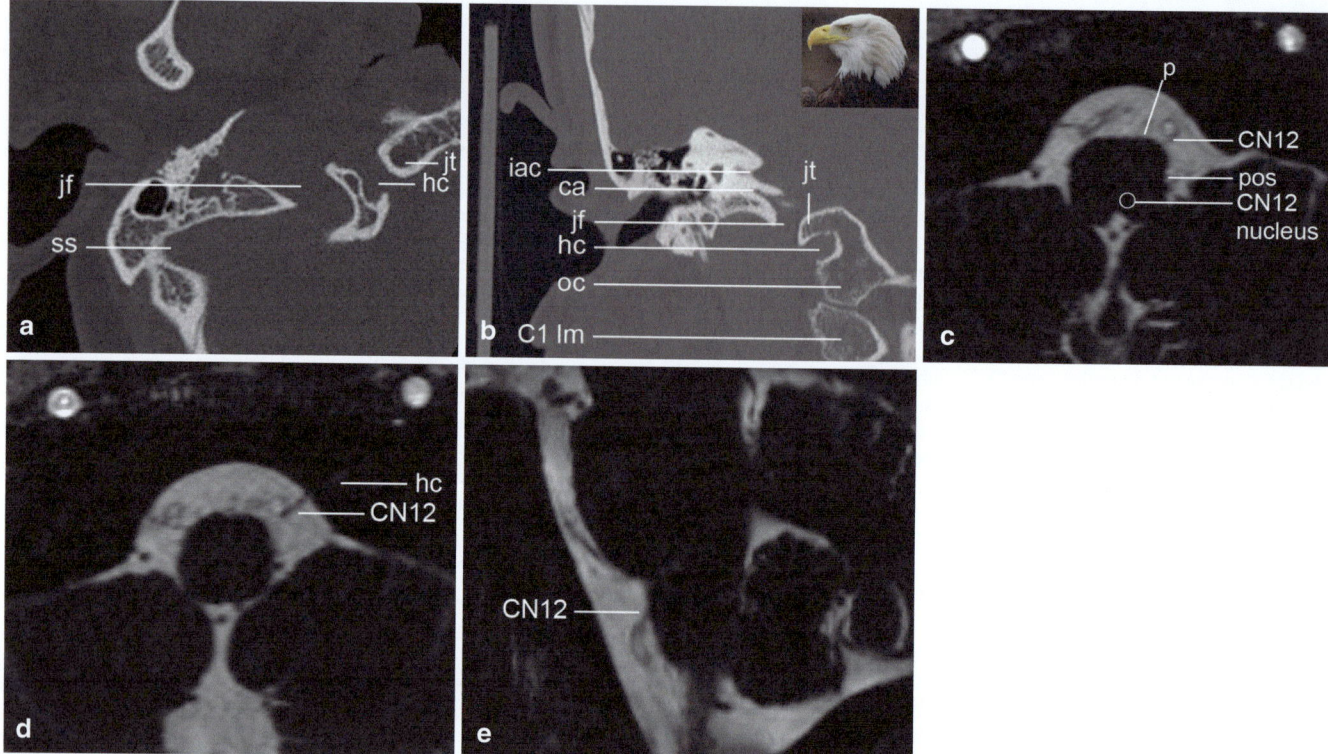

Fig. 34.4 Normal CT and MRI anatomy of the hypoglossal canal. (**a**) Axial and coronal (**b**) CT images with bony reformat at the level of the hypoglossal canal and JF. *ca* cochlear aqueduct, *c1 lm*: *hc* hypoglossal canal, *iac* internal auditory canal, *jf* jugular foramen, *jt* jugular tubercle, *oc* occipital condyle, *ss* sigmoid sinus. Please note the "eagle's head" appearance of the bony landmarks on coronal view (**b**), with the jugular tubercle forming the eagle's head and beak, the medial hypoglossal canal forming the neck and the occipital condyle forming the chest. (**c–e**) Axial (**c, d**) and sagittal (**e**) heavily T2-weighted CISS MR images of the hypoglossal canal shows the cisternal segment of the left hypoglossal nerve (CN12) exiting anterolaterally from the pre-olivary sulcus between the medullary pons and the olive. *hc* hypoglossal canal, *p* pons, *pos* post-olivary sulcus

Hypoglossal Canal Anatomy (Fig. 34.4)
- Located inferomedial to the jugular foramen.
- Separated from the jugular foramen and bordered superolaterally by the jugular tubercle, bordered inferiorly by the occipital condyle (Fig. 34.4a).
  - The jugular tubercle forms an important anatomic landmark of the hypoglossal canal on coronal view, demonstrating the classic "eagle's head" appearance (Fig. 34.4b).
- A fibrous or ossified septum may be present in the proximal canal and subdivide the hypoglossal rootlets in 16%

of cases. The roots of the hypoglossal nerve merge distally within the canal before exiting the skull base.
- Extends inferiorly/extra-cranially into the nasopharyngeal carotid space.
- Contains: hypoglossal nerve, surrounding venous plexus (Fig. 34.4c–e).

Cerebellopontine Angle/Internal Auditory Canal Lesions (Figs. 34.5, 34.6 and 34.7, e34.1 and e34.2)

(All electronic images (Figs. e34.1–e34.10) can be found on this chapter's website on SpringerLink: https://doi.org/10.1007/978-3-031-55124-6_34)

- Lesions can be subdivided based on their MR imaging signal characteristics (enhancement, T1 signal intensity) and location (intra- or extra-axial).
- CPA lesions are most commonly extra-axial in location.
- Most common CPA mass lesions are vestibular schwannoma (VS) (70–80%), meningioma (10–15%), and epidermoid cysts (5%).
  - CPA tumors constitute 6–10% of all intracranial tumors [5–8].
- The most common CPA lesions can be summarized under the mnemonic "SAME":
  - S: schwannoma.
  - A: arachnoid cyst, aneurysm.
  - M: meningioma, metastasis.
  - E: epidermoid cyst, ependymoma.

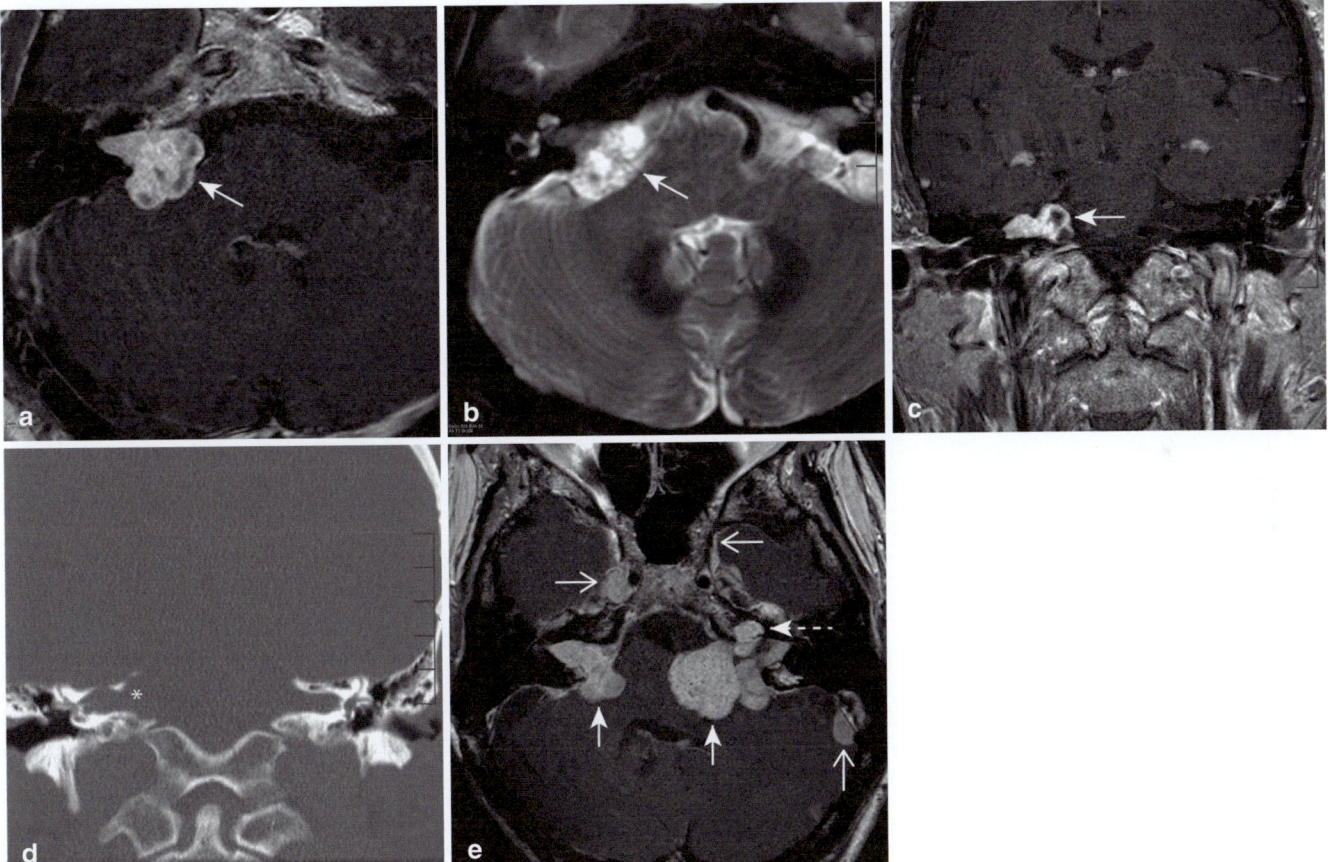

Fig. 34.5 CPA schwannoma. (**a**) Axial post-contrast T1WI MR image demonstrates a well-circumscribed, mixed cystic and solid mass (arrow) with heterogeneous, avid enhancement in the right CPA. It has the typical ice cream-on-a-cone or dumbbell-shaped appearance of a VS. Anterolaterally, the mass fills the entire right internal auditory canal to the fundus. Posteromedially, it extends into the right CPA cistern and abuts the right lateral middle cerebellar peduncle. There is mild mass effect and postomedial displacement of the right middle cerebellar peduncle. Multiple T2 hyperintense cystic components in this mass (**b**) are consistent with cystic degeneration. (**c**) Coronal, post contrast T1 MR image better delineates the cystic components of this mass lesion (arrow). (**d**) Coronal non-contrast CT bony reformat shows smooth widening of the right porus acusticus (*) and scalloping of the right IAC. (**e**) In a different patient with NF2, a similar appearing lesion in the right CPA (arrow) is consistent with a VS. Two additional well-circumscribed lesions in the left CPA are consistent with a left facial (dashed arrow) and a left VS (arrow). Note other well-circumscribed, homogenously enhancing extra-axial masses with dural tails along both right greater than left greater sphenoid wings, lateral walls of the cavernous sinuses and tentorium cerebelli, consistent with meningiomas (open arrows). Multiple ependymomas are also present in the cervical spine (not shown)

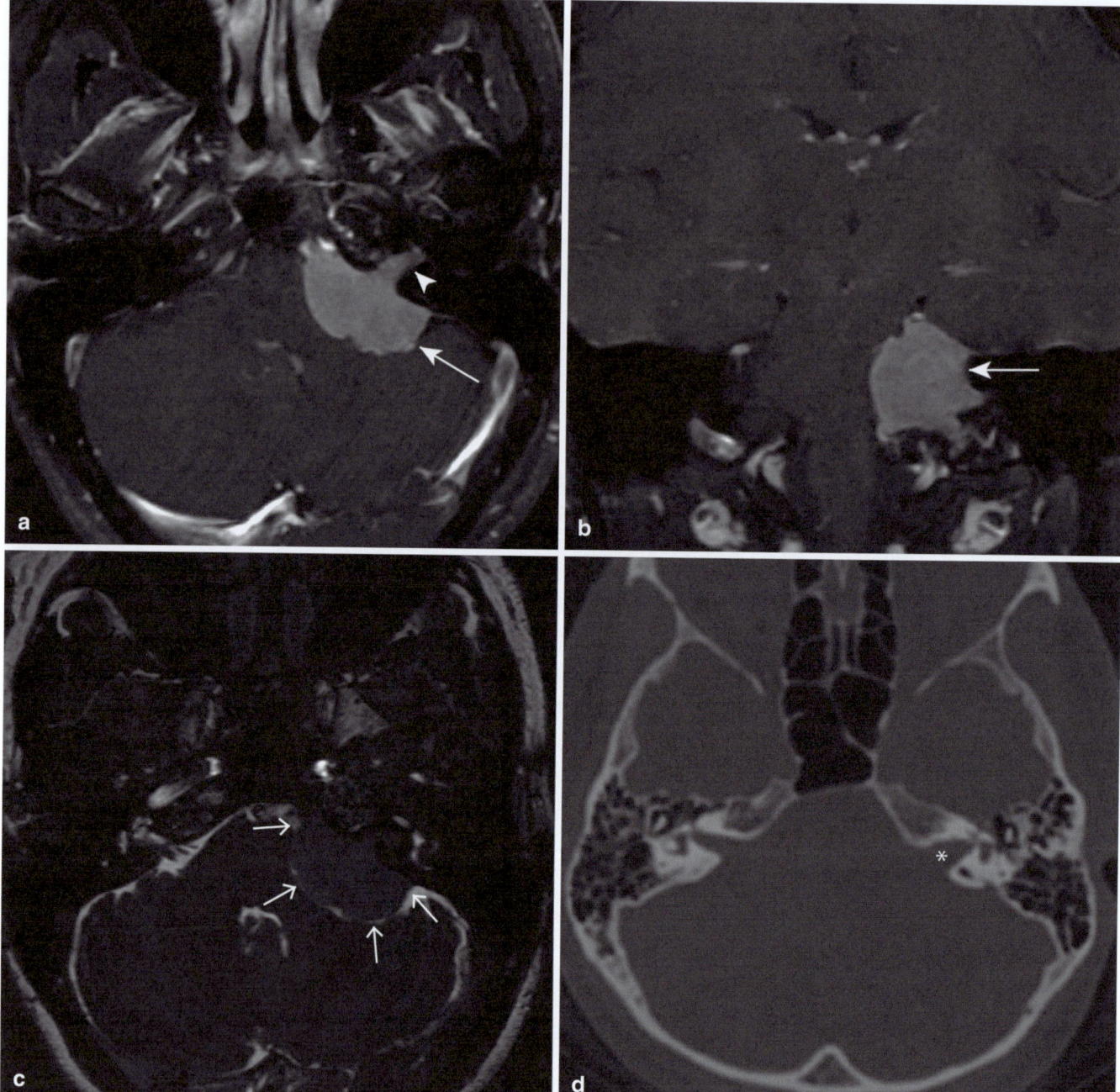

Fig. 34.6 CPA meningioma. (**a**) Axial and coronal (**b**) T1WI C+ MR images show a large, well-circumscribed extra-axial mass with broad dural base along the posterior wall of the left petrous temporal bone (arrow), consistent with a left CPA meningioma. Anterolaterally, it extends through the porus acusticus into and fills the left IAC (arrowhead). There is mass effect with medial displacement of the brainstem, middle cerebellar peduncle, and anterolateral left cerebellar hemisphere. (**c**) Axial CISS sequence at the level of the IAC demonstrates a thin CSF rim (open arrows) between this lesion and the pons, middle cerebellar peduncle and left cerebellar hemisphere, consistent with the "claw sign," confirming the extra-axial nature of this lesion. The dural tail (open arrows) is also best seen here. (**d**) Axial CT bony reformat shows mild smooth widening of the left porus acousticus (*)

- Clinical presentations include hearing loss, tinnitus, dizziness, facial pain or paresis, hemifacial spasm.
    - Clinical findings are not specific to the type of lesion, but secondary to cranial nerve involvement, brainstem or cerebellar compression.
- In the presence of bilateral VS, multiple CN schwannomas, intracranial meningiomas or ependymomas, suspect neurofibromatosis (NF) type 2 (NF2).
    - Mnemonic "MISME": multiple intracranial schwannomas, meningiomas, ependymomas.

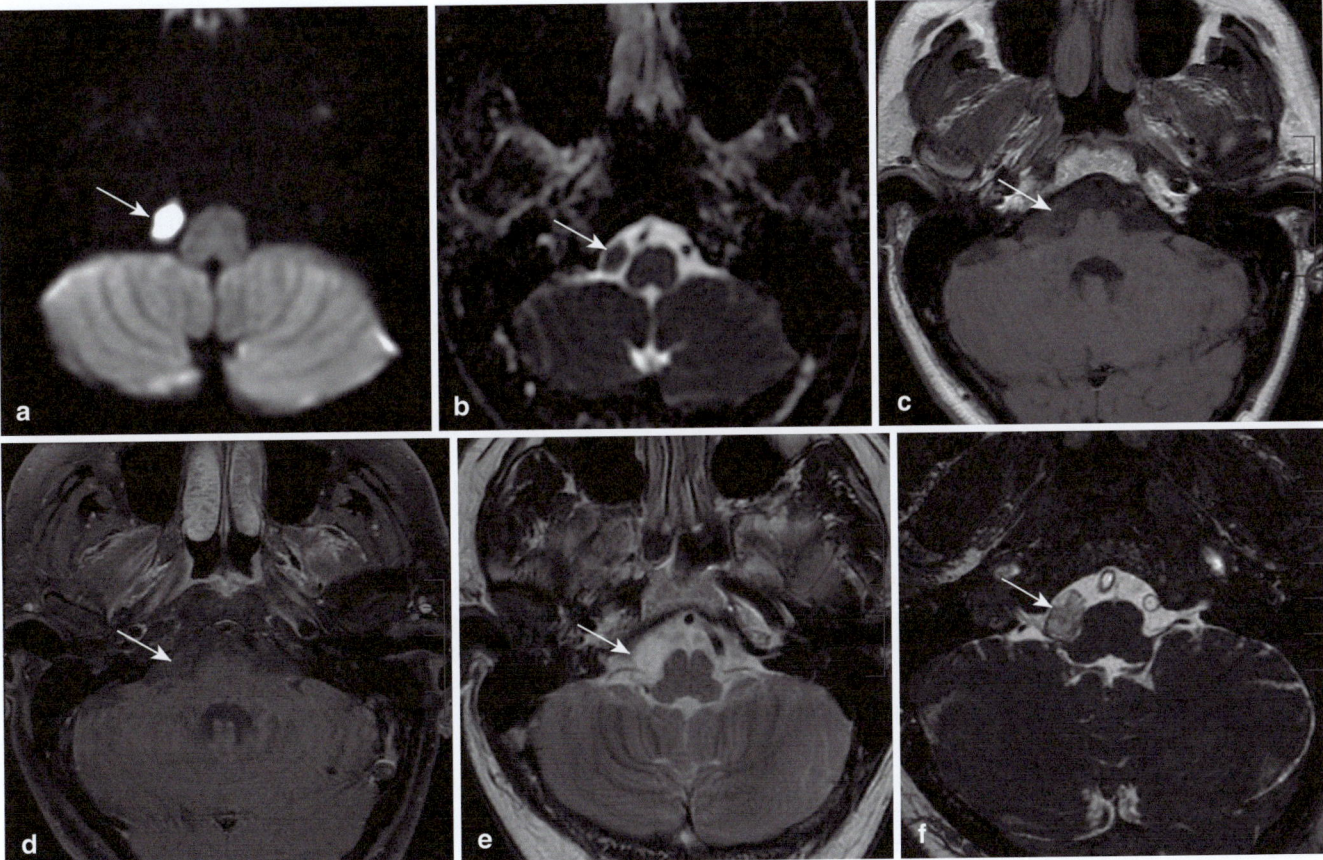

Fig. 34.7 CPA epidermoid cyst. (**a**) Axial DWI and ADC MR images (**b**) demonstrate a well-circumscribed ovoid mass in the right cerebellomedullary cistern (arrow) that restricts diffusion (**a**, **b**). On axial T2/FLAIR images, the lesion is iso- to hyperintense with incomplete fluid suppression (**c**), no enhancement on axial T1-weighted enhanced images (**d**). On axial T2-weighted images (**e**), its signal intensity is similar to CSF. (**f**) On the axial heavily T2-weighted (CISS) sequence, the lesion abuts the right post olivary sulcus, but does not displace the medulla. These findings are consistent with a CPA epidermoid cyst

- o Bilateral VS develops in 90–95% of patients with NF2 by the age of 30.

VESTIBULAR SCHWANNOMA (FIG. 34.5)

- Benign, slow-growing nerve sheath tumor originating from differentiated Schwann cells [6, 7, 9, 10].
- VS arising from CN VIII represents the most common extra-axial lesion and the most common contrast-enhancing lesion in the CPA cistern:
  - o Commonly originates from Schwann cells of the IVN in the IAC.
  - o Can be found anywhere along CN VIII from the IAC to its terminal ends within the vestibule, cochlea, or semicircular canals.
  - o Average growth rate: 1.2–1.9 mm/year [11].
  - o Other enhancing lesions including metastasis, lymphoma, and ependymoma each constitute less than 1% of all CPA mass lesions.
- Cystic VS:
  - o Distinct subtype; 4–24% of all VS [11].
  - o Larger at time of diagnosis.
  - o More rapid growth, lower rates of complete surgical resection.
- CT:
  - o Isodense lesion, enhances after contrast administration.
  - o Smooth enlargement of the porus acusticus.
  - o Typical "ice cream on cone" pattern.
- MRI:
  - o T1-weighted imaging:
    - Isointense relative to brainstem.
    - Heterogeneous T1 signal in larger tumors due to cystic or necrotic components.
  - o T2-weighted imaging: hyperintense lesion.
  - o T2* gradient echo sequences:
    - May present susceptibility artifacts due to intralesional hemorrhages.
  - o T1-weighted imaging, C(+):

- Strongly contrast enhancing.
- Cystic appearance (4–24%).
    - Axial thin heavily T2-weighted imaging (FIESTA, CISS, DRIVE):
        - Important sequence in the evaluation of the vestibulocochlear nerve and its branches.
        - Hypointense appearance, surrounded by hyperintense CSF.
    - T1-weighted 3D gradient-echo C+ imaging:
        - Provides better detection of small intracanalicular VS than CISS sequence [12].
        - Better identification of areas of necrosis [11].
    - Correlation between 3D MPRAGE and CISS sequences is required to reduce the risk of false-positive cases [11].
    - Treatment:
        - Surgery:
            - Preferred therapy for young patients, large (>3 cm) tumors, cystic VS, symptoms of mass effect [13].
        - Stereotaxic radiosurgery.
- Prevalence of schwannomas in the CPA: CN VIII >> CN V, VII > CN IX–XII:
    - CPA/IAC CN VII schwannoma may mimic VS. When present, involvement and enhancement of the labyrinthine facial nerve helps differentiate it from VS.

CPA MENINGIOMA (FIG. 34.6)

- Slow-growing neoplasm arising from meningothelial arachnoid cap cells of the CPA/IAC dura:
    - Second most common CPA mass.
    - 5–10% of intracranial meningiomas are located in the CPA.
- Risk factors: prior radiation exposure, hereditary syndromes (NF2, schwannomatosis), possible hormonal factors.
- Clinical presentation: mostly asymptomatic and found incidentally on brain MR imaging; <10% are symptomatic.
- Well-circumscribed, dural-based extra-axial enhancing mass in the CPA. Most commonly originating from the dura along the posterior wall of the petrous temporal bone with possible extension into the adjacent IAC. Less likely arising from the IAC dura.
- CT:
    - Isodense to hyperdense.
    - 25% of lesions are calcified.
    - Hyperostosis or permeative-sclerotic osseous changes in the surrounding skull base is possible.
    - IAC widening is rare in contrast to VS.

- MRI:
    - T1-weighted imaging: iso- to slightly hyperintense to gray matter.
    - T2-weighted imaging: isointense to slightly hypointense to gray matter. Focal or diffuse T2 hypointensity if calcified or fibrous.
        - CSF cleft: crescentic T2 hyperintense CSF between the brain parenchyma and meningioma.
        - Tumoral arterial feeders can be seen as intralesional flow voids.
    - T1-weighted imaging, C(+):
        - Avid uniform contrast enhancement.
        - "Dural tail" sign is reported in 60% of meningiomas but is also seen in solitary fibrous tumors, metastasis, lymphoma, or, less commonly, VS. More likely represents reactive change, rarely tumoral involvement.
- Treatment options:
    - Conservative: serial follow-up imaging for asymptomatic lesion or older patient.
    - Surgical resection: Less commonly associated with facial nerve palsy or hearing loss than VS [14, 15].
    - Stereotactic radiosurgery as adjunct treatment improves overall survival for patients with higher WHO-grade lesions [16].

CPA EPIDERMOID CYST (FIG. 34.7)

- Arises from congenital inclusion of ectodermal epithelial rests during neural tube closure:
    - Cyst wall is made up of an internal layer of stratified squamous epithelium surrounded by a fibrous capsule.
    - Contains desquamated stratified keratinized epithelium.
    - 50% of all intracranial epidermoid cysts occur in the CPA cistern.
- Third most common CPA mass lesion:
    - Most common non-enhancing CPA lesion.
- Well-circumscribed, expansile, cystic-appearing, non-enhancing lesion in the CPA cistern:
    - Encases CPA structures, including CN VII, VIII, and/or the anterior-inferior cerebellar artery.
- CT:
    - Well-circumscribed appearing lesion of CSF density with associated mass effect.
- MRI:
    - T1 and T2 are isointense or slightly hyperintense to CSF, similar to arachnoid cysts:
        - Rarely, T1 hyperintense "white epidermoid cysts" contain triglycerides and fatty acids.

- On heavily T2-weighted sequence, lesions demonstrate lobulated margins and are hypointense to CSF.
  o FLAIR: incomplete fluid signal suppression.
  o T1 C+: no enhancement. Enhancement is rare and may indicate malignant transformation into squamous cell carcinoma.
  o DWI: characteristic diffusion restriction helps differentiate it from other cystic CPA lesions, including arachnoid cyst, neurenteric cyst, or rarely, neurocysticercosis.
- Treatment:
  o Surgical removal.
  o Restricted diffusion on DWI on postsurgical follow-up MRI is key sequence for diagnosing recurrence.
- If the lesion involves the prepontine cistern, consider a neuroepithelial cyst in the differential diagnosis.

CPA ARACHNOID CYST [8, 17] (FIG. E34.1)

- Benign lesion arising from congenital splitting of the arachnoid layer and filling of the resulting intra-arachnoid pouch with CSF.
- Account for ~1% of all intracranial masses.
- 10–20% of intracranial arachnoid cysts are located in the posterior fossa, most commonly in the CPA cistern.
- Most commonly found incidentally. Larger arachnoid cysts in the CPA may be symptomatic due to direct compression of CN VII/VIII, brainstem, and/or the fourth ventricle and resulting hydrocephalus.
- Well-circumscribed ovoid or lentiform extra-axial cystic lesion with imperceptible walls. Cyst content follows CSF density in CT and CSF signal in all MR sequences.
- Mass effect results in displacement, but no engulfment of the surrounding structures. Together with absence of restricted diffusion, these features differentiate arachnoid cysts from epidermoid cysts.
- CT:
  o Homogenously hypointense lesion of CSF density.
- MR: follows CSF signal in all sequences.
  o T1 hypointense, T2 hyperintense.
  o FLAIR: complete fluid attenuation.
  o DWI: no diffusion restriction.
  o T1 C+: no enhancement.
- Treatment:
  o Most cases require no treatment.
  o Surgery for symptomatic lesions (increased intracranial pressure, seizure, focal neurological deficits, cognitive impairment).
    - Craniotomy with partial or complete cystectomy, fenestration, or cyst peritoneal shunting.

CPA LIPOMA (FIG. E34.2)

- Uncommon benign nonneoplastic mass of mature adipose tissue in the CPA/IAC region.
- Arises from developmental malformation of persistent meningeal precursor cells, meninx primitiva, that differentiate into fat [18–20].
- Represents <1% of all CPA lesions. Very slow growing.
- Well-circumscribed mass following fat signal characteristic encases rather than displaces CPA structures (CN VII, VIII, AICA loop):
  o May show concurrent intralabyrinthine lesion.
- Clinical presentation: most commonly found incidentally. Symptoms related to local mass effect.
- CT: homogenous fat density attenuation.
- MRI:
  o T1 is intrinsically hyperintense, with signal loss on fat suppression.
  o T1 C+: no enhancement.
- Treatment is surgical resection for symptomatic lesions.

Jugular Foramen Lesions

- Most lesions involving the JF are neoplasms: paraganglioma (50–80%), schwannoma, and meningioma (each ≤10%) [2, 21–23].
- Assessment of the surrounding bony changes and vector of lesion spread helps differentiate between these lesions:
  o Paragangliomas: Permeative erosive margins, superolateral vector of spread into the middle ear cavity.
  o Schwannomas: Smooth enlargement ("scalloping") of the JF with thin, sclerotic margins, superomedial vector of spread.
  o Meningiomas: Permeative sclerotic changes, centrifugal vector of spread.
- Due to the close proximity of CN IX–XI within the JF and to CN XII in the adjacent hypoglossal canal, lesions may result in complex cranial neuropathies [2, 4, 23]:
  o Imaging should include the entire intra- and extracranial course of the CN IX–XII.
- Lower cranial nerve syndromes:
  o Vernet syndrome: CN IX–XI neuropathy (location: jugular foramen).
  o Collet-Sicard syndrome: Vernet syndrome + CN XII neuropathy (location: jugular foramen + hypoglossal canal).
  o Villaret syndrome: Collet-Sicard syndrome + ipsilateral Horner syndrome (location: jugular foramen + hypoglossal canal + carotid canal, also assess nasopharyngeal carotid space).

- Imaging findings associated with CN IX–XII neuropathies:
  - CN X: Ipsilateral vocal cord paralysis: medialization of the true vocal cord, anteromedial rotation of the arythenoid cartilage, dilatation of the laryngeal ventricle (sail sign) and piriform sinus, medialization and thickening of the aryepiglottic fold.
  - CN XI: Chronic phase: atrophy of the ipsilateral trapezius and sternocleidomastoid muscles, compensatory hypertrophy of the ipsilateral levator scapulae muscle.
  - CN XII neuropathy: Acute phase: T2 hyperintensity and enhancement of the ipsilateral intrinsic tongue muscles. Chronic phase: fatty atrophy and absent enhancement of the ipsilateral intrinsic tongue muscles, posterior displacement of the ipsilateral hemitongue (Figs. 34.11 and e34.5).

JF PARAGANGLIOMA (FIG. 34.8)

- Paraganglioma (PGL) are highly vascular tumors arising from paraganglia:
  - Neuroendocrine cells are closely associated with the autonomic nervous system.
  - In head and neck, found in locations associated with cranial nerves and often referred to as "glomus" tumors.
- PGLs are named according to the location into which it extends:
  - A jugular foramen PGL is found in the jugular foramen:
    - Arises from paraganglia lining the adventitia of the jugular bulb along the tympanic branch of CN IX (Jacobson nerve) or the auricular branch of CN X (Arnold nerve) or superior ganglion of CN X [23, 24].
  - A tympanicum PGL is found in the tympanic cavity:
    - Arises from the Jacobson nerve:
    - Characteristically located medially against the cochlear promontory.
  - A jugulotympanicum PGL spans both the jugular foramen and middle ear:
    - Most common tumor in the jugular foramen.
    - The second most common temporal bone tumor after VS [25].
    - Comprise up to 80% of primary neoplasms in the jugular foramen.
- Most cases are sporadic:
  - Patients are between age 40 and 60 years:
    - Strong female predominance (M:F = 1:4).
  - One-third to one-half of cases are hereditary and associated with tumor syndromes, e.g., hereditary paraganglioma-pheochromocytoma syndrome, multiple endocrine neoplasia syndrome type 1 (MEN1) or NF type 1 (NF1) [26]:
    - Genetic testing and search for additional lesions are warranted upon identification of a tumor.
- Clinical presentation: Pulsatile tinnitus, conductive hearing loss, vascular retrotympanic mass on otoscopy.
- Most PGL are benign but locally aggressive tumors.
- Malignant paraganglioma are defined as pathologically proven tumor foci in distant sites including nodes and not by histopathology of the primary tumor [27].
- CT:
  - Appearance of the jugular foramen bone margin is the most important imaging feature to note when deciding whether there may be a jugular foramen PGL:
    - Classic mottled permeative-destructive bony changes along the jugular foramen margin, with erosion of the jugular or caroticojugular spine.

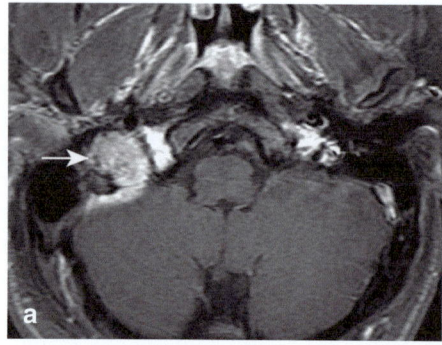 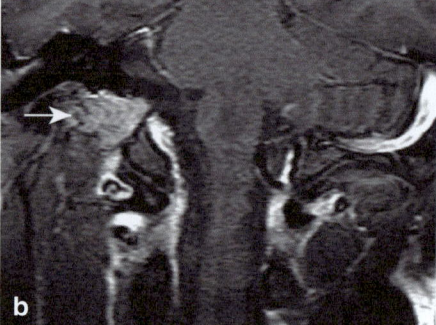 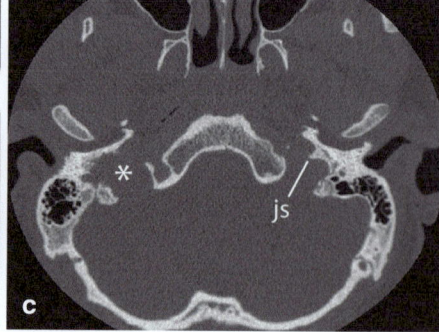

Fig. 34.8 Jugular foramen paraganglioma. (a) Axial T1WI C+ MR image shows a large, intensely enhancing mass in the right JF with internal flow voids, consistent with a JF paraganglioma (PGL) (white arrow). There is intracranial extension along the posterior wall of the right mastoid temporal bone without mass effect on the right cerebellar hemisphere. (b) Coronal T1WI C+ shows the typical superolateral vector of spread from the JF. (c) Axial CT in bone algorithm demonstrates permeative-destructive changes in the right JF wall (*) with erosion of the jugular spine. *Js* jugular spine

- o Tumor spread is typically in superolateral direction through the middle ear floor into the hypotympanum (=jugulotympanicum PGL):
  - Can be associated with ossicular or facial nerve canal erosion.
  - Less commonly:
    - Medial extension into the hypoglossal canal or jugular tubercle.
    - Spread toward the carotid sheath or posterior fossa.
- MRI:
  - o T1- and T2-weighted imaging:
    - Better delineates the highly vascular nature of the tumor.
    - Characteristic "salt and pepper" appearance more evident in larger lesions.
      - T1- and T2-hypointense "pepper" foci represent high-velocity flow voids.
      - Intrinsically T1-hyperintense "salt" foci are more rarely seen and represent subacute hemorrhage.
  - o T1-weighted imaging, C(+): Avidly enhancing mass.
- Nuclear medicine:
  - Indium 111-octreotide, F-18 FDG PET, and PET/CT imaging with Ga-68-labeled DOTA peptides:
    - Useful in detecting multifocal disease, recurrent disease [25], or metastatic or malignant paraganglioma.
- Treatment options:
  - o Surgical resection:
    - Possible preoperative angiography and embolization.
  - o Radiation therapy for unresectable or recurrent lesions [28].

JF SCHWANNOMA (FIG. 34.9)

- Benign, slow-growing nerve sheath tumor originating from differentiated Schwann cells [21–23]:
  - o Most commonly CN IX, less commonly CN X or XI.
- The second most common primary jugular foramen tumor:
  - o Mean age of presentation is 45 years.
- More than 90% of cases are sporadic:
  - o Bilateral or multiple tumors found in patients with NF2 or schwannomatosis [29, 30].
  - o Bilateral jugular foramen schwannomas are most commonly identified in NF2 patients.
    - 4% of NF2 patients develop jugular foramen schwannomas [31].
- Clinical presentation:
  - o Lower cranial nerve palsies (CN IX–XI).
  - o Sensorineural hearing loss when large:
    - May clinically mimic a VS.
- CT:
  - o Well-circumscribed, lobulated, low to intermediate attenuating, avidly enhancing lesions.
  - o Smooth expansion of the jugular foramen with preservation of the cortical margin.
  - o Bone remodeling can lead to blunting of the jugular tubercle.
  - o The vector of spread is along the cranial nerve superomedial toward the lateral brainstem and inferiorly into the post-styloid parapharyngeal space.
- MRI:
  - o Well-circumscribed, T1 isointense, T2 hyperintense mass with uniform and avid enhancement:
    - Fusiform or dumbbell-shaped.
    - Larger lesions can demonstrate cystic change.

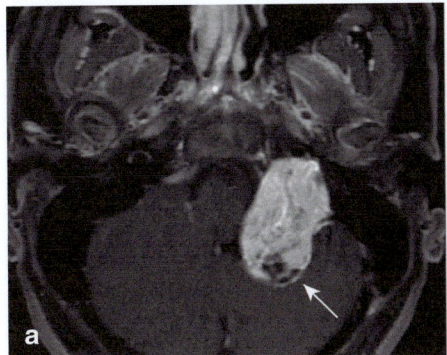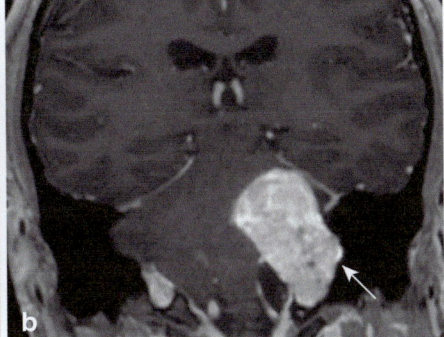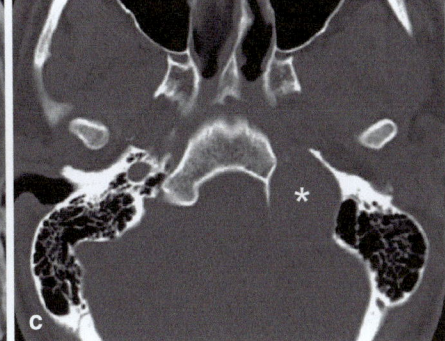

Fig. 34.9 Jugular foramen schwannoma. (a) Axial T1WI C+ MR image demonstrates a well-circumscribed, predominantly solid fusiform mass with avid homogenous enhancement (arrow), arising from either cranial nerve IX, X, or XI in the left jugular foramen and consistent with a JF schwannoma. The intralesional T1 hypointense, T2 hyperintense foci represent cystic degeneration. There is mass effect with medial displacement and flattening of the pons and posterior displacement of the left cerebellar hemisphere. (b) Coronal post-contrast T1 MR image best shows the typical superomedial vector of spread. (c) Axial bone CT shows smooth enlargement of the left JF with thin, sclerotic margins (*)

- Absent diffusion restriction [29].
- Flow voids or hemorrhage are typically absent, in contrast to jugular foramen paraganglioma.
• Treatment options:
- Microsurgical resection.
- Stereotactic radiosurgery may be used as primary or adjuvant treatment option [32].

JF MENINGIOMA (FIG. 34.10)

- The third most common jugular foramen mass:
  - Typically in females, 40–60 years old.
  - Most common presentation is progressive, unilateral CN IX–XI neuropathies.
- Benign neoplasm arising from arachnoid cap cells lining the jugular bulb.
- Primary jugular foramen meningiomas are defined as meningiomas centered in the jugular foramen:
  - Poorly circumscribed masses that infiltrate the adjacent skull base.
  - Diffuse centrifugal vector of spread into the hypotympanum, jugular tubercle, hypoglossal canal, nasopharyngeal carotid space, or dural sinus.
  - Differ in growth characteristics and imaging appearance from secondary meningiomas that arise from adjacent structures with extension into the jugular foramen [33]:
- Present as well-circumscribed extra-axial soft tissue masses extending into the foramen, with limited bone involvement.
• CT:
  - Hyperdense mass with extensive permeative-sclerotic changes and hyperostosis at the site of the infiltration.
  - Relative preservation of surrounding bone architecture.
  - Tumor calcification uncommon.
• MRI:
  - T1 iso- to hypointense, T2 intermediate hypointense mass with avid uniform contrast enhancement:
    • Dural tail is often present.
    • No internal flow voids.
• Treatment options:
  - Surgery is preferred option.
  - Radiotherapy or radiosurgery for older or poor-risk patients, or after subtotal resection.

JF MENINGOCELE (FIG. E34.3)

- CSF fistula extending into the jugular foramen.
- Uncommon, and described mainly in patients with NF1 [34, 35].
- CT: smooth widening of the jugular foramen.
- MRI: Well-circumscribed T1 hypointense, T2 hyperintense lesion contiguous with the subarachnoid CSF space and following CSF signal characteristics on all sequences.

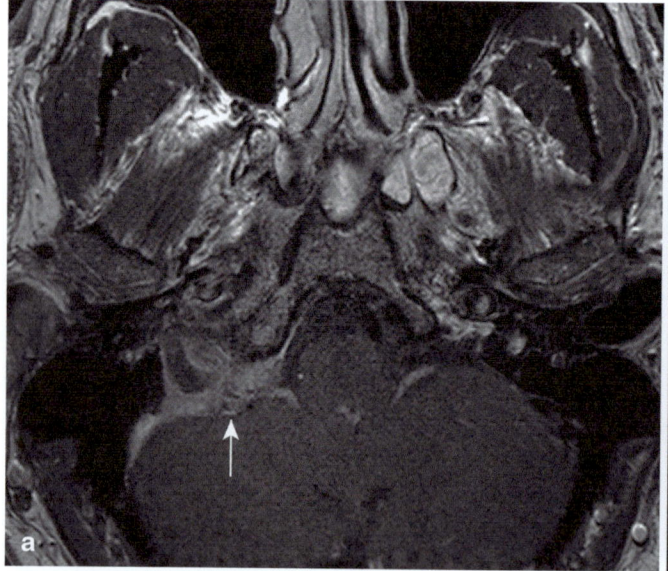 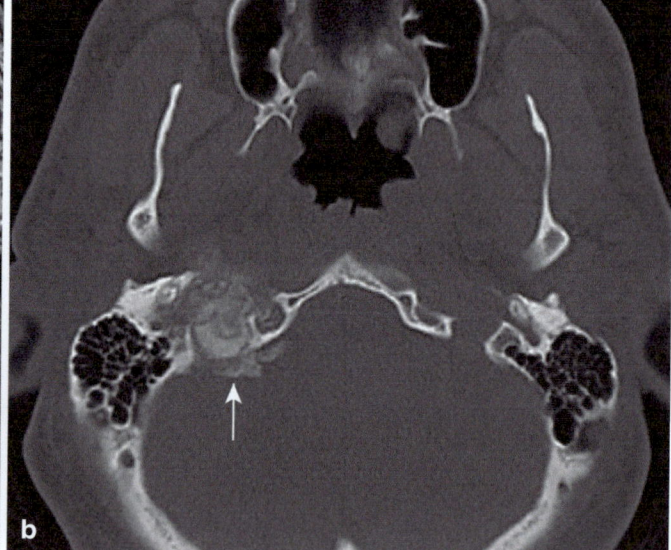

Fig. 34.10 Jugular foramen meningioma. (a) Axial T1WI C+ FS MR image shows a well-circumscribed, homogenously enhancing extra-axial mass in the right JF (arrow) with broad dural base along the posterior walls of the mastoid temporal bone and right occipital condyle. (b) On axial bone CT, there are permeative sclerotic changes in the right JF and lateral clivus walls and intralesional calcification. Note the centrifugal vector of spread. These findings are consistent with a JF meningioma

JUGULAR BULB DIVERTICULUM/DEHISCENCE (FIG. E34.4)

- Jugular bulb dehiscence:
  - Superolateral extension of a prominent jugular bulb toward the middle ear.
  - Accompanying dehiscence of bony covering separating the jugular bulb from the middle ear (sigmoid plate).
  - Can be congenital:
    - More commonly seen on the right side [36, 37].
  - Commonly associated with high-riding jugular bulb [38]:
    - Definition of the superior boundary that constitutes a high-riding jugular bulb varies, including the inferior tympanic annulus or the inferior margin of the basal turn of cochlea [23, 38].
  - Most cases of jugular bulb dehiscence are incidental findings:
    - Diagnosis should be considered in patients presenting with pulsatile tinnitus or conductive hearing loss and a blue retrotympanic mass on otoscopy.
  - CT:
    - Bone reformat:
      - Lobulated opacity bulging from the jugular foramen toward the middle ear.
      - Severe irregular thinning and dehiscence of the intervening bony covering.
    - Contrast-enhanced CT:
      - Contiguous with the adjacent sigmoid sinus and internal jugular vein and follows attenuation of the intracranial venous system.
      - Outside of the dehiscence site, the adjacent jugular foramen wall should remain intact and well-corticated:
        - Differentiates it from other jugular foramen masses such as a paraganglioma or metastasis.
  - MRI:
    - Flow phenomenon may demonstrate heterogeneous signal or uneven flow void in jugular bulb.
    - May mimic a soft tissue mass.
  - Treatment options:
    - Should be considered for symptomatic patients.
    - Options include surgical resection or ligation with reconstruction of the middle ear floor, or endovascular embolization.
    - In recent year, jugular bulb resurfacing with cement material has also been performed [39, 40].
- Jugular bulb diverticulum:
  - Anatomic variant where a focal outpouching protrudes beyond the jugular bulb into the adjacent bone, most commonly superomedially into the petrous temporal bone.
  - More commonly on the left side.
  - Imaging:
    - Focal outpouching is continuous with the jugular bulb.
    - Typically located posterior to the internal auditory canal and outlined by a well-corticated bony wall.
    - The jugular foramen wall is preserved, contrary to the permeative-destructive changes seen in jugular foramen PGL, or the permeative-sclerotic changes found in skull base meningiomas.

SIGMOID SINUS DIVERTICULUM/DEHISCENCE

- Sigmoid sinus diverticulum:
  - An anatomic variant in which there is a focal protrusion from the sigmoid sinus toward the mastoid portion of the temporal bone.
  - Can be seen with an intact, well-corticated remodeled sigmoid plate or in conjunction with a dehiscent sigmoid plate (sigmoid sinus dehiscence).
- Can cause pulsatile tinnitus [41].
- Increased prevalence of sigmoid sinus diverticulum/dehiscence in patients with idiopathic intracranial hypertension:
  - Not correlated with the pulsatile tinnitus described in these patients [42].
- CT:
  - Sigmoid sinus diverticulum.
    - Area of focal smooth bony remodeling and protrusion extending off of the sigmoid sinus toward the mastoid portion of the temporal bone.
    - Contrast-enhanced study is not necessary but can be confirmatory.
  - Sigmoid sinus dehiscence without diverticulum.
    - Focal bony thinning or demineralization overlying the sigmoid sinus where it interfaces with the posterior mastoid cells.
- MRI:
  - Often heterogeneous signal or uneven flow void within the diverticulum.
- Treatment:
  - Usually trans mastoid sigmoid sinus resurfacing or reshaping [43].

JUGULAR FORAMEN METASTASES

- Etiologies:
  - Secondary to hematogenous spread from systemic cancers. Most common primary malignancies include breast, lung, and prostate cancers.
  - Direct extension of local neoplasms arising from the external auditory canal, nasopharynx, skull base, or

temporal bone, e.g., chondrosarcoma, endolymphatic sac tumor [23, 44].
- Perineural spread of head and neck tumors, e.g., adenoid cystic carcinoma and mucoepidermoid carcinoma [45].
- Perineural spread:
  - Thickening and contrast-enhancement of the involved nerve.
  - On both CT and MR imaging, the jugular foramen appears eroded or enlarged, and there is infiltration or obliteration of the foraminal fat pad.
- Jugular foramen metastases especially from highly vascular primary malignancies (renal, thyroid cancer, and melanoma) may mimic PGL:
  - Metastases are typically lower in T2 signal and demonstrate centrifugal lesion spread.
  - Paragangliomas are hyperintense on T2-weighted images and spread in a superolateral direction.
  - No intratumoral flow voids.
- Treatment: palliative radiotherapy.

Hypoglossal Canal Lesions (Figs. 34.11, e34.5, e34.6, e34.7 and e34.8)

- Lesions arising or involving the hypoglossal canal include [46]:
  - Primary lesions arising from the hypoglossal nerve, e.g., schwannoma.
  - Primary skull base lesions (chordomas, chondrosarcomas, plasmacytomas, meningiomas), metastases, synovial cysts, congenital or acquired vascular structures (dural arteriovenous fistula, persistent hypoglossal artery), hypoglossal canal no enhancing cystic lesions.

HYPOGLOSSAL SCHWANNOMA (FIG. 34.11)

- Rare tumors, most often seen in association with NF2 [46].
- Imaging features similar to those described for other CN schwannomas:
  - Intradural tumors, associated with smooth enlargement of the hypoglossal canal.
  - MRI: well-circumscribed T2 hyperintense, avidly enhancing mass.
- Ipsilateral hemitongue atrophy may be seen.
- Should be differentiated from:
  - Skull base metastasis or direct invasion of the hypoglossal canal by nasopharyngeal carcinoma:
    - Eroded canal margins in these conditions.
  - Local spread to the hypoglossal canal from skull base meningioma or jugular foramen tumor:
    - Bulk of the tumor centered away from the hypoglossal canal.
- Treatment options:
  - Surgery or stereotactic radiotherapy.
  - Surveillance with follow-up imaging can be considered [46, 47].

HYPOGLOSSAL METASTASIS/PERINEURAL SPREAD (FIG. E34.5)

- Cancer spread along the course of the hypoglossal nerve is uncommon:
  - Mainly been reported in patients with squamous cell carcinoma affecting the base of tongue [45].
- MR imaging features are similar to those described for perineural spread to the jugular foramen.
- FDG-PET may prove helpful in estimating the tumor extent along the affected nerve [48].
- Treatment options:
  - Radiation therapy can provide local control of the perineural cancer spread.

HYPOGLOSSAL CANAL SYNOVIAL CYST (FIG. E34.6)

- Synovial cyst arising from an articular joint at the craniocervical junction with cephalad extension through the foramen magnum, encroaching on or extending into the hypoglossal canal.
- CT: May show smooth bone remodeling and enlargement of the hypoglossal canal.
- MRI: Well-circumscribed T2 hyperintense cystic lesion with thin peripheral and absent central enhancement arising from the adjacent craniocervical facet joint.
- Treatment is surgical resection.

HYPOGLOSSAL CANAL DURAL ARTERIOVENOUS FISTULA (FIG. E34.7)

- Uncommon posterior fossa dural arteriovenous fistula (dAVF), constitute 3.6–4.2% of all intracranial dAVF.
- dAVF involving the anterior condylar confluence (ACC) and/or anterior condylar vein (ACV) [49–51].
  - ACC [51, 52]:
    - Extracranial venous plexus located at the skull base, anterior to the extracranial hypoglossal canal aperture and medial to the internal jugular vein (IJV).

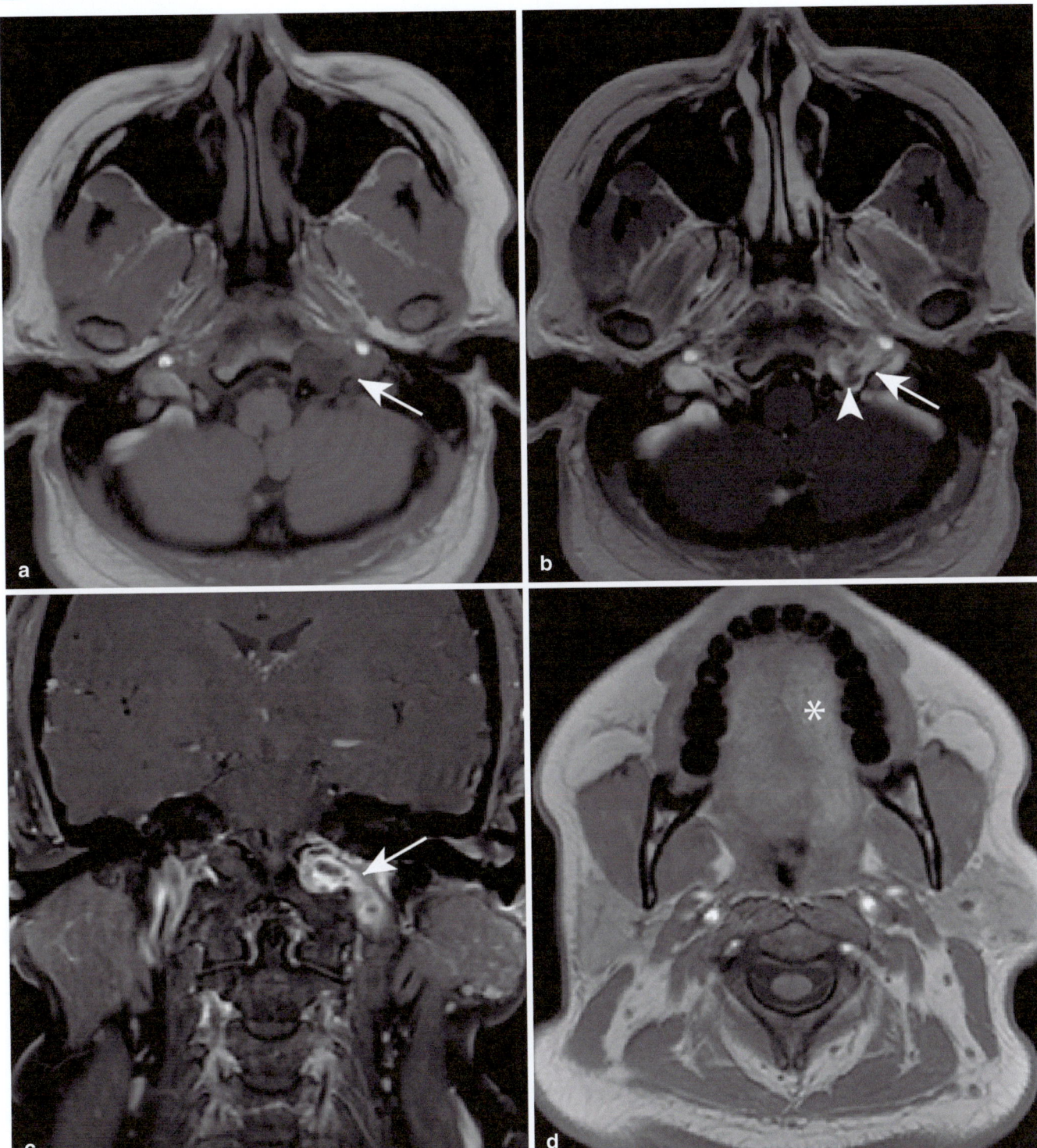

Fig. 34.11 Hypoglossal schwannoma. (**a**) Axial non-enhanced T1WI MR image shows an expansile well-circumscribed T1 isointense mass in the left hypoglossal canal (arrow). There is a widening of the left hypoglossal canal and scalloping of the left lateral clivus. Axial (**b**) and coronal (**c**) T1WI C+ MR images demonstrate avid enhancement of this lesion with internal foci of T1 hypointense (arrowhead), T2 hyperintense (not shown) cystic degeneration. These findings are consistent with a CN XII schwannoma. (**d**) More inferiorly, axial non-enhanced T1WI MR image at the level of the oral tongue shows fatty atrophy of the intrinsic muscles in the left hemitongue (*), consistent with chronic CN XII denervation

- Connects the cerebral venous system, internal and external vertebral venous plexuses (VVP) and IJV through complex communication with several venous networks.
    - Important structure in redirecting cerebral venous drainage into the internal and external VVP in upright position.
    - Cerebral venous drainage is predominantly through the IJV in supine position and the VVP in upright position.
- Communicates indirectly with the cavernous sinuses.
  o Anterior condylar vein (ACV):
    - Originates intracranially at the junction between the inferior petrosal sinus and the jugular bulb, then courses as a venous plexus around the hypoglossal nerve through the hypoglossal canal to connect to the ACC.
    - Contiguous inferiorly with the anterior internal VVP.
    - Communicates indirectly with the basilar plexus, cavernous sinuses, and anterior brainstem pial veins.

- Arterial feeders to dAVF: branches of the ascending pharyngeal artery, posterior auricular artery, petrous branch of the middle meningeal artery, or mastoid branch of the occipital artery.
- Absence of valves in the ACC, ACV, and their associated venous networks allows for multidirectional blood flow, and hypoglossal canal dAVFs can therefore be classified into three types based on their venous drainage pattern [51]:
  o Type 1 (62.5%): Dominant anterograde venous drainage into the IJV and/or VVP with or without reflux into the transverse, sigmoid, inferior petrosal or cavernous sinuses.
  o Type 2 (23.3%): Dominant retrograde drainage to the cavernous sinuses and/or orbital veins with or without anterograde drainage to the IJV and/or VVP or cortical venous reflux.
  o Type 3 (14.2%): Dominant or exclusive venous drainage to the cerebellar pial or perimedullary veins.
- Clinical presentation varies with each type:
  o Type 1: Pulsatile tinnitus, hypoglossal nerve palsy.
  o Type 2: Orbital symptoms mimicking cavernous sinus dAVF (chemosis, proptosis, and diplopia).
  o Type 3: Intracerebral hemorrhage, brainstem and/or upper spinal cord symptoms.
- Imaging:
  o CT bone reformat: Smooth widening of the hypoglossal canal.
  o MRI: Ill-defined T1 intermediate contrast-enhancing lesion near the jugular foramen involving the hypoglossal canal. Early filling and enhancement in the ACC and/or ACV.
  o MRA: Focus of flow-related signal near the jugular foramen, with early shunting into the ACC and/or ACV and draining veins.
  o Imaging appearance may mimic a jugular foramen tumor.
- Treatment:
  o Conservative therapy: Spontaneous regression may be observed in 5.8% of type 1 hypoglossal canal dAVF.
  o Endovascular transvenous embolization for types 1 and 2, endovascular trans arterial embolization or surgery for type 3.

PERSISTENT HYPOGLOSSAL ARTERY (FIG. E34.8)

- Second most common carotid-vertebrobasilar artery anastomosis after the persistent trigeminal artery [53, 54]:
  o Arises from the internal carotid artery at the levels of C1–C3.
  o Enters the posterior cranial fossa through the hypoglossal canal instead of the foramen magnum.
  o Anastomoses with the basilar artery.
- Estimated incidence is less than 0.1%; rarely bilateral.
- Most often represents an incidental finding in the setting of an enlarged hypoglossal canal with preserved cortical margins:
  o Can be associated with glossopharyngeal neuralgia or hypoglossal nerve palsy [55].
- Aneurysms are reported at the junction between the persistent hypoglossal artery and basilar artery in up to a third of cases:
  o Angiography studies should be planned when this diagnosis is suspected.

Foramen Magnum Lesions (Figs. 34.12, e34.9 and e34.10)

- Differential diagnoses include:
  o Intra-axial lesions: Cerebellar tonsillar descent (Chiari malformation, tonsillar herniation), metastases, posterior fossa tumors (cerebellar or brainstem tumors), hematoma, and demyelination.
  o Extra-axial lesions: Meningioma, peripheral nerve sheath tumors (schwannoma, neurofibroma), fourth ventricular lesions, ependymoma, congenital cysts (Blake pouch cyst, arachnoid cyst, neurenteric cyst, epidermoid cyst), and vascular (aneurysms, arteriovenous malformation).
  o Degenerative/inflammatory: rheumatoid arthritis, calcium pyrophosphate deposition disease, gout.

- Skull base lesions: plasmacytoma, metastases, chordoma, chondrosarcoma.
- Close proximity of the structures in the foramen magnum predisposes to high morbidity and mortality from mass effect:
  - Accurate diagnosis is therefore essential.

FORAMEN MAGNUM MENINGIOMA (FIG. 34.12)

- Most common benign tumors of the foramen magnum [56]:
  - Less than 3% of all meningiomas.
- Most often anterolateral location within the foramen magnum:
  - Posterolateral and posterior are less frequent [57].
- Mostly intradural.
- Average patient age at diagnosis is 57 years:
  - Mean time from onset of symptoms to diagnosis is 31 months.
  - Slow growth.
  - Mean tumor diameter is 3 cm.
  - More than 90% of tumors are WHO Grade I [56].
- Imaging:
  - Radiological features similar to meningiomas in other locations.
  - Important considerations when describing foramen magnum meningiomas:
    - Determine whether the origin of the meningioma is within the anatomical boundaries of the foramen magnum [57], or if it represents a spread from an adjacent location.
    - Identify which structures are displaced or encased by the meningioma:
      - Vertebral artery encasement occurs in about one-third of patients [56], more often with lateral foramen magnum meningiomas.
      - Displacement of adjacent lower CNs with lateral tumors.
      - Posterior displacement of spinal cord by anterior foramen magnum meningiomas.
- Treatment:
  - Surgical.
  - Gross total resection rate is approximately 40% [56].

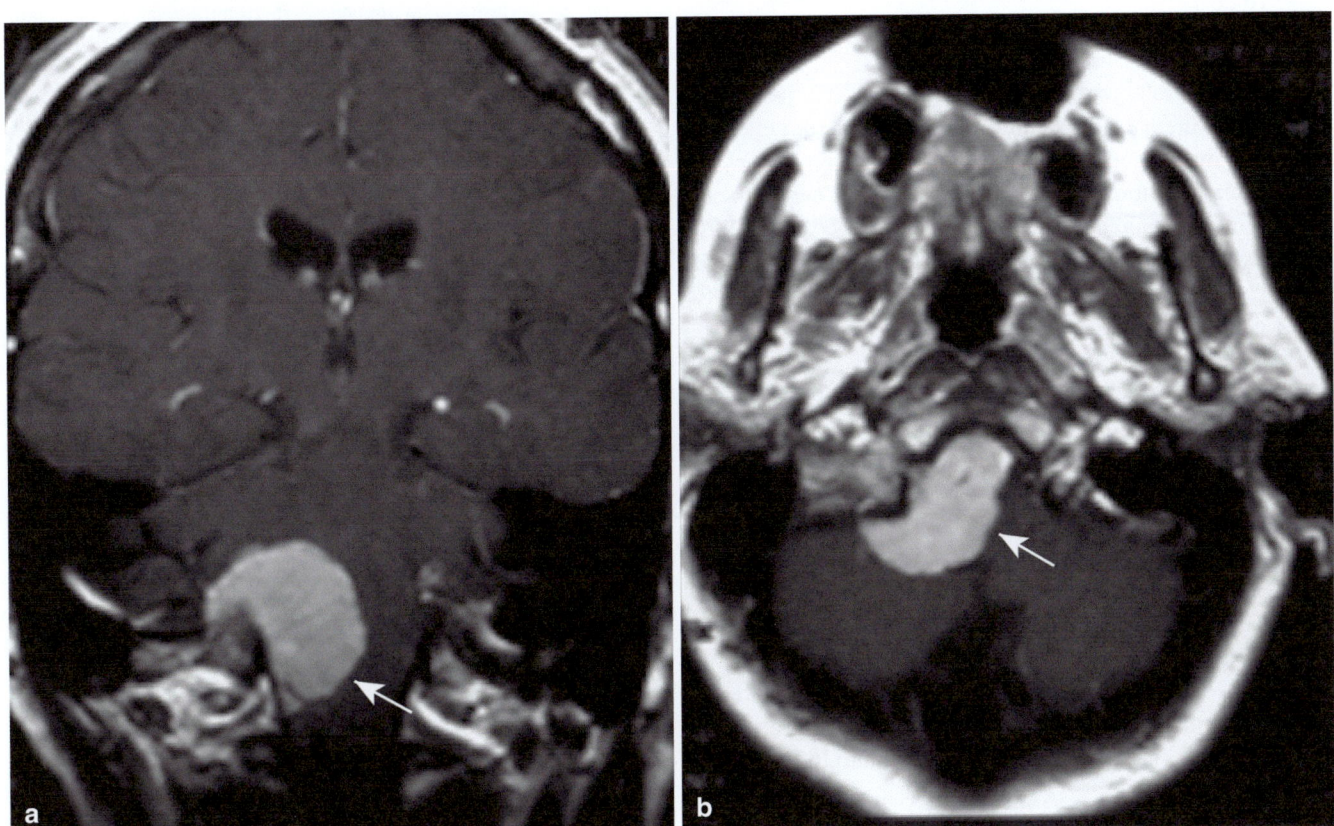

Fig. 34.12 Foramen magnum meningioma. Coronal (**a**) and axial (**b**) T1WI C+ MR images demonstrate a well-circumscribed homogenously enhancing extra-axial mass with broad dural base and dural tail along the posterior walls of the right mastoid temporal bone and clivus (arrow). The mass extends inferiorly into the right foramen magnum. These findings are consistent with a foramen magnum meningioma

FORAMEN MAGNUM SCHWANNOMAS

- Lower cranial nerve schwannomas are the second most common benign tumors of the foramen magnum:
  - Extension into the foramen magnum of schwannomas arising from the jugular foramen or the hypoglossal canal are most often seen.
  - Primary foramen magnum schwannomas are rare and represent less than 5% of intracranial schwannomas [29].
- CT and MR imaging appearances are similar to other cranial nerve schwannomas.

FORAMEN MAGNUM PLEXIFORM NEUROFIBROMAS (FIG. E34.9)

- Neurofibromas are benign peripheral nerve sheath tumors composed of a mixture of Schwann cells, perineurial cells, fibroblasts, and mast cells [58].
- Plexiform neurofibromas are focal or multifocal nodular lesions along a nerve:
  - Located in nerve fascicles of skin, subcutaneous or deep soft tissue, or along nerve roots.
- Found in 40–50% of patients with NF1. The presence of a plexiform neurofibroma constitutes a diagnostic criteria for NF1 [58, 59].
- MRI:
  - Multinodular enhancing masses with T2 peripheral hyperintensity, T2 central hypointensity (target sign), and mass effect on the surrounding structures.
  - Transformation to malignant peripheral nerve sheath tumors should be suspected in the presence of a painful expanding lesion, large lesion size, peripheral enhancement, perilesional edema, or intralesional cystic changes [60].
- Treatment:
  - Surgical resection.
  - Medical treatment (mammalian target of rapamycin (mTOR) or mitogen-activated protein kinase (MEK) inhibitors) in inoperable or subtotally resected symptomatic lesions [61].

BENIGN ENHANCING LESION OF THE FORAMEN MAGNUM (FIG. E34.10)

- Small, enhancing lesions posterior to and separate from the vertebral artery in the foramen magnum [62].
- MRI:
  - Relatively isointense to CSF on T1- or T2-weighted imaging:
    - May not be readily identifiable on routine imaging.
  - Typically hyperintense on fluid-attenuated inversion recovery sequences.
  - Enhance following contrast administration.
  - No restricted diffusion or susceptibility artifact.
  - Remain stable after prolonged imaging follow-up, which confirms their benign nature.
- Exact nature of these lesions remains uncertain:
  - Thought to represent bridging venous structures [62].

References

1. Baskin H, Chapman PR. Posterior skull base. In: Chapman PR, editor. Imaging anatomy: head and neck. Elsevier; 2018. p. 40–9.
2. Job J, Branstetter BF. Imaging of the posterior skull base. Radiol Clin N Am. 2017;55(1):103–21. https://doi.org/10.1016/j.rcl.2016.08.002.
3. Harnsberger HR, Vattoth S. CPA-IAC anatomy. In: Chapman PR, editor. Imaging anatomy: head and neck. Elsevier; 2018. p. 102–7.
4. Juliano AF, Ginat DT, Moonis G. Imaging review of the temporal bone: part I. Anatomy and inflammatory and neoplastic processes. Radiology. 2013;269(1):17–33. https://doi.org/10.1148/radiol.13120733.
5. Bonneville F, Sarrazin JL, Marsot-Dupuch K, Iffenecker C, Cordoliani YS, Doyon D, et al. Unusual lesions of the cerebellopontine angle: a segmental approach. Radiographics. 2001;21(2):419–38. https://doi.org/10.1148/radiographics.21.2.g01mr13419.
6. Bonneville F, Savatovsky J, Chiras J. Imaging of cerebellopontine angle lesions: an update. Part 2: intra-axial lesions, skull base lesions that may invade the CPA region, and non-enhancing extra-axial lesions. Eur Radiol. 2007;17(11):2908–20. https://doi.org/10.1007/s00330-007-0680-4.
7. Bonneville F, Savatovsky J, Chiras J. Imaging of cerebellopontine angle lesions: an update. Part 1: enhancing extra-axial lesions. Eur Radiol. 2007;17(10):2472–82. https://doi.org/10.1007/s00330-007-0679-x.
8. Fink JR. Imaging of cerebellopontine angle masses: self-assessment module. AJR Am J Roentgenol. 2010;195(3 Suppl):S15–21. https://doi.org/10.2214/AJR.09.7191.
9. Goldbrunner R, Weller M, Regis J, Lund-Johansen M, Stavrinou P, Reuss D, et al. EANO guideline on the diagnosis and treatment of vestibular schwannoma. Neuro-Oncology. 2020;22(1):31–45. https://doi.org/10.1093/neuonc/noz153.
10. Lin EP, Crane BT. The management and imaging of vestibular schwannomas. AJNR Am J Neuroradiol. 2017;38(11):2034–43. https://doi.org/10.3174/ajnr.A5213.
11. Dunn IF, Bi WL, Mukundan S, Delman BN, Parish J, Atkins T, et al. Congress of Neurological Surgeons systematic review and evidence-based guidelines on the role of imaging in the diagnosis and management of patients with vestibular schwannomas. Neurosurgery. 2018;82(2):E32–E4. https://doi.org/10.1093/neuros/nyx510.
12. Hakim A, Wagner F. An important pitfall in diagnosing intracanalicular vestibular schwannoma. AJNR Am J Neuroradiol. 2019;40(10):E58–E9. https://doi.org/10.3174/ajnr.A6192.
13. Hadjipanayis CG, Carlson ML, Link MJ, Rayan TA, Parish J, Atkins T, et al. Congress of Neurological Surgeons systematic review and evidence-based guidelines on surgical resection for the treatment of patients with vestibular schwannomas. Neurosurgery. 2018;82(2):E40–E3. https://doi.org/10.1093/neuros/nyx512.
14. Agarwal V, Babu R, Grier J, Adogwa O, Back A, Friedman AH, et al. Cerebellopontine angle meningiomas: postoperative outcomes

15. Batra PS, Dutra JC, Wiet RJ. Auditory and facial nerve function following surgery for cerebellopontine angle meningiomas. Arch Otolaryngol Head Neck Surg. 2002;128(4):369–74. https://doi.org/10.1001/archotol.128.4.369.
16. Kaye J, Zeller S, Patel NV, Herschman Y, Jumah F, Nanda A. Presentation, surgical management, and postoperative outcome of a fourth ventricular cavernous malformation: case report and review of literature. World Neurosurg. 2020;137:78–83. https://doi.org/10.1016/j.wneu.2020.01.185.
17. Osborn AG, Preece MT. Intracranial cysts: radiologic–pathologic correlation and imaging approach. Radiology. 2006;239(3):650–64. https://doi.org/10.1148/radiol.2393050823.
18. Christensen WN, Long DM, Epstein JI. Cerebellopontine angle lipoma. Hum Pathol. 1986;17(7):739–43. https://doi.org/10.1016/s0046-8177(86)80184-8.
19. Smirniotopoulos JG, Yue NC, Rushing EJ. Cerebellopontine angle masses: radiologic–pathologic correlation. Radiographics. 1993;13(5):1131–47. https://doi.org/10.1148/radiographics.13.5.8210595.
20. Friedmann DR, Grobelny B, Golfinos JG, Roland JT Jr. Nonschwannoma tumors of the cerebellopontine angle. Otolaryngol Clin N Am. 2015;48(3):461–75. https://doi.org/10.1016/j.otc.2015.02.006.
21. Caldemeyer KS, Mathews VP, Azzarelli B, Smith RR. The jugular foramen: a review of anatomy, masses, and imaging characteristics. Radiographics. 1997;17(5):1123–39. https://doi.org/10.1148/radiographics.17.5.9308106.
22. Eldevik OP, Gabrielsen TO, Jacobsen EA. Imaging findings in schwannomas of the jugular foramen. AJNR Am J Neuroradiol. 2000;21(6):1139–44.
23. Ong CK, Chong VFH. Imaging of jugular foramen. Neuroimaging Clin N Am. 2009;19(3):469–82. https://doi.org/10.1016/j.nic.2009.06.007.
24. El-Naggar A, Chan JKC, Grandis JR, Takata T, Slootweg PJ. WHO classification of head and neck tumors. IARC WHO classification of tumours series, vol. 9. 4th ed. Lyon: International Agency for Research on Cancer; 2017.
25. Touska P, Juliano AF. Temporal bone tumors: an imaging update. Neuroimaging Clin N Am. 2019;29(1):145–72. https://doi.org/10.1016/j.nic.2018.09.007.
26. Neumann HPH, Young WF Jr, Eng C. Pheochromocytoma and paraganglioma. N Engl J Med. 2019;381(6):552–65. https://doi.org/10.1056/NEJMra1806651.
27. Moskovic DJ, Smolarz JR, Stanley D, Jimenez C, Williams MD, Hanna EY, et al. Malignant head and neck paragangliomas: is there an optimal treatment strategy? Head Neck Oncol. 2010;2:23. https://doi.org/10.1186/1758-3284-2-23.
28. Gjuric M, Gleeson M. Consensus statement and guidelines on the management of paragangliomas of the head and neck. Skull Base. 2009;19(1):109–16. https://doi.org/10.1055/s-0028-1103131.
29. Skolnik AD, Loevner LA, Sampathu DM, Newman JG, Lee JY, Bagley LJ, et al. Cranial nerve schwannomas: diagnostic imaging approach. Radiographics. 2016;36(5):1463–77. https://doi.org/10.1148/rg.2016150199.
30. Thomas AK, Egelhoff JC, Curran JG, Thomas B. Pediatric schwannomatosis, a rare but distinct form of neurofibromatosis. Pediatr Radiol. 2016;46(3):430–5. https://doi.org/10.1007/s00247-015-3482-x.
31. Fisher LM, Doherty JK, Lev MH, Slattery WH 3rd. Distribution of nonvestibular cranial nerve schwannomas in neurofibromatosis 2. Otol Neurotol. 2007;28(8):1083–90. https://doi.org/10.1097/MAO.0b013e31815a8411.
32. Kano H, Meola A, Yang HC, Guo WY, Martinez-Alvarez R, Martinez-Moreno N, et al. Stereotactic radiosurgery for jugular foramen schwannomas: an international multicenter study. J Neurosurg. 2018;129(4):928–36. https://doi.org/10.3171/2017.5.JNS162894.
33. Macdonald AJ, Salzman KL, Harnsberger HR, Gilbert E, Shelton C. Primary jugular foramen meningioma: imaging appearance and differentiating features. AJR Am J Roentgenol. 2004;182(2):373–7. https://doi.org/10.2214/ajr.182.2.1820373.
34. Serindere M, Tasar M, Hamcan S, Bozlar U. Imaging findings of jugular foramen meningocele in a neurofibromatosis type 1 patient. Case Rep Radiol. 2017;2017:7047696. https://doi.org/10.1155/2017/7047696.
35. Siddiqui A, Connor S, Gleeson M. Jugular foramen meningocoele in a patient with neurofibromatosis type 1. J Laryngol Otol. 2008;122(2):213–6. https://doi.org/10.1017/S0022215107007244.
36. Atmaca S, Elmali M, Kucuk H. High and dehiscent jugular bulb: clear and present danger during middle ear surgery. Surg Radiol Anat. 2014;36(4):369–74. https://doi.org/10.1007/s00276-013-1196-z.
37. Friedmann DR, Eubig J, Winata LS, Pramanik BK, Merchant SN, Lalwani AK. A clinical and histopathologic study of jugular bulb abnormalities. Arch Otolaryngol Head Neck Surg. 2012;138(1):66–71. https://doi.org/10.1001/archoto.2011.231.
38. Park JJ, Shen A, Loberg C, Westhofen M. The relationship between jugular bulb position and jugular bulb related inner ear dehiscence: a retrospective analysis. Am J Otolaryngol. 2015;36(3):347–51. https://doi.org/10.1016/j.amjoto.2014.12.006.
39. DeHart AN, Shaia WT, Coelho DH. Hydroxyapatite cement resurfacing the dehiscent jugular bulb: novel treatment for pulsatile tinnitus. Laryngoscope. 2018;128(5):1186–90. https://doi.org/10.1002/lary.26711.
40. Lee SY, Song SK, Park SJ, Park HG, Choi BY, Koo JW, et al. Jugular bulb resurfacing with bone cement for patients with high dehiscent jugular bulb and ipsilateral pulsatile tinnitus. Otol Neurotol. 2019;40(2):192–9. https://doi.org/10.1097/MAO.0000000000002093.
41. Schoeff S, Nicholas B, Mukherjee S, Kesser BW. Imaging prevalence of sigmoid sinus dehiscence among patients with and without pulsatile tinnitus. Otolaryngol Head Neck Surg. 2014;150(5):841–6. https://doi.org/10.1177/0194599813520291.
42. Lansley JA, Tucker W, Eriksen MR, Riordan-Eva P, Connor SEJ. Sigmoid sinus diverticulum, dehiscence, and venous sinus stenosis: potential causes of pulsatile tinnitus in patients with idiopathic intracranial hypertension? AJNR Am J Neuroradiol. 2017;38(9):1783–8. https://doi.org/10.3174/ajnr.A5277.
43. Kim CS, Kim SY, Choi H, Koo JW, Yoo SY, An GS, et al. Transmastoid reshaping of the sigmoid sinus: preliminary study of a novel surgical method to quiet pulsatile tinnitus of an unrecognized vascular origin. J Neurosurg. 2016;125(2):441–9. https://doi.org/10.3171/2015.6.JNS15961.
44. Mitsuya K, Nakasu Y, Horiguchi S, Harada H, Nishimura T, Yuen S, et al. Metastatic skull tumors: MRI features and a new conventional classification. J Neuro-Oncol. 2011;104(1):239–45. https://doi.org/10.1007/s11060-010-0465-5.
45. Paes FM, Singer AD, Checkver AN, Palmquist RA, De La Vega G, Sidani C. Perineural spread in head and neck malignancies: clinical significance and evaluation with 18F-FDG PET/CT. Radiographics. 2013;33(6):1717–36. https://doi.org/10.1148/rg.336135501.
46. Weindling SM, Wood CP, Hoxworth JM. Hypoglossal canal lesions: distinctive imaging features and simple diagnostic algorithm. AJR Am J Roentgenol. 2017;209(5):1119–27. https://doi.org/10.2214/AJR.17.18102.
47. Santander XA, Cotua CE, Saldana C. Spontaneous regression of a hypoglossal neurinoma: case report and review of the literature. World Neurosurg. 2017;105(1033):e7–9. https://doi.org/10.1016/j.wneu.2017.06.004.

48. Lee H, Lazor JW, Assadsangabi R, Shah J. An Imager's guide to perineural tumor spread in head and neck cancers: radiologic footprints on ¹⁸F-FDG PET, with CT and MRI correlates. J Nucl Med. 2019;60(3):304–11. https://doi.org/10.2967/jnumed.118.214312.
49. Ernst R, Bulas R, Tomsick T, van Loveren H, Aziz KA. Three cases of dural arteriovenous fistula of the anterior condylar vein within the hypoglossal canal. AJNR Am J Neuroradiol. 1999;20(10):2016–20.
50. Liu JK, Mahaney K, Barnwell SL, McMenomey SO, Delashaw JB Jr. Dural arteriovenous fistula of the anterior condylar confluence and hypoglossal canal mimicking a jugular foramen tumor. J Neurosurg. 2008;109(2):335–40. https://doi.org/10.3171/JNS/2008/109/8/0335.
51. Spittau B, Millan DS, El-Sherifi S, Hader C, Singh TP, Motschall E, et al. Dural arteriovenous fistulas of the hypoglossal canal: systematic review on imaging anatomy, clinical findings, and endovascular management. J Neurosurg. 2015;122(4):883–903. https://doi.org/10.3171/2014.10.JNS14377.
52. San Millan Ruiz D, Gailloud P, Rufenacht DA, Delavelle J, Henry F, Fasel JH. The craniocervical venous system in relation to cerebral venous drainage. AJNR Am J Neuroradiol. 2002;23(9):1500–8.
53. Coulier B. Persistent hypoglossal artery. J Belg Soc Radiol. 2018;102(1):28. https://doi.org/10.5334/jbsr.1481.
54. Dimmick SJ, Faulder KC. Normal variants of the cerebral circulation at multidetector CT angiography. Radiographics. 2009;29(4):1027–43. https://doi.org/10.1148/rg.294085730.
55. Yilmaz E, Ilgit E, Taner D. Primitive persistent carotid-basilar and carotid-vertebral anastomoses: a report of seven cases and a review of the literature. Clin Anat. 1995;8(1):36–43. https://doi.org/10.1002/ca.980080107.
56. Magill ST, Shahin MN, Lucas CG, Yen AJ, Lee DS, Raleigh DR, et al. Surgical outcomes, complications, and management strategies for foramen magnum meningiomas. J Neurol Surg B Skull Base. 2019;80(1):1–9. https://doi.org/10.1055/s-0038-1654702.
57. Bruneau M, George B. Classification system of foramen magnum meningiomas. J Craniovertebr Junct Spine. 2010;1(1):10–7. https://doi.org/10.4103/0974-8237.65476.
58. Wang MX, Dillman JR, Guccione J, Habiba A, Maher M, Kamel S, et al. Neurofibromatosis from head to toe: what the radiologist needs to know. Radiographics. 2022;42(4):1123–44. https://doi.org/10.1148/rg.210235.
59. Mautner VF, Asuagbor FA, Dombi E, Funsterer C, Kluwe L, Wenzel R, et al. Assessment of benign tumor burden by whole-body MRI in patients with neurofibromatosis 1. Neuro-Oncology. 2008;10(4):593–8. https://doi.org/10.1215/15228517-2008-011.
60. Wasa J, Nishida Y, Tsukushi S, Shido Y, Sugiura H, Nakashima H, et al. MRI features in the differentiation of malignant peripheral nerve sheath tumors and neurofibromas. AJR Am J Roentgenol. 2010;194(6):1568–74. https://doi.org/10.2214/AJR.09.2724.
61. Solares I, Vinal D, Morales-Conejo M, Rodriguez-Salas N, Feliu J. Novel molecular targeted therapies for patients with neurofibromatosis type 1 with inoperable plexiform neurofibromas: a comprehensive review. ESMO Open. 2021;6(4):100223. https://doi.org/10.1016/j.esmoop.2021.100223.
62. McGuinness BJ, Morrison JP, Brew SK, Moriarty MW. Benign enhancing foramen magnum lesions: clinical report of a newly recognized entity. AJNR Am J Neuroradiol. 2017;38(4):721–5. https://doi.org/10.3174/ajnr.A5085.

Embryology and Anatomy of the Sella and Parasellar Region

Anil Vasireddi and Katie Suzanne Traylor

- Pituitary gland consists of an anterior adenohypophysis and posterior neurohypophysis.
  o Adenohypophysis.
    - Derived during fetal development from the Rathke pouch, cranially directed invagination of the primitive oral cavity.
    - Stalk-like connection between the primitive oral cavity and Rathke pouch obliterates by 6th–8th weeks of development [1].
    - Responsible for synthesis and secretion of growth hormone, follicle stimulating and luteinizing hormones, adrenocorticotropic hormone, thyroid stimulating hormone, and prolactin.
    - Individual parts of the adenohypophysis.
      - Pars intermedia: Located posterior to the adenohypophysis and separated from the pars distalis by thin hypophyseal cleft.
      - Pars distalis: Majority of the pituitary volume and hormone production.
      - Pars tuberalis: Encases the infundibulum.
  o Posterior neurohypophysis.
    - Derived from a caudally directed invagination of the diencephalon.
    - Secretes antidiuretic hormone and oxytocin, received from hypothalamus.
  o Pituitary infundibulum.
    - Attaches between adenohypophysis and neurohypophysis.
    - Extends caudally to the hypothalamus.
- Pituitary development is completed by the end of the first trimester.
- Pituitary vasculature.
  o Arterial supply.
    - Superior hypophyseal, inferior hypophyseal, posteroinferior hypophyseal, infundibular, and prechiasmal arteries.
  o Venous supply—hypophyseal veins provide venous drainage to regional sinuses including cavernous sinus.
- Pituitary gland positioned at midline within the sella turcica of the sphenoid bone.
  o Anteriorly—tuberculum sellae/planum spenoidale.
  o Anterolateral—anterior clinoid/optic nerves and foramina.
  o Posteriorly—dorsum sellae.
  o Posterolateral—posterior clinoid.
  o Superiorly—optic chiasm.
  o Laterally—cavernous sinuses/carotid arteries.
    - Cavernous sinus contained by meningeal and periosteal dura.
      - Cranial nerves III, IV, V1, and V2 are located along the lateral aspect of cavernous sinus.
      - Cranial nerve VI adjacent to the carotid artery.
        ♦ Given close approximation to the carotid artery, an intracerebral aneurysm here can rarely (7%) result in isolated abducens nerve palsy [2].
      - Anteriorly the cavernous sinuses communicate with the orbit via the superior orbital fissure.

Imaging of the Normal Pituitary Gland

- Anterior pituitary
  o Isointense to gray matter on T1. Posterior pituitary is T1 hyperintense (see Fig. e35.1a).
  o (All electronic images (Figs. e35.1–e35.15) can be found on this chapter's website on SpringerLink: https://doi.org/10.1007/978-3-031-55124-6_35)
- Posterior pituitary

Fig. 35.1 Pituitary stalk interruption syndrome. Sagittal (**a**) T1 non-contrast and (**b**) T2-weighted images demonstrate an absent pituitary infundibulum (white arrow). T1 bright spot (white arrowhead) located at the median eminence is compatible with ectopic location of the posterior pituitary. The anterior pituitary (black arrowhead) is appropriately within the sella

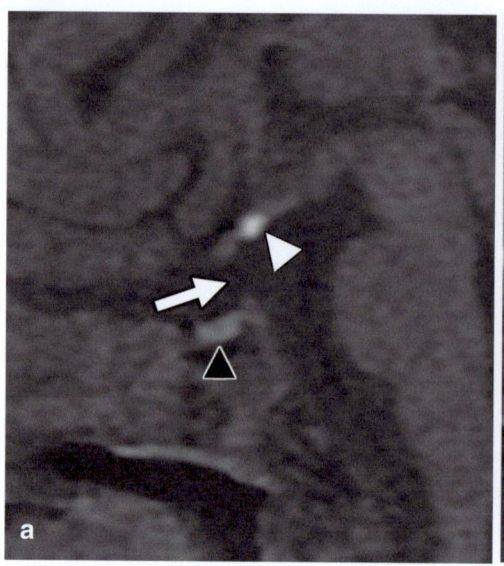
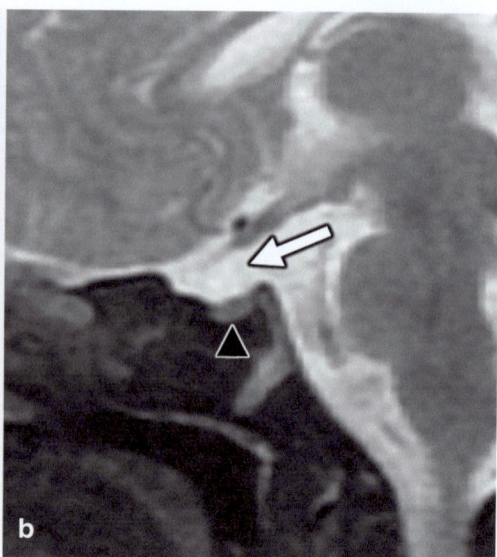

- Normal pituitary bright spot has intrinsic T1 hyperintensity.
    - T1-shortening effect of vasopressin neurosecretory granules or lipoid bodies (lysosomes) in pituicytes [1].
- Cavernous sinuses.
    - Contain CNs III, IV, V1, V2, VI, and internal carotid arteries (see Fig. e35.1b).
- Pituitary size is best evaluated utilizing coronal image and variables based on gender, race, and age (see Fig. e35.2).
    - After birth—serum growth hormone and prolactin decrease resulting in a small gland in the immediate postnatal period.
    - Childhood to Puberty—pituitary size gradually increases where it reaches maximum height at puberty due to rapid hormonal changes.
        - Pituitary gland can increase to 1.0–1.2 cm in height during puberty (and pregnancy) [1].
    - Puberty to Elderly—pituitary size begins to steadily decrease and volume being the lowest in the 70th decade.
- Infundibulum
    - Tapers superior to inferior—measuring approximately 3.25 ± 0.56 mm at optic chiasm and 1.91 ± 0.40 mm at insertion site at pituitary gland [3].
    - Avidly enhances secondary to lack of blood–brain barrier in the portal venous system.
    - Commonly can deviate slightly rather than being perfectly midline and does not necessarily imply disease.
    - Absence can result in ectopic posterior pituitary lobe as well as hypoplasia of the anterior pituitary lobe resulting in pituitary stalk interruption syndrome (Fig. 35.1).

Imaging Technique of the Sellar and Parasellar Region

- Best performed on minimum 1.5 Tesla MRI.
- CT is utilized where MRI is contraindicated, or bony landmarks need to be assessed.
- Dynamic MRI.
    - Useful for identifying microadenomas.
        - Tend to enhance more slowly than normal surrounding pituitary tissue with maximal contrast enhancement typically presenting around 1 min.
    - Acquired with a small field of view (12 cm × 12 cm) and thin 3 mm coronal slices around the pituitary.
        - Typical protocol includes the acquisition of 5 slices every 30 s for 3 min.
- MR angiography or CT angiography can be utilized in evaluating vascular disorders (e.g., aneurysm) when suspected.

Congenital Lesions

RATHKE CLEFT CYST

- True epithelial cystic remnant of the embryologic Rathke pouch.
- Calcification rare.
- Usually asymptomatic and incidental in up to 33% of pituitary glands at autopsy [4].
- Symptomatic presentation typically occurs around 30–60 years of age.
    - Typically presenting with headaches, endocrine dysfunction, and visual disturbances.
- Cyst often interposed between the pars distalis and pars intermedia, giving an *egg-in-cup* appearance.

- o Occasionally can extend superiorly along the anterior aspect of the infundibulum.
- Pituitary infundibulum midline.
- Imaging characteristics.
  - o MRI—variable signal and sometimes difficult to distinguish from adenomas (Fig. 35.2).
    - T1-weighted non-contrast—hyperintense represents protein or hemorrhage within the cyst.
    - T2-weighted.
      - Hyperintense—represents fluid within the cyst.
      - Hypointense—can represent mucinous intracystic nodules containing cholesterol or protein.
    - T1-weighted post-contrast—enhancement not typical.

ARACHNOID CYST

- Lined by arachnoid cells and filled with cerebrospinal fluid (CSF).
- Majority in the middle cranial fossa (34%) or retrocerebellar regions (33%) [5].
  - o Sellar/parasellar arachnoid cysts are only 1% of all cases [5].

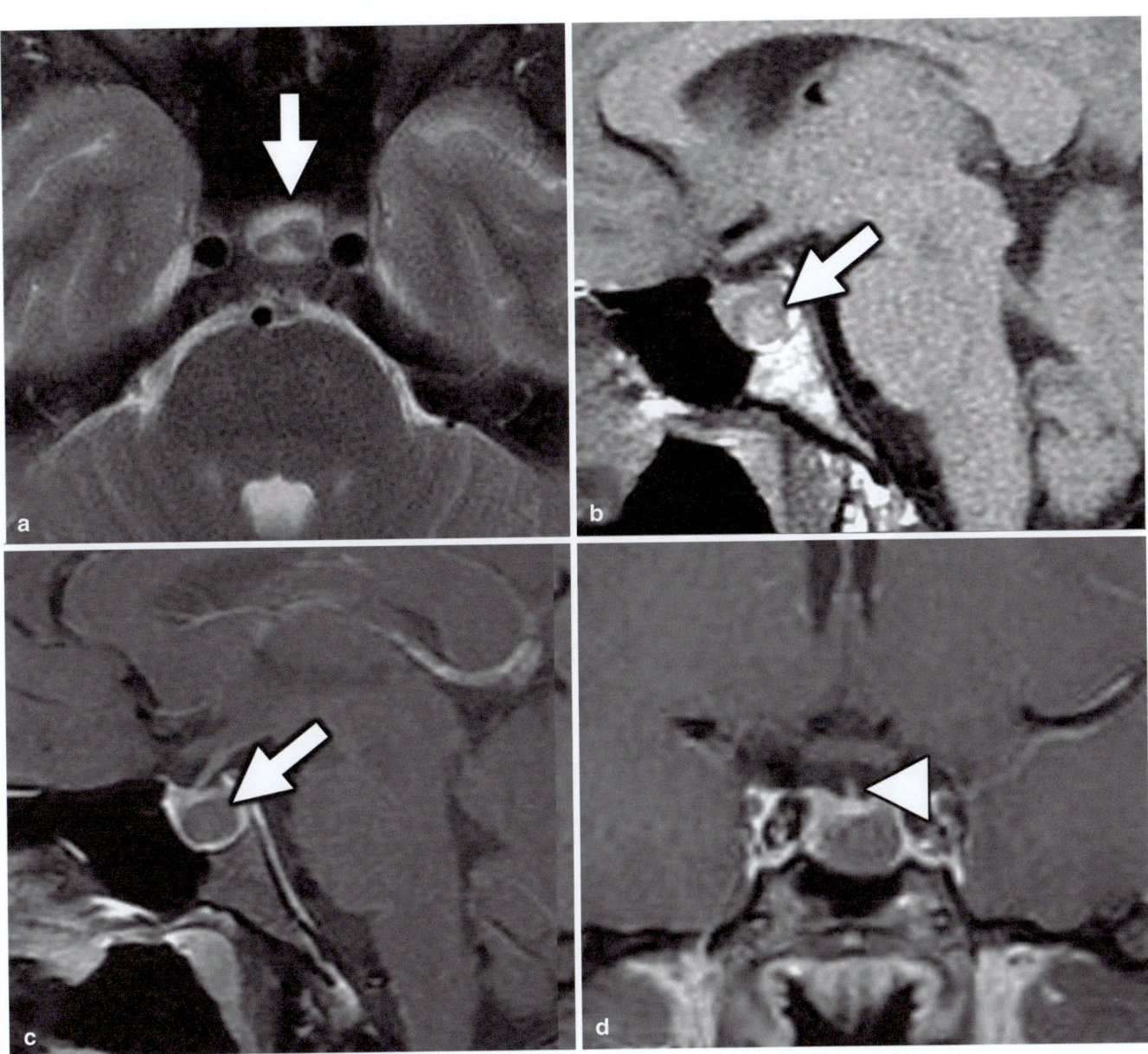

Fig. 35.2 Rathke's cleft cyst. (a) Axial T2-weighted image demonstrates a T2 hyperintense cystic lesion within the sella (white arrow). Cyst has proteinaceous debris corresponding to the central T2 hypointensity. Sagittal T1-weighted non-contrast (b) and post-contrast (c) images demonstrate the nonenhancing cystic lesion (white arrow). Coronal T1 post-contrast image (d) shows no deviation of the infundibulum (white arrowhead). Rathke's cleft cyst was surgically confirmed

- Thought to arise from flow of CSF through the diaphragma sella due to a ball-valve mechanism [1].
- Majority are asymptomatic but rarely can cause obstructive hydrocephalus, cranial neuropathies, seizures, and headaches.
- Pituitary can be displaced depending on size and location of the arachnoid cyst within the parasellar region.
- Imaging characteristics.
  - CT—Large cysts may result in smooth adjacent osseous remodeling of sella.
  - MRI—Follow CSF signal intensity on all sequences, including signal suppression on FLAIR (see Fig. e35.3).
  - Absent enhancement and calcification.

DERMOID AND EPIDERMOID

- Develop from retained ectodermal remnants during neural tube closure.
- Dermoid.
  - Contain dermal appendages made of macroscopic fat.
  - Typically midline.
  - Imaging characteristics.
    - Well-circumscribed.
    - CT—Fat attenuation (−140 to −20 Hounsfield units) (Fig. 35.3a) [6].
    - MRI—Hyperintense on both T1- and T2-weighted (Fig. 35.3b).
    - Thin peripheral rim enhancement can be present.

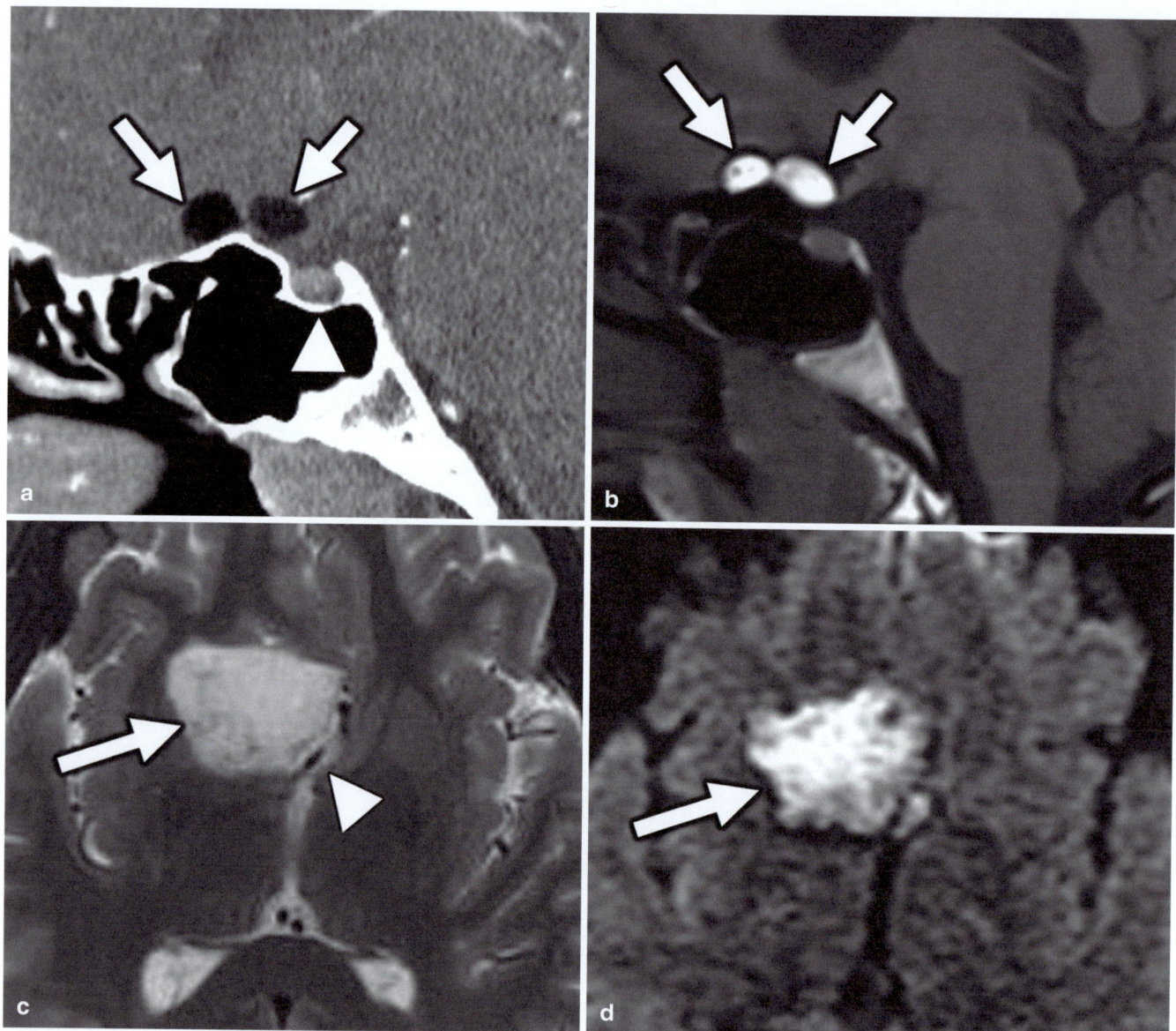

Fig. 35.3 Dermoid and epidermoid. (a) Sagittal post-contrast CT shows bilobed hypodense fat attenuating lesion (white arrows) straddled over the tuberculum sellae. Pituitary is enhancing within the sella (white arrowhead). (b) Sagittal non-contrast T1-weighted image shows the same lesion with intrinsic hyperintense T1 signal (white arrows), compatible with macroscopic fat in this case of this parasellar dermoid cyst. (c) Axial T2 in a different patient shows a T2 hyperintense cystic lesion (white arrow) exerting mass effect along the floor of the third ventricle (white arrowhead). (d) Axial diffusion-weighted image shows lesion with hyperintense diffusion signal (white arrow), characteristic of epidermoids

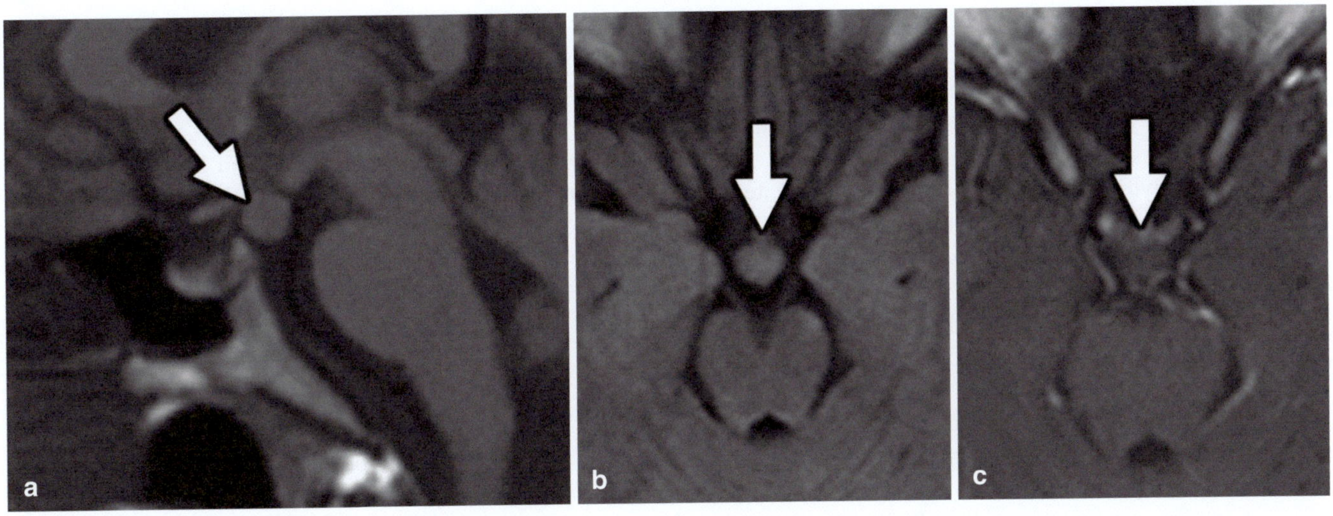

Fig. 35.4 Hypothalamic hamartoma. Sagittal (**a**) and axial (**b**) T1 non-contrast images demonstrate rounded enlargement of the tuber cinereum of the hypothalamus (white arrow). T1 signal is identical to surrounding brain parenchyma. (**c**) Post-contrast imaging shows no associated enhancement (white arrow)

- Epidermoid.
  - Does not contain macroscopic fat.
  - Typically occurs off-midline.
    - Most common location is the cerebellopontine angle (40–50%), 30% occur in parasellar region [7].
  - Imaging characteristics.
    - CT.
      - Typically, fluid attenuation (~0 HU).
      - The presence of hemorrhage, protein, and saponification may result in hyperdensity.
      - Calcification present in 10% [8].
    - MRI.
      - Follows fluid signal on MRI (T2 hyperintense, T1 hypointense).
      - Does NOT suppress on FLAIR (Fig. 35.3c).
      - Characteristic hyperintense signal on diffusion-weighted imaging (Fig. 35.3d).
      - Thin peripheral rim enhancement can be present.
    - Rare "white epidermoids" [9].
      - MRI—Demonstrate intrinsic hyperintense T1 signal and hypointense T2 signal secondary to proteinaceous material.
      - CT—Hyperdense.

HYPOTHALAMIC HAMARTOMA

- Benign lesions arise from the inferior hypothalamus or tuber cinereum.
- Usually found in pediatric patients.
- Consist of hamartomatous neuronal/glial tissue.
- Characteristic presentation—gelastic seizures, precocious puberty, developmental delay.
- Imaging characteristics.
  - MRI—similar to normal gray matter but slightly T1 hypointense and T2 hyperintense can occur from glial tissue (Fig. 35.4).
  - Absent enhancement.

Neoplasms

PITUITARY ADENOMA

- Make up 10–15% of all intracranial tumors [4].
- Prevalence of 17% was reported in a meta-analysis of autopsy and imaging data [10].
- Macroadenoma.
  - Defined as adenomas greater than or equal to 1 cm in diameter.
    - Considered "infiltrative" or "giant" if large and shows aggressive growth patterns into skull base, nasopharynx, and other cranial fossae.
  - Majority are nonfunctioning.
    - Most common functioning macroadenoma is the prolactinoma (25–41%), followed by adrenocorticotropic hormone (5%) and growth hormone (2.8%) secreting macroadenomas [4].
  - Infundibulum may be deviated away from the adenoma.
  - Extension superiorly through the diaphragma sellae can result in a *snowman* appearance of the adenoma due to extrinsic cinching of the tumor by the diaphragm.

- Imaging characteristics (Fig. 35.5).
  - MRI.
    - Variable T1 signal if intratumoral hemorrhage (T1 hyperintense) or necrosis (T1 hypointense) is present.
    - Growth hormone-producing adenomas tend to demonstrate T2 hypointensity.
    - Variable enhancement but typically homogeneous.
  - FDG PET—can be avid—do not mistake as metastasis.
- Complications:
  - Suprasellar extension resulting in compression of the optic chiasm, classically causing bitemporal hemianopsia.
  - Lateral extension may result in cavernous sinus invasion.
    - Cavernous sinus invasion is associated with increased surgical morbidity and mortality [11].
    - The Knosp–Steiner grading system (see Fig. e35.4) classifies macroadenomas by lateral extent of the tumor and has been shown to be predictive of likelihood of cavernous sinus invasion identified during surgery and on histology, ranging from 0 (Grade 0) to 100% (Grade 4).
      - Grade 0: Medial to intracavernous internal carotid artery.
      - Grade 1: Extends to the medial margin of intracavernous internal carotid artery.
      - Grade 2: Extends to between medial and lateral margins of intracavernous internal carotid artery.
      - Grade 3: Extends beyond lateral margin of intracavernous internal carotid artery.
      - Grade 4: Completely encases the intracavernous internal carotid artery [12, 13].
  - Macroadenomas can outgrow their blood supply and undergo spontaneous infarction and/or hemorrhage (see pituitary apoplexy).
- Microadenoma
  - Defined as adenomas smaller than 1 cm in diameter.
  - Dynamic contrast-enhanced MRI can aid in the diagnosis of microadenomas.
    - Adenomatous tissue tends to enhance more slowly than normal pituitary parenchyma allowing the microadenoma to be better detected.
    - Maximal contrast between normal tissue and microadenoma typically present at ~1 min [4].
    - Can rarely enhance earlier than pituitary tissue if direct arterial supply to the adenoma.
  - Imaging characteristics (see Fig. e35.5).
    - Typically discrete lesions are hypointense in comparison to the surrounding homogeneously enhancing pituitary gland.
    - Often infundibulum will be deviated away from the adenoma.

MENINGIOMA

- Most common intracranial neoplasm and second most common sellar/parasellar tumor (tuberculum sellae) [1].
- Most commonly in adults and three times more common in females versus males [14].
- Risk factors for meningiomas include genetic disorders (neurofibromatosis type II), radiation history, family history, and hormonal factors (e.g., obesity, pregnancy, and breast cancer).
- Arise from arachnoid cap cells of the leptomeninges.
- Vast majority (90%) are benign (Grade I) while the remainder are classified as anaplastic (Grade II) or malignant (Grade III) [4].

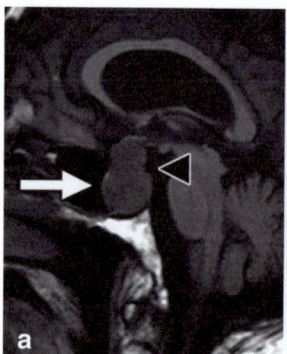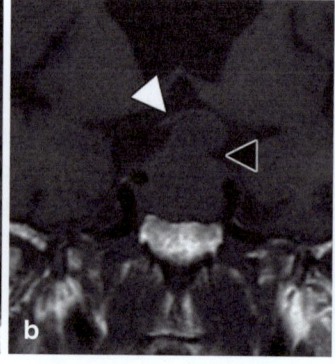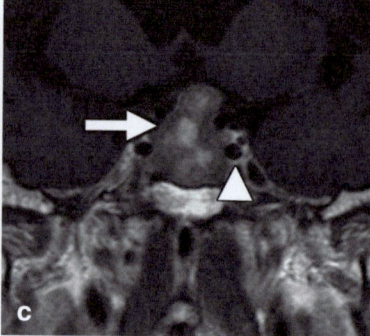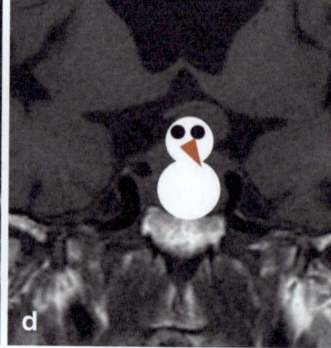

Fig. 35.5 Macroadenoma. Sagittal (**a**) and coronal (**b**) non-contrast T1 sequences demonstrate a sellar mass (white arrow) with suprasellar extension (white arrow) and significant mass effect on the optic chiasm (white arrowhead). The slight "waist" appearance is due to the extrinsic cinching by the diaphragma sellae (black arrowhead). (**c**) Coronal post-contrast T1 (white arrow) shows a heterogeneously enhancing pituitary mass. The internal carotid arteries (white arrowhead) are also visualized and not narrowed. (**d**) Coronal non-contrast T1 image with an illustration of a snowman at the level of the mass, an appearance that can often occur

- o Approximately 1–3% can transform into malignant meningiomas.
- Rarely, cystic meningiomas can be difficult to differentiate from metastatic lesion or glioma.
- Sphenoid wing is the most common location for anterior skull base meningioma (9.8% of all meningiomas).
  - o Other typical (less common) locations include tuberculum sellae/planum sphenoidale/anterior clinoid process (7.6%), cavernous sinus (2.9%), and clival/petroclival region (1.9%) [15].
- Enlarging parasellar meningiomas can extend into the optic canals, cavernous sinuses, and sella.
- o Smaller field of view skull base protocol MRI may be of benefit to better evaluate these small structures and better delineate the meningioma extent.
- Since many meningiomas are asymptomatic, often managed with close observation and imaging follow-up. Symptomatic patients, on the other hand, may need surgery.
- Imaging characteristics (Fig. 35.6).
  - o CT
    - Typically are isodense/hyperdense to cerebral cortex.
    - Intratumoral calcification may be present.

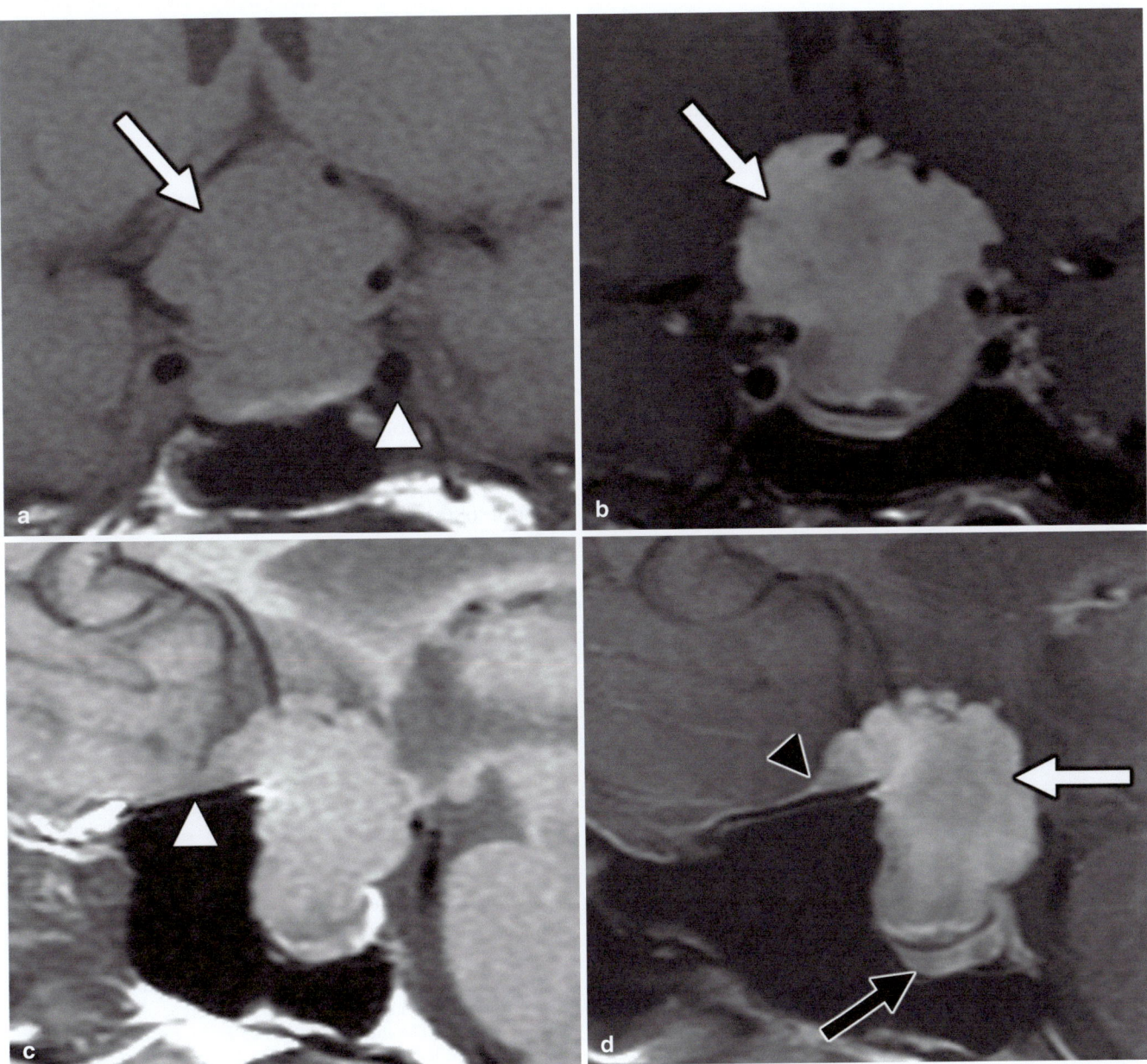

Fig. 35.6 Meningioma. Coronal T1 (**a**) pre-contrast and (**b**) post-contrast MRI with an enhancing extra-axial sellar/suprasellar mass (white arrow) without narrowing of the carotid arteries (white arrowhead). Sagittal T1 (**c**) pre-contrast and (**d**) post-contrast showing tuberculum sellae (white arrowhead) mass with a thin enhancing dural tail (black arrowhead). Mass (white arrow) extends into the sella exerting mass effect on the superior aspect of the pituitary (black arrow), depressing the thickened diaphragma sellae

- Presence of hyperostosis of the subjacent bone is extremely helpful in diagnosis and helps clinch the diagnosis.
  o MRI
    - Shows well-circumscribed mass, typically with avid homogeneous enhancement.
    - Dural tail may be visible.
  o Conventional angiogram.
    - Have quick arterial enhancement persisting into venous phase of imaging—referred to as *"mother-in-law"* sign as these lesions "come early and stay late."

CRANIOPHARYNGIOMA

- Benign tumors arising from squamous epithelial rests along the craniopharyngeal duct [1].
- Make up 2–5% of all primary intracranial neoplasms.
- Divided into two primary histopathological groups: adamantinomatous and papillary.
- Bimodal distribution:
  o Pediatric population.
    - Most commonly in patients aged 5–16 years [1].
    - Predominantly adamantinomatous subtype (~20 times more likely than papillary subtype among patients aged <20 years of age).
    - >90% are suprasellar [1].
  o Older adult population
    - Most commonly in patients aged 45–75 years [1].
  - Both adamantinomatous and papillary subtypes are seen (~2:1 predominance for adamantinomatous subtype) [16].
  o Imaging characteristics
    - Adamantinomatous craniopharyngioma (Fig. 35.7).
      - CT—Calcifications common.
      - MRI—Mixed cystic and solid mass where signal of the cystic component can be variable depending on presence of protein, cholesterol, and/or hemorrhage while solid components have enhancement and along the cyst margins.
    - Papillary craniopharyngioma.
      - Tend to be more solid with strong contrast enhancement.
      - CT—Calcifications less common.

GERM CELL TUMOR

- Subdivided into germinomas or nongerminomatous.
- Primarily diagnosed in pediatric patients, where the majority are diagnosed between 5 and 14 years [4].
- Make up ~4% of all pediatric intracranial tumors [17].
- Typically midline, usually occurring in the suprasellar region and/or pineal regions.
- Disruption of the infundibulo-neurohypophyseal system may result in the absence of the normal pituitary bright spot on MRI, often the earliest imaging finding.
- Tendency to disseminate via CSF, therefore, full neuraxis imaging is warranted to evaluate the full disease extent prior to treatment.

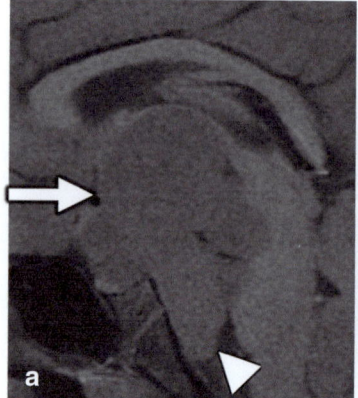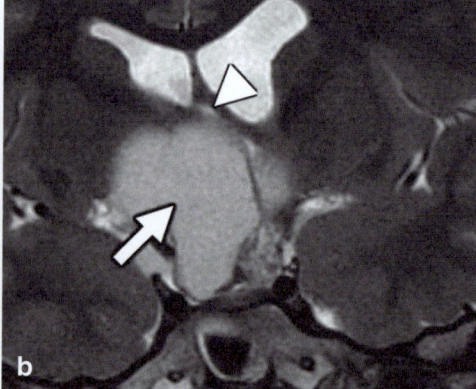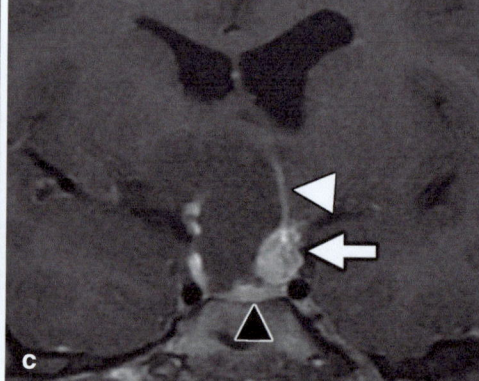

Fig. 35.7 Craniopharyngioma. (**a**) Sagittal T1 non-contrast image demonstrates suprasellar mass (white arrow) extending in the sella and retroclival regions (white arrowhead) resulting in mass effect on the ventral pons. There is an intermediate T1 signal, likely a result of a combination of cholesterol and hemorrhage. (**b**) Coronal T2-weighted image demonstrates the mass with a predominantly T2 hyperintense cystic (white arrow) portion extending superiorly to the level of the third ventricle (white arrowhead). (**c**) Coronal T1 post-contrast image demonstrates some nodular enhancing solid components (white arrow) within the mass. The infundibulum is severely stretched, thinned, and deviated to the left (white arrowhead). There is a mass effect on the otherwise normal-appearing pituitary gland (black arrowhead). Surgical pathology confirmed adamantinomatous craniopharyngioma

- Elevated serum and CSF AFP or β-hcg can aid in diagnosis.
- Imaging characteristics (see Fig. e35.6).
  - CT.
    - Hyperdense due to hypercellularity.
    - Calcifications uncommon.
  - MRI.
    - DWI—Hyperintense on diffusion-weighted imaging and hypointense on corresponding ADC map.
    - T1-weighted.
      - Variable depending on the degree of hemorrhage.
      - Cystic changes may be present with Isointense.
    - T2-weighted—Cystic components can be hyperintense.
    - T1 post-contrast—Typically avid, homogeneous enhancement but can be variable if hemorrhagic components are present.

PITUICYTOMA, SPINDLE CELL ONCOCYTOMA, GRANULAR CELL TUMOR

- Rare, low-grade tumors of the pituitary gland/infundibulum with distinct histological features but grouped together under the fifth edition of WHO classification of CNS tumors.
- All three demonstrate expression of the thyroid transcription factor 1 [18].
- Often misdiagnosed as pituitary adenomas but tend to be more vascular and at increased risk of bleeding during surgical resection.
- Most often present with visual disturbances (60%) followed by headaches and hypopituitarism [19].
  - Diabetes insipidus or galactorrhea/hyperprolactinemia are rare manifestations of pituitary dysfunction (unlike pituitary adenomas).
- Location
  - Pituicytomas and granular cell tumors are of neurohypophyseal origin.
  - Spindle cell oncocytomas arise from the adenohypophysis.
  - Granular cell tumors and spindle cell oncocytomas often have a suprasellar component but are rarely strictly intrasellar.
  - Pituicytomas may be intrasellar, suprasellar, or both.
- Imaging
  - CT—Granular cell tumors are usually hyperdense to brain parenchyma.
  - MRI.
    - T2-weighted.
      - Pituicytomas typically hyperintense to gray matter.
      - Granular Cell Tumors typically isointense to gray matter.
    - T1-weighted—typically isointense to gray matter (all three tumors).
    - T1 post-contrast.
      - Pituicytomas: Homogeneous enhancement.
      - Spindle cell oncocytomas and granular cell tumors: homogeneous or heterogeneous enhancement.

SCHWANNOMA

- Slow-growing neoplasms arising from Schwann cells of cranial nerves.
- Vast majority of intracranial Schwannomas involve CN VIII (90%) [4].
- CN V is the most commonly affected cranial nerve in the parasellar region.
  - Typically involves Gasserian ganglion in Meckel's Cave, located near the trifurcation of the trigeminal nerve where the nerve branches into the ophthalmic (V1), maxillary (V2), and mandibular (V3) divisions.
  - Less commonly, postganglionic, cisternal segments, or cavernous sinus (V1 and V2) may be affected.
- Imaging characteristics
  - MRI.
    - T1-weighted—typically isointense/hypointense.
      - Melanotic schwannoma, a rare subtype, is T1 hyperintense due to melanocytes.
    - T2-weighted—typically hyperintense.
    - T1 post-contrast—avid contrast enhancement present.
  - Signal may be atypically heterogeneous depending on cystic changes, hemorrhage, or calcification.

OPTIC GLIOMA

- Primarily found in the pediatric population, where the majority are diagnosed in patients aged less than 20 [4].
- 1/3rd of all optic gliomas associated with Neurofibromatosis Type I.
  - Neurofibromatosis Type I associated optic gliomas tend to be lower grade than sporadic subtypes. May be result of earlier identification of tumors among asymptomatic patients with Neurofibromatosis Type I due to regular imaging screening.
- Occurs anywhere along the optic nerves (more common in patients with Neurofibromatosis Type I) or optic chiasm/post-chiasmatic optic tract (more common in patients with sporadic optic gliomas).

- Best assessed on MRI and characterized by fusiform enlargement of the optic nerve, chiasm, and optic tract.
- Imaging characteristics (Fig. 35.8).
  - MRI.
    - Well circumscribed.
    - T1-weighted—isointense/hypointense.
    - T2-weighted—hyperintense.
    - T1 post-contrast—variable enhancement.
  - Calcifications and hemorrhage are not typical but cystic change may be seen and more common in sporadic tumors.

LANGERHANS CELL HISTIOCYTOSIS

- Characterized by abnormal proliferation of Langerhans' cells, a type of dendritic cell.
- May involve multiple organ systems including bones, lungs, hypothalamic-pituitary axis, liver, spleen, and lymph nodes.
- Most commonly affects children with a peak age of incidence of 1–3 years [20].
- Multisystem langerhans cell histiocytosis is associated with up to 20% mortality rate and early diagnosis is important [20].
- Involvement of the hypothalamic-pituitary axis has been reported in 5–50% of children [20].
- Most common endocrine manifestation is posterior pituitary dysfunction resulting in diabetes insipidus (17–25%) [20].
- Imaging Characteristics (Fig. 35.9).
  - Pituitary stalk/infundibulum thickening (>3.5 mm).
  - Homogeneously enhancing infundibulum.
  - Absence of posterior pituitary bright spot.

CHORDOMA

- Locally aggressive tumors derived from embryonic notochord remnants.
- Peak incidence in the 50th to 60th decades and twice as common in males as females [21].
- Three histological subtypes:
  - Conventional subtype—most common.
  - Chondroid subtype contains cartilaginous elements.
  - Dedifferentiated subtype—least common with the worst prognosis.
- 50% of chordomas occur in the sacrococcygeal region the most common location where 33% occur in the skullbase [4].
  - Most often midline at the spheno-occipital synchondrosis.
  - Chondroid subtype chordomas tend to arise more laterally at the petroclival junction.
- Imaging Characteristics (see Fig. e35.7)
  - CT—can see bony sequestra given the extradural location.
  - MRI.
    - T2-weighted.
      - Characteristically hyperintense.
      - Interlobular septa within the tumor are typically hypointense, consisting of epithelioid cells.
    - T1 post-contrast—variable enhancement.

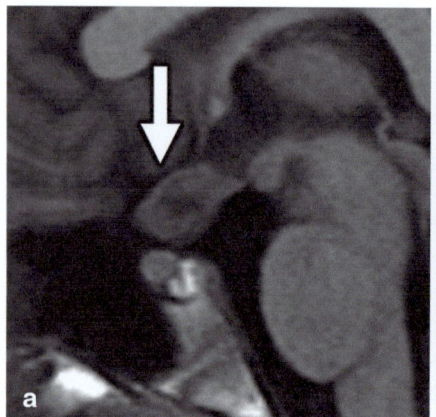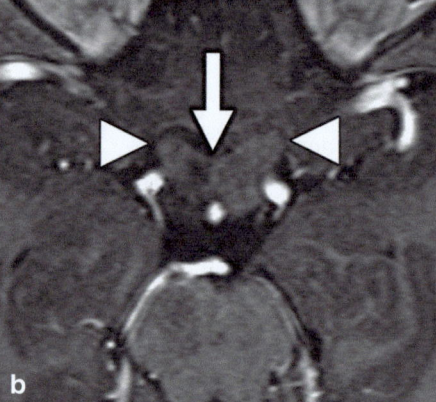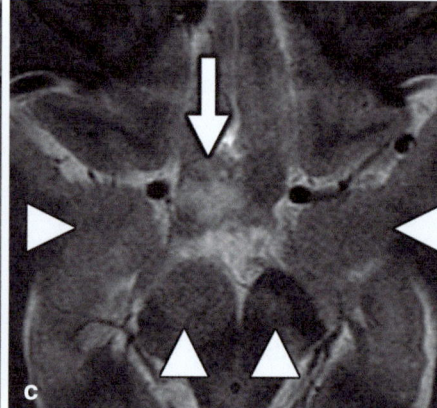

Fig. 35.8 Optic glioma. (a) Sagittal T1 pre-contrast image demonstrates a suprasellar mass isointense to gray matter within the optic chiasm (white arrow). (b) Axial T1 post-contrast image shows no associated enhancement (white arrow). Both optic nerves can be seen extending anteriorly from the mass (white arrowheads). Findings are consistent with an optic pathway glioma in this patient with neurofibromatosis type I. (c) Axial T2-weighted image shows a patchy hyperintense signal within the tumor (white arrow). Additional focal areas of abnormal T2 hyperintense signal within the brainstem and mesial temporal lobe may represent dysmyelinating lesions typical of neurofibromatosis type I (white arrowheads)

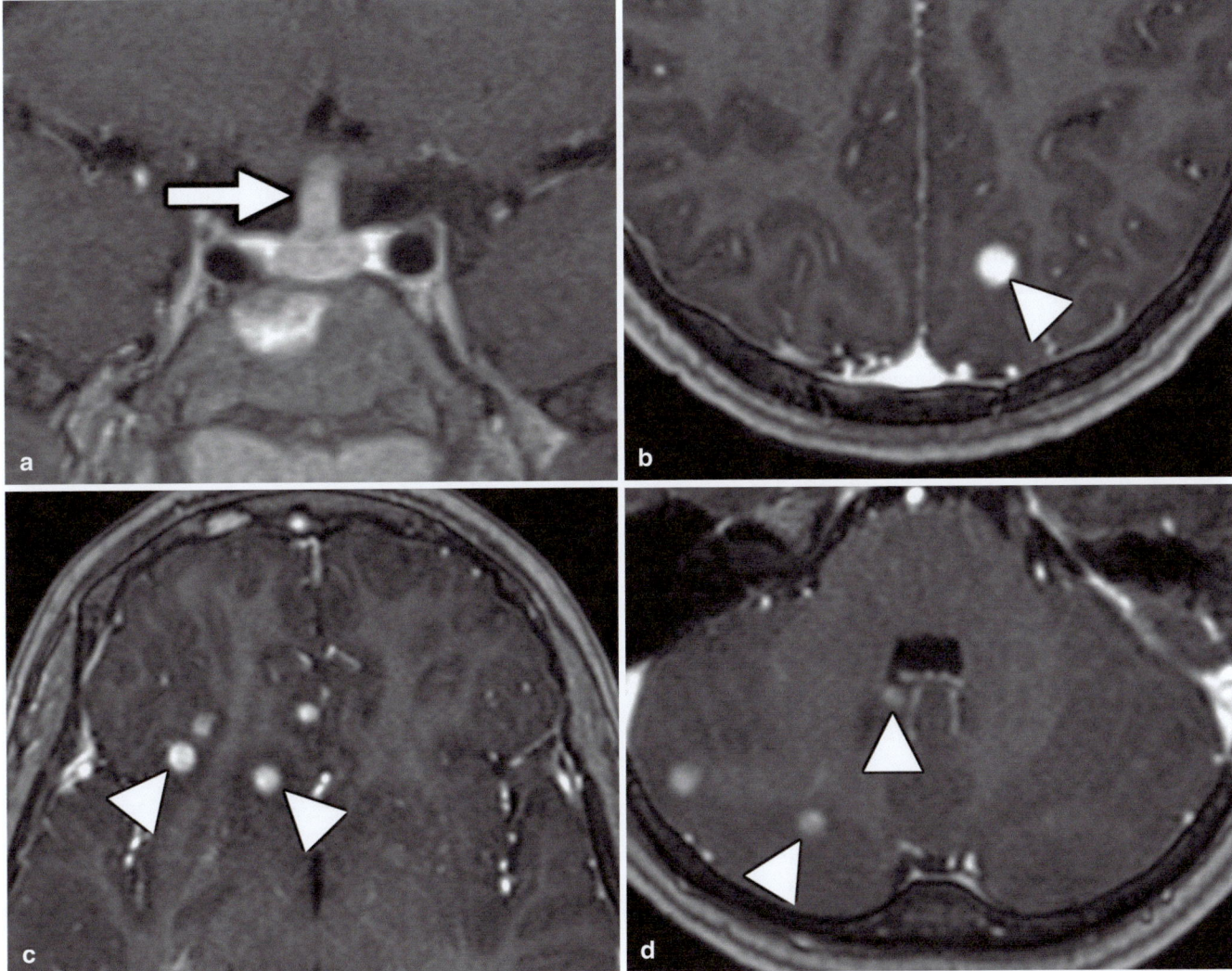

Fig. 35.9 Langerhans cell histiocytosis. (**a**) Coronal MRI T1 post-contrast FSPGR sequence demonstrating thickening and solid enhancement of the infundibulum (white arrow). (**b–d**) Axial post-contrast images through different levels of the brain show areas of nodular parenchymal enhancement (white arrowheads), which may also be seen in this disease

- - Adjacent blood vessels tend to be displaced or encased without stenosis.
  - May extend through the dura into the subarachnoid space.

CHONDROSARCOMA

- Rare, slow-growing tumors arising from mesenchyme developing into transformed cartilage cells.
- Six percent of all skull base tumors [4].
- Most often arise from cartilage at the petroclival, spheno-occipital, sphenopetrosal synchondroses, and typically off-midline, unlike chordomas which are typically midline.
- Present around fourth to fifth decades of life, often with symptoms of ophthalmoplegia [4].
- Imaging characteristics (Fig. e35.8).
  - CT
    - Typical chondroid matrix (rings and arcs) or nonspecific foci of amorphous calcification.
    - May erode through adjacent bone.
  - MRI
    - T2-weighted—hyperintense but less so than chordoma.
    - T1 post-contrast—heterogeneous enhancement.
    - DWI—tend to have the higher ADC map values ($2051 \pm 261 \times 10^{-6}$ mm^2/s) versus classic chordomas ($1474 \pm 117 \times 10^{-6}$ mm^2/s).

METASTASIS

- Occur via hematogenous spread, through Batson venous plexus, perineural spread (CN V most typically), direct extension.
- Prostate cancer, breast cancer, lymphoma, and lung cancer most common to metastasize to skull base [22].
- Osseous metastases can result in parasellar syndrome, characterized by neuropathies of cranial nerves III and V.
- Pituitary metastases (see Fig. e35.9).
  - Uncommon.
  - Most common—breast cancer, lung cancer, followed by renal and colorectal cancer [23].
  - Early findings may be loss of normal posterior pituitary bright spot on T1-weighted imaging.
  - Difficult to distinguish from a pituitary adenoma on imaging so pathology is often required.
- Imaging characteristics
  - CT—sclerotic or lytic lesions.
  - MRI.
    - T1-weighted—geographic areas of hypointensity in the bone marrow.
    - DWI—often restricts diffusion.
  - Can be difficult to distinguish from other pituitary lesions.

PLASMOCYTOMA

- Defined as a discrete plasma cell neoplasm, not necessarily seen as part of the systemic disease (e.g., multiple myeloma).
- Most common locations for plasmacytomas in the skull base—sphenoclival region (59.5%), nasopharynx (21.2%), petrous apex (10.6%), and orbital roof (8.5%) [24].
- Typically presents with headache and vision changes.
  - Cranial nerve palsies may occur from direct compression or involvement of disease—CN VI palsy is most common [25].
- Imaging characteristics
  - MRI
    - Homogeneous T1 hyperintense, T2 iso-/hyperintense mass.
    - Tends to be more T2 hypointense, unlike some other skull base tumors (e.g., chordomas, chondrosarcomas), when compared to the T1 signal in plasmacytomas.
      - Likely due to the densely packed cells resulting in relatively low water content.
    - Avid, homogeneous enhancement.

INFECTIOUS/INFLAMMATORY PROCESSES

LYMPHOCYTIC HYPOPHYSITIS

- Inflammatory disorder typically occurs in pregnant or postpartum patients but is also linked to autoimmune diseases and the drug ipilimumab, a common treatment in melanoma and other malignancies (see Fig. e35.10).
- Results in pituitary dysfunction and can affect the infundibulum, anterior or posterior pituitary.
  - Impaired adrenocorticotropic hormone secretion is the earliest and most common dysfunction.
    - Found in up to 65% of patients with lymphocytic hypophysitis and endocrine dysfunction [20].
- Chronic inflammation can lead to fibrosis, followed by gland atrophy or possible apoplexy.
- Imaging characteristics (see Fig. e35.11).
  - MRI
    - T1-weighted—loss of posterior pituitary bright spot.
    - T1 post-contrast—best modality for evaluation where the affected portions of the pituitary/infundibulum demonstrate thickening and avid enhancement.

SARCOIDOSIS

- 25% of patients with systemic sarcoidosis found to have subclinical central nervous system involvement on autopsy [4].
- May involve any portion of the brain, but most commonly manifests as leptomeningeal enhancement, typically with nodular enhancement of the basilar meninges.
- Involvement of the hypothalamus and pituitary infundibulum may sometimes be seen with basilar leptomeningeal involvement or be an isolated finding [26].
- Involvement of the pituitary gland itself is rare.
- Imaging (see Fig. e35.12).
  - MRI
    - T1-weighted
      - Lesions isointense to brain parenchyma.
      - Absence of posterior pituitary bright spot.
    - T1 post-contrast—lesions show enhancement.

TUBERCULOSIS

- CNS involvement is seen in 1% of all patients with tuberculosis globally [27].

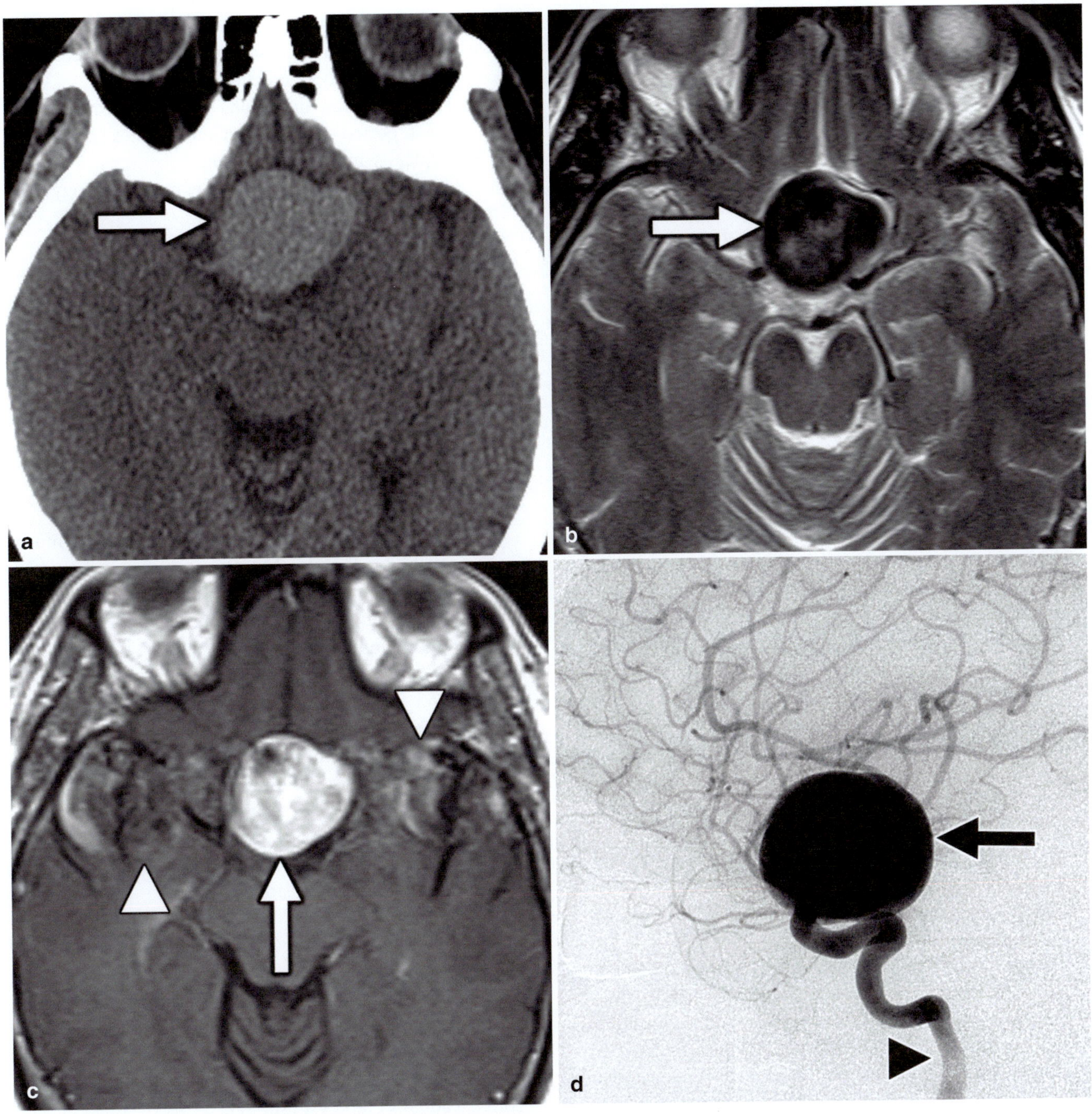

35 Embryology and Anatomy of the Sella and Parasellar Region

Fig. 35.10 Aneurysm. (a) Axial non-contrast CT showing large round hyperdense mass (white arrow) in the suprasellar region. (b) Axial T2-weighted image showing the mass (white arrow) being predominantly T2 hypointense related to flow void in the aneurysm. (c) Axial T1 post-contrast image showing homogeneous enhancement of the lesion (white arrow) with the addition of pulsation artifact confirming it is arterial in nature (white arrowheads). (d) Cerebral angiogram following a left internal carotid artery (black arrowhead) injection confirms the aneurysm (black arrow)

- Intrasellar involvement is extremely rare, typically manifesting as a tuberculoma, a mass-like caseating granuloma—Less than 110 reported cases [27].
- Majority of reported cases of pituitary tuberculosis were in India [27].
- Clinical symptoms.
  - Common—headache, visual disturbances, low-grade fever, and vomiting.
  - Other reported symptoms of endocrine dysfunction include hyperprolactinemia/galactorrhea, amenorrhea, and central diabetes insipidus.

- Imaging characteristics.
  - Thickening and nodularity along the pituitary stalk.
  - Tuberculomas tend to be T2 hyperintense.
  - Ring enhancement from central caseation.

TOLOSA-HUNT SYNDROME

- Diagnosis of exclusion—episodes of recurrent painful ophthalmoplegia secondary to granulomatous inflammation of cavernous sinus.
- Suspected clinically with the following triad—unilateral orbital pain, cranial nerve palsies, headache—symptoms improve with systemic corticosteroids [28].
- Imaging characteristics (see Fig. e35.13).
  - MRI is typically most useful.
    - T1-weighted—isointense Inflammatory soft tissue within the cavernous sinuses when compared to gray matter.
    - T2-weighted—isointense/hypointense to gray matter.
    - T1 post-contrast - strong enhancement.
  - Angiographic imaging—irregular narrowing or displacement of the cavernous internal carotid artery.
  - Resolution of imaging findings with steroid therapy lags improvement in clinical symptoms [28].
  - Soft tissue can extend to ipsilateral orbital apex, sphenoid sinus, and middle cranial fossa.

INVASIVE FUNGAL SINUSITIS

- Characterized by invasion of fungal infection into the mucosa, submucosa, bones, and blood vessels from paranasal sinuses.
- Parasellar extension is typically seen in cases of sphenoid sinusitis with direct extension into the cavernous sinuses.
- Complications include—cavernous sinus thrombosis, carotid artery occlusion, and pseudoaneurysm [29, 30].
- Invasive fungal sinusitis is classified into three subtypes:
  - Acute invasive or fulminant fungal sinusitis.
    - Rapid progression over days to weeks [31].
    - Immunocompromised patients (80% infected with Aspergillus) [29].
    - Poorly controlled diabetes (80% infected with Zygomycetes) [29].
  - Chronic invasive fungal sinusitis.
    - More prolonged course lasting >12 weeks [31].
    - Immunocompetent or mildly immunocompromised patients.
    - Typically have a chronic history of rhinosinusitis.
    - *Aspergillus fumigatus* is the most common etiology [31].
  - Granulomatous invasive fungal sinusitis.
    - Formation of a noncaseating granuloma in response to chronic fungal infection.
    - Primarily seen in Sudan, southeast Asia—only a few reported cases in the United States [29].
    - Typically immunocompetent.
    - *Aspergillus flavus* is the most common etiology [31].
- Imaging characteristics
  - CT
    - Acute invasive subtype demonstrates more hypodense mucosal thickening/soft tissue.
    - Chronic invasive and granulomatous subtypes show hyperdense soft tissue within the paranasal sinuses, sometimes with foci of calcification.
    - Bone destruction/erosions—may be subtle, especially in acute invasive subtype.
    - Chronic/granulomatous sinusitis can result in sclerotic change within adjacent bones.
  - MRI
    - Retro-antral fat infiltration in setting of sinus mucosal thickening should raise suspicion for invasive sinusitis.
    - T1-weighted—fungal hyphae are isointense/hypointense.
    - T2-weighted—fungal hyphae are hypointense.
    - DWI—can demonstrate diffusion restriction.
    - T1 post-contrast.
      - Enhancement of mucosal disease/invading soft tissue.
      - Absence of paranasal sinus mucosal enhancement can also be seen with necrosis.
      - Leptomeningeal enhancement can be seen with intracranial invasion.

PITUITARY ABSCESS

- Extremely rare but may occur spontaneously (2/3rd) or secondary (1/3rd) to a preexisting pituitary lesion that becomes infected such as an adenoma, craniopharyngioma, Rathke's cleft cyst [20, 32].
- Infection can be due to hematogenous seeding or direct extension from infections in the sphenoid sinus or cavernous sinus.
- Typical presenting symptoms include those of anterior pituitary dysfunction, headache, and vision changes.
- Staphylococcus and Streptococcus are most isolated from the abscess [32].
- *Aspergillus fumigatus* is the most common in secondary pituitary abscesses [32].
- Timely diagnosis and treatment with excision and drainage and antibiotics are paramount for decreasing mortality.

- o Mortality rate can be 30–50% if course is complicated by meningitis [20].
- Imaging characteristics.
  - o MRI.
    - T1-weighted—centrally hypointense.
    - T2-weighted—hyperintense cystic or partially cystic mass.
    - T1 post-contrast—rim enhancement.
    - DWI—centrally restricted diffusion.

Vascular Lesions

ANEURYSM

- Represent 1–2% of all intracranial aneurysms, relatively rare in the parasellar region [1].
- May mimic a parasellar mass—accurate diagnosis is mandatory to avoid a catastrophic biopsy.
- May result in osseous remodeling of the skull base.
- Most common presenting symptoms among patients with unruptured sellar aneurysms –headaches or visual field defects (61%), endocrinopathies (57%), symptomatic hyponatremia (21%), cranial nerve paresis (excluding CN II) (18%) [33].
  - o Hyperprolactinemia and gonadotropin deficiency are most common endocrinopathies.
- Categorized into two groups based on location.
  - o Infradiaphragmatic aneurysm—arises from cavernous/clinoid internal carotid artery and extends medially into the sella.
  - o Supradiaphragmatic aneurysm—arises from ophthalmic segment of internal carotid artery or from the anterior communicating artery and extends inferomedially into the sella.
- Imaging characteristics (Fig. 35.10).
  - o CT—well-circumscribed hyperdense/isodense mass with or without the presence of mural calcification.
  - o MRI.
    - Variable heterogenous signal related to calcification and thrombus formation.
    - T2-weighted—hypointense central flow void.
  - o Pulsation artifact in the phase encoding direction can help differentiate from other pathologies.
  - o Post-contrast angiography—opacification of the mass confirms diagnosis.

PITUITARY APOPLEXY

- Infarction and/or hemorrhage within the pituitary gland.
  - o Typically within a pituitary macroadenoma that has outgrown blood supply.
    - Complication found in 1–3% of macroadenomas [34].
- Can occur in Peripartum females.
- Most common presentation is acute onset headache, decreasing mental status, visual deficits [34].
  - o Considered a neurosurgical/medical emergency.
- Imaging characteristics (see Fig. e35.14).
  - o CT—can demonstrate the underlying macroadenoma within the sella with hyperdense blood products.
  - o MRI is ideal for diagnosis.
    - Signal follows that of blood degradation products.
      - T1-weighted—hyperintense in subacute phase.
      - T2-weighted—hypointense in the acute and subacute phases.
    - T1 post-contrast—may be heterogeneous, sometimes with the presence of a peripheral rim-like enhancement pattern.
    - DWI—diffusion restriction may be present within areas of infarcted pituitary tissue.
  - o Fluid levels with debris and blood products may be present layering along the dependent portion with varying signal appearance due to age of the blood products.
    - Sphenoid mucosal swelling can be an ominous sign [34].

CAVERNOUS SINUS THROMBOSIS

- Complication of bacterial or fungal infection within adjacent structures (e.g., paranasal sinuses, orbits, and skull base).
- Typical presentation—acute onset ophthalmoplegia, exophthalmos, and vision loss [35].
- More common among patients with diabetes or immunocompromised status.
- Imaging characteristics (see Fig. e35.15).
  - o Filling defects within the cavernous sinus on contrast-enhanced imaging (CT or MRI).
  - o Mass effect from thrombus may result in convex configuration of the lateral wall of the cavernous sinus. Look for asymmetry between the bilateral cavernous sinuses which may raise suspicion.
  - o In acute stages, thrombus may demonstrate restricted diffusion.
  - o Increased back pressure and stasis within the superior ophthalmic vein can result in engorgement or thrombosis of this vein.

References

1. Kirsch CFE. Imaging of sella and parasellar region. Neuroimaging Clin N Am. 2021;31(4):541–52.

2. Nguyen DQ, Perera L, Kyle G. Recurrent isolated sixth nerve palsy secondary to an intracavernous carotid artery aneurysm. Eye (Lond). 2006;20(12):1416–7.
3. Simmons GE, Sucknicki JE, Rak KM, Damiano TR. MR Imaging of Pituitary size shape and enhancement pattern. AJR Am J Roentgenol. 1992;159(2):375–7.
4. Zamora C, Castillo M. Sellar and parasellar imaging. Neurosurgery. 2017;80(1):17–38.
5. Al-Holou WN, Terman S, Kilburg C, Garton HJ, Muraszko KM, Maher CO. Prevalence and natural history of arachnoid cysts in adults. J Neurosurg. 2013;118(2):222–31.
6. Bertot B, Steele WJ, Boghani Z, Britz G. Diagnostic dilemma: cerebellopontine angle lipoma versus dermoid cyst. Cureus. 2017;9(11):e1894.
7. Nagasawa DT, Choy W, Spasic M, Yew A, Trang A, Garci FM, et al. An analysis of intracranial epidermoid tumors with malignant transformation: treatment and outcomes. Clin Neurol Neurosurg. 2013;115(7):1071–8.
8. Nagasawa D, Yew A, Saface M, Fong B, Gopen Q, Parsa AT, et al. Clinical characteristics and diagnostic imaging of epidermoid tumors. J Clin Neurosci. 2011;18(9):1158–62.
9. Osborn AG, Preece MT. Intracranial cysts: radiologic–pathologic correlation and imaging approach. Radiology. 2006;239(3):650–64.
10. Ezzat S, Asa SL, Couldwell WT, Barr CE, Dodge WE, Vance ML, et al. The prevelance of pituitary adenomas: a systemic review. Cancer. 2004;101(3):613–9.
11. Micko AS, Wohrer A, Wolfsberger S, Knosp E. Invasion of the cavernous sinus space in pituitary adenomas: endoscopic verification and its correlation with an MRI-based classification. J Neurosurg. 2015;122(4):803–11.
12. Knosp E, Steiner E, Kitz K, Matula C. Pituitary adenomas with invasion of the venous sinus space: a magnetic resonance imaging classification compared with surgical findings. Neurosurgery. 1993;33(4):610–7. discussion 617-8
13. Hwang J, Seol HJ, Nam DH, Lee JI, Lee MH, Kong DS. Therapeutic strategy for cavernous sinus-invading non-functioning pituitary adenomas based on the modified Knosp grading system. Brain Tumor Res Treat. 2016;4(2):63–9.
14. Dolecek TA, Dressler EV, Thakkar JP, Liu M, Al-Qaisi A, Villano JL. Epidemiology of meningiomas post-Public Law 107-206: The Benign Brain Tumor Cancer Registries Amendment Act. Cancer. 2015;121(14):2400–10.
15. Sun C, Dou Z, Wu J, Jiang B, Iranmanesh Y, Yu X, et al. The preferred locations of meningioma according to different biological characteristics based on voxel-wise analysis. Front Oncol. 2020;10:1412.
16. Zacharia BE, Bruce SS, Goldstein H, Malone HR, Neugut AI, Bruce JN. Incidence, treatment and survival of patients with craniopharyngioma in the surveillance, epidemiology and end results program. Neuro-Oncology. 2012;14(8):1070–8.
17. Ostrom QT, de Blank PM, Kruchko C, Peterson CM, Liao P, Finlay JL, et al. Alex's Lemonade stand Foundation Infant and Childhood Primary Brain and Central Nervous System Tumors Diagnosed in the United States in 2007–2011. Neuro Oncol. 2015;16(Suppl10):x1–x36.
18. Cole TS, Potla S, Sarris CE, Przybylowski CJ, Baranoski JF, Mooney MA, et al. Rare thyroid transcription factor 1-positive tumors of the sellar region: Barrow Neurological Institute Retrospective Case Series. World Neurosurg. 2019;129:e294–302.
19. Covington MF, Chin SS, Osborn AG. Pituicytoma, spindle cell oncocytoma, and granular cell tumor: clarification and meta-analysis of the world literature since 1893. AJNR Am J Neuroradiol. 2011;32(11):2067–72.
20. Carpinteri R, Patelli I, Casanueva FF, Giustina A. Pituitary tumours: inflammatory and granulomatous expansive lesions of the pituitary. Best Pract Res Clin Endocrinol Metab. 2009;23(5):639–50.
21. Jahangiri A, Jian B, Miller L, El-Sayed IH, Aghi MK. Skull base chordomas: clinical features, prognostic factors, and therapeutics. Neurosurg Clin N Am. 2013;24(1):79–88.
22. Laigle-Donadey F, Taillibert S, Martin-Duverneuil N, Hildebrand J, Delattre JY. Skull-base metastases. J Neurooncol. 2005;75(1):63–9.
23. Go JL, Rajamohan AG. Imaging of the sella and parasellar region. Radiol Clin N Am. 2017;55(1):83–101.
24. Na'ara S, Amit M, Gil Z, Billan S. Plasmacytoma of the skull base: a meta-analysis. J Neurol Surg B Skull Base. 2016;77(1):61–5.
25. Siyag A, Soni TP, Gupta AK, Sharma LM, Jakhotia N, Sharma S. Plasmacytoma of the skull-base: a rare tumor. Cureus. 2018;10(1):e2073.
26. Smith JK, Matheus MG, Castillo M. Imaging manifestations of neurosarcoidosis. AJR Am J Roentgenol. 2004;182(2):289–95.
27. Kumar T, Nigam JS, Jamal I, Jha VC. Primary pituitary tuberculosis. Autopsy Case Rep. 2021;11:e2020228.
28. Dutta P, Anand K. Tolosa-Hunt syndrome: a review of diagnostic criteria and unresolved issues. J Curr Ophthalmol. 2021;33(2):104–11.
29. Aribandi M, McCoy VA, Bazan C 3rd. Imaging features of invasive and noninvasive fungal sinusitis: a review. Radiographics. 2007;27(5):1283–96.
30. Zhang H, Jiang N, Lin X, Wanggou S, Olson JJ, Li X. Invasive sphenoid sinus aspergillosis mimicking sellar tumor: a report of 4 cases and systematic literature review. Chin Neurosurg J. 2020;6:10.
31. Kim TH, Jang HU, Jung YY, Kim JS. Granulomatous invasive fungal rhinosinusitis extending into the pterygopalatine fossa and orbital floor: a case report. Med Mycol Case Rep. 2012;1(1):107–11.
32. Liu Y, Liu F, Liang Q, Li Y, Wang Z. Pituitary abscess: report of two cases and review of the literature. Neuropsychiatr Dis Treat. 2017;13:1521–6.
33. Hanak BW, Zada G, Nayar VV, Thiex R, Du R, Day AL, et al. Cerebral aneurysms with intrasellar extension: a systematic review of clinical, anatomical, and treatment characteristics. J Neurosurg. 2012;116(1):164–78.
34. Boellis A, di Napoli A, Romano A, Bozzao A. Pituitary apoplexy: an update on clinical and imaging features. Insights Imaging. 2014;5(6):753–62.
35. Mahalingam HV, Mani SE, Patel B, Prabhu K, Alexander M, Fatterpekar GM, et al. Imaging spectrum of cavernous sinus lesions with histopathologic correlation. Radiographics. 2019;39(3):795–819.

Facial and Skull Base Fractures

Suehyb G. Alkhatib, Francis Deng,
Dan Cohen-Addad, and Suyash Mohan

- CT of the face without contrast is usually appropriate as initial imaging for evaluation of suspected facial injury following the primary trauma survey. The role of radiography is limited.
- CT of the temporal bones without contrast is usually appropriate when lateral skull base fracture is suspected based on a physical exam or incompletely characterized on initial face and/or head CT. Dedicated thin-section, bone algorithm, and small field-of-view reconstructions offer better spatial resolution than standard head CT.
- Multiplanar reconstructions and 3D volume rendering improve detection and classification of fracture patterns. Fractures that course roughly parallel to one plane are best depicted in an orthogonal plane.
- Let the soft tissues and air spaces augment your evaluation. If you see soft tissue contusions/hematomas or emphysema, or fluid/fluid levels in the sinuses or tympanomastoid cavities, carefully evaluate the adjacent bones for a fracture.
- Employing a systematic framework for evaluating facial and skull base fractures will prevent you from missing the finite number of clinically important fractures.
- Additional vascular imaging is warranted in some cases. All skull base fractures, displaced Le Fort II or III midfacial fractures, and mandibular fractures warrant neck CT angiography to evaluate for blunt cerebrovascular injury. Skull base fractures that traverse the grooves for the lateral or transverse sinus or the jugular foramen are an indication for head CT venography to evaluate for injury to dural venous sinuses.

Fracture Classification

- The facial skeleton is split into thirds, which is helpful for organizing your report in cases of panfacial fracture (involving all thirds) as repairs are sequenced bottom-up or top-down:
  - **Upper third (5%):** frontal bone (including frontal sinuses and upper orbits).
  - **Middle third (70%):** midface (including maxilla, nasal skeleton, palate, lower orbits, and zygoma).
  - **Lower third (25%):** mandible.
- The lower two-thirds of the facial skeleton can also be conceptualized as a system of structurally important ***buttresses*** (4 paired vertical and 4 horizontal), most of which are targets for repair to restore "form" (cosmesis) and masticatory "function" (see Fig. e36.1):
  (All electronic images (Figs. e36.1–e36.5) can be found on this chapter's website on SpringerLink: https://doi.org/10.1007/978-3-031-55124-6_36)
  - **Three vertical buttresses of the maxilla:** *medial maxillary* (nasomaxillary), *lateral maxillary* (zygomaticomaxillary), and *posterior maxillary* (*pterygomaxillary*).
  - **Two horizontal buttresses of the maxilla:** *upper transverse maxillary* and *lower transverse maxillary*.
  - **One vertical buttress of the mandible:** *posterior mandibular*.
  - **Two horizontal buttresses of the mandible:** *upper transverse mandibular* and *lower transverse mandibular*.

- Skull base fractures are divided by region (Fig. e36.2):
  - **Anterior skull base:** central (cribriform plate and ethmoido-sphenoidal planum) and lateral (orbital roof).
  - **Middle skull base:** central (sellar/parasellar region) and lateral (petrous temporal bones).
  - **Posterior skull base:** central (clivus) and lateral (lateral and squamous occipital bone).
- **Simple** (isolated) fractures involve a single bone or osseous plate in isolation, whereas **complex** fractures involve multiple bones within a region. One possible search pattern starts by looking for fractures that are characteristic of the complex midfacial fracture patterns, then looking for the simple midfacial fractures, and finally evaluating for fractures of the frontal sinuses, mandible, and skull base.
- To facilitate communication with surgeons, complex facial fractures should be expressed in terms of familiar patterns and regional units rather than a laundry list of bones or buttresses broken. Skull base fractures should be described in anatomic detail to help predict or explain complications such as CSF leak, neurologic deficit, or vascular compromise. As with fractures elsewhere in the body, facial and skull base fractures should also be described by the presence of comminution (fragmentation), displacement, and/or bone loss [1–3].

Simple Fractures

FRONTAL SINUS FRACTURES (FIG. 36.1)

- Fractures may involve the anterior (outer) table, posterior (inner) table, both anterior and posterior tables, and/or (naso)frontal recess. Specify the involvement of each, the degree of comminution, and significant displacement (>2 mm), as they have different management implications.

- Displaced anterior table fractures create a cosmetic deformity that may require open reduction and internal fixation and, if severely comminuted, obliteration of the sinus.
- Displaced posterior table fractures are a risk for CSF leak that may require obliteration or, if severe, cranialization of the sinus with dural repair.
- Fractures that injure the frontal recess create an unsafe sinus at risk of mucocele and infection that may require obliteration or functional endoscopic sinus surgery.
- Carefully inspect the underlying intracranial contents for extra-axial hemorrhage or cerebral contusion. Pneumocephalus is a clue to posterior table fracture and subarachnoid pneumocephalus indicates a dural tear.

ORBITAL FRACTURES (FIGS. 36.2 AND 36.3)

- Pure (isolated) orbital fractures involve the orbital roof, medial or lateral orbital walls, or orbital floor, but spare the orbital rims. They are also called "blow-out" fractures when fracture fragments extend beyond the

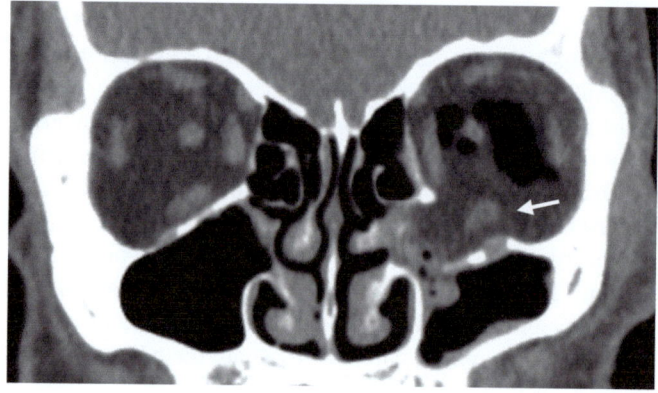

Fig. 36.2 Orbital floor blow out fracture. Coronal CT through the orbits demonstrates a blow-out fracture of the left orbital floor with displacement of the fracture fragment and abnormal morphology of the inferior rectus muscle herniating through the fracture defect (white arrow). Note extensive intraconal locules of gas. This patient had a small hematoma near the orbital apex

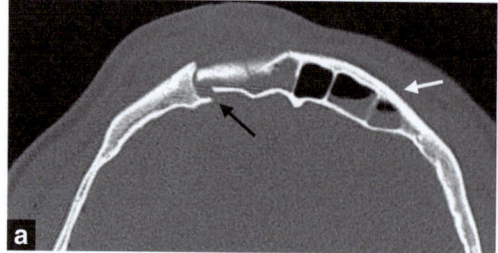
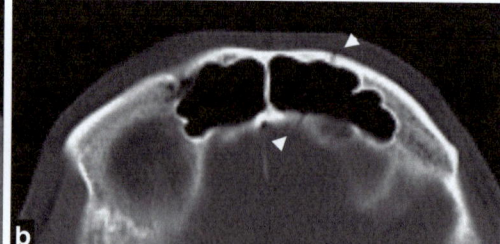

Fig. 36.1 Frontal sinus fracture. Axial CT through the frontal sinus of two separate patients. (**a**) Comminuted anterior table fracture with depression, mildly displaced fracture of the posterior table (black arrow). Note layering fluid in the sinus (white arrow). This can be a sign of fracture when the fracture is subtle and nondisplaced. This fracture extended to involve the nasofrontal recess and naso-orbitoethmoid complex (not shown). (**b**) Nondisplaced frontal sinus fracture involving inner and outer table (white arrowheads). On a lower slice, this fracture extended into the anterior skull base (cribriform plate, not shown)

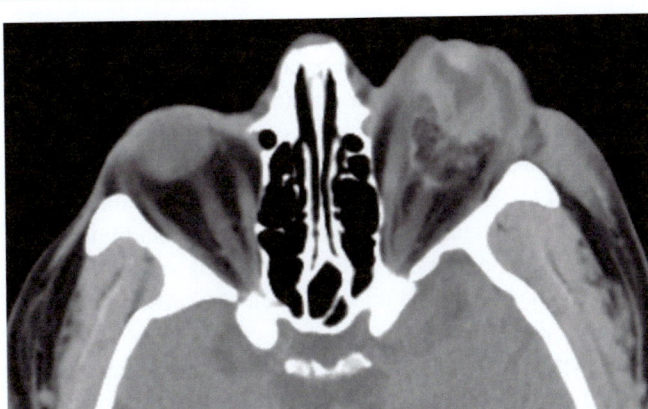

Fig. 36.3 Globe rupture and retrobulbar hematoma. Axial CT of the orbits in a patient who fell from a ladder with rupture of the left globe. There is proptosis and stranding of the intraconal fat behind the ruptured globe representing a retrobulbar hematoma

confines of the orbit (outwardly displaced) and "blow-in" fractures when fracture fragments buckle into the orbit (inwardly displaced). Impure orbital fractures involving the rims, in contrast, are usually part of more complex fracture patterns (e.g., Le Fort II or III, zygomaticomaxillary complex, or naso-orbitoethmoid fractures) and *should not* be called blow-out or blow-in fractures.

- The *most common* pure orbital fractures involve the medial orbital wall (lamina papyracea) followed by the orbital floor as they are more vulnerable. The lateral orbital wall and orbital roof are thicker and sturdier and rarely fracture in isolation. The names of the bones that make up each side are less important.
- Describe the size of the fracture. Critical-sized orbital defects (e.g., defect involving more than half the orbital floor area, or herniated orbital volume of more than 1.5–2 mL) are likely to result in significant malposition of the globe (e.g., enophthalmos or hypoglobus), which may not be evident in the acute setting due to swelling. These fractures will commonly undergo operative repair.
- Carefully evaluate for a range of soft tissue injuries:
  1. Globe rupture—increased or decreased anterior segment depth, *"flat tire"* or *"mushroom"* sign of irregular globe contour indicating hypotony, or intraocular gas or foreign body.
  2. Intraocular injuries—e.g., lens subluxation or dislocation, cataract, hemorrhage, or retinal detachment.
  3. Retrobulbar hemorrhage—ranging from fat stranding to hematoma with frank mass effect.
  4. Orbital emphysema.
  5. Displaced fracture involving the orbital apex or infraorbital nerve canal, often associated with orbital neuropathy and/or vascular injury and therefore CT angiography should be recommended.
  6. Orbital compartment syndrome—significant mass effect (proptosis, tenting of the posterior globe (*"guitar-pick" sign*), and stretching of the optic nerve), although orbital compartment syndrome is primarily a "clinical diagnosis".
  7. Extraocular muscle entrapment—rounding/swelling, differential attenuation, or displacement through a fracture defect, although entrapment remains primarily a clinical diagnosis.
- Muscle entrapment mostly occurs in the pediatric population due to a *"trapdoor"* fracture, where a fracture fragment swings open on one side and then back closed, incarcerating orbital tissue through the narrow defect. A high index of suspicion is needed to identify these at CT as they can look nondisplaced but should have surrounding soft tissue changes, emphasizing the importance of careful evaluation of soft tissue window settings in the coronal plane. Lack of herniation of the muscle does not rule out entrapment, which can occur through tethering of fascial septae along with orbital fat prolapse alone.

NASAL SKELETON FRACTURES (FIG. 36.4)

- Fractures of the nasal pyramid and septum are the most common facial fractures but are often not reduced unless there is an external deformity or airway obstruction. Nasal fractures are usually isolated but can occur in naso-orbitoethmoid complex or Le Fort II or III fractures, which should be reported together.
- Fractures may involve the paired nasal bones, frontal processes of the maxillae, anterior nasal spine of the maxilla, and/or nasal septum.
- Evaluate for significant septal hematomas as they require drainage to prevent necrosis.

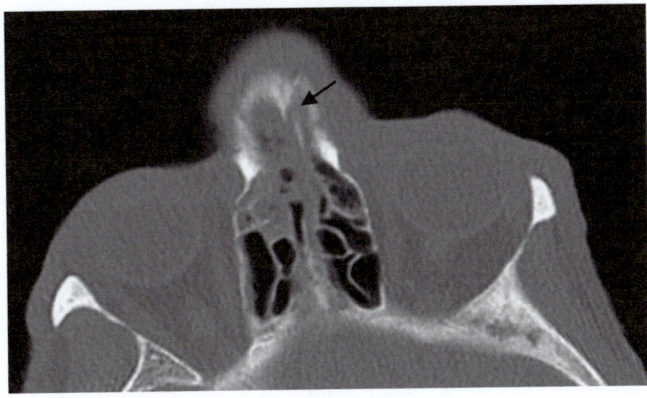

Fig. 36.4 Nasoseptal fracture. Axial CT through the nasal bones demonstrates mildly displaced fractures of the nasal bones and anterior bony nasal septum (black arrow). There was moderate soft tissue swelling and frothy secretions in the nasal cavities. This patient went on to have a closed reduction and required drainage of a septal hematoma

PALATOALVEOLAR FRACTURES

- The hard palate is made of two bones but should be considered as a single midline structure, which is fractured usually in conjunction with other midfacial fractures. A consistent search pattern is needed to avoid missing a palatal fracture.
- When present, examine and describe any involvement of the maxillary alveolar process and teeth. Fracture extension to a tooth socket should be highlighted in the report as these are considered open (contaminated) fractures. Evaluate the teeth for fractures or luxation, though these should be apparent on intraoral exam unless there is trismus.

MANDIBLE FRACTURES (FIG. 36.5)

- Mandibular fractures are the second most common facial fractures and the most frequently encountered fracture requiring operative repair [4].
- The mandible simulates a ring, so fractures most commonly (but not always) occur in pairs or a fracture-dislocation combination.
    1. When a fracture is identified, carefully evaluate the remainder of the mandible to identify any additional site of fracture.
    2. Evaluate the temporomandibular joint (TMJ). Note: The mandibular condyle may be anterior to the glenoid fossa in the open mouth position or with intubation. If the condyle is anterior to the articular eminence, the TMJ is likely to be dislocated.
- Flail mandible—trifocal, parasymphyseal and bicondylar fractures, bilateral angle fractures, and bilateral body fractures can result in posterior displacement of the tongue, sublingual and submandibular hematomas, and intraoral bleeding may contribute to airway compromise. Identifying flail mandible and associated soft-tissue injuries risk of airway compromise is critical, as failure to protect the airway after facial trauma is a common factor causing the death of the patient. When mandibular fractures and soft-tissue swelling prevent oral intubation, fiberoptic nasal intubation or even tracheostomy may be necessary.
- Describe mandibular fractures by their specific location. The mandible is segmented on each side into the mandibular condyle/subcondylar region, coronoid process, ramus, angle, body, and parasymphyseal region (fracture line in between mandibular canines) (Fig. e36.3).
    1. The hemimandibles meet in the midline at the symphysis menti.
    2. The parasymphysis and body are separated at the canine.
    3. The body and angle are separated at the third molar.
    4. The condyle is subdivided into the head, neck, and base (subcondylar area).
    5. The outer and inner surfaces are referred to as buccal and lingual cortices, respectively.
    6. The tooth-bearing aspect is the alveolar bone/ridge/process, and the inferior non-tooth-bearing aspect is the basal bone.
- As with maxillary/palatal fractures, fracture extension to a tooth socket should be highlighted in the report as they are considered open fracture. Evaluate the teeth for fractures or luxation as well. Displaced fracture involvement of the inferior alveolar nerve canal should be described.

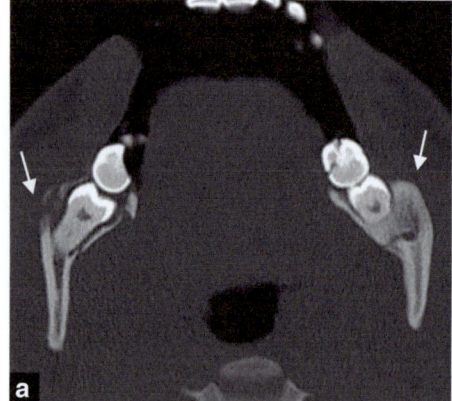 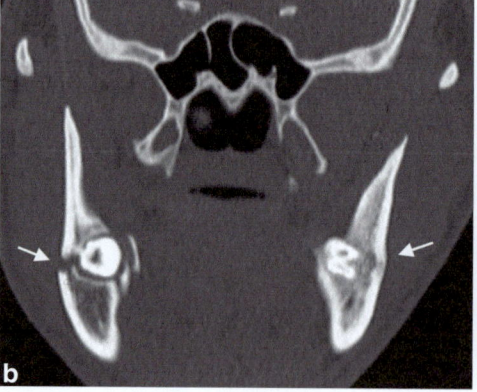 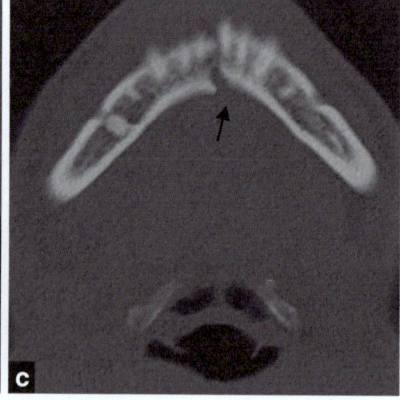

Fig. 36.5 Flail mandibular fracture. (**a**) Axial and (**b**) coronal CT demonstrates bilateral angle fractures (white arrows) and (**c**) axial CT demonstrates a parasymphyseal fracture (black arrow). A pattern called "trifocal" fracture, which is specifically at risk for airway compromise as the tongue can be displaced posteriorly and it is often associated with sublingual and submandibular hematomas

Complex Midfacial Fractures

LE FORT FRACTURES (FIGS. 36.6 AND E36.4)

- The Le Fort fracture patterns are transfacial fractures that extend to the pterygoid plates/processes of the sphenoid bone (posterior maxillary/pterygomaxillary buttress). *It is important to remember if there is no fracture of the pterygoid plate, a Le Fort pattern is not present.* Conversely, pterygoid plate fractures can occur *without a Le Fort*, but they are almost always associated with additional fractures of the facial skeleton or skull base. If you find a pterygoid plate fracture, you should carefully search for associated fractures that comprise the Le Fort spectrum.
  1. **Le Fort I**—low horizontal maxillary fracture resulting in a *floating palate deformity*. Look for fracture extension involving all walls of the maxillary sinus to the **nasal pyriform aperture/nasal septum**.
  2. **Le Fort II**—oblique fracture resulting in a pyramidal *floating maxilla or "dish-face" deformity*. Look for fracture extension from the lateral wall of the maxillary sinus to the **inferior orbital rim** and continuing into the naso-orbitoethmoid region.
  3. **Le Fort III**—high transverse fracture resulting in a *floating face* (craniofacial disjunction). Look for fracture extension from the **zygomatic arch** and **lateral orbital wall/rim** through the orbit and continuing into the naso-orbitoethmoid region.
- Different Le Fort fracture patterns can occur on the left and right sides of the face, and multiple Le Fort fractures can be described in combination on the same side. However, a bilateral Le Fort I, II, and III combination fracture pattern can be equivalently described (and managed surgically) as five regional units: a bilateral Le Fort I fracture, a zygomaticomaxillary complex (ZMC) fracture on each side, and a naso-orbitoethmoid (NOE) fracture on each side.
- The lowest Le Fort level is managed to restore a functional occlusion (usually via intermaxillary fixation) and additional regions are reduced and fixated to restore the preinjury midfacial contour and alignment. See the following sections for site-specific considerations [3, 5].

NASO-ORBITOETHMOID (NOE) FRACTURE (FIG. 36.7)

- The NOE fracture involves the upper medial midface from the nasal pyriform aperture to the inferomedial orbit and disrupts the confluence of the medial maxillary and upper transverse maxillary buttresses, along at least 4 of 5 cardinal tracts [3, 5]:

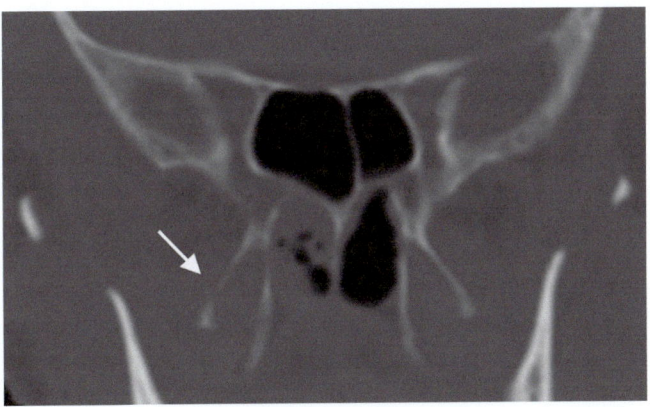

Fig. 36.6 Pterygoid plate fracture. Coronal CT through the level of the pterygoid plates demonstrating a mildly displaced fracture through the lateral process of the right pterygoid plate (white arrow). Although the presence of a pterygoid plate fracture is indicative of a Le Fort pattern injury, these can also occur in isolation, no other facial fracture was identified in this patient

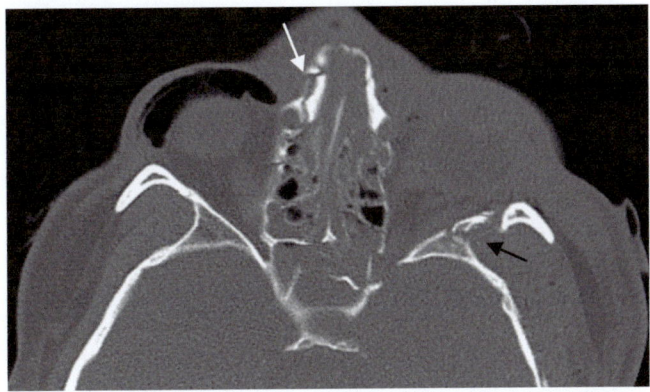

Fig. 36.7 Naso-orbitoethmoid (NOE) Fracture. Axial CT demonstrating a mildly displaced comminuted fracture of the right nasal bones and frontal process of the maxilla involving the right lacrimal fossa (white arrow) in a naso-orbitoethmoid complex pattern. Note fracture of the lateral orbital wall (black arrow). This patient also had a left ZMC fracture (see Fig. 36.8)

1. Frontomaxillary suture (frontal process of maxilla and nasal part of frontal bone).
2. Nasomaxillary suture (nasal bone and frontal process of maxilla).
3. Lateral nasal wall (medial maxillary buttress).
4. Inferior orbital rim and orbital floor.
5. Medial orbital (ethmoid) wall.

- The central fragment contains the lacrimal fossa (made of the frontal process of maxilla and lacrimal bone), which is where the medial canthal tendon inserts after it splits around the lacrimal sac. Disruption of this insertion results in telecanthus.
- Describe the extent of fracture displacement and comminution. NOE fractures are most commonly graded by the Markowitz and Manson classification:

- **Type I:** intact central fragment (outlined by cardinal fracture tracts).
- **Type II:** comminuted central fragment but the insertion of the medial canthal tendon is maintained.
- **Type III:** comminuted central fragment where the insertion of the medial canthal tendon is disrupted or avulsed.

A preoperative distinction of type II and III NOE fractures may be difficult as the medial canthal tendon is not directly visualized on CT, so it may suffice to simply note the degree of comminution. Note, a heavily comminuted NOE fracture with marked lateral deviation of the globe, is indicative of a medial canthal ligament avulsion, and type III fracture.

- Mention involvement of the nasolacrimal duct as this predisposes to obstruction with chronic epiphora, dacryocystocele formation, or dacryocystitis.
- Describe the extent of displaced orbital fracture involvement such as the orbital volume change, which may necessitate orbital reconstruction.
- Evaluate for fracture extension to the anterior skull base or frontal sinus (see separate sections for details) including adjacent intracranial hemorrhage.
- An NOE fracture that extends to the ipsilateral pterygoid plates will be part of a Le Fort II or III complex fracture.

ZYGOMATICOMAXILLARY COMPLEX (ZMC) FRACTURE (FIG. 36.8)

- The ZMC fracture pattern, also known as a zygomatic or orbitozygomatic fracture, involves disruption of upper transverse maxillary buttress and lateral vertical maxillary buttress. It is a spectrum of injuries ranging from isolated zygomatic arch fracture to a "tetrapod fracture" involving all four articulations of the zygoma [3, 5]:
  1. zygomaticotemporal suture (along zygomatic arch).
  2. zygomaticofrontal suture (along lateral orbital rim).
  3. zygomaticomaxillary buttress (through maxillary sinus walls, usually extending into the inferior orbital rim and floor including through the infraorbital nerve foramen/canal).
  4. zygomaticosphenoid suture (along lateral orbital wall).
- Describe the components of the ZMC that are fractured and displaced. Mention the degree of comminution of the zygoma and evaluate whether bone fragments are lost or displaced into the maxillary sinus.
- Describe the extent of displaced orbital fracture involvement such as extraocular muscle herniation and orbital volume change, which may necessitate orbital reconstruction.
- A ZMC fracture that extends to the ipsilateral pterygoid plates will be part of a Le Fort III complex fracture.

Skull Base Fractures

TRANSSPHENOIDAL BASILAR SKULL FRACTURES (FIG. E36.5)

- Some severe skull base fractures have common patterns of propagation through the sphenoid, which can guide your search for subtle fracture involvement once one component is identified [3, 6].
- Anterior transverse transsphenoidal basilar skull fractures are due to lateral impacts near the pterion. The fracture extends through the sphenoid greater and lesser wings on one side, through the planum sphenoidale or posterior ethmoid roof, and out the other sphenoid wings. The frac-

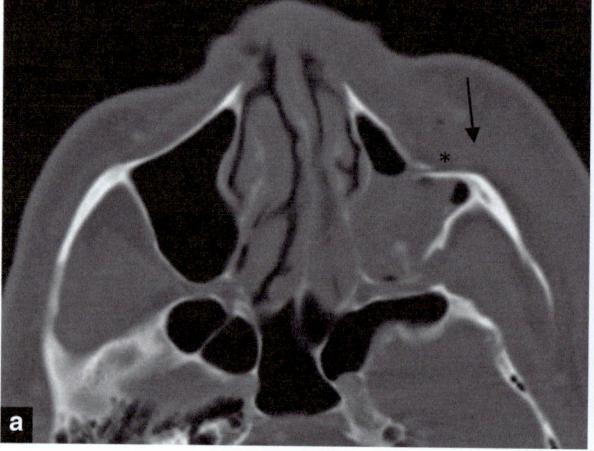
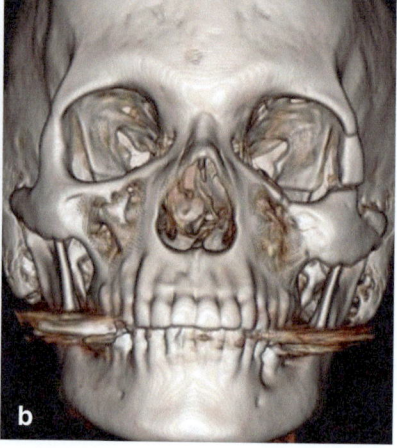

Fig. 36.8 Zygomaticomaxillary complex fracture. Axial maxillofacial CT (**a**) partially demonstrates a left ZMC fracture. Note, the loss of the malar projection (black arrow) and the displace left zygomaticomaxillary buttress fracture (asterisk). (**b**) 3D reconstruction shows the malar eminence asymmetry. Note, three out of the four components of the ZMC fracture, including the lateral orbital rim, the zygomatic arch, and the inferior orbital rim as well as the maxillary sinus

ture can sometimes extend down through the sphenoid body to the pterygoid plates.
- Posterior transverse transsphenoidal basilar skull fractures are due to lateral impacts near the ear. The fracture extends through one petrous temporal bone longitudinally, along the sphenopetrosal suture or carotid canal, transversely through the clivus/posterior sphenoid sinus wall, and out the contralateral side through the sphenopetrosal suture or carotid canal and the petrous temporal bone.
- Lateral frontal diagonal transsphenoidal basilar skull fractures are due to impacts to the side of the forehead. The fracture extends through the orbital roof (lateral anterior skull base), across the sphenoid body, and out the contralateral side through the sphenopetrosal suture or carotid canal and the petrous temporal bone.
- Mastoid diagonal transsphenoidal basilar skull fractures are due to impacts to the lateral back of the head. The fracture extends through the posterior skull base at the occipitomastoid suture to the jugular foramen, along the petrooccipital fissure, obliquely through the sphenoid body, and out the anterior skull base.

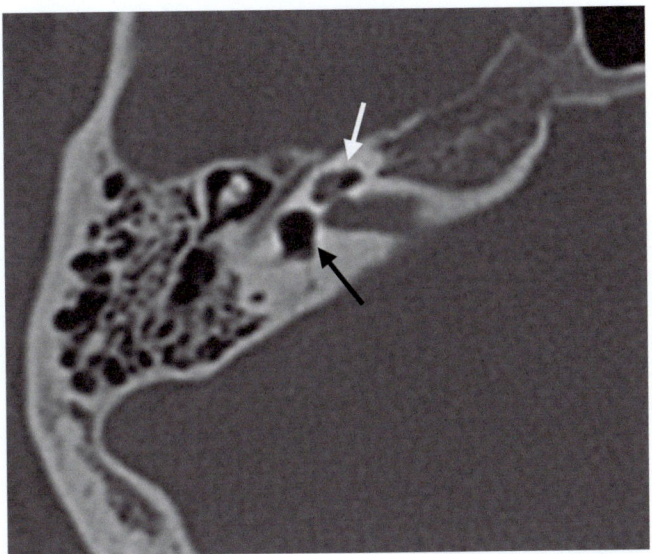

Fig. 36.9 Pneumolabyrinth in a trauma patient. Axial high-resolution multidetector CT image of the right temporal bone shows small foci of air within the vestibule (black arrow) and basal turn of the cochlea (white arrow). There was a nondisplaced occipital bone fracture and bifrontal parenchymal contusions (not shown) but no temporal bone fracture or ossicular disruption was identified

ANTERIOR SKULL BASE (FRONTOBASAL) FRACTURES

- Fractures that involve the central anterior skull base, including cribriform plates, ethmoid roof (fovea ethmoidalis), or sphenoid roof (planum sphenoidale), present a risk for CSF leak and meningitis. While these are often managed conservatively, these should be reported if there is a large bony defect or large volume pneumocephalus, which portends a higher risk of persistent CSF leak requiring subsequent operative repair [6].
- Fractures that involve the lateral anterior skull base, essentially representing the orbital roofs, can impinge on neurovascular structures at the orbital apex (optic canal, superior orbital fissure, and inferior orbital fissure). Report if there are displaced bone fragments or a large hematoma.
- Carotid artery and/or cavernous sinus injury is possible, necessitating CTA for further evaluation.

TEMPORAL BONE (LATERAL SKULL BASE) FRACTURES (FIGS. 36.9, 36.10 AND 36.11)

- Temporal bone fractures were traditionally classified anatomically as longitudinal or transverse, but fractures can be mixed and the clinical relevance of the fracture is not dependent on the orientation of the fracture. A more current and clinically relevant framework for temporal bone fractures is primarily based on *violation of the otic capsule*, the dense bone surrounding the cochlea, vestibule, and semicircular canals. Most fractures are longitudinal and otic capsule-sparing, while transverse and otic-capsule-violating fractures are more severe [6].
- Opacification of the mastoid air cells and middle ear cavities should increase your scrutiny of the temporal bone for a possible fracture. Also look for air in the inner ear structures (pneumolabyrinth, Fig. 36.9), extradural air along the inner table of the temporal bone, or soft tissue emphysema overlying the mastoid.
- Once a temporal bone fracture is identified, the following should be carefully evaluated and reported:
  1. Otic capsule violating or sparing (predicts risk of persistent CSF leak and hearing loss).
  2. Ossicular chain discontinuity or fracture (e.g., incudomalleolar separation, Fig. 36.10b).
  3. Tegmen tympani/mastoideum fracture involvement and displacement or bone loss (possible route of CSF leak).
  4. Facial nerve canal fracture involvement (always trace from the stylomastoid foramen to the internal acoustic meatus, ideally on reconstructions dedicated to the temporal bone), most commonly impinged at the geniculate ganglion and labyrinthine segment.
  5. Vascular channel fracture involvement at the carotid canal, groove for the sigmoid sinus, or jugular foramen (warranting CTA and/or CTV to evaluate for vascular injury, Fig. 36.11).

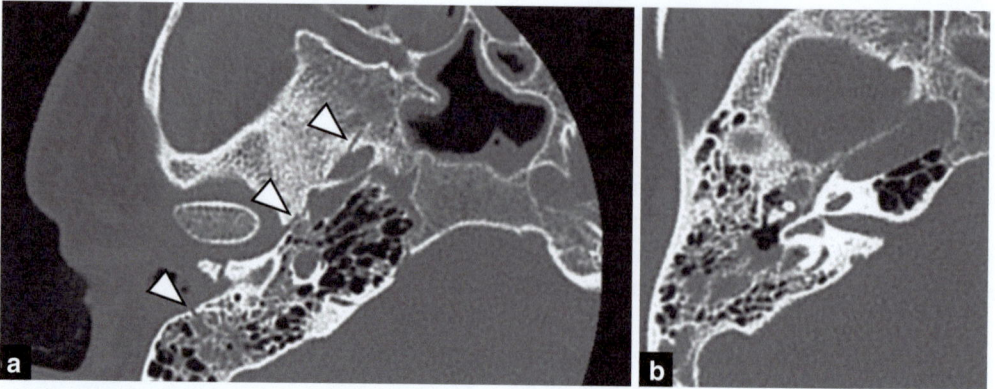

Fig. 36.10 Otic-capsule sparing longitudinal right temporal bone fracture. (**a**) Multiplanar reformatted CT of the right temporal bone showing fracture line through (arrowheads) the temporal bone extending into the greater wing of the sphenoid and crossing foramen spinosum and ovale. (**b**) Axial image at the level of the incudomalleolar articulation showing separation of the malleus head from its articulation with the incus

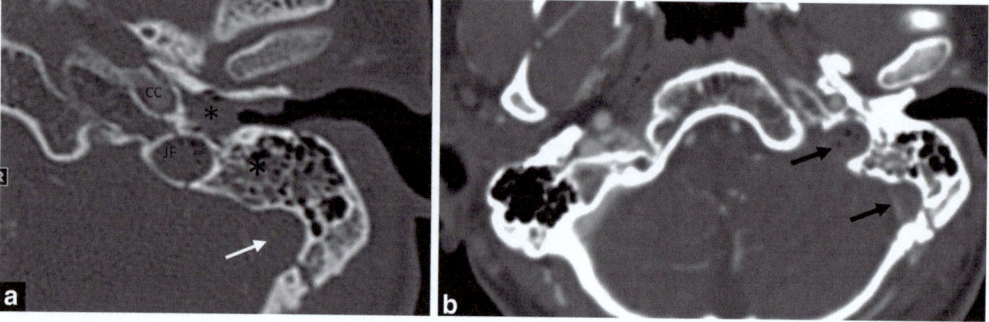

Fig. 36.11 Complex temporal bone fracture. Axial high-resolution multidetector CT image of the left temporal bone (**a**) shows comminuted oblique fracture involving the left mastoid and petrous segments, left jugular foramen (JF), and left carotid canal (CC). Partial opacification of the left mastoid air cells and middle ear cavity (asterisks) from posttraumatic hemorrhage. Gas locules and hypodensity are seen along the course of the left transverse and sigmoid sinuses (white arrow). Axial source images of the CT angiogram (**b**) demonstrate venous thrombosis of the left transverse and sigmoid sinuses, extending to the proximal left internal jugular vein (black arrows)

POSTERIOR SKULL BASE FRACTURES

- Posterior skull base fractures involve the occipital bone and can extend into the temporal or sphenoid bones [6].
- Cranial nerve palsies are common but generally managed conservatively. Fractures through the clivus can injure cranial nerves 3–6, those through the jugular foramen can injure cranial nerves 9–11, and fractures through the occipital condyle can injure cranial nerve 12.
- Occipital condyle fractures are commonly missed on both head and cervical spine CTs. When detected, evaluate for displacement of the fracture fragment and malalignment of the occiput-C1–C2 joint complex. MRI may be reasonable to directly evaluate the integrity of the key ligaments at the craniocervical junction: tectorial membrane, alar ligaments, and transverse atlantal ligament.
- Displaced sagittal fractures of the clivus can injure or impinge the basilar artery. Fractures of the lateral or squamous occipital bone can cause traumatic dural venous sinus thrombosis if the fracture line extends to the jugular foramen or through the course of the transverse/sigmoid sinuses. These merit CTA/CTV for further evaluation.

Grant Funding/Disclosures/Acknowledgements The authors have no relevant disclosures.

References

1. Follmar KE, Baccarani A, Das RR, Erdmann D, Marcus JR, Mukundan S. A clinically applicable reporting system for the diagnosis of facial fractures. Int J Oral Maxillofac Surg. 2007;36(7):593–600.
2. Gómez Roselló E, Quiles Granado AM, Artajona Garcia M, Juanpere Martí S, Laguillo Sala G, Beltrán Mármol B, et al. Facial fractures: classification and highlights for a useful report. Insights Imaging. 2020;11(1):49.
3. Fraioli RE, Branstetter BF, Deleyiannis FW-B. Facial fractures: beyond Le fort. Otolaryngol Clin N Am. 2008;41(1):51–76.
4. Dreizin D, Nam AJ, Tirada N, Levin MD, Stein DM, Bodanapally UK, et al. Multidetector CT of mandibular fractures, reductions, and complications: a clinically relevant primer for the radiologist. Radiographics. 2016;36(5):1539–64.
5. Dreizin D, Nam AJ, Diaconu SC, Bernstein MP, Bodanapally UK, Munera F. Multidetector CT of midfacial fractures: classification systems, principles of reduction, and common complications. Radiographics. 2018;38(1):248–74.
6. Dreizin D, Sakai O, Champ K, Gandhi D, Aarabi B, Nam AJ, et al. CT of skull base fractures: classification systems, complications, and management. Radiographics. 2021;41(3):762–82.

Neck Infections

Emma Lindsey, Parth Vaghasia, and Evan G. Stein

- The goal of imaging in the setting of suspected neck infections should be to delineate the extent of infection, look for evidence of a source, identify drainable collections, and assess for complications.
- The most common cause of neck infections in adults is odontogenic, related to the teeth; in children, neck infections often result from tonsillitis.
- It is important to determine what mucosal compartment or deep space of the neck the infection involves and if the infection involves multiple spaces (trans-spatial).
- One should always look for related complications, including airway compromise, osteomyelitis of the adjacent bone, and vascular complications such as thrombosis or pseudoaneurysm.

Oral Cavity

- The oral cavity is defined as the mucosal compartment anterior to the tonsillar pillars or the junction of the hard and soft palates.
- It includes the lips, anterior 2/3 of the tongue, maxillary and mandibular teeth, gingiva, hard palate, buccal mucosa, and floor of mouth.
- The most common origin of infection in the oral cavity is odontogenic, but infections may also arise from salivary gland duct obstruction, most often secondary to a calculus.

ABSCESS

- An abscess is a walled-off collection of infected fluid and debris.
- Odontogenic abscess usually arises in the setting of periodontal disease, inflammation of the gingiva, and/or alveolar bone (Fig. 37.1).
  - Bacteria from dental caries can extend into the central pulp of the tooth and cause an infected periapical or radicular cyst. Untreated infection can then spread to the subperiosteal space of the maxilla or mandible and cause an adjacent abscess (Figs. e37.1, e37.2, e37.3, e37.4 and e37.5).
  - (All electronic images (Figs. e37.1–e37.17) can be found on this chapter's website on SpringerLink: https://doi.org/10.1007/978-3-031-55124-6_37)
- Imaging:
  - On CECT an abscess appears as a focal area of central low density with a peripherally enhancing rim.
    - Other noninfectious cystic lesions may appear similarly such as ranula, which is a painless postinfectious or post-traumatic sublingual or minor salivary gland retention cyst, which may have a thin enhancing wall. However, these will lack surrounding signs of inflammation and will have a different clinical presentation.
  - Associated local inflammatory changes include infiltration of the surrounding fat (so-called fat stranding), thickening of the adjacent fascial planes, and ipsilateral enlarged reactive lymph nodes.

Supplementary Information The online version contains supplementary material available at https://doi.org/10.1007/978-3-031-55124-6_37.

E. Lindsey · E. G. Stein (✉)
NYU Grossman School Medicine, New York, NY, USA
e-mail: Emma.Lindsey@nyulangone.org; evan.stein@nyulangone.org

P. Vaghasia
Maimonides Medical Center, Brooklyn, NY, USA
e-mail: pavaghasia@maimonidesmed.org

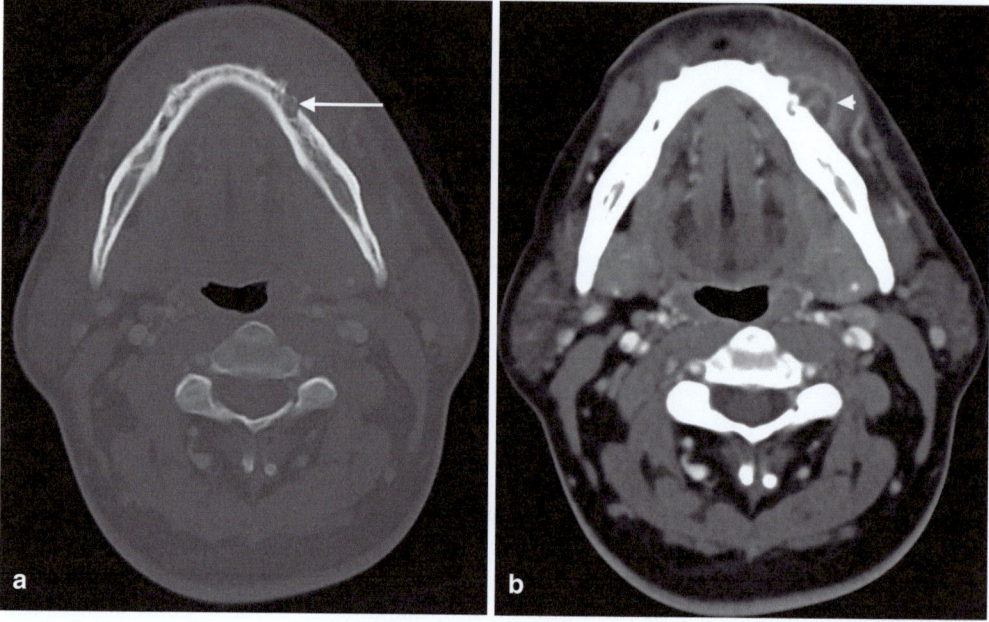

Fig. 37.1 Dental abscess. Axial contrast-enhanced CT on soft tissue (**a**) and bone (**b**) windows through the mandible shows a semicircular region of central heterogeneous but predominantly low density with peripheral enhancement and overlying fat infiltration and swelling (arrowhead) with a broad base along the left mandible body centered over a region of cortical erosion (arrow) compatible with a dental abscess

- o On MRI an abscess will also be peripherally enhanced with internal high signal intensity on T2-weighted imaging and low signal intensity on T1-weighted imaging and will often show central restricted diffusion.
- o Odontogenic abscess may be more easily identified by first looking at the teeth for dental caries and periapical/radicular lucency then closely examining the surrounding soft tissues for a hypodense rim-enhancing collection.

CELLULITIS

- Cellulitis is an infiltrative soft tissue infection, which causes inflammation of the skin, fascia, and fat.
- Patients present with signs and symptoms of inflammation: pain, swelling, warmth, and redness of the area as well as symptoms more specific to oral cavity infections including trismus (inability to open the mouth fully) and dysphagia or odynophagia.
- Imaging:
  - o Skin thickening, fat infiltration with obscuration of expected fat planes, mucosal edema, and hyperenhancement (Fig. 37.2).
    - On non-contrast CT (NCCT) or contrast-enhanced CT (CECT) there will be increased fat density.
    - On MRI edema will appear as abnormal hyperintensity on T2-weighted imaging and as hypointensity on T1-weighted sequences.
  - o Edema and thickening of the adjacent fascia, muscles, or glands may also be present, which may indicate concomitant fasciitis, myositis, and/or adenitis, depending on their degree of involvement.

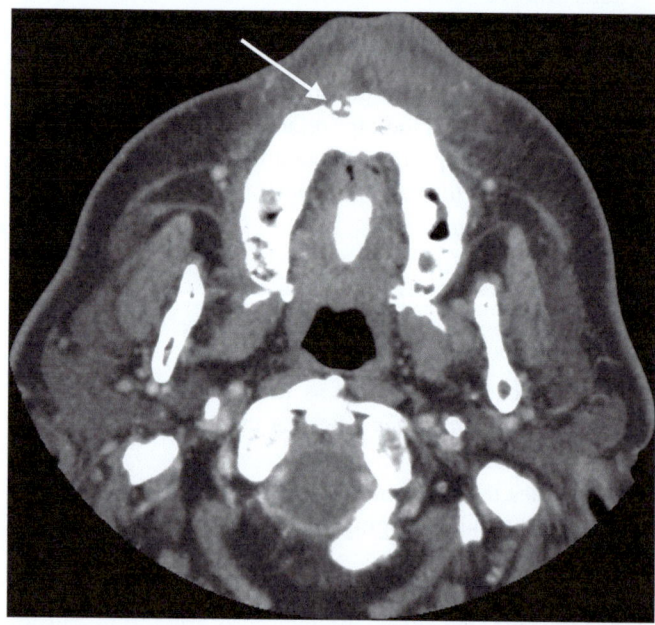

Fig. 37.2 Cellulitis. Axial contrast-enhanced CT through the maxilla shows a focus of cortical erosion to the right of midline (arrow) there is swelling of the overlying soft tissues and infiltration of the fat with thickening of the skin overlying the frenulum which presented clinically as a cellulitis

LUDWIG'S ANGINA

- A specific type of rapidly progressive cellulitis involving the floor of the mouth is called Ludwig's Angina.
  - o The "floor of mouth" refers to the sublingual space, which is inferiorly demarcated by the mylohyoid muscular sling.

- The infection typically spreads trans-spatially to involve the sublingual and submandibular spaces bilaterally. Infection can also spread into the parapharyngeal and retropharyngeal spaces, with the potential to extend into the mediastinum by tracking inferiorly and extending into the danger space.
- Patients present with pain in the mouth and neck, dysphagia, and dysphonia usually accompanied by systemic signs of infection such as fever and chills.
- The tongue may be enlarged and elevated secondary to sublingual edema, which can compromise the airway and make intubation difficult. Therefore, it is considered a medical emergency. Patients may be observed in the ICU, and IV antibiotics are usually administered.
- Imaging:
  - Imaging findings include those of typical cellulitis with swelling and edema of the tongue and floor of the mouth (Figs. e37.6 and e37.7).
  - The tongue may be superiorly displaced, and the oropharyngeal airway may be narrowed.
  - Abscess or soft tissue emphysema may be present at later stages but is not required for the diagnosis.
  - Lymphadenopathy may also be absent because of the rapid progression of the infection.

SIALOLITHIASIS AND SIALOADENITIS

- Sialolithiasis refers to the formation of salivary gland calculi, which can become lodged within the salivary ducts and cause obstruction and stasis of secretions.
  - Most commonly affects the submandibular glands because of the more viscous and alkaline secretions paired with a narrow distal opening and upward course of Wharton's duct. Parotid gland sialolithiasis can also occur. Calculi rarely form in the sublingual glands.
  - Patients may be asymptomatic or have periprandial pain related to increased saliva production.
  - Sialodochitis refers to inflammation of the salivary duct.
- Sialoadenitis is inflammation of the salivary glands and may be acute or chronic.
  - The most common cause of acute sialadenitis is duct obstruction from sialolithiasis, commonly with superimposed bacterial infection secondary to salivary stasis.
  - Other causes include viral infection or autoimmune conditions.
  - Chronic sialoadenitis may cause atrophy or fibrosis of the gland and stenosis and pruning of the ductal system.
    - Kuttner tumor is a term that refers to chronic sclerosing sialadenitis, usually of the submandibular gland. It is associated with IgG4 disease.

- Imaging:
  - Salivary gland calculi (sialoliths) are most often calcified and hyperdense to surrounding tissues on plain films and CT. On T2 weighted MRI sequences, a focal area of signal void surrounded by T2 hyperintense saliva may be seen.
  - Sialectasis, ductal dilation, upstream to the calculus may be present.
    - On CT, a dilated duct appears as a tubular hypodense structure along the expected course of the salivary gland duct.
    - On MRI, sialectasis appears as an elongated T2 hyperintense collection.
  - Sialography may be performed, with contrast injection or high-resolution T2-weighted MRI, if there is concern for noncalcified sialoliths, which appear as filling defects or signal voids.
  - Sialoadenitis causes enlargement of the gland (submandibular or parotid).
  - The gland is usually lower density on NCCT because of edema and hyperenhancing on CECT (Fig. 37.3).

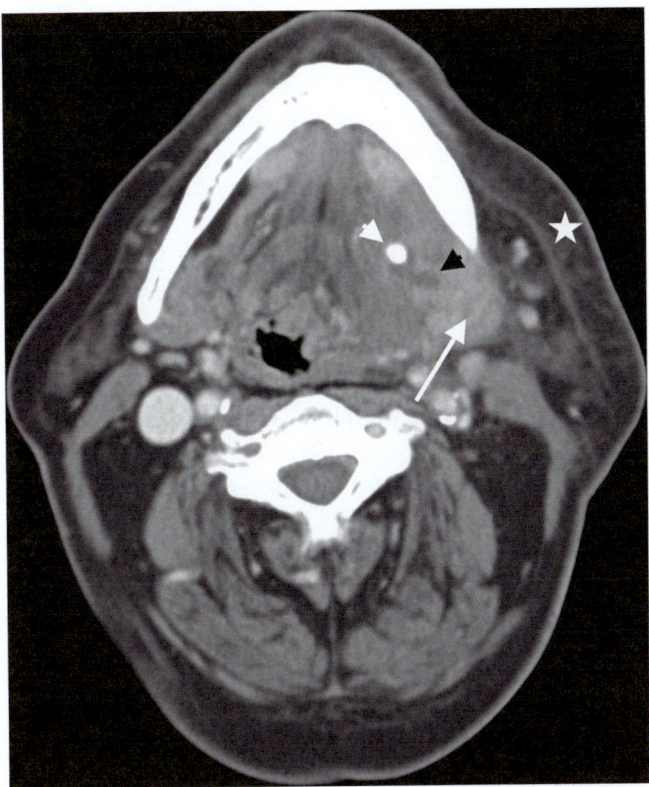

Fig. 37.3 Sialoadenitis. Contrast-enhanced imaging through the floor of mouth and the submandibular space demonstrate swelling and enhancement of the left submandibular gland (arrow) with infiltration of the surrounding fat and swelling of the adjacent floor of mouth structures. There is also infiltration of the fat and platysma overlying the left submandibular space (star). There is a hyperdense sialolith (white arrowhead) in the floor of mouth with proximal sialoectasis (black arrowhead)

- On MRI, the gland is hyperintense on T2-weighted imaging and enhances.
- There is often stranding of the fat around the gland and thickening of the overlying muscle (platysma) and skin.

Pharynx

- The pharynx is divided cranio-caudally into three parts—the nasopharynx, the oropharynx, and the hypopharynx.
  - The nasopharynx is the posterior extension of the nasal cavity via the posterior choanae. It extends from the skull base superiorly to the level of the hard palate inferiorly.
  - The oropharynx is contiguous with and immediately posterior to the oral cavity. It extends from the level of the hard palate to the level of the superior aspect of the hyoid bone body.
  - The hypopharynx extends from the inferior border of the oropharynx to the bottom of the cricoid cartilage; the hypopharynx continues inferiorly as the cervical esophagus.
- The pharyngeal mucosal space refers to the mucosal surface of the pharynx and the associated contents including lymphatic tissue/tonsils (Waldeyer ring), minor salivary glands, and the pharyngeal muscles.
- The pharyngeal mucosal space is superficial to the middle layer of the deep cervical fascia.
- The retropharyngeal space lies deep to the pharyngeal mucosal space, and the parapharyngeal space/fat lies laterally.

RETROPHARYNGEAL INFECTIONS

- The retropharyngeal space is a potential space lined anteriorly by the middle layer of deep cervical fascia and posteriorly by the alar fascia. It extends from the skull base to between C6 and T4 (usually C7) where the two fascial layers fuse. The space is bounded laterally by the deep layer of the deep cervical fascia (Cloisson sagitale fascia).
- The danger space is a space between the alar fascia and the deep layer of the deep cervical fascia that invests in the prevertebral muscles and is also known as the prevertebral fascia. The danger space extends inferiorly to

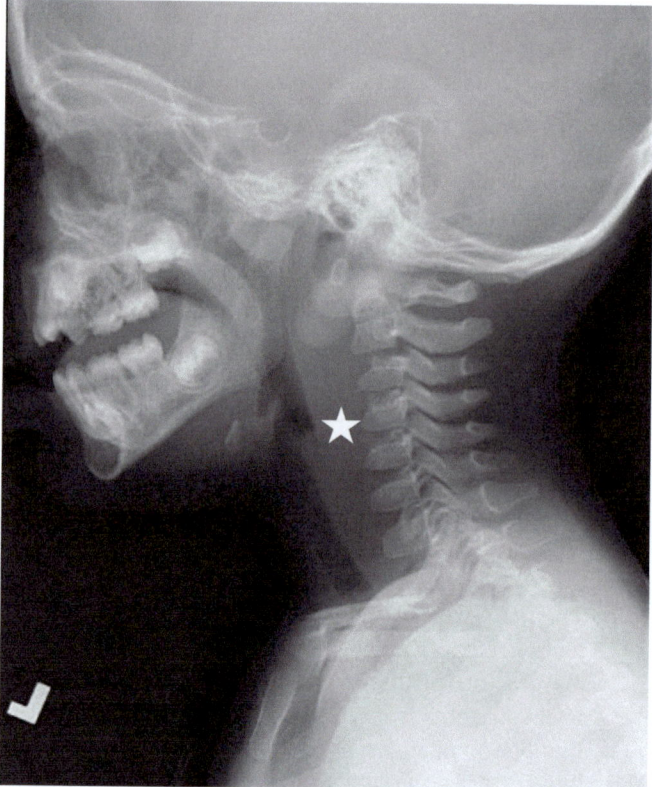

Fig. 37.4 Retropharyngeal abscess. Lateral radiograph of the neck in a 2 years old with cough and odynophagia demonstrating marked thickening of the retropharyngeal soft tissues (star)

just above the diaphragm where the alar and middle layer of deep cervical fascia then fuse with the deep layer of deep cervical fascia. Infection high in the neck can spread inferiorly via the danger space (Figs. 37.4 and 37.5).

- Imaging:
  - The earliest sign of a retropharyngeal abscess during an imaging work-up may be on a lateral radiograph of the neck with thickening of the prevertebral soft tissues. Many mnemonics are used to remember the normal width of the prevertebral soft tissues. One of the easiest to remember is that the soft tissues should not be wider than the vertebral body. Another is that the soft tissues should be less than 7 mm thick at C2 and less than 2 cm thick at C7 ("7 at 2, 2 at 7"). Gas is sometimes also seen on the lateral radiograph and, in combination, gas, and swelling are highly specific for abscess.

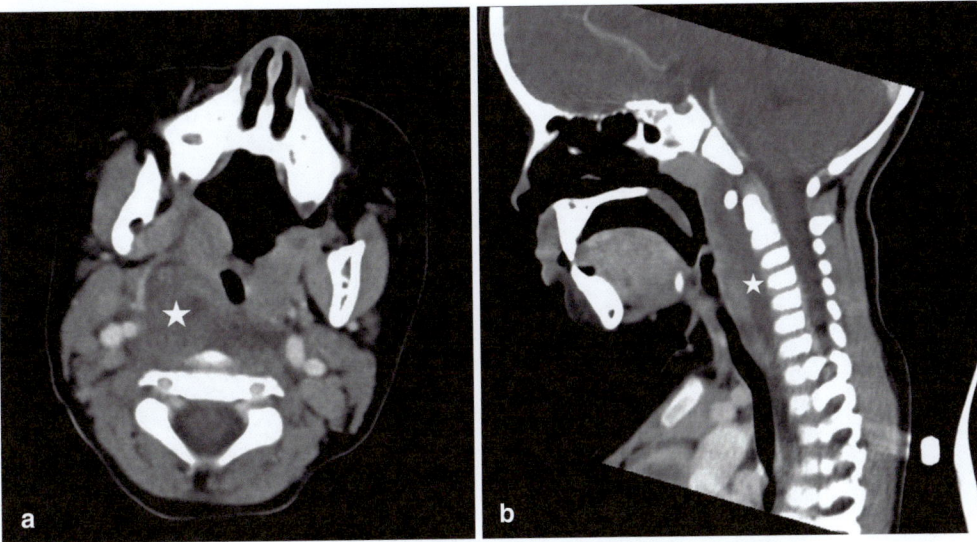

Fig. 37.5 Retropharyngeal abscess. Axial (**a**) and sagittal (**b**) CECT images demonstrate a low-density collection with subtle peripheral enhancement in the retropharyngeal space (star) extending caudally to C7

- On CECT, there will be marked thickening of the retropharyngeal space by a peripherally enhancing fluid collection. Enhancement may be subtle at first but, as the abscess evolves, the wall enhancement becomes thicker and more conspicuous. There is infiltration of the surrounding fat and the adjacent muscles often become edematous (Fig. e37.8).
- The findings on MRI will parallel the CECT findings with a rim-enhancing T2 hyperintense collection in the retropharyngeal space. Signal intensity on T1-weighted imaging can be variable because of the content of protein and pus. MRI is not usually used for diagnosis because of the tenuous nature of these patients but MRI can be very sensitive for residual abscess after drainage and it is sometimes necessary to differentiate a retropharyngeal abscess from a prevertebral abscess.

TONSILLAR OR PERITONSILLAR ABSCESS

- When the palatine tonsils become infected, they enlarge and enhance with a striated pattern.
- As the infection progresses, the tonsil may develop a well-defined low-density collection with a thick, enhancing wall. Sometimes the collection will be multiloculated or septated.
- The fascia that covers the lateral wall of the palatine tonsil is a very loose connective tissue and the abscess will grow laterally from the tonsil into the parapharyngeal space or masticator space to become a peritonsillar abscess.
- Imaging:
  - CECT will show a well-defined low-density space surrounded by a thick-walled enhancing capsule. The mass effect from the abscess and surrounding edema may narrow the oropharyngeal airway and, if it extends inferiorly, the hypopharyngeal and laryngeal airways (Fig. 37.6).
  - MRI is not commonly performed for this indication. On MRI, the pus filling the abscess is usually low signal on T1-weighted imaging, high signal on T2-weighted imaging, and diffusion restricting. The capsule vividly enhances, and there is often hyperintense signal on T2-weighted imaging and patchy enhancement in the surrounding tissues either as a consequence of phlegmon formation or reactive inflammation.

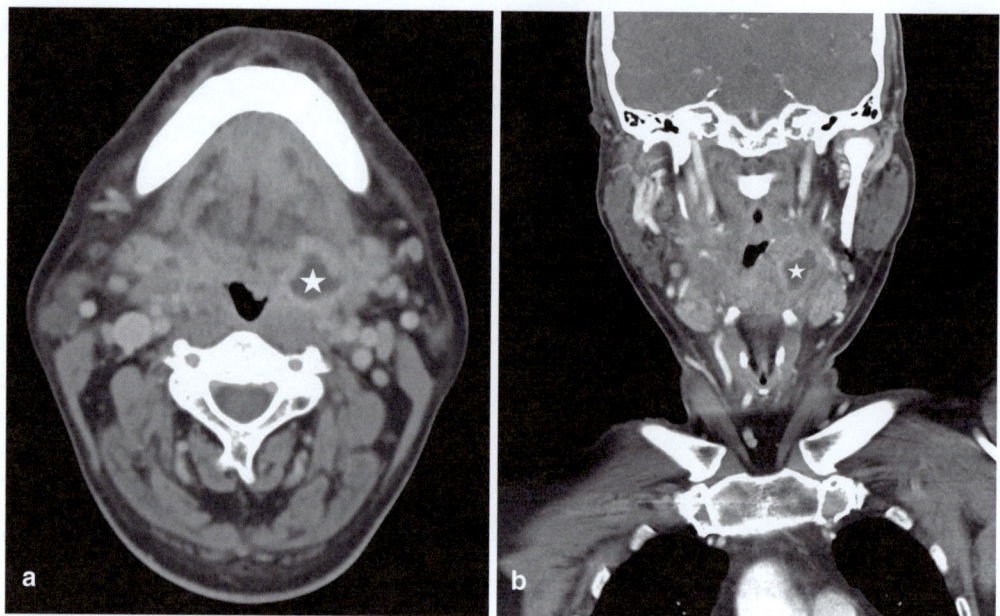

Fig. 37.6 Tonsillar abscess. Axial (**a**) and coronal (**b**) contrast-enhanced CT images through the oropharynx demonstrate a low-density collection with a thick enhancing wall (star) in the left palatine tonsil. There is a mild mass effect on the adjacent structures and oropharyngeal airway

Larynx

- Detailed review of the anatomy of the larynx can be found elsewhere in this text (see Chap. 41).
- For the purposes of evaluating infections of the larynx, it is important to remember the division of the larynx into three levels, the supraglottis, the glottis, and the subglottis.

CROUP

- Croup is the consequence of a viral infection (usually parainfluenza) that causes subglottic edema.
- The diagnosis of croup is usually made clinically:
  - Age—6 months to 3 years.
  - Season—while croup CAN occur in any season, it is most common in late autumn and early winter.
  - Onset—accompanied by a low-grade fever, cough, and rhinorrhea.
  - Presentation—barking cough.
- Imaging is reserved for identifying other causes of symptoms: foreign body aspiration, epiglottitis, angioedema.
- While croup is usually self-limited and results in a barky cough and stridor, it can worsen to respiratory failure with cyanosis and altered mental status.
- Imaging:
  - The diagnosis can often be made on frontal and lateral plain radiographs of the soft tissue neck.
  - Frontal radiographs will show narrowing of the subglottic airway with an upside-down "V" or "steeple" configuration as the narrowed subglottic airway widens into the trachea. The normal subglottic airway configuration has "shoulders" that are lost in croup.
  - Lateral radiographs show a normal epiglottis and aryepiglottic folds. You may also see overdistension of the hypopharynx and haziness of the subglottic trachea (Fig. 37.7).

EPIGLOTTITIS

- Epiglottitis is a life-threatening inflammation of the supraglottic soft tissues—the epiglottis and the aryepiglottic folds—leading to airway obstruction and intubation.
- Epiglottitis is usually caused by *Haemophilus influenzae* type b (Hib) and the incidence has dropped since the introduction of vaccination against Hib.
- Currently, epiglottitis is more rare and is caused by staph and strep, as well as herpes viruses such as HSV, EBV, and VZV. Cases have been reported in association with COVID-19. It can also be caused by allergic reactions and trauma.
- Imaging:
  - Diagnosis is made with plain radiography of the neck. Prolonged supine positioning for CT can be life-threatening in a child with epiglottitis.
  - Lateral radiograph shows an enlarged and thickened epiglottis, termed the "Thumb Sign," and thickened aryepiglottic folds.
  - On CECT and MRI the epiglottis and aryepiglottic folds will be enlarged and edematous—low density on

Fig. 37.7 Croup. Frontal (**a**) and lateral (**b**) radiographs of the neck show narrowing of the airway (arrow) just beneath the cords. There is loss of the usual subglottic "shoulders" and haziness of the subglottic airway walls (arrowhead). The dilation of the hypopharynx was not seen in this patient

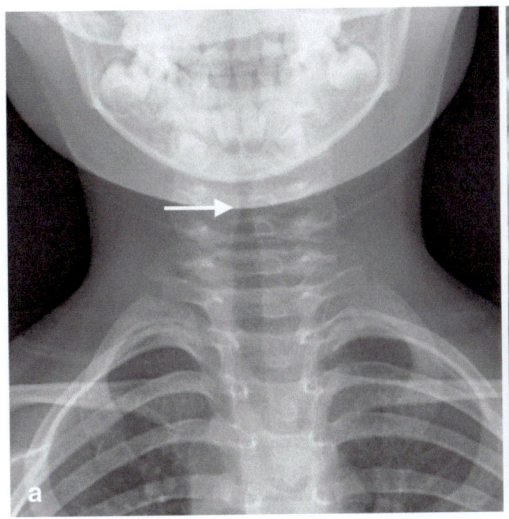
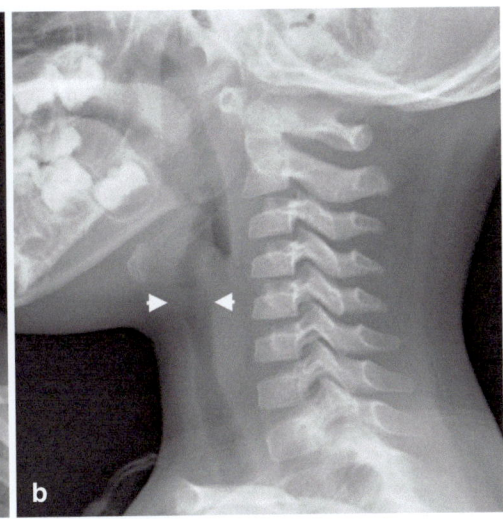

CT, hyperintense on T2-weighted imaging (Figs. e37.9 and e37.10).
- When it is severe, the inflammation may extend into the subglottic larynx and imitate Croup on imaging, however; croup will NOT have an enlarged epiglottis or aryepiglottic folds.

SUPRAGLOTTITIS

- Also known as adult-onset epiglottitis.
- It comes with all of the same risks and ramifications as epiglottitis in children—airway compromise, respiratory arrest.
- Because of Hib vaccination, Supraglottitis is now more common than Epiglottitis in children and is usually caused by staph and strep.
- Imaging:
  - Contrast-enhanced neck CT is the imaging modality of choice.
  - Thickening of the epiglottis and the aryepiglottic folds as well as enlarged enhancing palatine and lingual tonsils.
  - CECT is also very important if there is a suspicion of an abscess in the soft tissues.
  - Unlike in children, supraglottitis in adults has highly variable involvement of the epiglottis which makes radiographs less sensitive.

LARYNGOCELE/MUCOCELE/PYOCELE

- The laryngeal ventricle is the air-filled space between the false vocal folds and the true vocal folds.
- If a mass or adhesion forms in that space then gas, fluid, or secretions can accumulate in that space and expand the space over time resulting in a laryngocele or mucocele.

The space can become so large that it herniates through the thyrohyoid membrane and is called a mixed laryngocele.
- If the secretions become super-infected then it is a pyolaryngocele or pyocele.
- Laryngocele is most commonly found in older adults and is almost exclusively unilateral.
- Imaging:
  - CECT demonstrates a well-defined air- or fluid-filled lesion within the laryngeal ventricle or paralaryngeal space. Depending on the material filling the lesion, density can vary (Figs. e37.11, e37.12 and e37.13). They can be black when air-filled and range from fluid to soft tissue density depending on the protein and mucus content of the fluid. If super-infected, pyolaryngoceles demonstrate peripheral enhancement and surrounding inflammatory changes.
  - MR is better for soft tissue discrimination and to detect communication with the laryngeal airway. Like with CECT, signal varies based on content. The lesion can be iso- to hypointense on T1-weighted imaging and is usually hyperintense on T2-weighted imaging or STIR with little to no enhancement. As on CECT, if super-infected, pyolaryngoceles demonstrate thick peripheral enhancement (Figs. e37.14 and e37.15).

Soft Tissue Infections of the Neck

CELLULITIS

- Cellulitis is a superficial infection of the neck starting at the skin with local inflammatory changes before penetrating deeper when untreated.
- Infections may be transpatial and reviewing the deep spaces of the neck can be helpful when describing the extent of infection.

- Imaging:
  - CECT.
    - Thickening of the skin and superficial fascia with subcutaneous fat stranding and septations.
  - MRI.
    - Thickening of the skin and superficial fascia with soft tissue edema as ill-defined or linear hyperintensity on T2/STIR more prominently in the hypodermis.
    - Post-contrast imaging demonstrates enhancement of affected tissue.

ABSCESS

- An abscess is a walled-off collection caused by an infection, most commonly bacterial.
  - An abscess within the soft tissues of the neck is a serious, potentially fatal, condition.
  - Most commonly seen in children and adolescents, but can also be seen in immunocompromised patients.
  - Abscesses within the soft tissues of the neck usually begin as pharyngeal infections and spread either directly or through lymphatic drainage with resulting suppurative adenitis (Fig. 37.8).
- Imaging:
  - CECT shows a central low-density portion with thick rim enhancement and adjacent inflammatory changes including fat stranding or loss of fat planes, entirely.
  - MRI demonstrates central high signal intensity on T2-weighted imaging and low signal intensity on T1-weighted imaging with thick rim enhancement. The central, non-enhancing region, also often demonstrates a high signal on DWI and low signal on the corresponding ADC map indicating restricted diffusion.

SUPPURATIVE ADENOPATHY

- More common in children than adults:
  - Cervical adenitis is any inflammation of lymph nodes due to infectious process and is most common neck mass in pediatric patients following infection.
  - Suppurative adenopathy, also known as intranodal abscess formation, is when the inflamed lymph nodes undergo liquefactive necrosis, most commonly occurs with bacterial infections (Figs. e37.16 and e37.17).
- Almost always stays within nodal borders, but can rupture and cause an extranodal abscess.
- TB adenopathy (scrofula) has a similar imaging presentation but is usually painless and often calcified.
- Nontuberculous mycobacterial adenopathy can produce very large lymph nodes (often solitary) with no surrounding signs of inflammation.
- Imaging:
  - CECT shows homogeneous lymph node enlargement with enhancing peripheral nodal tissue and central hypodense collection and adjacent fat stranding indicating perinodal inflammatory changes.
  - MRI demonstrates central T1-hypointensity, T2-hyperintensity with peripheral enhancement. High DWI values and low ADC values have been seen in suppurative lymph nodes indicating restricted diffusion.

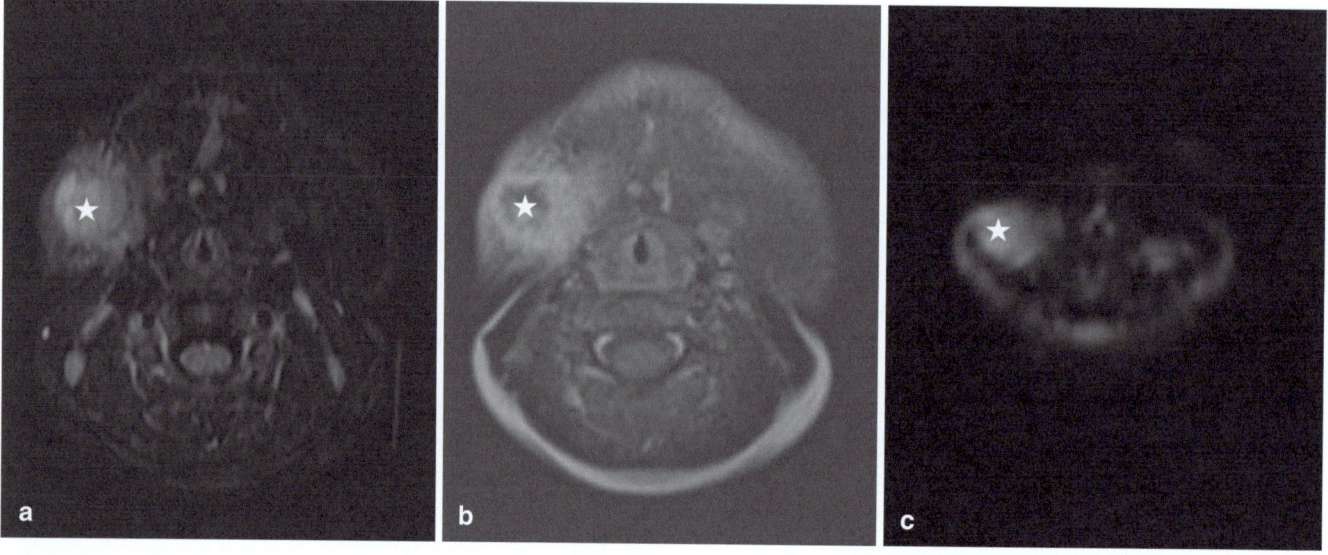

Fig. 37.8 Abscess. Axial STIR (**a**) demonstrates a round hyperintense mass in the right neck (star) with thick rim enhancement on contrast-enhanced T1-weighted imaging (**b**) and bright signal on diffusion-weighted imaging (**c**) all compatible with an abscess in this febrile child

37 Neck Infections

NECROTIZING FASCIITIS

- Cervical necrotizing fasciitis is a rare, complex infection with tissue invasion and necrosis. It requires a high degree of clinical suspicion and aggressive treatment.
- The hallmark of necrotizing fasciitis is the presence of gas dissecting along fascial planes. In the absence of penetrating trauma or recent intervention, soft tissue gas should raise suspicion for a necrotizing infection.
- Imaging:
  - CECT generally demonstrates multispatial collections, including poorly or non-enhancing fluid and gas collections. Isolated non-gas-containing fluid collections may also be seen but are less common. Other findings include thickening and enhancement of the fascial planes, myonecrosis, and cellulitis (Fig. 37.9).
  - MRI demonstrates diffuse T2 hyperintense thickening of fascial planes, often both superficial and deep. However, CT is the modality of choice for this diagnosis.

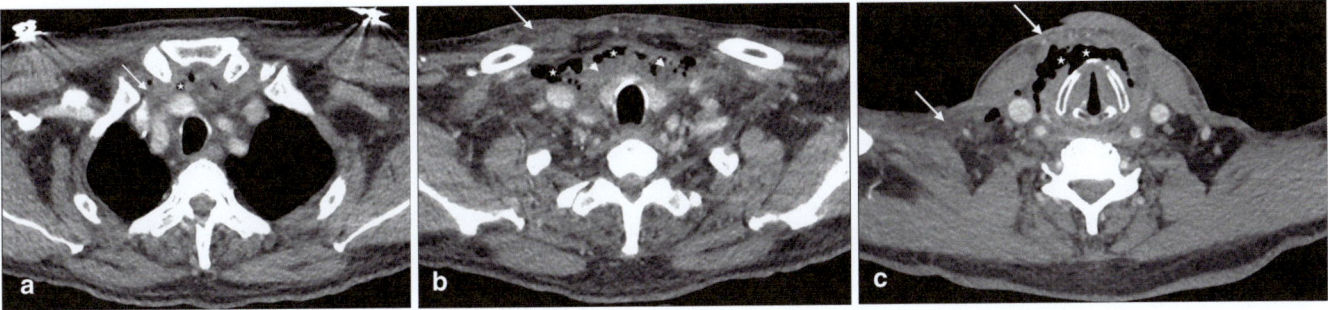

Fig. 37.9 Necrotizing fasciitis. Axial CECT images through the lower neck (**a**), glottis (**b**), and hyoid (**c**) all demonstrate gas (star), fluid (arrowhead), and inflammatory changes (arrow) including fat infiltration, myositis, and cellulitis. Aggressive debridement is necessary

Further Readings

1. Som PM, Curtin HD, editors. Head and neck imaging. 4th ed. St. Louis: Mosby; 2003. p. 1507–9.
2. StatPearls [Internet]. Treasure Island (FL): StatPearls Publishing; 2022. https://www.ncbi.nlm.nih.gov/books/NBK430685/.
3. Gonzalez-Beicos A, Nunez D. Imaging of acute head and neck infections. Radiol Clin N Am. 2012;50:73–83.
4. Capps EF, Kinsella JJ, Gupta M, et al. Emergency imaging assessment of acute, nontraumatic conditions of the head and neck. Radiographics. 2010;30:1335–52.

Imaging of Neck Spaces

Shehanaz K. Ellika, Anthony Portanova, Devanshi Mistry, and Edward Lin

Key Points

- The neck is anatomically complex but can be organized into multiple spaces, based on the three layers of the deep cervical fascia which allows segmentation of pathology into well-defined fascially enclosed spaces.
- The neck spaces can be broadly divided into the suprahyoid or infrahyoid compartments, with some spaces, such as the carotid, retropharyngeal, danger, and perivertebral spaces, spanning both levels.
- Placing a pathologic process within a neck space is the first step in generating an appropriate differential diagnosis. Next, its relationship to the surrounding spaces and structures is evaluated. A differential diagnosis is then generated based on the unique anatomic contents of each space.
- Displacement of the parapharyngeal fat can help determine the site of origin of suprahyoid neck masses.
- Squamous cell carcinoma is the most common malignancy of the pharyngeal mucosal space. The role of imaging is to characterize the submucosal extent of disease, involvement of adjacent spaces and evaluate nodal spread.
- The parotid gland is the only salivary gland to contain lymph nodes; lymphadenopathy must be considered in the differential diagnosis of any parotid space mass.
- The CS spans the suprahyoid and infrahyoid neck, with all three layers of the DCF contributing to the carotid sheath. It serves as a route for travel of infection or malignancy from the neck into the mediastinum.
- Retropharyngeal collections that have entered the danger or prevertebral spaces can descend to the mediastinum or as far inferiorly as the coccyx.
- The visceral space is the only space contained entirely in the infrahyoid neck. US is the main imaging modality for the evaluation of thyroid gland inflammatory disease and thyroid nodules. Cross-sectional imaging is used when there is a concern for extrathyroidal extension of tumor to evaluate airway compression or substernal extension.

Introduction

- In head and neck imaging, anatomy plays a major role.
- Just like identifying whether an intracranial lesion is located in the intra-axial or extra-axial compartments, or if a spinal lesion is located in the extradural versus intradural/extramedullary versus intramedullary compartments; in the head and neck, lesions need to be placed into spaces/compartments to accurately localize the lesion and generate an appropriate differential diagnosis.
- Report the precise anatomy and provide a short differential diagnosis to the clinician.
- Add clinical history to give the report relevance.
- Use CT for skull base/vertebral involvement and MRI to assess intracranial or intraspinal involvement.
- CT is helpful in acute infections, stones, trauma, and osseous disease processes.

Layers Of Cervical Fascia

- Superficial cervical fascia (SCF) consists of the subcutaneous tissues of the head and neck [1, 2].
- Deep cervical fascia is subdivided into superficial, middle, and deep layers (Fig. 38.1) [1, 2].
  o Superficial layer of deep cervical fascia (SLDCF) (Fig. 38.1).

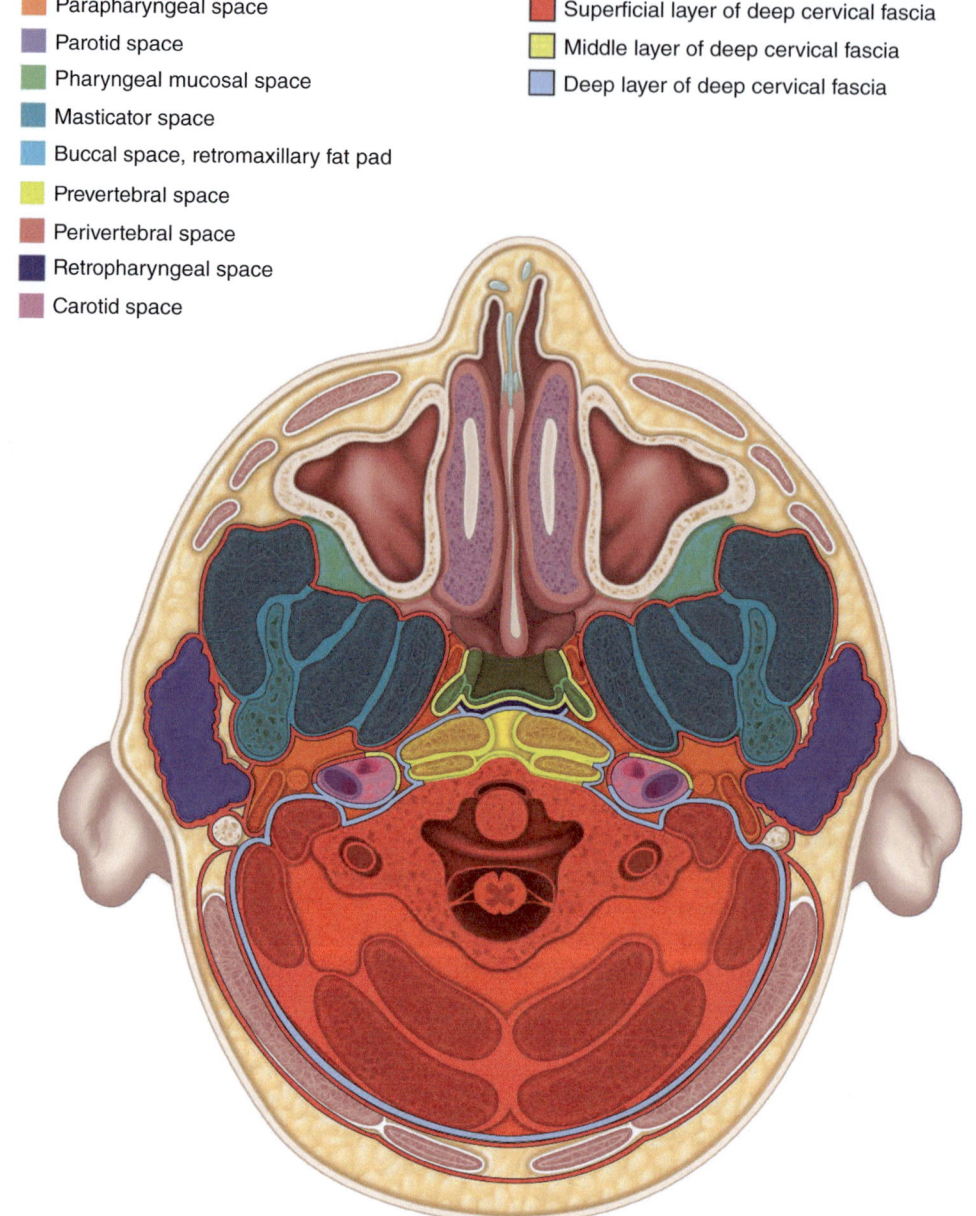

Fig. 38.1 Axial graphic at the C2 vertebral level, depicting the suprahyoid neck spaces. Each space is separated and contained within the investing fascial layers. The paired MS (teal) surrounds the PMS (green). Posterior to the MS are the paired PS (purple) and, medially, the CS (pink). Nestled between the MS, PMS, and CS lies the triangular-shaped PPS (orange)

- Parapharyngeal space
- Parotid space
- Pharyngeal mucosal space
- Masticator space
- Buccal space, retromaxillary fat pad
- Prevertebral space
- Perivertebral space
- Retropharyngeal space
- Carotid space
- Superficial layer of deep cervical fascia
- Middle layer of deep cervical fascia
- Deep layer of deep cervical fascia

- Invests parotid, submandibular, and masticator spaces.
- Invests the sternocleidomastoid and trapezius muscles.
- "Rule of twos": SLDCF encloses two glands (submandibular and parotid) and two muscles (sternocleidomastoid and trapezius) [2].

○ Middle layer of deep cervical fascia (MLDCF) (Figs. 38.1 and 38.2).
- Extends from the skull base to the mediastinum.
- Divided into a muscular layer investing the strap muscles and a visceral layer investing the larynx, pharynx, trachea, esophagus, and thyroid [2].

○ Deep layer of deep cervical fascia (DLDCF) (Figs. 38.1 and 38.2).
- Surrounds the vertebral column and paravertebral muscles.
- Two distinct components: Alar and prevertebral fascia; alar fascia forms the posterior and lateral walls of the retropharyngeal space (Fig. e38.1).
- (All electronic images (Figs. e38.1–e38.3) can be found on this chapter's website on SpringerLink: https://doi.org/10.1007/978-3-031-55124-6_38) and prevertebral layer encloses the paraspinal muscles [2].
- Carotid sheath is composed of all three layers of DCF.

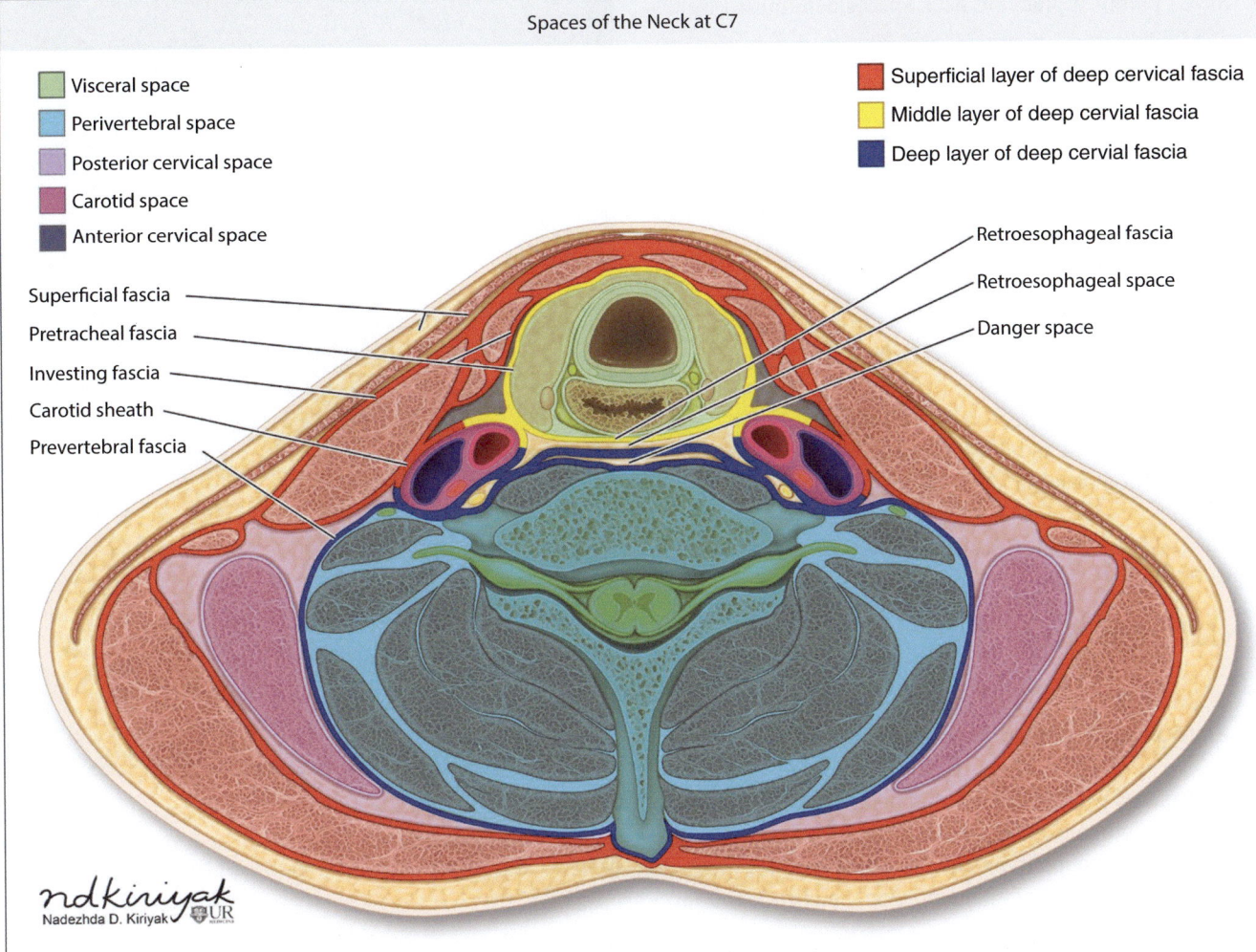

Fig. 38.2 Axial graphic of the infrahyoid neck demonstrating the layers of the deep cervical fascia and the enclosed spaces including the VS (light green), PVS (blue), CS (pink), anterior (grey), and posterior (lavender) cervical spaces

- o Pharyngobasilar fascia.
  - Aponeurosis between pharyngeal mucosal space and MLDCF/pharyngeal constrictors.

Cervical Spaces

- Anterior and posterior cervical spaces are two well-defined spaces that are not enclosed by their own fascia, extending from the skull base to the clavicles and composed predominantly of fat (Fig. 38.2) [3, 4].
- Anterior cervical space is a small space in the anterolateral neck located lateral to the visceral space and anterior to the carotid space (Fig. 38.2) [4].
- Posterior cervical space lies posterolateral to the carotid space and lateral to the paraspinal space and contains fat, spinal accessory nerve, and spinal accessory chain of deep cervical lymph nodes (Fig. 38.2) [4].

Global Head And Neck Anatomy

- Neck spaces are determined by fascial planes: superficial, middle, and deep layers of the deep cervical fascia (Figs. 38.1 and 38.2).
- Broadly the neck is divided into suprahyoid (SHN) and infrahyoid (IHN) compartments [2].
- Hyoid bone provides central fascial attachment for the deep cervical fascia and thus used as a landmark for this broad division.
- Some head and neck spaces transgress both the SHN and IHN, including the carotid, retropharyngeal, and perivertebral spaces.

Suprahyoid Neck Spaces

- Extend from the base of skull to the hyoid bone, excluding the orbits, paranasal sinuses, and oral cavity [1, 2].

- Seven purely suprahyoid neck spaces determined by fascial planes:
  - Pharyngeal mucosal space (PMS)
  - Parapharyngeal space (PPS)
  - Parotid space (PS)
  - Masticator space (MS)
  - Buccal space (BS)
  - Submandibular space (SMS)
  - Sublingual space (SLS)

Spaces Spanning Shn And Ihn

- Carotid space (CS).
- Retropharyngeal and danger space (RPS/DS).
- Perivertebral space (PVS).

Spaces In Ihn

- Visceral space (VS).

Pharyngeal Mucosal Space (Pms)

- Surrounded by the MLDCF and pharyngobasilar fascia.
- Divided into nasopharynx and oropharynx (some also include the hypopharynx and oral cavity) [5–8].
- Abuts clivus, floor of sphenoid sinus, and foramen lacerum at skull base.
- PMS located anteromedial to the PPS and anterior to the RPS [5].
- PPS displaced posterolaterally by PMS mass lesions [2].
- CONTENTS:
  - Squamous mucosa of nasopharynx and oropharynx.
  - Lymphatic tissue/Waldeyer's ring (adenoids, palatine, and lingual tonsils).
  - Minor salivary glands.
  - Superior and middle constrictor, levator palatini, palatoglossus, palatopharyngeus, and salpingopharyngeus muscles [9].
  - Torus tubarius/cartilaginous Eustachian tube.
- PATHOLOGY:
  - Pseudomass: Normal lymphoid tissue (involutes with age).
  - Squamous cell carcinoma, nasopharyngeal carcinoma.
  - Lymphoma.

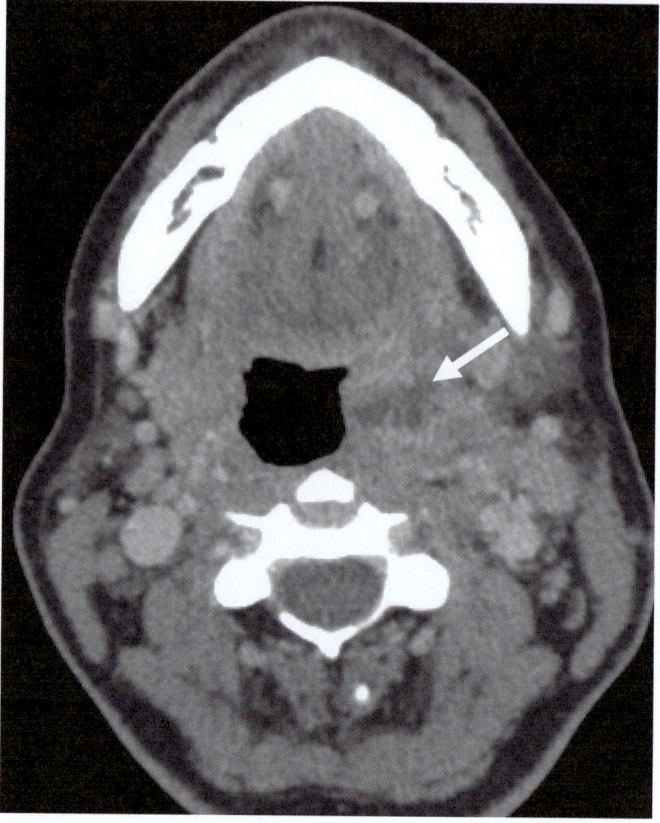

Fig. 38.3 Peritonsillar abscess. Axial contrast-enhanced CT of the neck in a 43-year-old female presenting with sore throat and dysphagia, demonstrating prominent palatine tonsils and left peritonsillar abscess (white arrow)

  - Minor salivary gland tumors.
  - Tonsillitis/pharyngitis (Fig. 38.3).
  - Congenital: Thornwalt cyst (notochordal remnant, midline mass).
  - Squamous cell carcinoma (SCCa) is the most common tumor of the PMS. Lymphoma and submucosal minor salivary gland neoplasms may arise from the Waldeyer's ring and minor salivary glands, respectively.
  - Clinical information indicating the site of mucosal lesion evident on endoscopy/visual inspection may be very helpful at the time of image review [10].
  - Mucosal lesions are visualized with greater accuracy by the referring otorhinolaryngologist. The role of imaging in guiding treatment decisions in SCCa is to correctly characterize the submucosal extent of the mass, including invasion into adjacent spaces and evaluating nodal spread. Review of the most current American Joint Committee on Cancer staging criteria

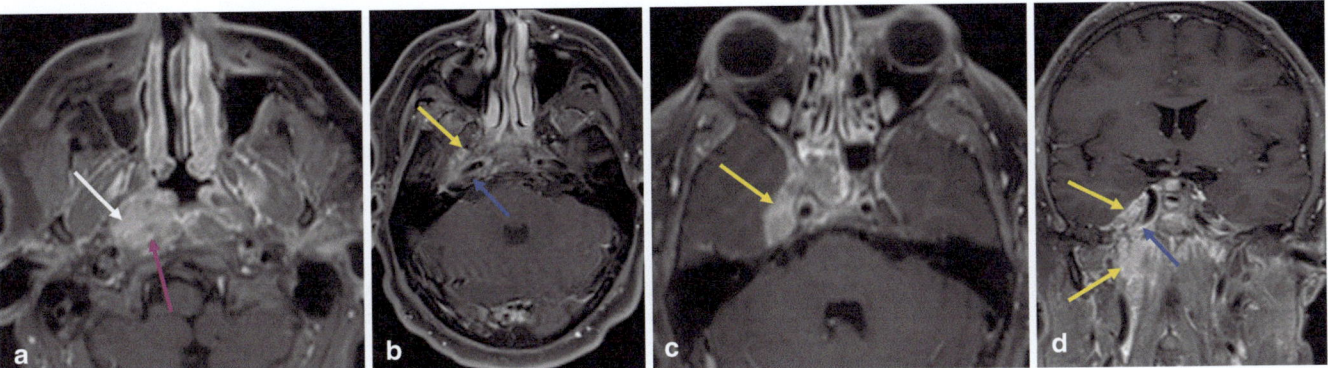

Fig. 38.4 Nasopharyngeal Carcinoma. Axial (**a–c**) and coronal (**d**) post-contrast T1WI's in a 44-year-old male presenting with diplopia, demonstrating a right nasopharyngeal carcinoma (white arrow) posteriorly infiltrating the prevertebral muscles (pink arrow) and extending superiorly to involve the foramen lacerum (blue arrows). Additionally, there is a perineural tumor spread along the mandibular division of the right trigeminal nerve (yellow arrows)

allows radiologists to note the important sites of disease spread to aid clinical staging [10].
- The relationship between the PMS and the skull base is important in the setting of nasopharyngeal carcinoma (NPC). NPC has a propensity for early intracranial spread due to its proximity to the foramen lacerum (Fig. 38.4). Tumors can invade through the foramen's cartilaginous floor and travel along the ICA to invade the cavernous sinus. NPC may also spread via perineural tumor spread into the skull base and cavernous sinus (Fig. 38.4) [10].

Parapharyngeal Space (Pps)

- Also called prestyloid PPS. PPS is divided into two compartments by fascia that join the styloid process to the tensor veli palatini: prestyloid and poststyloid compartments [11, 12].
- The post-styloid PPS is designated as the carotid space and prestyloid PPS is considered the true PPS [13, 14].
- Not actually bounded by its own fascia but is limited by the surrounding fascially defined spaces (Fig. 38.1) [3].
- Easily identified triangular space extending from skull base to hyoid bone, lateral to the PMS (Fig. e38.2).
- Bounded laterally by the MS and PS, medially by the PMS, and posteriorly by the CS (Figs. 38.1 and e38.2).
- Communicates laterally with the PS through the stylomandibular tunnel and inferiorly with the SMS.
- Displacement of this space helps in the localization of large SHN lesions; PPS fat displacement anteromedially by PS lesions, posteromedially by MS lesions, laterally by PMS, and anteriorly by CS lesions (Fig. 38.5) [2].
- CONTENTS:
  - Fat.
  - Ectopic rests of minor salivary glands.
  - Pterygoid venous plexus, internal maxillary, and ascending pharyngeal arteries.
  - Nerves.
- PATHOLOGY: Table 38.1
  - Lipoma.
  - Minor salivary gland tumors.
  - Pseudomass: Pterygoid venous plexus.
  - Venous vascular malformations (Fig. 38.6).
  - Invasion by malignancy or infection.

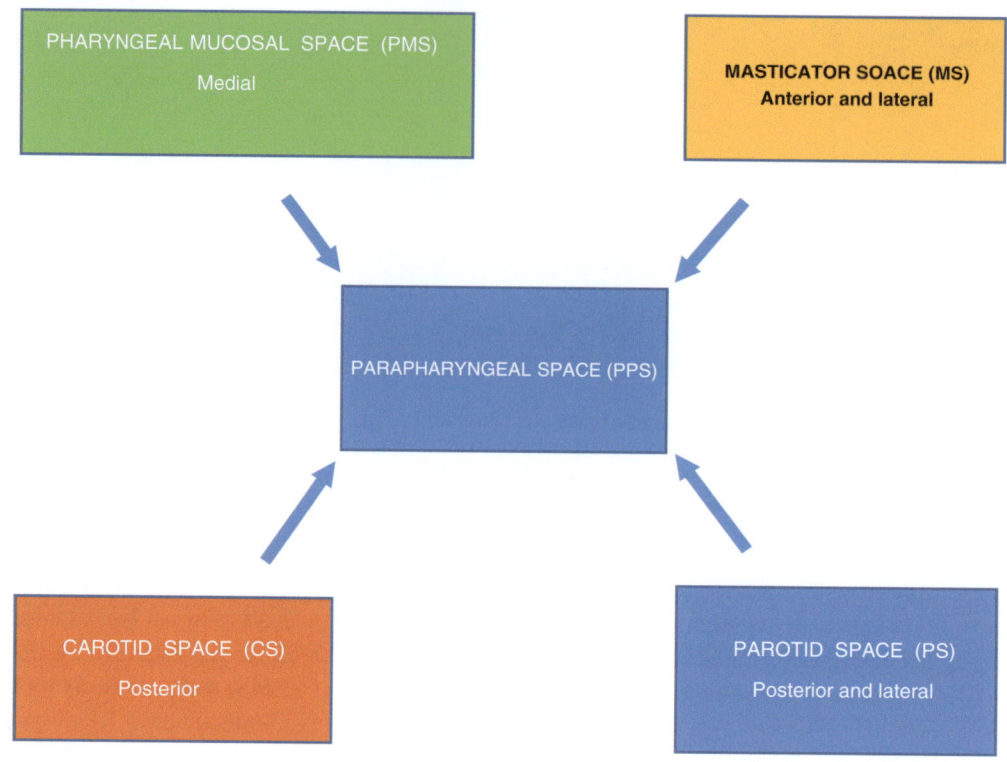

Fig. 38.5 Diagram demonstrating the relationship between the suprahyoid neck spaces and parapharyngeal fat. A mass or pathologic process displaces the fat in a predictable pattern, allowing for correct identification of the space of origin

Table 38.1 Differential diagnosis for parapharyngeal lesions

Fat: Lipoma
Minor salivary gland: Tumors
Pterygoid venous plexus: Pseudomass with asymmetric prominence of the plexus
Secondary extension into PPS: Deep lobe parotid tumors

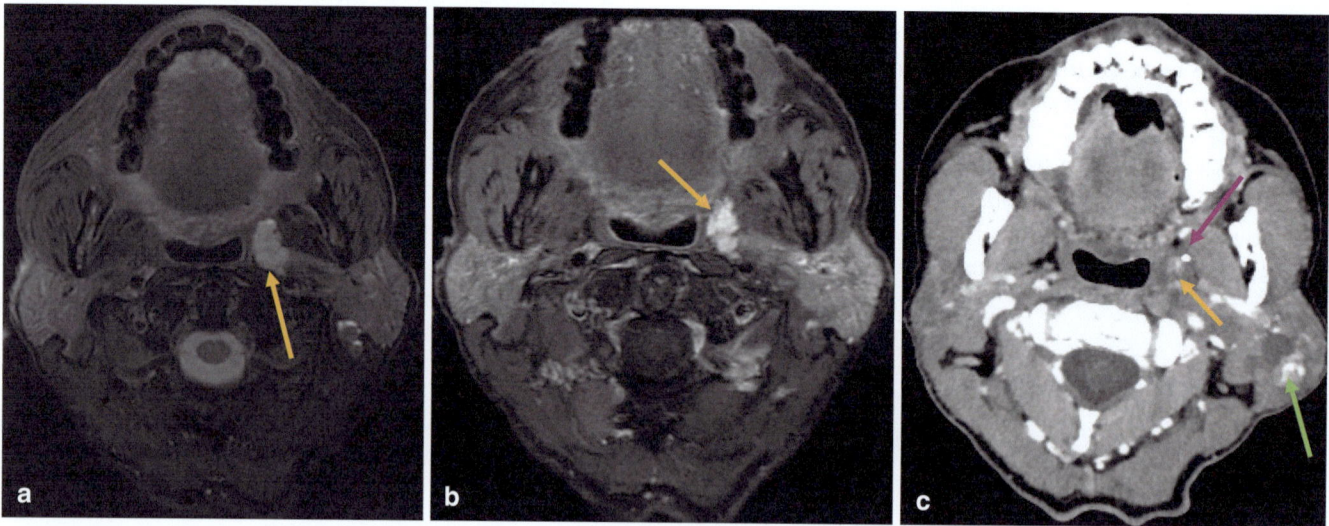

Fig. 38.6 Venous vascular malformation in the PPS. Axial T2WI (**a**), post-contrast T1WI (**b**), and contrast-enhanced CT (**c**) demonstrating a T2 hyperintense, enhancing lesion (yellow arrows) with internal phleboliths (pink arrow) in the left PPS, consistent with a venous vascular malformation. Additional venous malformation is also seen in the left parotid gland. (green arrow)

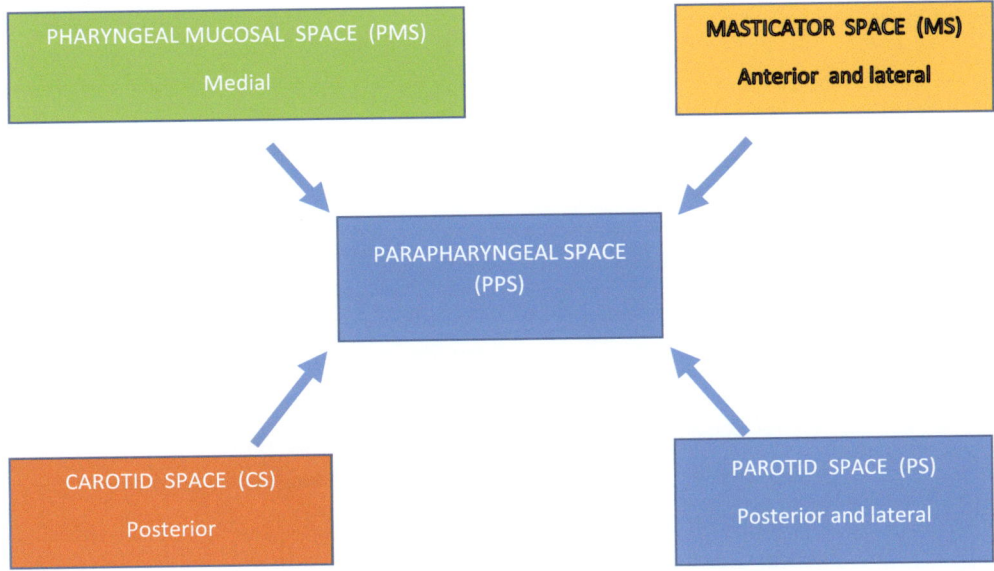

Parotid Space (Ps)

- Extends from external auditory canal to the angle of the mandible [15].
- Lateral to PPS and CS, posterior to MS and invested by SLDCF (Fig. 38.1).
- No fascia at superomedial aspect of the gland, allowing direct communication with the PPS [3, 15].
- PPS displaced anteromedially by PS mass lesions (Fig. 38.5) [2, 10].
- Parotid gland is divided into superficial and deep lobes by the facial nerve.
- Identifying the facial nerve in the parotid gland is difficult on imaging and the adjacent retromandibular vein, which is located medial to the facial nerve is used as a landmark on cross-sectional imaging (Fig. 38.7) [10].
- Localization of lesions into superficial and deep lobes is important to prevent inadvertent facial nerve injury during resection [10].
- The parotid gland is the only salivary gland to contain lymph nodes; lymphadenopathy must be included in the differential diagnosis for any PS mass lesion [2, 10].
- CONTENTS:
  o Superficial and deep lobes of the parotid gland.
  o Intraparotid lymph nodes (normal finding due to embryologically late encapsulation of the gland) [10].
  o Facial nerve.
  o External carotid artery branches and retromandibular vein.
- PATHOLOGY: Table 38.2
  o Benign and malignant salivary neoplasms (70% benign).

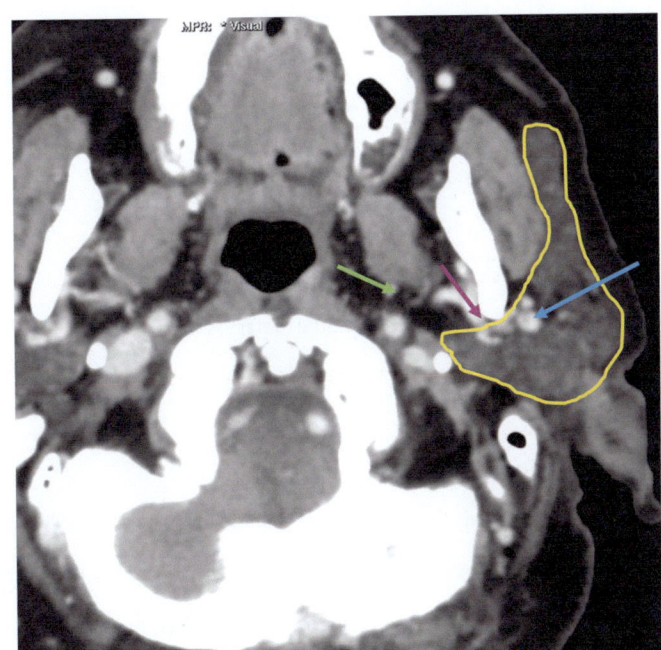

Fig. 38.7 Axial contrast-enhanced CT demonstrating the left parotid space (yellow line) with the deep lobe of parotid gland projecting through stylomandibular tunnel (pink arrow) to abut the PPS fat (green arrow). Identifying the facial nerve is difficult on imaging and the retromandibular vein (blue arrow), which is located medial to the facial nerve is used as a landmark on cross-sectional imaging

  o Metastases to intraparotid lymph nodes from skin squamous cell carcinoma and melanoma.
  o Lymphoma.
  o Parotitis, sarcoidosis, Sjogrens, juvenile recurrent parotitis.
  o Hemangioma, type I branchial cleft cyst.

Table 38.2 Differential diagnosis for parotid space lesions

Parotid gland:
Neoplastic: Primary benign (BMT/PA and Warthins tumors) and malignant tumors (mucoepidermoid carcinoma, adenoid cystic carcinoma, acinic cell carcinoma, oncocytoma, carcinoma ex pleomorphic adenoma, etc.)
Inflammatory/infectious: Parotitis, abscess, HIV with lymphothelial lesions, juvenile recurrent parotitis
Vascular tumors and vascular malformations: Hemangioma, lymphatic malformation, venous malformation
Lymph nodes: Metastases from skin cancer, melanoma and lymphoma
Facial nerve: Perineural spread of tumor and neurogenic tumors
Congenital lesion: Type I branchial cleft cyst

Table 38.3 Parotid space inflammatory pathology

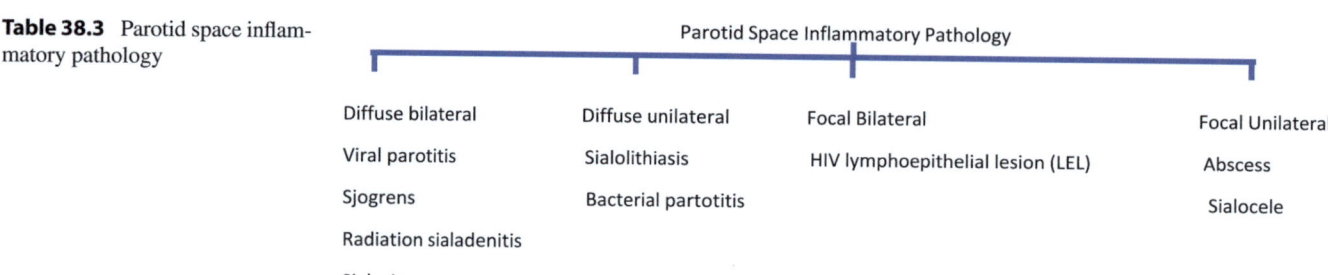

Table 38.4 Parotid space focal masses

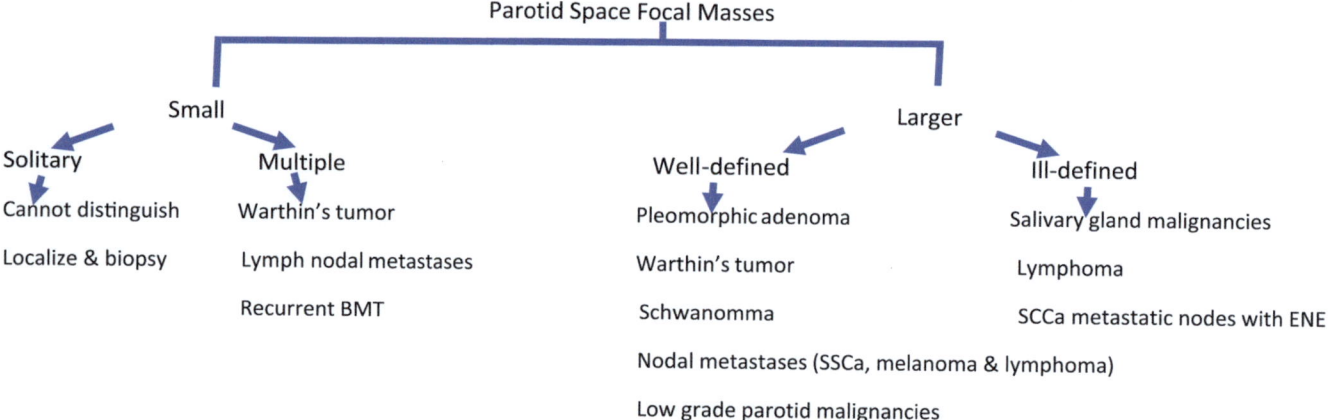

Multiple unilateral parotid lesions with ipsilateral cervical lymph nodes: Think nodal metastases

Multiple bilateral parotid lesions with bilateral cervical lymph nodes: Think of lymphoma

Multiple bilateral cystic and solid parotid lesions, no cervical lymph nodes: Think Warthin tumor

Multiple unilateral, very T2 hyperintense parotid lesions: Think recurrent BMT

- The purpose of imaging PS masses is not to provide an exact diagnosis given the diverse neoplastic histology of this space, a specific diagnosis cannot be reliably predicted based on cross-sectional imaging [2].
- Key imaging considerations include well-defined versus ill-defined margins, unifocal versus multifocal location, solid versus cystic, and homogeneous versus heterogeneous appearance (Tables 38.3 and 38.4) [10].
- Malignant lesions may appear well-defined and benign on cross-sectional imaging [10]. An ill-defined appearance more likely suggests malignancy or infection (Fig. 38.8) [10].
- Multiplicity is also helpful in the differential diagnosis of parotid pathology with differentials including non-Hodgkin lymphoma, HIV with lymphoepithelial lesions, Sjogren's disease, and Warthin's tumor (Fig. e38.3) (Tables 38.3 and 38.4) [10].

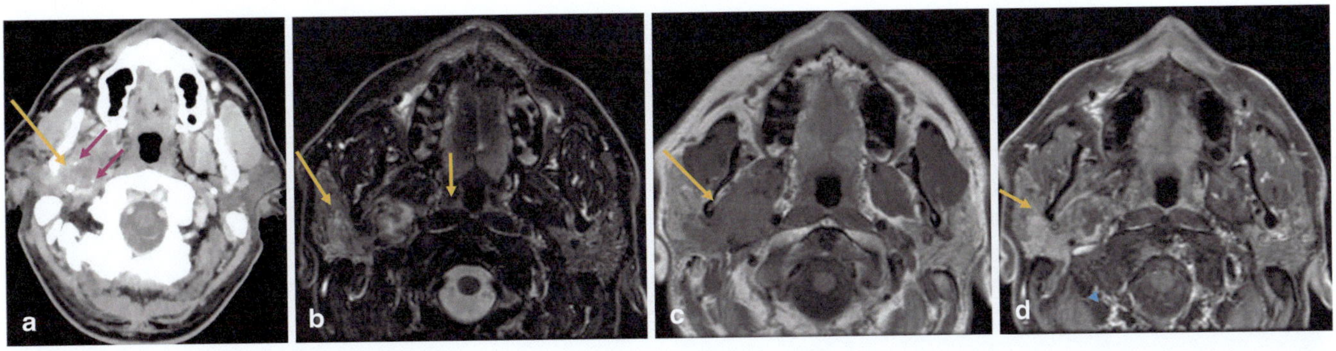

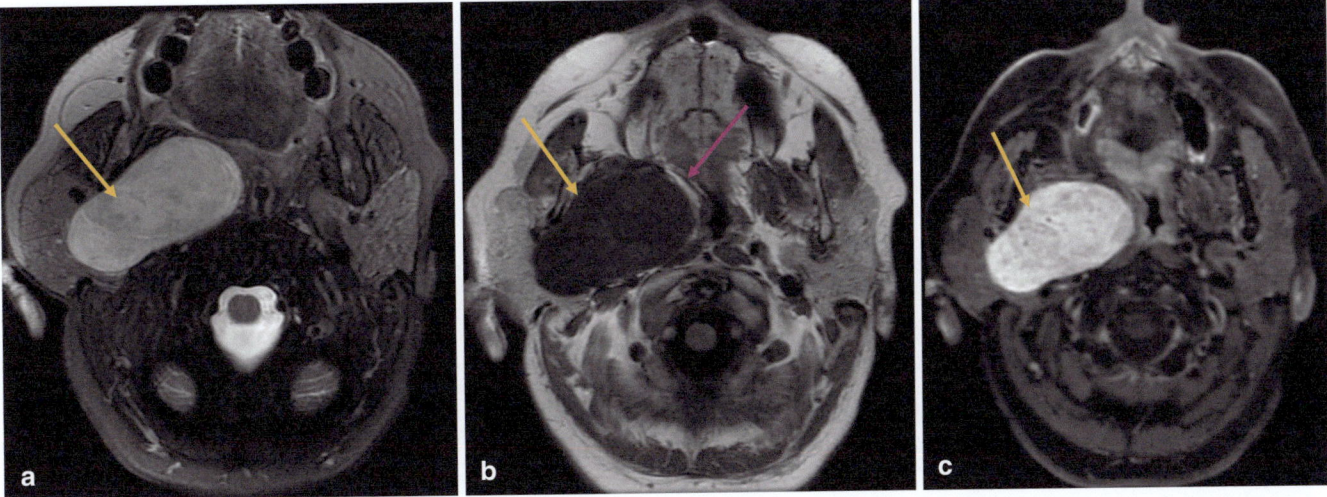

Fig. 38.8 Parotid Malignancy. Contrast-enhanced CT (**a**), axial T2WI with fat saturation (**b**), axial T1WI (**c**), and axial post-contrast T1WI with fat saturation (**d**) images in a 63-year-old female presenting with right facial paralysis, demonstrating an ill-defined, heterogenous T2 signal, heterogeneously enhancing mass (yellow arrows) with scattered punctate calcifications (pink arrows) in the superficial and deep lobes of the right parotid gland with perineural spread along the right facial nerve (blue arrows). Imaging findings are consistent with a malignant parotid mass. Pathology was consistent with carcinoma ex pleomorphic adenoma

Fig. 38.9 Pleomorphic Adenoma. Axial T2WI (**a**), T1WI (**b**) and post-contrast T1WI (**c**) images demonstrating a large, very T2 hyperintense, enhancing lesion (yellow arrows) arising from the deep lobe of the right parotid gland, causing anteromedial displacement right PPS fat (pink arrow). Imaging findings are typical for pleomorphic adenoma which was confirmed on pathology

- The parotid lymph nodes represent the first echelon drainage for cancers of the external auditory canal as well as skin cancers of the scalp and face.
- Most common primary salivary neoplasms is benign mixed tumor (BMT) or pleomorphic adenoma (PA) and characteristically demonstrates very high signal on T2-weighted and ADC scans (Fig. 38.9) [2, 16]. Although these lesions are benign, they are often surgically removed for cosmetic reasons and potential risk of malignant degeneration. Complete resection at the time of initial surgery is critical as residual tumor can create multiple daughter lesions that are difficult to resect (Fig. 38.10) [10].
- Acute parotitis may occur due to obstruction by calculi, retrograde migration of oral flora secondary to poor salivary flow, or hematogenous viral infection [2].
- Chronic parotitis is typically bilateral and reflects underlying systemic disease such as Sjogren syndrome or sarcoidosis [2].

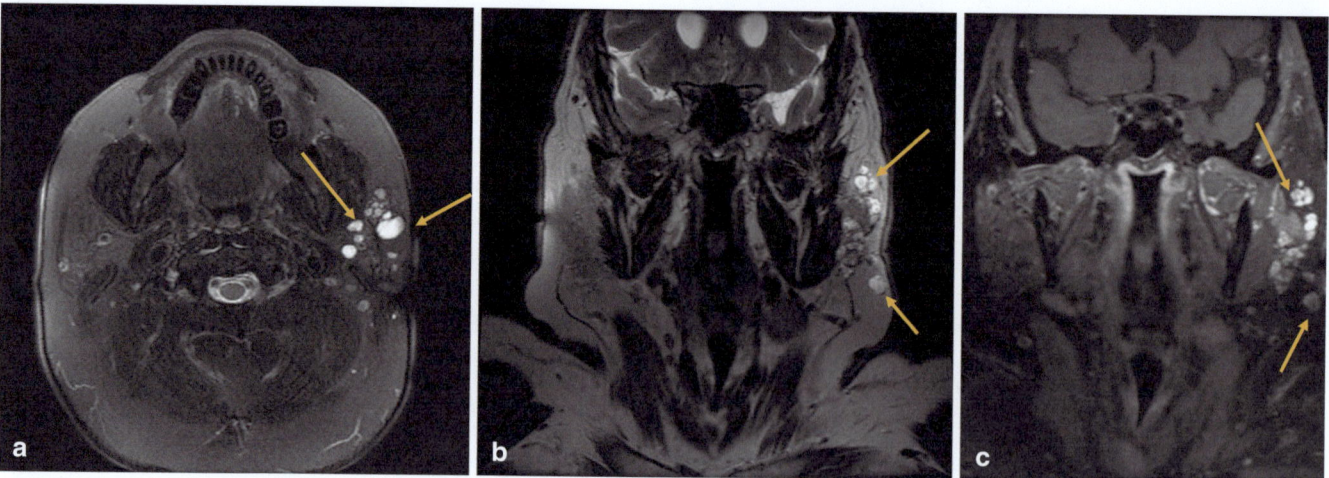

Fig. 38.10 Recurrent Pleomorphic Adenoma. Axial T2WI with fat saturation (**a**), coronal T2WI (**b**), and coronal post-contrast T1WI (**c**) images in a 69-year-old female with history of left parotid pleomorphic adenoma, status post excision in the 1980s, demonstrating cluster of multiple, well-defined, very T2 hyperintense, enhancing lesions (yellow arrows) within the operative bed and adjacent soft tissues, compatible with recurrent pleomorphic adenoma

Masticator Space (Ms)

- Largest suprahyoid neck space extending craniocaudally from skull base to the inferior mandible [10].
- Divided into suprazygomatic and infrazygomatic portions [10].
- Anterior to PS, lateral to the PPS, and invested by the SLDCF (Fig. 38.2).
- Broad attachment superiorly to skull base contacting foramen ovale (containing mandibular division of fifth cranial nerve) and foramen spinosum (containing the middle meningeal artery) [10].
- PPS displaced posteromedially by MS mass lesions (Fig. 38.5) [2].
- Most pathology of the MS arises in the neighboring spaces, with the most common being odontogenic infection arising from molar teeth (Fig. 38.11) [2].
- CONTENTS:
  - Mandible.
  - Muscles of mastication.
  - Mandibular division of trigeminal nerve and inferior alveolar nerve.
- PATHOLOGY: Table 38.5
  - Odontogenic infections.
  - Sarcoma lives here; common neoplastic lesion in an adult is leiomyosarcoma or malignant fibrous histiocytoma, whereas rhabdomyosarcoma is the most common MS space neoplasm in a child [10].
  - Perineural tumor spread along V3, neurogenic tumors.
  - Venous vascular malformations.
  - Accessory parotid tissue on surface of masseter muscle.

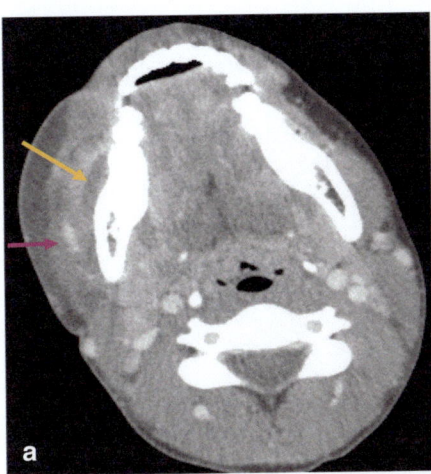
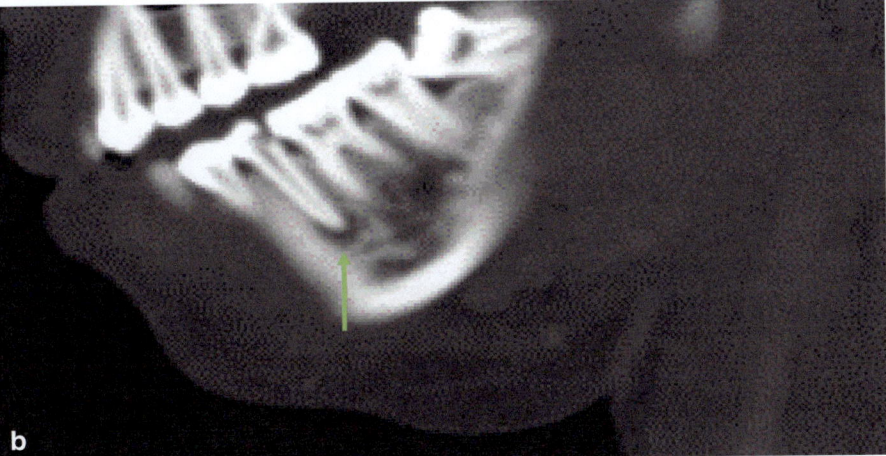

Fig. 38.11 Odontogenic Abscess. Axial contrast-enhanced CT (**a**) and sagittal CT reconstruction (**b**), in a 29-year-old female presenting with right facial swelling, demonstrating a fluid collection in the right masticator space (yellow arrow) and inflammatory enlargement of the right masseter muscle (pink arrow), representing an odontogenic abscess arising from the right mandibular premolar tooth (green arrow)

Table 38.5 Differential diagnosis for masticator space lesions

Muscles of mastication: Sarcomas arising from muscle, bone, and other soft tissues, lymphoma, benign masseteric hypertrophy, denervation atrophy, myositis ossificans
Mandibular division of V3: Perineural spread of tumor, neurogenic tumors
Mandible: Osteomyelitis, odontogenic lesions, primary jaw tumors, metastases
Secondary extension into MS: Deep spread of SCC from oropharynx or retromolar trigone, inferior extension of intracranial or skull base lesions.
Congenital/developmental lesions: Hemangioma, lymphatic malformation, venous malformation

Sublingual Space (Sls)

- Also called the floor of the mouth.
- Horse shoe-shaped space parallel to the mandibular body.
- Bordered anteriorly by the mandible, medially by the midline genioglossus/geniohyoid muscle complex, inferolaterally by the mylohyoid muscle and superomedially by the mucosa of the floor of the mouth and intrinsic tongue muscles (Fig. 38.12) [17].
- The right and left SLS communicate anteriorly under the frenulum of the tongue [18].
- Majority of neoplasms in this region are squamous cell carcinomas originating from the oral mucosa.
- Salivary epithelial tumors may arise from the major salivary glands (sublingual and submandibular glands) or from minor salivary glands in the SLS.
- Obstruction of the sublingual gland or submucosal minor salivary gland duct may result in the formation of a ranula (epithelial-lined cyst) in the SLS. When ranulas rupture, they form pseudocysts that may "dive" or "plunge" behind the posterior free edge of the mylohyoid muscle into the SMS (Fig. 38.13).
- CONTENTS
  - Sublingual gland and duct, deep portion of the submandibular gland and duct.
  - Lingual artery and vein.
  - Lingual nerve (branch of CN V), branches of glossopharyngeal (IX) and hypoglossal (XII) nerves.
- PATHOLOGY
  - Sialadenitis, sialocele.
  - Ludwigs angina.
  - Sublingual gland neoplasm (30% benign).
  - Ranula.
  - Squamous cell carcinoma of floor of mouth and oral tongue.
  - Obstructed submandibular gland duct (Wharton's duct).
  - Sialolithasias.
  - Dermoid and epidermoid inclusion cyst.
  - Venous and lymphatic malformation.

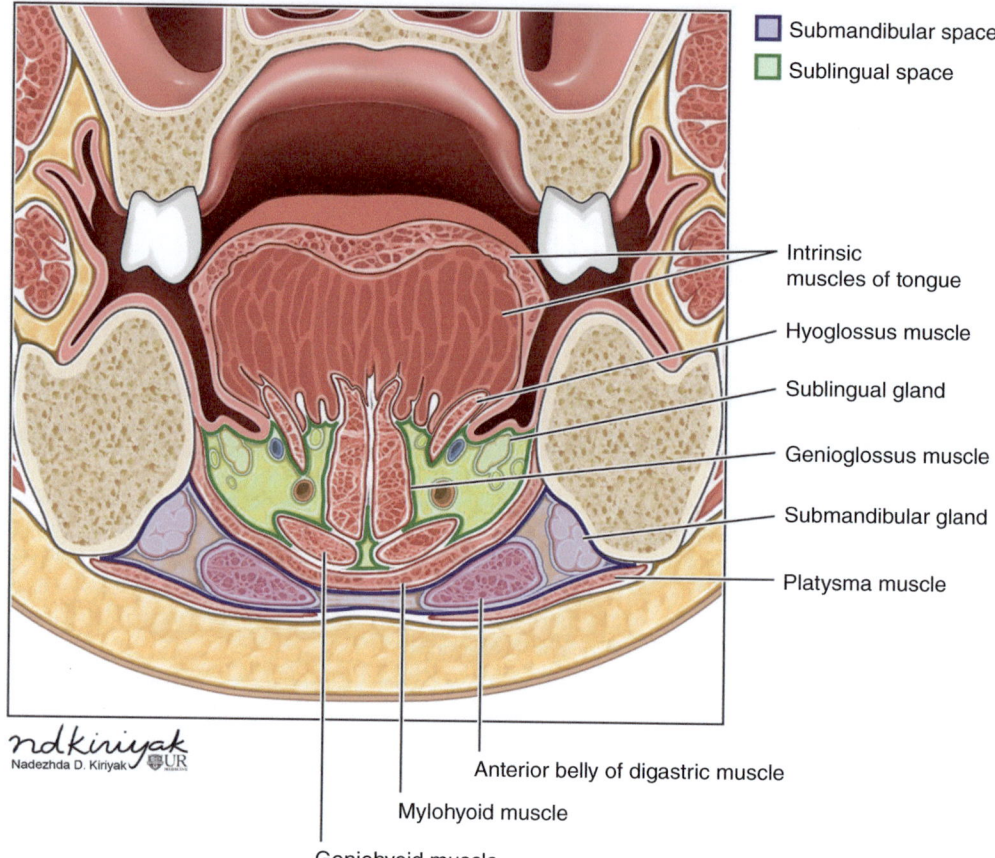

Fig. 38.12 Coronal graphic demonstrating the sling-like mylohyoid muscle separating the SLS (green) from the SMS (blue)

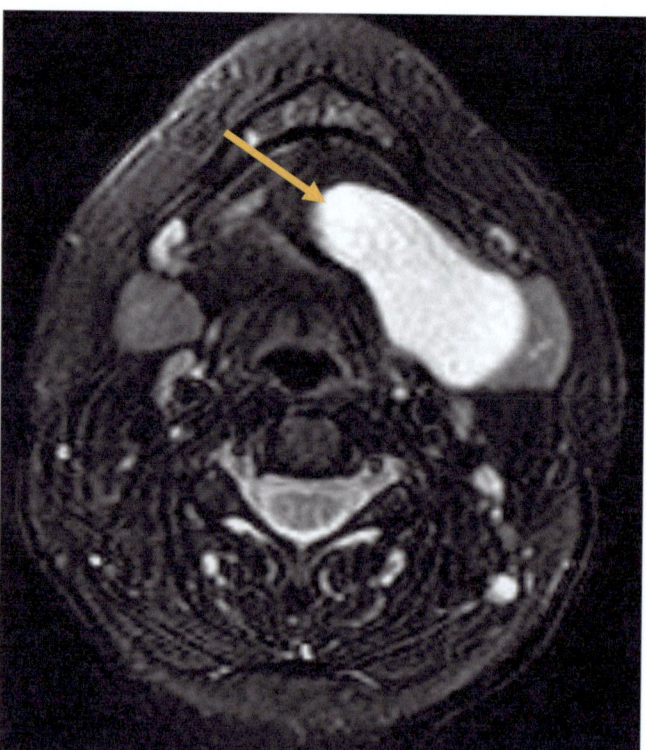

Fig. 38.13 Plunging Ranula. Axial T2WI demonstrating a "diving" or "plunging" ranula (yellow arrow), extending from the SLS to the SMS behind the posterior free margin of the mylohyoid muscle

Submandibular Space (Sms)

- Horseshoe-shaped space, orthogonal to the mandible.
- Located deep to the platysma and inferior and lateral to the mylohyoid muscle [19].
- Bound anteriorly and laterally by the mandible, medially by the anterior belly of the digastric muscles, superiorly by the mylohyoid muscle, and inferiorly by the hyoid bone (Fig. 38.12) [17, 19, 20].
- Enclosed by the superficial layer of deep cervical fascia except along the posterior margin of the mylohyoid muscle, permitting continuity with the SLS and communication with the PPS.
- The teeth and salivary glands are important sources of inflammation/infection in the SLS and SMS [2].
- CONTENTS:
    - Superficial portion of the submandibular gland.
    - Anterior belly of the digastric muscles.
    - Fat.
    - Lymph nodes.
    - Facial artery and facial vein.
    - Inferior loop of the hypoglossal nerve.
- PATHOLOGY:
    - Sialadenitis/abscess.
    - Ludwigs angina.
    - Diving ranula.
    - Salivary gland neoplasm (50% benign).
    - Minor salivary gland tumors.
    - Sialolithasias.
    - Lymph nodal metastases, lymphoma, TB, cat scratch disease, reactive lymph nodes.
    - Venous and lymphatic malformations.
    - Second branchial cleft cyst.

Buccal Space (Bs)

- Does not have complete fascial coverings.
- Located lateral to the buccinator muscle and deep to the zygomaticus major muscle and bordered posteriorly by the MS (Fig. 38.14) [21].
- It is separated from the subcutaneous tissues of the face by the plane formed by the superficial muscle of facial expression and the investing fascia [22].
- CONTENTS:
    - Fat.
    - Minor salivary glands.
    - Parotid duct.

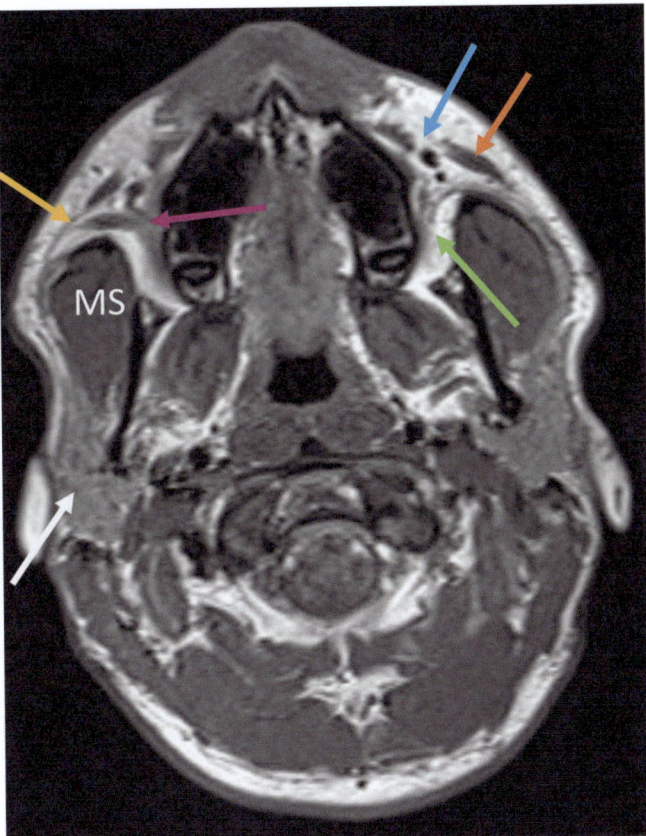

Fig. 38.14 Axial T1WI demonstrates the parotid gland (white arrow) and parotid duct (yellow arrow) running over the masseter muscle (MS) to pierce the buccinator muscle (pink arrow). Buccal space (green arrow) is seen anterior to the masticator space, lateral to the buccinator muscle (pink arrow), and deep to the zygomaticus major muscle (orange arrow). The facial vein (blue arrow) is located within the buccal space

-
    - Lymph nodes.
    - Facial vein and facial and buccal arteries.
    - Buccal branches of the VII and V cranial nerves.
- PATHOLOGY:
    - Lipoma.
    - Squamous cell carcinoma (direct extension or nodal metastases), lymphoma, minor salivary gland tumors, and sarcoma.
    - Hemangioma, venous vascular malformations (Fig. 38.15).
    - Obstructed duct, accessory parotid tissue.
    - Sebaceous cysts.
    - Cellulitis and abscess.

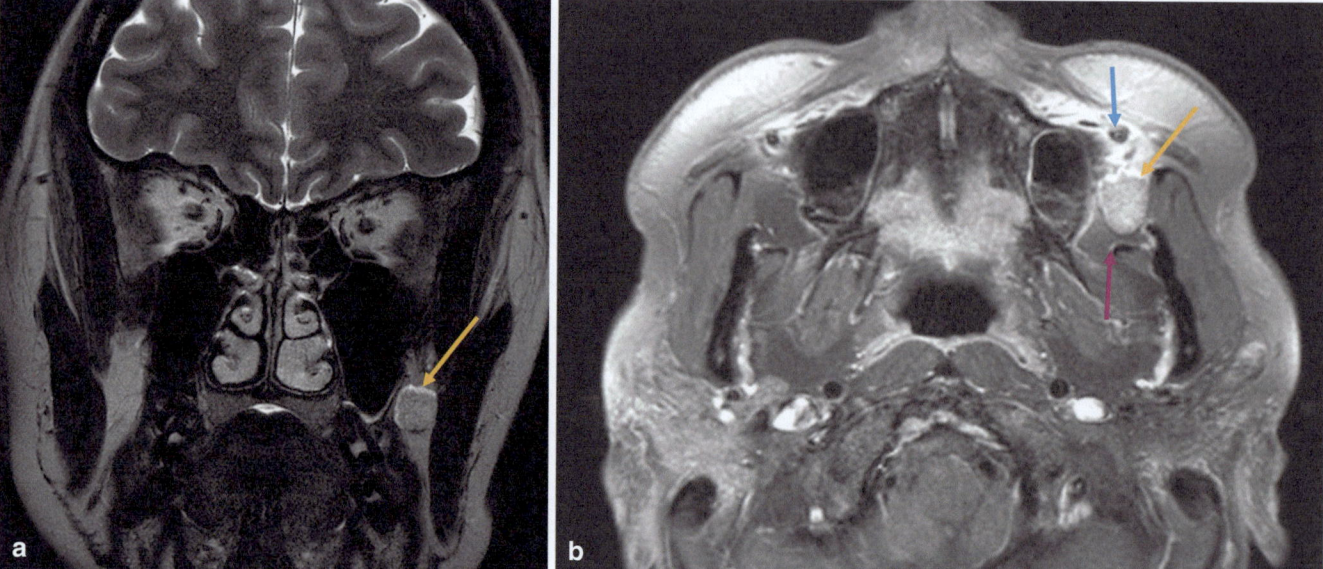

Fig. 38.15 Incidental left buccal space venous vascular malformation. Coronal T2WI (**a**) and axial post-contrast T1WI (**b**), demonstrating a well defined, lobulated, T2 hyperintense, enhancing venous malformation in the right buccal space (yellow arrows), located posterior to the left facial vein (blue arrow) and anterior to the left lateral pterygoid muscle (pink arrow)

Carotid Space (Cs)

- Spans the suprahyoid and infrahyoid neck, extending from the skull base to the aortic arch.
- All three layers of the deep cervical fascia contribute to the carotid sheath (Fig. 38.16) [23].
- The fascia is incomplete above the angle of the mandible, so the CS contents lie within the area of the PPS [13]. Also sometimes referred to as the post-styloid PPS [24].
- Can be subdivided into nasopharyngeal, oropharyngeal, cervical, and mediastinal components [3, 11].
- The suprahyoid CS abuts the MS and PPS anteriorly, PMS anteromedially, PS laterally, RPS medially, and PVS posteriorly (Fig. 38.1) [25]. The CS abuts the carotid canal, hypoglossal canal, and jugular foramen at the skull base.
- The infrahyoid CS abuts the anterior cervical space anteriorly, VS and RPS medially and posterior cervical space, and PVS posteriorly (Fig. 38.2).
- CONTENTS:
  - Suprahyoid CS: Carotid artery, internal jugular vein (IJV), IX-XII cranial nerves, sympathetic chain, and lymph nodes.
  - Infrahyoid CS: Carotid artery, IJV, and X cranial nerve as all cranial nerves have exited except the vagus nerve (Williams DW III & Fruin M). The internal jugular nodal chain is associated with but not in the infrahyoid CS.
  - Within the carotid sheath, the carotid artery is located medially, IJV laterally, vagus nerve posteriorly along the vessels, and sympathetic chain posteromedially within the sheath (Fig. 38.16).
- CS space masses push adjacent structures in different directions depending on the level (Table 38.6).
- Carotid space is the so-called Lincoln Highway of the neck and serves as a route for travel of infection or malignancy from the neck into the mediastinum [26].
- CT and MR angiography or venography are studies of choice for vascular lesions/pathologies (Table 38.7) [2].
- Attention should be paid to the carotid space to exclude dissection in any patient presenting with Horner's syndrome (Table 38.7).
- IJV thrombophlebitis caused by an extension of oropharyngeal or odontogenic infection is called Lemierre syndrome (Fig. 38.17).
- Glomus vagale and carotid body paragangliomas arise in the carotid space. Carotid body tumors are located at the carotid bifurcation in the infrahyoid neck and splay the internal and external carotid arteries (Fig. 38.18). The rare glomus vagale is located in the high nasopharyngeal carotid space within 2 cm of the skull base (Fig. 38.21).
- On MRI, paragangliomas intensely enhance and demonstrate classic "salt and pepper" appearance with the "salt" representing microhemorrhages on T1-weighted images and the pepper representing flow voids on T2-weighted images (Fig. 38.18).

Fig. 38.16 Axial graphic showing the contribution of all three layers of the deep cervical fascia to the carotid sheath. Within the carotid sheath, the carotid artery is located medially, IJV laterally, vagus nerve posteriorly along the vessels, and sympathetic chain posteromedially within the sheath

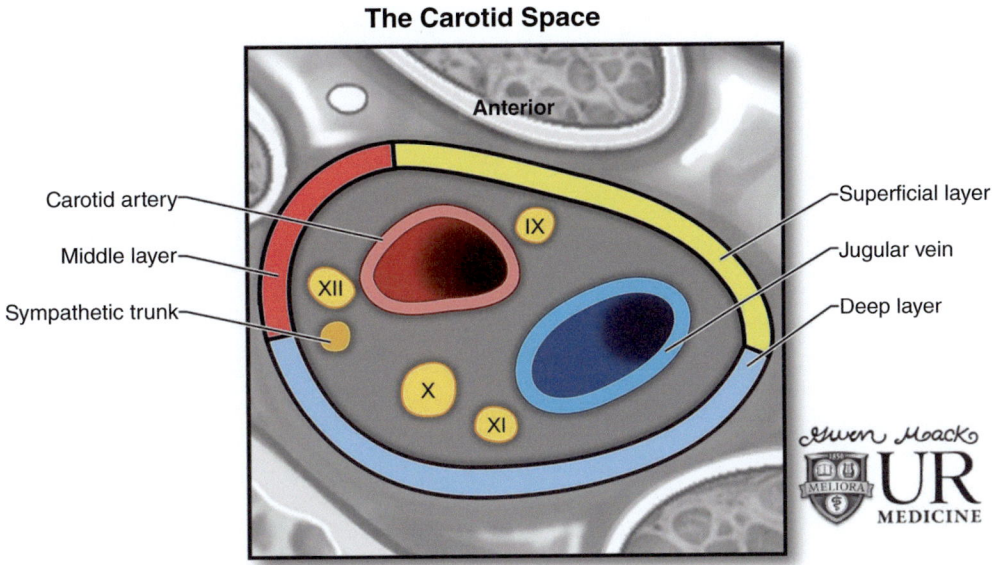

Table 38.6 Displacement of adjacent spaces and structures by CS mass lesions

Nasopharyngeal level: Displaces PPS anteriorly, styloid process anterolaterally, and splays the carotid and IJV, often displacing ICA anteriorly and IJV posterolaterally
Oropharyngeal level: Displaces PPS anteriorly, posterior belly of the digastric muscle anterolaterally and may splay the ECA-ICA bifurcation
Infrahyoid level: Intimate relation to the carotid artery and IJV

Table 38.7 Differential diagnosis for carotid space lesions

Carotid artery: Atherosclerosis, aneurysm, pseudoaneurysm, dissection, thrombosis, fibromuscular dysplasia, carotidynia, encasement by direct spread of SCCa, ectatic arteries and retropharyngeal course
Jugular vein: Asymmetric enlarged jugular vein, thrombosis, thrombophlebitis
Lymph nodes: Metastatic cervical adenopathy, inflammatory adenopathy, lymphoma
Cranial nerves (IX-XII and sympathetic chain): Neurogenic tumors (Schwanomma, neurofibroma)
Neoplasm: Paraganglioma (carotid body tumor and glomus vagale), meningioma (inferior extension of jugular foramen meningiomas or rarely, primary extradural meningiomas arising from embryologic arachnoid rests

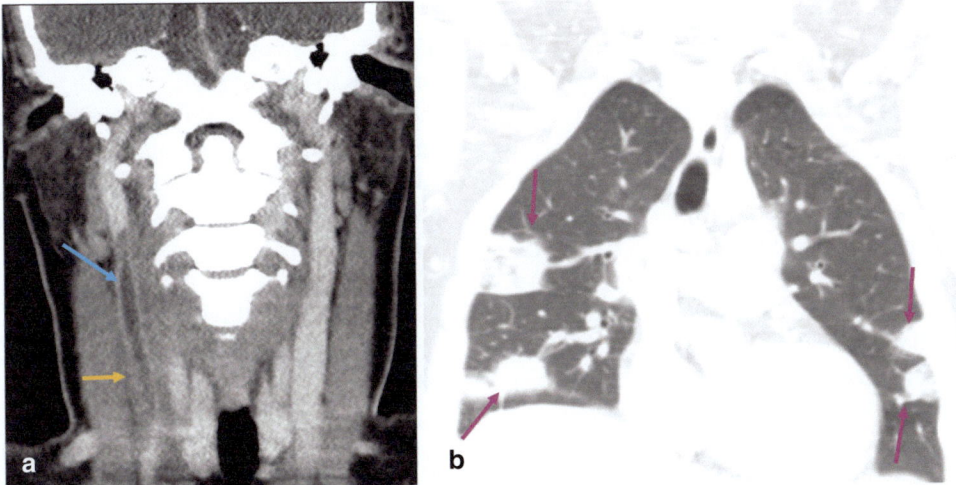

Fig. 38.17 Lemierre Syndrome. Coronal contrast-enhanced CT (**a**) demonstrates an occlusive thrombus in the right internal jugular vein (blue arrow) with surrounding inflammatory changes (yellow arrows), consistent with thrombophlebitis. Coronal CT (**b**) through the chest demonstrates multiple nodular opacities in bilateral lungs (pink arrows), some of which demonstrate central cavitation consistent with septic emboli. This patient was found to have pharyngitis with resulting septic thrombophlebitis caused by Fusobacterium necrophorum, seen with Lemierre syndrome

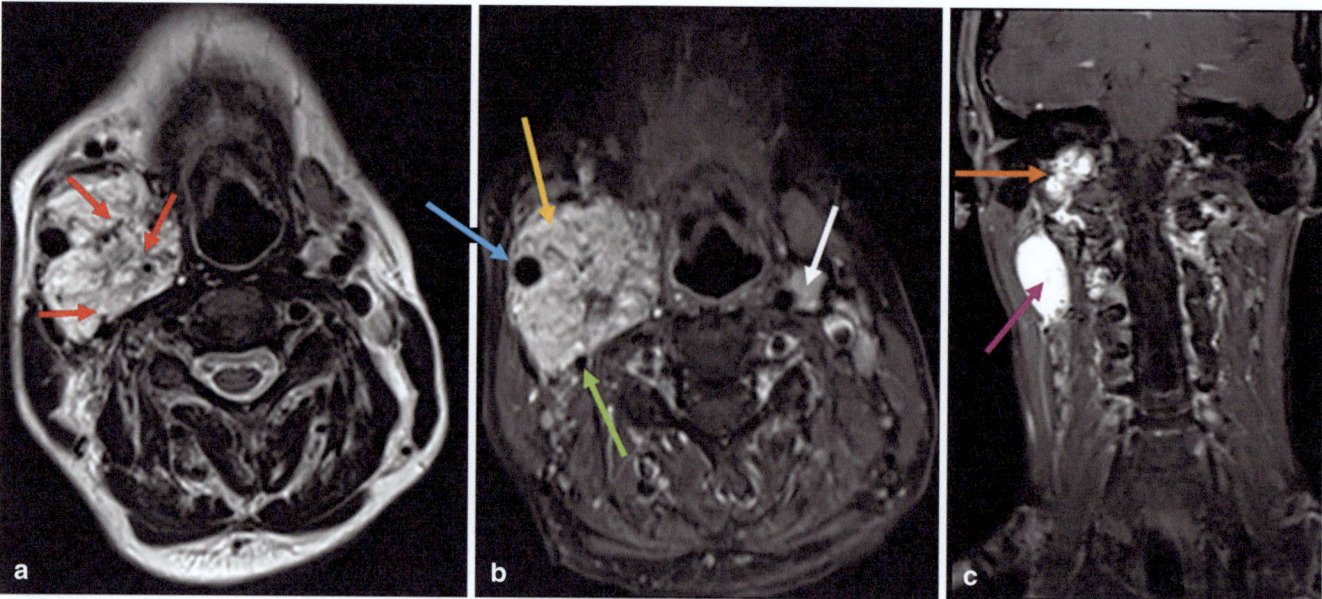

Fig. 38.18 Neck Paragangliomas. Axial T2WI (**a**), axial (**b**), and coronal (**c**) post-contrast T1WI's demonstrating a classic right glomus carotid paraganglioma with multiple internal flow voids (red arrows) and avid enhancement (yellow arrow), causing splaying of right ECA (blue arrow) and right ICA (green arrow). Additional right vagal (pink arrow), right jugular (orange arrow), and left carotid (white arrow) paragangliomas are also identified

- Structures within the CS are displaced depending on the pathology which serves as a differentiating imaging characteristic. Vagal and sympathetic schwannomas share the same imaging appearance but a vagal schwannoma splays ICA anteromedially and IJV posterolaterally whereas a sympathetic schwannoma displaces both structures anteriorly [27].
- In children the most common primary malignancy of the carotid sheath is a neuroblastoma [22].

Retropharyngeal And Danger Spaces (Rps/Ds)

- RPS is a fat-filled space between the MLDCF anteriorly and alar fascia posteriorly and laterally (Fig. e38.1) [9, 11, 28].
- DLDCF has two components: Alar and prevertebral fascia which results in the formation of three posterior neck spaces, RPS between visceral and alar fascia, DS between alar and prevertebral fascia, and PVS between the prevertebral fascia and the vertebral periosteum.
- Bordered anteriorly by the PMS, posteriorly by the PVS, laterally by the PS, and limited medially by a median raphe. The median raphe divides the RPS into two halves and is difficult to identify with imaging.

Table 38.8 Differential diagnosis for retropharyngeal space lesions

Inflammatory: Cellulitis, nodes, abscess
Neoplasm: Direct invasion by PMS SCCa
Lymph nodes: Nodal spread from Nasopharyneal carcinoma, PMS SCCa's, PMS lymphoma, sarcomas, thyroid tumors
Congenital: Lymphatic malformation, venous malformations, hemangiomas
Pseudomasses: Retropharyngeal course of carotid artery

- RPS terminates at the T3 vertebral level, DS extends more inferiorly to a point just above the diaphragm, and PVS continues to the coccyx.
- These spaces cannot be distinguished separately on imaging; however, it is important to track posterior neck space collections inferiorly, recognizing that they may extend to the chest or below.
- CONTENTS:
  - Fat.
  - Retropharyngeal lymph nodes (lateral retropharyngeal node = nodes of Rouviere).
- Pathology: Table 38.8
  - Edema/fluid, cellulitis and abscess.
  - RPS lymph nodes: Reactive adenopathy, suppurative adenitis (Fig. 38.19), metastatic adenopathy and lymphoma.
  - Secondary extension into the RPS: direct extension from squamous cell carcinoma.

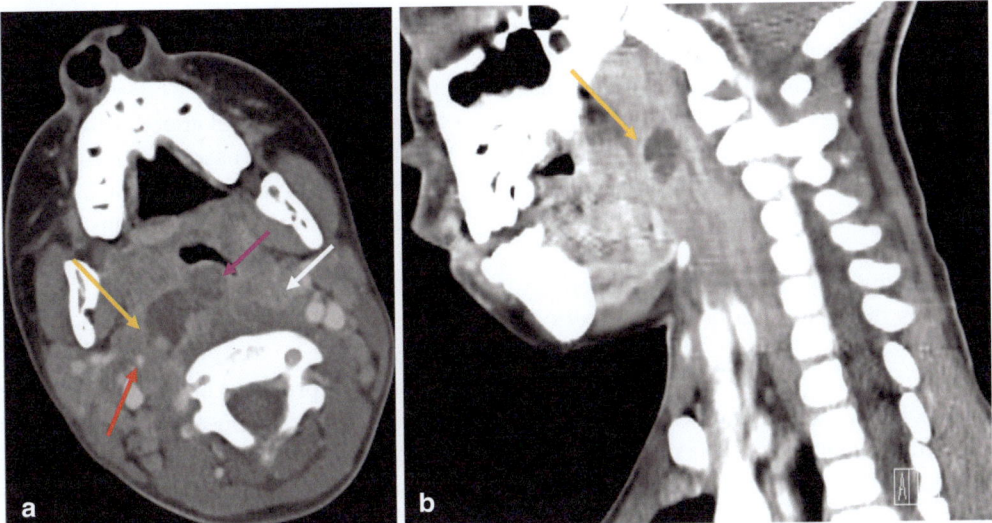

Fig. 38.19 Suppurative right retropharyngeal adenitis/abscess. Axial (**a**) and sagittal (**b**) contrast-enhanced CT images in a 5-year-old male presenting with fever and right-sided neck pain, demonstrating suppurative right retropharyngeal lymphadenopathy (yellow arrows) that has ruptured medially forming a retropharyngeal abscess (pink arrows). Additionally, there is spasm of the right ICA adjacent to the suppurative right RPS nodes (red arrow). Prominent left RPS nodes are also seen (white arrow)

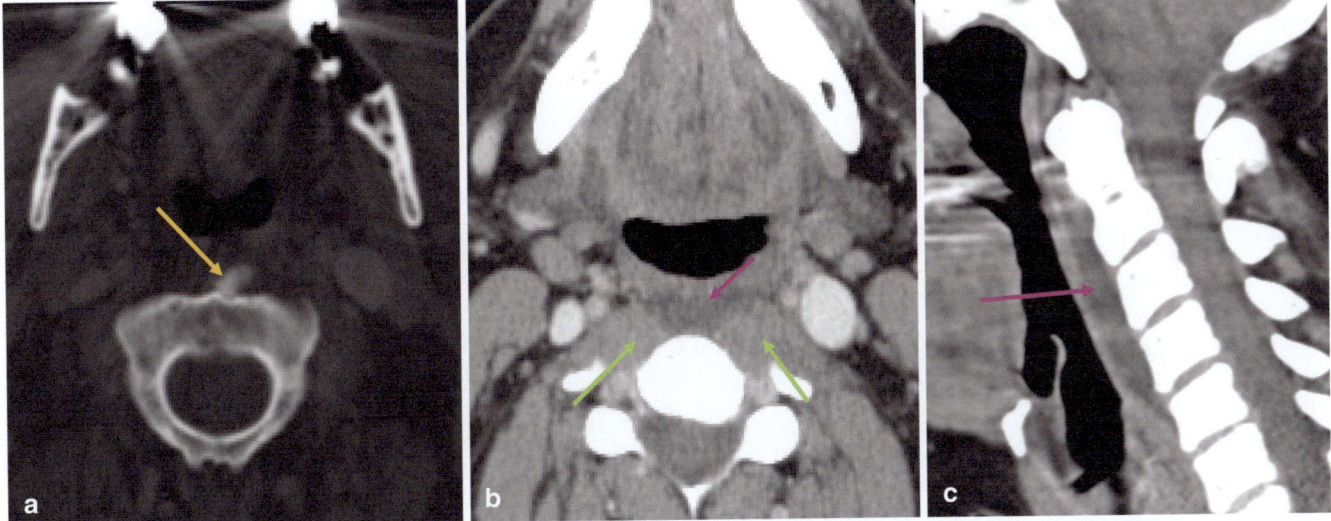

Fig. 38.20 Acute calcific longus colli tendinitis. 51-year-old female with progressively worsening neck pain over 2 days. Axial CT in bone (**a**) and soft tissue windows (**b**) and sagittal CT (**c**), demonstrates calcification in the prevertebral musculature (yellow arrow) with a sympathetic retropharyngeal effusion (pink arrows), consistent with acute calcific longus colli tendinitis. Note that the retropharyngeal effusion is located anterior to the prevertebral muscles (green arrows)

- o Tortuous carotid artery.
- o Lipoma.
- o Hemangioma.
- RPS Edema or effusion may occur due to wide variety of disease processes, including pharyngitis, lymphatic or venous obstruction, angioedema, longus colli tendinitis (Fig. 38.20) and radiation therapy [29].

Perivertebral Space (Pvs)

- Cylindrical space around the vertebral column, traversing the SHN and IHN, extending from the skull base to the mediastinum (T4 level) (Figs. 38.1 and 38.2).
- Invested in the DLDCF which is interrupted by traversing brachial plexus nerve roots.

- The DLDCF divides the PVS into an anterior prevertebral space and posterior paraspinal space [30, 31].
- RPS lies anterior and paired carotid spaces lie anterolateral to the PVS (Fig. 38.1).
- The prevertebral muscles are invested in the anterior deep layer of the DCF, known as the "carpet" by surgeons. It is tough and serves as a barrier to infection and neoplasm [2].
- PVS lesions displace the prevertebral muscles anteriorly, whereas RPS lesions displace these muscles posteriorly [2].
- CONTENTS:
  - Vertebral bodies, intervertebral discs.
  - Musculature: Prevertebral and scalene muscles.
  - Vertebral arteries in foramen transversarium.
  - Phrenic nerve.
- PATHOLOGY: Table 38.9
  - Degenerative: anterior disk herniation, diffuse idiopathic skeletal hyperostosis, and osteophytes.
  - Inflammatory/infectious: Discitis osteomyelitis, abscess, calcific tendinitis.
  - Bone tumors: Primary bone tumors and metastases.
  - Vascular: Vertebral artery aneurysm, dissection.
  - Extension from nasopharyngeal carcinoma, squamous cell carcinoma and lymphoma.
  - Majority of pathologic lesions in the PVS are centered in the vertebral bodies and disc spaces with pyogenic discitis/osteomyelitis (Fig. 38.21) and bone metastasis being the most common pathologies found in this space [2].
  - Certain primary bone tumors have characteristic locations and appearance such as chordomas which can be suggested when a vertebral lesion demonstrates characteristic bright T2 signal and enhancement [2].
  - The most common PVS malignancy in children is a rhabdomyosarcoma.

Table 38.9 Differential diagnosis for perivertebral space lesions

Degenerative: anterior disc herniation, DISH, osteophytes
Inflammatory: Discitis osteomyelitis, abscess, calcific tendinitis
Bone tumors: Primary bone tumors and metastases
Vascular: vertebral artery tortuosity, aneurysm, dissection
Secondary extension into the PVS: Direct extension from nasopharyngeal carcinoma, squamous cell carcinoma, and lymphoma

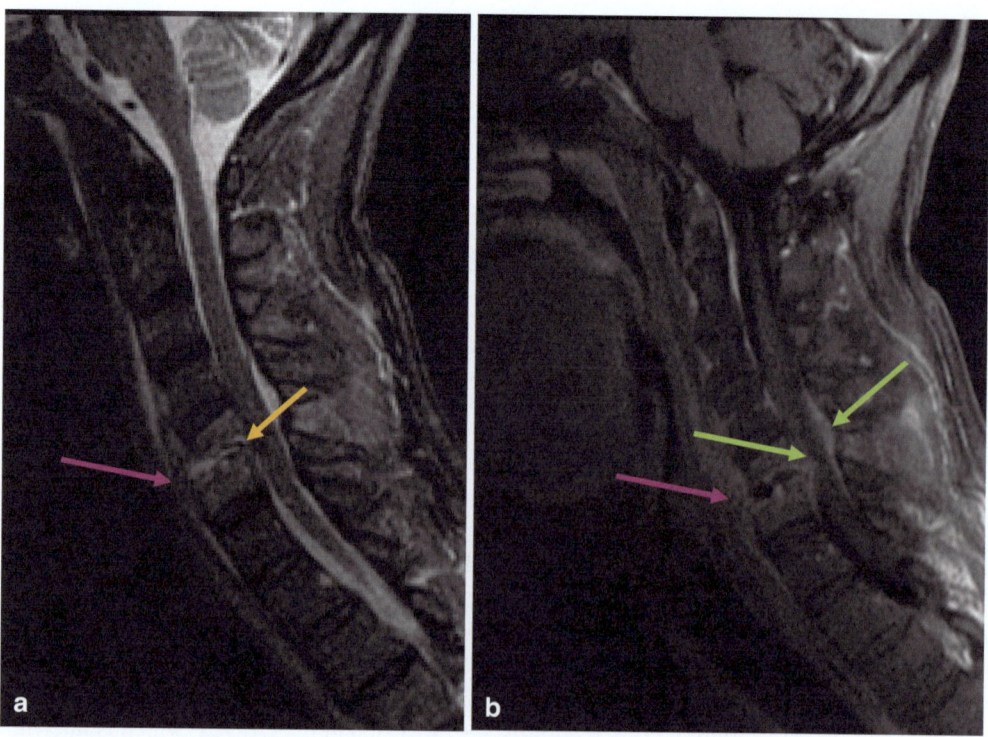

Fig. 38.21 Discitis osteomyelitis. Sagittal T2WI (**a**) and sagittal post-contrast T1WI (**b**), demonstrating C5-C6 discitis osteomyelitis (yellow arrow) with prevertebral (pink arrows) and epidural (green arrow) phlegmonous changes

Visceral Space (Vs)

- Cylindrical, central, infrahyoid space enclosed by the middle layer of deep cervical fascia (Fig. 38.2).
- Largest space in the infrahyoid neck and the only space that is found entirely in the IHN [32].
- The VS extends from the hyoid bone down into the mediastinum [33].
- It is bordered posteriorly by the RPS, posterolaterally by the CS, and laterally by the anterior cervical spaces (Fig. 38.2) [32, 33].
- CONTENTS:
  - Thyroid and parathyroid glands.
  - Larynx, trachea, hypopharynx, esophagus [33].
  - Recurrent laryngeal nerve: On the left recurs at the aortic arch and passes through the aortopulmonary window and on the right recurs around the right subclavian artery in the tracheoesophageal groove up to the larynx [19].
  - Level VI groups of lymph nodes (paratracheal, prelaryngeal, and pretracheal nodes).
  - Infrahyoid strap muscles.
- PATHOLOGY:
  - Infectious or inflammatory thyroiditis, thyroid nodules, thyroid cancer, parathyroid adenoma.
  - Mucosal squamous cell carcinoma, submucosal masses including minor salivary gland tumors, sarcomas, and lymphoma.
  - Parathyroid adenoma and carcinoma.
  - Schwanommas of the recurrent laryngeal nerve.
  - Chondrosarcoma of the laryngeal cartilages.
  - Congenital lesions: Infrahyoid thyroglossal duct cysts and ectopic thyroid tissue.
- Thyroid gland abnormalities are a major indication for imaging the VS. In general, ultrasound is the main imaging modality for inflammatory or infectious thyroiditis and intrathyroidal nodules (colloid cysts, adenomas, differentiated thyroid cancer, and metastases).
- Several ultrasound classification systems exist to risk stratify thyroid nodules and decide on biopsy, including American Thyroid Association (ATA), Society of Radiologists in Ultrasound (SRU), European (EU-TIRADS), and American College of Radiology Thyroid Imaging and Reporting Data System (ACR TIRADS) [34, 35].
- Thyroid cancer includes differentiated thyroid carcinomas (papillary and follicular), medullary and anaplastic carcinomas and non-Hodgkin lymphoma. Cross-sectional imaging is appropriate if there is a concern for extrathyroidal extension of tumor [36, 37].
- Thyroglossal duct cysts (TDC) are the most common congenital neck masses; present as movable mass that may fluctuate in size after upper respiratory tract infection. Characteristically midline when suprahyoid and often para-midline when infrahyoid.
- Parathyroid adenomas are hypervascular, demonstrate rapid wash-in on early arterial phase and relatively rapid wash-out on the on venous phase multiphase contrast-enhanced CT (Fig. 38.22) [38].

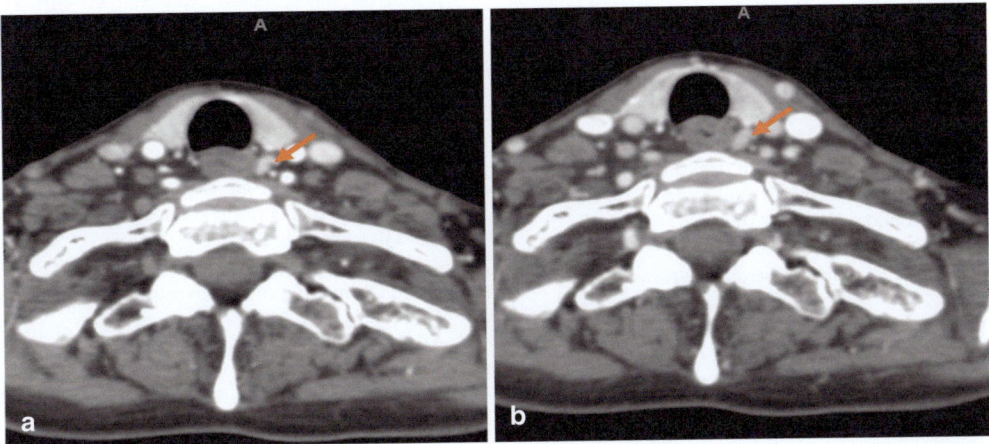

Fig. 38.22 Axial images of a 4D CT study in the arterial (**a**) and venous (**b**) phases demonstrating a parathyroid adenoma (orange arrows) posterior to left thyroid lobe. On the venous phase (**b**) there is washout of this adenoma when compared to the thyroid gland

Conclusion

- The neck is anatomically complex but can be organized into compartments or "spaces" in order to simplify the approach to neck masses [2].
- Each space has common and unusual pathology, based on the normal contents of the space [2]. Once a lesion is accurately localized to the correct space, the imaging features and clinical information are used to provide a clinically useful imaging differential diagnosis.
- Displacement of the PPS fat can help determine site of origin of a suprahyoid mass.
- Minor salivary gland tumors can be seen anywhere in the suprahyoid neck!

References

1. Warshafsky D, Goldenberg D, Kanekar SG. Imaging anatomy of deep neck spaces. Otolaryngol Clin N Am. 2012;45:1203–21.
2. Aiken AH, Shatzkes DR. Approach to masses in head and neck spaces in diseases of the brain, head and neck. In: Hodler J, Kubik-Huch RA, von Schulthess GK, editors. Spine 2020–2023: diagnostic imaging [Internet]. Cham: Springer; 2020.
3. Williams DW III. An Imager's guide to normal neck anatomy. Semin Ultrasound CT MR. 1997;18(3):157–81.
4. Parker G, Harnsberger H, Smoker W. The anterior and posterior cervical spaces. Semin Ultrasound CT MR. 1991;12(3):257–73.
5. Parker GD, Harnsberger HR, Jacobs JM. The pharyngeal mucosal space. Semin Ultrasound CT MR. 1990;11(6):460–75.
6. Guidera AK, Dawes PJ, Fong A, Stringer MD. Head and neck fascia and compartments: no space for spaces. Head Neck. 2014;36(7):1058–68.
7. Wippold FJ. Head and neck imaging: the role of CT and MRI. J Magn Reson Imaging. 2007;25(3):453–65.
8. Koch BL, Hamilton BE, Hudgins PA, Harnsberger HR. Diagnostic imaging: head and neck e-book; 2016.
9. Cummings C, Flint P. Cummings otolaryngology—head and neck surgery, revision. 5th ed. Philadelphia: Mosby Elsevier; 2010. p. 201–8.
10. Gamss C, Gupta A, Chazen JL, Phillips CD. Imaging evaluation of the suprahyoid neck. Radiol Clin North Am. 2015;53:133–44.
11. Brown W, Gleeson M. Scott-Brown's otolaryngology, head and neck surgery. 7th ed. London: Hodder Arnold; 2008.
12. Babbel R, Harnsberger H. The parapharyngeal space: the key to unlocking the suprahyoid neck. Semin Ultrasound CT MR. 1990;11(6):444–59.
13. Yousem D. Suprahyoid spaces of the head and neck. Semin Roentgenol. 2000;35(1):63–71.
14. Stambuk HE, Patel SG. Imaging of the parapharyngeal space. Otolaryngol Clin N Am. 2008;41:77–101.
15. Pollei S, Harnsberger H. The radiologic evaluation of the parotid space. Semin Ultrasound CT MR. 1990;11(6):486–503.
16. Heaton CM, Chazen JL, van Zante A, et al. Pleomorphic adenoma of the major salivary glands: diagnostic utility of FNAB and MRI. Laryngoscope. 2013;123(12):3056–60.
17. Patel S, Bhatt AA. Imaging of the sublingual and submandibular spaces. Insights Imaging. 2018;9:391–401.
18. Harnsberger HR. Diagnostic imaging: head and neck. 2nd ed. Philadelphia: Amirsys; 2011. p. 2.
19. Gervasio A, D'Orta G, Mujahed I, et al. Sonographic anatomy of the neck: the suprahyoid region. J Ultrasound. 2011;14(3):130–5.
20. Moore K, Dalley A, Agur A. Clinically oriented anatomy. 6th ed. Philadelphia: Wolters Kluwer; 2010.
21. Tart RP, Kotzur IM, Mancuso AA, Glantz MS, Mukherji SK. CT and MR imaging of the buccal space and buccal space masses. Radiographics. 1995;15:531–50.
22. Mukherji SK, Castillo M. A simplified approach to the spaces of the suprahyoid neck. Radiol Clin North Am. 1998;36(5):761–80.
23. Kuwada C, Mannion K, Aulino JM, Kanekar SG. Imaging of the carotid space. Otolaryngol Clin N Am. 2012;45(6):1273–92.
24. Chong V, Mukherji S, Goh C. The suprahyoid neck: normal and pathological anatomy. J Laryngol Otol. 1999;113:501–8.
25. Fruin M, Smoker W, Harnsberger H. The carotid space in the suprahyoid neck. Semin Ultrasound CT MR. 1990;11(6):504–19.
26. Kono T, Kohno A, Kuwashima S, et al. CT findings of descending necrotizing mediastinitis via the carotid space ('Lincoln Highway'). Pediatr Radiol. 2001;31(2):84–6.
27. Anil G, Tan TY. Imaging characteristics of schwannoma of the cervical sympathetic chain: a review of 12 cases. AJNR Am J Neuroradiol. 2013;34:628–33.
28. Davis W, Smoker W, Harnsberger H. The normal and diseased retropharyngeal and prevertebral spaces. Semin Ultrasound CT MR. 1990;11(6):520–33.
29. Bhatt AA. Non-traumatic causes of fluid in the retropharyngeal space. Emerg Radiol. 2018;25(5):547–51.
30. Harnsberger H. Perivertebral space anatomy—imaging issues. Diagnostic imaging. III-10-2-3. Diagnostic imaging head and neck. Manitoba (Canada): Amirsys Publishing; 2004.
31. Mills MK, Shah LM. Imaging of the perivertebral space. Radiol Clin North Am. 2015;53(1):163–80.
32. Babbel R, Smoker W, Harnsberger H. The visceral space: the unique infrahyoid space. Semin Ultrasound CT MR. 1991;12(3):204–23.
33. Smoker W. Normal anatomy of the infrahyoid neck. Semin Ultrasound CT MR. 1991;12(3):192–203.
34. Tessler FN, Middleton WD, Grant EG, et al. ACR thyroid imaging, reporting and data system (TI-RADS): white paper of the ACR TI-RADS Committee. J Am Coll Radiol. 2017;14(5):587–95.
35. Russ G, Bonnema SJ, Erdogan MF, Durante C, Ngu R, Leenhardt L. European thyroid association guidelines for ultrasound malignancy risk stratification of thyroid nodules in adults: the EU-TIRADS. Eur Thyroid J. 2017;6(5):225–37.
36. Loevner LA, Kaplan SL, Cunnane ME, Moonis G. Cross-sectional imaging of the thyroid gland. Neuroimaging Clin N Am. 2008;18(3):445–61.
37. Aiken AH. Imaging of thyroid cancer. Semin Ultrasound CT MR. 2012;33(2):138–49.
38. Phillips CD, Shatzkes DR. Imaging of the parathyroid glands. Semin Ultrasound CT MR. 2012;33(2):123–9.

Imaging of the Nasopharynx

Harry Griffin and Amy Juliano

Anatomy

- The nasopharynx is part of the suprahyoid head and neck. Specific anatomic landmarks and contents define its boundaries.
- The nasopharynx is the uppermost portion of the aerodigestive tract, located posterosuperior to the hard palate. The oropharynx and nasopharynx are in direct continuity, separated by a horizontal plane along the hard and soft palates.
- Posterosuperiorly, the nasopharynx is bound by the floor of the sphenoid sinuses, clivus, the upper cervical vertebrae, and associated prevertebral soft tissues.
- Anteriorly, the nasopharynx communicates with the nasal cavity; these two regions are separated by the nasal choanae.
- Laterally, the nasopharynx is bordered by the medial pterygoid and the tensor and levator veli palatini muscles. The lateral nasopharyngeal wall contains the torus tubarius, an area of elevated mucosa under which is the cartilaginous portion of the Eustachian tube (Fig. 39.1).
    - Importantly, the lateral wall also contains the fossa of Rosenmüller, located posterior and lateral to the torus tubarius.
    - The fossa of Rosenmüller is the most common site of primary nasopharyngeal carcinoma.
- The upper nasopharynx is lined by respiratory epithelium (pseudostratified ciliated columnar epithelium). The lower nasopharynx is lined by stratified squamous epithelium. The underlying submucosa contains an abundance of minor salivary glands and prominent lymphoid tissue. The lymphoid component is particularly prominent in the fossa of Rosenmüller and upper posterior wall where it constitutes the adenoids.
- The mucosa and submucosa are invested by the pharyngobasilar fascia, a tough aponeurosis that represents the superior extension of the superior constrictor muscle that extends from the medial pterygoid plate to the skull base, medial to the tensor veli palatini.
    - Eustachian tube pierces through a defect in the pharyngobasilar fascia (sinus of Morgagni), which can serve as a potential route for tumor spread from the nasopharynx laterally.
- Lateral retropharyngeal nodes of Rouviere represent the primary nodes in nasopharyngeal lymphatic drainage, located anterior to the prevertebral musculature and medial to the carotid sheath. Lymphatic drainage continues into the adjacent cervical lymph nodes.

H. Griffin
Department of Radiology, Massachusetts General Hospital, Boston, MA, USA

Harvard Medical School, Boston, MA, USA
e-mail: hgriffin1@mgh.harvard.edu

A. Juliano (✉)
Department of Radiology, Massachusetts Eye and Ear, Boston, MA, USA

Harvard Medical School, Boston, MA, USA
e-mail: amy_juliano@meei.harvard.edu

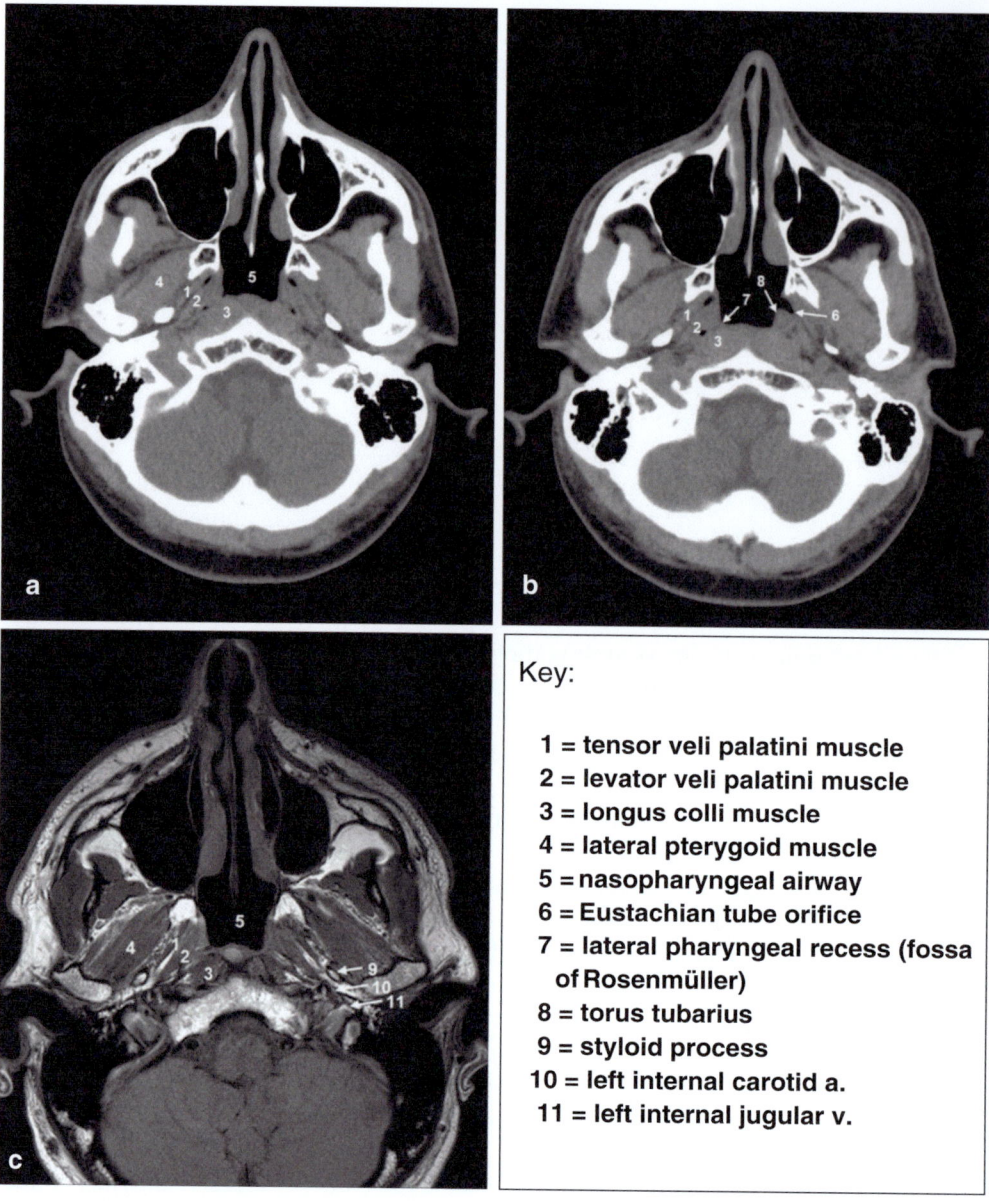

Fig. 39.1 (a, b) Normal imaging anatomy of the nasopharynx on noncontrast axial CT scan, and (c) axial noncontrast T1-weighted MR image

Adenoid Tissue

- Aggregate of mucosal lymphoid tissue in the posterior superior wall and roof of the nasopharynx.
- Enlarge during early childhood, reaching maximum size in children aged 3–7 years after which they typically undergo appreciable atrophy [1]. The absence of visible adenoidal tissue in a child should raise concern for an underlying immunodeficiency, most commonly Bruton (X-linked) agammaglobulinemia [2].
- Adenoid enlargement may be due to benign lymphoid hyperplasia and can persist or recur secondary to inflammatory or infectious processes.
- Enlarged adenoids can contribute to significant airway obstruction and lead to obstructive sleep apnea, particularly in children. Adenoid hypertrophy can contribute to chronic Eustachian tube dysfunction and resultant chronic otitis media, hearing loss, and/or delayed speech development.
- Distinguishing between benign nasopharyngeal thickening and neoplasm such as lymphoma or early nasopharyngeal carcinoma can be challenging.
    - Features suggestive of benign lymphoid hyperplasia include a vertically aligned striped appearance on T1-weighted gadolinium-enhanced MR imaging and midline symmetry in the thickness of the adenoids and mucosal (Fig. 39.2).

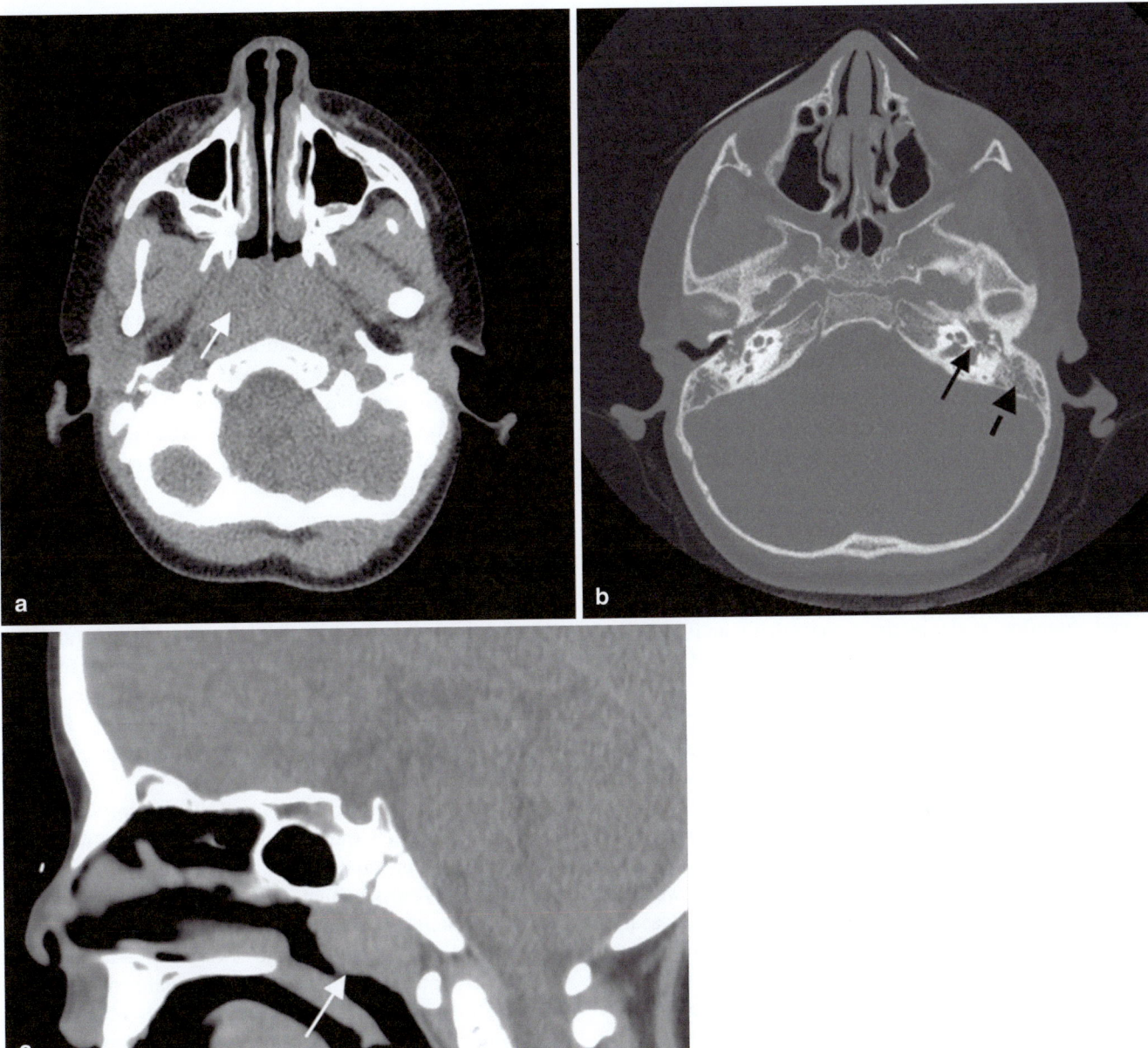

Fig. 39.2 Adenoid hypertrophy. (**a**) Axial noncontrast CT scan of the head in a child with adenoid hypertrophy. The adenoids (white arrow) appear as homogeneous soft tissue filling the posterior nasopharynx that is isodense to adjacent musculature. (**b**) Bone windows better show opacification of the middle ear cavity (black arrow) and mastoid air cells (dashed arrow) secondary to obstruction of the Eustachian tube by the mass. (**c**) Sagittal CT illustrates the degree of nasopharyngeal airway narrowing caused by the enlarged adenoid tissue (white arrow)

- Abnormal causes of adenoid enlargement include nasopharyngeal carcinoma, lymphoma, aggressive infectious processes such as skull base osteomyelitis, and minor salivary gland malignancies (e.g., adenoid cystic carcinoma).
- Lymphoma arising from the adenoidal lymphoid tissue may present as a bulky midline mass with loss of the internal enhancing stripes, often accompanied by regional and distant nodal involvement.

Inflammatory Sinonasal Disease

- Chronic rhinosinusitis is characterized by a combination of polyps, retention cysts, sinus wall osteitis, and mucocele formation. Polyps and mucus retention cysts are histologically distinct but clinically and radiographically indistinct but for location; polyps are generally located in the nasal cavity, while retention cysts are in sinus spaces. Both may be solitary or numerous.
- Sinonasal polyposis is the presence of numerous polyps and retention cysts in the nasal cavity and paranasal sinuses, potentially resulting in obstruction of the nasal passage.
- Characteristic CT features of sinonasal polyposis include multiple polypoid lesions within the nasal cavity and paranasal sinuses. Smooth osseous remodeling may be present in severe cases.
- On MRI, polyps, retention cysts, and fluid may demonstrate various complex signal intensities. Fresh mucus has high water content, appearing hypointense on T1-weighted images and hyperintense on T2-weighted images; as protein concentration increases with time, the T1-weighted signal intensity increases, and the T2-weighted signal intensity decreases. Markedly inspissated mucus may appear as a signal void on T2-weighted signal such that it mimics an aerated sinus1.
- Contrast-enhanced images may show thin peripheral mucosal enhancement without a central enhancing component.

Tornwaldt Cyst

- Benign congenital cyst along the midline posterior mucosa that results from focal adhesion of pharyngeal mucosa to the notochord during development [3].
- Common incidental finding and usually asymptomatic, although can become obstructed or infected.
- Well-circumscribed, thin-walled cystic structure along the posterior nasopharyngeal mucosa between the prevertebral muscles.
- CT typically demonstrates a well-defined cyst with hypodense mucoid attenuation. May be isodense to soft tissue if there is increased protein content within the cyst.
- MR is most sensitive for detection, with characteristic hyperintense signal on T2-weighted sequences. T1-weighted signal intensity can vary depending on the protein content [4, 5].

Nasochoanal Polyp

- Large polyp in the nasal cavity that protrudes through the nasal choana into the nasopharynx. When there is involvement of the maxillary sinus through the maxillary infundibulum, this is termed an antrochoanal polyp. Patients may present with sinonasal symptoms or with an obstructed nasal passage.
- Histologically identical to other inflammatory sinonasal polyps, in which there is nonneoplastic inflammatory swelling of the mucosa that buckles to form polypoid lesions [6]. Antrochoanal polyps may have a narrow stalk in the maxillary sinus; there is potential for vascular compromise with hemorrhage or organizing hematoma.
- CT will typically demonstrate a well-defined mass with mucin density in the nasal cavity, variably involving the maxillary sinus, and extending into the nasopharynx with smooth expansile remodeling of the maxillary ostium (Fig. 39.3). The narrow stalk is typically not evident [7].
- Regions of internal high-attenuation secondary to inspissated mucus or fungal colonization may be present.

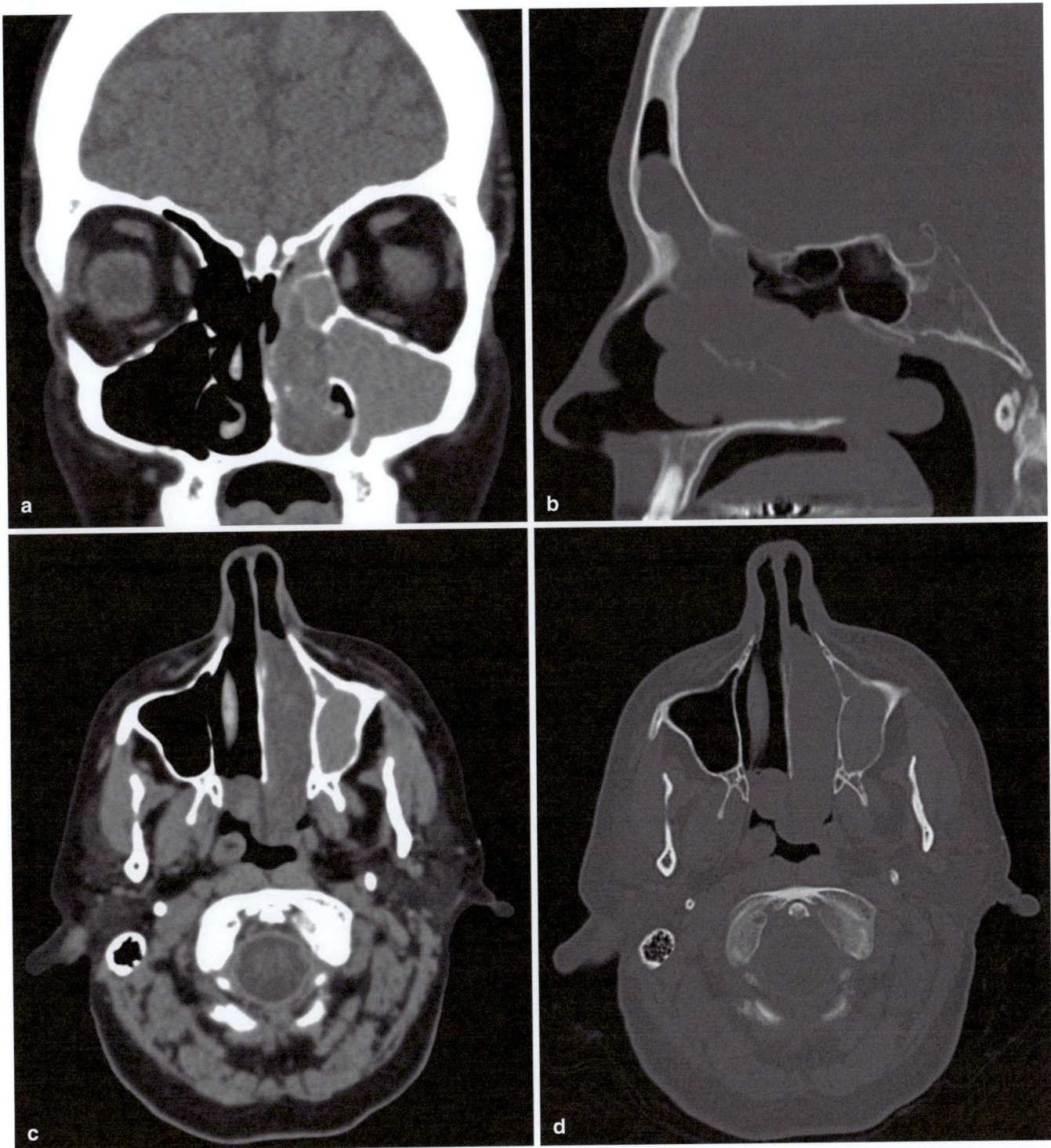

Fig. 39.3 (a) Coronal, (b) sagittal, (c and d) axial noncontrast CT images of the nasopharynx in a 56-year-old female demonstrate multiple polypoid lesions within the left frontal sinus, left ethmoids, and left maxillary sinus obstructing the left nasal passage

Inverted Papilloma

- The upper nasopharyngeal mucosa is formed by ciliated pseudostratified columnar epithelium, termed Schneiderian respiratory membrane, and contains mucus-secreting glands called Bowman's glands [8].
- This mucosa can give rise to papillomas formed by a hyperplastic zone of basement membrane enclosing epithelium that falls inward on itself.
- There are three papilloma subtypes based on the histologic and morphologic appearance: fungiform papilloma, oncocytic papilloma, and inverted papilloma [9]. Inverted papilloma is more common than the other two subtypes.
- Inverted papilloma is a rare, locally aggressive benign neoplasm more commonly seen in middle-aged men. Although benign, there is a 15% rate of malignancy most often due to degeneration into squamous cell carcinoma9.
- Inverted papilloma classically arises from the lateral nasal wall in the region of the middle turbinate or ethmoid recesses, commonly with local extension into the maxillary or ethmoid sinuses. Extension into the nasopharynx is common, making differentiation from inflammatory and antrochoanal polyps difficult by CT.
- On CT, inverted papillomas appear as lobulated soft tissue density masses, most commonly arising from the middle meatus and projecting into the nasal cavity.
- MRI typically demonstrates a polypoid mass that is isointense to hyperintense on T1-weighted images and hyperintense on T2-weighted images relative to muscle with heterogeneous enhancement on postcontrast images, in a classic "cerebriform pattern" that can be seen on T2- and contrast-enhanced T1-weighted images (Fig. 39.4).

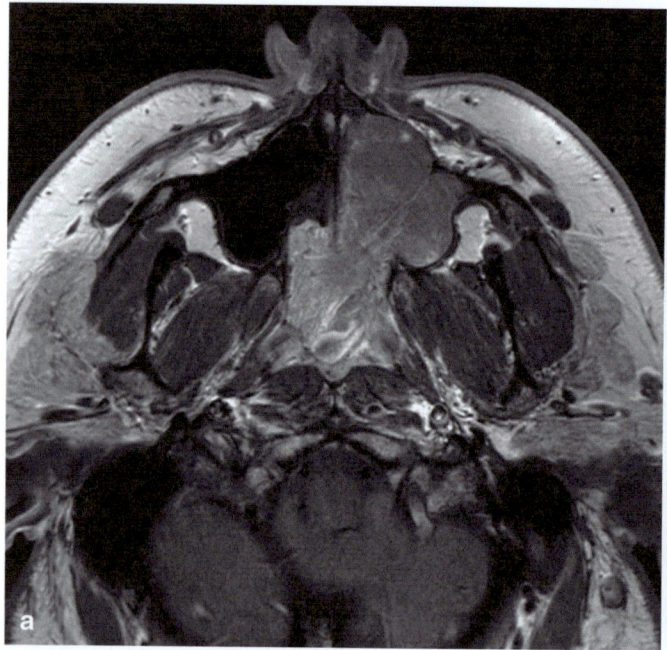
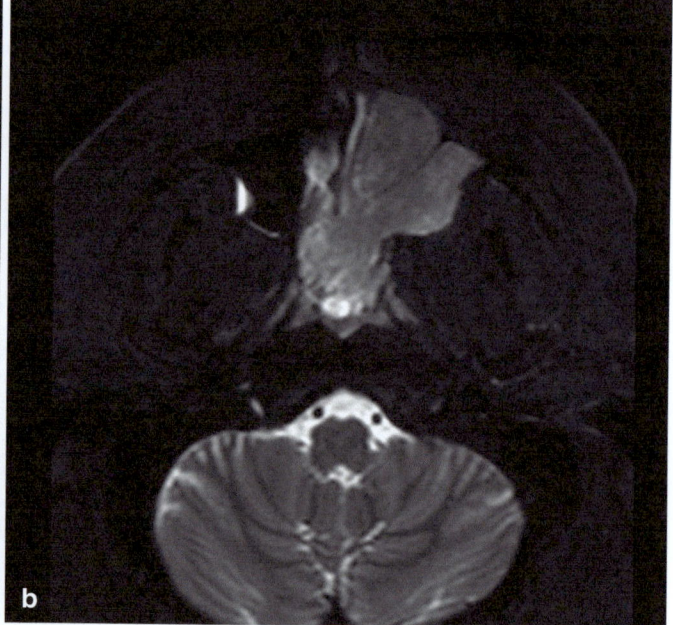

Fig. 39.4 (a) Axial T1-weighted MR image demonstrates a heterogeneously hyperintense mass opacifying the left maxillary sinus and nasal cavity, with erosion through the medial wall of the maxillary sinus. (b) Axial T2-weighted MR image MR image with fat suppression better illustrates the high signal intensity mass filling the nasal cavity, maxillary sinus, and nasopharynx

Skull Base Osteomyelitis

- Skull base osteomyelitis is a rare and potentially life-threatening infection of the sphenoid, occipital, or temporal bones, most often a complication of advanced otogenic or sinonasal infection.
- Immunosuppressed patients or elderly patients with diabetes are most at risk. Other risk factors include small vessel disease, radiation exposure, and malignancy 10.
- Typical skull base osteomyelitis is the most common form, resulting from necrotizing otitis externa (NOE) or other otologic infections spreading through natural gaps in the cartilaginous external auditory canal (fissures of Santorini), and classically in elderly patients with uncontrolled diabetes. The spread of infection from the external auditory canal results in localized osteomyelitis, which can spread anteromedially to the infratemporal soft tissues, petrous apex, and clivus.
    - o Symptoms of typical osteomyelitis related to NOE include otorrhea and severe otalgia. Involvement of the stylomastoid foramen may result in facial nerve palsy. Extension into the petrous apex can produce Gradenigo syndrome, characterized by facial pain, cranial nerve VI palsy, and persistent otorrhea [10].
- Atypical (or central) skull base osteomyelitis predominantly involves the basiocciput and basisphenoid, often secondary to regional infections of the sinuses, nasopharyngeal cavity, or face, or from medial extension of temporal bone infection. Involvement of the preclival or nasopharyngeal space soft tissues should raise concern for nasopharyngeal neoplasm.
    - o Most commonly occurs in elderly patients in immunocompromised states such as HIV, chronic steroid use, and diabetes. Other risk factors include previous radiation therapy, Paget disease, and osteoporosis.
- CT with bone reconstruction algorithm is the initial test of choice. Imaging features of osteomyelitis include cortical bone erosion and periostitis 10. Attention to the bony EAC, mastoid tip, petrous apex, petro-occipital suture, clivus, and foramina of the skull base is recommended. CT findings can be helpful for identifying the underlying etiology, such as opacification, mucosal thickening, and fluid in the pneumatized portions of the temporal bone and sinuses (Fig. 39.5).
- Contrast-enhanced CT may demonstrate inflammatory changes in the soft tissues. Asymmetric soft tissue thickening in the nasopharynx is common and can mimic nasopharyngeal neoplasm.
- MR imaging is superior for the full evaluation of the skull base and surrounding structures. Osteomyelitis replaces the normal marrow fat signal resulting in T1-signal hypointensity and T2/STIR signal hyperintensity. Heterogeneous marrow enhancement or peripherally enhancing collections on post-contrast sequences confirm the diagnosis (Fig. 39.6).

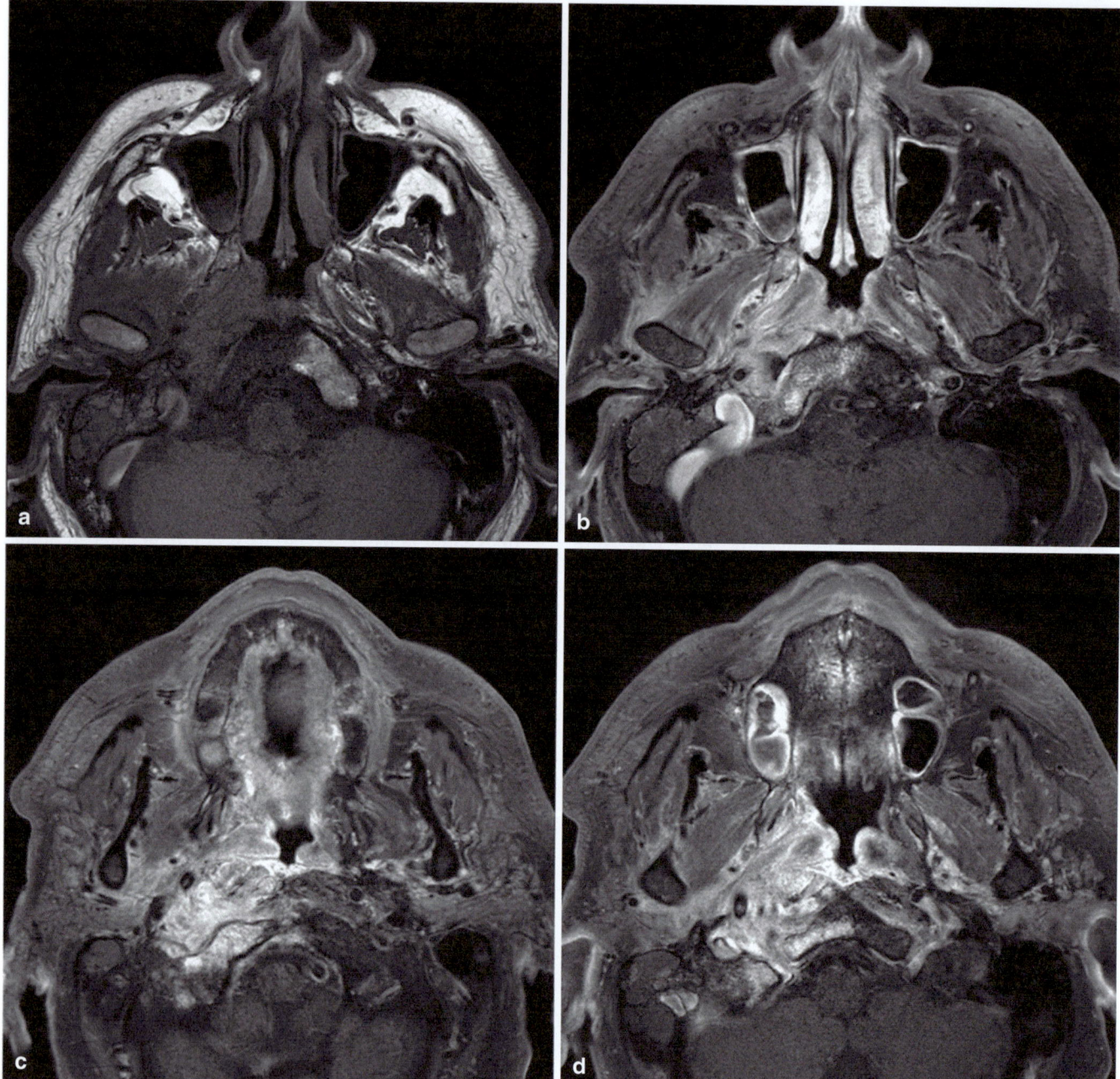

Fig. 39.5 Skull base osteomyelitis in a 74-year-old male with a history of chronic sinusitis and nasal polyps. (**a**) Axial noncontrast T1-weighted MR image of the nasopharynx shows loss of the normal hyperintense signal from the intramedullary fat in the clivus and right parapharyngeal space. (**b–d**) Axial post-contrast enhanced T1-weighted images with fat suppression demonstrate enhancement in the right nasopharyngeal mucosa, parapharyngeal space, and the tensor and levator veli palatini and pterygoid muscles. There is enhancing tissue in the prevertebral space and the right side of the clivus, confirming skull base involvement

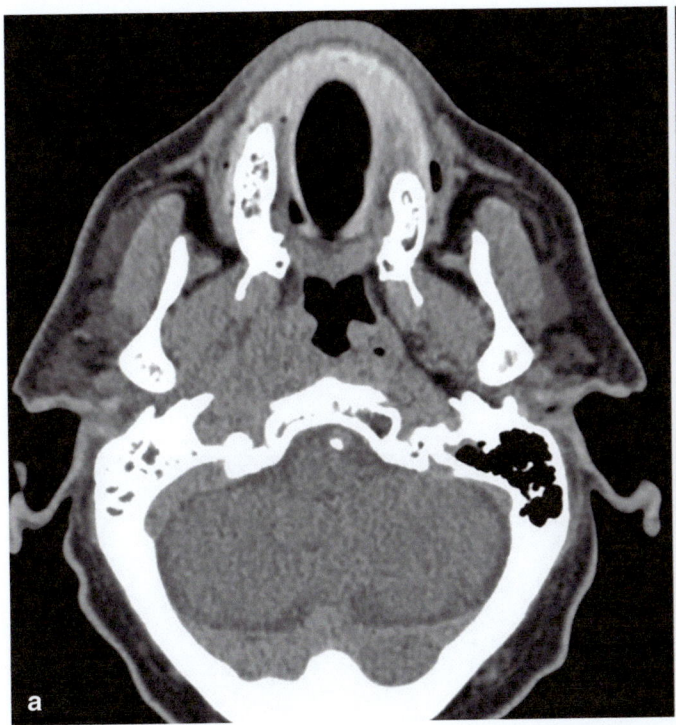 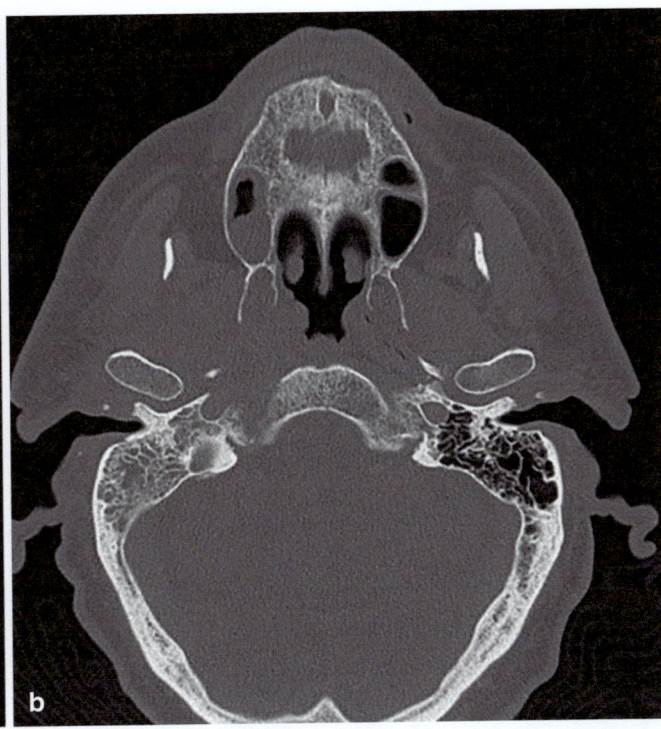

Fig. 39.6 Skull base osteomyelitis in the same patient. Axial noncontrast CT in soft tissue (**a**) and bone (**b**) windows. There is asymmetry of the parapharyngeal soft tissues with obliteration of the fat in the parapharyngeal space. There is erosion and subtle sclerosis of the clivus. Opacification of the right mastoid air cells represents sequela of Eustachian tube obstruction

Nasopharyngeal Carcinoma

- Nasopharyngeal carcinoma (NPC) is the most common primary nasopharyngeal malignancy, accounting for 70% of all primary malignancies. The incidence is highest in patients from southern China and southeast Asia [11]. Additional risk factors include nitrosamine-rich salted foods, cigarette and alcohol use, chronic sinonasal infection, and prior infection with human papillomavirus (HPV) and Epstein–Barr virus (EBV).
- Although often asymptomatic, symptoms of early stage disease include postnasal drip, nasopharyngeal irritation, middle ear fullness/effusion, and otitis media. Later-stage disease can present with epistaxis or cranial nerve involvement. Cervical lymphadenopathy is frequently a presenting symptom.
- Squamous cell carcinoma is subdivided into three histologic subtypes recognized by the World Health Organization (WHO) [12]:
  o Keratinizing SCC (25%).
  o Nonkeratinizing carcinoma (12%).
  o Undifferentiated carcinomas (63%).
- Keratinizing NPC is analogous to squamous cell carcinoma elsewhere in the pharynx and is associated with cigarette and alcohol use11.
- Undifferentiated and nonkeratinizing NPC are more strongly associated with prior EBV infection.
- Early stage tumors appear as asymmetrical thickening of the superficial nasopharyngeal mucosa, most commonly in the fossa of Rosenmüller. Key imaging features to differentiate from physiologic asymmetry include:
  o Obliteration of the fat stripe between the tensor and levator veli palatini.
  o Ipsilateral middle ear and mastoid opacity related to effusion or otomastoiditis, suggestive of Eustachian tube dysfunction.
  o Cervical lymphadenopathy, especially enlarged ipsilateral lateral retropharyngeal nodes (of Rouviere), with low to intermediate T1-weighted and high T2-weighted signals.
- Classic imaging features of more advanced nasopharyngeal malignancy include a bulky invasive mass arising from the mucosa of the superolateral nasopharyngeal wall with infiltration of the deep fascia and spaces around the nasopharynx3.
- Nasopharyngeal carcinoma staging follows the American Joint Committee on Cancer (AJCC) eighth edition staging manual (Fig. 39.7).
- CT findings include a soft tissue mass involving the fossa of Rosenmüller. Submucosal spread and deep infiltration

into the parapharyngeal space can be seen; however, there is often no significant enhancement within the tumor, rendering differentiation of tumor from uninvolved nearby structures such as the adenoid tonsils and prevertebral muscles difficult11.
- MR imaging is superior at delineating NPC from uninvolved surrounding structures. NPC typically shows intermediate signal intensity on T2-weighted images relative to muscle, and low signal intensity on T1-weighted images relative to normal mucosa. T1-weighted sequences are useful for detecting abnormal infiltration and replacement of normal high-signal fat by tumor in the skull base and neck spaces (Fig. 39.8).
- Fat-suppressed postcontrast T1-weighted sequences are useful for defining the extent of tumor infiltration into the marrow of the skull base while maintaining good contrast between the enhancing tumor and adjacent muscles [3, 11].

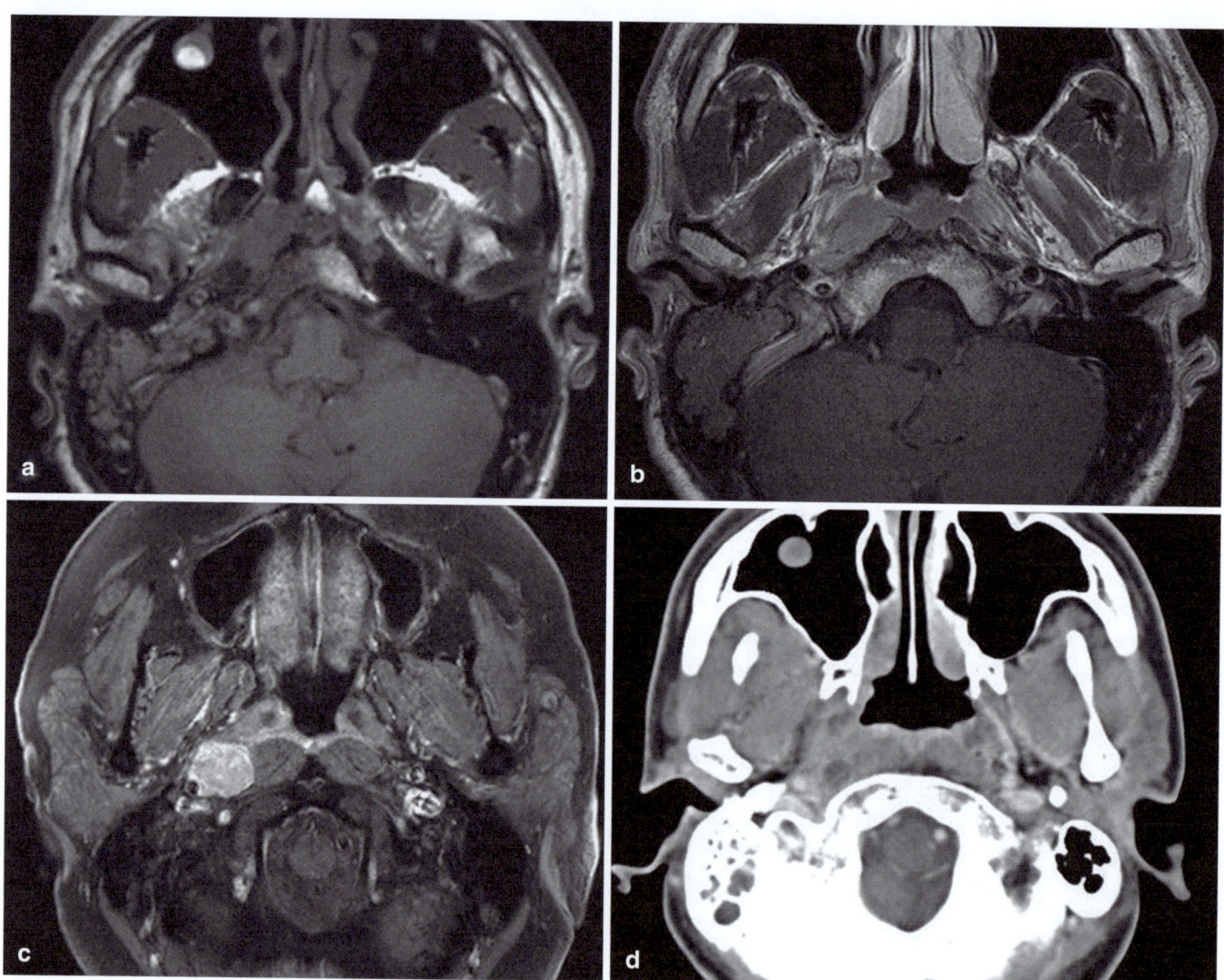

Fig. 39.7 Nasopharyngeal carcinoma. (**a** and **b**) Axial noncontrast and contrast-enhanced T1-weighted images of the nasopharynx. Images demonstrate a T1-isointense soft tissue mass producing subtle asymmetry in the fossa of Rosenmüller. There is a loss of fat signal between the levator and tensor veli palatini muscles, indicative of involvement of the parapharyngeal space. Ipsilateral middle ear and mastoid effusion are indicative of Eustachian tube obstruction. Loss of the normal fat marrow signal in the clivus is suggestive of skull base involvement. (**c**) Axial post-contrast T1-weighted fat-suppressed and (**d**) axial noncontrast CT images in a different patient with nasopharyngeal carcinoma (primary lesion not shown). These images demonstrate a typical appearance of an enlarged and rounded lateral retropharyngeal node (of Rouviere), consistent with lymph node metastasis

Fig. 39.8 Nasopharyngeal Cancer AJCC eighth edition TNM Staging [13]

T Category	T Criteria
TX	Primary tumor cannot be assessed
T0	No tumor identified, but EBV-positive cervical node(s) involvement
Tis	Tumor in situ
T1	Tumor confined to nasopharynx or extension to oropharynx and/or nasal cavity without parapharyngeal involvement
T2	Tumor with extension to parapharyngeal space, and/or adjacent soft tissue involvement (medial pterygoid, lateral pterygoid, prevertebral muscles)
T3	Tumor with infiltration of bony structures at skull base, cervical vertebra, pterygoid structures, and/or paranasal sinuses
T4	Tumor with intracranial extension, involvement of cranial nerves, hypopharynx, orbit, parotid gland, and/or extensive soft tissue infiltration beyond lateral surface of lateral pterygoid muscle
N Category	N Criteria
NX	Regional nodes cannot be assessed
N0	No regional lymph node metastasis
N1	Unilateral metastasis in cervical node(s) and/or unilateral or bilateral metastasis in retropharyngeal node(s), 6 cm or smaller in greatest dimension, above the caudal border of cricoid cartilage
N2	Bilateral metastasis in cervical nodes(s), 6 cm or smaller in greatest dimension, above the caudal border of cricoid cartilage
N3	Unilateral or bilateral metastasis in cervical lymph node(s), larger than 6 cm in greatest dimension, and/or extension below the caudal border of cricoid cartilage
M Category	M Criteria
M0	No distant metastasis
M1	Distant metastasis

References

1. Bhatia KSS, King AD, Vlantis AC, Ahuja AT, Tse GM. Nasopharyngeal mucosa and adenoids: appearance at MR imaging. Radiology. 2012;263(2):437–43.
2. Vogler RC, Li FJ wippold, Pilgram TK (2000) Age-specific size of the normal adenoid pad on magnetic resonance imaging. Clin Otolaryngol 25(5):392–395.
3. Haaga JR. CT and MR imaging of the whole body. Philadelphia, PA: Mosby/Elsevier; 2009.
4. Ben Salem D, Duvillard C, Assous D, Ballester M, Krausé D, Ricolfi F. Imaging of nasopharyngeal cysts and bursae. Eur Radiol 16(10):2249–2258.
5. Ikushima I, Korogi Y, Makita O, Komohara Y, Kawano H, Yamura M, Arikawa K, Takahashi M. MR imaging of Tornwaldt's cysts. AJR Am J Roentgenol. 1999;172(6):1663–5.
6. Eggesb H. Radiological imaging of inflammatory lesions in the nasal cavity and paranasal sinuses. Eur Radiol. 2006;16(4):872–88.
7. Tatekawa H, Shimono T, Ohsawa M, Doishita S, Sakamoto S, Miki Y. Imaging features of benign mass lesions in the nasal cavity and paranasal sinuses according to the 2017 WHO classification. Jpn J Radiol. 2018;36(6):361–81.
8. Mafee M. Nasopharynx, parapharyngeal space, and base of skull. Imaging of the head and neck: Thieme, Stuttgart; 1995. p. 339.
9. Chawla A, Shenoy J, Chokkappan K, Chung R. Imaging features of Sinonasal inverted papilloma: a pictorial review. Curr Probl Diagn Radiol. 2016;45(5):347–53.
10. Chapman PR, Choudhary G, Singhal A. Skull Base osteomyelitis: a comprehensive imaging review. AJNR Am J Neuroradiol. 2021;42(3):404–13.
11. Razek AAKA, King A. MRI and CT of nasopharyngeal carcinoma. Am J Roentgenol. 2012;198(1):11–8.
12. Brennan B. Nasopharyngeal carcinoma. Orphanet J Rare Dis. 2006;1(1):23.
13. Amin MB, Greene FL, Edge SB, Compton CC, Gershenwald JE, Brookland RK, Meyer L, Gress DM, Byrd DR, Winchester DP. The eighth edition AJCC cancer staging manual. CA Cancer J Clin. 2017;67(2):93–9.

Imaging of the Oral Cavity and Oropharynx

Jennifer M. Watchmaker, Laura B. Eisenmenger, and Jacqueline C. Junn

Basic Anatomy of Oral Cavity and Oropharynx

ORAL CAVITY

- The anatomic borders of the oral cavity are depicted in Fig. 40.1.
- The oral cavity can be divided into distinct subsites which include the lip, hard palate, gingiva, buccal mucosa, oral tongue, floor of the mouth (FOM), upper and lower alveolar ridges, and the retromolar trigone.
- The sublingual and submandibular spaces lie beneath the oral tongue.
- The sublingual space is bounded by the mandible (anterior), genioglossus/geniohyoid (medial), mylohyoid (inferolateral), and the floor of the mouth mucosa (superior) (Fig. e40.1).
- (All electronic images (Figs. e40.1–e40.15) can be found on this chapter's website on SpringerLink: https://doi.org/10.1007/978-3-031-55124-6_40).

- The submandibular space is bounded by the mandible (anterior), anterior belly of the digastric (medial), mylohyoid (superior), and hyoid bone (inferior).
- Focal discontinuity in the right mylohyoid muscle, an anatomic variant, allows the sublingual gland to protrude from the sublingual space into the submandibular space and is known a *Boutonniere Deformity* (Fig. e40.2).

OROPHARYNX

- The oropharynx is the midportion of the muscular tube created by the pharyngeal constrictor muscles, between the nasopharynx superiorly and hypopharynx inferiorly.
- The oropharynx is bounded by the base of tongue/lingual tonsil (anterior), pharyngeal wall (lateral and posterior), tonsillar complex (lateral), and the soft palate (superior), and inferior boundary is at the hyoid bone (Fig. 40.2).
- In addition to the aforementioned spaces, there are additional spaces of the head and neck, some of which are defined by fascial planes and may communicate with the oral cavity in the setting of disease. Of relevance to the contents of this chapter is the retropharyngeal space (Fig. e40.3).

Supplementary Information The online version contains supplementary material available at https://doi.org/10.1007/978-3-031-55124-6_40.

J. M. Watchmaker
Department of Diagnostic, Molecular and Interventional Radiology, Icahn School of Medicine at Mount Sinai, New York, NY, USA
e-mail: jennifer.watchmaker@mountsinai.org

L. B. Eisenmenger
Department of Radiology, University of Wisconsin School of Medicine and Public Health, Madison, WI, USA
e-mail: LEisenmenger@uwhealth.org

J. C. Junn (✉)
Department of Radiology and Imaging Sciences, Emory School of Medicine, Atlanta, GA, USA
e-mail: jjunn@emory.edu

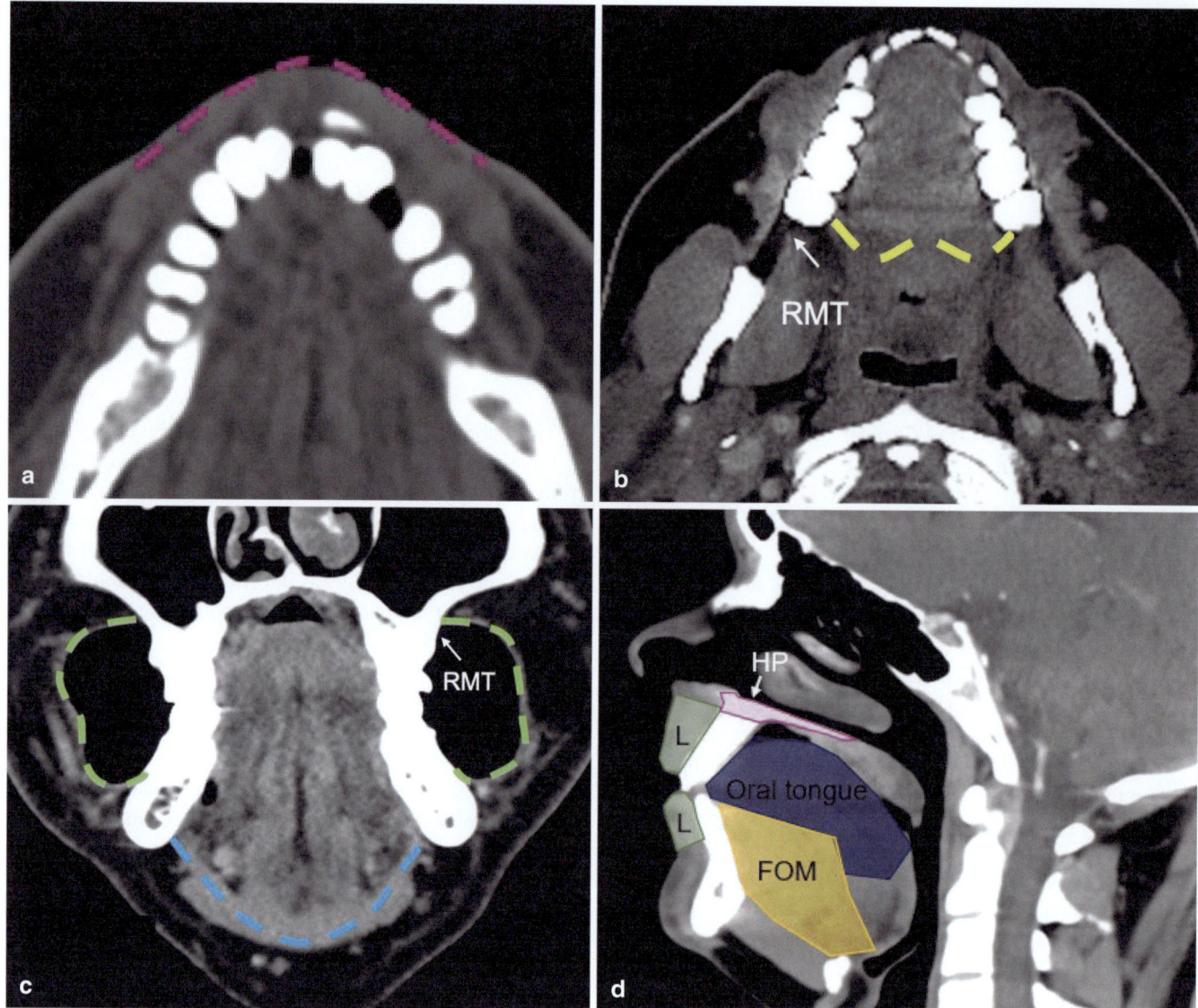

Fig. 40.1 Anatomical boundaries of oral cavity. Axial (**a** and **b**), coronal (**c**), and sagittal (**d**) images of the oral cavity with the boundaries outlined. The anterior border is at the vermillion border of the lips (pink line), posterior border along the imaginary line drawn at the circumvallate papillae (yellow line); lateral border along the gingivobuccal region (green line), inferiorly along the mylohyoid (blue line), and superiorly along the hard palate (HP). The retromolar trigone (RMT) is an important mucosal line subsite of the oral cavity located posterior to the third mandibular molar. The oral cavity subsites including lips (L), gingiva (G), and floor of mouth (FOM) are additionally annotated on sagittal view

40 Imaging of the Oral Cavity and Oropharynx

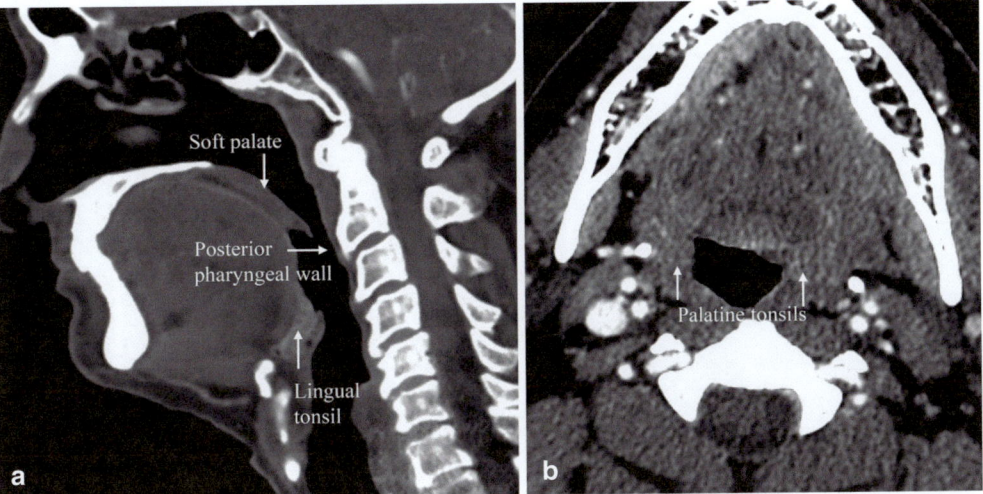

Fig. 40.2 Oropharynx. Sagittal (**a**) and axial (**b**) contrast-enhanced CT of the neck. The sagittal image shows soft palate (superior border), posterior pharyngeal wall (posterior border), and lingual tonsils. The axial CT shows bilateral palatine tonsils

Infection/Inflammation

DENTAL INFECTIONS

- Dental abscesses (periapical lucency) are infections around the tooth root due to apical periodontal or pulpal disease.
- Tooth abscess involving the second and third mandibular molars spread to the submandibular space and masticator space. Their roots are below the insertion of the mylohyoid muscle.
- Imaging
- Lucency surrounding the tooth root and may be related with surrounding periosteal abscess or myositis (Fig. 40.3).

LUDWIG'S ANGINA

- Ludwig's angina is a life-threatening cellulitis of the floor of the mouth (Fig. e40.4). It usually starts with a dental infection/procedure and can quickly spread into the parapharyngeal space. It can extend inferiorly via the "danger space" and result in mediastinitis; this is a surgical emergency.

Imaging
- Diffuse floor of mouth edema. There may be associated abscesses. Tongue may be elevated.

SIALOCELE

- **Sialocele is** a collection of saliva containing cystic space from a salivary gland. It can occur secondary to an obstructing stone, post-trauma, postinfectious, or after surgery. Clinically, they can be asymptomatic or present as a fluctuant mass and may have surrounding swelling.

Imaging
- Well-marginated fluid collection associated with salivary gland. Low attenuation on CT with thin walls if any.
- T_2 hyperintense on MRI and little to no enhancement on postcontrast images. No restricted diffusion.

SIALADENITIS

- Inflammation of the salivary glands and most often acute in presentation with patients presenting with a painful, swollen gland.

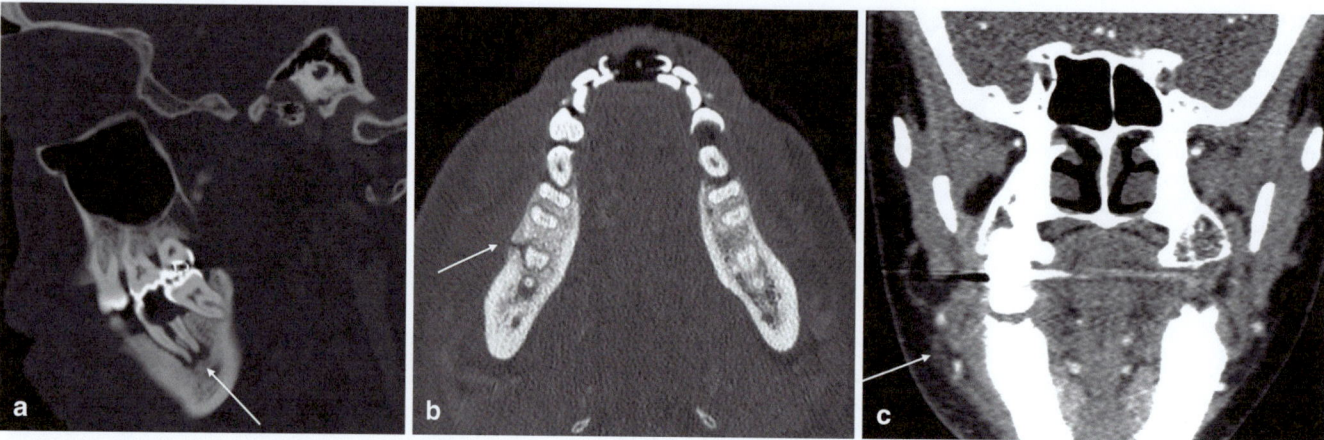

Fig. 40.3 Periapical abscess, myositis, and cellulitis. Right mandibular second molar periapical lucency (**a**) with buccal cortical defect (**b**) and surrounding soft tissue swelling and fat stranding (**c**)

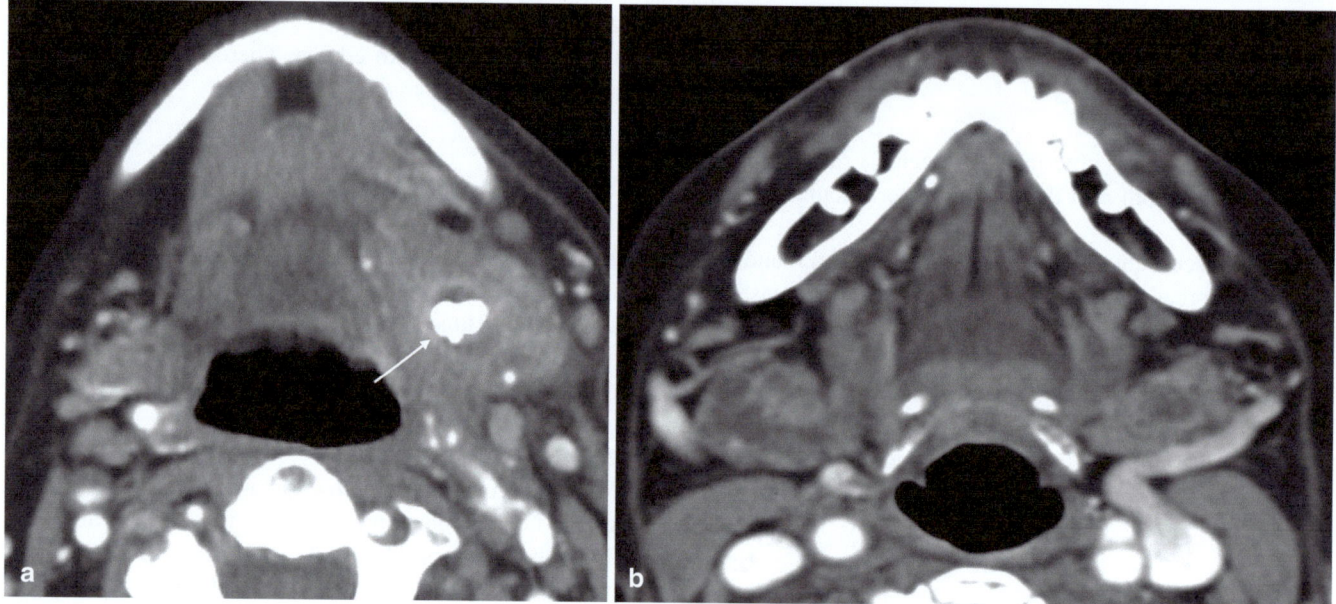

Fig. 40.4 Sialadenitis. A calculus in the left submandibular gland with the left submandibular gland enlargement and enhancement, compatible with acute sialadienitis (**a**); Chronic sialdenitis with atrophic bilateral submandibular glands with sialectasis (**b**)

- The most common cause of sialadenitis is Staphylococcus aureus and can result from ductal obstruction or decreased flow secondary to ductal stone or stenosis, respectively.
- In the chronic phase, the gland will be atrophied with fatty replacement.
- Patients with Sjogren syndrome (autoimmune destruction of exocrine glands) and Mikulicz syndrome (IgG4 related) can suffer from chronic sialadenitis.
- Küttner tumor (otherwise known as chronic sialadenitis) is a benign fibroinflammatory condition affecting the submandibular gland.
- Iodine-131/radiation-induced and HIV-associated sialadenitis are additional etiologies, typically presenting as bilateral parotid swelling.

Imaging
- Acute: Enlarged salivary glands with enhancement with or without surrounding soft tissue stranding (Fig. 40.4a). May see ductal dilatation and sialolith. T_1 hypointensity and T_2 hyperintensity.
- Chronic: Atrophic gland with fibrosis (Fig. 40.4b). MR may show heterogeneous T_1 signal and T_2 hypointensity depending on the degree of fibrosis.

TONSILLITIS

- Inflammation of the tonsils.
- Most common head and neck infection in adolescents and young adults.

- Typically caused by group A beta-hemolytic *Streptococci*.
- Untreated tonsillitis can result in spread of infection to adjacent spaces including retropharyngeal, parapharyngeal, masticator, or submandibular space.

Imaging
- Tonsillar enlargement that may touch each other (kissing tonsils).
- Linear, striped postcontras t enhancement (tiger stripe sign) (Fig. e40.5a).
- Complication of tonsillitis is peritonsillar abscess with internally hypodense collection with peripherally enhancing rim (Fig. e40.5b).

ADENOIDITIS

- Inflammation/infection of the pharyngeal tonsils (adenoids).
- Infections of the tonsils and pharyngeal tonsils are referred to as "tonsillopharyngitis."
- Common causes of adenoiditis include viral infections such as common cold, influenza, or mononucleosis.

Imaging
- Enlarged adenoids with linear enhancement (Fig. e40.6).

SUPERFICIAL NECK ABSCESS

- Odontogenetic and tonsillar infections can result in abscesses of the neck.
- Infections can spread between neck spaces, and careful inspection of surrounding bone for erosive changes is important.

RETROPHARYNGEAL ABSCESS

- Purulent fluid collection in retropharyngeal space.
- Retropharyngeal abscesses most frequently occur in children less than 5 years of age.
- Most commonly caused by *Staphylococcus aureus*, *Hemophilus*, and *Streptococcus*.
- Complications: jugular vein thrombosis, pseudoaneurysm, vasospasm, and airway narrowing.

Imaging
- Plain radiographs show enlarged prevertebral soft tissue (Fig. 40.5a). Best when imaged on inspiration with neck extended.
- CT shows distended, fluid-filled collection with enhancing wall in retropharyngeal space (Fig. 40.5b) that may have accompanying prevertebral muscle edema.

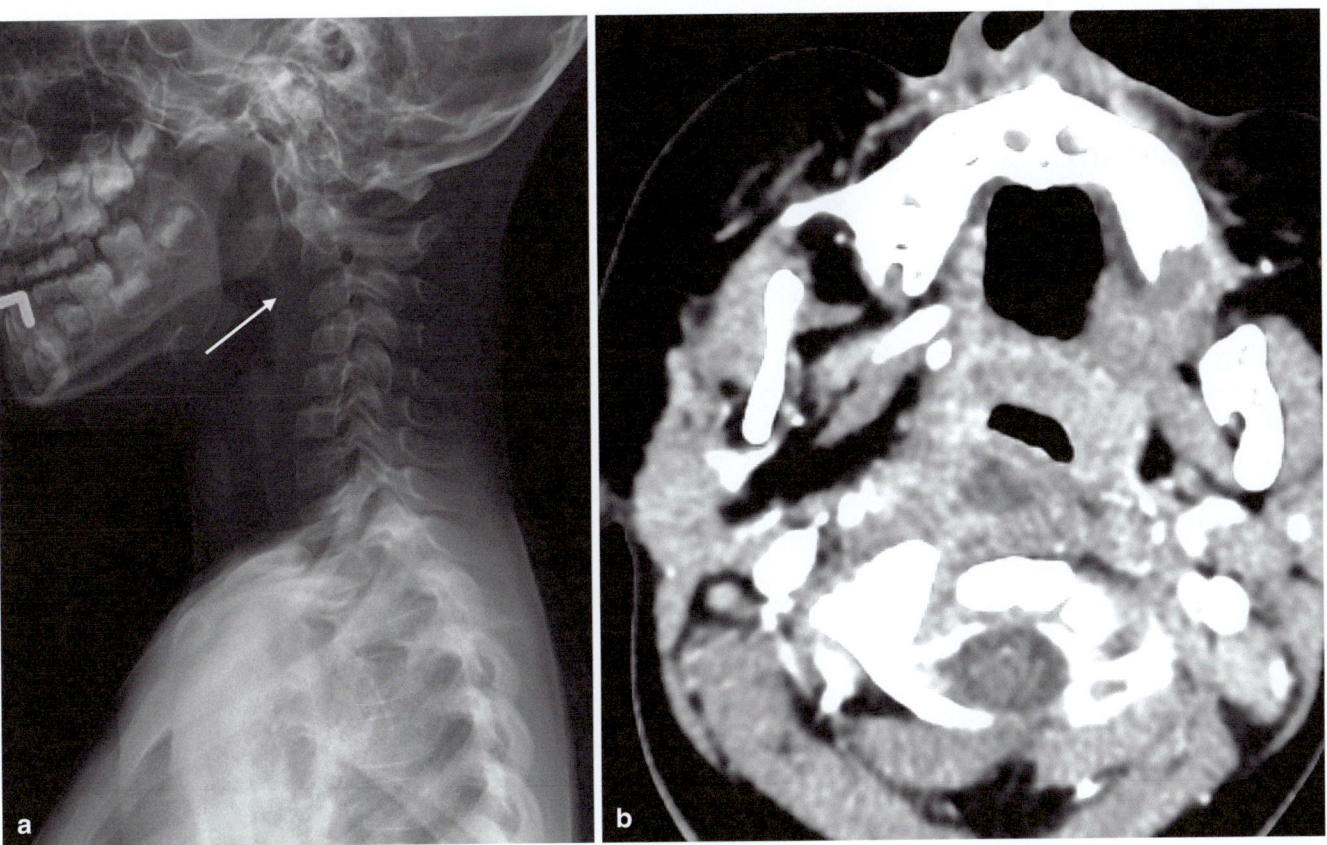

Fig. 40.5 Retropharyngeal abscess. Lateral x-ray shows enlarged prevertebral soft tissue (**a**). Axial CT neck with contrast shows hypodense fluid collection in the retropharyngeal space to the right of midline (**b**)

ACUTE CALCIFIC LONGUS COLLI TENDONITIS

- Inflammatory response to calcium hydroxyapatite deposition in the longus colli tendon.
- Self-limited and treated with NSAIDS.

Imaging

- Calcium is present in prevertebral space at C1–2 level.
- CT: Diffuse retropharyngeal and muscle edema (Fig. e40.7).
- MR: T_2 hyperintense retropharyngeal edema. May show inflammation of prevertebral muscle. No rim-enhancement.

Lymphadenopathy

NONNEOPLASTIC LYMPHADENOPATHY

- Level I: Submental nodes (Ia) located between anterior belly of digastric; submandibular nodes (Ib) in the submandibular space (Fig. e40.8).
- Level II: IIa nodes are posterior to the submandibular gland and anterior to the posterior border of the internal jugular vein. IIb nodes are posterior to the internal jugular vein and anterior to the posterior border of the sternocleidomastoid muscle. They are above the inferior margin of the hyoid bone (Fig. e40.8).
- Reactive lymphadenopathy of the cervical lymph node is a common finding in patients with infections of the oral cavity and oropharynx.

CERVICAL ADENITIS

- Inflammation of lymph node.
- Presentation: painful cervical mass.
- Mostly secondary to upper respiratory infections.

Imaging

- Enlarged lymph nodes with preservation of fatty hilum. May have adjacent soft tissue stranding.
- Complication: suppuration with central necrosis with central hypodensity (Fig. 40.6). It may progress to abscess formation with peripheral rim enhancement.

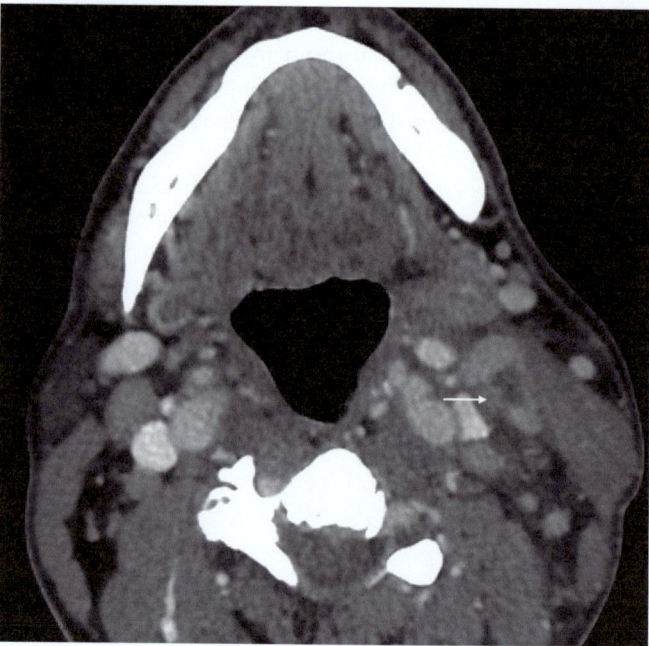

Fig. 40.6 Suppurative adenitis. Centrally necrotic left IIa node and enlarged IIb nodes with surrounding fat stranding

Tumors and Tumor-Like Conditions

MALIGNANT ADENOPATHY

- Metastatic disease and lymphoma can cause malignant neck lymphadenopathy.
- Squamous cell carcinoma in the head and neck follows the expected pattern.
- Oral cavity squamous cell carcinoma: levels I–III.
- Oropharyngeal squamous cell carcinoma: II, III, retropharyngeal.
- The extranodal extension is when there is infiltration beyond the lymph node capsule into adjacent tissue.
- HPV-related oropharyngeal carcinoma: multiple nodes, cystic nodes particularly at level II.
- Lymphoma: lymphadenopathy in addition to B-symptoms including weight loss, night sweats, and fever. PET-CT is used for initial staging and re-staging of lymphoma.

Imaging

- Heterogeneously enhancing, enlarged lymph nodes with loss of fatty hilum (Fig. e40.9).
- Hypermetabolic on PET-CT.

SQUAMOUS CELL CARCINOMA OF THE NECK

- Head and neck squamous cell carcinoma (SCC) is the sixth most common cancer worldwide.
- SCC can arise from both the oral cavity and oropharynx and early nodal involvement.
- Oral cavity SCC: Associated with smoking and alcohol.
- Oropharyngeal squamous cell carcinoma is commonly associated with HPV.

Imaging

- CT: Variably enhancing lesion (Fig. 40.7) may show ulceration.
- MR: Variable enhancement pattern. Typically, T_2 hyperintense.
- PET-CT: Often metabolically active.

MINOR SALIVARY GLAND NEOPLASMS

- May be benign or malignant; the majority of tumors within the parotid gland.
- Large salivary gland neoplasms are more likely to be benign with increasing incidence of malignancy with decreasing gland size.
- Minor salivary glands are small unnamed glandular tissues located in the oral cavity and oropharynx and can be sites of origin for salivary gland tumors.
- Imaging is used to assess tumor extent is considered more relevant rather than subtype differentiation.
- Most common: Adenoid cystic carcinoma or mucoepidermoid carcinoma.

Imaging

- Location: Hard palate is most common.
- Usually well-defined with homogeneous enhancement and T_2 hyperintensity (Fig. e40.10).

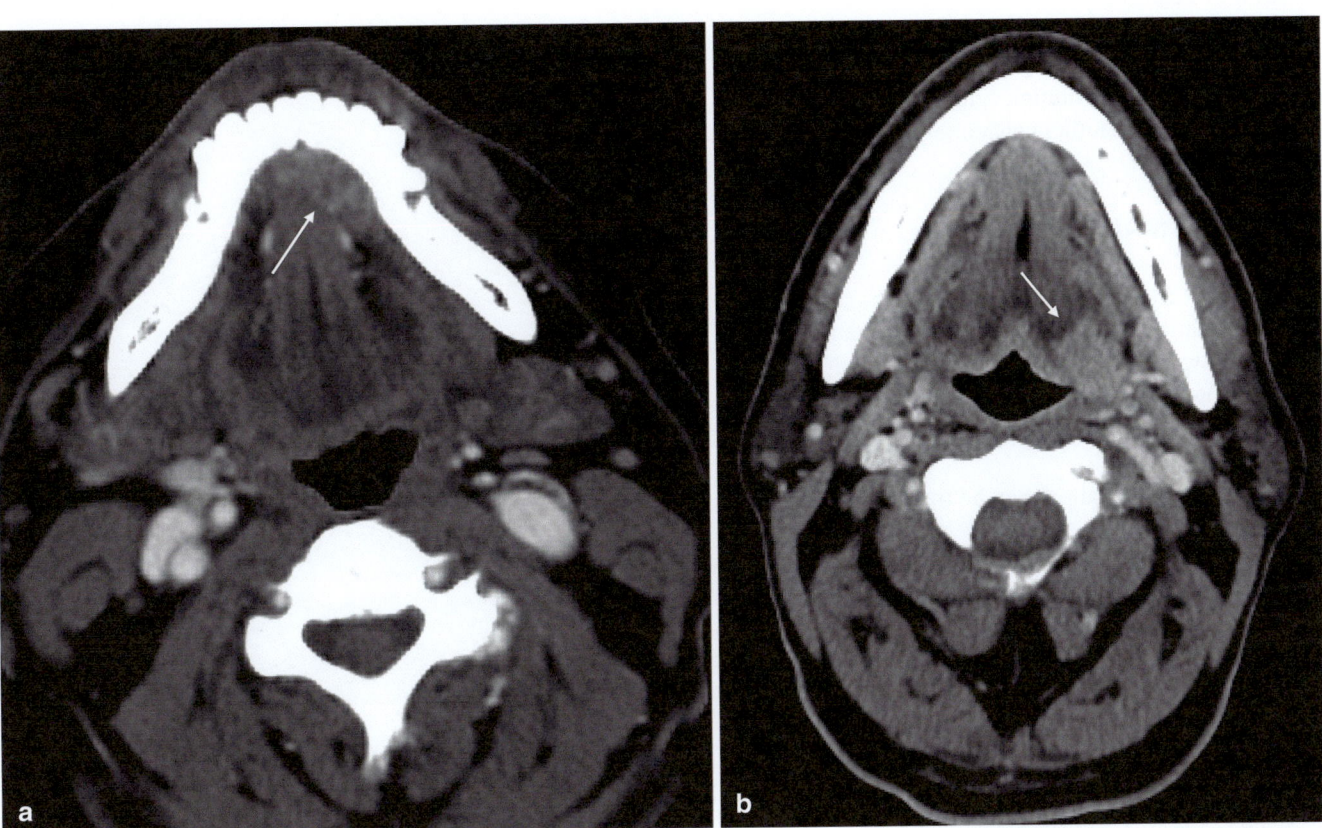

Fig. 40.7 Oral cavity squamous cell carcinoma. Anterior floor of mouth squamous cell carcinoma (**a**) and left base of tongue/glossotonsillar sulcus squamous cell carcinoma (**b**). Enhancing lesions is appreciated in both cases

Vascular Lesions

VASCULAR NEOPLASMS

Infantile hemangioma

- Benign vascular neoplasm due to endothelial cell proliferation.
- Positive for GLUT1 immunohistochemistry marker.
- Typically not apparent at birth.
- PHACES association (Posterior fossa/supratentorial brain malformations, Hemangioma, Arterial anomalies, Cardiovascular defects, Eye abnormalities, Supraumbilical raphe/sternal clefts).
- Fatty replacement during the involuting phase.

Imaging
- US Doppler shows high-flow vessels within or adjacent to the mass (proliferative phase).
- Low-resistance arterial waveforms on spectral tracing.
- Well-defined mass with avid post-contrast enhancement.

Congenital Hemangioma (RICH/SICH/PICH/NICH)
- Benign vascular tumor present at birth.
- GLUT1 negative.
- RICH: Rapidly involuting congenital hemangioma.
- SICH: Slowly involuting congenital hemangioma.
- PICH: Partially involuting congenital hemangioma.
- NICH: Non-involuting congenital hemangioma.

VASCULAR MALFORMATIONS

- Includes arteriovenous malformation (AVM), venous malformation (VM), lymphatic malformation (LM).
- High flow: AVM.
- Low flow: VM, LM.
- Most of them are present at birth. AVM can result post-trauma.
- Vascular malformations can be trans-spatial (more than 1 compartment).
- VM: Abnormal collection of venous channels, fat with degenerated muscle matrix.
- LM: Abnormal collection of lymphatics. Two forms (macrocystic and microcystic).

Imaging
- Venous malformations: Usually well-circumscribed, lobulated mass. T_2 hyperintense with avid post-contrast enhancement. CT can show phleboliths (pathognomonic) (Fig. e40.11).
- Lymphatic malformation: cystic, multiseptated mass where enhancement is limited to capsule or septae. Prone to internal hemorrhage with fluid-fluid level (Fig. e40.12).

Congenital Lesions in the Head and Neck

BRANCHIAL CLEFT CYST

- Second branchial cleft cyst: most commonly posterior to the submandibular gland. Lateral to carotid space and anterior and medial to sternocleidomastoid.
- Cervical sinus of His remnant.
- Can be confused with cystic metastatic lymph node (e.g., HPV-associated oropharyngeal SCC).
- Can get superinfected.

Imaging
- Well-circumscribed cystic, non-enhancing mass posterior to the submandibular gland, lateral to carotid space, and anteromedial to sternocleidomastoid (Fig. 40.8).

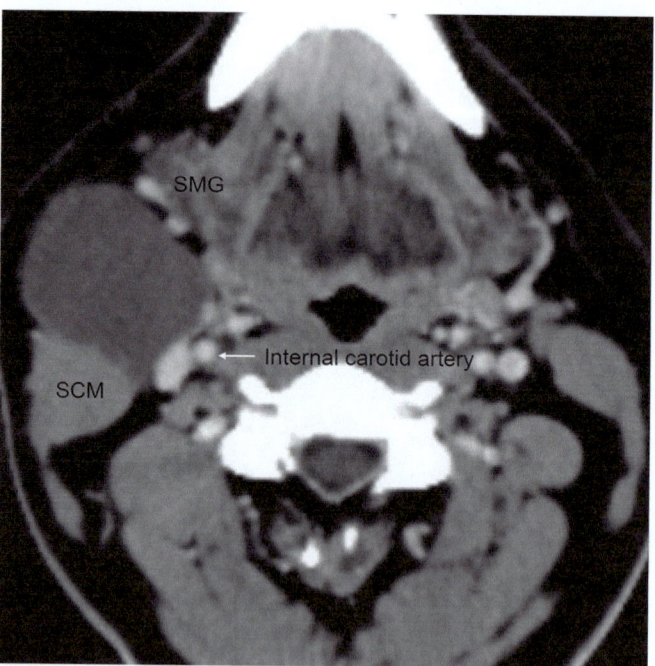

Fig. 40.8 Second branchial cleft cyst. Well-circumscribed non-enhancing cystic lesion posterior to the submandibular gland (SMG), anterior to sternocleidomastoid (SCM), and lateral to the carotid space

THYROGLOSSAL DUCT CYST (TGDC)

- Thyroglossal duct remnant: Midline cystic lesion that can be seen anywhere from the foramen cecum (tongue base) to the thyroid bed.
- Locations: suprahyoid, hyoid, and infrahyoid.

Imaging

- Well-circumscribed cystic midline neck mass. May have thin peripheral wall enhancement (Fig. e40.13).

ECTOPIC THYROID

- Thyroid tissue rests along the thyroglossal duct.
- Most common location: Base of tongue (lingual thyroid).
- Maybe the only thyroid tissue present.

Imaging

- CT: Hyperdense mass on noncontrast-enhanced CT.
- MR: T_1 hyper to isointense to muscle. Shows homogeneous avid postcontrast enhancement (Fig. 40.9).

RANULA

- Sublingual gland or minor salivary gland retention cyst.
- Simple ranula is contained in sublingual space.
- Diving ranula pierces through mylohyoid defect into submandibular space.

Imaging

- Well-circumscribed cystic mass in sublingual gland. CT shows low-density mass (Fig. e40.14a).
- T_2 hyperintense. Little to no peripheral rim enhancement (Fig. e40.14b).

DERMOID/EPIDERMOID

- Cystic mass due to epithelial inclusion or rest.
- Epidermoid: Only epithelial elements.
- Dermoid: Epithelial elements and dermal appendages (e.g., fat, calcium).

Imaging

- Epidermoid: CT shows well-circumscribed cystic lesion.
- Dermoid: Well-circumscribed lesion that may also show fat or calcifications. Density may vary depending on the fluid content (Fig. 40.10).
- MR: Restricted diffusion, may show "stack of marbles" intralesional fat. T_1 signal varies depending on the protein content (increasing intensity with increasing protein content). Little to no peripheral rim enhancement.

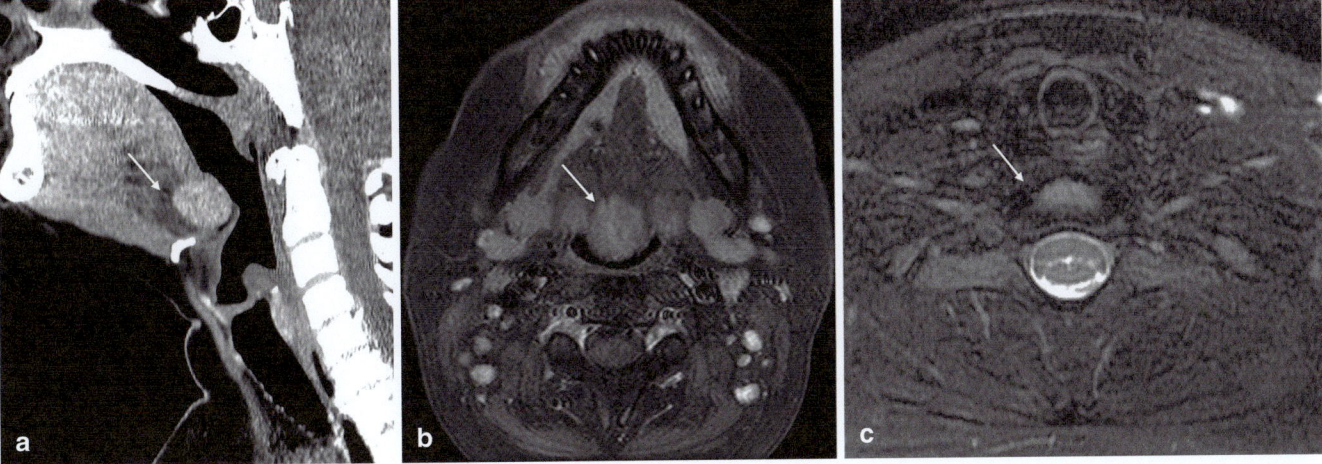

Fig. 40.9 Ectopic thyroid. Sagittal post-contrast CT (**a**) and axial post-contrast MRI (**b**) show an avidly enhancing, well-circumscribed lesion at base of tongue. No thyroid tissue was seen in the thyroid bed (**c**)

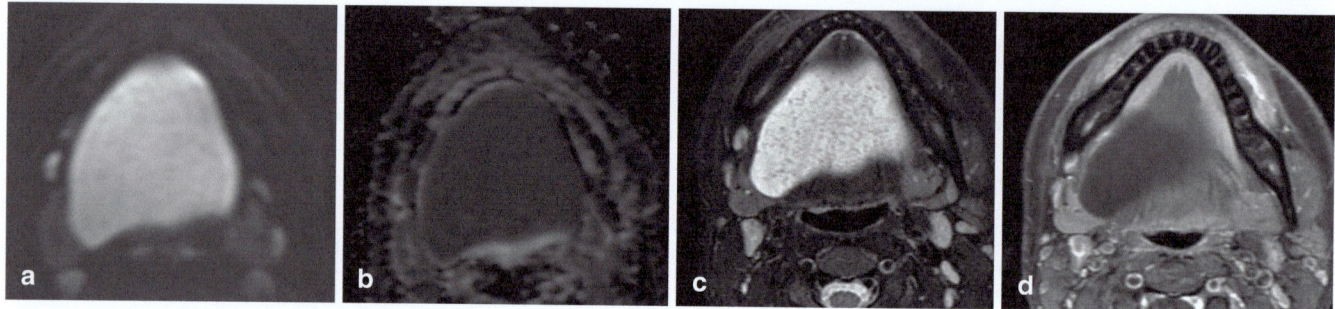

Fig. 40.10 Dermoid. A well-circumscribed mass with restricted diffusion (**a** and **b**). The lesion is T_2 hyperintense with intralesional T_2 hypointense fat lobules on axial T_2 fat-saturated image (**c**). There is no enhancement (**d**)

Trauma

- Dedicated imaging of the maxilla, temporal bone, and face can be obtained in the setting of trauma and suspected fracture.
- The majority (~60%) of mandibular fractures are multifocal, as the mandible and base of the skull create a bony ring, articulated via the temporomandibular joints (Fig. e40.15).

Bibliography

1. Law CP, Chandra RV, Hoang JK, Phal PM. Imaging the oral cavity: key concepts for the radiologist. Br J Radiol. 2011;84(1006):944–57.
2. Chapman MC, Soares BP, Li Y, et al. Congenital oral masses: an anatomic approach to diagnosis. Radiographics. 2019;39(4):1143–60.
3. Loureiro RM, Naves EA, Zanello RF, Sumi DV, Gomes RLE, Daniel MM. Dental emergencies: a practical guide. Radiographics. 2019;39(6):1782–95.
4. Brahmbhatt AN, Skalski KA, Bhatt AA. Vascular lesions of the head and neck: an update on classification and imaging review. Insights Imaging. 2020;11(1):19.
5. Capps EF, Kinsella JJ, Gupta M, Bhatki AM, Opatowsky MJ. Emergency imaging assessment of acute, nontraumatic conditions of the head and neck. Radiographics. 2010;30(5):1335–52.

Imaging of the Larynx and Hypopharynx

Kevin Byunghoon Oh and Xin Cynthia Wu

General Anatomy

- The hyoid bone divides the neck into the suprahyoid and infrahyoid neck.
- The larynx and hypopharynx are aerodigestive tract subsites that are located within the infrahyoid visceral space and serve as conduits between the oropharynx and trachea as well as the oropharynx and esophagus, respectively [1, 2].
- Cartilage structures (Fig. 41.1; Table 41.1), attached ligaments, and fascial planes demarcate boundaries between the larynx, hypopharynx, and adjacent structures, which are important for understanding patterns of spread for pathology (Table 41.2).

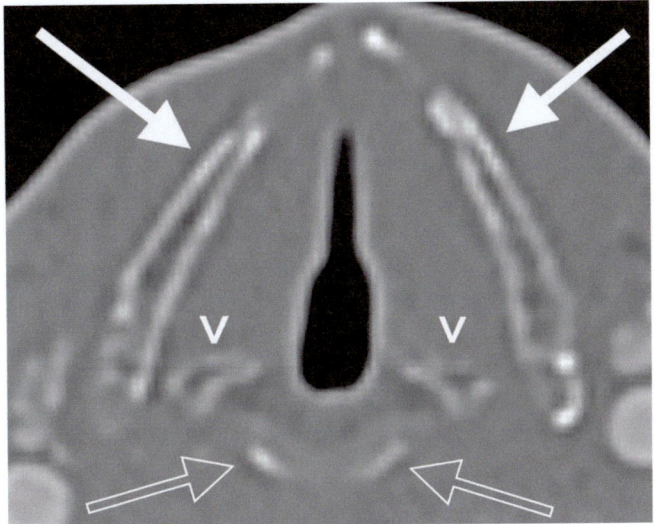

Fig. 41.1 Cartilage structures of the larynx. Axial CT image showing the thyroid cartilage (*solid arrow*), which lies anterior to the cricoid cartilage (*arrow outline*). The arytenoid cartilages (*arrowheads*) articulate with the lateral edges of the cricoid. The cartilages are partially calcified, a process that begins around the second decade of life

Table 41.1 Laryngeal cartilages [3]

Thyroid cartilage	Cricoid cartilage	Arytenoid cartilage
Ventral to the larynx	Dorsal to the thyroid cartilage	Paired small cartilages articulating with the dorsal and superolateral edges of the cricoid
"Protects" more dorsal structures	Helps maintain airway patency. Only laryngeal cartilage forms a complete ring	Attaches to the true vocal cords

Supplementary Information The online version contains supplementary material available at https://doi.org/10.1007/978-3-031-55124-6_41.

K. B. Oh
Department of Radiology and Imaging Sciences, Emory University School of Medicine, Atlanta, GA, USA
e-mail: kevin.byunghoon.oh@emory.edu

X. C. Wu (✉)
Neuroradiology Division, Department of Radiology and Biomedical Imaging, University of California San Francisco, San Francisco, CA, USA
e-mail: xin.wu@ucsf.edu

Table 41.2 Laryngeal membranes [3]

Thyrohyoid membrane	Quadrangular membrane	Conus elasticus
Connects the superior cornua of thyroid cartilage to the body and greater cornua of the hyoid bone	Connects the lateral margin of the epiglottis to the arytenoid cartilage	Connects the cricoid cartilage with the thyroid cartilage; also known as the cricovocal/cricothyroid membrane
Only membrane completely external to the laryngeal lumen	Internal membrane within the laryngeal mucosa, serving as the medial border of the paraglottic space	Consists of an *anterior* cricothyroid ligament and *lateral* cricothyroid ligaments in the inferior larynx
The superior laryngeal nerve and artery pass through this membrane	Two additional important ligaments form its borders: aryepiglottic ligament (cranial) and vestibular ligament (caudal)	The lateral cricothyroid ligaments are thickened and help form the vocal ligaments, which help make up the true vocal cords

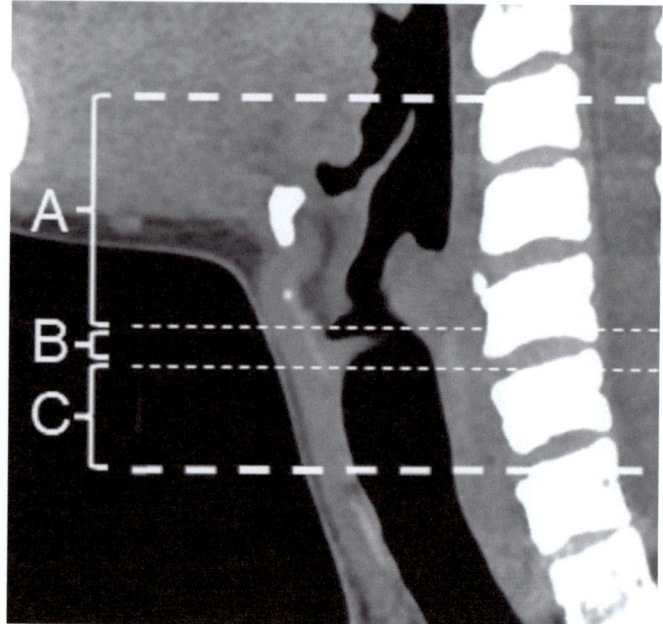

Fig. 41.2 Sagittal view of the laryngeal subregions. On this sagittal CT image, the epiglottis approximates the region of the supraglottic larynx (*A*) followed by the glottic larynx (*B*). The region approximately 1 cm below true vocal cords (*C*) is the subglottic larynx

Anatomy of the Larynx

- The larynx connects the oropharynx cranially to the trachea caudally.
    - Extends from approximately the level of the hyoid bone down to the cricoid cartilage.
    - Functions in airway protection and phonation.
- Bordering structures of the larynx.
    - Cranial—tongue base and vallecula.
    - Caudal—trachea.
    - Dorsal—hypopharynx.
    - Lateral—carotid spaces.
- The larynx is divided into three subregions: the supraglottic, glottic, and subglottic larynx (Fig. 41.2); each subregion contains different structures and affects the prognosis and staging for cancers depending on location within these different subregions.

SUPRAGLOTTIC LARYNX (Figs. 41.3 and 41.4; Figs. e41.1 and e41.2)

(All electronic images (Figs. e41.1–e41.9) can be found on this chapter's website on SpringerLink: https://doi.org/10.1007/978-3-031-55124-6_41)

- The most cranially located subregion interfaces with the oropharynx as well as the hypopharynx (Table 41.3).
- The *pre-epiglottic space* and the *paraglottic space* are important fat-filled structures that should be identified when evaluating for malignancy in the supraglottic lar-

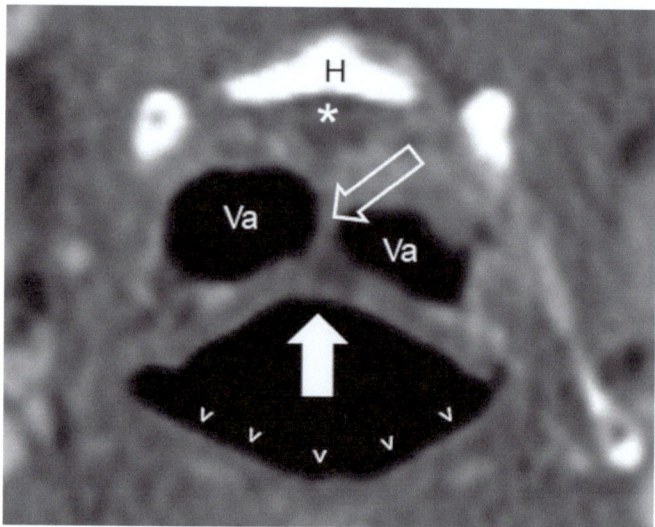

Fig. 41.3 Supraglottic larynx. Axial CT image of the supraglottic larynx, visualized around the level of the hyoid bone (H). The vallecula (Va) are spaces belonging to the oropharynx located ventral to the free epiglottis (solid arrow) and are divided by the median glossoepiglottic fold (arrow outline). The posterior pharyngeal wall is seen dorsal to the epiglottis (arrowheads). The pre-epiglottic space (*) can be seen in this image as the fat-filled space dorsal to the hyoid bone

ynx, as their involvement affects cancer staging (Table 41.4).
- The pre-epiglottic space is contiguous with the paraglottic space inferiorly and laterally [5].

41 Imaging of the Larynx and Hypopharynx

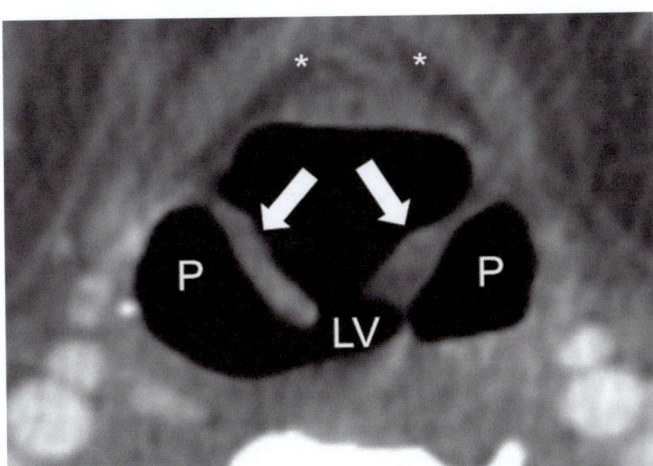

Fig. 41.4 Aryepiglottic folds. Axial CT image of the more caudal aspect of the supraglottic larynx, where the aryepiglottic folds (solid arrows) can be seen with the pyriform sinuses (P), which belong to the hypopharynx, sitting dorsally. The beginning of the laryngeal vestibule (LV), which leads into the glottic larynx through the vestibular folds, is also seen. The paraglottic space (*) is partially visualized

Table 41.3 Structures in the supraglottic larynx

Epiglottis	Structure consisting of cartilage covered by a mucosal membrane, connecting to the hyoid bone (via the hyoepiglottic ligament) and the thyroid cartilages (via the thyroepiglottic ligaments). Consists of a *fixed margin* and a *free margin* which folds down to protect the airway during swallowing
Glossoepiglottic fold	Connects the epiglottis to the tongue, consisting of median and lateral folds
Aryepiglottic folds	Connects the arytenoid cartilages with the lateral edges of the epiglottis, primarily functioning to protect the airway during swallowing. Also forms the superior border of the quadrangular membrane
Vestibular folds (false vocal cords)	Fixed membranes which protect caudally located structures, not involved in phonation (unlike the *true vocal cords*). Paraglottic fat deep to the false vocal cords can separate them from the true vocal cords
Laryngeal vestibule	Air-filled lumen within the supraglottic larynx
Laryngeal ventricles	Slit-like cavities between the true and false vocal cords, lined by laryngeal saccules are thought to provide lubrication

Table 41.4 Borders of the pre-epiglottic and paraglottic spaces [4]

Pre-epiglottic space		Paraglottic space	
Cranial	Hyoepiglottic ligament	Cranial	Pre-epiglottic space
Caudal	Petiole of the epiglottis	Caudal	Conus elasticus
Dorsal	Thyrohyoid membrane	Dorsal	Pyriform sinus
Ventral	Free margin of the epiglottis	Medial	Quadrangular membrane
Lateral	Paraglottic space	Lateral	Thyrohyoid membrane and thyroid cartilage

GLOTTIC LARYNX (Fig. 41.5)

- The middle subregion of the larynx containing the true vocal cords can be approximately identified when all the laryngeal cartilages (thyroid, cricoid, and arytenoids) are seen together on an axial image.
- The primary structures in the glottic larynx are the true vocal cords and their supporting cartilages.
- The vocal folds (true vocal cords) are the primary structure involved in phonation, manipulated by intrinsic laryngeal muscles (Table 41.5).
- The true vocal cords consist of a free edge, which vibrates in phonation, and the vocal ligament, a segment of connective tissue on the conus elasticus stretching along the medial aspect of this free edge.

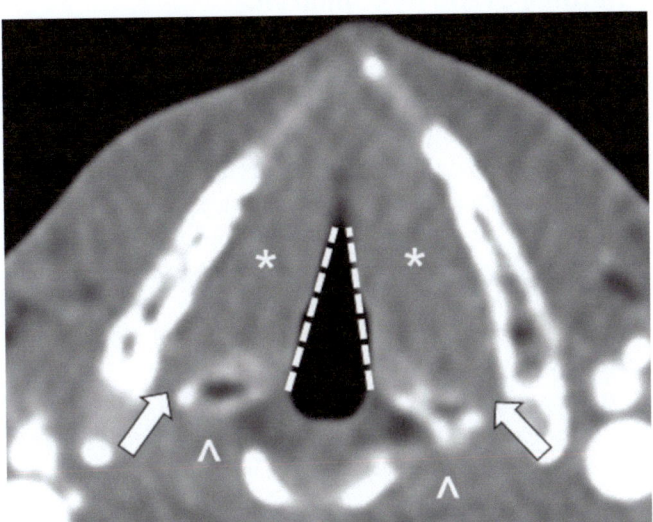

Fig. 41.5 Glottic larynx. Axial CT showing the glottic larynx, which can be approximated visually when all 3 cartilages are seen. The true vocal cords are seen with the thyroarytenoid, or vocalis muscles (*), bounded medially by the vocal ligaments (dotted lines). The lateral cricoarytenoid muscles (solid arrows) and posterior cricoarytenoid muscles (arrowheads) adduct and abduct the true vocal cords, respectively

Table 41.5 Intrinsic laryngeal muscles [5, 6]

Lateral cricoarytenoid	Attach onto the lateral aspects of the cricoid cartilage and onto the muscular process of the arytenoid cartilages	Principal adductors of the true vocal cords
Interarytenoid muscles	Attach onto the medial aspects of the arytenoid cartilages	Adductors of the arytenoid cartilages
Thyroarytenoid (vocalis)	Attach onto the inner thyroid cartilage and vocal processes of the arytenoid cartilages	Relax the vocal ligaments
Posterior cricoarytenoid	Attach onto the posterior cricoid cartilage and onto the muscular processes of the arytenoid cartilages	Abduct and open the true vocal cords

- The spaces ventral and dorsal to the true vocal cords are known as the anterior and posterior commissure (Fig. e41.3).
- The superior and recurrent laryngeal nerves, branches of the vagus nerve, innervate the true vocal cords.

SUBGLOTTIC LARYNX

- This most caudal aspect of the larynx extends below the vocal folds to the inferior border of the cricoid cartilage, continuous with the trachea inferiorly.
- On imaging, the subglottic subregion begins approximately 1 cm caudal to the free edge of the vocal ligament.

Anatomy of the Hypopharynx

- The hypopharynx interfaces with the oropharynx cranially and the esophagus caudally, forming a part of the alimentary tract (Fig. 41.6).
- Located directly dorsal to the larynx and ventral to the retropharyngeal and prevertebral spaces [2].
- Important subregions within the hypopharynx are the *pyriform sinuses*, *postcricoid region*, and *posterior hypopharyngeal wall*.
- Shared regions of the larynx and hypopharynx are as follows:
  - Aryepiglottic folds—boundary between the supraglottic larynx ventromedially and pyriform sinuses dorsolaterally.
  - Postcricoid region—space with borders formed by the cricoid cartilage ventrally and hypopharyngeal wall dorsally [4].

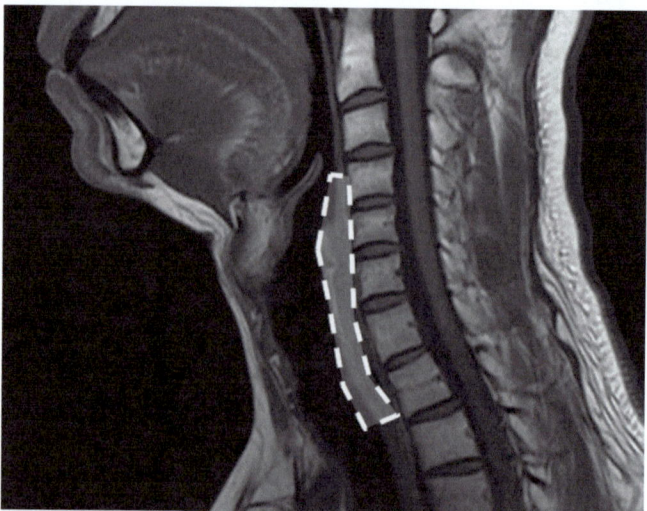

Fig. 41.6 Hypopharynx. A view of the hypopharynx (*outline*) is illustrated on a sagittal T1 weighted MR image of the neck

IMAGING MODALITIES

- Contrast-enhanced CT is the primary tool for imaging the larynx and hypopharynx; the patient should engage in quiet breathing during image acquisition to prevent abduction of the true vocal cords.
- MRI is a complementary tool that provides superior anatomical resolution for certain pathologies and indications, such as cartilaginous invasion in the setting of malignancy; however, MR is more time-consuming and prone to motion artifact from swallowing and breathing.
- PET/CT with FDG is widely used to assist in staging and monitoring of malignancies.
- Application of ultrasound to the larynx is currently limited due to artifact from cartilaginous structures and user variability [7].

Developmental and Congenital Pathology

THYROGLOSSAL DUCT CYST

- The most common congenital neck cyst and pediatric neck mass, making up to 70% of all congenital neck lesions.
- Thyroglossal duct cysts result from abnormalities in embryological thyroid gland development.
  - At gestational week 3, the thyroid gland begins its development by descending from the level of the foramen cecum, through the anterior neck inside the thyroglossal duct.
  - By gestational week 8–10, the thyroid completes its migration, and the thyroglossal duct closes.
  - Remnant thyroglossal duct tissue following duct closure can continue to produce secretions from its epithelial lining, resulting in cyst formation.
- Approximately 75% are located at or below the level of the hyoid bone.
- CT demonstrates well-circumscribed, thin-walled lesions with fluid attenuation, most often located in the *midline* infrahyoid neck (Fig. 41.7) [8].

BRANCHIAL CLEFT CYST

- Branchial cleft cysts result from abnormal embryologic development of the branchial apparatus, which grows between the fourth and sixth weeks of gestation and gives rise to the adult head and neck.
  - The branchial apparatus consists of five branchial clefts.
  - The first branchial cleft gives rise to the external auditory canal.

- o The second, third, and fourth branchial clefts do not form normal adult structures.
- o The branchial cleft involved dictates the location of the anomaly.
- Third and fourth branchial cleft cysts are the rarest but occur at the level of the larynx and hypopharynx.
- Third branchial cleft cysts are found in the posterolateral neck, deep to the sternocleidomastoid muscle.
- Fourth branchial cleft cysts course between the pyriform sinus and thyroid bed and often occur in the left neck, commonly presenting as a superinfection and/or recurrent thyroiditis (Fig. 41.8).

LARYNGOCELE

- Abnormal dilatation of the saccule within the laryngeal ventricle.
- Laryngoceles can be confined to the larynx (internal), extended through the thyrohyoid membrane (external), or mixed.
- Can be congenital or acquired, commonly associated with chronically raised intralaryngeal pressure such as in woodwind or brass instrument players.
- CT demonstrates smooth, well-defined borders with air or fluid attenuation (Fig. 41.9) [9].

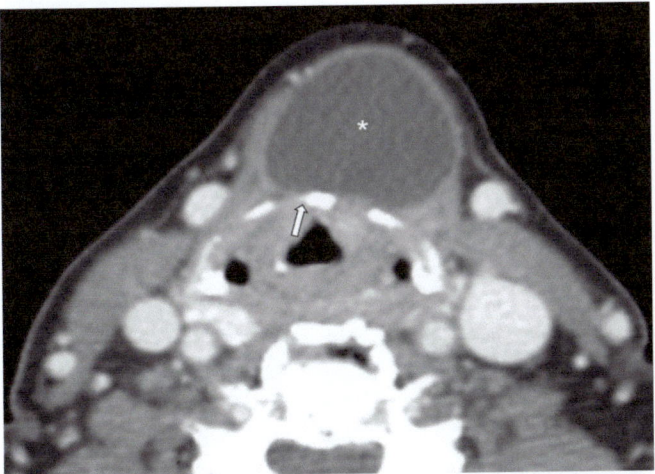

Fig. 41.7 Thyroglossal duct cyst. Axial CT in the soft tissue window demonstrates a well-circumscribed, thin-walled lesion with fluid attenuation (*) at the level of the supraglottic larynx. Located midline and ventral to the thyroid cartilage (solid arrow), this is compatible with a thyroglossal duct cyst

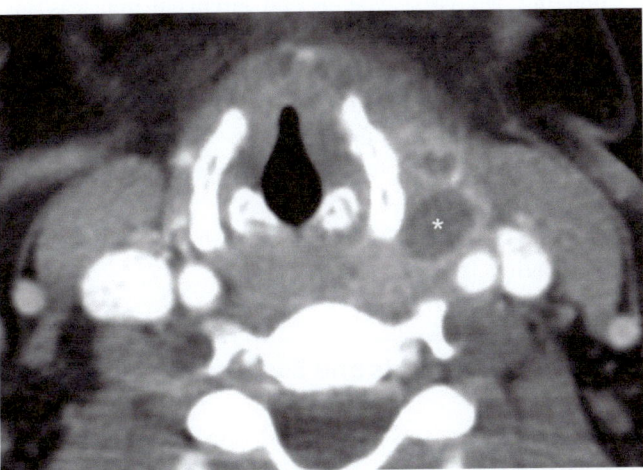

Fig. 41.8 Fourth branchial cleft cyst. Axial CT in the soft tissue window at the level of the glottic larynx demonstrates a fluid-attenuating lesion in the left neck just above the thyroid bed (*). Mild rim enhancement and surrounding inflammatory changes are compatible with superinfection of the fourth branchial cleft cyst

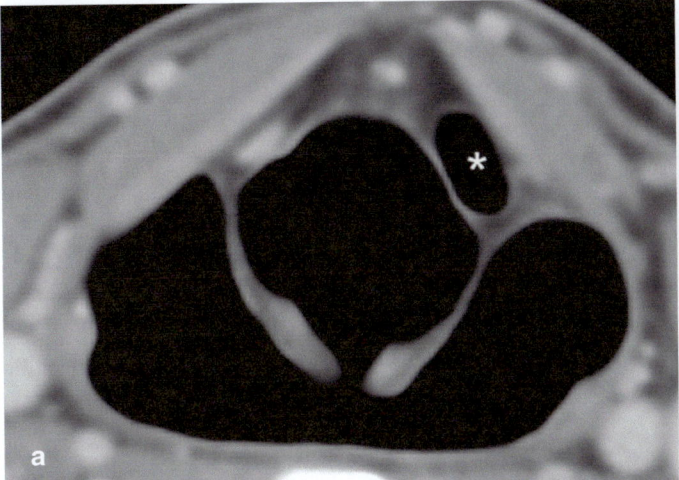

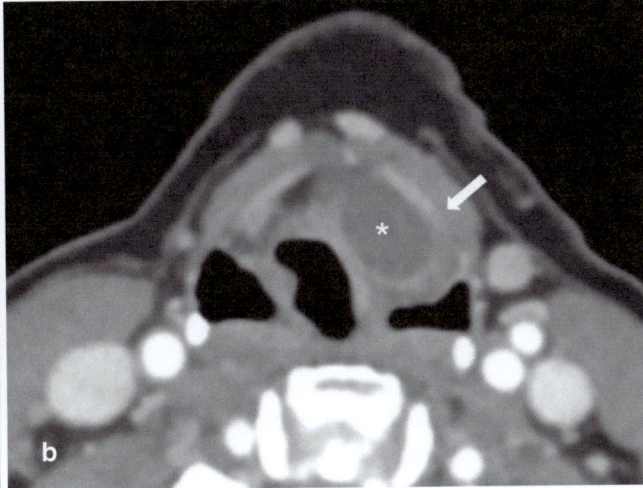

Fig. 41.9 Air and fluid-filled laryngoceles. (**a**) Axial CT image in the soft tissue window at the level of the supraglottic larynx shows a well-circumscribed, smooth-walled lesion (*) filled with air in the left paraglottic fat, compatible with an internal laryngocele. (**b**) A well-circumscribed, fluid-filled laryngocele in the supraglottic larynx (*) dorsal to the thyroid cartilage (solid arrow)

- When identified, secondary causes, including inflammation, trauma, or compression from malignancy, must be ruled out.

Trauma

- Though relatively rare, blunt traumatic injury to the anterior neck, as in motor vehicle accidents, clothesline injury, strangulation, or sports injuries, is associated with high morbidity and mortality [10].
- Laryngeal trauma can lead to airway obstruction and may present clinically as hoarseness, subcutaneous emphysema, or palpable fractures in the anterior neck.
- Imaging can assist when occult laryngeal injury is suspected, most commonly performed with noncontrast CT (Figs. e41.4 and e41.5).
- Injuries can manifest in endolaryngeal soft tissues as edema, hematoma, or emphysema.
- The hyoid bone and laryngeal cartilages can be fractured or dislocated [11].
- Ingested or inhaled foreign bodies can also be visualized on imaging.

Vocal Cord Paralysis and Dysfunction

- Vocal cord paralysis can present with symptoms such as hoarseness, but up to 40% of individuals are asymptomatic.
- The most common CT findings include:
  - Medial positioning and thickening of the ipsilateral aryepiglottic fold.
  - Ipsilateral pyriform sinus dilatation.
  - Ipsilateral laryngeal ventricle dilatation, also known as the "sail sign" (Figs. 41.10 and 41.11) [12].
- Vocal cord paralysis can result from injury to the recurrent laryngeal nerve, caused by surgery (such as thyroidectomies or neck dissections), malignancy, infection, or other compressive lesions.
- The right and left recurrent laryngeal nerves, branches of the vagus nerve (cranial nerve X), share similar courses intracranially, at the skull base, and within the neck, but have differing courses at the level of the superior mediastinum.
- As the left nerve is longer in length (12 cm) than the right (5–6 cm), it is more prone to injury.
- The recurrent laryngeal nerves initially begin by following the course of the vagus nerve as it exits the medulla and leaves the skull base through the jugular foramen, descending through the carotid sheath in the neck into the mediastinum (Table 41.6).

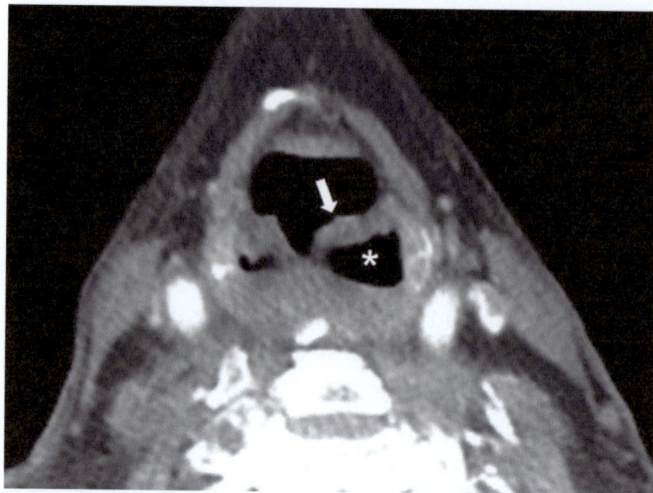

Fig. 41.10 Vocal cord paralysis. Axial CT image of the supraglottic larynx in the soft tissue window demonstrating asymmetric thickening and medialization of the left aryepiglottic fold (*solid arrow*) with dilatation of the ipsilateral pyriform sinus (*), which suggests vocal cord paralysis

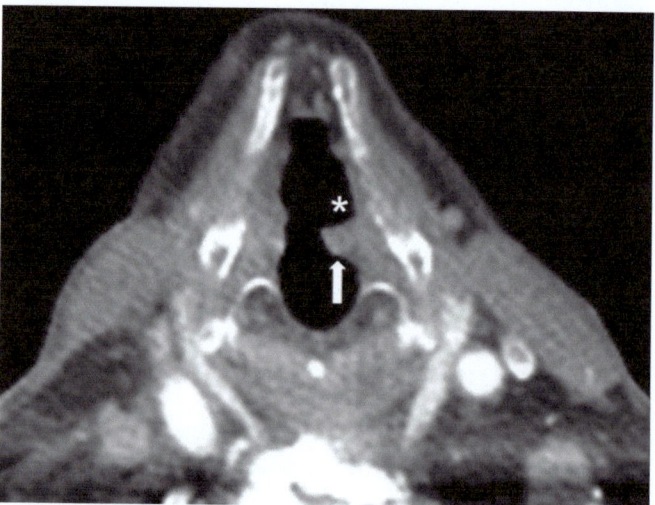

Fig. 41.11 Sail sign. Axial CT image in the soft tissue window demonstrating asymmetric dilatation of the left laryngeal ventricle (*) with a medialized vocal cord margin (*solid arrow*) at the glottic larynx, also known as the "sail sign"

- After identifying imaging signs of vocal cord paralysis, it is important to evaluate the courses of the recurrent laryngeal nerves to identify the etiology of injury, such as malignancy along the respective courses of these nerves [13].
- Treatment of vocal cord paralysis includes laryngoplasty, where high-density material is injected into the paralyzed vocal fold to medialize and improve contact with the contralateral fold during phonation.

41 Imaging of the Larynx and Hypopharynx

Table 41.6 Mediastinal course of the recurrent laryngeal nerves

Right	Left
Exit the carotid sheath ventral to the subclavian artery	Exit the carotid sheath lateral to the thoracic aorta
Loop dorsal to the right brachiocephalic artery	Loop dorsally through the aortic arch and aortopulmonary (AP) window
Ascend cranially and enter the right tracheoesophageal groove	Ascend cranially in the superior mediastinum into the left tracheoesophageal groove
Ascend cranially to the larynx	Ascend cranially to the larynx

- On CT, this can be seen as autologous fat or high-density material (up to 280 to 700 HU) within the vocal fold (Fig. e41.6) [14].

Infection

- Acute epiglottitis, known as supraglottitis in adults, is an infection of the supraglottic epiglottis which can lead to upper airway edema and rapid death.
- The most common pathogens involved are *Haemophilus influenzae Type B* (Hib), especially in children younger than the age of 5.
  - However, since the introduction of the Hib vaccine in 1985, the incidence of epiglottis in children has decreased dramatically.
  - Adults are now more commonly affected, especially in the setting of immunocompromise with pathogens such as Streptococcus pyogenes, Streptococcus pneumoniae, and Staphylococcus aureus [15].
- Commonly made as a clinical diagnosis and with direct inspection on laryngoscopy, imaging can assist in excluding sources of other infections in the soft tissues of the neck as well as identify potential complications such as abscess formation.
- On lateral neck radiographs, epiglottitis can present as the "thumb sign" in the setting of epiglottic enlargement as well as prevertebral soft tissue swelling.
- Contrast-enhanced CT can demonstrate supraglottic edema, effaced fat planes, and thickening of the platysma muscle and prevertebral fascia (Fig. 41.12) [16].

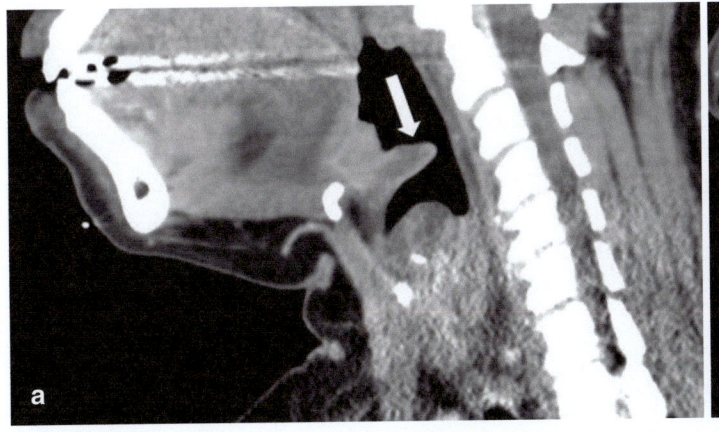
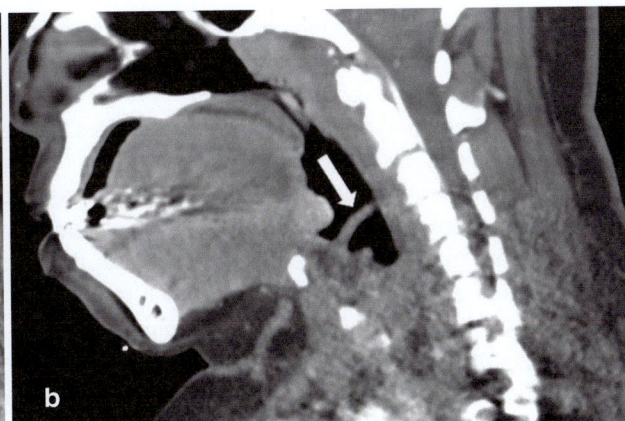
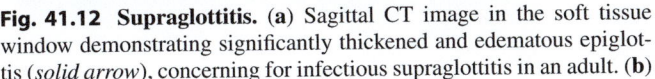

Fig. 41.12 Supraglottitis. (**a**) Sagittal CT image in the soft tissue window demonstrating significantly thickened and edematous epiglottis (*solid arrow*), concerning for infectious supraglottitis in an adult. (**b**) Following treatment with antibiotics and steroids, there is a significant improvement in previously seen thickening and edema of the epiglottis (*solid arrow*)

Vascular Variations

- Retropharyngeal carotid arteries are an important anatomical variant present in 2.6% of patients, resulting from both congenital normal anatomy and developed from long-standing atherosclerosis or hypertension [17].
- Symptoms include fullness, dysphagia, or a pulsatile mass in the back of the mouth.
- Complications include potentially lethal hemorrhage from injury during surgical procedures, such as tonsillectomy or peritonsillar abscess drainage.
- Imaging demonstrates carotid arteries that course medial to the uncovertebral joints (Fig. e41.7) [18].

Neoplasms

LARYNGEAL NEOPLASMS

- The larynx is the second most frequent subsite of head and neck cancers after the oral cavity.
- The most common laryngeal neoplasm is *squamous cell carcinoma*.
- Risk factors include tobacco and alcohol consumption, male sex, >55 years of age, and HPV (present in up to 20–30% of laryngeal cancers) [19].
- Clinical presentation of laryngeal cancer includes hoarseness, dysphonia, dyspnea, and dysphagia.
- Diagnosis is a multidisciplinary effort requiring both direct inspection and biopsy with laryngoscopy and clinical imaging to determine the extent of disease; the invasion pattern and submucosal extent of the tumor play a critical role in staging and treatment planning [20].
- Contrast-enhanced CT is the major imaging modality for staging disease, supplemented by PET-CT for restaging disease and MRI for increasing sensitivity for detecting cartilaginous invasion [21].
- The subsite location of the tumor within the larynx (Figs. 41.13, 41.14, 41.15; Table 41.7) affects the staging algorithm and prognosis of disease (Figs. 41.16 and 41.17; Table 41.8), as the lymphatic drainage differs between each region and affects the local metastatic spread.
- Glottic cancers have the best 5-year relative survival with a higher percentage of patients presenting with localized disease.
- Clinical findings of impaired vocal cord and laryngeal function may override imaging findings when staging laryngeal and hypopharyngeal cancers.
- Treatment options include chemoradiation therapy and surgical removal with the goal of preserving the larynx if still functional; however, for advanced tumors, patients would require total laryngectomy.

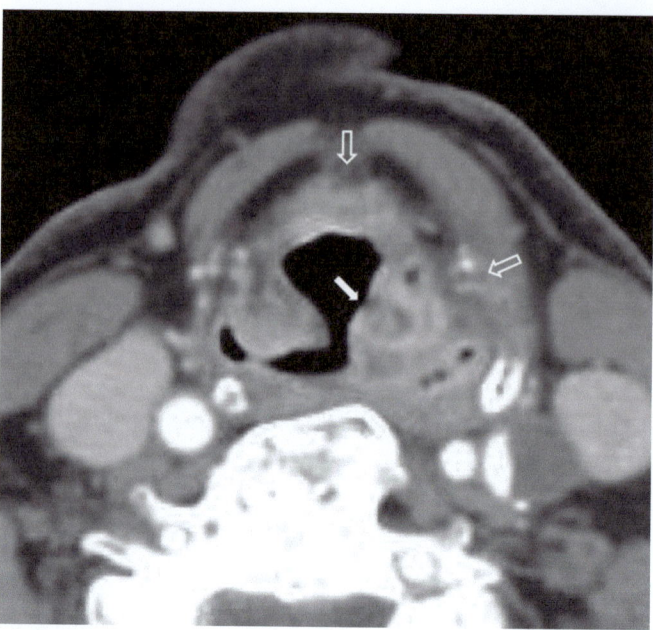

Fig. 41.13 Supraglottic laryngeal carcinoma. Axial CT image in the soft tissue window demonstrating an enhancing lesion of the supraglottic larynx (*arrow outlines*), particularly involving the left aryepiglottic fold (*solid arrow*)

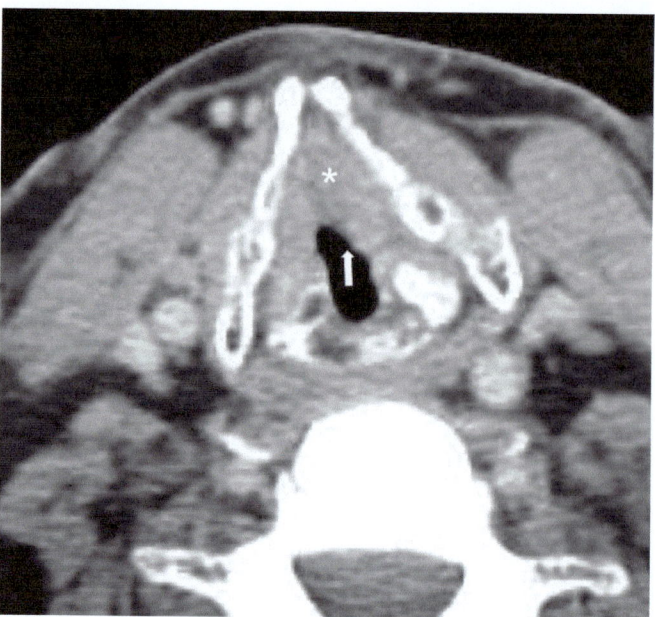

Fig. 41.14 Glottic laryngeal carcinoma. Axial CT image of the glottic larynx demonstrating mildly enhancing, asymmetric soft tissue thickening of the true vocal cords (*solid arrow*) with significant thickening of the anterior commissure (*)

- Total laryngectomy resects all structures from the hyoid bone to the cricoid cartilage, including the epiglottis, aryepiglottic folds, true and false vocal cords, and subglottis (Fig. e41.8).

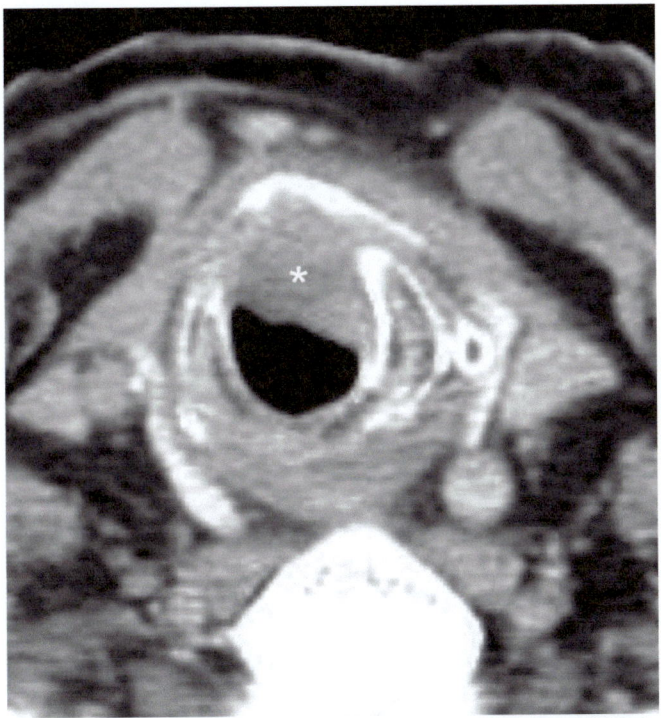

Fig. 41.15 Subglottic laryngeal carcinoma. Axial CT image of the subglottic larynx with significant soft tissue thickening on the ventral aspect of the larynx (*). Normally, the soft tissue abutting the cricoid cartilage is nearly imperceptible at this level

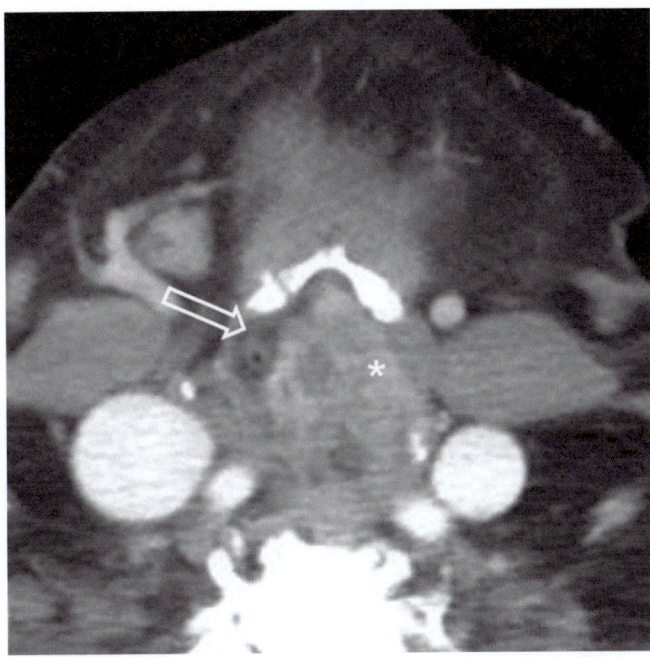

Fig. 41.16 Supraglottic laryngeal carcinoma invading the paraglottic fat spaces. Axial CT image in the soft tissue window showing a supraglottic laryngeal cancer effacing the paraglottic fat spaces on the left (*), compared with the normal paraglottic fat space on the right (*arrow outline*)

Table 41.7 Subsite locations of laryngeal squamous cell carcinoma [22]

	Supraglottic	Glottic	Subglottic
Relative incidence	35%	60%	5%
5-year relative survival rate	46%	77%	53%

- Typical post-total laryngectomy imaging shows a smooth, rounded appearance of the esophagus due to "loss" of the laryngeal structures which normally compress it [23].
- Depending on the extent of invading tumor into the adjacent hypopharynx, a surgical flap is required to form a neoalimentary tract during total laryngectomy if significant resection of the hypopharyngeal wall is required.
- Subsequent surveillance imaging is performed to determine tumor response and recurrence.
- Postradiation complications in the larynx include radiochondronecrosis, which may lead to decline in laryngeal function and eventually require total laryngectomy, even in the absence of tumor recurrence (Fig. e41.9).
- Imaging findings of radiochondronecrosis include heterogeneously enhancing, destructive changes centered in the

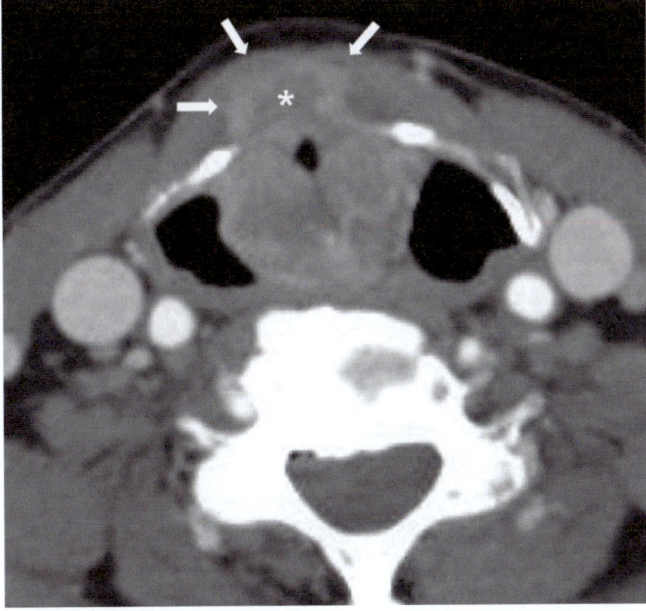

Fig. 41.17 Extra-laryngeal extension of glottic carcinoma. Axial CT image showing a glottic laryngeal cancer (*) extending through the thyroid cartilage (*solid arrows*), a finding that will result in increased TNM staging per the AJCC eighth edition guidelines

Table 41.8 Major imaging features that affect AJCC eighth edition primary site staging of laryngeal cancers

Tumor involvement of multiple laryngeal subregions
Invasion into the pre-epiglottic or paraglottic fat spaces
Cartilaginous invasion and extra-laryngeal extension beyond the thyroid cartilage
Prevertebral or mediastinal invasion
Carotid encasement

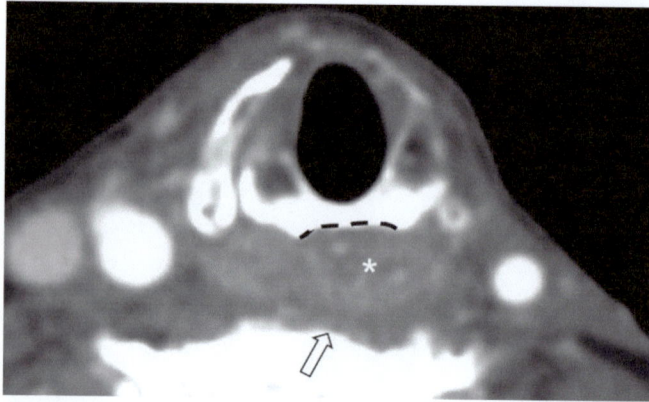

Fig. 41.19 Hypopharyngeal carcinoma. Axial CT image demonstrating mildly enhancing soft tissue in the postcricoid region (*solid arrow*), compatible with a hypopharyngeal carcinoma. Of note, there is scalloping of the dorsal aspect of the cricoid cartilage (*dotted lines*), suggesting tumor invasion

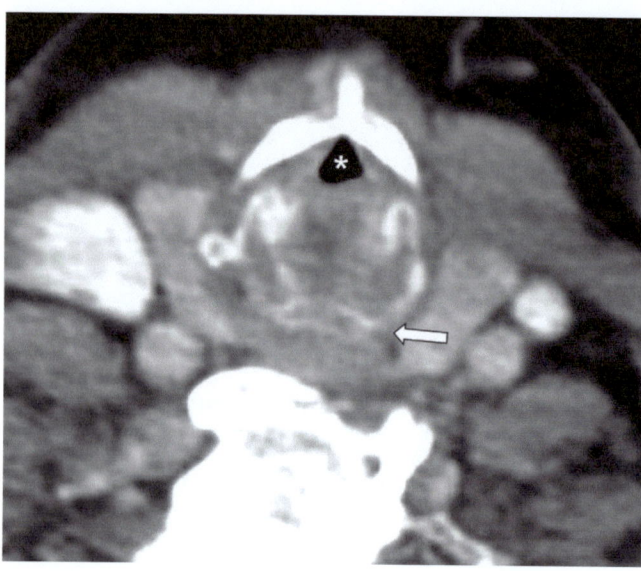

Fig. 41.18 Chondrosarcoma of the cricoid cartilage. Axial CT image in the soft tissue window exhibiting an expansile mass (*solid arrow*) arising from the cricoid cartilage, exerting mass effect on the adjacent subglottic larynx (*)

cartilaginous structures which can be difficult to distinguish from disease recurrence.
- Other tumors that may also rarely affect the larynx, including *chondroid tumors* or *non-Hodgkin's lymphomas*.
- *Chondroid tumors* can arise from any cartilage tissue including the laryngeal cartilages, though only 10% of all chondrosarcomas occur in the head and neck region and make up less than 1% of all laryngeal malignancies [24].
- The most common location for chondroid tumors is the cricoid cartilage, seen on CT as well-circumscribed, expansile masses with smooth walls and coarse calcifications in the cartilage with resultant mass effect (Fig. 41.18) [25] [24].
- *Non-Hodgkin's lymphoma* can also rarely arise from the larynx as a primary site and most commonly involves the supraglottic larynx [26].

HYPOPHARYNGEAL NEOPLASMS (Fig. 41.19, 41.20, 41.21, and 41.22)

- Hypopharyngeal squamous cell carcinomas comprise approximately 7% of all cancers in the aerodigestive tract.

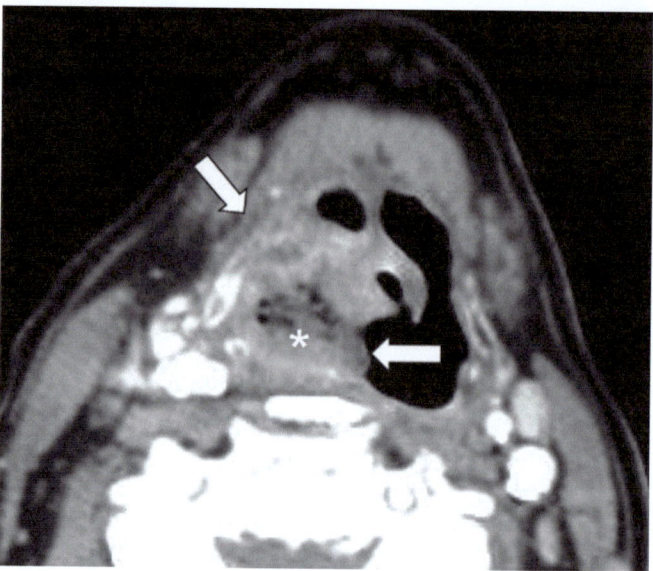

Fig. 41.20 Pyriform sinus carcinoma. Axial CT image showing an enhancing mass within the right pyriform sinus (*solid arrow*), associated with foci of internal gas and decreased tissue enhancement, suggesting necrosis (*)

- Clinical symptoms are vague and can present initially with dysphagia, globus sensation, and otalgia; upon growing large, symptoms include aspiration, hoarseness, and respiratory compromise.
- Overall 5-year survival rate is poor, ranging from 25% to 40%.
- Risk factors include tobacco and alcohol consumption and nutritional deficiency in iron and vitamin C [27].
- The rich lymphatic and vascular drainage in the hypopharynx results in high potential for local and distant metastasis.

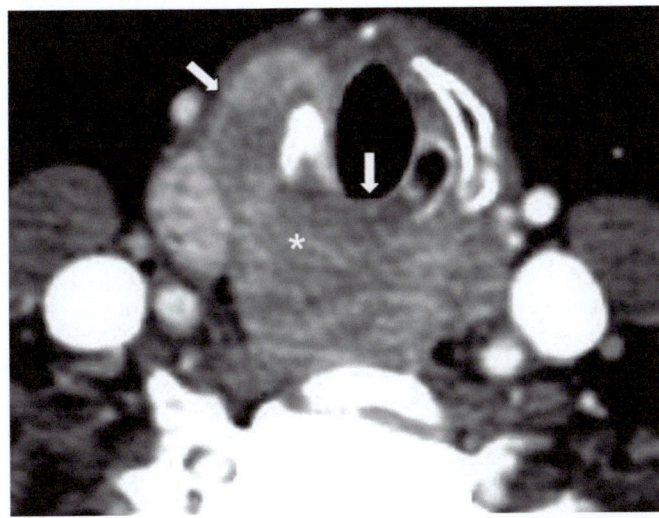

Fig. 41.21 **Extension of carcinoma beyond the hypopharynx.** Axial CT image demonstrating a large, enhancing hypopharyngeal carcinoma (*) extending into the thyroid, strap muscles, and cricoid cartilage (*solid arrows*)

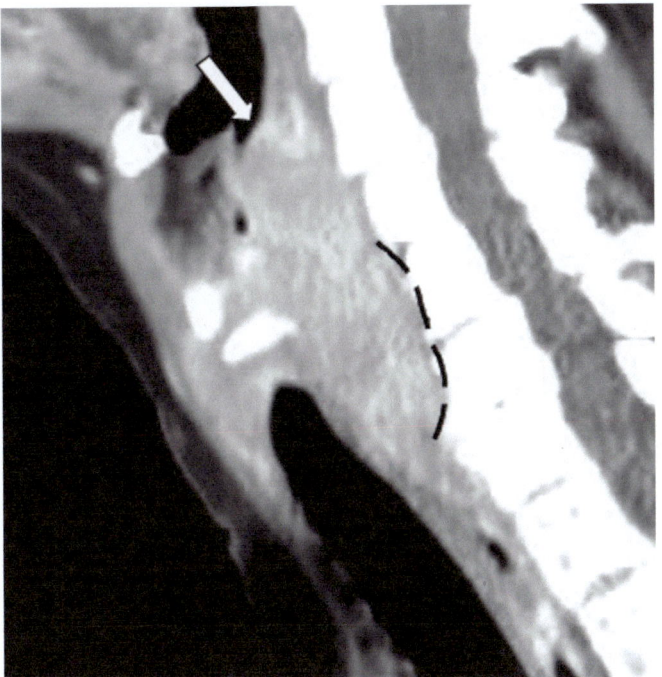

Fig. 41.22 **Prevertebral extension of hypopharyngeal carcinoma.** Sagittal CT image demonstrating a mildly enhancing hypopharyngeal carcinoma (*solid arrow*) with invasion of the prevertebral space, extending into the vertebral bodies (*dotted line*)

- The most common location in the hypopharynx is the pyriform sinus. Primary disease staging criteria are dependent on both tumor size and extent of tumor invasion into surrounding structures (Table 41.9).

Table 41.9 Major imaging features that affect AJCC eighth edition primary site staging of hypopharyngeal cancers

Size of tumor: <2 cm, 2–4 cm, >4 cm
Extension of tumor beyond the hypopharynx, such as into the carotid sheath or spine
Cartilaginous invasion
Invasion of adjacent soft tissue or fat spaces

References

1. Anderson JC, Homan JA. Radiographic correlation with neck anatomy. Oral Maxillofac Surg Clin North Am. 2008;20:311–9.
2. Branstetter BFT, Weissman JL. Normal anatomy of the neck with CT and MR imaging correlation. Radiol Clin North Am. 2000;38(925–40):ix.
3. Netter FH. Atlas of human anatomy. Philadelphia, PA: Elsevier Inc; 2019.
4. Strandring S. Gray's anatomy. Elsevier; 2021.
5. Flint PW. Cummings otolaryngology: head and neck surgery. Philadelphia, PA: Elsevier Inc; 2021.
6. Vahabzadeh-Hagh AM, Pillutla P, Zhang Z, Chhetri DK. Dynamics of intrinsic laryngeal muscle contraction. Laryngoscope. 2019;129:E21–5.
7. Becker M, Burkhardt K, Dulguerov P, Allal A. Imaging of the larynx and hypopharynx. Eur J Radiol. 2008;66:460–79.
8. Ahuja AT, Wong KT, King AD, Yuen EH. Imaging for thyroglossal duct cyst: the bare essentials. Clin Radiol. 2005;60:141–8.
9. Glazer HS, Mauro MA, Aronberg DJ, Lee JKT, Johnston DE, Sagel SS. Computed tomography of laryngoceles. Am J Roentgenol. 1983;140:549–52.
10. Becker M, Duboe PO, Platon A, Kohler R, Tasu JP, Becker CD, Poletti PA. MDCT in the assessment of laryngeal trauma: value of 2D multiplanar and 3D reconstructions. AJR Am J Roentgenol. 2013;201:W639–47.
11. Gamaliel L, Peterson RB, Hudgins PA. Laryngeal trauma: common findings and imaging pearls. Neurographics. 2013;3:92–9.
12. Chin SC, Edelstein S, Chen CY, Som PM. Using CT to localize side and level of vocal cord paralysis. Am J Roentgenol. 2003;180:1165–70.
13. Paquette CM, Manos DC, Psooy BJ. Unilateral vocal cord paralysis: a review of CT findings, mediastinal causes, and the course of the recurrent laryngeal nerves. Radiographics. 2012;32:721–40.
14. Vachha BA, Ginat DT, Mallur P, Cunnane M, Moonis G. "Finding a Voice": imaging features after phonosurgical procedures for vocal fold paralysis. AJNR Am J Neuroradiol. 2016;37:1574–80.
15. Allen M, Meraj TS, Oska S, Spillinger A, Folbe AJ, Cramer JD. Acute epiglottitis: analysis of U.S. mortality trends from 1979 to 2017. Am J Otolaryngol. 2021;42:102882.
16. Smith MM, Mukherji SK, Thompson JE, Castillo M. CT in adult supraglottitis. AJNR Am J Neuroradiol. 1996;17:1355–8.
17. Ozgur Z, Celik S, Govsa F, Aktug H, Ozgur T. A study of the course of the internal carotid artery in the parapharyngeal space and its clinical importance. Eur Arch Otorrinolaringol. 2007;264:1483–9.
18. Lukins DE, Pilati S, Escott EJ. The moving carotid artery: a retrospective review of the retropharyngeal carotid artery and the incidence of positional changes on serial studies. AJNR Am J Neuroradiol. 2016;37:336–41.

19. Steuer CE, El-Deiry M, Parks JR, Higgins KA, Saba NF. An update on larynx cancer. CA Cancer J Clin. 2017;67:31–50.
20. Kuno H, Onaya H, Fujii S, Ojiri H, Otani K, Satake M. Primary staging of laryngeal and hypopharyngeal cancer: CT, MR imaging and dual-energy CT. Eur J Radiol. 2014;83:e23–35.
21. Guenette JP. Radiologic evaluation of the head and neck cancer patient. Hematol Oncol Clin North Am. 2021;35:863–73.
22. Bradford CR, Ferlito A, Devaney KO, Makitie AA, Rinaldo A. Prognostic factors in laryngeal squamous cell carcinoma. Laryngosc Investig Otolaryngol. 2020;5:74–81.
23. Mukherji SK, Weadock WJ. Imaging of the post-treatment larynx. Eur J Radiol. 2002;44:108–19.
24. Wang SJ, Borges A, Lufkin RB, Sercarz JA, Wang MB. Chondroid tumors of the larynx: computed tomography findings. Am J Otolaryngol. 1999;20:379–82.
25. Wippold FJ 2nd, Smirniotopoulos JG, Moran CJ, Glazer HS. Chondrosarcoma of the larynx: CT features. AJNR Am J Neuroradiol. 1993;14:453–9.
26. Siddiqui NA, Branstetter BFT, Hamilton BE, Ginsberg LE, Glastonbury CM, Harnsberger HR, Barnes EL, Myers EN. Imaging characteristics of primary laryngeal lymphoma. AJNR Am J Neuroradiol. 2010;31:1261–5.
27. Wycliffe ND, Grover RS, Kim PD, Simental A, JR. Hypopharyngeal cancer. Top Magn Reson Imaging. 2007;18:243–58.

Vascular Lesions of the Head and Neck

Yang M. Jiang and Alok A. Bhatt

Introduction

- It is important to correctly classify and diagnose vascular lesions of the head and neck as this affects treatment. Important considerations include patient age and clinical history.
- This chapter will use the International Society for the Study of Vascular Anomalies (ISSVA) 2018 classification to review common vascular lesions.
- Vascular lesions are broadly classified into vascular tumors or vascular malformations. Vascular tumors are true proliferative neoplasms, whereas vascular malformations are defects in morphogenesis.

Vascular Tumors

- Vascular tumors are true proliferative neoplasms. They are further classified as benign, locally aggressive (borderline), or malignant. What follows is a discussion of the more commonly encountered vascular tumors in radiology; this is not an inclusive discussion of all the possible vascular tumors.

BENIGN

- Hemangiomas:
  - There are two types of hemangiomas, infantile and congenital. These lesions are differentiated by the age of presentation and clinical course. Infantile hemangiomas are glucose transporter protein-1 (GLUT-1) positive, whereas congenital hemangiomas are not.
  - Infantile hemangiomas are usually diagnosed in the first year of life and undergo rapid growth followed by eventual fatty involution.
  - Congenital hemangiomas are present at birth. Like infantile hemangiomas, they initially undergo rapid growth, however, unlike infantile hemangiomas these lesions then either rapidly involute, partially involute, or remain unchanged.
  - On imaging, hemangiomas are highly vascular, well-circumscribed lesions that demonstrate progressive enhancement and delayed washout. On MRI, they are usually T2 hyperintense (fibrofatty tissue makes these lesions less T2 hyperintense than cerebral spinal fluid) with serpiginous flow voids from feeding and draining vessels on T1 and T2 (Fig. 42.1).
  - Infantile hemangiomas are associated with PHACE syndrome, which is a neurocutaneous syndrome consisting of posterior fossa malformations (P), hemangiomas (H), arterial anomalies (A), coarctation of the aorta and cardiac defects (C), and eye abnormalities (E).

LOCALLY AGGRESSIVE (BORDERLINE)

- Kaposiform hemangioendothelioma:
  - Kaposiform hemangioendothelioma is the most common locally aggressive vascular tumor. Approximately 20% of lesions are found in the head and neck, with the remainder of lesions found in the extremities.
  - On imaging, the lesion is T2 hyperintense with heterogeneous enhancement on T1. The lesion displays aggressive features such as infiltration of fascial planes, subcutaneous fat stranding and may hemorrhage causing fluid–fluid levels and residual hemosiderin deposits (Fig. 42.2).

Y. M. Jiang · A. A. Bhatt (✉)
Mayo Clinic, Jacksonville, FL, USA
e-mail: jiang.yang@mayo.edu; bhatt.alok@mayo.edu

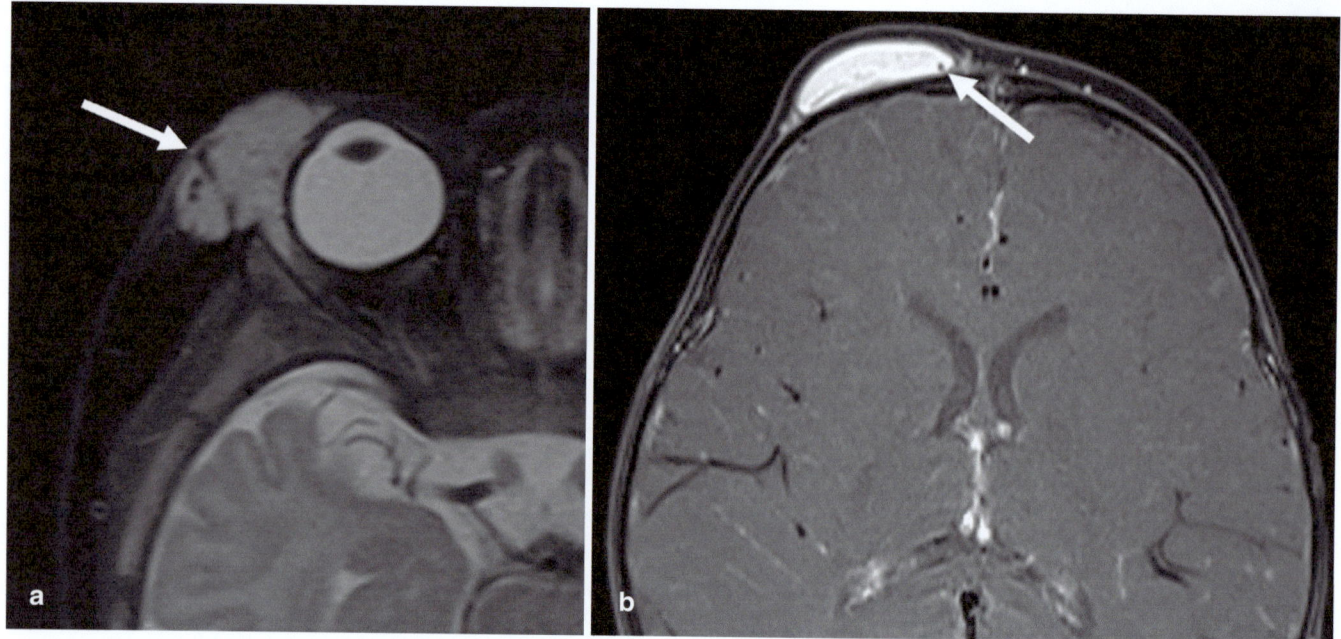

Fig. 42.1 Hemangioma. (**a**) Axial T2-weighted image demonstrates a T2 hyperintense mass centered in the right periorbital region. Note the relative lower T2 signal of the mass compared to the cerebral spinal fluid. (**b**) Axial T1 post-contrast fat-saturated image demonstrates avid enhancement of the lesion. Serpiginous low signal from feeding and draining vessels are seen on both T2 and T1 images (arrow)

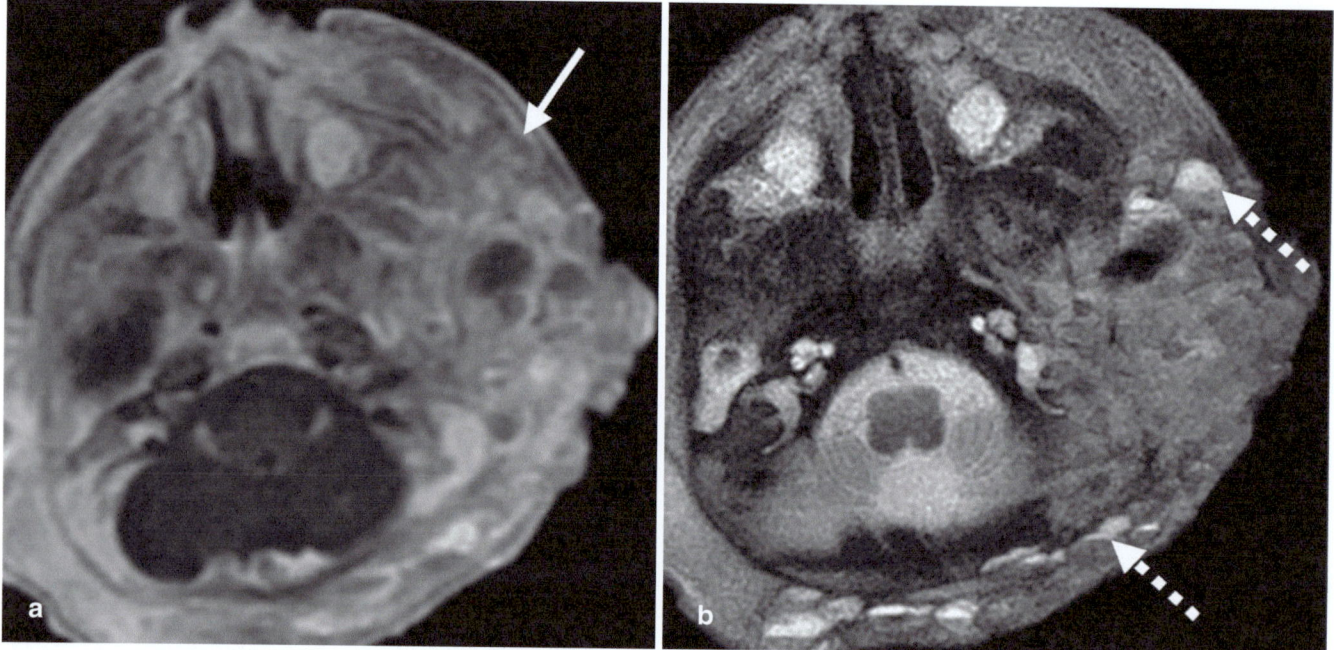

Fig. 42.2 Kaposiform hemangioendothelioma. (**a**) Axial T1-weighted post-contrast image demonstrates an infiltrative mass (multiple fascial planes) within the left face and upper neck with heterogenous enhancement. Note the subcutaneous fat stranding along the peripheral margins of the lesion (solid arrow). (**b**) Axial T2-weighted image demonstrates layering of T2 signal due to hemorrhage (dashed arrows)

- Associated with Kasabach–Merritt syndrome, a life-threatening condition in which rapid proliferation causes consumptive coagulopathy leading to microangiopathic hemolytic anemia, thrombocytopenia, and pain.
- Kaposi's sarcoma:
  - Four variants: classic, endemic, iatrogenic, and epidemic.
  - Iatrogenic is commonly associated with chronic drug-induced immunosuppression in post-organ transplantation. The allograft and lungs are commonly involved.
  - Epidemic or acquired immunodeficiency syndrome (AIDS)-related is associated with human herpesvirus 8 (HHV8) infection.
  - Iatrogenic and AIDS-related are the most aggressive forms, commonly presenting with disseminated disease.
  - Majority of lesions are cutaneous and present as multifocal, purple macules or papules that coalesce, ulcerate, or cause mass effect. Remainder of the lesions involve the oral and laryngeal-pharyngeal mucosa or present with isolated lymphadenopathy.
  - On imaging, these lesions are infiltrative and multinodular with avid enhancement on T1 and hyperintense on T2.

MALIGNANT

- Angiosarcoma:
  - Angiosarcoma is a rare and aggressive vascular lesion. It can occur at any age but commonly presents in the seventh to eighth decade of life. Risk factors include chronic lymphedema and prior radiation.
  - Most lesions occur in the scalp and commonly present as an enlarging bruise or discolored nodule which ulcerates. Remainder of the lesions occur in the deep soft tissue, peritoneum/retroperitoneum and parenchymal organs, breast, bone, and liver. These lesions metastasize via hematogenous spread, most commonly to the lung and bone.
  - On imaging, an angiosarcoma appears as an avid, heterogeneously enhancing soft tissue mass with indistinct borders, often with invasion into adjacent structures. On MRI, the lesion contains serpentine flow voids on T1 and T2 weighted sequences (Fig. 42.3).
- Epithelioid Hemangioma:
  - Epithelioid hemangiomas are very rare, accounting for only 1% of all vascular malignancies. Although it most commonly affects the lungs, bones, or liver, epithelioid hemangiomas can also occur in the head and neck.

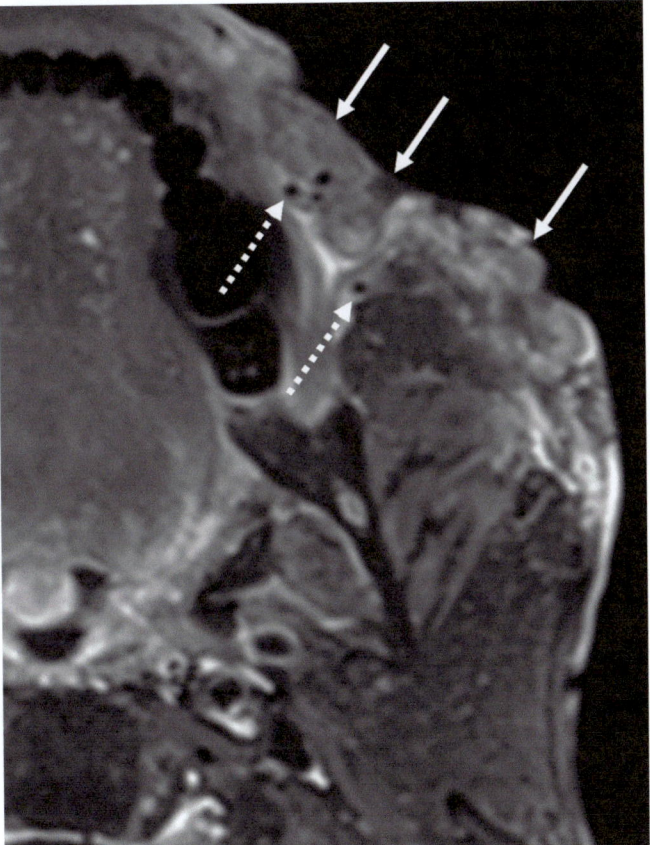

Fig. 42.3 Angiosarcoma. Axial T1-weighted post-contrast image demonstrates a heterogenously enhancing, lobulated ulcerative mass (solid arrows) within the soft tissues overlying the left mandible with several internal void flows (dashed arrows)

  - Often incidentally diagnosed occurs between 30 and 50 years of age.
  - Bony involvement demonstrates well-circumscribed lucent lesions on radiographs. On MRI, they display T1 signal hyperintensity greater than that of muscle and heterogeneous high T2 signal.

Vascular Malformations

- Vascular malformations are defects in morphogenesis.
- They are classified as simple, combined, malformation of major vessels, or by their association with other anomalies.
- Physiologically they can be classified as slow-flow, high-flow, or combined/mixed type.
- Careful evaluation of internal appearance on imaging can help accurately characterize these lesions (Fig. 42.4).

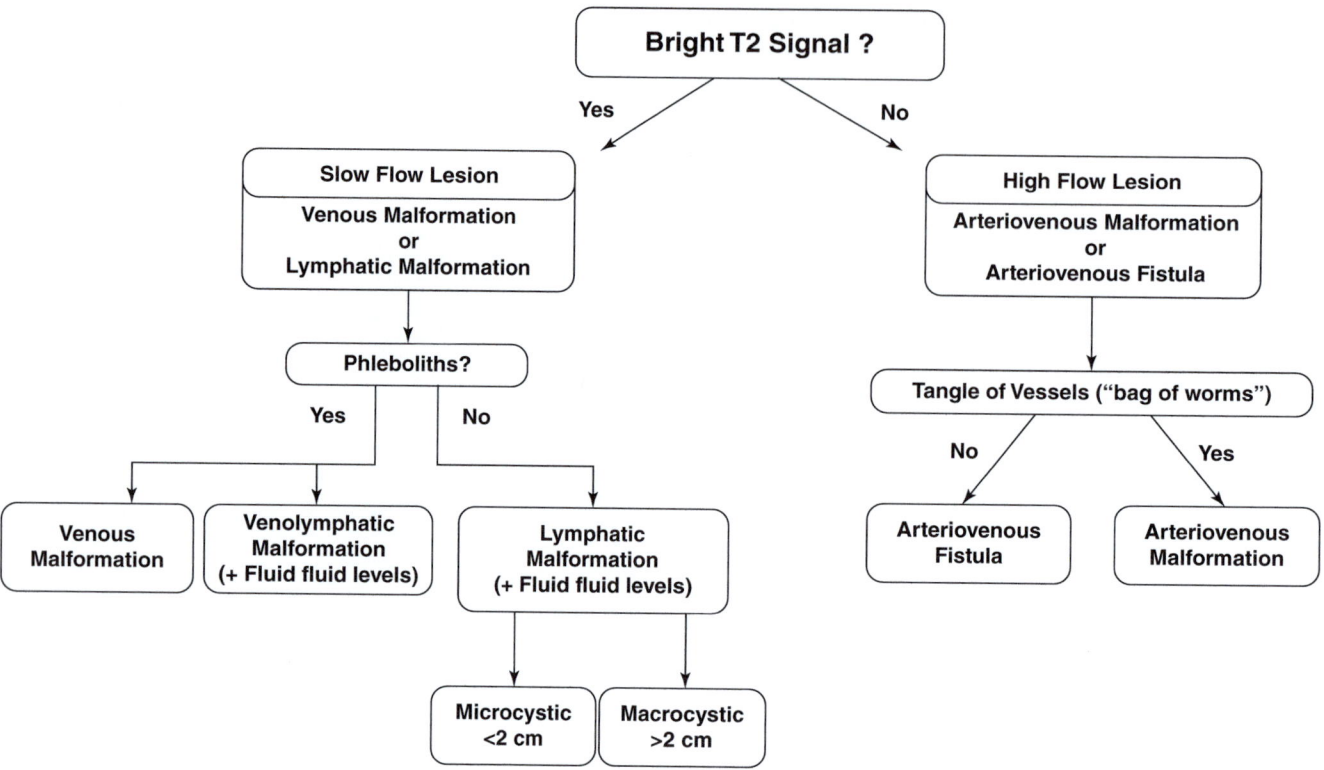

Fig. 42.4 **Vascular malformations.** Flow chart for imaging characterization of vascular malformations

SLOW FLOW LESIONS

- Capillary malformations:
  - Cutaneous lesions confined to the dermis and follow dermal pattern; diagnosed clinically as a "port wine stain."
  - Limited utility of imaging unless concurrent syndromes such as Sturge–Weber or CLAPO is suspected (see below).
  - Sturge–Weber syndrome is a neurocutaneous syndrome consisting of a port wine stain in the ophthalmic division of the trigeminal nerve and leptomeningeal angioma occurring in isolation or combination.
  - CLAPO syndrome: Capillary vascular malformation of the lower lip (C), lymphatic malformations of the head and neck (L), Asymmetry (A), and Partial (P) or generalized Overgrowth (O).
- Venous malformations:
  - Most common vascular malformation.
  - On physical exam, present as a nonpulsatile, compressive soft tissue prominence or discrete mass with a blueish-purple hue.
  - On imaging, lesions demonstrate delayed, avid enhancement with multiple phleboliths due to their slow flow and propensity to thrombose. On MRI, they are serpiginous tubules of T2 hyperintensity (similar signal to cerebral spinal fluid) with scattered internal punctate foci of hypointensity (phleboliths) (Fig. 42.5a). CT demonstrates the phleboliths as calcifications (Fig. 42.5b).
- Lymphatic malformations:
  - Overall, rare vascular malformations, but majority occur in the head and neck. Present at birth or by 2 years of age.
  - Further characterized based on the size of their internal cystic structures: macrocystic (greater than 2 cm) and microcystic (less than 2 cm).
  - Macrocystic:
    - Present as soft, large translucent nontender mass.
    - No internal enhancement.
  - Microcystic:
    - Present as several small, raised sacs on the skin.
    - May demonstrate enhancement of the walls and septa.
  - On imaging, lesions are trans-spatial, multiloculated, cystic masses often with fluid–fluid levels (due to internal hemorrhage). On MRI, there are variable signal on T1 and hyperintense on T2, no internal enhancement (Fig. 42.6).

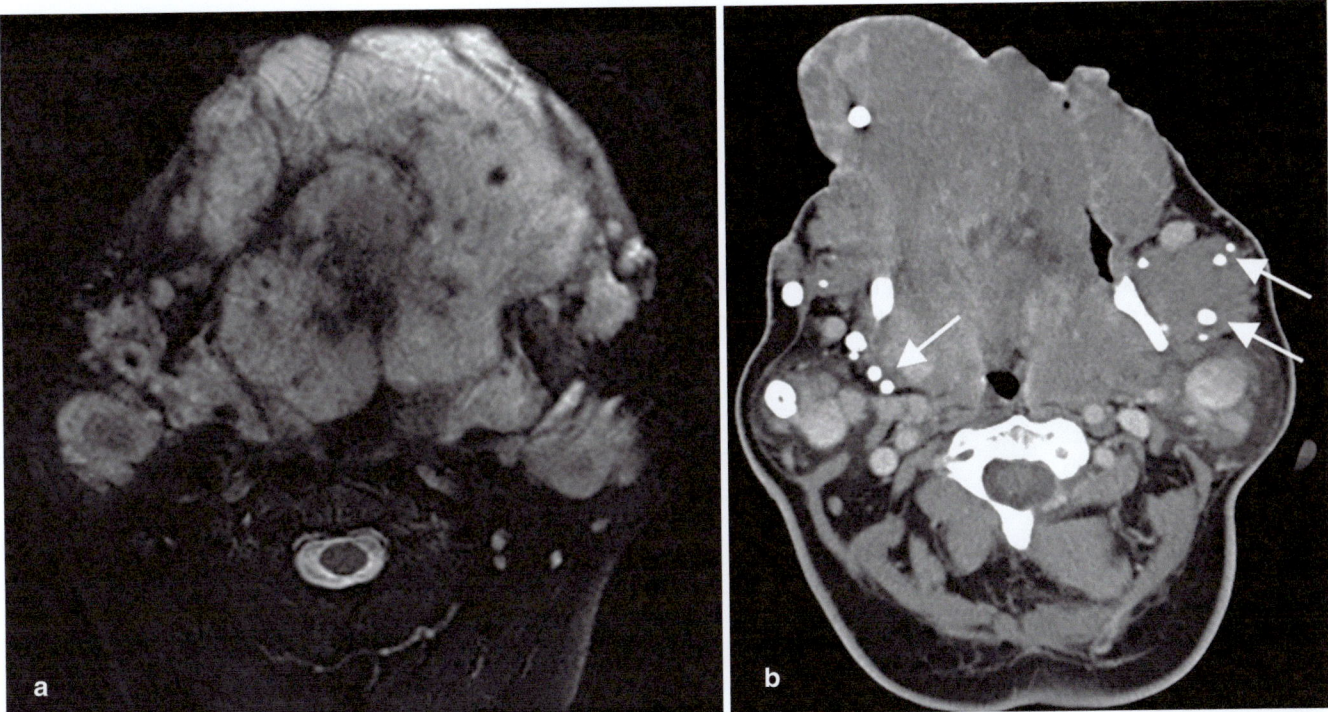

Fig. 42.5 Venous Malformation. (**a**) Axial T2-weighted fat-saturated image demonstrates a large T2 hyperintense trans-spatial mass involving the face and oral cavity. Note the similar T2 hyperintensity relative to cerebral spinal fluid. (**b**) Axial contrast-enhanced CT at the same level demonstrates multiple scattered internal phleboliths (arrows) with the lesion

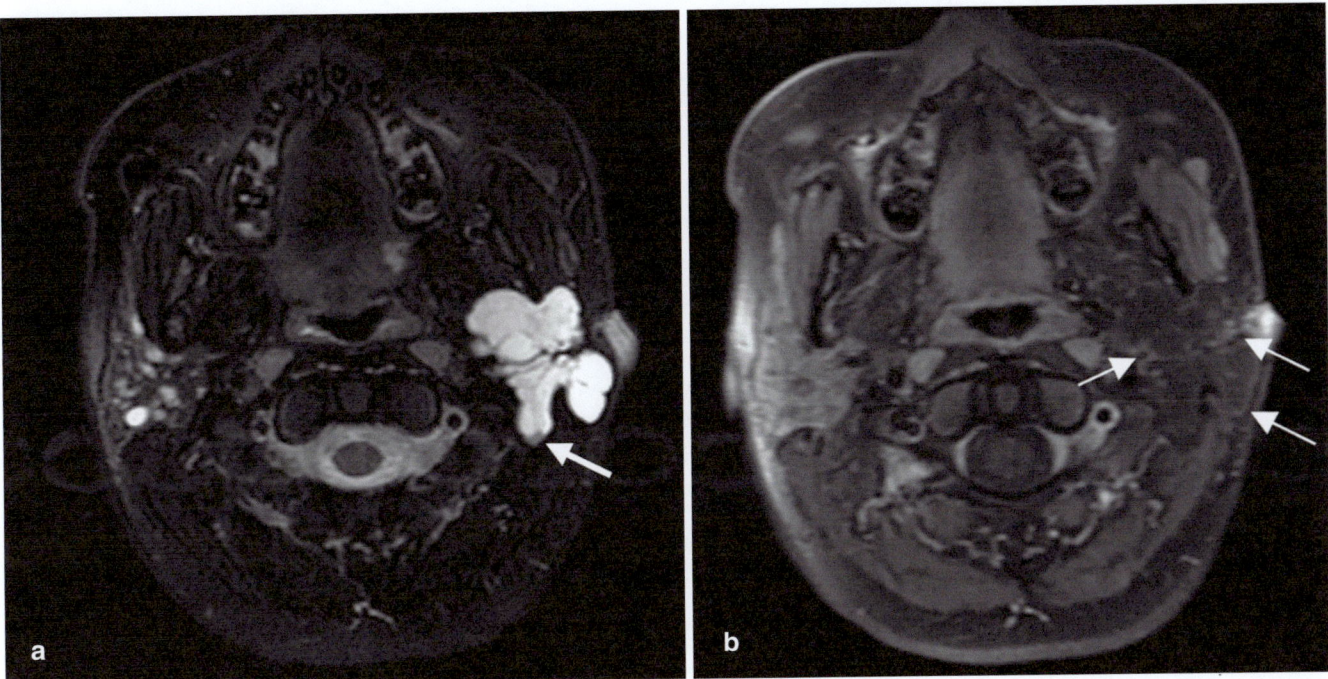

Fig. 42.6 Lymphatic malformation. (**a**) Axial T2-weighted image demonstrates a predominantly high signal mass in the left face; subtle fluid-fluid level at the posterior aspect (arrow). (**b**) Axial T1-weighted post-contrast fat-saturated image demonstrates no internal enhancement. Trace enhancement of the internal septa and peripheral walls (arrows)

HIGH FLOW LESIONS

- Arteriovenous malformation:
  - Lesions lack a normal capillary bed between their arterial inflow and venous outflow, and therefore, may be pulsatile on exam with symptoms of congestive heart failure, venous congestion, arterial steal syndrome, pain, or bleeding.
  - On imaging, serpiginous tangle of vessels, "bag of worms" appearance, with avid enhancement. Often identifiable feeding artery(ies), a nidus with serpentine flow voids, and early enhancement of the dilated draining vein(s) (Fig. 42.7).
- Arteriovenous fistula:
  - Abnormal connection between an artery and vein. Symptoms depend on location of the lesion with some lesions remaining asymptomatic.
  - Best characterized on MR angiogram or conventional angiogram with early venous enhancement and early filling of the markedly dilated vein due to chronic high arterial inflow (Fig. 42.8).

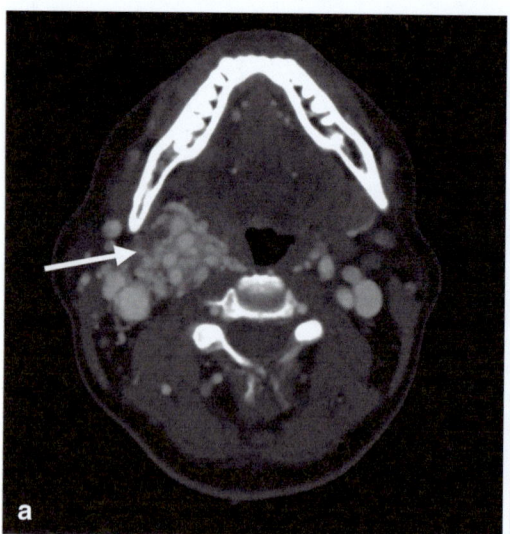 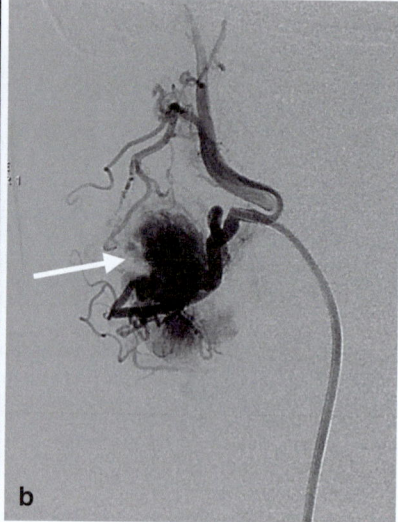 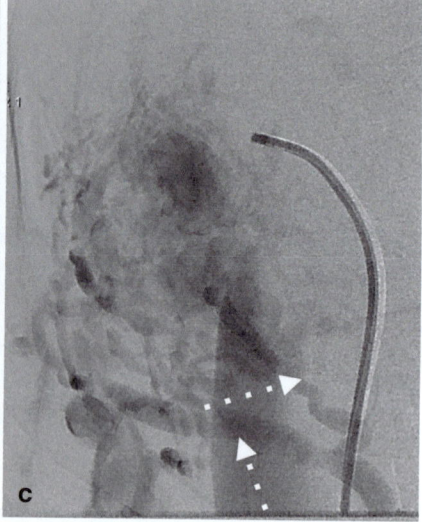

Fig. 42.7 Arteriovenous Malformation. (**a**) CTA of the neck demonstrates a tangle of vessels in the deep right neck, representing the nidus (arrow). (**b**) Conventional angiographic images in the arterial phase demonstrates the nidus (solid arrow) fed by dilated arteries. (**c**) The venous phase demonstrates marked distended draining veins (dashed arrows)

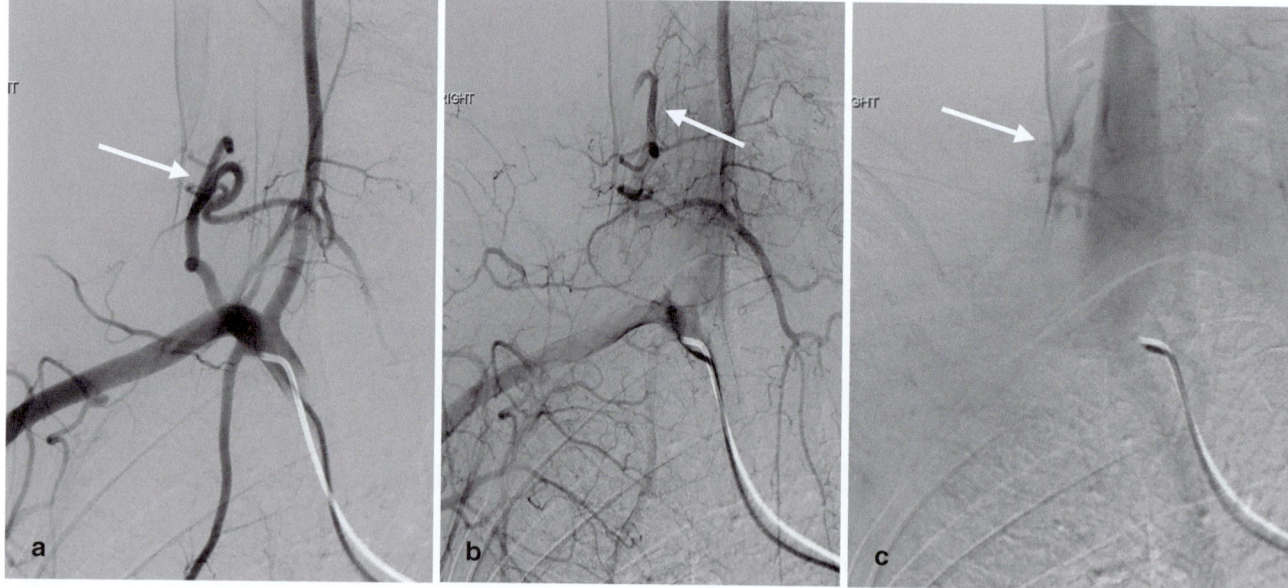

Fig. 42.8 Arteriovenous fistula. Conventional angiogram of the neck with catheter tip in the distal brachiocephalic artery. (**a**) Arterial phase demonstrates a dilated thyrocervical trunk and transverse cervical branch (arrow). (**b**) Late arterial phase demonstrates early venous filling of a dilated vein (arrow). (**c**) Early venous phase demonstrates abnormally dilated and tortuous veins due to chronic high arterial inflow (arrow)

MIXED/COMBINED VASCULAR MALFORMATION

- Complex, which includes more than one type of malformation, can be difficult to diagnose; important to determine if lesion is slow or high flow or a combination. Most common is the venolymphatic malformation.
- Venolymphatic malformation:
  o Displays characteristics of both lymphatic and venous malformations.
  o On imaging, appear as a multiloculated cystic mass with fluid–fluid levels and enhancement on delayed phase. The venous component will have multiple scattered phleboliths due to slow flow and propensity to thrombose (Fig. 42.9).

Conclusion

- Appropriate classification and imaging diagnosis of head and neck vascular lesions is important to guide correct treatment.
- Vascular lesions consist of vascular tumors and vascular malformations.
- Vascular tumors are further classified as benign, locally aggressive (borderline), or malignant.
- Vascular malformations can be further characterized by their flow rate into slow flow lesions (capillary malformation, venous malformation, lymphatic malformation, or combination of the above) and high flow lesions (arteriovenous malformation and arteriovenous fistula).

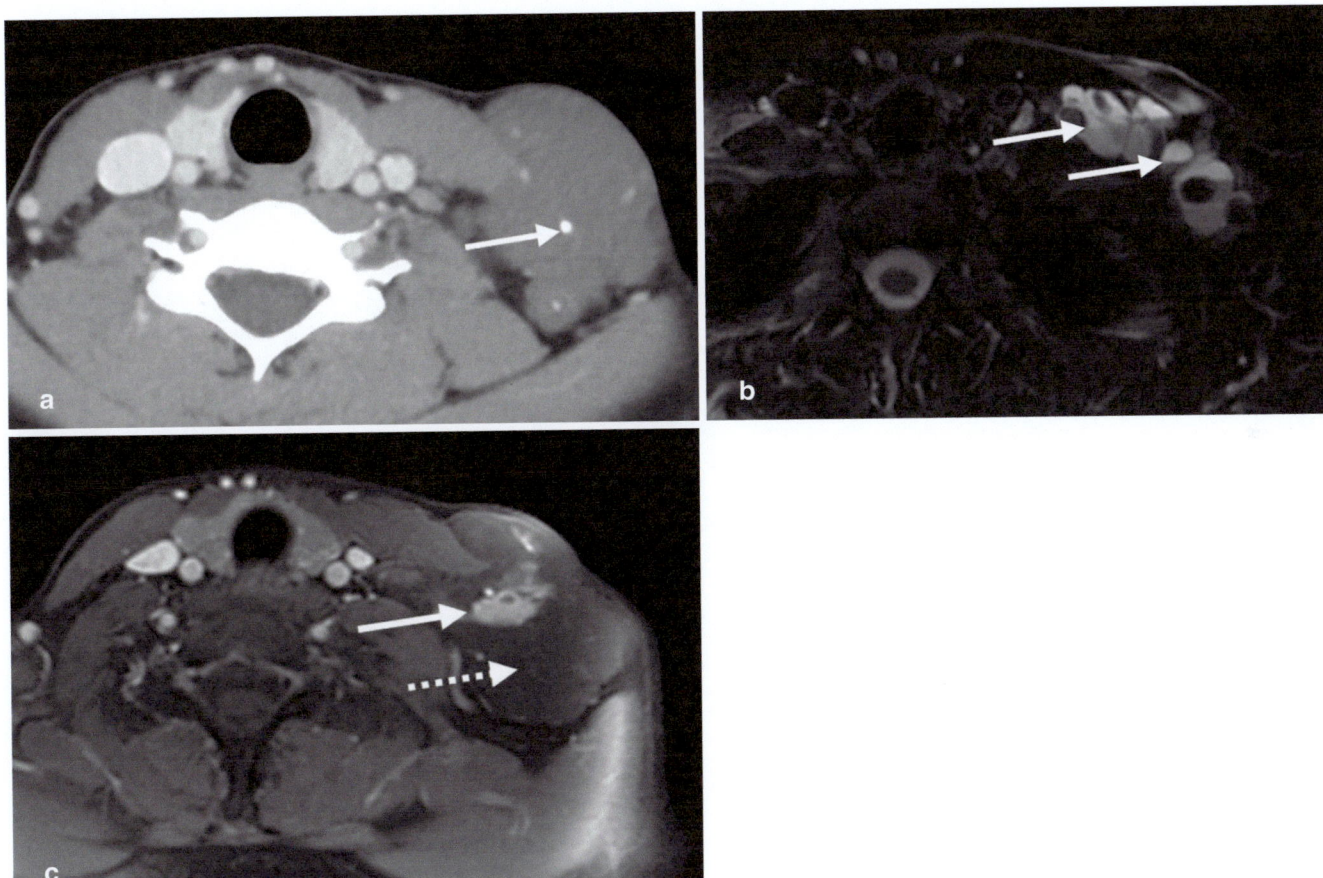

Fig. 42.9 Venolymphatic malformation. (**a**) Axial CT post-contrast image demonstrates a cystic lesion at the left neck base with internal phleboliths (venous component, arrow). (**b**) Axial T2-weighted image demonstrates fluid-fluid levels within the lesion (lymphatic component, arrows). (**c**) Axial T1-weighted post-contrast image demonstrates enhancing (venous component, solid arrow) and non-enhancing components (lymphatic component, dashed arrow)

Further Reading

1. Brahmbhatt AN, Skalski KA, Bhatt AA. Vascular lesions of the head and neck: an update on classification and imaging review. Insights Imaging. 2020;11(1):19. https://doi.org/10.1186/s13244-019-0818-3.
2. Metry D, Heyer G, Hess C, et al. Consensus statement on diagnostic criteria for Phace syndrome. Pediatrics. 2009;124:1447–56.
3. Flors L, Leiva-Salinas C, Maged IM, et al. MR imaging of soft-tissue vascular malformations: diagnosis, classification, and therapy follow-up. Radiographics. 2011;31:1321–40.
4. Guneyli S, Ceylan N, Bayraktaroglu S, Acar T, Savas R. Imaging findings of vascular lesions in the head and neck. Diagn Interv Radiol. 2014;20:432–7.
5. ISSVA. Classification for vascular anomalies. https://www.issva.org/UserFiles/file/ISSVA-Classification-2018.pdf. Accessed 31 Jan 2022.
6. Rodriguez-Laguna L, Ibañez K, Gordo G, et al. CLAPO syndrome: identification of somatic activating PIK3CA mutations and delineation of the natural history and phenotype. Genet Med. 2018;20:882–9.
7. Restrepo CS, Martínez S, Lemos JA, Carrillo JA, Lemos DF, Ojeda P, Koshy P. Imaging manifestations of Kaposi sarcoma. Radiographics. 2006;26:1169–85.

Cystic Neck Masses

Kathryn E. Dean and Oren Jaspan

Introduction

- Cystic neck masses are commonly encountered on imaging as either the primary indication for the study or entirely incidental.
- Patient age and clinical presentation may narrow the differential, but imaging characteristics are often key to diagnosis.
- Computed tomography (CT) is the workhorse modality for imaging of the neck soft tissues. Ultrasound and Magnetic Resonance Imaging (MRI) are useful adjuncts.
- Cystic neck masses can broadly be categorized as either *congenital* or *acquired*.

Congenital Cystic Neck Masses

THYROGLOSSAL DUCT CYST (TDC)

- Most common congenital cystic neck mass.
- Remnant of the thyroglossal duct, which extends from the foramen cecum (at the tongue base) to the thyroid bed in the lower neck. Failure of in-utero obliteration of the thyroglossal duct may result in TDC formation or ectopic thyroid tissue at any point along the course of the duct in the anterior neck soft tissues.
  - ~25% suprahyoid, ~50% at the level of the hyoid, ~25% infrahyoid neck [1].

Supplementary Information The online version contains supplementary material available at https://doi.org/10.1007/978-3-031-55124-6_43.

K. E. Dean (✉)
Weill Cornell Medical College, New York, NY, USA
e-mail: ked9042@med.cornell.edu

O. Jaspan
NewYork-Presbyterian Weill Cornell, New York, NY, USA
e-mail: onj9002@nyp.org

  - Termed *lingual* or *intralingual TDC* when at the tongue base.
- ~90% present by age 10 as a compressible and painless midline/paramidline neck mass.
  - Usually asymptomatic, but may cause dysphagia, stridor, or dysphonia [2].
  - May occasionally become superinfected.
- Very rarely develop superimposed thyroid cancer.
- Imaging is important to confirm diagnosis, define anatomic relationships, identify the presence of ectopic/orthotopic thyroid tissue, and evaluate for evidence of superimposed malignancy/infection.

Imaging

- General—Midline or paramidline cystic mass in the anterior neck soft tissues, anywhere along the course of the thyroglossal duct and often intimately related to the hyoid bone.
  - Infrahyoid TDCs may be embedded within the strap muscles.
- Ultrasound—Circumscribed, anechoic cyst with posterior acoustic enhancement; occasionally more complicated with low-level echoes (*pseudosolid* appearance) or septations if cyst contains proteinaceous debris/hemorrhage.
- CT—Circumscribed, hypodense, fluid—attenuation mass (Fig. 43.1).
- MRI—T2 hyperintense mass. T1 signal is variable depending on internal contents.
- CT and MRI—Thin, non-enhancing, or faintly enhancing walls. Wall thickening and/or avid rim enhancement is suggestive of superimposed infection.
  - Solid/nodular enhancing components or internal calcifications are suspicious for malignancy.
- Nuclear Scintigraphy—May aid in identifying ectopic thyroid tissues when suspected.

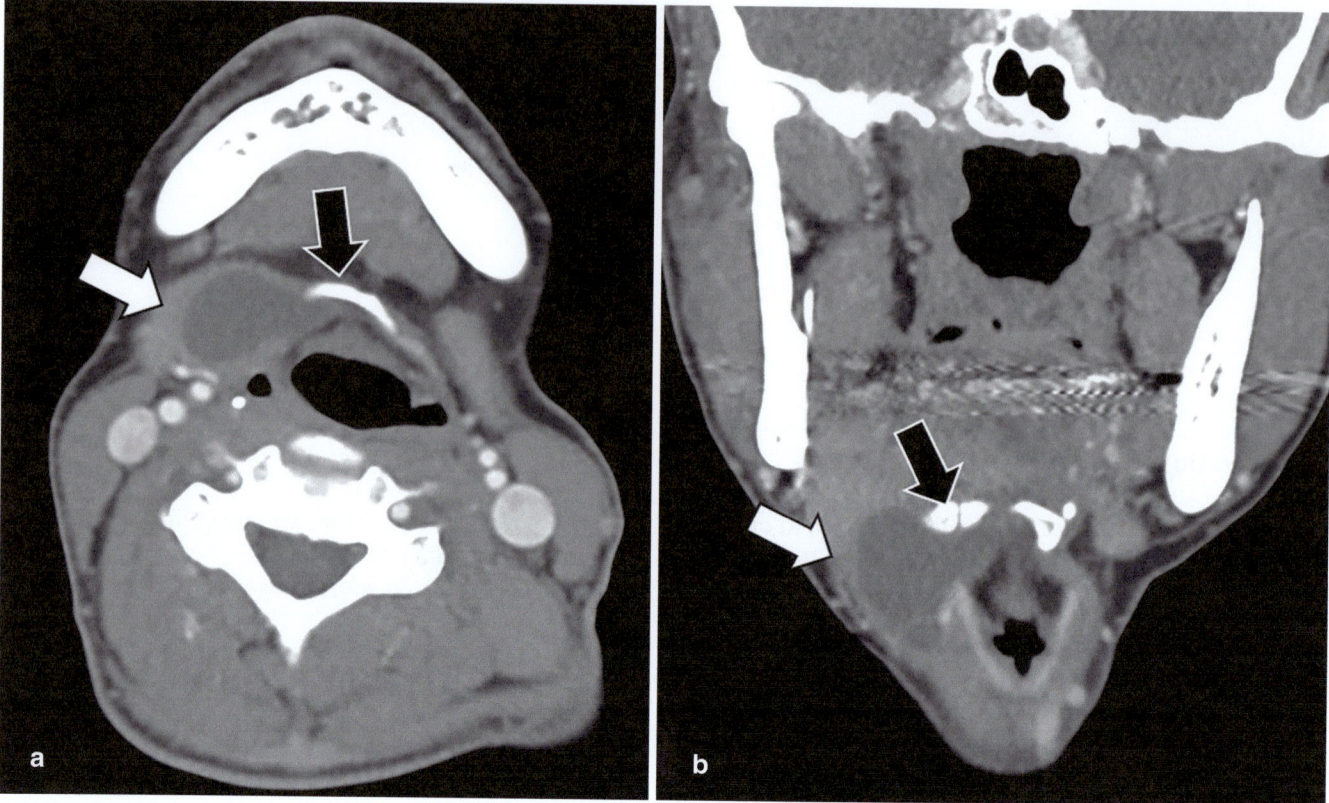

Fig. 43.1 Thyroglossal duct cyst. (**a**) Axial and (**b**) coronal contrast-enhanced CT (CECT) images demonstrate a right, paramidline, well-defined cystic mass with thin, non-enhancing walls (white arrows) insinuating along the inferior surface of the hyoid bone (black arrows)

BRANCHIAL CLEFT ANOMALIES

- Branchial cleft cysts (BCC), sinus tracts, and fistulas form due to incomplete in-utero obliteration of the branchial clefts in the fetal neck.
- BCCs tend to present in the second or third decades, while sinus tracts and fistulas tend to present earlier in the first decade of life [3].
- *First branchial cleft cysts* (5–8%) occur above the level of the mandible in or adjacent to the external auditory canal or in close association with the parotid gland.
  - May present with chronic otorrhea or recurrent parotid abscesses.
- *Second branchial cleft cysts* are by far the most common branchial cleft anomaly (95%) [3]. They may be subdivided based on precise location but occur most frequently within the submandibular space along the anteromedial surface of the sternocleidomastoid muscle, posterior to the submandibular gland, and lateral to the carotid space.
  - Classically presents as a soft painless neck mass adjacent to the mandibular angle. May demonstrate slow progressive growth and intermittent episodes of pain and inflammation corresponding to instances of infection.
  - Caution must be exercised if invoking this diagnosis for a newly discovered cystic lesion in an adult, which may represent a cystic or necrotic head and neck squamous cell carcinoma metastasis.
- *Third branchial cleft cysts* are exceedingly rare lesions that arise in the posterior triangle of the neck and present as painless soft masses that may become distended in the setting of a viral upper respiratory tract infection.
- *Fourth branchial cleft anomalies* are very rare and usually present as sinus tracts or fistulae. They arise from the pyriform sinus (usually on the left), insinuate laterally through the thyrohyoid membrane, and course inferiorly into the mediastinum along the tracheoesophageal groove toward the thyroid gland.
  - May result in recurrent abscesses in or anterior to the left thyroid lobe.

Imaging

- First BCC—Round or ovoid cystic mass along the external auditory canal or in close association with the parotid gland. Often indistinguishable from other cystic parotid masses by imaging alone.

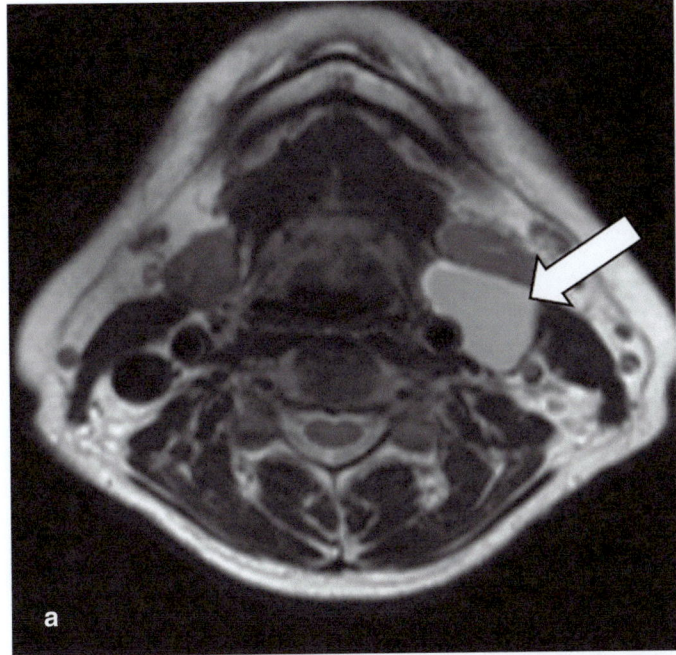 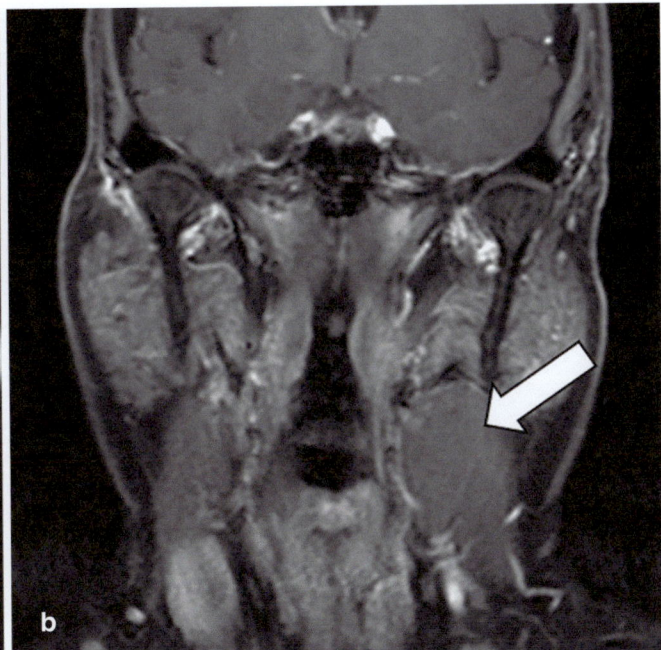

Fig. 43.2 Second branchial cleft cyst. (**a**) Axial T2 and (**b**) coronal T1 post-contrast fat-saturated MR images demonstrate a T1-intermediate/T2-hyperintense and non-enhancing cyst (white arrows) in the left submandibular space, along the anteromedial aspect of the left sternocleidomastoid muscle and immediately posterior to and contacting the left submandibular gland. The superior aspect of the mass is adjacent to the left angle of the mandible

- Second BCC—Cystic mass, classically within the submandibular space along the anteromedial surface of the sternocleidomastoid muscle, posterior to the submandibular gland (Fig. 43.2).
  - Ultrasound—Circumscribed, compressible, usually anechoic mass with posterior acoustic enhancement, but may contain debris.
  - CT—Circumscribed, typically homogeneously hypodense mass with a thin wall.
  - MRI—T2 hyperintense mass with variable T1 signal depending on proteinaceous/hemorrhagic contents.
- Third BCC—Usually a unilocular cystic mass in the posterior cervical space, posterior to the sternocleidomastoid muscle. May be difficult to distinguish from a fourth branchial cleft anomaly.
- Fourth branchial cleft sinus tract/fistula—Typically left-sided fluid collection extending inferiorly from the pyriform sinus toward the left thyroid lobe.
  - CT and MRI—Avid rim enhancement will develop in the setting of abscess formation. Abscess may form within the associated thyroid parenchyma.
  - Fluoroscopy—A sinus tract extending from the pyriform sinus to the lower neck may be demonstrated after barium swallow.

LYMPHATIC MALFORMATION

- Type of congenital low-flow vascular malformation due to abnormal development of lymphatic vessels.
- Generally detected in the perinatal period or in early childhood (90% by 2 years of age) [1].
- Usually presents as a soft, compressible, and painless mass in the head, neck, or axilla.
  - Most symptoms are due to mass effect on nearby structures.
  - May rapidly enlarge or become painful with internal hemorrhage or infection.
- Frequently seen in combination with other low-flow vascular malformations (e.g., venous malformation).
- May be classified based on size of cystic lesions: *macrocystic* (>1 cm), *microcystic* (<1 cm), or *mixed*.

Imaging

- General—Lobulated, multicystic mass of variable size and often trans-spatial (crossing tissue planes and midline; involving multiple deep spaces). The lesion may encase normal blood vessels.

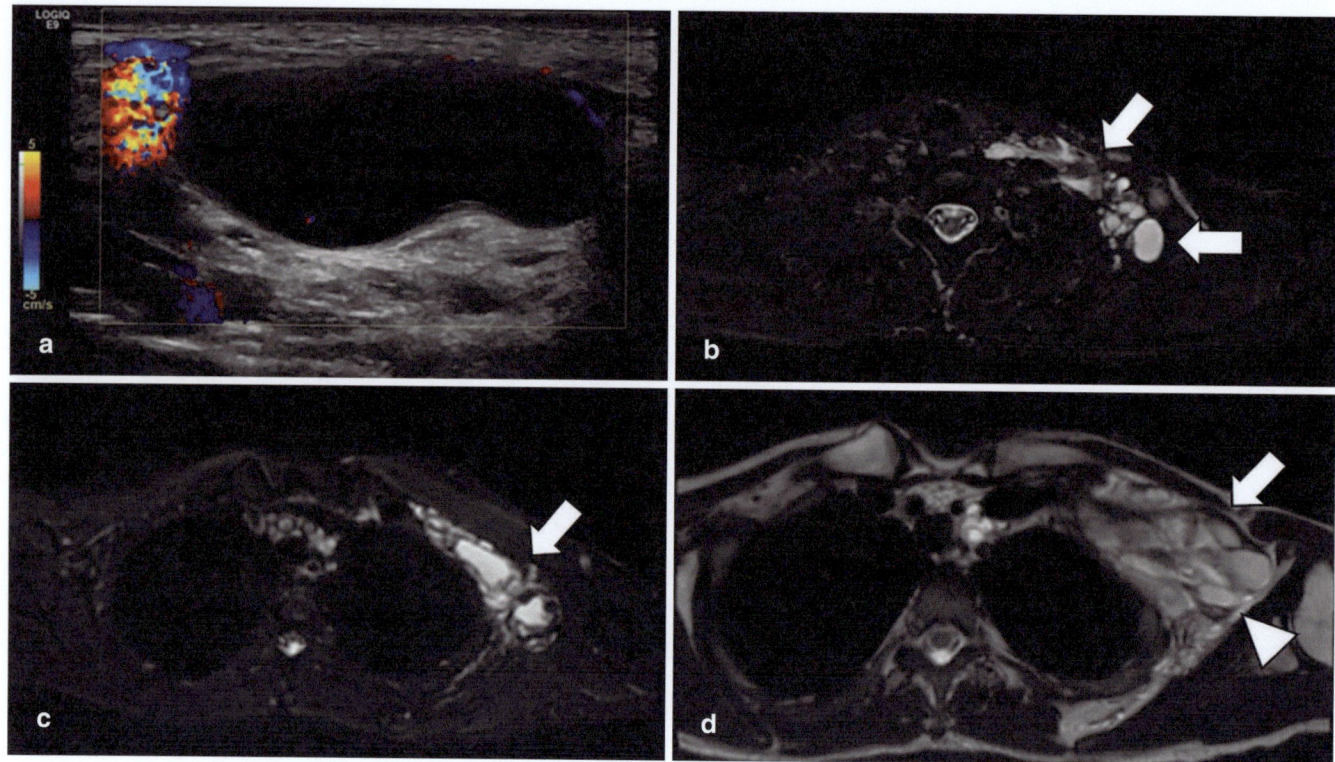

Fig. 43.3 Lymphatic malformation. (a) Transverse color Doppler ultrasound of the left supraclavicular region demonstrates a thin-walled, anechoic, cystic mass with posterior acoustic enhancement and without internal vascularity. (b, c) Axial short tau inversion recovery (STIR) and (d) T2 MR images reveal a corresponding large, multilobulated, transspatial, T2-hyperintense mass (white arrows) with a small internal fluid-fluid level (white arrowhead)

- Ultrasound—Compressible, thin-walled, predominantly anechoic (if macrocystic), cystic mass without internal vascularity on Doppler imaging (Fig. 43.3a). May contain septations and internal hemorrhagic or proteinaceous debris.
- CT—Multilobulated, hypodense fluid-attenuation mass. May contain hyperdense hemorrhagic or proteinaceous material, or fluid-fluid levels.
- MRI—Multilobulated, T2-hyperintense, with possible fluid levels if hemorrhagic (Fig. 43.3b–d). Usually, T1-hypointense, but blood, protein, or chyle may result in T1-hyperintensity.
    - Macrocystic lesions may demonstrate thin-rim enhancement.
    - Microcystic lesions may demonstrate more confluent, infiltrative enhancement.

CERVICAL THYMIC CYST (THYMOPHARYNGEAL DUCT CYST)

- Cystic remnant of the thymopharyngeal duct in the neck.
    - The thymus develops from the third pharyngeal pouch and descends the neck via the thymopharyngeal duct to its normal location in the anterior superior mediastinum.
    - Sequestration of thymic tissue and failure of involution of the thymopharyngeal duct may lead to cyst formation [4].
- Presents as a solitary neck mass at any level along the course of thymic descent from the level of the hyoid to the mediastinum. They are usually left-sided and ~ 50% communicate directly with the thymus in the mediastinum [5].
- Usually detected in the first decade of life.
- Very rare—less than 1% of all cystic neck masses.
- Definitive diagnosis usually requires the identification of thymic cells on histology.

Imaging
- Solitary thin-walled cystic mass adjacent to the carotid sheath, often paralleling the course of the sternocleidomastoid in the infrahyoid neck (Fig. e43.1).
- (All electronic images (Figs. e43.1–e43.7) can be found in this chapter's website on Springer Link: https://doi.org/10.1007/978-3-031-55124-6_43).
- Often indistinguishable from fourth branchial cleft anomalies and lymphatic malformations on imaging.
- CT or MRI may demonstrate continuity with the thymus in the mediastinum, which is pathognomonic.

FOREGUT DUPLICATION CYST

- Benign congenital anomaly arising from heterotopic rests of foregut-derived epithelium, the embryologic precursor to the lower respiratory tract, pharynx, and upper gastrointestinal tract. The result is a cystic mass containing foregut epithelium communicating with foregut-derived tissue and covered by a layer of smooth muscle.
- Subtypes include:
  o Bronchogenic cysts.
  o Esophageal duplication cysts.
  o Enteric duplication cysts.
- Typically diagnosed in infancy or early childhood.
- Usually develops in the thorax and abdomen but may rarely manifest in the head and neck.
- Most frequently involve the tongue or anterior floor of mouth when present in the head and neck.
- Presenting symptoms include feeding difficulties, odynophagia, speech difficulties, stridor, and tongue edema [6].

Imaging
- Cystic lesion in an infant, involving the tongue or anterior floor of mouth.
- Appearance is nonspecific and may be difficult to distinguish from other congenital or acquired cystic lesions including TDCs, dermoid/epidermoid cysts, and ranulas.

TORNWALDT CYST

- Benign developmental cyst in the midline of the nasopharynx. Formed from a notochord remnant.
- Usually detected incidentally as they are almost invariably asymptomatic.
  o Rarely the cyst can develop chronic infection, resulting in halitosis.

Imaging
- General—Circumscribed, unilocular cyst along the midline, posterior nasopharyngeal wall. Bounded anteriorly by the nasopharyngeal mucosa and posteriorly by the longus colli muscles.
- CT—Hypodense cyst, possibly with mild rim enhancement.
- MRI—T2-hyperintense cyst, with variable T1 signal depending on protein content (Fig. e43.2).

EPIDERMOID AND DERMOID CYSTS

- Congenital inclusion cysts consisting of ectopic epithelial cell rests.
  o *Epidermoid*—Only epithelial constituents.
  o *Dermoid*—Epithelial AND dermal constituents (e.g., sebaceous glands, hair follicles, fat).
- May occur anywhere in the body. In the head and neck, epidermoid and dermoid cysts have a predilection for the oral cavity, orbit, nose (often associated with a dermal sinus tract, with or without intracranial extension), and the midline anterior neck.
- Present as painless masses which may grow very slowly over time. May rarely rupture, resulting in rapid growth and inflammation.
- Orbital and nasal lesions tend to present in childhood, while oral cavity lesions are more common in adolescence and early adulthood [1].

Imaging
- Epidermoid—Fluid-filled, often proteinaceous.
  o Ultrasound—circumscribed mass containing homogeneous low-level internal echoes or a *pseudosolid* appearance due to protein and posterior acoustic enhancement.
  o CT—Circumscribed, simple-appearing, hypodense, fluid-attenuation mass (Fig. 43.4a, b).
  o MRI—Homogeneously T2-hyperintense, often T1-iso to hyperintense depending on protein content. Classically restricts diffusion due to protein.
- Dermoid—Contains mixture of fluid, protein, fat, and calcifications.
  o Ultrasound—Circumscribed mass with heterogeneous internal echogenicity depending on contents. Fat and calcium contents will result in echogenic foci. Calcium causes posterior acoustic shadowing.
  o CT—Mixed-density mass depending on contents. If pure fluid contents, may be indistinguishable from epidermoid. May cause adjacent bony remodeling.
  o MRI—Heterogeneously T2-hyperintense. T1-signal corresponds to fatty contents. Signal dropout on fat-saturated sequences is helpful to confirm the presence of internal fat. The "sack of marbles" sign is suggestive of a dermoid cyst in the head and neck region (Fig. 43.4c, d).

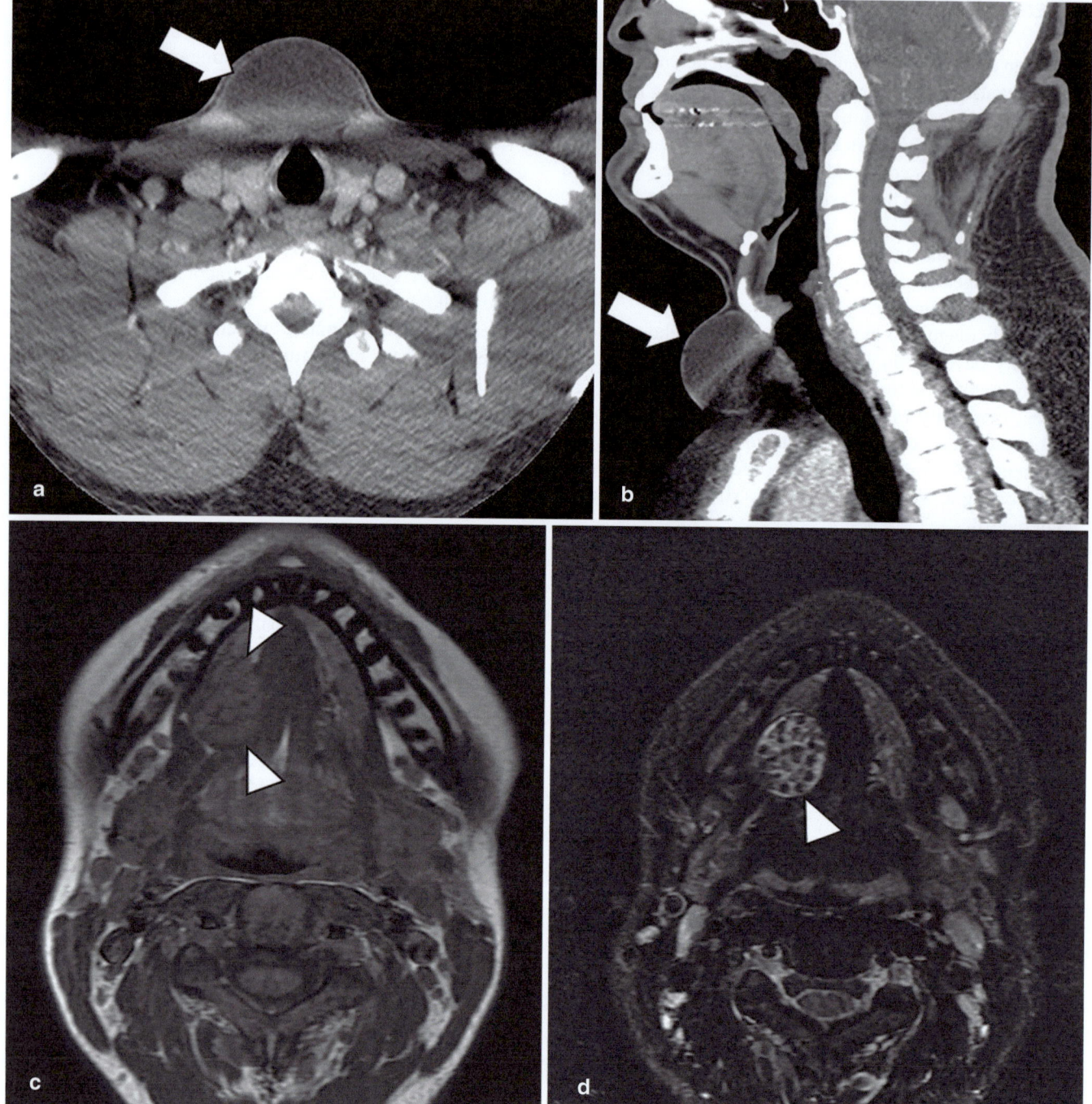

Fig. 43.4 Epidermoid and dermoid cysts. (**a**) Axial and (**b**) sagittal CECT images of an *epidermoid cyst* demonstrate a unilocular cystic mass (white arrows) in the midline anterior neck soft tissues, superficial to the strap muscles. While this may appear similar to an infrahyoid thyroglossal duct cyst, the precise midline location and position superficial to the strap muscles are more typical of epidermoid cysts. Diffusion restriction on MRI would be diagnostic. (**c**) Axial T1 and (**d**) T2-weighted fat-suppressed MR images of a *dermoid cyst* in a different patient demonstrate a well-defined, ovoid, cystic mass in the right sublingual space with a "sack of marbles" appearance (white arrowheads). Internal T1-hyperintense foci within the cyst that saturate out on the fat-saturated sequence represent fat globules floating within a cyst

NASOLABIAL CYST

- Rare congenital cyst that develops between the upper lip and the nasal vestibule (opening) but does not usually manifest until adulthood.
- Also known as *nasoalveolar* or *Klesdadt cyst*.
- Classically presents in women in the fourth and fifth decades.
- Patients often present with cosmesis concerns with obliteration of the ipsilateral nasolabial fold, with or without nasal obstruction, and/or localized pain in the setting of superimposed infection [7].

Imaging

- General—extraosseous, paramedian, soft tissue mass between the upper lip and nasal ala, usually unilateral.
- CT—Isodense to hyperdense soft tissue mass without contrast enhancement. When large, may cause bony scalloping of subjacent maxilla (Fig. 43.5).
- MRI—Uniformly T2-hyperintense mass with intermediate to hyperintense T1 signal due to proteinaceous contents.

NASOPALATINE DUCT CYST

- Also known as an incisive canal cyst.
- Congenital cyst arising from the nasopalatine duct within the incisive canal in the midline maxilla.
- Usually asymptomatic and detected incidentally in the 4th–fifth decades. May occasionally become infected, resulting in pain. May also cause swelling of the maxilla and extend to the floor of the nasal cavity when large.

Imaging

- General—Circumscribed, smooth expansion of the maxillary incisive canal, posterior to the central maxillary incisors. Incisive canal diameter > 1 cm is essentially diagnostic of nasopalatine duct cyst.
- CT—Smooth, hypodense expansion of the incisive canal, with possible thinning and dehiscence of the palatal (posterior) cortex of the maxilla, posterior to the central maxillary incisors. When large, the cyst may extend to the floor of the nasal cavity (Fig. e43.3).
- MRI—T2-hyperintense expansion of the incisive canal with intermediate to hyperintense T1 signal.

VALLECULAR CYST

- Congenital cyst arising in the vallecula, thought to represent retention cyst of a minor salivary gland.
- Typically presents as inspiratory stridor and airway obstruction in infants. Usually diagnosed with laryngoscopy.
- Arises within the vallecula at the base of tongue and anterior to the epiglottis. Can enlarge to fill the vallecula, posteriorly displace the epiglottis, and result in airway narrowing.

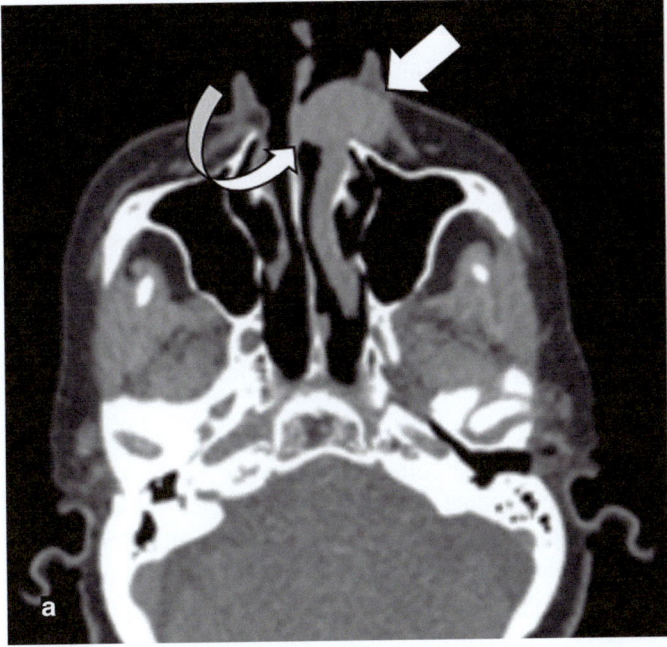
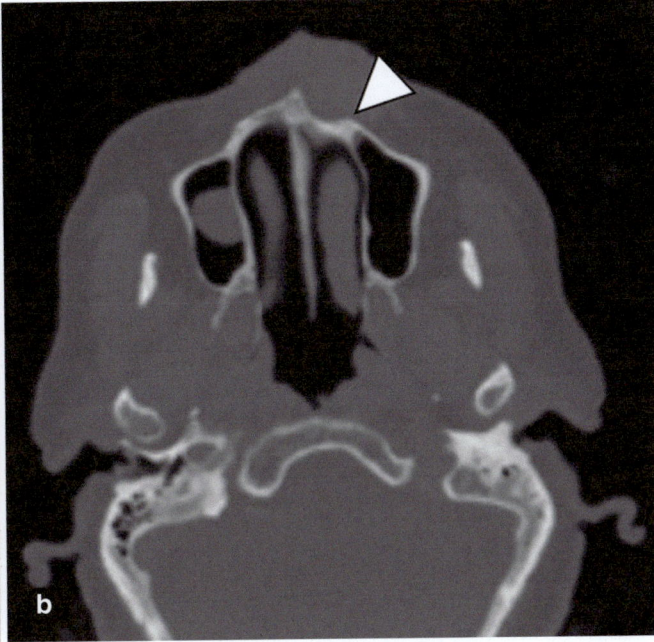

Fig. 43.5 Nasolabial cyst. (**a**) Non-contrast axial CT image demonstrates an extraosseous, paramidline, isodense, soft tissue mass arising near the left nasal ala (white arrow) and narrows the left nasal vestibule (curved white arrow). (**b**) Non-contrast axial CT image in bone window reveals the related scalloping of the underlying maxillary bone (white arrowhead)

Imaging
- Radiography—Lateral projection may demonstrate a well-defined soft tissue mass within the vallecula and posteriorly deflecting the epiglottis.
- CT—Circumscribed, hypodense, and non-enhancing cystic mass filling the vallecula.
- MRI—Circumscribed, T2-hyperintense, and T1-hypointense mass in the vallecula (Fig. e43.4).

Acquired Cystic Neck Masses

LARYNGOCELE

- Abnormally dilated laryngeal saccule, which may be filled with air or fluid.
  - If superinfected and filled with pus, may be referred to as *pyolaryngocele*.
- *Primary laryngoceles* are caused by chronically elevated intraglottic pressures (e.g., wind instrument players). An extremely rare congenital variant also exists.
- *Secondary* laryngoceles (~5–15%) are caused by laryngeal tumors which obstruct the laryngeal ventricle [1].
- Further categorized based on anatomic extent [8]:
  - Internal laryngocele (~40%)—dilated saccule confined to the larynx.
  - Mixed laryngocele (~45%)—dilated saccule extends laterally through the thyrohyoid membrane into the inferior submandibular space.
  - External laryngocele (~15%)—dilated lateral component of the saccule communicating with a non-dilated component that has extended through the thyrohyoid membrane.
- Most commonly in adults >50; males > females.
- May present with hoarseness or stridor when large.

Imaging
- Thin-walled air or fluid-filled mass communicating with the laryngeal ventricle best defined on CT.
- Internal laryngoceles are confined to the supraglottic paraglottic space.
- Mixed laryngoceles extend laterally from the paraglottic space through the thyrohyoid membrane with a waist (*isthmus*) at the thyrohyoid membrane (Fig. e43.5).
- Thick enhancing walls suggest superinfection (pyolaryngocele).
- Secondary laryngoceles will usually be seen in association with an enhancing glottic or inferior supraglottic laryngeal mass obstructing the laryngeal ventricle. This is important to exclude whenever a laryngocele is identified.

RANULA
- Saliva-containing retention cyst of the sublingual gland or a minor salivary gland within the sublingual space.
  - Usually results from trauma or inflammation of the involved salivary gland [1].
  - Congenital variant is much rarer.
- May be confined to the sublingual space (*simple* ranula) or rupture inferiorly into the submandibular space (*diving* or *plunging* ranula), either posteriorly around the free margin of the mylohyoid sling or through a defect in the mylohyoid muscle (mylohyoid boutonniere).
- Presents as a painless floor of mouth mass or swelling. May become secondarily infected.
- Most commonly detected in young adults, with increased incidence in Maori and Pacific Islander populations.

Imaging
- *Simple ranula*—Circumscribed unilocular ovoid or lenticular cystic mass in the sublingual space (Fig. 43.6a, b).
- *Diving ranula*—Unilocular cystic mass in the submandibular space with *tail* extending superiorly into the ipsilateral sublingual space around the posterior margin of the mylohyoid or via a mylohyoid defect (Fig. 43.6c, d).
  - T2 fat-saturated MRI is most sensitive for detecting subtle T2-hyperintense *tail* sign.
- Wall thickening and enhancement suggest active or recent infection.

SIALOCELE (SALIVARY MUCOCELE)

- Saliva-containing fluid collection caused by extravasation from a ruptured salivary gland duct.
  - Occurs most frequently in the sublingual space due to damage to the submandibular duct.
- Duct obstruction by a stone (sialolith) is the most common etiology. Surgery and trauma are less frequent causes.
- Presents as a soft painless mass in the setting of sialolithiasis, recent oral cavity surgery, or a history of trauma. They may progressively enlarge if not treated.

Imaging
- General—Fluid collection along the course of the submandibular duct in the sublingual space, which may be difficult to distinguish from a simple ranula if no stone is identified or provided history of recent surgery or trauma.
- CT—Hypodense, fluid collection in the sublingual space, possibly seen in conjunction with a dilated submandibular duct and/or an obstructing stone (Fig. 43.7).

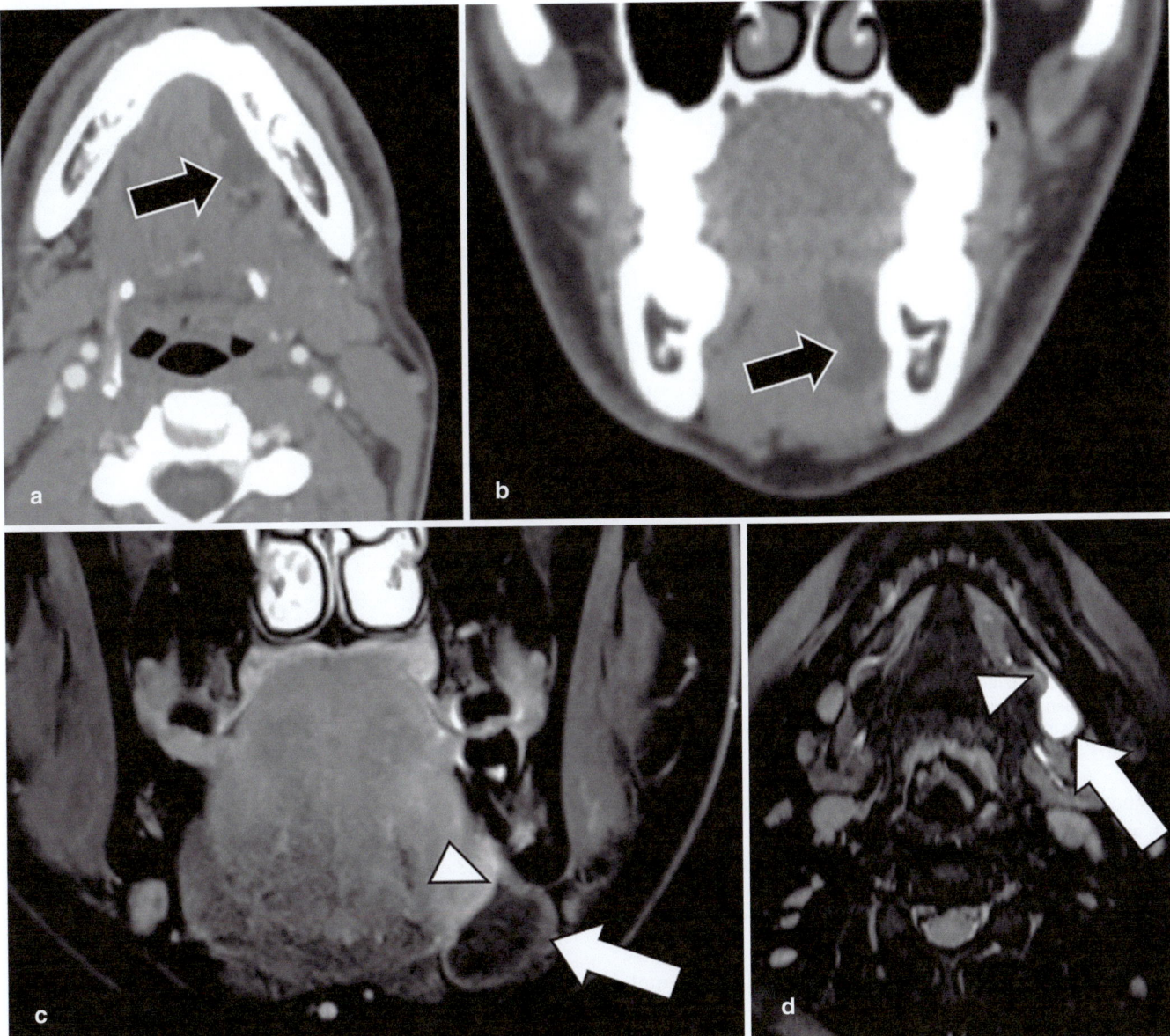

Fig. 43.6 Ranula. (**a**) Axial and (**b**) coronal CECT images demonstrate a lobulated, hypodense, cystic mass confined to the left sublingual space, compatible with a *simple ranula* (black arrows). (**c**) Coronal T1 post-contrast fat-saturated and (**d**) axial T2 fat-saturated MR images in a different patient reveal a unilocular T1-hypointense/T2-hyperintense cystic mass centered within the left submandibular space (white arrows). A thin "tail" (white arrowheads) can be seen coursing anterosuperiorly around the posterior margin of the left mylohyoid muscle, extending into the left sublingual space, consistent with a *diving* or *plunging ranula*

- MRI—T1-hypointense and T2-hyperintense fluid collection in the sublingual space along the course of the submandibular duct with or without an associated A T1/T2-hypointense sialolith.
- CT and MRI—Contrast enhancement of the surrounding soft tissues and/or submandibular gland suggests acute sialocele formation. Atrophy of the ipsilateral submandibular gland is suggestive of prior sialadenitis.

BENIGN LYMPHOEPITHELIAL LESIONS

- Cystic lesions most frequently identified within the parotid glands of patients with HIV or Sjögren syndrome.
  - Limited to the parotid glands as they are the only salivary glands to contain lymphoid tissue.
- Hypertrophy of intrinsic lymphoid tissue causes lymphoid aggregates (solid lesions). Subsequent obstruction

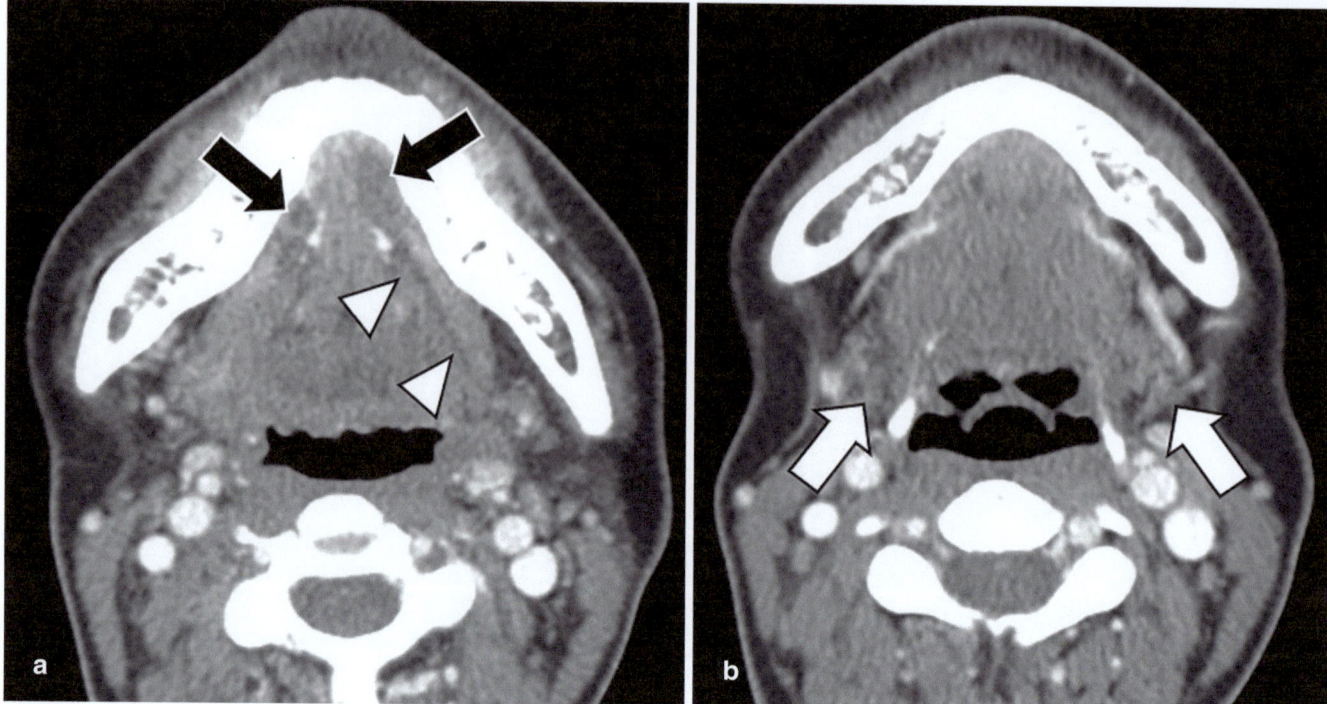

Fig. 43.7 Sialocele. (a, b) Axial CECT images of a patient with floor of mouth swelling demonstrate small hypodense collections with in the left greater than right sublingual spaces (black arrows). While differentiating these sublingual cystic lesions from bilateral simple ranulas is difficult given the lack of associated sialoliths, the associated findings of bilateral submandibular gland atrophy (white arrows) suggestive of prior submandibular duct inflammation and a slightly dilated left submandibular duct (white arrowheads) favor the diagnosis of sialoceles

and dilatation of intraglandular ducts result in purely as well as cystic and solid lesions.
- Patients present with painless parotid gland enlargement, often bilateral. Concurrent findings of lymphoid activation such as tonsillar hypertrophy and enlarged cervical lymph nodes are often present.
- Lesions are benign but may very rarely undergo lymphomatous transformation.
- Presentation may occur before HIV diagnosis is made, so identification of these lesions should prompt HIV testing.
  - 5% of HIV patients develop benign lymphoepithelial lesions, although prevalence has decreased with antiretroviral therapy [1].

Imaging
- General—Enlarged parotid glands typically contain multiple mixed solid and cystic lesions. Solitary unilateral cystic lesions are also possible, which may complicate the diagnosis and make differentiation from first branchial cleft cysts difficult.
- CT—Bilateral enlarged, hyperdense parotid glands containing multiple, circumscribed, hypodense, cystic lesions or mixed cystic, and solid lesions. The lesions may contain septations and mural nodules.
- MRI—T1-hypointense/T2-hyperintense, mixed solid and cystic lesions within enlarged parotid glands (Fig. 43.8a, b).
- CT and MRI—Tonsillar hypertrophy, cervical lymphadenopathy, and bone marrow signal changes support the diagnosis.
  - Cysts may demonstrate rim enhancement, and any solid components may enhance (Fig. 43.8c).

WARTHIN TUMOR

- Benign tumor of the parotid gland derived from lymphoid tissue.
- Second most common benign parotid tumor after pleomorphic adenoma, representing 5–10% of all parotid tumors.
- Multicentric (multiple unilateral or bilateral) in ~20% of cases.
  - Classically occurs in the parotid tail.
  - If predominantly cystic, they may be challenging to differentiate from pleomorphic adenoma (especially if solitary) or benign lymphoepithelial lesions. Clinical history and other imaging findings are key for differentiation.

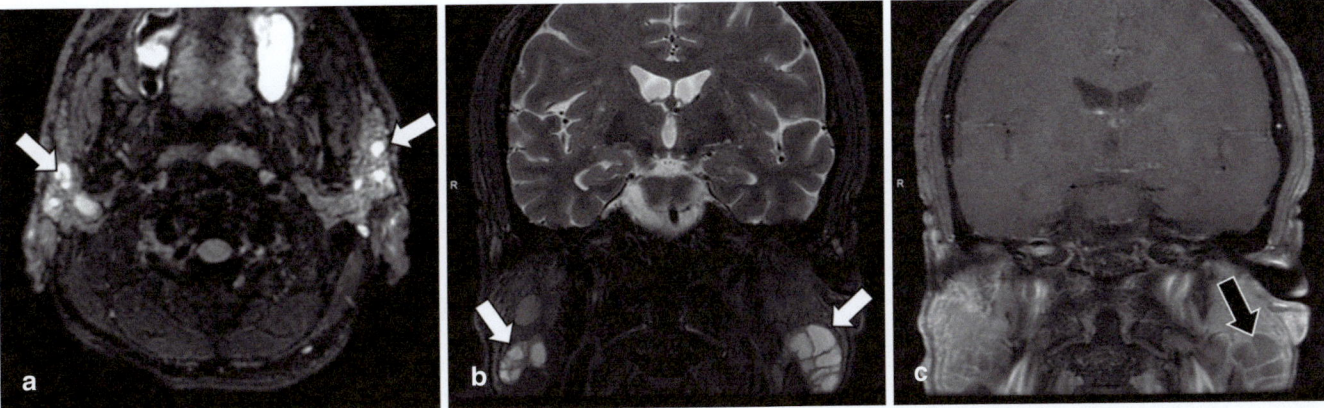

Fig. 43.8 Benign lymphoepithelial lesions. (a) Axial and (b) coronal T2-weighted fat-saturated MR images in a patient with HIV demonstrate numerous septated cysts within the bilateral enlarged parotid glands (white arrows). (c) Coronal T1 post-contrast fat-saturated MR image shows thin enhancement along the septations (black arrow). No frank solid or mixed cystic and solid lesions are demonstrated here but can be seen with benign lymphoepithelial lesions representing lymphoid aggregates. Also not demonstrated here but often associated is tonsillar hypertrophy or cervical lymph node enlargement

- Classically presents as a painless mass or masses in the parotid gland of elderly male smokers.
   o 90% of patients with Warthin tumors smoke [1].
   o Radiation exposure is an additional risk factor.

Imaging
- General—Classically a well-defined parotid tail mass, which may have cystic component in ~30% of cases.
- CT—Small, circumscribed masses in the superficial parotid lobe with or without hypodense fluid-attenuation cystic component. Solid component does not typically enhance strongly. Well-defined margins help differentiate from malignant tumors.
- MRI—Circumscribed, typically T1-hypointense and T2-intermediate to hyperintense masses with or without T2-hyperintense cystic components. Cystic components may be T1-variable depending on hemorrhage and proteinaceous content. Warthin tumors may demonstrate lower ADC values, aiding in differentiating them from benign mixed tumors.
- CT and MRI—Minimal enhancement of solid components. Dynamic post-contrast imaging classically shows rapid enhancement and wash-out.
- Nuclear Medicine—Usually FDG-avid on positron emission tomography (PET) scans and uptake Technetium 99-m due to mitochondrial-rich oncocytes (Fig. e43.6).

METASTATIC LYMPHADENOPATHY

- Metastatic disease is a common cause of both cystic and necrotic lymph nodes in adults.
- Cystic nodal metastases are most frequently associated with head and neck malignancies, particularly HPV-positive squamous cell carcinomas (SCCs) and papillary thyroid cancers.
   o HPV-positive head and neck SCCs generally portend favorable outcomes compared to HPV-negative head and neck SCCs [9, 10].
- Necrotic nodal metastases are a result of the metastatic lesion outgrowing its vascular supply leading to cellular hypoxia and are often seen with extra-nodal extension (ENE), a poor prognostic factor.
- Cystic or necrotic nodal metastasis should always be a consideration for a new cystic head and neck mass in an adult.

Imaging
- General—Distribution of metastatic nodes is generally dependent on location of primary tumor.
- *Cystic metastatic lymph nodes* are generally defined as being mostly cystic with a capsule no thicker than 2 mm. Punctate calcific foci are highly suspicious for metastatic papillary thyroid cancer (Fig. 43.9).
   o Ultrasound—Loss of the normal reniform morphology with central hypoechoic central degeneration with posterior acoustic enhancement.
   o CT and MRI—Enlarged lymph nodes with loss of normal reniform morphology with well-defined, cystic components. Some nodes may be nearly entirely cystic.
- *Necrotic metastatic lymph nodes* have a more irregular and nodular soft tissue component.

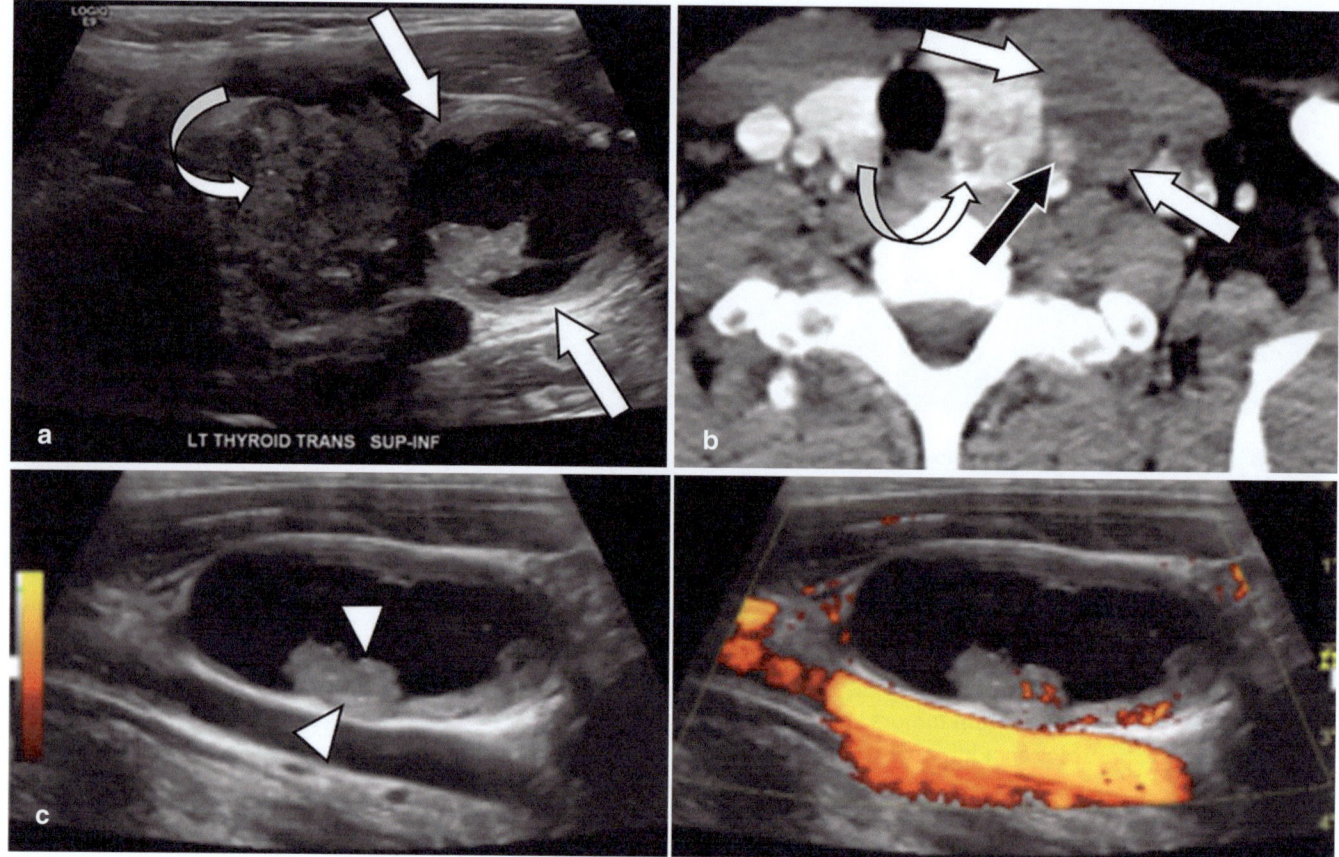

Fig. 43.9 Metastatic lymphadenopathy. (**a**) Transverse ultrasound and (**b**) axial CECT images at the level of the left thyroid lobe demonstrate a cystic and solid mass (white arrows), concerning for an abnormal lymph node, adjacent to an enlarged and heterogenous left thyroid lobe (curved white arrows). Note the solid component of the partially cystic mass is apparently enhancing on CT (black arrow). (**c**) Additional longitudinal ultrasound images redemonstrate the abnormal partially cystic lymph node adjacent to the left thyroid lobe with the solid component demonstrating punctate internal hyperechoic foci (white arrowheads), possibly macrocalcifications, and internal vascularity. Subsequent biopsy confirmed metastatic papillary thyroid carcinoma

- ○ Ultrasound—Loss of normal reniform morphology with thickened irregular cortex and central heterogeneously hypoechoic necrosis. Solid portions of the node usually demonstrate increased vascularity on Doppler imaging.
- CT and MRI—Enlarged nodes with irregular cortex and central necrotic component.
  - ○ Findings suggestive of ENE include indistinct nodal margins or infiltration of the surrounding fat [11].

INFECTIOUS LYMPHADENOPATHY

- Infections are a more common cause of cystic or necrotic lymphadenopathy in the younger population.
- Head and neck infections can lead to bacterial infection/pus formation within draining lymph nodes, which can progress to frank intranodal abscess formation (suppurative lymphadenitis).
  - ○ Subsequently, there is a risk of extra-nodal rupture into either the superficial or deep spaces of the neck depending on the involved lymph node.
  - ○ *Staphylococcus* and *Streptococcus* are the most common causal organisms particularly in children <5 years old.
  - ○ Primary infectious sources include dental infection, pharyngitis, or tonsilitis.
- Tuberculous cervical lymphadenitis (*scrofula*) classically results in necrotic/cystic lymph node masses related to central caseation.
  - ○ Most common manifestation of extrapulmonary tuberculosis.
  - ○ Common cause of cystic/necrotic cervical lymphadenopathy in children and young adults in the developing world and in immunocompromised populations.

Imaging
- Suppurative lymphadenopathy will begin as enlarged, heterogenous nodes with increased vascularity/enhancement and progress to demonstrate a defined central hypoechoic/hypoenhancing necrotic center.
  - ○ Ultrasound—Best defines the drainability of the intranodal phlegmon versus abscess.

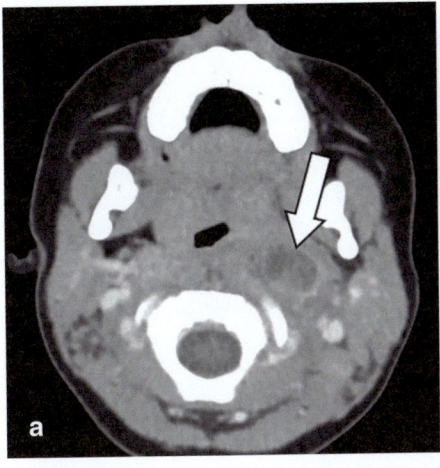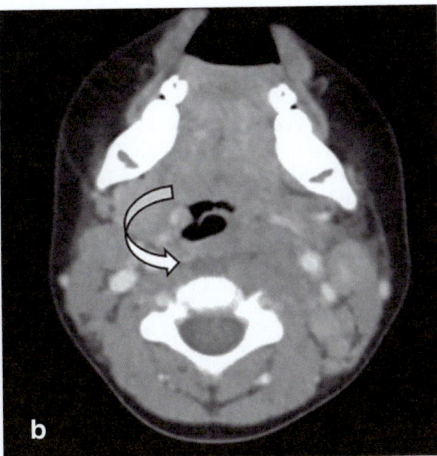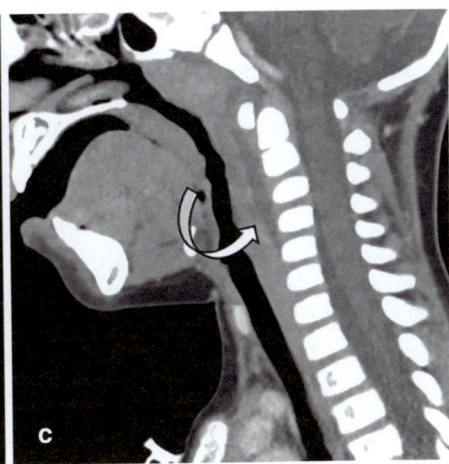

Fig. 43.10 Infectious lymphadenopathy. (a) Axial CECT image of a febrile child demonstrates an enlarged, rim-enhancing, left retropharyngeal lymph node with central hypodensity, compatible with intranodal abscess/suppurative lymphadenitis (white arrow). There is a mild mass effect upon the oropharynx. (b) More inferior axial and (c) midline sagittal CECT images from the same exam demonstrate hypodensity retropharyngeal fluid with early marginal enhancement, concerning for retropharyngeal phlegmon/developing abscess (curved white arrows)

- CECT—Best defines the extent of the infection, identifies extra-nodal decompression, complications (retropharyngeal abscess, thrombophlebitis, etc.), as well as aids in defining the infectious source (Fig. 43.10).
- MRI—Enlarged, peripherally enhancing lymph node with central T2 hyperintense and non-enhancing phlegmon/abscess and surrounding inflammation.
- Tuberculous lymphadenitis images similarly to suppurative lymphadenitis with central cystic changes being variable depending on the degree of caseation. As such, history is key.
  - Predilection for the cervical lymph nodes in the posterior triangle.

DEEP NECK SPACE ABSCESS

- Abscesses commonly develop within many of the deep neck spaces, including the parapharyngeal space, retropharyngeal space, masticator space, and floor of mouth (sublingual, submandibular, and submental spaces).
  - Wide-ranging etiologies include oropharyngeal infections, pharyngitis, sialadenitis, and penetrating trauma.
- *Parapharyngeal/retropharyngeal space* abscess—most common in children and adolescents.
  - Typically caused by oral cavity or pharyngeal infections.
  - Can be a result of direct spread or via lymphatic drainage.
  - May occur with or without suppurative lymphadenitis.
  - Often rapidly progressive. Patients usually appear very sick with systemic signs of infection, sore throat, hoarse or altered (hot potato) voice, and trismus. A large abscess can exert a mass effect on and compromise the airway.
- *Masticator space and floor of mouth* abscess—most common in adults. Typically caused by contiguous spread of odontogenic infection (Fig. e43.7).
  - *Ludwig angina* refers to a rapidly progressing floor of mouth cellulitis, typically related to odontogenic infection. May be associated with abscess formation. Floor of mouth swelling can result in proximal asphyxia.

Imaging

- Typically imaged on CECT of the neck to define the extent of the infection and rim-enhancing fluid collection (abscess), identify etiology (odontogenic, sialadenitis, etc.), and define complications (airway compromise, thrombophlebitis, etc.).
- Enlarged retropharyngeal or cervical lymph nodes are often present.
- If tonsillitis is present, tonsils will appear enlarged and enhance heterogeneously or with a striated, *tiger-stripe*, appearance.

References

1. Koch BL, Hamilton B, Hudgins P, Harnsberger HR. Diagnostic imaging: head and neck. 3rd ed. Elsevier; 2016. p. 1352.
2. Zander DA, Smoker WRK. Imaging of ectopic thyroid tissue and Thyroglossal duct cysts. Radiographics. 2014;34(1):37–50.
3. Koeller KK, Alamo L, Adair CF, Smirniotopoulos JG. From the archives of the AFIP—congenital cystic masses of the neck: radiologic-pathologic correlation. RadioGraphics. 1999;19(1):121–46. https://doi.org/10.1148/radiographics.19.1.g99ja06121.

4. Tovi F, Mares AJ. The aberrant cervical thymus. Embryology, pathology, and clinical implications. Am J Surg. 1978 Nov;136(5):631–7.
5. Saggese D, Ceroni Compadretti G, Cartaroni C. Cervical ectopic thymus: a case report and review of the literature. Int J Pediatr Otorhinolaryngol. 2002;66(1):77–80.
6. Kieran SM, Robson CD, Nosé V, Rahbar R. Foregut duplication cysts in the head and neck: presentation, diagnosis, and management. Arch Otolaryngol Neck Surg. 2010;136(8):778–82.
7. Marcoviceanu MP, Metzger MC, Deppe H, Freudenberg N, Kassem A, Pautke C, et al. Report of rare bilateral nasolabial cysts. J Cranio-Maxillo-fac Surg. 2009;37(2):83–6.
8. Glazer HS, Mauro MA, Aronberg DJ, Lee JK, Johnston DE, Sagel SS. Computed tomography of laryngoceles. AJR Am J Roentgenol. 1983;140(3):549–52.
9. Goldenberg D, Begum S, Westra WH, Khan Z, Sciubba J, Pai SI, et al. Cystic lymph node metastasis in patients with head and neck cancer: an HPV-associated phenomenon. Head Neck. 2008;30(7):898–903.
10. Weiss D, Koopmann M, Rudack C. Prevalence and impact on clinicopathological characteristics of human papillomavirus-16 DNA in cervical lymph node metastases of head and neck squamous cell carcinoma. Head Neck. 2011;33(6):856–62.
11. Glastonbury CM. Critical changes in staging of head and neck cancer. Radiol: Imaging Cancer. 2020;2(1):e190022.

Noninterpretive Skills Including Quality and Safety

Syed S. Hashmi and Tarik F. Massoud

CORE ELEMENTS OF PROFESSIONALISM

FUNDAMENTAL PRINCIPLES OF MEDICAL PROFESSIONALISM [1]

- *Primacy of patient welfare*—serving the interest of the patient is paramount.
- *Patient autonomy*—patients should be empowered to make informed decisions that must then be respected.
- *Social justice*—physicians must strive to ensure fair distribution of healthcare resources and eliminate healthcare discrimination.

TEN PROFESSIONAL RESPONSIBILITIES OF THE MEDICAL PROFESSIONAL [1]

- *Commitment to professional competence*—emphasis on lifelong learning to ensure quality patient care.
- *Commitment to honesty with patients*—patients are thoroughly informed for decision-making. Medical errors should be honestly communicated to patients when injury has occurred. Physicians should be committed to report and analyze medical errors to develop prevention strategies.
- *Commitment to patient confidentiality*—physicians must safeguard patient information and privacy. However, considerations of public interest may override this commitment such as when patients endanger others.
- *Commitment to maintaining appropriate relations with patients*—physicians should never exploit patients for sexual advantage, personal financial, or other gain.
- *Commitment to improving quality of care*—emphasis on reducing medical errors, improving patient safety, and optimizing clinical outcomes.
- *Commitment to improving access to care*—commitment to promoting public health and preventative medicine while striving to reduce various barriers to equitable healthcare.
- *Commitment to a just distribution of finite resources*—develop evidence-based guidelines for effective and judicious use of healthcare resources while avoiding unnecessary tests and procedures.
- *Commitment to scientific knowledge*—uphold scientific standards, promote research, and create new medical knowledge based on scientific evidence and physician experience.
- *Commitment to maintaining trust by managing conflicts of interest*—obligation to recognize and disclose conflicts of interest that may arise through interactions with for-profit organizations, especially when physicians are determining criteria for conducting and reporting clinical trials, writing therapeutic guidelines, or serving as editors of scientific journals.
- *Commitment to professional responsibilities*—members of the profession should define the educational standards that should be met for current and future members to provide quality patient care. Physicians must participate in processes of self-regulation including remediation and discipline of members who fail to meet the defined professional standards.

ETHICAL CONSIDERATIONS SPECIFIC TO RADIOLOGY PER THE ACR BYLAWS [2]

- *Professional limitations*—radiologists should be aware of their limitations, seek suitable consultations in clinical situations, and appropriately disclose limitations to patients and referring physicians.

S. S. Hashmi (✉)
Division of Neuroimaging and Neurointervention, Stanford University School of Medicine, Stanford, CA, USA
e-mail: hashmi@stanford.edu

T. F. Massoud
Department of Radiology, School of Medicine, Stanford University, Stanford, CA, USA
e-mail: tmassoud@stanford.edu

- *Reporting illegal or unethical conduct*—report perceived illegal or unethical conduct of medical professionals to the appropriate governing body.
- *Report signature*—a radiologist should not claim credit for imaging interpretation or sign a report rendered by another independent radiologist.
- *Participation in quality and safety activities*—radiologists who actively interpret imaging should partake in quality assurance, technology assessment, utilization review, and other matters of policy affecting quality and safety of care.
- *Self-referral*—one should not refer patients to healthcare facilities in which they have a financial interest when it is not in the best interest of the patient and may violate the Rules of Ethics.
- *Harassment*—demonstrate mutual respect with other members of the healthcare team and refrain from unfair discriminatory behavior or harassment.
- *Undue influence*—ensure their practice setting does not unduly influence the selection and performance of appropriate imaging studies or therapeutic interventions.
- *Agreements for provision of high-quality care*—radiologists must not enter into an agreement that prohibits the provision of medically necessary care or leads to delivery of substandard care.
- *Misleading billing arrangements*—radiologists should not participate in fraudulent billing arrangements that mislead patients or payers.
- *Expert medical testimony*—when called for, radiologists must provide nonpartisan, clinically accurate, and scientifically correct testimony. Compensation solely linked to the outcome of litigation is unacceptable.
- *Research integrity*—research must be performed and reported in honesty.
- *Plagiarism*—claiming others' work or intellectual property as one's own without appropriate attribution is unethical.
- *Misleading publicizing*—radiologists should not promote themselves through any medium or forum of public communication in an untruthful, misleading, or deceptive manner.

CORE CONCEPTS OF QUALITY

- In the Radiology realm, quality is defined as "the extent to which the right procedure is done in the right way, at the right time, and the correct interpretation is accurately and quickly communicated to the patient and referring physician. The goals are to maximize the likelihood of desired health outcomes and to satisfy the patient."
- Quality is defined by two important parameters—excellence and consistency.
- Performance must be measurable and monitored to ensure consistent quality.
- Quality control (QC)—involves measuring and testing elements of performance to ensure that standards are met and correcting instances of poor quality. Example—correcting dictation errors before finalizing a report [3].
- Quality assurance (QA)—process for monitoring and *maintaining* performance quality set by the organization itself to reduce errors. QA assumes that the quality of work is adequate in the first place and seeks to maintain that high quality. Example—utilizing standardized report templates to minimize errors accompanied by auditing to ensure compliance [3].
- Quality improvement (QI)—activities designed to *improve* performance quality in an organization in a systemic and sustainable manner. QI assumes that the quality is not as good as baseline and strives to improve it. Example—radiologists agree to improve reporting consistency, implement standardized radiology report templates, implement those templates, monitor radiology reports, make necessary adjustments, and ensure consistency through feedback mechanisms and accountability [3].
- The Institute of Medicine (IOM) states that healthcare should be safe, effective, patient-centered, timely, efficient, and equitable [4].

- *Six core competencies for physicians as defined by the Accreditation Council for Graduate Medical Education (ACGME)* [5]:
    o *Practice-based Learning and Improvement*—demonstrate the ability to investigate healthcare practices and assimilate scientific evidence to improve the practice of medicine.
    o *Patient Care and Procedural Skills*—provide compassionate, appropriate, and effective care.
    o *Systems-Based Practice*—demonstrate awareness of the larger context and systems of healthcare and be able to utilize system resources to allow for optimal patient care.
    o *Medical Knowledge*—demonstrate knowledge of established and evolving biomedical, clinical, and cognitive sciences, and their application in patient care.
    o *Interpersonal and Communication Skills*—demonstrate skills that result in effective information exchange and teaming with patients, their families, and other healthcare professionals.
    o *Professionalism*—demonstrate a commitment to carrying out professional responsibilities, adhering to ethical principles, and being sensitive to diverse patient populations.

CORE CONCEPTS OF SAFETY

- Quickly establishing a correct diagnosis is critical to the provision of safe and effective patient care.
- Per the IOM's 2015 report, Improving Diagnosis in Healthcare, a diagnostic error is defined as "the failure to establish an accurate and timely explanation of the patient's health problem(s) or communicate that explanation to the patient."
- Eight specific recommendations made by the report authors for improving diagnostic processes [6].
   o Facilitate more effective teamwork among healthcare professionals, patients, and their families. Radiologists and pathologists are an integral part of the diagnostic team.
   o Enhance healthcare professional education and training in the diagnostic process.
   o Ensure that health information technologies support patients and healthcare professionals.
   o Develop and deploy organizational approaches to identify, learn from, and reduce diagnostic errors and near misses in clinical practice.
   o Establish a work system and culture that supports the diagnostic process and improvements in performance. This may include redesigning payment structures since fee-for-service (FFS) payments lack incentives to coordinate care among team members, such as communication among treating clinicians, pathologists, and radiologists about diagnostic test ordering, interpretation, and subsequent decision-making.
   o Develop a reporting environment and medical liability system that facilitates improvement.
   o Design a payment and care delivery environment that supports the diagnostic process. Specifically, oversight bodies should require that healthcare organizations have programs in place to monitor the diagnostic process and identify, learn from, and reduce diagnostic errors and near misses in a timely fashion.
   o Provide dedicated funding for research on the diagnostic process and diagnostic errors.
- The 2015 IOM report identified failures in communication as a significant contributor to diagnostic errors with respect to Radiology. Communication is defined as the meaningful exchange of information between individuals or groups and is often bi—or multidirectional and is successful when it results in a shared understanding of meaning. It consists of two major parts—A. *conveyance*—transmission of information from a sender to a receiver, B. *convergence*—verification, discussion, and clarification until both parties recognize that they mutually agree or fail to agree on the meaning of the information. The 2015 IOM report made the following recommendations in regard to improving communication [6].
   o Standardize communication policies and definitions across networked organizations.
   o Ensure clear identification of the patient's care team to facilitate contact by the radiology team.
   o Implement effective results management and tracking processes.
   o Develop shared quality and reporting metrics.
- Human factors are a major contributor to errors in medical practice. Human factors engineering (HFE) attempts to identify and address these problems in a systematic manner, considering human strengths and limitations in the design of interactive systems that involve people, equipment, technology, and work environments to ensure safety, effectiveness, and ease of use [7].
- HFE emphasizes the role of standardization of equipment and processes whenever possible to increase reliability, improve information flow, minimize cross-training needs, and overall reduce medical errors.7
- High-Reliability Organization (HRO) is defined as an organization that, despite operating in a high-stress, high-risk, complex environment, continually manages its environment mindfully, adopting a constant state of vigilance that results in the fewest number of errors. Such organizations anticipate and monitor unexpected events and focus on containing the impact of errors when they occur [7].
- A commonly used classification scheme for human errors is the "skill-rule-knowledge" (SRK) model, which refers to the cognitive mode in which the individual is operating when he/she commits an error [7].
   o Actions that are performed automatically, such as tying one's shoes, are considered skill-based actions. In light of HFE, these errors are amenable to behavior-shaping constraints that make it harder to perform the wrong actions; for example, a microwave oven cannot be operated with the door open.
   o Actions that require an intermediate level of attention, such as deciding which clothes to wear, are considered rules-based actions. Errors relating to these types of actions are amenable to increased supervision, additional training and coaching, deliberate practice, and intelligent decision support.
   o Actions requiring a high level of concentration, usually in the setting of new situations, such as playing a sport for the first time, are knowledge-based actions and are addressed in a similar fashion as rule-based actions, as stated earlier.

CULTURE OF SAFETY

A culture of safety is key to reducing human errors and achieving the high level of functioning and commitment to safety achieved by high-reliability organizations. Steep authority gradients, especially where there is fear of punish-

Table 44.1 Three manageable behaviors of the just culture model

Behavior or event	Human error	At-risk behavior	Reckless behavior
Definition	A product of our current system design and behavioral choices	A choice where the risk is believed to be insignificant or justified	A conscious disregard for a substantial and unjustifiable risk
Management strategies	• Modify available choices • Change processes/workflows • Improve training programs • Redesign system/facility	• Counsel individual • Better incentivize correct behavior • Modify training and processes as needed	• Remediate or remove from the environment • Take punitive action as warranted
Recommended approach to the individual	Console	Coach	Punish/sanction

Outline of the just culture model. Adapted from Marx 2009 [8]

ment for errors, undermine a culture of safety. The cornerstones of a culture of safety are the following [7]:

- Acknowledgment of the high-risk nature of an organization's activities and the determination to achieve consistently safe operations.
- A blame-free environment where individuals are able to report errors or near misses without fear of reprimand or punishment.
- Encouragement of collaboration across ranks and disciplines to seek solutions to patient safety problems.
- Organizational commitment of resources to address safety concerns.

JUST CULTURE

The just culture model balances the need for individual accountability for errors while reducing the sole focus on blame itself, which has historically been shown to impair the advancement of a safety culture. [7, 8] In this model, the response to an error or near miss is predicated on the type of behavior associated with the error and not the outcome/severity of the event itself. See Table 44.1.

PRACTICAL QUALITY AND SAFETY APPLICATIONS IN HEALTHCARE

PRACTICAL QUALITY APPLICATIONS IN HEALTHCARE

- Quality improvement activities can be categorized into either defined and dedicated improvement projects addressing specific areas of performance improvement, or frequent small improvement efforts focused on the management and quality assurance of day-to-day clinical operations.
- Examples of frequent small improvement efforts include daily management systems that seek to solve small problems as they arise, and tiered huddles that assess quality efforts at different levels of the organization [7, 9].
- Continuous problem solving is a foundational element of such regular quality improvement efforts. Problems are documented on the visibility board, along with an "owner" of the problem and an expected resolution date. These problems are regularly followed up to ensure resolution or escalation to a higher tier [7, 9].
- Problems that are too difficult to solve using routine daily problem-solving methods may be more amenable to dedicated improvement projects.
- There are certain core elements to a well-structured and organized quality improvement project [10].
  o The problem driving the improvement project has to be clearly identified and stated.
  o A dedicated team should be organized and include the project sponsor, project leader, participants, and a project coach who is an expert in improvement methods and can guide the team during the process.
  o Assessing the current state of quality and gaining a deeper sense of the problem at hand by directly observing the workplace is an essential first step.
  o It is of utmost importance to develop or define performance metrics to measure the current state as well as assess change after interventions are put in place. Performance can be monitored with a *run chart*.
  o The project team should establish a performance goal. A commonly used acronym to describe the attributes of the goal is "SMART," meaning that the goal should be specific, measurable, achievable, relevant, and timebound. The goal should state the beginning performance, the end performance, and the date (i.e., "from what, to what, by when").
  o After establishing a measure and a goal, and having observed the processes in detail, the team should document the causes of the problem at hand. Various tools can be utilized to achieve this including a cause-and-effect fishbone diagram. A tally sheet of the frequencies of the causes contributing to a problem can be kept with a Pareto chart.
  o Solutions to problems can be developed through iterative testing, refining, and validating process changes, known as the Plan-Do-Study-Act (PDSA) cycle.

- o Because the effects of process changes are not known in advance, initial changes are typically tested on as small a scale as possible and in a relatively protected environment. Changes are tested on a larger scale only after they have been proven successful on a smaller scale. The final determination of whether the changes are effective in practice is if they result in improved performance. Hence, it is critical to continuously monitor performance throughout the life of an improvement project.
- o Without deliberate mechanisms to sustain improvements after the defined quality improvement project concludes, performance usually reverts to the initial state. Process owners should be clearly identified at the conclusion of the QI project and regular check-ins can facilitate maintenance of high quality.

PRACTICAL SAFETY APPLICATIONS IN HEALTHCARE

- Patient identifiers — at least two identifiers that can include patient name, assigned medical record number, telephone number, date of birth, government-issued ID card, and last four digits of the social security number can be used to ensure that the right patient receives the right medical intervention or procedure, as well as to reduce the chance of unnecessary radiation exposure [11, 12].
- Patient assessment—before sedation can be performed, a patient must be assessed and approved for the level of sedation that is deemed appropriate for a specific intervention/procedure. Assessment includes documenting recent oral intake, illnesses, cardiopulmonary status, vital signs, level of consciousness, any additional appropriate workup, and monitoring [11, 12].
- *Sedation*—The Joint Commission and the American Society of Anesthesiologists have defined four levels of sedation, analgesia, and anesthesia [12]:
  - o Minimal Sedation or Anxiolysis—a drug-induced state, created by the administration of medications to reduce anxiety, during which the patient responds to verbal commands—in this state, cognitive function and coordination may be impaired, but ventilatory and cardiovascular functions are unaffected.
  - o Moderate Sedation/Analgesia—mildly depressed level of consciousness, induced by the administration of pharmacologic agents, in which the patient retains a continuous and independent ability to maintain protective reflexes and a patent airway and to be aroused by physical or verbal stimulation.
  - o Deep Sedation/Analgesia –a drug-induced depression of consciousness during which the patient cannot be easily aroused but responds purposefully after repeated or painful stimulation. Independent ventilatory function may be impaired. The patient may require assistance in maintaining a patent airway. Cardiovascular function is usually maintained.
  - o General Anesthesia—a controlled state of unconsciousness in which there is a complete loss of protective reflexes, including the ability to maintain a patent airway independently and to respond appropriately to painful stimulation.
- The patient's American Society of Anesthesiologists (ASA) Physical Status Classification should also be assessed. This is a six-level classification as follows [13]:
  - o Class I—A normal healthy patient.
  - o Class II—A patient with mild systemic disease.
  - o Class III—A patient with severe systemic disease.
  - o Class IV—A patient with severe systemic disease that is a constant threat to life.
  - o Class V—A moribund patient who is not expected to survive without the operation.
  - o Class VI—A declared brain-dead patient whose organs are being removed for donor purposes.
  - o Patients in Classes III and IV or with other significant risk factors may require a consultation with anesthesiology or the performance of sedation by an anesthesiologist or anesthetist. Patients in Class V should not be sedated by non-anesthesiologists.
- When sedation is performed under the supervision of a radiologist, there must be a separate qualified healthcare professional whose primary focus is the monitoring, medicating, and care of the patient. The patient must have intravenous access. Continuous monitoring should include, at a minimum, level of consciousness, respiratory rate, pulse oximetry, blood pressure (as indicated), heart rate, and cardiac rhythm [11, 12].
- It is recommended that consciousness and vital signs return to acceptable levels and remain at those levels for a period of 2 h from the time the reversal agent was administered before monitoring ends and the patient is discharged [11, 12].
- *Informed Consent*—required for invasive image-guided procedures. Patients have the right to be informed about the procedures they undergo and may request to speak with a radiologist even when local policy does not require the radiologist to initiate an informed consent process [12].
- Consent can also be documented by a note in the patient's medical record, by a recording on videotape, or by another similar permanent modality. Consent should be obtained from the patient or the patient's legal representative by a physician or other healthcare provider performing the procedure [12].
- Elements of informed consent include (1) the purpose and nature of the intended procedure, (2) the method by which

the procedure will be performed, (3) likely risks, complications, and expected benefits, (4) risks of not proceeding, (5) any reasonable alternatives to the proposed procedure, and (6) the right to decline the proposed procedure [12].
- An exception to these steps exists when a delay in treatment would jeopardize the health of a patient who is unable to provide informed consent (e.g., an unconscious trauma patient for whom family has not yet been identified). Since the patient must be able to understand the consent process for it to be valid, consent must be obtained before procedure-related sedation is administered. When the patient is not able to give valid consent because of short-term or long-term mental incapacity, whether from pain medications or otherwise, or when the patient has not achieved the locally recognized age of majority, consent should be obtained from the patient's appointed healthcare representative, legal guardian, or appropriate family member [12].
- In emergency situations when the patient needs immediate care, the patient's predetermined wishes are not known or appropriately documented, and consent cannot be obtained from the patient's representative, the physician may provide treatment or perform a procedure "to prevent serious disability or death or to alleviate great pain or suffering" [12].
- *Minors' Rights in Medical Decision Making* [14].
  o States and courts have never allowed children younger than 12 years to make medical decisions and exercise self-determination, whereas adolescents between ages 12 and 18 (or 19 in some states) experience a gradual transition to self-determination. Factors that impact the determination of adolescents' rights include the following:
    - Legal determination of maturity, such as married status, parenthood, self-sufficiency, or active duty in the armed services.
    - Evidence that the child is sufficiently mature to make his or her own decisions, such as age greater than 14 years; evidence that the minor has the ability to understand the implications of treatment, including risks, benefits, likely short—and long-term consequences, and alternatives; and evidence that the minor can make an informed decision without coercion.
    - Conditions exempting parental consent, such as seeking testing or treatment for sexually transmitted diseases, including HIV; seeking contraception, prenatal care, or abortion; or seeking mental health treatment, emergency care, or treatment of alcohol or drug abuse after the age of 12 years.
- *Universal Protocol* [15].
  o Refers to the three-part process of conducting a pre-procedure verification, marking the procedure site, and performing a pre-procedure time out.
- *Hand Hygiene* [12, 16].
  o Should be performed (1) before eating, (2) before and after having direct contact with a patient's skin, (3) after contact with blood, body fluids or excretions, mucous membranes, non-intact skin, or wound dressings, (4) after contact with inanimate objects in the immediate vicinity of the patient, (5) if hands will be moving from a contaminated-body site to a clean—body site during patient care, (6) after glove removal, and (7) after using a restroom. When hands are cleaned with soap and water, the soap and water should cover all surfaces of the hands and fingers. When alcohol-based hand sanitizer is used, the product should cover all surfaces as hands are rubbed together. Adequate cleansing can be achieved in about 20 s via either route.
- *Root Cause Analysis (RCA)* [17].
  Structured method of analyzing serious adverse events with a goal of identifying active errors as well as latent, systemic errors that could increase the likelihood of adverse events. An analysis of the collected data as well as objective narrative of the events can identify the active errors as well as latent issues in the system, and lead to a corrective plan that can limit similar events in the future.

PRACTICAL SAFETY APPLICATIONS SPECIFIC TO RADIOLOGY

MRI SAFETY [18, 19]

Because the strong static magnetic field of the MR scanner is always on, safety must be ensured for all people working in that environment including patients, technologists, nurses, cleaning personnel, support and administrative staff, and visitors.

- MRI safety is managed by people in three specific roles—MR Medical Director for MR Safety (MRMD) who is ultimately responsible for a site's operational safety and may be filled by a radiologist. The MR Safety Officer (MRSO) is typically filled by a technologist who ensures that policies and procedures are followed. The MR Safety Expert (MRSE), typically a physicist, renders expert guidance and recommendations for safe and appropriate scanning of patients, including those with implanted devices.
- *MRI Safety Zoning.*
  o Zone I—unrestricted access– includes all areas freely accessible to the public.
  o Zone II—interface between zone I and III—includes areas that are used to screen patients and obtain histories. This area is under the supervision of MR personnel.

- o Zone III—scanner control room with strictly restricted access, under the supervision of MR personnel and with physical restrictions in place such as locks. There is potential danger of serious injury or death for unscreened people.
- o Zone IV—defined as the MR scanner room itself and is considered the highest-risk area. This area is clearly demarcated as potentially hazardous and under the direct supervision of MR personnel. In the case of a medical emergency during the exam, the patient should be urgently moved to a magnetically safe location when feasible.
- MR personnel working within Zone III and Zone IV should have specific education on MR safety and pass an MR safety screening process.
- *MRI Screening.*

  Focused history to identify potential metallic foreign implants and objects that can be supplemented by the review of existing radiographs, CT, or MRI, as well as operative reports and review of implanted device information within the medical records. All MR sites should have a handheld magnet for testing purposes and ferromagnetic objects should be restricted from entering Zone III.

  Screening is more difficult when the patient is unconscious or otherwise unable to provide a reliable history. In such cases, screening should be performed as effectively as possible from other sources, such as family members and the medical record, and the urgency of the examination should be balanced with the level of uncertainty of the screening process. An examination by trained MR personnel should be performed to assess for surgical scars that may warrant additional evaluation. Radiography may be required to assess for foreign bodies, implants, or devices.
- MR Safe—objects that are nonhazardous in all MR environments, such as plastic tubing.
- MR Unsafe—those objects that are contraindicated such as a ferromagnetic clip.

  MR conditional—devices that can be safely scanned provided certain conditions are met, including suitable magnetic field strength, permissible coils, and specific absorption rate (SAR). Detailed scanning requirements are generally available on the product manufacturer's website.
- *MRI and Pregnancy.*

  MR exposure without the administration of gadolinium-based contrast has not shown to have any detrimental effects on the developing fetus. However, since it is impossible to completely exclude the mere possibility of any risk, clinicians and patients should weigh the benefits of scanning during pregnancy versus delaying until the end of pregnancy.
- *MRI-induced Burns.*

Thermal injury is attributed to the radiofrequency (RF) fields. Physical contact alone with the inner surface of the bore can produce burns, and insulating pads are necessary to keep skin at least 1–2 cm from the surface. Commercial padding is recommended to prevent skin-to-skin contact, of which obese patients are at a higher risk, in order to avoid a "closed loop" that can lead to the induction of currents within the body and lead to burns. The ACR Committee on MR Safety recommends that all MR patients be changed into MR-safe gowns/scrubs to minimize risk of burns from metallic fibers found in patient street clothes. Certain transdermal patches may contain metal and can lead to RF burns, and hence should be removed prior to the scan. Large tattoos are also at risk of undergoing heating and causing burns; application of a cold compress or ice pack may be necessary in such a scenario.

MANAGEMENT OF INTRAVASCULAR CONTRAST MEDIA [20]

Nonionic low-osmolality agents are considered the safest and approved for intravascular contrast administration in the United States. Only one iso-osmolality contrast agent, iodixanol (Visipaque), has been approved for use. Ionic, high-osmolality agents are not approved for use in the United States owing to the higher rates of adverse reactions.

- Adverse Reactions to Iodinated Contrast Media
  - o Uncommon, reported in about 3% of patients administered nonionic contrast agents.
  - o Allergic-like contrast reactions are poorly understood and in most patients, these reactions do not incite an IgE response seen in typical allergic reactions.
  - o Idiosyncratic reactions can occur at any volume of contrast media and without prior contrast exposure.
  - o Severe life-threatening allergic-like reactions are extremely rare, with the incidence of such reactions estimated to be 0.01% to 0.04% of injected patients.
  - o Patients with a prior allergic-like reaction to iodinated contrast media are at five times the risk of the general population.
  - o Patients with other allergies and asthma are two to three times as likely to react to contrast media.
  - o Allergies to shellfish, other iodine-containing products such as povidone-iodine, or gadolinium-based MR contrast agents do not place patients at a higher risk for a reaction to iodinated intravascular contrast.
- Examples of some reactions of different types and severity as summarized in the ACR Manual on Contrast Media are as follows:
  - o *Mild Reactions*: Signs and symptoms are self-limited and without progression. (1) Mild Physiologic

Reactions: Nausea, vomiting, flushing, warmth, chills, headache, anxiety, altered taste, mild hypertension, and spontaneously resolving vasovagal reaction. (2) Mild Allergic-like Reactions: Few hives, pruritus, limited cutaneous edema, itchy/scratchy throat, nasal congestion, repetitive sneezing, stuffy nose.
- *Moderate Reactions*: Signs and symptoms are more pronounced and commonly require medical management.
  - Moderate Physiologic Reactions: Protracted nausea, chest pain, vasovagal reaction that requires and is responsive to treatment.
  - Moderate Allergic-like Reactions: Diffuse hives, diffuse erythema (with stable vital signs), facial edema without dyspnea, wheezing with mild or no hypoxia.
- *Severe Reactions*: Signs and symptoms are potentially life-threatening and can result in permanent morbidity or death if not managed appropriately. (1) Severe Physiologic Reactions: Vasovagal reaction resistant to treatment, arrhythmia, seizures, hypertensive crisis, pulmonary edema, cardiopulmonary arrest. (2) Severe Allergic-like Reactions: Diffuse edema or facial edema with dyspnea, erythema with hypotension, laryngeal edema with stridor and/or hypoxia, wheezing with hypoxia, severe hypotension and tachycardia, pulmonary edema, cardiopulmonary arrest.

- Patients with thyroid cancer or hyperthyroidism should not receive iodinated contrast 4–6 weeks prior to radioactive iodine treatment since the nonradioactive iodine can saturate the thyroid gland and render the treatment ineffective.
- Premedication can be considered for patients at a higher risk for an allergic-like reaction to iodinated contrast. The ACR Manual on Contrast Media (2020) suggests consideration of premedication only for patients who have had a prior allergic-like or unknown-type reaction to the same class of contrast media as that to be administered. Various premedication regimens are available and widely accepted. One common adult regimen involves oral administration of 50 mg of prednisone 13, 7, and 1 h before contrast media injection, and oral administration of 50 mg of diphenhydramine (Benadryl®) 1 h before injection.

POSTCONTRAST ACUTE KIDNEY INJURY AND CONTRAST-INDUCED NEPHROPATHY [20]

Postcontrast acute kidney injury (PC-AKI) is a general, broad term used to describe a sudden deterioration in renal function that occurs after the intravascular administration of iodinated contrast media, regardless of whether contrast injection led to the kidney injury as causation is difficult to prove in many cases given the clinical complexity. Contrast-induced nephropathy (CIN), a subset of PC-AKI, is defined as a sudden deterioration in renal function directly *caused* by intravascular administration of iodinated contrast media.

Many large retrospective studies have shown that true CIN is much less common than previously thought, and if CIN occurs at all, it is most likely to develop in patients who have severe chronic kidney disease (CKD) (estimated glomerular filtration rate [eGFR] < 30 mL/min/1.73 m^2) or AKI. CIN occurring in patients with an eGFR of 45 mL/min/1.73 m^2 or higher is very unlikely, and it is questionable in patients with an eGFR between 30 and 45 mL/min/1.73 m^2. As a result, special precautions for administering intravascular iodinated contrast media are advised only for patients with severe CKD or AKI.

The Acute Kidney Injury Network (AKIN) has suggested that, regardless of the cause, AKI should be diagnosed whenever there is (1) an absolute serum creatinine increase of at least 0.3 mg/dL; or (2) a percentage increase in serum creatinine of at least 50% (1.5-fold above baseline); or (3) a reduction in urine output to 0.5 mL/kg/h for at least 6 h.

The usual clinical course of PC-AKI (including CIN) is a rise in serum creatinine beginning within 24 h of contrast media administration, peaking at about 4 days and then usually returning to baseline by 7–10 days. Most affected patients do not have oliguria. Permanent renal dysfunction is uncommon.

Although patients with end-stage renal disease who are on chronic hemodialysis could experience additional renal function compromise (resulting in a further decrease in any remaining urine output that might be helpful for managing electrolyte balance), such a risk is theoretical. Many nephrologists agree to inject these patients with intravascular contrast media if a contrast-enhanced study is necessary.

Because iodinated contrast media have no significant toxicity if retained in the body after injection, there is no requirement that chronic hemodialysis be timed to occur either immediately before or immediately after contrast media administration.

The most widely accepted strategy for minimizing the risk of PC-AKI in at-risk patients is IV volume expansion with isotonic fluids, such as 0.9% saline or Lactated Ringer's solution.

Metformin itself is not a risk factor for the development of CIN, but patients who develop renal failure while taking metformin are at risk of developing lactic acidosis.

IODINATED CONTRAST MEDIA IN PREGNANCY AND WOMEN WHO ARE BREASTFEEDING [20]

Although iodinated contrast crosses the placenta, there is no evidence that maternal exposure to contrast media is harmful to the fetus. Only 1% of contrast enters breast milk of which only a negligible amount is absorbed by the infant's GI tract. There is no evidence that this tiny amount of contrast has any adverse effect on the infant.

CONTRAST EXTRAVASATION [20]

The reported overall rate of extravasation with power injection for CT ranges from 0.1% to 1.2%.

Most patients complain of swelling or tightness and/or stinging or burning pain at the site of extravasation. Edema, erythema, and tenderness may be found on physical examination.

In total, 98% of extravasation injuries resolve with no adverse sequelae. Contrast media can damage the regional tissues, likely owing to a combination of direct toxic effects and its hyperosmolality, seen in about 2% of cases. Adverse effects are usually self-limited, most commonly consisting of prolonged pain or swelling.

Severe extravasation injuries occur in <1% of patients. The most common and most potentially devastating severe injuries after extravasation of nonionic contrast media are compartment syndromes, which result from mechanical compression, presenting early on with severe/progressive pain.

Cold compresses or ice packs can be applied to the site of extravasation. Surgical consultation should be obtained after an extravasation whenever there is concern for a developing compartment syndrome or tissue necrosis.

GADOLINIUM-BASED CONTRAST MEDIA (GBCM) [18–20]

Acute adverse reactions to GBCM occur approximately two to four times less frequently than acute adverse reactions to iodinated contrast media.

In general, the physiologic and allergic-like reactions that occur after GBCM administration are similar to those that occur after injection of iodinated contrast agents. For this reason, the treatment of contrast reactions to GBCM is similar to that of contrast reactions to iodinated contrast media.

Rash, hives, and urticaria are the most frequent allergic-like symptoms; however, respiratory and cardiovascular reactions can occur. Fatal contrast reactions have been reported but are exceedingly rare.

It should be noted that the FDA-approved package insert for one GBCM (gadobenate dimeglumine [MultiHance®]) states that use of this GBCM is specifically contraindicated in patients who have had prior allergic-like contrast reactions to ANY GBCM. Another preventive measure is premedicating patients with corticosteroids and antihistamines (using a regimen identical to that used for prophylaxis of adverse reactions to iodinated contrast media) before injection. The effectiveness of premedication before GBCM has not yet been determined.

GBCM IN PREGNANCY

These agents pass through the placental barrier and enter the fetal circulation. They are then filtered by the fetal kidneys and excreted into the amniotic fluid, where they may remain for a prolonged period which could theoretically increase the risk of dissociation from the chelate of the potentially toxic gadolinium ion. GBCM should only be administered to pregnant patients in carefully selected situations in which the benefit is thought to outweigh the potential risk.

GBCM IN WOMEN WHO ARE BREASTFEEDING

Only tiny amounts (0.04%) of administered GBCM are excreted into the milk of breastfeeding mothers, and only a tiny percentage of this (1%) GBCM is absorbed through an infant's gastrointestinal tract. This is much less than the allowed GBCM dose, when a contrast-enhanced imaging study is needed in an infant. There is no evidence that the tiny amount of absorbed GBCM has any adverse effect on a breastfed infant. Therefore, there is no need for a mother to stop breastfeeding after a GBCM-enhanced study.

NEPHROGENIC SYSTEMIC FIBROSIS (NSF)

NSF is a fibrosing disease, without an effective treatment, most evident in the skin and subcutaneous tissues, but it also may involve other organs, such as the lungs, esophagus, heart, and skeletal muscles. Symptoms and signs may progress rapidly, with some affected patients developing contractures and joint immobility, and can occasionally be fatal. NSF occurs nearly exclusively in patients with severe CKD (eGFR <30 mL/min/1.73 m^2) or in patients with AKI who have been exposed to GBCM. Symptom onset can occur from days to years after GBCM administration.

NSF has been encountered almost exclusively after patient exposure to several specific linear GBCM, with the high-risk agents being gadodiamide (Omniscan®), gadoversetamide (OptiMark®, no longer manufactured), and gadopentetate dimeglumine (Magnevist®). Higher doses and multiple doses of the higher-risk GBCM are believed to increase the likelihood of NSF, although cases have occurred after only a single administration of a standard dose of GBCM. Hence these agents are absolutely contraindicated by the Food and Drug Administration in patients with severe CKD (eGFR <30 mL/min/1.73 m^2).

Few, if any, cases of unconfounded NSF have been reported with the lower-risk agents, which include gadobenate dimeglumine (MultiHance®), gadobutrol (Gadavist®), gadoterate meglumine (Dotarem® and Clariscan®), and gadoteridol (ProHance®). Gadoxetate disodium (Eovist®) is a newer agent with limited information about its association with NSF; however, the risk of NSF developing after gadoxetate disodium administration is probably very low.

TREATMENT OF ACUTE CONTRAST REACTIONS [20, 21]

Hives

- No treatment in most cases.
- Diphenhydramine (Benadryl®), 25 to 50 mg orally (PO), intramuscularly (IM), or intravenously (IV) can be administered in symptomatic cases.

Diffuse Erythema

- Normotensive patient—observe only.
- Hypotensive patient—give O$_2$, 6–10 L/min (via mask), administer 1 L IV fluids rapidly.
- Continue to monitor vitals and maintain IV access.
- Epinephrine IV (1 mg/10 mL) (1:10,000), 1 mL (0.1 mg) can be infused slowly with IV fluids if hypotension does not respond to IV fluid bolus.

Laryngeal Edema

- Give O$_2$, 6–10 L/min (via mask). Continue to monitor vitals and maintain IV access.
- Administer epinephrine IM (1:1000), 0.3 mL (0.3 mg), or IM EpiPen or equivalent (0.3 mL, 1:1000 dilution fixed), or, especially if hypotensive, epinephrine IV (1:10,000), 1 mL (0.1 mg) slowly into a running infusion of IV fluids.
- Repeat epinephrine as needed up to a maximum of 1 mg.
- Consider calling an emergency response team or 911 based on the severity of the reaction and the completeness of patient response to treatment.

Bronchospasm

- Give O$_2$, 6–10 L/min (via mask). Continue to monitor vitals and maintain IV access.
- Give beta-agonist inhaler albuterol, 2 puffs (90 mcg per puff); can repeat up to three times. In cases in which bronchospasm is severe and/or unresponsive to an inhaler, consider adding epinephrine IM (1 mg/mL) (1:1000), 0.3 mL (0.3 mg), or IM EpiPen or equivalent (0.3 mL, 1 mg /mL 1:1000 dilution fixed), or epinephrine IV (1 mg/10 mL) (1:10,000), 1 mL (0.1 mg) slowly into a running infusion of IV fluids.
- Repeat epinephrine as needed up to a maximum of 1 mg.
- Consider calling an emergency response team or 911 based on the completeness of patient response to treatment.

Hypotension (systolic BP < 90 mm Hg)

- Give O$_2$, 6–10 L/min (via mask). Continue to monitor vitals and maintain IV access.
- Elevate legs at least 60 degrees (Trendelenburg position).
- Consider rapid administration of 1 L of IV fluids.

Hypotension with Bradycardia (pulse <60 bpm) (Vagal Reaction)

- If mild, no additional treatment is usually needed beyond that listed above for any cause of hypotension.
- If severe (patient remains unresponsive to above measures), give atropine, 0.6–1.0 mg IV, into a running infusion of IV fluids.
- May repeat atropine up to a total dose of 3 mg.
- Consider calling an emergency response team or 911.

Hypotension with Tachycardia (pulse >100 bpm) (Allergic-like Reaction)

- If hypotension persists after the basic treatment listed above for any cause of hypotension, give epinephrine IV (1 mg/10 mL) (1:10,000), 1 mL (0.1 mg) slowly into a running infusion of IV fluids. Can repeat as needed up to 10 mL (1 mg) total. Alternatively, IM epinephrine (1 mg/mL) (1:1000) could be given, 0.3 mL (0.3 mg), or IM EpiPen or equivalent (0.3 mL, 1 mg/mL 1:1000 dilution fixed). IM epinephrine may be repeated up to 1 mg total.
- Consider calling an emergency response team or 911 based on the severity of the reaction and the completeness of patient response to treatment.

Unresponsive and Pulseless

- Check for responsiveness.
- Activate the emergency response team or call 911.
- Perform CPR per American Heart Association protocols.
- Defibrillate as indicated if the equipment is available.
- May administer epinephrine IV 1 mg/10 mL) (1:10,000), 10 mL (1 mg), between 2-min cycles of CPR.

REIMBURSEMENT, REGULATORY COMPLIANCE, AND LEGAL CONSIDERATIONS IN RADIOLOGY

PRINCIPLES GUIDING HEALTHCARE REIMBURSEMENT [22, 23]

- Shift from a fee-for-service to a value-based payment model that requires attaining certain quality measures.
- Each service or procedure rendered by a physician is assigned a unique code, called a Current Procedural Terminology (CPT) code that is assigned a specific reimbursement value. CPT codes are maintained by the American Medical Association (AMA) Editorial Panel.
- Each CPT code is assigned a value called a Relative Value Unit (RVU); this is a relative value in comparison to other services/procedures within the specialty as well as services rendered by other specialties.
- Work RVU—reflects time, effort, and skill of physician providing the service—measures physician productivity.
- Practice expense RVU—reflects costs of maintaining a practice such as equipment, supplies, and nonphysician staff.
- Professional liability RVU—reflects expenses related to maintaining malpractice insurance.
- A multiplier called the Conversion Factor (CF), set annually by the Center for Medicare Management (CMS), is used to determine the actual reimbursement. Payment = RVU × CF.
- Preauthorization for reimbursement of elective outpatient advanced imaging may be required by Medicare and other private payers.

PATIENT PRIVACY AND HIPAA [24]

- Protected Health Information (PHI) includes names, dates, geographic subdivisions smaller than a state, phone, and fax numbers, vehicle identification and license numbers, email addresses, Social Security numbers, medical record numbers, health plan beneficiary numbers, biometric identifiers such as finger—and voice-prints, full face photographs, any other unique identifiers.
- An individual's PHI cannot be disclosed to anyone other than the individual without that individual's authorization. Exceptions include information disclosed or transmitted when necessary for (1) the delivery of care or treatment, (2) payment activities, and (3) healthcare operations involving quality or competency assurance, fraud or abuse detection, or compliance. In addition, when required by law, information can be released (1) to public health authorities, (2) during the investigation of abuse, neglect, or domestic violence, (3) to oversight agencies, (4) for judicial and administrative proceedings, (5) for law enforcement purposes, and (6) for worker's compensation.

HUMAN SUBJECTS RESEARCH [25]

- The Institutional Review Board (IRB) for a particular entity is responsible for the oversight of research involving human subjects.
- An IRB has the authority to approve, require modifications in order to secure approval, or deny approval for proposed research protocols.
- IRBs are required to ensure a "diversity of members, including consideration of race, gender, cultural backgrounds, and sensitivity to such issues as community attitudes" and to register with the Department of Health and Human Services (HHS).
- The research informed consent process involves (1) providing adequate information about a study to potential subjects, (2) providing an adequate opportunity for subjects to consider all options, (3) responding adequately to all subject questions, (4) ensuring that the subject comprehends all necessary information, (5) obtaining the subject's voluntary agreement to participate, and (6) providing ongoing information as the subject or situation so requires.
- In the case of retrospective review of imaging or quality improvement projects, an IRB may waive the requirement for informed consent when the research involves no more than minimal risks to participants, and cannot be practically carried out without such a waiver.

MALPRACTICE AND RISK MANAGEMENT [26, 27]

- Approximately 7% of all radiologists are named in a medical malpractice lawsuit each year.
- Malpractice insurance is mandated as a condition for state licensure and hospital credentialing.
- Four elements that comprise a medical malpractice lawsuit:
  o Established duty of the physician to the patient.
  o Failure to meet the standard of care leads to a breach of this duty.
  o Causation of the breach resulting in injury must be established.
  o The negligence must result in damages.
- Claims of negligence against radiologists generally fall into 3 categories. The most common claims are related to diagnostic errors, followed by procedural complications, and then communication deficiencies [27].
- Negligent diagnosis claims can be categorized as related to (1) failures of perception (i.e., not identifying a finding), (2) failures of interpretation (i.e., identifying a finding but not appropriately appreciating or adequately communicating its significance), or (3) combinations of both.
- Diagnostic errors can also be categorized as (1) cognitive errors (e.g., not identifying a lung nodule when interpreting

a chest radiograph), which are usually errors of visual perception (scanning, recognition, and interpretation), or (2) system errors (e.g., failure to adequately communicate the presence of that nodule), which are usually attributed to health system issues or context of care delivery problems.
- Routine communication—final signed radiology reports.
- Nonroutine communication—situations warranting preliminary reports and results of an urgent, life-threatening, or other significantly important nature.
- Critical result—defined as "any result or finding that may be considered life threatening or that could result in severe morbidity and require urgent or emergent clinical attention."
- Direct verbal communication of critical results is required by the interpreting radiologist to the requesting or responding clinician or another licensed healthcare provider responsible for that patient's care, and generally expected to occur within 60 min. Critical results may be directly communicated to the patient when the ordering clinician cannot be contacted immediately.

CORE CONCEPTS OF IMAGING INFORMATICS [28, 29]

- The Digital Imaging and Communications in Medicine (DICOM) standard (http://dicom.nema.org) is the international standard that specifies protocols for display, transfer, storage, and processing of medical images.
- DICOM transactions enable data to be queried, retrieved, and transmitted between systems in an organized fashion.
- The radiology information system (RIS) is a software application that manages all aspects of an imaging exam, including order reconciliation, patient scheduling and tracking, communication with modalities, and PACS (picture archiving and communications system), reporting, results notification, and billing. The RIS may be a stand-alone application or a component of the electronic medical record (EMR) application.
- The PACS is the radiologist's primary tool for imaging viewing and interpretation. Basic components of PACS include a workstation, display, short-term storage, and long-term archive. PACS communicates with imaging modalities using DICOM transactions, and with the RIS and/or EMR using HL7 transactions that are translated to and from DICOM.

ARTIFICIAL INTELLIGENCE IN RADIOLOGY [30]

- Artificial intelligence (AI) is the field of computer science that gives computers the ability to mimic human intelligence.
- Machine learning (ML) is a subfield of AI that enables computers to learn a task without being given an explicit set of instructions.
- Deep learning (DL) uses multi-layered neural networks with weighted connections to analyze images and text.
- Generating training data for radiology requires experts to label images or text.
- Supervised ML exposes an algorithm to a set of training data and then evaluates how well the resulting model has "learned" the task using a different set of "test" data. It is important that the testing data are completely separate from the training data, in order to fairly evaluate the performance of the model.
- Major challenges in deploying AI for radiology include understanding how the model produces its results, ensuring that the model performs reliably in all potential applied settings and conditions, and efficiently integrating the model into the clinical workflow.
- Once deployed, model performance should be monitored to identify data drift, in which model performance degrades over time owing to gradual changes in the data it processes.
- Additionally, the way that radiologists interact with AI should be monitored to guard against automation bias, in which the computer is always assumed to be more correct than the human practitioner.

References

1. ABIM Foundation. American Board of Internal Medicine; ACP-ASIM Foundation. American College of Physicians-American Society of Internal Medicine; European Federation of Internal Medicine. Medical professionalism in the new millennium: a physician charter. Ann Intern Med. 2002;136(3):243–6. https://doi.org/10.7326/0003-4819-136-3-200202050-00012. Accessed 22 Mar 2022.
2. American College of Radiology. Code of Ethics. American College of Radiology Website. https://www.acr.org/MemberResources/CommissionsCommittees/Ethics. Accessed 22 Mar 2022.
3. Kruskal JB, Anderson S, Yam CS, Sosna J. Strategies for establishing a comprehensive quality and performance improvement program in a radiology department. Radiographics. 2009;29(2):315–29.
4. Committee on quality of health Care in America; for the Institute of Medicine. Crossing the quality chasm: a new health system for the 21st century. Washington, DC: National Academy Press; 2001.
5. A Trusted Credential: Based on Core Competencies. American Board of Medical Specialties Website. www.abms.org/boardcertification/a-trusted-credential/based-oncore-competencies. Accessed 22 Mar 2022.
6. Balogh EP, Miller BT, Ball JR, editors. Board on health care services, Institute of Medicine. Improving diagnosis in health care. Washington, DC: The National Academy of Sciences, The National Academies Press; 2015.
7. Larson DB, Kruskal JB, Krecke KN, Donnelly LF. Key concepts of patient safety in radiology. Radiographics. 2015;35(6):1677–93.
8. Marx D. Console, coach, or punish? In: Whacka-mole: the price we pay for expecting perfection. Plano, TX: By Your Side Studios; 2009. p. 47–55.

9. Donnelly LF. Daily management systems in medicine. Radiographics. 2014;34(2):549–55.
10. Larson DB, Mickelsen LJ. Project management for quality improvement in radiology. AJR Am J Roentgenol. 2015;205(5):W470–7.
11. American College of Radiology, Society of Interventional Radiology. ACR-SIR practice parameter for sedation/analgesia. American College of Radiology, Society of Interventional Radiology. https://www.acr.org/-/media/ACR/Files/Practice-Parameters/sedanalgesia.pdf. Accessed 22 Mar 2022.
12. Kohi MP, Fidelman N, Behr S, Taylor AG, Kolli K, Conrad M, Hwang G, Weinstein S. Periprocedural Patient Care. Radiographics. 2015;35(6):1766–78.
13. American Society of Anesthesiologists (ASA). Physical Status Classification. American Society of Anesthesiologists. https://www.asahq.org/standards-and-guidelines/asa-physical-status-classification-system. Accessed 22 Mar 2022.
14. Hickey K. Minors' rights in medical decision making. JONAS Healthc Law Ethics Regul. 2007;9(3):100–4.
15. The Joint Commission. Speak UP. The Joint Commission Website. https://www.jointcommission.org/-/media/tjc/documents/standards/universal-protocol/up_poster1pdf.pdf. Accessed 22 Mar 2022.
16. Centers for Disease Control and Prevention. Hand hygiene in healthcare settings. Centers for Disease Control and Prevention Website. http://www.cdc.gov/handhygiene/providers/index.html. 2022 Noninterpretive Skills Study Guide 32 Accessed 22 Mar 2022.
17. Brook OR, Kruskal JB, Eisenberg RL, Larson DB. Root cause analysis: learning from adverse safety events. Radiographics. 2015;35(6):1655–67.
18. ACR Manual on MR Safety https://www.acr.org/-/media/ACR/Files/Radiology-Safety/MRSafety/Manual-on-MR-Safety.pdf. Accessed 22 Mar 2022.
19. Tsai LL, Grant AK, Mortele KJ, Kung JW, Smith MP. A practical guide to MR imaging safety: what radiologists need to know. Radiographics. 2015 Oct;35(6):1722–37.
20. American College of Radiology. ACR Manual on Contrast Media (version 10.3). American College of Radiology Website. https://www.acr.org/-/media/ACR/Files/Clinical-Resources/Contrast_Media.pdf. Accessed 22 Mar 2022.
21. Lasser EC, Berry CC, Mishkin MM, Williamson B, Zheutlin N, Silverman JM. Pretreatment with corticosteroids to prevent adverse reactions to nonionic contrast media. AJR Am J Roentgenol. 1994;162(3):523–6.
22. Lam DL, Medverd JR. How radiologists get paid: resource-based relative value scale and the revenue cycle. AJR Am J Roentgenol. 2013;201:947–58.
23. Thorwarth WT Jr. From concept to CPT code to compensation: how the payment system works. J Am Coll Radiol. 2004;1:48–53.
24. Schoppmann MJ, Sanders DL. HIPAA compliance: the law, reality, and recommendations. J Am Coll Radiol. 2004;1:728–33.
25. Cooper JA. Responsible conduct of radiology research: part II. Regulatory requirements for human research. Radiology. 2005;236:748–52.
26. American College of Radiology. ACR Practice Parameter for Communication of Diagnostic Imaging Findings. https://www.acr.org/-/media/ACR/Files/Practice-Parameters/ communicationdiag.pdf. Accessed 22 Mar 2022.
27. Whang JS, Baker SR, Patel R, Luk L, Castro A 3rd. The causes of medical malpractice suits against radiologists in the United States. Radiology. 2013;266:548–54.
28. American College of Radiology. ACR– AAPM–SIIM technical standard for electronic practice of medical imaging. 2017. https://www.acr.org/-/media/ACR/Files/Practice-Parameters/elec-practice-medimag.pdf. Accessed 22 Mar 2022.
29. Horii SC. Primer on computers and information technology. Part four: a nontechnical introduction to DICOM. Radiographics. 1997;17(5):1297–309.
30. Thrall JH, Li X, Li Q, et al. Artificial intelligence and machine learning in radiology: opportunities, challenges, pitfalls, and criteria for success. JACR. 2018;15(3):504–8.

Advanced Imaging Techniques

Brian Dang, Max Wintermark, Behroze A. Vachha, and Michael Iv

Introduction

This chapter introduces basic concepts and principles as well as clinical applications of advanced imaging techniques used in neuroradiology. Imaging techniques covered include CT perfusion, MR perfusion, task-based functional MRI, diffusion tensor imaging, MR spectroscopy, and nuclear scintigraphy. An emphasis is placed on describing the utility of each technique for problem solving in routine clinical practice. Technical challenges such as artifacts and pitfalls are also briefly reviewed so that readers have a better sense of the limitations for each technique. The goal of this chapter is to highlight the power of advanced imaging in current clinical care.

CT Perfusion

Basic Principles and Technique [1]

- Acquisition and postprocessing of CT perfusion images are performed by monitoring the first pass of iodinated contrast agent bolus through the cerebral circulation with continuous imaging for 45–60 s over the same volume of tissue.

- During dynamic contrast administration, there is transient hyperattenuation of brain tissue, which is proportional to the amount of contrast material in the vessels and blood in that region.
- Time-attenuation (proportional to time-concentration) curves are generated for an arterial region of interest (ROI) placed within a proximal major intracranial artery (arterial input function) and a venous ROI placed within the superior sagittal sinus (venous output function), both of which are important in mathematical modeling used to derive perfusion parameters from the time-concentration curve.
- Individual hemodynamic perfusion metrics acquired include cerebral blood volume (CBV), cerebral blood flow (CBF), mean transit time (MTT), and time-to-maximum (Tmax).
- While CBV represents the area under the time-concentration curve, the other parameters are calculated by defining the arterial input function and venous output function and through a mathematical technique called deconvolution.

Radiation Dose Considerations

- A comprehensive stroke CT protocol that includes an unenhanced and postcontrast head CT, perfusion CT, and CT angiography (CTA) of the cervical and intracranial arteries can deliver a mean effective dose up to six times that of a standard unenhanced head CT.
- Perfusion CT studies should be performed at 80 kVp and no more than 200 mAs so the effective dose associated with a single slab perfusion CT study is equivalent to an unenhanced head CT [2].

B. Dang
Radiology Resident, Stanford University, Stanford, CA, USA
e-mail: dangb@stanford.edu

M. Wintermark
MD Anderson Cancer Center, Houston, TX, USA

B. A. Vachha
UMass Chan Medical Center, UMass Memorial Medical Center, Worcester, MA, USA
e-mail: Behroze.Vachha@umassmemorial.org

M. Iv (✉)
Department of Radiology (Neuroradiology), Stanford University, Center for Academic Medicine, Palo Alto, CA, USA
e-mail: miv@stanford.edu

© The Author(s), under exclusive license to Springer Nature Switzerland AG 2024
B. A. Vachha et al. (eds.), *What Radiology Residents Need to Know: Neuroradiology*, What Radiology Residents Need to Know, https://doi.org/10.1007/978-3-031-55124-6_45

Derived Perfusion Metrics [1]

- CBV is the blood volume within the tissue vessel and can be a measure of collateral flow (measured in mL blood/100 g tissue).
- CBF is the speed of blood through tissue (measured in mL blood/100 g tissue/min).
- MTT is the average transit time for a tracer particle to traverse the capillary bed (e.g., transit time of blood from an arteriole to a venule measured in seconds).
- Tmax is the delay of bolus from the proximal vasculature to tissue (measured in seconds) and is used as a marker of transit time like MTT.
- By convention, on color maps, lower values are coded blue, higher values are coded red, and intermediate values are coded shades on the blue-green-yellow-red (low-high) spectrum (Fig. 45.1).

Clinical Applications [3, 4]

- Acute Stroke Imaging.
    - Most commonly used application for CTP and is valuable for triaging patients to interventions such as thrombolysis or thrombectomy.
    - Allows differentiation between salvageable ischemic brain tissue (penumbra) and unsalvageable infarct core.
    - Mismatch concept refers to the volume difference (mismatch) between the perfusion deficit and ischemic core.
    - Perfusion fundamentals of stroke imaging: infarct core is characterized by increased MTT or Tmax, markedly decreased CBF (<30% relative to normal brain tissue), and markedly decreased CBV, while penumbra is characterized by increased MTT or Tmax, moderately reduced CBF (>30% relative to normal brain tissue), and normal or increased CBV (Fig. 45.2).
    - DEFUSE 3 (stroke trial) defined the values for determining which patients should receive endovascular therapy as follows: cervical or intracranial ICA or MCA-M1 occlusion AND Target Mismatch Profile on CT perfusion or MRI (ischemic core volume < 70 mL, mismatch ratio > 1.8 and mismatch volume > 15 mL). Of note, the size of penumbra was estimated from the volume of tissue with Tmax>6 s [5].
    - Hypoperfusion intensity ratio (the ratio of volume of tissue with a Tmax>10 s divided by the volume of tissue with a Tmax >6 s) is a good predictor for collateral flow and infarct growth.

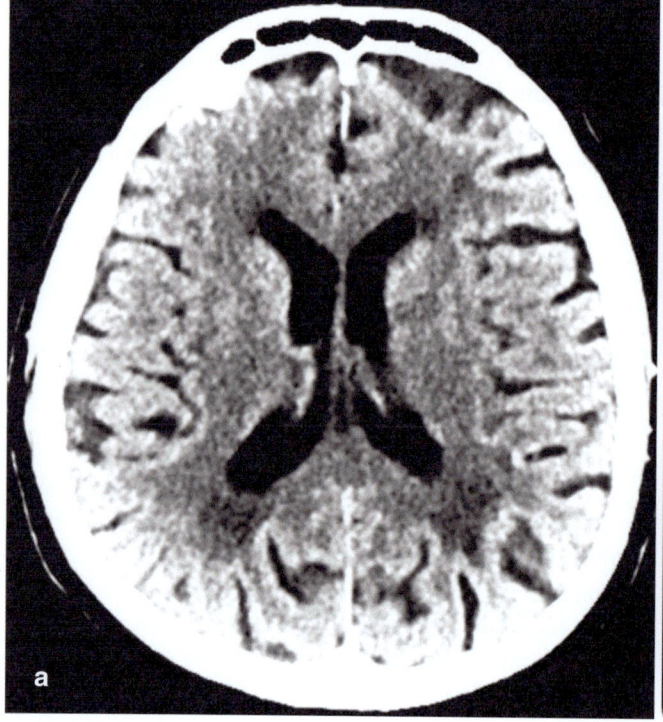
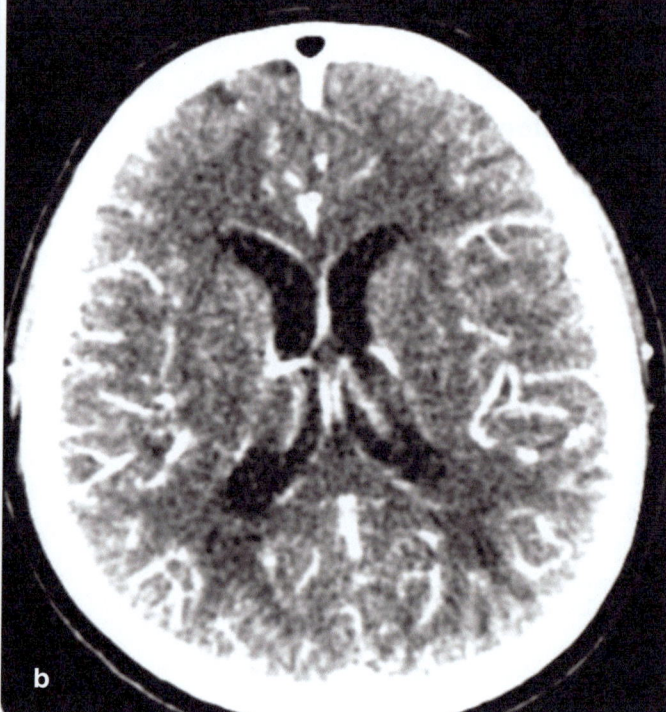

Fig. 45.1 Noncontrast CT (NECT) and CT perfusion. (**a**) NECT: Normal appearance of the brain without loss of gray-white differentiation. (**b**) CT perfusion raw image. (**c**) Perfusion color maps demonstrate normal appearance of the derived variables. (**d**) Perfusion summary map: Normal perfusion without any area of significant Tmax delay (defined as Tmax>6 s)

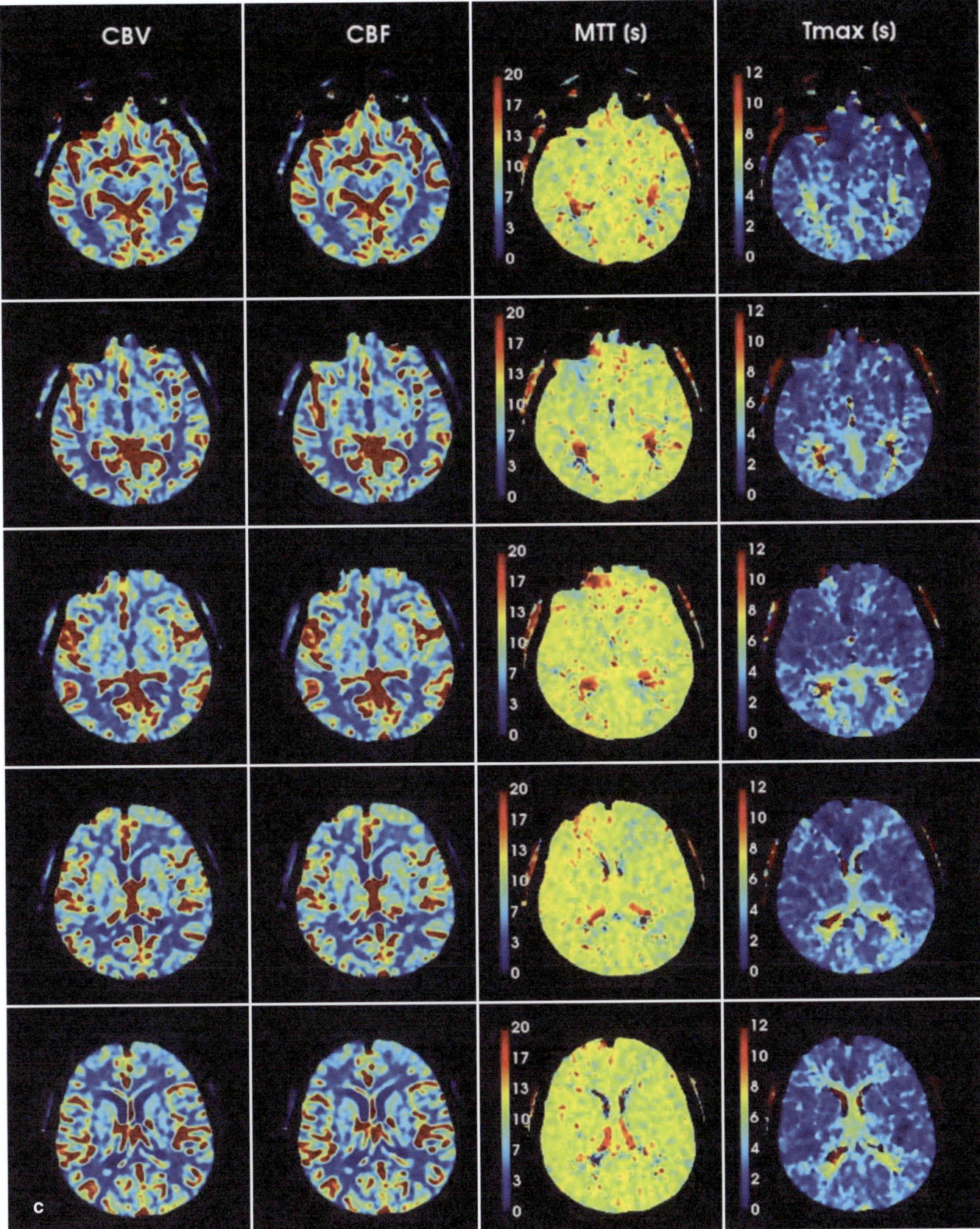

Fig. 45.1 (continued)

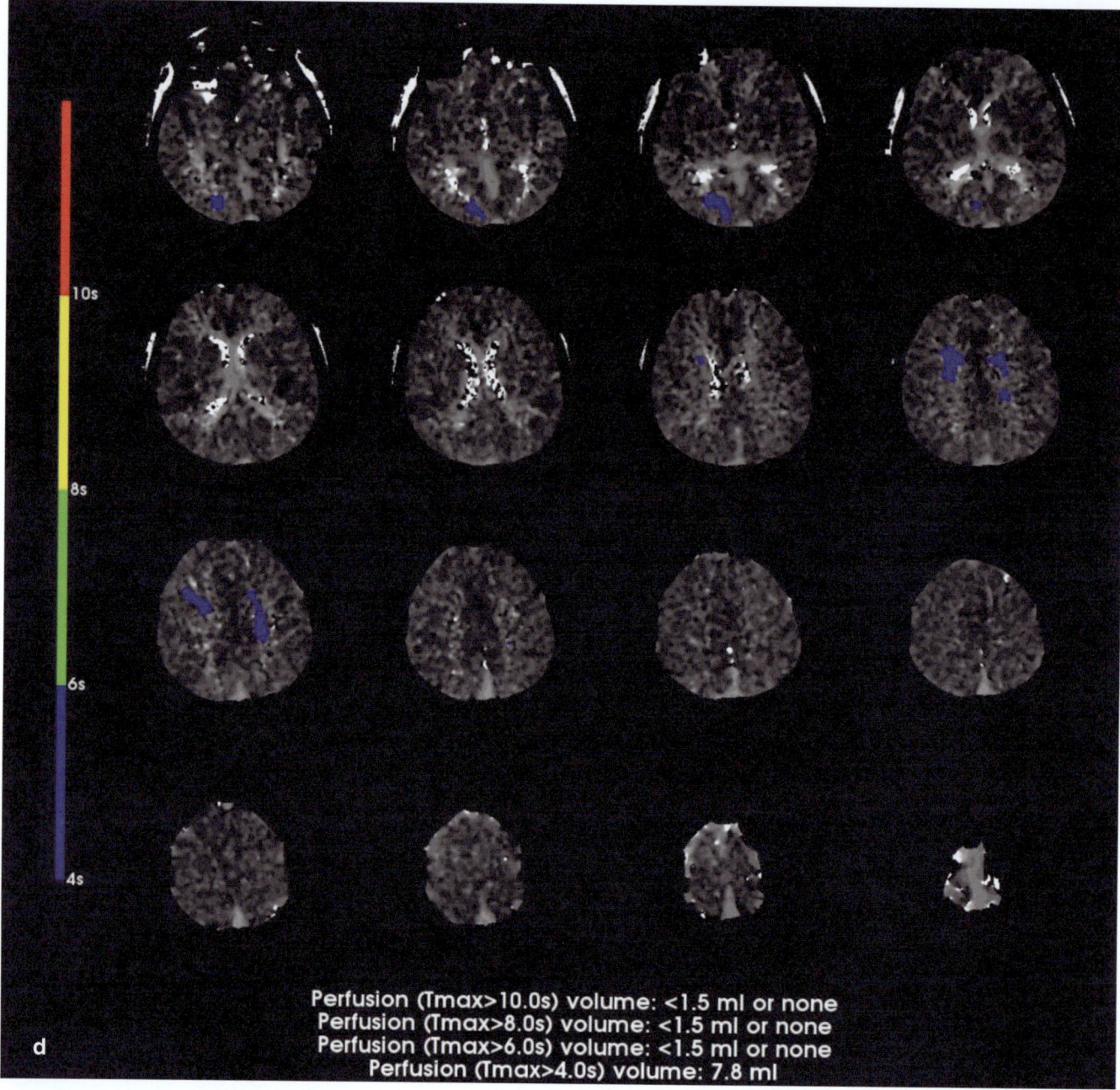

Fig. 45.1 (continued)

- Cerebrovascular reserve (CVR).
  - CVR is the compensatory ability of cerebral arteries to vasodilate to maintain CBF at a normal level in the setting of chronic steno-occlusive disease.
  - CVR imaging can be performed using an acetazolamide challenge.
  - Acetazolamide causes vasodilation of normal cerebral arteries and increases CBF in the corresponding territory, but patients with impaired CVR are already maximally dilated due to autoregulatory mechanisms and, as a result, there is unchanged or even decreased CBF ("steal" phenomenon) [6].
  - Look for the following changes after an acetazolamide challenge: increase in CBF 20–40% over baseline is considered normal augmentation; increase of <5% over baseline indicates relative hemodynamic insufficiency; and decrease of 5% from baseline ("steal" phenomenon) indicates tissue at higher risk of stroke.
- Epilepsy/seizures.
  - Status epilepticus and postictal paralysis are both mimickers of acute stroke.
  - CTP can show asymmetric perfusion with ictal areas of the brain showing hyperperfusion and interictal areas of the brain showing hypoperfusion.

45 Advanced Imaging Techniques

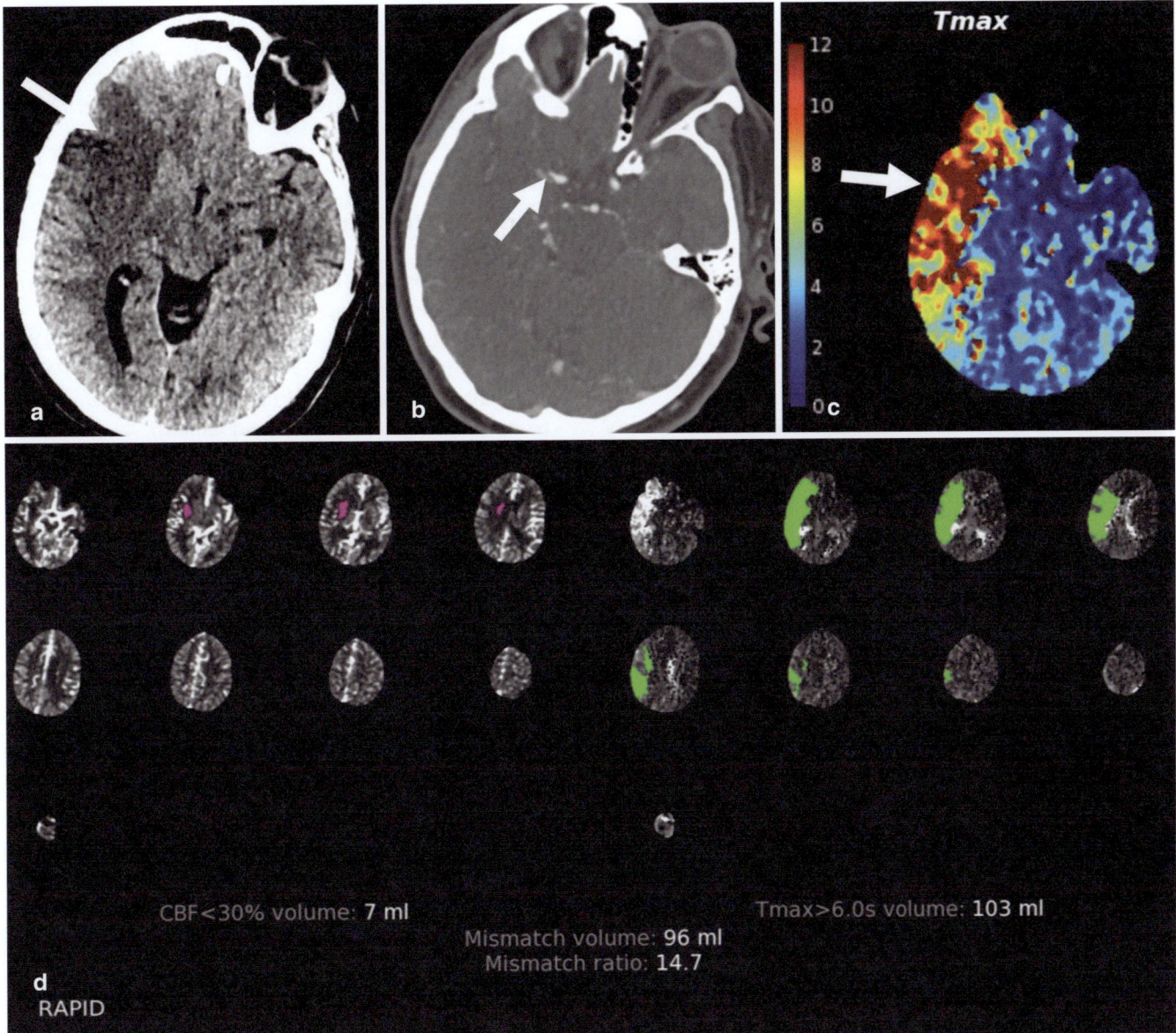

Fig. 45.2 Acute Stroke Imaging. (**a**) NECT: Loss of gray-white differentiation in the right middle cerebral artery (MCA) territory involving the right basal ganglia, frontal lobe, and insula consistent with acute infarct (white arrow). (**b**) CTA Head: Right M1 MCA occlusion (white arrow) with minimal distal filling of the distal M2 and M3 segments. (**c**) Tmax color map demonstrates significant Tmax delay (Tmax>6 s) within the entire right MCA territory (red) (white arrow). (**d**) Perfusion summary maps show small core infarct defined as CBF <30% relative to the contralateral side (7 mL) (purple), significant Tmax delay >6 s within the entire right MCA territory (103 mL) (green). When comparing the degree of core infarct and Tmax delay, there is a mismatch volume of 96 mL and mismatch ratio of 14.7, compatible with sizeable penumbra

- o Perfusion abnormalities in epilepsy can be mistaken for ischemia.
- o Key: look for nonvascular territory involvement with epilepsy.
- Brain tumors.
  - o MRI is superior for brain tumor evaluation because of its higher soft tissue resolution, but CTP can also be helpful.
  - o Hypervascular tumors such as meningiomas, hypervascular metastases (e.g., lung, breast, renal cell, melanoma, and thyroid), and malignant gliomas demonstrate high CBF and CBV.
  - o High-grade gliomas (WHO grade 3 and 4 tumors) demonstrate higher CBF and CBV than low-grade gliomas (WHO grade 1 and 2 tumors) [7].
  - o Can be used to differentiate between aggressive tumors, tumefactive demyelinating lesions, and infectious abscesses, as demyelinating lesions and abscesses tend to have low central CBF and CBV [7].
  - o Can be used to differentiate between recurrent or progressive tumor and radiation necrosis in previously irradiated tumors, as tumor tends to have higher CBF and CBV [7].

Artifacts, Pitfalls, and Limitations [3, 8]

- Lacunar or small subcortical infarcts are not usually detected using CTP thresholds.
- It is sometimes difficult to differentiate between acute and chronic tissue at risk; for example, increased MTT or Tmax is the most consistent CTP abnormality in hemodynamically significant extracranial carotid stenosis. Acuity of clinical symptoms is important in this scenario!
- Poststenotic areas can mimic or overestimate areas of acute ischemic penumbra.
- Steno-occlusive disease can also mask areas of true infarct.
- Vasospasm can mimic areas of penumbra in the setting of acute stroke syndrome.
- Severe vasospasm has been correlated with transiently increased MTT and CBF.

MR Perfusion

Basic Principles

- Exogenous and endogenous methods exist to assess regional cerebral hemodynamics and perfusion.
- Exogenous methods such as dynamic susceptibility contrast (DSC) and dynamic contrast-enhanced (DCE) imaging require the intravenous administration of gadolinium.
- Endogenous methods such as arterial spin labeling (ASL) imaging do not require contrast and instead exploit the spins of labeled water protons to measure perfusion.
- MR perfusion techniques can be used to evaluate the same conditions (e.g., ischemia and brain tumors) as CTP, although MRI allows for better soft tissue resolution and visualization.

Dynamic Susceptibility Contrast (DSC) [9, 10]

- Principles of DSC MR perfusion are similar to those of CT perfusion (CTP), except DSC estimates the concentration of gadolinium contrast agent from the signal of gadolinium using T2- or T2*- weighted imaging.
- T2-weighted DSC is more sensitive to signal changes from contrast passing through small vessels, while T2*-weighted DSC is more sensitive to larger vessels.
- DSC measures transient signal changes (susceptibility effect) in the local magnetic field of the surrounding tissue induced by a bolus of paramagnetic contrast agent (gadolinium) passing through the organ capillary network.
- The signal–time course data is converted into a relative tissue contrast concentration-time curve on a pixel-by-pixel basis, which can subsequently be analyzed to determine various tissue hemodynamic parameters such as CBF, CBV, MTT, and Tmax.
- Semiquantitative or relative values of a region of interest can be obtained using an internal standard of reference (e.g., normal contralateral white matter).
- In MRI, DSC is the most commonly used method to measure brain perfusion.

Dynamic Contrast Enhancement (DCE) [9]

- DCE MR perfusion is based on T1-weighted dynamic imaging, in contrast to DSC which is based on T2- or T2*-weighted dynamic imaging; in other words, DCE measures the T1 relaxivity effects instead of the T2/T2* susceptibility effects of an intravenous injected dose of paramagnetic contrast agent (gadolinium).
- DCE measures increases in T1 signal intensity over time to calculate a time–signal intensity curve, which can then be used to derive several semiquantitative parameters.
- The DCE curve depicts the wash-in, plateau, and washout contrast kinetics of tissue and can provide information about tissue microvascular properties.
- Ktrans, a measure of blood-brain barrier permeability and (in tissues with very high permeability) flow, is the most frequently used parameter.
- DCE is less clinically used than DSC in neuroimaging, in large part due to the complex pharmacokinetic modeling required and lack of clinical validation in various pathologies.

Arterial Spin Labeling (ASL) [9]

- ASL does not require contrast administration and can be performed in patients with renal insufficiency.
- In ASL, water protons in inflowing arterial blood are magnetically labeled ("tagged") by the application of radiofrequency pulses designed to invert spins in a thick slab proximal to the slice of interest.
- By measuring signal changes between tagged images and baseline untagged images, qualitative or quantitative images of CBF can be obtained.
- CBF measurements derived from ASL correlate well with CBF measurements derived from DSC.
- Normal CBF values are variable and can range from 30 to 70 (average 50) mL/100 g/min in healthy adults.

Clinical Applications

- Acute Stroke Imaging.
  - The utility of MR perfusion such as DSC and CT perfusion is similar in acute stroke imaging, as the main purpose is to identify infarct and penumbra (Fig. 45.3).

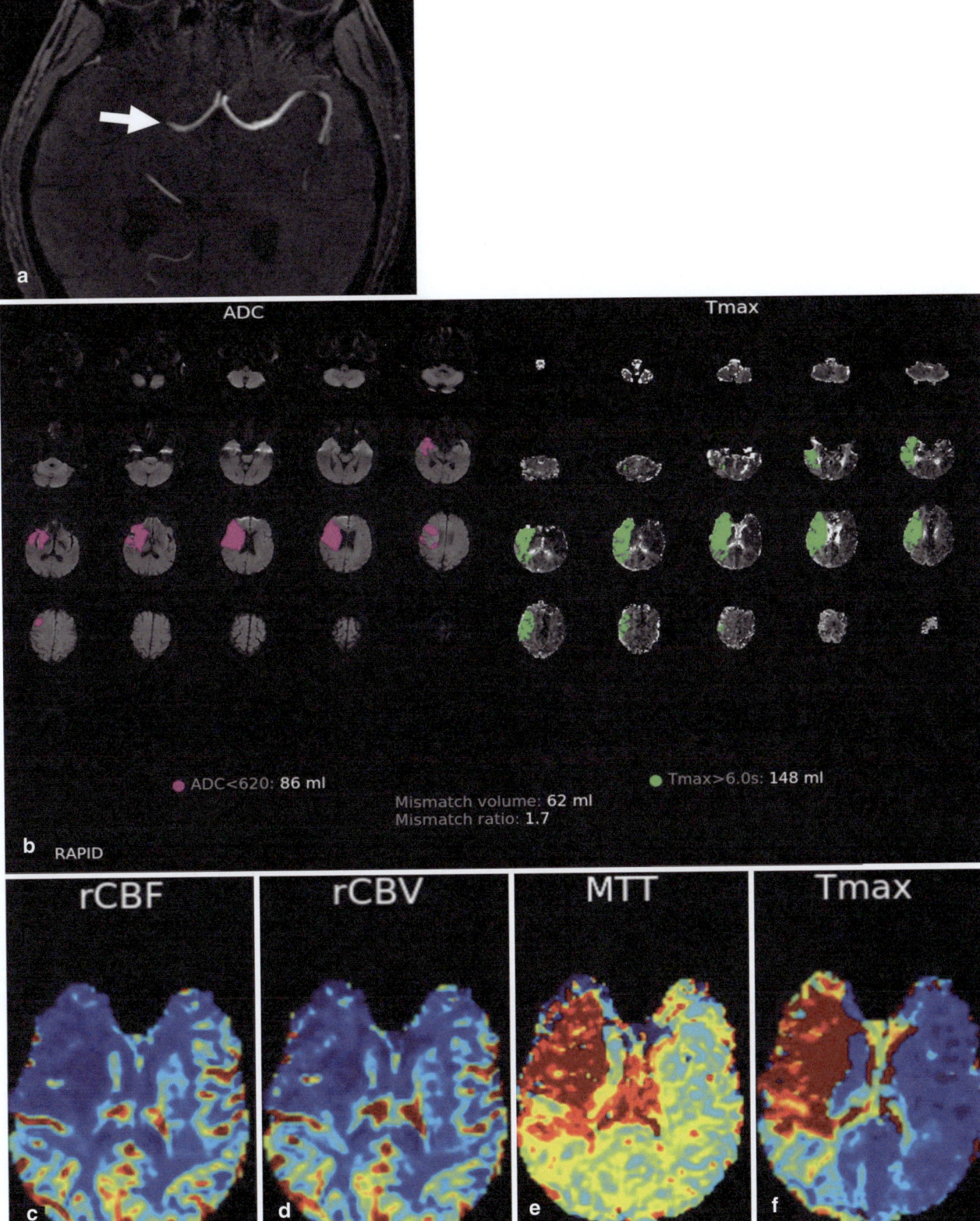

Fig. 45.3 Large acute right M1 MCA infarct. (a) Axial MRA images demonstrate abrupt right M1 MCA cutoff (white arrow). (b) Perfusion summary map demonstrates infarct core of 86 mL (magenta), Tmax>6 s of 148 mL (green), and mismatch volume of 62 mL. (c–f) Colored perfusion parameter maps demonstrate markedly reduced cerebral blood flow (CBF) (dark blue) and cerebral blood volume (CBV) in the low right MCA territory (dark blue) as well as markedly increased mean transit time and Tmax (red). The volume of Tmax abnormality is larger than the volume of diffusion (as shown by the mismatch volume calculation) and CBF and CBV abnormality (not shown), consistent with core infarct and surrounding penumbra

- Diffusion imaging is more accurate for the estimation of core infarct than CTP.
- Mismatch between perfusion and diffusion abnormalities can provide important information about potentially salvageable ischemic tissue at risk (penumbra).
- In the setting of subacute infarction, DSC and ASL can be used to evaluate for the presence of luxury perfusion, which represents reperfusion either spontaneously or following intravenous or endovascular treatment (look for increased CBV or CBF in the periinfarct region).
- Cerebrovascular Reserve (CVR).
  - MR perfusion and CT perfusion in CVR imaging provide similar information.
  - Pharmacologic vasodilation is used as an indirect means of measuring CVR [9].
  - DSC and ASL can be used to assess CBV and/or CBF changes before and after a vasodilatory challenge using agents such as carbon dioxide or carbonic anhydrase inhibitor (acetazolamide).
- Brain Tumors.
  - CBF and CBV can be used to assess tumor vascularity, as increased vascularity (and therefore increased CBF and/or CBV) is often associated with greater malignant potential, higher tumor grade, and poorer prognosis (Fig. 45.4).
  - Benign hypervascular tumors such as meningiomas and hemangioblastomas can also show high CBF and CBV.
  - CBV is the most commonly used perfusion metric in brain tumor imaging.
  - CBV can help to guide surgical tissue sampling, as areas of increased intratumoral CBV may provide better diagnostic yield [11].
  - CBV can help to differentiate between treatment effect (radiation necrosis) and recurrent tumor in previously irradiated tumors: elevated CBV is typically higher in recurrent tumor than in radiation necrosis (of note: it may be difficult to differentiate between low-grade or hypovascular tumors and radiation necrosis because both may have low CBV).
- Other Disorders.
  - Perfusion can help to differentiate tumor from tumor mimics such as tumefactive demyelinating lesions or pyogenic abscesses, as the latter conditions tend to show low central CBF and CBV [12].
  - A unilateral hemispheric decrease in CBV and CBF is seen during the aura phase in patients with hemiplegic migraines.
  - Decreased CBV in the temporal and parietal lobes has been reported in Alzheimer's patients.

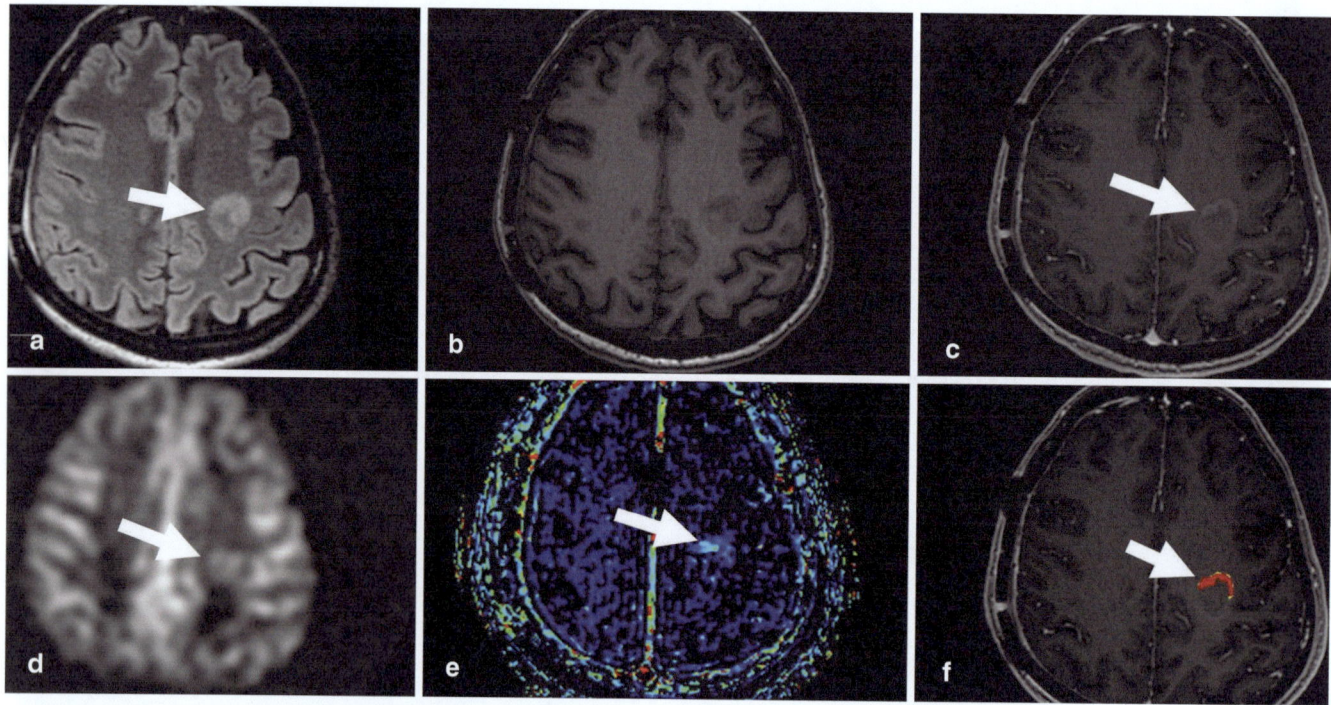

Fig. 45.4 MR perfusion of biopsy-proven left centrum semiovale anaplastic astrocytoma. (**a**) Nodular T2/FLAIR hyperintense lesion in the left centrum semiovale (white arrow). (**b** and **c**) The lesion demonstrates peripheral enhancement anteriorly (white arrow). (**d–f**) The lesion also shows increased cerebral blood flow on ASL, ktrans on DCE, fractional tumor burden (red), and cerebral blood volume on DSC, supporting the diagnosis of a higher-grade tumor (white arrows)

o High venous signal intensity on ASL can indicate abnormal arteriovenous shunting, typically seen with an arteriovenous malformation or dural arteriovenous fistula.

Artifacts, Pitfalls, and Limitations [11]

- DSC limitations include: requirement of an arterial input function measurement for absolute quantification; complexity of T1, T2, or T2* leakage effects in tissues with increased blood-brain barrier permeability; prone to susceptibility and motion artifacts.
- DCE limitations include complexity of pharmacokinetic modeling, postprocessing, and perfusion parameter quantification; lack of clinical validation and standardization.
- ASL limitations include: intrinsically low signal-to-noise ratio (SNR); technique can underestimate CBF in cases of severe ischemia due to relaxation of spin labels from prolonged arterial transit times; prone to motion artifacts.

Task-Based Functional MRI

Basic Principles

- Functional magnetic resonance imaging (fMRI) is a noninvasive method of assessing brain function.
- The most common method of functional MRI (fMRI) uses the blood oxygenation level-dependent (BOLD) effect [13].
- The magnitude of the BOLD signal is an indirect measure of neuronal activity which reflects an interplay between changes in regional cerebral blood flow (CBF), cerebral blood volume (CBV), cerebral metabolic rate of oxygen ($CMRO_2$), and blood oxygenation. This is called neurovascular coupling [14, 15].

- The BOLD effect takes advantage of the intrinsic magnetic susceptibility contrast induced by the difference between oxygenated hemoglobin and deoxygenated hemoglobin.
- Magnetic susceptibility is the degree to which a material develops magnetization of its own when placed in an external magnetic field.
- Deoxyhemoglobin (dHb) is paramagnetic and produces a large magnetic susceptibility effect.
- Oxyhemoglobin (HbO_2) is diamagnetic with a small magnetic susceptibility effect.
- T2*-weighted images are used in BOLD fMRI to investigate brain function.
- Key physiologic contributions to the T2*-weighted BOLD signal start with increased neural activity, which increases local $CMRO_2$, CBV, and CBF.
- Increased $CMRO_2$ results in increased local oxygen extraction from vessels decreasing the HbO_2: dHb ratio. A relative increase in dHb concentration in blood results in a corresponding increase in local magnetic field nonuniformity due to the magnetic susceptibility effect. This results in a net reduction in the local MR signal due to more rapid T2* dephasing which is described as the T2* effect or reduction in the apparent transverse relaxation time [13, 14].
- After a few seconds increased neural activity also increases CBF and CBV.
- Increased CBV augments the volume fraction of capillaries and venules more than arterioles and results in a decrease in the HbO_2: dHb ratio.
- Increased CBF increases the influx of oxygenated blood and increases the HbO_2:dHB ratio.
  On balance, the CBF increase is disproportionately higher than the increase in $CMRO_2$ and CBV resulting in a net increase in HbO_2: dHb ratio, dilution of the dHb, less dephasing of the T2 signal and increased T2*weighted fMRI BOLD signal (Fig. 45.5) [13, 14].
- This change over time in the BOLD fMRI signal, which is a function of the properties of the local vascular network,

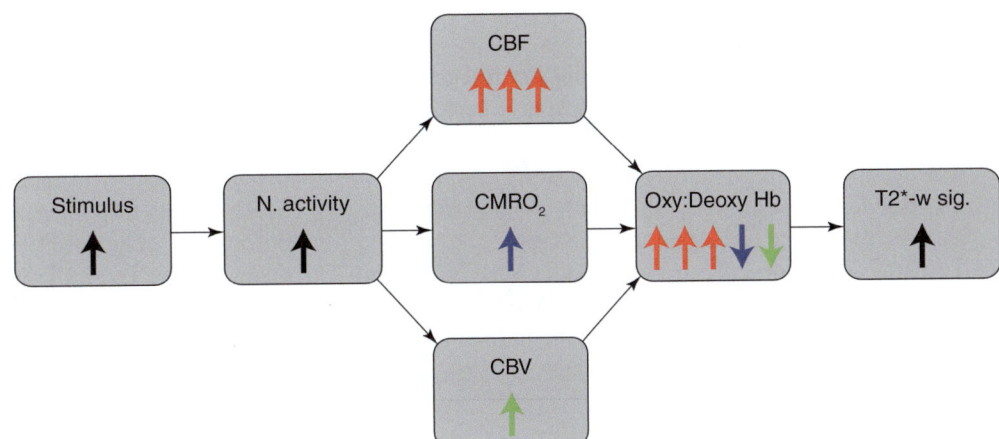

Fig. 45.5 Schematic figure summarizing key physiological contributions to the T2*-weighted BOLD signal. (copyright permission obtained from **Atlas, Scott W**. Magnetic Resonance Imaging of the Brain and Spine. Fifth edition. ed. Philadelphia: Wolters Kluwer, 2017. Print)

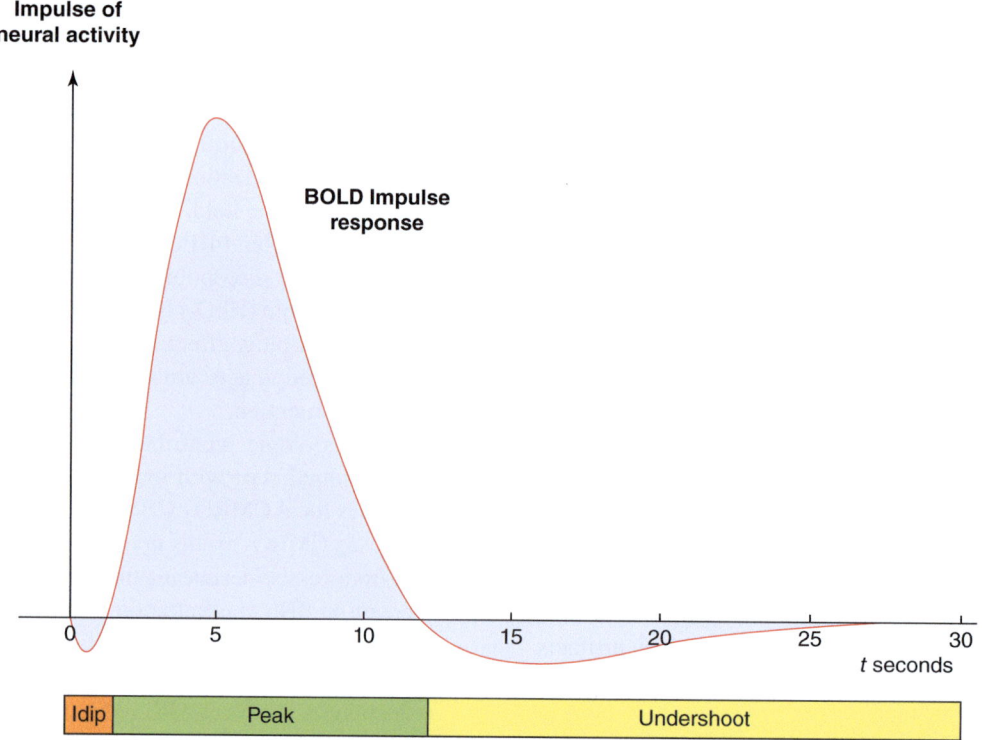

Fig. 45.6 Schematic time course of BOLD hemodynamic/metabolic impulse response. At time 0, there is a brief impulse of neural activity. The time course of the BOLD impulse is divided into three phases. The initial dip lasts 1–2 s and is likely due to a burst of oxidative metabolism that precedes the rise in CBF and associated influx of oxygen. Subsequently, CBF increases disproportionately to $CRMO_2$ and CBV, dHb declines, and BOLD signal rises to a peak at approximately 5–6 s. Bold signal declines toward baseline as CBF and $CRMO_2$ responses dissipate. Afterward, the signal typically falls below baseline to form the poststimulus undershoot. This undershoot peaks at approximately 15 s. (copyright permission obtained from Atlas, Scott W. Magnetic Resonance Imaging of the Brain and Spine. Fifth edition. Ed. Philadelphia: Wolters Kluwer, 2017. Print)

is termed the hemodynamic response function (HRF). Figure 45.6 demonstrates the different parts of the HRF. The initial dip in signal is related to the increase in $CMRO_2$ and therefore increase in dHb, decrease in $dHbO_2$ and resultant decrease in BOLD signal (Fig. 45.6).

Types of fMRI

- Task-based fMRI (tb-fMRI): Identifies brain regions that are functionally involved in a specific task performance (e.g., motor, language, or memory tasks).
- Resting-state fMRI (rs-fMRI): Measures spontaneous low-frequency fluctuations in the BOLD signal to investigate the functional architecture of the brain.
- Tb-fMRI is traditionally used in clinical settings and has billing codes associated with it. Rs-fMRI is predominantly used in research settings, although there has been recent interest in using it clinically to complement tb-fMRI.

Imaging Protocol/Acquisition

- The most frequently used sequence for fMRI is a T2*-weighted gradient-recall echo (GRE) sequence with echo planar imaging (EPI) readout.
- The advantage of using this sequence is (1) its sensitivity to magnetic field inhomogeneities influencing the speed of dephasing, i.e., T2* contrast; (2) its ability to scan the whole brain with adequate spatial (2–3 mm) and temporal (2–3 s) resolution.
- Structural MRI images of the brain have a long acquisition time in order to obtain high-resolution images.
- In contrast, in BOLD fMRI the goal is to measure changes in signal intensity in each voxel over short periods so one needs to scan the entire brain very quickly multiple times during the acquisition to capture the signal intensity changes over shorter periods of time (order of 2 to 4 s). Each voxel in the resulting scan produces a time series that is subsequently analyzed.
- For tb-fMRI, the patient performs language, motor, or less likely memory tasks while in the scanner. The goal is

to determine whether the change in signal intensity over time matches the task/paradigm.
- For rs-fMRI: The subject typically is asked to lie still in the scanner with eyes fixated on a crosshair or eyes closed without presentation of a task stimulus.

Tb-fMRI Paradigms

- A paradigm is the activity performed or stimulus received by the subject while in the MRI scanner.
- Both clinical and research tb-fMRI rely on the effective design of paradigms to activate specific brain regions of interest.
- There are two types of functional paradigms:
  o Block design: The typical task/paradigm employed in clinical fMRI is known as a "box-car" paradigm during which the subject performs a task alternating with a control/baseline condition or rest condition. For example, a bilateral finger-tapping paradigm can be used to generate motor and premotor activity in which the subject taps the fingers of both hands for about 20 s and alternates this with 30 s of finger relaxation/no movement for several repeating cycles. Block designs are preferred over event-related designs (described below) in clinical fMRI as they are more robust with relatively large BOLD signal changes compared to baseline and have increased statistical power [16].
  o Event-related design: In this type of design, discrete and short-duration events are presented with randomized timing and order. Event-related designs have advantages over block designs in that they allow for analysis of individual response to trials and therefore reduce subject's expectation effects. However, for the reasons described above it is mainly used in research with block designs preferred for clinical fMRI [13].

Clinical Care Points

- A detailed patient interview before the actual fMRI to determine patient strengths and weaknesses will help to tweak the selected paradigms to best answer the question for the individual patient and will also help ensure the patient's cooperation during the scan.
- Monitoring for patient compliance during the tb-fMRI will improve the overall diagnostic quality of the fMRI scans.

Data Processing [13, 14]

- After the images are acquired, the time series data must be processed to obtain maps of brain activation.

- For both tb-fMRI and rs-fMRI, the data undergoes a number of preprocessing steps to reduce artifact and noise-related signal components.
- This is followed by statistical data analysis to infer neuronal activation.
- Several different methods of statistical analyses ranging from simple to complex have been described for both tb-fMRI and rs-fMRI; a description of these is beyond the scope of this chapter.
- Common methods of analyses of clinical tb-fMRI data include correlation analyses and General Linear Model analysis.
- Correlation analysis computes the correlation coefficient between the observed BOLD response obtained during the stimulus period and the modeled hemodynamic response.
- Simply put, for tb-fMRI the signal intensity time curve for each voxel in the brain is generated.
- This signal intensity time curve is compared with the stimulus/task to determine if there is a correlation between the two.
- If the signal correlates significantly with the task/paradigm for a particular voxel then it means that the voxel is considered active for that task/paradigm.
- The final fMRI-imaging map is a correlational map of signal intensity changes in the fMRI imaging paradigms.

Anatomic Landmarks

- Anatomical landmarks pertaining to the most commonly assessed brain functions in clinical neuroradiology, including motor, language, and vision are discussed in Chap. 3.

Clinical Application: Presurgical Mapping

- The most common clinical application of tb-fMRI is as a preoperative planning tool for brain tumor and epilepsy surgery.
- The main goal is to optimize resection of brain lesions/epileptogenic zone while preserving functionally relevant brain structures, i.e., eloquent cortices such as language and motor regions.
- tb-fMRI is used to (1) identify eloquent cortices (mainly language and motor) and determine their proximity to the brain lesion and (2) determine the hemispheric dominance for language [13, 14].
- Three CPT codes are now available for tb-fMRI.
- Rs-fMRI can be used as a complement to tb-fMRI in presurgical planning particularly in young pediatric patients or patients with cognitive challenges who cannot adequately perform tb-fMRI but its role in clinical fMRI remains limited.

Challenges in Interpretation of Tb-Fmri [13, 14]

- False negatives.
  - Poor task performance may be seen in young patients or patients with cognitive challenges such that the lack of activation may simply reflect that the patient was not able to complete the task appropriately.
- Susceptibility related BOLD signal decrease.
  - Susceptibility artifacts represent one of the major limitations of BOLD fMRI performed using T2*EPI sequences.
  - Susceptibility artifacts resulting in reduced signal loss can be seen in brain regions close to an air–bone interface (e.g., orbitofrontal cortex, medial temporal cortex), a post-surgical resection cavity, craniotomy hardware, vascular clips, stent grafts, dental work or blood products related to surgery or intralesional hemorrhage.
  - This is why it is important to implement a general quality control step in clinical fMRI to visually inspect the raw EPI images to identify areas that may be affected by susceptibility artifacts as these areas may result in false-negative BOLD signal loss.
- Neurovascular uncoupling (NVU).
  - NVU refers to a decreased or absent BOLD signal in a task-activated brain network despite intact neural activity.
  - It is believed to be due to altered tumor neovasculature such that the tumor neovasculature loses the ability to autoregulate. Therefore, an increase in neuronal activity does not lead to increase in blood flow and this results in a decreased BOLD signal [17].
  - This is rarely seen in healthy volunteers with normal hemodynamics but can be seen in patients with brain tumors or arteriovenous malformations with altered regional hemodynamic responses.
  - Different methods have been used to identify NVU such as breath-hold cerebrovascular reactivity mapping and several techniques have been proposed to overcome NVU. Detailed descriptions of these topics are beyond the scope of this text.
- False positives.
  - Venous Effect: false positive effects can be caused by an area of activation adjacent to a large draining vein such as cortical veins or the superior sagittal sinus.
  - Reviewing the high-resolution images to look for presence of large draining veins will help identify the cause of this false positive signal.
- True negatives.
  - Tumor-induced destruction of eloquent cortex: the eloquent cortex may be infiltrated by tumor so that the lack of activation may reflect the fact that there is no functional region available to be activated.
  - Cortical reorganization: neural plasticity and cortical reorganization can result in true negatives.

DTI and Fiber Tractography

Basic Principles

- Axonal cellular membranes and myelin serve as microstructural barriers to diffusion of water resulting in preferential diffusion of water along the long axis of axons (anisotropy).
- Isotropy refers to uniform diffusion of water in all directions.
- Diffusion tensor imaging (DTI) is a variant of DWI, which utilizes a tissue water diffusion rate for image production.
- DTI is primarily used to image white matter tracts allowing imaging of orientation, location, and anisotropy of the tracts to be measured and evaluated.
- Tractography entails the reconstruction of white matter pathways from a single in vivo scan.

Imaging Protocol/Acquisition/Data Processing

- MRI gradients are employed which are sensitive to diffusion in a particular direction and repeated in multiple directions to estimate a 3D diffusion model (the tensor) [16].
- The information contained in the tensor is condensed into one number (a scalar) or into four numbers (to give an RGB color and brightness value).
- Commonly used scalar quantities are reflective of diffusion magnitude and anisotropy measures: fractional anisotropy (most commonly used DTI metric), mean diffusivity, axial diffusivity, and radial diffusivity [18].
  - Fractional anisotropy (FA) quantifies the directionality of diffusivity in a summative manner and is highly sensitive to change in microstructure. FA values are numerical values based on the anisotropy of water along the axon, which reflects the health of the axon;

therefore, abnormal FA values indicate axonal damage.
  - Mean diffusivity quantifies cellular and membrane density whereas an increase in mean diffusivity indicates disease processes such as edema or necrosis.
  - Radial (perpendicular) diffusivity quantifies myelin neuropathology and increases with demyelination.
  - Axial (parallel) diffusivity quantifies axonal degeneration and increases with brain maturation.
- 3D reconstructions of the tensor tracts are accomplished with computer modeling and can illustrate the fiber tracts, identify pathology, and aid neurosurgeons in intraoperative planning.
- Color coding convention applied to the direction of fiber streamlines in tractography imaging are as follows: red (left-right fiber streamlines), green (anterior–posterior fiber streamlines), blue (superior–inferior fiber streamlines) [19].
- Fibers with oblique orientations are represented by colors on the red, green, and blue color spectrum (e.g., magenta = red + blue; yellow = green + red; cyan = green + blue) [19].

Technical Considerations

- Algorithm works poorly when more bundles of fibers coexist or where multiple fibers cross, approach, converge, or diverge.
- As a result, postprocessed images can show tracts that do not actually exist (false positive) or fail to show tracts that do exist (false negative).

Clinical Applications

- DTI and tractography are most commonly used for surgical planning in the presence of a focal lesion such as a brain tumor or vascular malformation (e.g., arteriovenous malformation or cavernous malformation) (Figs. 45.7 and 45.8).
  - DTI and tractography provide an in-depth visualization of neuroanatomy and specific eloquent white matter tracts in relation to a focal brain lesion, which can help to minimize damage to critical tracts during surgery and can help to preserve vital functions such as motor capabilities, language, and vision.
- Epilepsy: DTI and tractography can be helpful in specific pediatric patient groups with temporal lobe epilepsy or for planning of epilepsy surgery.
- Traumatic Brain Injury/Diffuse Axonal Injury: diffuse axonal injury is closely correlated with decreased FA values in specific brain regions. However, while results are promising, it is challenging to extrapolate and apply results from a population to an individual; as such, DTI is not yet routinely used in the clinical setting for this condition.
- Extracranial DTI applications: largely investigational at this time but DTI has been used for imaging and mapping out peripheral nerve fibers.

Artifacts, Pitfalls, and Limitations [20]

- DTI has low SNR, which may increase scanning times and result in patient motion artifact.
- Diffusion anisotropy will only show on DTI when all structures course a voxel aligned on a microscopic (microstructure, myelin sheath, and protein filaments) and macroscopic (axons and dendrites) scale.
- Limitations are as follows: (1) assumes that fibers at each voxel are well described by a single orientation estimate so it performs poorly in regions of fiber crossing, complexity, or with small or tortuous vessels; (2) a single voxel is typically a few millimeters cubed so a single voxel could contain tens of thousands of axons; (3) inability to differentiate anterograde and retrograde connections, to detect the presence of synapses, or to determine whether a pathway is functional; (4) false positives and negatives will occur so the presence of absence of a particular pathway in a tractography result should always be interpreted with care.

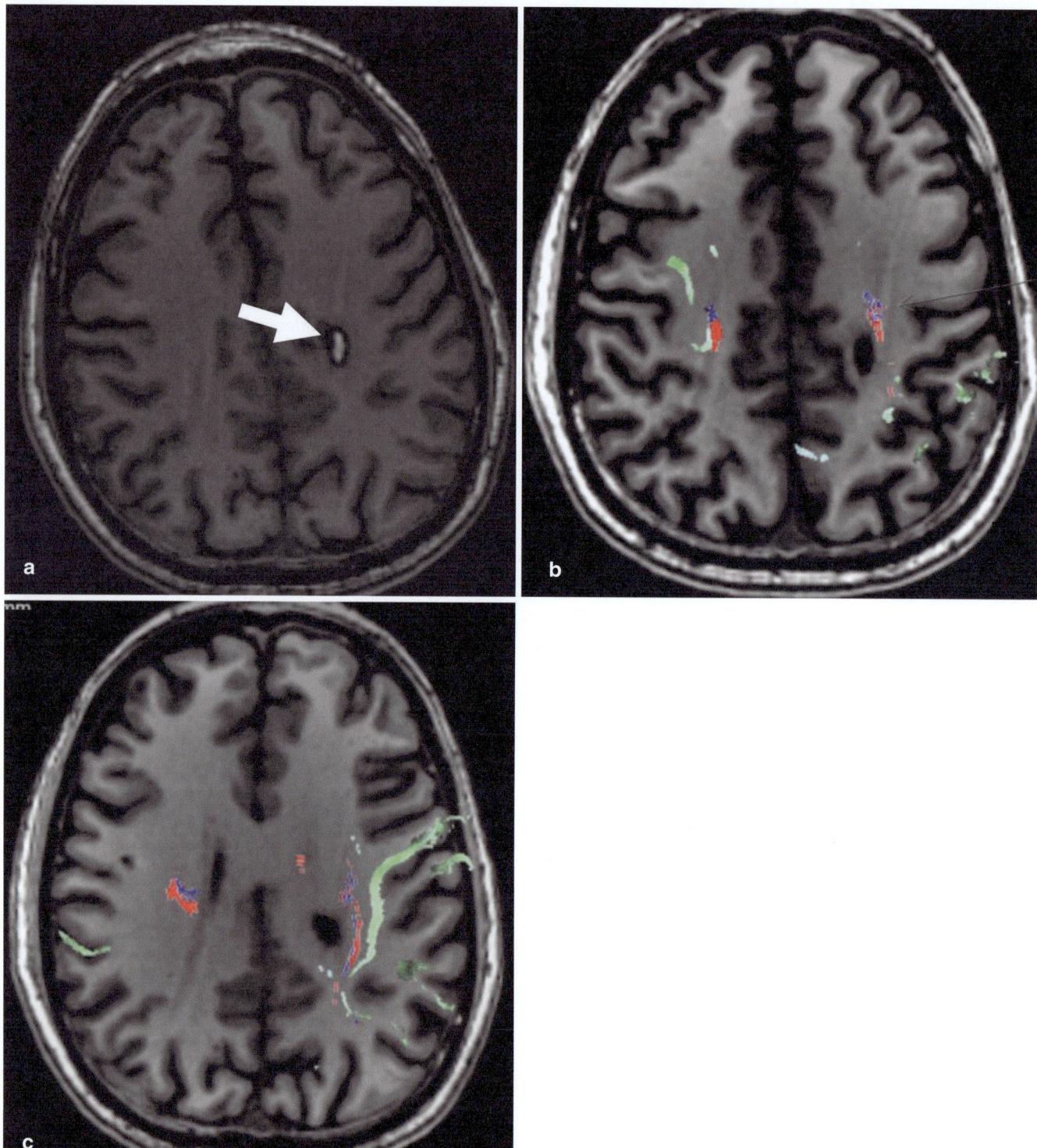

Fig. 45.7 DTI and tractography performed for surgical planning. (**a**) Small hemorrhagic cavernous malformation in the left centrum semiovale (white arrow). (**b**) Tractography image shows that the left corticospinal tract (CST) (red-blue) streamline is anterior and lateral to the cavernous malformation. (**c**) The superior longitudinal fasciculus (SLF) streamline is lateral to the cavernous malformation and CST streamline

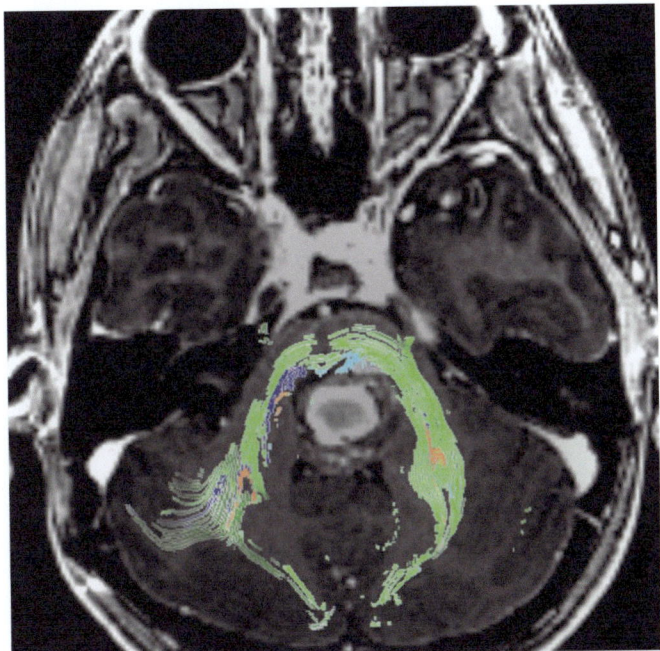

Fig. 45.8 Axial tractography image of a large hemorrhagic pontine cavernous malformation acquired for presurgical planning. The following streamlines are color coded as follows: right corticospinal tract: dark blue; left corticospinal tract: light blue; transverse pontine fibers: orange; right middle cerebellar peduncle: dark green; left middle cerebellar peduncle: light green. The cavernous malformation is located posterior to the pontine corticospinal tract streamlines. The lesion intimately abuts the left corticospinal tract streamline along its left ventral aspect. The right corticospinal tract is in very close proximity to the lesion but no definite contact is clearly identified. The cavernous malformation also abuts and possibly incorporates fiber projections of the transverse pontine fibers and left middle cerebellar peduncle

MRS

Basic Principles

- In vivo 1H MR spectroscopy is a technique that adds complementary clinically relevant information about metabolites in certain brain abnormalities and can help to differentiate between different pathologies based on tissue composition [3].

Technical Considerations [21]

- Pulse sequence and parameters are often dictated by the disease.
    o Single-voxel spectroscopy can be used when the affected region is well-defined (i.e., used to identify metabolites in a small area for diagnosis).
    o Multi-voxel imaging is used when the lesion is undefined, multiple, or heterogenous, or there is diffuse disease.
- MR spectrogram typically shows resonance frequency of the metabolite (measured in parts per million, ppm) on the x-axis and height of the molecule peak, which is dependent on concentration and the available 1H, on the y-axis.
- The minimum technical requirements to ensure that a 1H MR spectrum is clinically interpretable:
    o SNR > 3 for major resonances such as high Cho and low NAA in tumors.
    o SNR > 2 for detection only of important indicator metabolites such as lactate.
    o Spectral resolution: Full-width half maximum (FWHM) of metabolites <0.1 ppm.
    o Line shape: symmetric.
    o Water suppression >98%.
    o No lipid contamination from the scalp.
    o Artifacts, such as chemical shift artifact, ghosting, patient motion, eddy currents, and volume averaging, are absent or minor.
- Short TE (e.g., 20–40 ms) shows more metabolites but has a fluctuating baseline, while intermediate TE (e.g., 135–144 ms) shows more defined peaks because of a flatter baseline.
- Higher magnet strength offers better-defined metabolite peaks.

Common Metabolites Biomarkers and their Clinical Significance [21]

- Choline (Cho) is a marker for cell membranes (cellular turnover).
- N-acetyl aspartate (NAA) is a marker of neuronal density/integrity.
- Creatine (Cr) is the internal standard because it is evenly distributed in many types of cells.
- Elevated myo-inositol (MI) is a sugar most concentrated in glial cells and is a marker for gliosis.
- Elevated lactic acid (Lac) indicates anaerobic glycolysis; lactate doublet is inverted with long TE scans.
- Choline, creatine, and N-acetyl aspartate are located at 3.2, 3.0, and 2.0 ppm, respectively.
- The typical way to analyze a clinical spectrum is to look at the metabolite ratios (Fig. 45.9).
    o NAA/Cr ratio < 1.6 is abnormal and suggests neuronal loss or damage such as radiation necrosis or demyelinating disorders.
    o Cho/Cr > 1.5 is abnormal and indicates an active metabolic process such as a brain tumor.

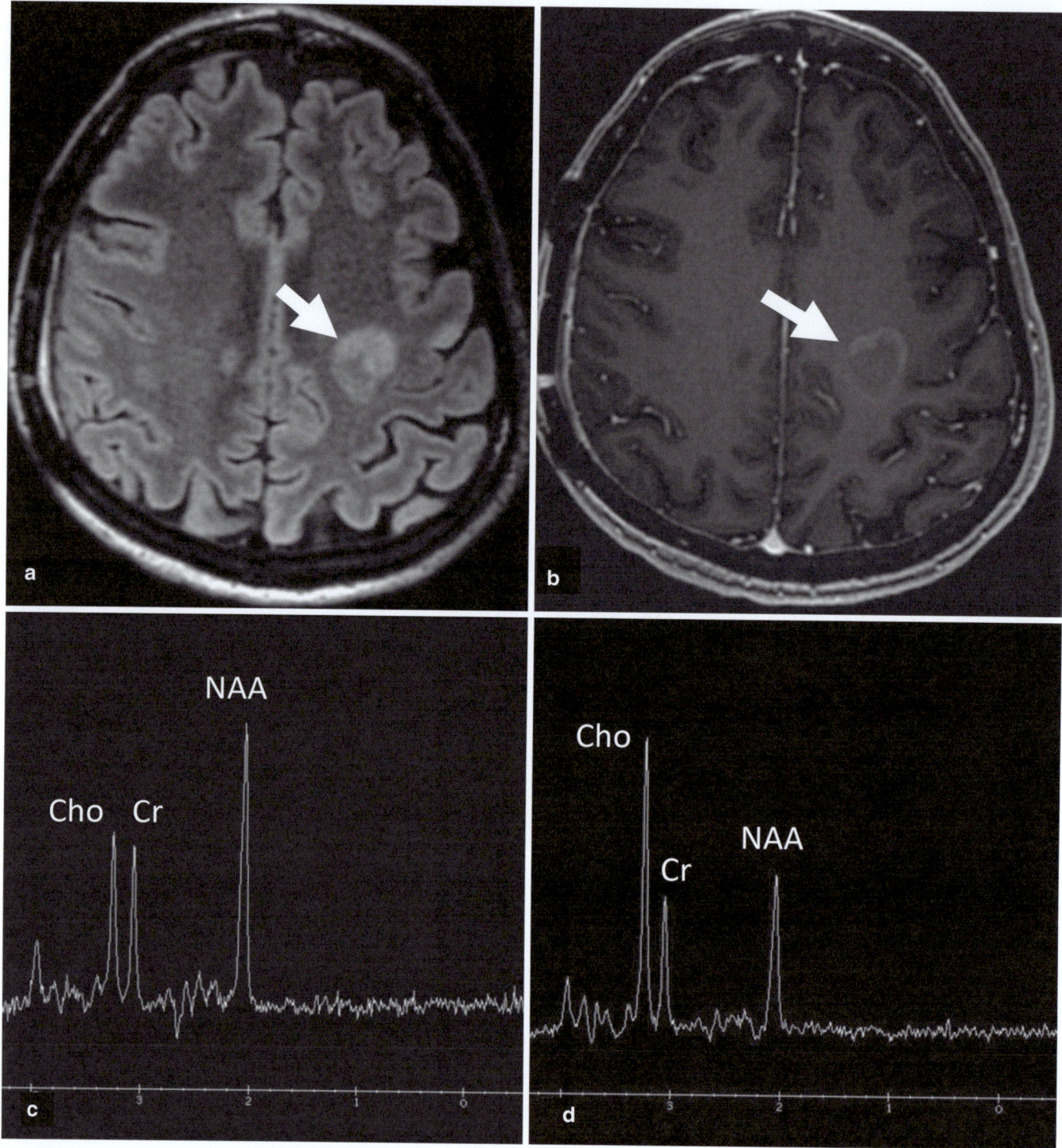

Fig. 45.9 Biopsy proven anaplastic astrocytoma. (**a** and **b**) T2/FLAIR hyperintense lesion in the left centrum semiovale with peripheral irregular enhancement (white arrows). (**c**) MR Spectroscopy performed in a normal region of brain parenchyma demonstrates normal choline, creatine, and NAA peaks. (**d**) MR Spectroscopy of the lesion demonstrates elevated choline and decreased NAA peaks, consistent with a metabolically active process such as tumor

Clinical Applications [21, 22]

- Brain Tumors.
  - MRS can assist in differentiating tumor from other focal lesions (such as demyelinating lesions), help in preprocedural planning and intraoperative resections, and can be helpful in postoperative and post-treatment follow-up.
  - Cho/NAA ratio can help to differentiate areas of solid tumor with the highest cell density from edema.
  - An increased Cho/NAA ratio in the peritumoral region reflects tumor invasiveness and can be used to differentiate high-grade gliomas from brain metastases, as metastases characteristically show a near-normal spectrum in the peritumoral region.
  - Differentiating treatment-induced changes and recurrent tumor: Cho/Cr ratio can help to distinguish radiation necrosis from recurrent tumor or infection, as a common diagnostic feature of brain tumors is elevated Cho and decreased NAA.
  - Nonneoplastic lesions often demonstrate elevated amino acids and lipids.
  - Other metabolites observed in brain neoplasms: elevated taurine in primitive neuroectodermal tumors; elevated alanine in meningiomas; elevated glycine in high-grade pediatric tumors; elevated 2-hydroxyglutarate in isocitrate dehydrogenase-1 mutated gliomas.
- Hypoxia-Ischemia: elevated Lac due to hypoxia-ischemia is one of the earliest imaging signs of clinical brain injury and persistence of high Lac is associated with poor outcomes.
- Inherited Metabolic Diseases.
  - These metabolic disorders result in the accumulation of metabolites that are either neurotoxic or interfere with normal function.
  - Pyruvate plus Lac and/or alanine is an early indication of pyruvate dehydrogenase complex deficiency.
  - Elevated succinate indicates succinate dehydrogenase deficiency.
  - Elevated glycine is observed in nonketotic hyperglycinemia, although intracerebral hemorrhage can confound the interpretation of high glycine levels.
  - Grossly elevated NAA is a hallmark of Canavan disease.
- Demyelinating Diseases.
  - MRS plays an integral role in evaluating hereditary leukoencephalopathies but is of limited clinical utility in multiple sclerosis.
  - MRS is used to monitor the onset of demyelination in asymptomatic patients with X-linked adrenoleukodystrophy and indicates the need for hematopoietic stem cell transplantation, which is the only treatment currently.
- Focal Infections.
  - Succinate, acetate, alanine, leucine, isoleucine, and valine are biomarkers that are specific to pyogenic abscesses.
  - Parasitic cysts also contain succinate and acetate but the absence of amino acids helps to differentiate them from anaerobic abscesses.
  - Tuberculous abscesses demonstrate lactate and lipid signals without any cytosolic amino acids.
- Neurodegenerative diseases.
  - A hallmark finding of neurodegenerative disorders is decreased NAA localized to regions affected by the degenerative process.
  - NAA/Cr ratio tends to be lower in subjects with mild cognitive impairment who convert to dementia compared to those who remain stable.
  - Elevated mIns level may be associated with glial or microglial activation, a characteristic feature in neurodegenerative disorders.
- Epilepsy.
  - MRS can aid in localizing epileptogenic foci when MR imaging is negative or ambiguous.
  - Decreased NAA and NAA/Cr ratios are the most common findings at epileptogenic zones.

Artifacts, Pitfalls, and Limitations [23]

- The value of MRS can be limited as it often lacks specificity and therefore may not add much to diagnostic yield.
- Clinical MRS is not reimbursed by all insurance companies, so the cost to patients is a consideration!
- Additional time is needed for MRS imaging.

Clinical Nuclear Medicine Neuroimaging

Planar Brain Imaging [24]

- Planar brain imaging is primarily performed for evaluation of brain death.
- Two types of perfusion agents: 1) transient: technetium-99 m [99mTc]-diethylenetriamine pentaacetic acid [DTPA], 99mTc-pertechnetate; 2) lipophilic agents extracted by the brain on first pass: 99mTc–hexamethylpropyleneamine oxime [HMPAO], 99mTc–ethylene l-cysteinate dimer [ECD].
- Angiographic phase and delayed static images are obtained following administration of the radiolabeled perfusion agent.
- A normal examination demonstrates prompt symmetric perfusion in the bilateral middle cerebral arteries and

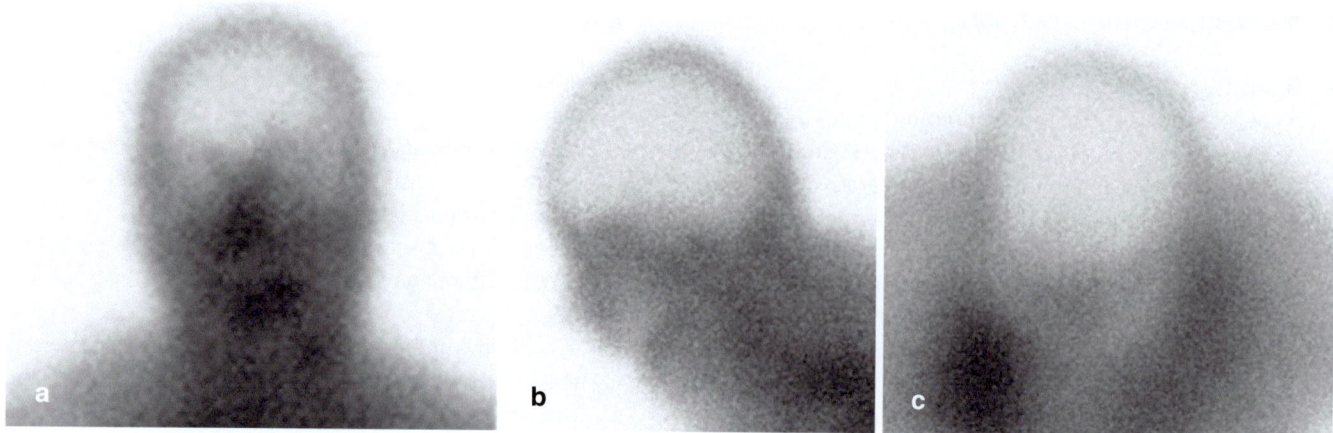

Fig. 45.10 Brain Death. (a–c) Anterior, lateral, and vertex images demonstrate the absence of cerebral radiotracer uptake, compatible with brain death

anterior cerebral arteries in the anterior projection, which resembles a trident.
- Brain death is suggested when there is absent intracranial carotid blood flow (Fig. 45.10).
- Angiographic flow images may demonstrate the "hot-nose" sign, which represents increased perfusion over the nasal region due to increased or collateral flow through the maxillary branch of the external carotid artery in the setting of absent intracranial carotid blood flow.

SPECT Brain Perfusion Imaging [24]

- SPECT perfusion imaging uses lipophilic radiopharmaceuticals that commonly cross the BBB to localize normal brain tissue and pathologic processes in proportion to regional cerebral blood flow.
- Types of lipophilic agents: 99mTc-HMPAO (exametazime); 99mTc-ECD (bicisate); Thallium-201 chloride (very little thallium is concentrated in normal brain tissue so an increase in thallium indicates the presence of viable tumor).
- Imaging technique: (1) SPECT images obtained 15–20 min after injection of tracer agent; (2) Minimize external sensory stimuli, patient motion, and cognitive functions (eg reading) at time of injection and localization to prevent interfering increased activity in the corresponding sensory cortex.
- Clinical Applications.
    o Brain Death: The absence of perfusion on the angiographic phase and lack of cerebral activity on subsequent static planar or SPECT images support the diagnosis of brain death.
    o Cerebral infarction: The acute phase (first 2–3 h) demonstrates reduced blood flow to the affected area; there is decreased sensitivity for detecting subacute phase of stroke (1–3 weeks) due to luxury perfusion.
    o Transient Ischemic Attacks: can use pharmacologic cerebrovascular vasodilatation using acetazolamide (Diamox), a carbonic anhydrase inhibitor, in conjunction with SPECT brain perfusion imaging to evaluate cerebrovascular reserve: relative Diamox-induced regional perfusion defect on SPECT brain perfusion images compared with surrounding normal regions because the autoregulatory vasodilatation is already maximal.
- Brain tumors.
    o Primary and metastatic brain lesions manifest as localized defects that correspond to mass lesions.
    o Radiation necrosis versus tumor recurrence: Thallium-201 activity is a marker of viability; 99mTcHMPAO images demonstrates focal defect in the region of abnormality for both necrotic tissue and recurrent tumor or both; High degree of increased Thallium-201 uptake in a region of 99mTcHMPAO images defect is indicative of tumor recurrence.

PET Metabolic Brain Imaging [24]

- PET with 18F-fluorodeoxyglucose (FDG) allows evaluation of local cerebral metabolism in various clinical conditions discussed below.
- The gray matter of the cortex, basal ganglia, and thalami normally demonstrate the highest concentration of 18F-FDG.
- There are numerous normal areas of focal hypermetabolism such as the posterior cingulate cortex, posterior superior temporal lobe (Wernicke region), frontal eye fields, and the posterior parietal lobes.

- Clinical Applications.
  o Brain tumors: High FDG uptake is commonly associated with high-grade aggressive lesions; lymphoma is typically very hypermetabolic.
  o Cerebellar diaschisis manifests as focal areas of hypoperfusion and hypometabolism in the cerebellar hemisphere contralateral to a supratentorial lesion.
  o Temporal lobe epilepsy: Ictal studies demonstrate focal temporal lobe hypermetabolism while interictal studies demonstrate focal hypometabolism.
  o Certain glucose metabolism patterns are suggestive of specific neurodegenerative disorders.
  o Symmetric hypometabolism in the posterior temporal and parietal lobes with relative sparing of the primary sensorimotor and visual cortices as well as the thalamus, basal ganglia, and cerebellum is suggestive of Alzheimer's Disease (AD).
  o Multiple bilateral asymmetric areas of hypometabolism scattered throughout the cortex and deep structures are suggestive of multi-infarct dementia.
  o Areas of hypometabolism in the frontal and frontotemporal regions are suggestive of Pick Disease (frontotemporal dementia).
  o Parkinson Disease demonstrates hypometabolism similar to AD with more mesiotemporal and less visual cortical sparing.
  o Hypometabolism in the basal ganglia, particularly in the caudate head and lentiform nuclei, is suggestive of Huntington disease.
  o Dementia with Lewy bodies demonstrates a similar pattern to AD, but with less sparing of the occipital cortex and greater involvement of the posterior parietal and occipital cortices.
  o Acquired Immunodeficiency Syndrome Dementia Complex can present as multifocal or patchy cortical areas of decreased uptake in the frontal, temporal, and parietal lobes.

Cerebrospinal Fluid Imaging [24]

- Radionuclide cisternography can be performed by imaging the spinal canal and basal cisterns following intrathecally administering a radionuclide (most commonly Indium-111 labeled DPTA).
- Clinical Applications1.
  o Cerebrospinal fluid leaks: Images are obtained at the suspected site of the leak (commonly in the ear, paranasal sinuses, or nose) then differential activity in pledgets placed deep into each nostril or ear is measured.
  o Shunt patency: Radiotracer is injected into the shunt reservoir or tubing and serial images are obtained throughout the course of the shunt to evaluate for areas of partial or complete obstruction in the distal limb.
  o Communicating hydrocephalus: Normal pressure hydrocephalus classically presents as early lateral ventricular entry, persistence of lateral ventricular activity at 24–48 h, and delayed activity in the superior cerebral convexities.

Parathyroid Imaging [24]

- Hyperfunctioning parathyroid adenomas can be evaluated with nuclear medicine imaging techniques using Technetium-99 m sestamibi (Fig. 45.11).
- Images of the chest and neck are obtained sequentially over the course of 2–3 h following intravenous administration of the radiotracer.
- Radiotracer activity persists in parathyroid adenomas while radiotracer activity in normal thyroid tissue and thyroid adenomas significantly decrease over time.
- Radiologists must recognize that atypical thyroid adenomas and thyroid cancers can produce false-positive examinations.

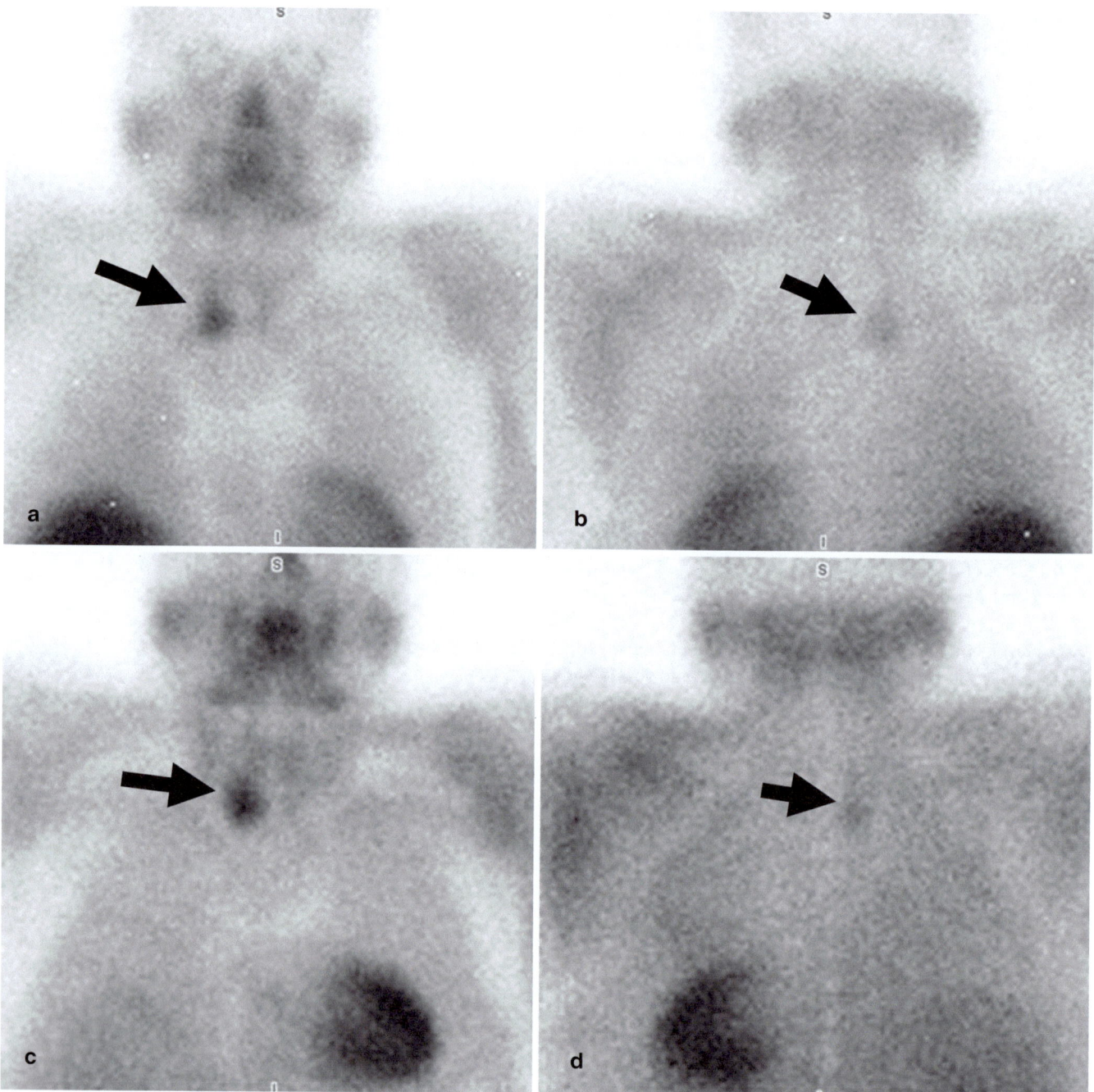

Fig. 45.11 Right parathyroid adenoma. (**a** and **b**) Anterior and posterior early phase images demonstrate focal radiotracer uptake in the region of the right lower lobe of the thyroid gland (black arrows). (**c** and **d**) Anterior and posterior delayed phase images demonstrate persistent focal uptake, consistent with a parathyroid adenoma (black arrows)

References

CT Perfusion

1. de Lucas EM, et al. Ct protocol for acute stroke: tips and tricks for general radiologists. Radiographics. 2008;28(6):1673–87. Print.
2. Wintermark M, Lev MH. Fda investigates the safety of brain perfusion Ct. AJNR Am J Neuroradiol. 2010;31(1):2–3. Print.
3. Lui YW, et al. Evaluation of Ct perfusion in the setting of cerebral ischemia: patterns and pitfalls. AJNR Am J Neuroradiol. 2010;31(9):1552–63. Print.
4. Demeestere J, et al. Review of perfusion imaging in acute ischemic stroke: from time to tissue. Stroke. 2020;51(3):1017–24. Print.
5. Albers GW, et al. Thrombectomy for stroke at 6 to 16 hours with selection by perfusion imaging. N Engl J Med. 2018;378(8):708–18. Print.
6. Vagal AS, et al. The acetazolamide challenge: techniques and applications in the evaluation of chronic cerebral ischemia. AJNR Am J Neuroradiol. 2009;30(5):876–84. Print.
7. Yeung TP, et al. Dynamic perfusion Ct in brain tumors. Eur J Radiol. 2015;84(12):2386–92. Print.
8. Allmendinger AM, et al. Imaging of stroke: part 1, perfusion Ct—overview of imaging technique, interpretation pearls, and common pitfalls. AJR Am J Roentgenol. 2012;198(1):52–62. Print.

MR Perfusion

9. Petrella JR, Provenzale JM. Mr perfusion imaging of the brain: techniques and applications. AJR Am J Roentgenol. 2000;175(1):207–19. Print.
10. Welker K, et al. Asfnr recommendations for clinical performance of Mr dynamic susceptibility contrast perfusion imaging of the brain. AJNR Am J Neuroradiol. 2015;36(6):E41–51. Print.
11. Wong JC, Provenzale JM, Petrella JR. Perfusion Mr imaging of brain neoplasms. AJR Am J Roentgenol. 2000;174(4):1147–57. Print.
12. Al-Okaili RN, et al. Advanced Mr imaging techniques in the diagnosis of intraaxial brain tumors in adults. Radiographics. 2006;26(Suppl 1):S173–89. Print.

Task-Based fMRI

13. Ogawa S, et al. Brain magnetic resonance imaging with contrast dependent on blood oxygenation. Proc Natl Acad Sci USA. 1990;87(24):9868–72. Print.
14. Atlas SW. Magnetic resonance imaging of the brain and spine. 5th ed. Philadelphia: Wolters Kluwer; 2017. Print.
15. Stippich C, Blatow M. Clinical functional Mri: presurgical functional neuroimaging, Medical Radiology Diagnostic Imaging. Berlin; New York: Springer; 2007. Print.
16. Hagmann P, et al. Understanding diffusion Mr imaging techniques: from scalar diffusion-weighted imaging to diffusion tensor imaging and beyond. Radiographics. 2006;26(Suppl 1):S205–23. Print.
17. Agarwal S, Sair HI, Pillai JJ. The problem of neurovascular uncoupling. Neuroimaging Clin N Am. 2021;31(1):53–67. Print.

DTI and Fiber Tractography

18. Soares JM, et al. A Hitchhiker's guide to diffusion tensor imaging. Front Neurosci. 2013;7:31. Print.
19. O'Donnell LJ, Westin CF. An introduction to diffusion tensor image analysis. Neurosurg Clin N Am. 2011;22(2):185–96, viii. Print.
20. Jones DK, Cercignani M. Twenty-five pitfalls in the analysis of diffusion Mri data. NMR Biomed. 2010;23(7):803–20. Print.

MRS

21. Oz G, et al. Clinical proton Mr spectroscopy in central nervous system disorders. Radiology. 2014;270(3):658–79. Print.
22. Zhu H, Barker PB. Mr spectroscopy and spectroscopic imaging of the brain. Methods Mol Biol. 2011;711:203–26. Print.
23. Gillard JH, Waldman AD, Barker PB. Clinical Mr neuroimaging : physiological and functional techniques. 2nd ed. Cambridge: Cambridge University Press; 2010. Print.

Clinical Nuclear Medicine

24. Mettler FA, Guiberteau MJ. Essentials of nuclear medicine and molecular imaging. 7th ed. Philadelphia, PA: Elsevier; 2019. Print.

Correction to: What Radiology Residents Need to Know: Neuroradiology

Behroze A. Vachha, Gul Moonis, Max Wintermark, and Tarik F. Massoud

---

Correction to:
B. A. Vachha et al. (eds.), *What Radiology Residents Need to Know: Neuroradiology*, What Radiology Residents Need to Know,
https://doi.org/10.1007/978-3-031-55124-6

There was an inconsistency in the editor's name, which has now been updated to "Behroze A. Vachha" throughout the book. In addition, the copyright year has been corrected to 2024 in the revised publication.

The updated version of this book can be found at
https://doi.org/10.1007/978-3-031-55124-6

© The Author(s), under exclusive license to Springer Nature Switzerland AG 2025
B. A. Vachha et al. (eds.), *What Radiology Residents Need to Know: Neuroradiology*, What Radiology Residents Need to Know,
https://doi.org/10.1007/978-3-031-55124-6_46

Index

A

Aberrant carotid artery, 417
    internal, 416
Abscess, 210, 226
Accreditation Council for Graduate Medical Education (ACGME), 576
Acquvired cystic neck masses, 568–573
Acquired toxoplasmosis, 224
ACR Manual on Contrast Media, 581
Acute calcific longus colli tendinitis, 515
Acute calcific longus colli tendonitis, 536
Acute disseminated encephalomyelitis (ADEM), 203, 363
Acute flaccid myelitis, 357
Acute hyperammonemia, 234
Acute invasive fungal sinusitis, 401, 402
Acute Kidney Injury Network (AKIN), 582
Acute rhinosinusitis, 399, 401
Acute sinusitis, 400
Acute stroke imaging, 590, 593, 594
Adenocarcinoma, 408, 409
Adenohypophysis, 465
Adenoid cystic carcinoma, 409
Adenoid enlargement, 520
Adenoid hypertrophy, 521
Adenoiditis, 535
Adrenoleukodystrophy, 187, 188
Adrenomyeloneuropathy (AMN), 187
Adult-type diffuse gliomas, 207
    astrocytoma, isocitrate dehydrogenase (IDH) mutant, 207, 208
    glioblastoma, IDH-wildtype, 210
    oligodendroglioma, IDH-mutant and 1p/19q co-deleted, 209, 210
Advanced imaging techniques
    clinical applications, 589
    CT perfusion, 589
    diffusion tensor imaging, 589
    MR perfusion, 589
    MR spectroscopy, 589
    in neuroradiology, 589
    nuclear scintigraphy, 589
    task-based functional MRI, 589
Aging, normal, 245, 246
Agreements for provision of high-quality care, 576
Alajouanine syndrome, 371
Alar ligament, 280
Alexander disease, 190, 191
Allergic fungal sinusitis, 402, 403
Alpha-fetoprotein (AFP), 293
Alzheimer disease (AD), 246, 247
American Joint Committee on Cancer (AJCC) eighth edition staging manual, 527
American Medical Association (AMA) Editorial Panel, 585
American Society of Anesthesiologists (ASA) Physical Status Classification, 579
Amyotrophic lateral sclerosis (ALS-FTD), 248
Aneurysm, 477
Aneurysmal bone cyst (ABC), 337, 340
Aneurysmal SAH (aSAH), 109, 110
Angiosarcoma, 555
Ankylosing spondylitis, 330
Anterior cerebral artery (ACA), 38
Anterior cervical space, 501
Anterior condylar vein (ACV), 460
Anterior cord or total cord infarct patterns, 364
Anterior cord syndrome, 315
Anterior cranial fossa, 427
Anterior inferior cerebellar artery loop, 447
Anterior longitudinal ligament, 278
Anterior meningocele, 295
Anterior skull base (ASB), 423, 425, 427, 429, 431
    anatomy, 423–425
Anterior spinal artery, 364
Anti-MOG encephalomyelitis, 184, 185
Antiretroviral therapy, 355
Antrochoanal polyp, 402–404
Antronasal polyps, 403
Apical ligament, 280
Apparent diffusion coefficient (ADC), 10, 225
Arachnoid cysts, 263, 264, 467, 468
Arachnoiditis, 359
Arachnoid mater, 284
Arcuate foramen, 283
Arrested pneumatization of sphenoid sinus, 433
Arterial ischemia, 364
Arterial spin labeling (ASL) imaging, 594
    limitations, 597
Arterio-venous fistula, 348, 373, 558
Arteriovenous malformation (AVM), 103, 104, 348, 373, 538, 558
Artery of Adamkiewicz, 285
Arthritides, 319
Arthrosis, 323
Artificial intelligence (AI), 586
ASL, *see* Arterial spin labeling (ASL) imaging
Aspergillus, 174, 175
Aspergillus ventriculitis, 259
Astrocytoma, 340, 341
    isocitrate dehydrogenase (IDH) mutant, 207, 208, 210
Asymmetric pneumatization of petrous apex, 433
Asymmetric sacroiliitis, 329
Atlanto-axial subluxation, 314
Atlantodental interval, 280
Atlanto-occipital and atlantoaxial joints, 278
Atlanto-occipital dissociation, 313

Atypical (central) skull base osteomyelitis, 525
Atypical teratoid/rhabdoid tumor, 221
Axial (parallel) diffusivity, 601
Axial tractography, 603

B

Bacterial CNS infection
    bacterial meningitis (*see* Bacterial meningitis)
    tuberculosis (*see* Tuberculosis)
Bacterial discitis/osteomyelitis, 349–350
Bacterial meningitis
    brain abscess, 160–162
    cerebritis, 160–162
    clinical features, 159
    empyema, 163
    imaging, 159, 160
    overview, 159
    ventriculitis, 162
Balanced fast field echo, BFFE, 257
Basal ganglia (BG), 250–252
Basion-dens interval, 282
Behavioral variant FTD (bvFTD), 248
Benign congenital anomaly, 565
Benign congenital cyst, 522
Benign enhancing lesion of foramen magnum, 462
Benign fibro-osseous lesion, 339, 406
Benign lymphoepithelial lesions, 569–571
Benign pineal cyst, 222
Benign vertebral body fracture, 312
Bilateral facet dislocation, 313
Billing arrangements, 576
Binswanger disease, 204, 205
Biopsy proven anaplastic astrocytoma, 604
Black hole sign, 97
BOLD fMRI signal, 597
BOLD hemodynamic/metabolic impulse response, 598
Bones, 273
    reconstruction algorithm, 525
    tumors, 346
Bony spine tumor mimics, 339
Boutonniere deformity, 531
Brachial plexus, 285, 286
    injury, 317
Brain abscess, 160–162
Brain death, 606
Brain interstitial fluid, 255
Brainstem glioma, 221
Brain tumors, 596
    evaluation, 593
    tumor and epilepsy surgery, preoperative planning tool, 599
Branchial cleft cysts (BCC), 538–539, 562, 563
Bronchospasm, 584
Brown tumor, 340
Brown-Sequard syndrome, 315
Buccal space (BS), 511
Burst fracture, 309
Butterfly glioblastoma, 210

C

Calvarial fractures
    complex calvarial fractures, 128
    diastatic skull fracture, 128
    morphology, and characteristics, 127
    posttraumatic leptomeningeal cyst, 128
    types, 127
Calvarial tuberculosis, 166
Canavan disease, 192
Cancer staging criteria, 502
Candida subdural empyema, 352
Capillary malformations, 556
Carbon monoxide (CO) toxicity, 237, 238
Caroticocavernous fistulae (CCF), 134
    clinical presentation, 118
    epidemiology, 118
    imaging characteristics, 118–120
    overview, 118
Carotid space (CS), 512, 514
Carotid-vertebrobasilar artery anastomosis, 460
Cauda equina/filum terminale, 342
Cauda equina syndrome, 316
Caudal regression syndrome (CRS), 301, 302
Cavernous carotid fistula, 390
Cavernous malformation, 348
    clinical presentation, 121
    epidemiology, 120, 121
    imaging characteristics, 121–123
Cavernous sinus thrombophlebitis, 401
Cavernous sinus thrombosis, 386, 479
Cavernous sinuses, 466
Cavernous venous malformation (hemangioma), 396
Cavum velum interpositum cyst, 263
Cellulitis, 390
Center for Medicare Management (CMS), 585
Central cord syndrome, 315
Central neurocytoma, 213, 216, 219
Central skull base, 433, 435–438, 442, 444
Cephaloceles, 64, 65
Cephoceles, 428
Cerebellar atrophy, 252
Cerebellar degeneration, 252
Cerebellar pilocytic astrocytoma, 221
Cerebellopontine angle (CPA)/internal auditory canal lesions, 446, 447, 449, 450
    arachnoid cyst, 453
    epidermoid cyst, 451–453
    lipoma, 453
    meningioma, 450, 452
    schwannoma, 449
Cerebral amyloid angiopathy (CAA), 102, 103, 183
Cerebral amyloid angiopathy-related inflammation (CAA-RI), 183, 184
Cerebral aneurysm, 105, 106
Cerebral autosomal dominant arteriopathy with subcortical infarcts and leukoencephalopathy (CADASIL), 203, 204
Cerebritis, 160–162
    and abscess, 165
Cerebrospinal fluid (CSF), 255
    alteration in pressure/volume, 260
        IIH, 260
        leaks/spontaneous intracranial hypotension, 261, 262
    CSF-filled bony canal, 446
    fistula, 421
    hydrocephalus, 256, 257
    imaging technique, 255, 607
    leaks, 261, 262
    phase contrast imaging, 256
    shunts and complications, 257
Cerebrovascular reserve (CVR), 592, 596

Index

Cervical adenitis, 536
Cervical and lumbar enlargements, 284
Cervical spaces, 501
Cervical spine, 274, 276, 279–281
    imaging, 307
    MRI, 287
Cervical thymic cyst, 564
Cervicothoracic lipomas, 296
Chalk (or carrot) stick fractures, 311
Chance fracture, 310
Chemical meningitis, 177–179
Chemotherapy-associated PRES, 239
Chiari I malformation (C1M), 63
Chiari II malformation (C2M), 63, 64
Chiari III malformation (C3M), 64
Childhood to puberty, 466
Cholesteatoma, 417, 418, 436
Cholesterol granuloma (chocolate cyst), 418
Chondroblastoma, 335
Chondrosarcoma, 335, 411, 438, 475
Chordoma, 337, 338, 438, 474, 475
Choroid plexus, 255
Choroid plexus cyst, 267
Choroid plexus papilloma, 213, 218, 219, 221, 258
Choroid plexus tumors
    classifications, 219
    differential considerations, 219
    imaging patterns, 219
    subtypes, 219
Chronic rhinosinusitis, 522
Chronic sinusitis, 401
Chronic subdural haematoma (CSDH), 146
Circle of Willis (COW), 39
Circumscribed astrocytic gliomas
    pilocytic astrocytoma, 210, 211
    pleomorphic xantoastrocytoma, 213
    SEGA, 213
Classic X-linked adrenoleukodystrophy (X-ALD), 187, 188
Clay-shoveler fracture, 310
Clinical assessment, 291
Clinical nuclear medicine neuroimaging, 605–608
Closed spinal dysraphism (CSD), 289, 291, 295
    clinical presentation, 295
    vs. open spinal dysraphism, 292
    prognosis, 295
    with subcutaneous mass
        lipomas with a dural defect, 295, 297
        meningocele, 295
        myelocystoceles, 295
    without subcutaneous mass, 296
        dermal sinus tract, 297, 298, 300
        filar fibrolipoma, 296, 299
        intradural lipoma, 296
        intraspinal lipoma, 296, 299
        midline notochordal integration, disorder of, 298–301
        notochordal formation, disorder of, 301, 302
        persistent terminal ventricle, 297
        tight filum terminale, 297
Coagulopathy, 105
Coalescent mastoiditis, 420
Coccygeal fractures, 311
Coccyx, 283
Colloid cyst, 267, 268
Color coding convention, 601
Communicating hydrocephalus, 257

Complex cysts, 263
Complicated mastoiditis, 420
    acute, 420
Comprehensive stroke CT protocol, 589
Compression and burst fractures, 308
Compressive myelopathy, 348
Computed tomography (CT)
    cervical spine, 287
    CTDI, 3
    CT perfusion, 589, 590, 592, 594
    dual energy, 2, 3
    ICH, 97, 98
    lumbosacral spine, 287
    principles, 1, 2
    radiation dose, 3
    spinal dysraphism, 291
    thoracic spine, 287
Congenital aqueductal stenosis, 256
Congenital brain malformations
    cephaloceles, 64, 65
    cysts, 65
    embryology, 53
    head circumference, 68
    hindbrain malformations, 63
        C1M, 63
        C2M, 63, 64
        C3M, 64
        DWC, 64
        Joubert syndrome, 64
        RES, 64
    HPE
        alobar HPE, 53
        classification, 53, 54
        definition, 53
        etiology, 53
        lobar HPE, 55
        middle interhemispheric variant, 55
        semilobar HPE, 55
        septo-optic dysplasia, 55
        septopreoptic HPE, 55
    MCD
        cobblestone malformation, 60–62
        FCD, 59, 60
        GMH, 57, 58
        HMEG, 59
        non-MCD pathologies, 62
        pachygyria, 58, 59
        PMG, 59–61
    midline commissures, 55–57
    myelination, 68
    phakomatosis
        NF1, 65, 66
        NF2, 66
        SWS, 67, 68
        TSC, 66, 67
        VHL, 66
    three-dimensional isotropic imaging, 68
Congenital hemangioma (RICH/SICH/PICH/NICH), 538, 553
Congenital inclusion cysts, 565
Congenital low-flow vascular malformation, 563
Congenital midline lesions, 426
Congenital rubella syndrome (CRS), 156
Congenital spinal malformation by stage of embryogenesis, 290
Connatal cyst, 272
Connective tissue periosteum lining the orbit, 377

Constructive interference in steady state CISS, 257
Contrast extravasation, 583
Conus medullaris syndrome, 291, 316
Conversion factor (CF), 585
Copper deposition, 238
Cord infarction, 348
Cord injury, 316
Cord trauma, 315
Coronavirus 2019 (COVID 19), 168–170
Corpus callosum (CC), 55
Correlation analysis, 599
Cortical-based lesions, 226
Cortical dementias, 247, 248
Cortical reorganization, 600
Cortical venous/venous sinus thrombosis, 104, 105
Corticobasal degeneration (CBD), 248
CPT codes, see Current Procedural Terminology (CPT) codes
Cranial leaks, 261
Craniocervical junction injuries, 280
Craniopharyngioma, 472
Creutzfeldt-Jakob disease (CJD), 93
Crista falciformis, horizontal bony crest, 446
Cruciate ligaments, 280
Cruciform (cruciate) ligament, 282
Cryptococcus, 174, 175
CT Dose Index (CTDI), 3
Culture of safety, 577
Currarino syndrome, 301
Currarino triad, 295
Current Procedural Terminology (CPT) codes, 585, 599
Cystic metastatic lymph nodes, 571
Cystic neck masses, 561
    BCC, 562, 563
    lymphatic malformation, 563, 564
    TDC formation, 561, 562
Cytomegalovirus (CMV), 149, 150, 167
    polyradiculomyelitis, 354
    polyradiculopathy, 355
Cytomegalovirus polyradiculopathy, 355

D

Dandy-Walker Continuum (DWC), 64
Data processing, 599
Deep brain stimulation (DBS), 148
Deep cervical fascia, 499
Deep layer of deep cervical fascia (DLDCF), 500
Deep learning (DL), 586
Deep neck space abscess, 573
DEFUSE 3 (stroke trial), 590
Degenerative changes and arthritides, intervertebral disc, 319
Degenerative disc disease, 319, 347
Dementia with Lewy bodies (DLB), 247, 249
Demyelination process, 226, 361
    diseases, 605
Dens fractures, 308, 310
Dental abscesses (periapical lucency), 533
Dental infections, 533
Deoxyhemoglobin (dHb), 597
Derived perfusion metrics, 590
Dermal sinus tract (DST), 297, 298, 300
Dermoid/epidermoid, 226, 390, 391, 468, 539–540
    cysts, 265, 266, 347, 565, 566
Diabetic striatopathy, 240
Diastematomyelia (DMM), 293, 299, 301
Diffuse axonal injury (DAI), 129, 131, 601

Diffuse erythema, 584
Diffuse idiopathic skeletal hyperostosis (DISH), 328, 329
Diffusion tensor imaging (DTI), 10, 600
Diffusion-weighted imaging (DWI), 9, 10
Digital Imaging and Communications in Medicine (DICOM) standard, 586
Disc bulge/herniation, 322
Disc degeneration, 320
Disc desiccation, 319
Discitis osteomyelitis, 516
Disseminated necrotizing encephalopathy, 236
Distinctive bony and ligamentous anatomy
    cervical spine, 279, 280
    coccyx, 283
    craniocervical junction, 280
    lumbar spine, 282
    sacrum, 282
    thoracic spine, 282
    variant anatomy, 283
Diving ranula, 568
DNET, see Dysembryoplastic neuroepithelial tumor (DNET)
Dorsal enteric fistula, 298
Dorsal roots, 284
Dose-Length Product (DLP), 3
DTI and tractography, 601, 602
Duct obstruction, 568
Dura Mater, 283
Dural arteriovenous fistulae (dAVF)
    clinical presentation, 116
    epidemiology, 115
    history, 116
    imaging characteristics, 116, 117
    overview, 115
Dural arteriovenous fistulae (DAVF), 104
Dural metastasis, 223
Dural-based lymphoma, 223
Dynamic contrast enhancement (DCE), 594
Dynamic contrast-enhanced (DCE) imaging, 594
Dynamic susceptibility contrast (DSC), 594
Dysembryoplastic neuroepithelial tumor (DNET), 210, 215, 217, 218
Dysplastic cerebellar gangliocytoma, 217
Dysplastic megalencephaly (DMEG), 59

E

Early-stage tumors, 527
Ecchordosis physaliphora, 434
Echo-planar imaging, 9
Ectopic thyroid, 539
Elevated intracranial pressure, 260
Embryogenesis, 290
Embryonal tumors
    ETMR, 221
    medulloblastoma, 219–221
    PENT, 221
Embryonal tumors with multilayered rosettes (ETMR), 221
Empyema, 163
Encephalocele, 421
Endolymphatic sac tumor, 422
Endoscopic third ventriculostomy (ETV), 260
Endovascular embolization using liquid embolic agents, 371
Enlarged cavernous sinuses, 400
Enlarged perivascular spaces, 272
Enostosis (Bone island), 333

Enterovirus, 156, 157
Entry slice phenomenon, 287
Eosinophilic granuloma, 336
Ependymal cyst, 267
Ependymal tumors, 218
    posterior fossa ependymoma, 218
    subependymoma, 219
Ependymoma, 213, 216, 219, 221, 341, 342
Epidermal growth factor receptor (EGFR) gene amplification, 210
Epidermoid cysts, 264, 265, 347, 468, 469, 539–540, 565, 566
Epidural abscess, 359
Epidural hematomas, 314
Epidural or extradural hemorrhage (EDH), 99, 100, 129, 130
Epidural space, 283
Epilepsy/seizures, 592, 601, 605
Epithelioid hemangiomas, 555
Esthesioneuroblastoma, 409–410
Ewing sarcoma, 337
Extension teardrop fractures, 308, 310
Extracranial DTI applications, 601
Extracranial injury, 128, 129
Extradural tumors, 346
Extramedullary hematomas, 314
Extraocular muscles, 377
Extra-ventricular (communicating) hydrocephalus, 257
Extra-ventricular neurocytoma, 216
Extremely rare spinal canal/cord tumors, 347

F
Face of giant panda sign, 238
Facet (zygapophyseal) joints, 279
    degenerative arthrosis, 323
    effusions, 323
    tropism, 279
Facet malalignment, 313
Fahr disease/syndrome, 240, 250
False vocal folds, 381
Fast Imaging Employing Steady-state Acquisition (FIESTA), 257
Fast Spin Echo (FSE), 7
Fibrous dysplasia (FD), 339, 405, 406, 434
Fiducial markers, 148
Filar fibrolipoma, 296, 299
Finite resources, 575
Flexion teardrop fracture, 308, 310
Flip angle, 4
Fluid-attenuated inversion recovery (FLAIR) images, 208
Focal cortical dysplasia (FCD), 59, 60, 217, 218
    type II, 216
Focal discontinuity in right mylohyoid muscle, 531
Focal infections, 605
Foix-Alajouanine syndrome, 370
Foramen magnum lesions, 460
Foramen magnum meningioma, 461, 462
Foramen magnum plexiform neurofibromas, 462
Foramen magnum schwannomas, 462
Foraminal stenosis, 323
Foregut duplication cyst, 565
Fossa of Rosenmuller, 381
Fractional anisotropy (FA), 600
Freidrich's ataxia, 252
Frontal bone osteomyelitis, 400
Frontal dominant FTD (fd-FTD), 248
Frontotemporal dementia (FTD), 247, 248
Frontotemporal lobar degeneration (FTLD), 246

FTD (frontotemporal dementia), 247, 248
Functional anatomy
    sensorimotor system
        fiber tracts, 45, 46
        overview, 43
        PMC, 44
        SMA, 43, 45
        somatosensory cortex, 44
    speech and language system
        fiber tracts, 47, 48
        IFG, 46, 47
        overview, 46
        SMA, 47
        supramarginal gyrus, 47
        ventral stream, 48–50
        vPMC, 47
    vision
        overview, 50
        primary visual cortex, 50, 51
Functional magnetic resonance imaging (fMRI), 597
Fungal infection, 351
Fungus balls, 402

G
Gadolinium-based contrast media (GBCM), 583
    in pregnancy, 583
    in women, breastfeeding, 583
Gangliocytoma, 217
Ganglioglioma, 210, 214, 216, 217, 347
Germ cell tumors (GCT), 222, 472, 473
    germinoma, 225
    teratomas, 225, 226
Germinoma, 222, 223, 225
Giant cell tumor (GCT), 339
Giant perivascular spaces, 272
Giant tumefactive perivascular spaces, 272
Glioblastoma, 217, 225
    IDH-wildtype, 208, 210
Glioependymal cyst., 270
Glioneural and neuronal tumors
    central neurocytoma, 216
    DNET, 215
    dysplastic cerebellar gangliocytoma, 217
    extraventricular neurocytoma, 216
    gangliocytoma, 217
    ganglioglioma, 214
    MVNT, 217, 218
Globe, 377
Globoid cell leukodystrophy, 193, 194
Gradenigo syndrome, 421
Gradient-recalled echo (GRE), 8, 9
Granular cell tumors, 473
Granulomas, 223
Granulomatosis with polyanigiitis (GPA), 405
Granulomatous disease, 390
Graves ophthalmopathy, 388
Gray matter, 285
Gray matter heterotopia (GMH), 57, 58
Gunshot wounds, 131, 132

H
Hand Hygiene, 580
Hangman's fracture, 308, 309
Harassment, 576

Head trauma
    acute effects, 133
    calvarial fractures
        complex calvarial fractures, 128
        diastatic skull fracture, 128
        morphology, and characteristics, 127
        posttraumatic leptomeningeal cyst, 128
        types, 127
    complications, 134, 135
    extracranial injury, 128, 129
    long-term sequelae, 134
    NAT, 132
    overview, 127
    traumatic hemorrhage
        extra axial, 129, 130
        intraparenchymal, 129–132
Hemangioblastoma, 213, 218, 224, 341, 343
Hemangioma, 395, 396
    congenital, 553
    infantile, 553
Hematolymphoid tumors, primary CNS lymphoma, 224, 225
Hematoma, 347
Hemimegalencephaly (HMEG), 59
Hemimyelocele, 293
Hemimyelomeningocele, 293
Hemodynamic response function (HRF), 598
Hemorrhagic metastases, 227
Hemorrhagic transformation (HT), 106, 107
Hepatic encephalopathy, 232, 234
Hepatolenticular degeneration, 250
Herpes simplex virus (HSV), 152, 153
Herpes zoster oticus, 421
High-grade gliomas, 593
High-reliability organization (HRO), 577
HIV, 154
    HIV myelitis, 354
Hives, 584
Holoprosencephaly (HPE)
    alobar HPE, 53
    classification, 53, 54
    definition, 53
    etiology, 53
    lobar HPE, 55
    middle interhemispheric variant, 55
    semilobar HPE, 55
    septo-optic dysplasia, 55
    septopreoptic HPE, 55
Hot cross bun sign, 250
Human factors engineering (HFE), 577
Human Herpesvirus (HHVs), 166, 167
Hummingbird sign, 250
Huntington disease, 250
Hydrocephalus, 256
    extra-ventricular (communicating), 257
    intraventricular (obstructive), 256, 257
    NPH, 257
    overproduction, 257
Hydromyelia, 289
Hyoid bone, 501
Hyperammonemia, 232
Hyperfunctioning parathyroid adenomas, 607
Hypernatremia, 233, 234
Hypertension, 102
Hypervascular tumors, 593
Hypoglossal canal, 448
    anatomy, 448–449
    dural arteriovenous fistula, 458–460
    lesions, 458–460
    synovial cyst, 458
Hypoglossal metastasis/perineural spread, 458
Hypoglossal schwannoma, 458, 459
Hypoglycemic encephalopathy, 232
Hypoperfusion intensity ratio, 590
Hypopharynx, 383
Hypotension, 584
    with bradycardia, 584
    with tachycardia, 584
Hypothalamic hamartoma, 469, 470
Hypoxic ischemic encephalopathy, 232, 233, 605

I
Idiopathic hypertrophic pachymeningitis, 223
Idiopathic intracranial hypertension, 261
Idiopathic orbital inflammation (IOI), 389, 390
Iliolumbar ligaments, 282
Immune Reconstitution Inflammatory Syndrome (IRIS), 355
Immunocompromised conditions, 353
Inborn errors of metabolism, 253
Incidental left buccal space venous vascular malformation, 512
Incisive canal cyst, 567
Inclusion cysts, 347
Infantile hemangiomas, 538, 553
Infection of osseous spine, 349–352, 354–357, 359
Infectious lymphadenopathy, 572, 573
Infectious myelitis, 364, 365
Inferior frontal gyrus (IFG), 46, 47
Inflammatory demyelinating disease, 361
Inflammatory disorder, 476
Inflammatory sinonasal disease, 522
Informed consent, 579
Infrahyoid neck, 501
Infundibulum, 466
Inherited metabolic diseases (IMD), 605
    adrenoleukodystrophy, 187, 188
    Alexander disease, 190, 191
    Canavan disease, 192
    globoid cell leukodystrophy, 193, 194
    metachromatic leukodystrophy, 188, 189
    Pelizaeus-Merzbacher Disease, 194
Institute of Medicine (IOM), 576
    2015 IOM report, 577
Institutional Review Board (IRB), 585
Internal auditory canal anatomy, 446–447
Internal cerebral artery (ICA), 36–38
International Society for the Study of Vascular Anomalies (ISSVA)
    2018 classification, 553
Interpersonal and communication skills, 576
Interspinous ligament, 278
Intervertebral discs, 279, 320
    injuries, 315
Intestinal type adenocarcinoma, 408
Intracranial aneurysms, 479
    epidemiology, 110
    imaging, 112, 113
    morphologies, 110
    risk factors, 110, 111
Intracranial arteriovenous malformations (AVM)
    clinical presentation, 114
    epidemiology, 114
    history, 114
    imaging characteristics, 114–116

Index

Intracranial cysts
    extra-axial lesions
        arachnoid cysts, 263
        cavum velum interpositum cyst, 263
        choroid plexus cyst, 267
        colloid cyst, 267
        dermoid cyst, 265
        ependymal cyst, 267
        epidermoid cyst, 264, 265
        neurenteric cyst, 265
        pineal cyst, 268
        Rathke cleft cyst, 269
    imaging characteristics of, 263
    intra-axial lesions
        connatal cyst, 272
        enlarged perivascular spaces, 272
        neuroglial cyst, 270
        porencephalic cyst, 271, 272
    location, 263
Intracranial hemorrhage (ICH)
    AVM, 103, 104
    basal ganglia hemorrhage, 101, 102
    CAA, 102, 103
    cerebellar hemorrhage, 101
    cerebral aneurysm, 105, 106
    coagulopathy, 105
    computed tomography, 97, 98
    cortical venous/venous sinus thrombosis, 104, 105
    DAVF, 104
    extra-axial hemorrhage
        EDH, 99, 100
        SAH, 100, 101
        SDH, 101
    hemorrhagic transformation, 106, 107
    hypertension, 102
    IVH, 101
    lobar hemorrhage, 101
    MRI, 97, 99, 102
    pontine hemorrhage, 101
    trauma, 102, 103
    tumors, 105
    vasculitis/vasculopathy, 106
Intradural/extramedullary tumor, 343, 346
Intradural lipoma, 296
Intramedullary abscess, 356
Intramedullary vascular malformations, 374
Intraspinal lipoma, 296, 299
Intraventricular cyst, 267
Intraventricular hemorrhage (IVH), 101, 132
Intraventricular (obstructive) hydrocephalus, 256, 257
Intraventricular metastases, 216, 219
Invasive EEG monitoring, 148
Invasive fungal sinusitis, 478
Invasive intracranial pressure monitoring, 147, 148
Inversion recovery, 8
Inverted papilloma, 524
In vivo 1H MR spectroscopy, 603, 605
Iodinated contrast media, 581
    in pregnancy and women, 583
Ischemic stroke
    cardioembolism, 88–92
    classification system, 84
    large artery atherosclerosis, 84–88
    small vessel occlusion, 88
Isotropy, 600

J
Jefferson fracture, 308
JF meningioma, 456
JF meningocele, 456
JF paraganglioma, 454–455
JF schwannoma, 455–456
Joubert syndrome, 64
Jugular bulb dehiscence, 457
Jugular bulb diverticulum, 457
Jugular foramen, 448
    anatomy, 447
    lesions, 453, 454
    metastases, 457–458
Jugular foramen meningioma, 456
Jugular foramen paraganglioma, 454
Jugular foramen schwannoma, 455
Just culture model, 578
Juvenile nasopharyngeal angiofibroma, 407

K
Kaposiform hemangioendothelioma, 553
Kaposi's sarcoma, 555
Keratinizing NPC, 527
Klesdadt cyst, 567
Krabbe disease, 193, 194

L
Labyrinthitis, 421
Lacrimal gland, 379
    mass, 397, 398
Lacrimal gland epithelial neoplasm, 398
Lacunar or small subcortical infarcts, 594
Langerhans cell histiocytosis (LCH), 182, 183, 474, 475
Larmor frequency, 4
Laryngeal edema, 584
Laryngocele, 568
Larynx, 381
Lateral recess, 279
Lateral retropharyngeal nodes of Rouviere, 519
Leigh syndrome, 253
Lemierre syndrome, 513
Lentiform fork sign, 240
Leptomeningeal disease/neuritis, 357, 358
Leptomeningeal metastases, 346
Leptomeningeal tuberculosis, 258
Lhermitte-Duclos disease, 217
Ligament, 278
Ligamentum flavum, 278
Limbus fracture, 311
Limbus vertebra, 283, 313
Lipoma, 226
    with dural defect, 295
Lipomyelocele (LMC), 295, 297
Lipomyelomeningocele, 296
Listeria cord abscess, 358
Lobular capillary hemangioma, 407–408
Localizing disc herniations, 279
Lower cranial nerve schwannomas, 462
Ludwig's angina, 533
Lumbar spine, 275, 282
Lumbosacral spine
    MRI, 287
Lyme neuritis, 357, 358

Lymphadenopathy, 536
Lymphatic malformations, 556, 557, 563, 564
Lymphocytic hypophysitis (LH), 180
Lymphoma, 337, 347, 396, 442, 522
    and lymphoproliferative disorders, 390
Lymphoproliferative disorders, 396, 397

M
Machine learning (ML), 586
Macroadenoma, 469, 470
Magnetic resonance imaging (MRI)
    cervical spine, 287
    DWI, 9, 10
    echo-planar, 9
    exposure, and pregnancy, 581
    flow-related enhancement, 10
    gradients, 4
    GRE, 8, 9
    ICH, 97, 99, 102
    lumbosacral spine, 287
    magnetic field, 4, 5
    magnetic susceptibility, 4
    MRI-induced burns, 581
    net magnetization, 4
    perfusion techniques, 594
    relaxation, 4
    RF energy, 4
    safety, 3, 4, 580
        zoning, 580
    screening, 581
    spinal dysraphism, 291
    spin echo
        FSE, 7
        half-Fourier acquisitions, 7, 8
        inversion recovery, 8
        PDw, 6
        RF excitation, 5
        T1 weighted (T1w), 5, 6
        T2 weighted (T2w), 6
        ultrafast spin echo, 7, 8
    SWI, 9
    thoracic spine, 287
    tissue magnetization, 4
Malformations of cortical development (MCD)
    cobblestone malformation, 60–62
    FCD, 59, 60
    GMH, 57, 58
    HMEG, 59
    non-MCD pathologies, 62
    pachygyria, 58, 59
    PMG, 59–61
Malignant adenopathy, 536–537
Malignant melanotic nerve sheath tumor, 346
Malignant peripheral nerve sheath tumor (MPNST), 345
Malignant vertebral body fractures, 312
Malpractice and risk management, 585, 586
Malpractice insurance, 585
Maple syrup urine disease, 240, 241
Marchiafava-Bignami disease, 242, 243
Marfan syndrome, 295
Masticator space (MS), 508, 509
    and floor of mouth abscess, 573
Mean diffusivity, 601
Medical decision making, minors' rights in, 580
Medical Professionalism, principles, 575

Medical testimony, 576
Medulloblastoma, 211, 218–221
Melanocytic tumors, 347
MELAS, 93
Meningeal tumors, meningioma, 223
Meningioma, 216, 219, 223, 343, 346, 422, 427, 438, 470, 471
Meningocele, 295, 298
Mesenchymal, nonmeningothelial tumors
    hemangioblastoma, 224
        solitary fibrous tumor, 223, 224
Metabolic abnormalities, 231
Metabolic disorders, imaging appearances of, 231
Metachromatic leukodystrophy, 188, 189
Metastasis, 219, 222, 224, 226, 342, 439
Metastatic disease, 210, 339
Metastatic lymphadenopathy, 571, 572
Metformin, 582
Methanol, 238, 239
Methotrexate toxicity, 236
Metronidazole toxicity, 241, 242
Microadenoma, 470
Middle cerebral artery (MCA), 38
Middle layer of deep cervical fascia (MLDCF), 500
Midline notochordal integration, disorder of, 298–301
Miliary tuberculosis, 165, 166
Minor salivary gland neoplasms, 537
Misleading publicizing, 576
Modic types, 320, 321
Modified Thrombolysis in Cerebral Infarction (mTICI)
    grading, 84
Monro-Kelly doctrine, 255
MR Medical Director for MR Safety (MRMD), 580
MR perfusion of biopsy-proven left centrum semiovale anaplastic
    astrocytoma, 596
MR Safety Expert (MRSE), 580
MR Safety Officer (MRSO), 580
MSUD edema, 240
Mucoceles, 404
Mucosal lymphoid tissue, 520
Multinodular and vacuolating neuronal tumor (MVNT), 216–218
Multiple myeloma/plasmacytoma, 337, 442
Multiple sclerosis (MS), 361, 362
    differential diagnosis, 199
    imaging, 197–200
    optic neuritis, 200
    overview, 197
    tumefactive MS, 198, 199
    variants, 199, 200
Multiple systems atrophy (MSA), 250
Myelitis, 355, 356
Myelocele, 293, 294
Myelocystoceles, 295
Myelomeningocele, 293, 294
Myelopathies
    acute, 364
    systemic inflammatory and immune-mediated diseases, 363, 364
Mylohyoid muscle, 510
Myxopapillary ependymoma, 342, 344

N
NAA/Cr ratio, 605
Nasoalveolar cyst, 567
Nasochoanal polyp, 522
Nasolabial cyst, 567
Nasopalatine duct cyst, 567

Index

Nasopharyngeal Cancer AJCC 8th edition TNM Staging, 529
Nasopharyngeal carcinoma (NPC), 503, 527, 528
    staging, 527
Nasopharynx, 381
    anatomy, 519, 520
Natural aging of brain, 246
Neck paragangliomas, 514
Necrotic metastatic lymph nodes, 571
Necrotizing (malignant) external otitis, 419
Necrotizing otitis externa (NOE), 419, 525
Nephrogenic systemic fibrosis (NSF), 583
Nerve sheath tumors, 342
Neural arch, 273
Neural foraminal stenosis, 326
Neural placode, 289, 293
Neurenteric cyst, 265, 266, 298
Neuroanatomy
    arteries
        ACA, 38
        basilar, 39
        COW, 39
        ICA, 36–38
        MCA, 38
        middle meningeal artery, 39
        PCA, 39
        vertebral, 38, 39
    brainstem, 29, 31–33
    central deep brain
        basal ganglia, 24–26
        capsules, 25
        claustrum, 25
        pituitary gland, 25
        thalamus, 25
    cerebellum, 33
    cerebrum, 17
        fissures, lines and central sulcus, 17–19
        frontal lobe, 19–21
        insular lobe, 23
        limbic lobe, 24
        occipital lobe, 23
        parietal lobe, 22, 23
        perirolandic cortex, 24
        perisylvian cortex, 24
        secondary auditory cortex, 24
        temporal lobe, 20–22
    cisterns, 33, 34
    cranial nerves
        abducens nerve (CN VI), 35
        facial nerve (CN VII), 35
        glossopharyngeal nerve (CN IX), 36
        hypoglossal nerve (CN XII), 36
        oculomotor nerve (CN III), 35
        olfactory nerve (CN I), 34
        optic nerve (CN II), 34, 35
        spinal accessory nerve (CN XI), 36
        trigeminal nerve (CN V), 35
        trochlear nerve (CN IV), 35
        vagus nerve (CN X), 36
        vestibulocochlear nerve (CN VIII), 35, 36
    deep venous system, 42
    extra-axial spaces, 17
    extracranial venous system, 42
    meninges
        leptomeninges, 15–17
        pachymeninx, 15–17
    skull
        anterior cranial fossa, 14
        calvarium, 12
        ethmoid bone, 14
        foramen lacerum, 14
        frontal bone, 12, 13
        inferior orbital fissure, 14
        jugular foramen, 14
        middle cranial fossa, 15
        occipital bone, 12
        occiput, 15
        parietal bones, 12
        posterior cranial fossa, 15
        skull base, 12
        sphenoid bone, 14
        sutures, 15
        synchondrosis, 15
        temporal bone, 12–14
        vertex, 14
    superficial venous system, 40–42
    ventricles, 28–30
    white matter
        anterior commissure-posterior commissure line, 28
        centrum semiovale, 28
        commissures, 28
        corona radiata, 28
        long-range fibers, 28
        projection fibers, 25–28
        short-range fibers, 28
Neurocutaenous syndrome with etiology, 391
Neurocysticercosis (NC), 353
    extra parenchymal stages, 171
    overview, 171
    parenchymal stages, 171, 172
    vasculitis, 171
Neurodegeneration with brain iron accumulation (NBIA), 250
Neurodegenerative disorders, 245, 605
    aging, 245, 246
    Alzheimer disease, 246, 247
    basal ganglia (BG), 250–252
    cerebellar degeneration, 252
    characteristic patterns, 245
    clinical and imaging manifestations, 245
    cortical dementias, 247, 248
    Inborn errors of metabolism, 253
    Parkinson disease, 249
    Parkinson-plus syndromes, 249, 250
Neuroenteric cyst, 347
Neuroepithelial cyst, 270
Neurofibroma (NF), 344
Neurofibromatosis type 1 (NF1), 65, 66, 391
Neurofibromatosis type 2 (NF2), 66
Neuroforamen, 273
Neuroglial cyst, 270
Neuromyelitis optica (NMO), 200, 201
Neuromyelitis optica spectrum disorder (NMOSD), 361, 362
Neurosarcoid, 363
Neurovascular uncoupling (NVU), 600
Nexus (National Emergency X-Radiography Utilization Study) criteria, 307
NMOSD optic neuritis, 387
Nonaccidental trauma (NAT), 132
Non-intestinal type adenocarcinomas, 408
Nonionic low-osmolality agents, 581
Nonneoplastic lymphadenopathy, 536
Normal pressure hydrocephalus (NPH), 257, 259
Notochordal formation, disorder of, 301, 302

Notochordal process, 290
Nuchal ligament, 279

O
Obstructive pineal germinoma, 257
Ocular melanoma, 392, 393
Odontogenic abscess, 509
Odontogenic sinusitis, 401
Odontoid/dens variants, 313
Olfactory groove meningiomas, 427
Oligodendroglioma, 209, 217, 347
    IDH-mutant and 1p/19q co-deleted, 209, 210
Omphalocele-extrophy-imperforate anus-spinal defects (OEIS) complex, 295
Open spinal dysraphism (OSD), 289, 291, 293
    vs. closed spinal dysraphism, 292
    diastematomyelia, 293
    imaging, 293
    myelocele, 293, 294
    myelomeningocele, 293, 294
Opioid-induced leukoencephalopathy, 235
Optic gliomas, 473, 474
Optic nerve, 377
    sheath meningioma, 213, 394, 395
Optic neuritis (ON), 213, 387, 388
    in multiple sclerosis, 388
Optic pathway glioma (OPG), 393, 394
    in NF1, 394
Optic pathway pilomyxoid astrocytoma, 213
Oral cavity, 381
    anatomical boundaries, 531, 532
    squamous cell carcinoma, 537
    sublingual space, 531
    submandibular space, 531
Orbital abscess, 386
Orbital cavernous venous malformation, 395, 396
Orbital cellulitis, 400
Orbital imaging
    first line emergency imaging modality, 385
    localized lesions, 385
    pathologic patterns, 385
Orbital infection, 386, 387
Orbital lymphoma, 397
Orbital pseudotumor, 389
Orbits, 377
Oropharynx, 381, 531, 533
Osmotic demyelination, 242
Osmotic myelinolysis, 236, 237
Os odontoideum, 283
Osseous metastases, 476
Ossification of the posterior longitudinal ligament (OPLL), 327, 328
Ossifying fibroma, 406
Osteoblastoma, 333
Osteodural defects, 435
Osteoid osteoma, 333, 334
Osteoma, 405
Osteopetrosis, 340
Osteosarcoma, 334, 411–412
Otomastoiditis, 420–421
Otospongiosis, 421
Oxyhemoglobin (HbO_2), 597

P
Pachygyria, 58, 59
PACS (picture archiving and communications system), 586
Paget disease, 339
Pantothenate kinase-associated neurodegeneration (PKAN), 250
Papillomas, 406
Paraganglioma, 342, 422
Paraganglioma (PGL), 454
Paranasal sinuses, 379, 381
Parapharyngeal/retropharyngeal space abscess, 503, 573
Parasitic cysts, 605
Parasitic infections, 351, 353
Parathyroid adenomas, 517, 608
Parathyroid dysfunction disorder, 239
Parathyroid imaging, 607–609
Parinaud syndrome, 222, 225
Parkinson disease (PD), 249
Parkinson disease dementia (PDD), 249
Parkinson-plus syndromes, 249, 250
Parotid malignancy, 507
Parotid space (PS), 505, 507
Pars articularis, 273
Pars interarticularis defect, 308
Pars nervosa, 447
Pars vascularis, 447
Participation in quality and safety activities, 576
Patient care and procedural skills, 576
Patient confidentiality, 575
Pelizaeus-Merzbacher Disease, 194
Perfusion CT studies, 589
Perfusion fundamentals of stroke imaging, 590
Perineural tumor spread (PNTS), 442
Peripheral nerve sheath tumors, 343, 346
    spectrum, 346
Peritonsillar abscess, 502
Perivertebral space (PVS), 515–517
Persistent hypoglossal artery, 460
Persistent ossiculum terminale, 283
Persistent stapedial artery, 415, 416
Persistent terminal ventricle, 297
PET metabolic brain imaging, 606–607
PET with 18F-fluorodeoxyglucose (FDG), 606
Petrous apex effusion, 437
Petrous apex-specific entities, 436–437
Petrous apicitis, 421, 437
Phakomatosis
    NF1, 65, 66
    NF2, 66
    SWS, 67, 68
    TSC, 66, 67
    VHL, 66
Pharyngobasilar fascia, 501
Pia mater, 284
Pick's disease, 248
Pilocytic astrocytoma, 210, 211, 217, 224, 341
Pineal apoplexy, 268
Pineal cyst, 268
Pineal parenchyal tumors, 225
    of intermediate differentiation, 222
Pineal region meningioma, 222
Pineal tumors, 222
    pineoblastoma, 222
    pineocytoma, 222, 223
Pineoblastoma, 222, 225
Pineocytoma, 222, 223, 225, 473
Pituitary abscess, 478, 479
Pituitary adenoma, 469, 470, 473
Pituitary apoplexy, 479
Pituitary gland, 465
Pituitary infundibulum, 465

Pituitary metastases, 476
Pituitary stalk interruption syndrome, 466
Pituitary vasculature, 465
Placode–lipoma interface, 295
Plagiarism, 576
Plain radiograph
    cervical spine, 286
        lumbosacral spine, 286
        thoracic spine, 286
Planar brain imaging, 605
Planum sphenoidale and olfactory groove meningiomas, 427
Plasmacytoma, 336, 412
Plasmocytoma, 476
Plastic tumors, 218
Pleomorphic adenoma, 507
Pleomorphic xanthoastrocytoma (PXA), 210, 213
Pleomorphic xanthoastryctoma, 216
Plunging ranula, 510
Pneumocephalus, 142, 143
Polymicrogyria (PMG), 59–61
Polyomavirus or John Cunningham Virus (JC Virus), 167, 168
Porencephalic cyst, 271, 272
Postcontrast acute kidney injury (PC-AKI), 582
Posterior cerebral arteries (PCAs), 39, 247
Posterior cervical space, 501
Posterior cord syndrome, 316
Posterior fossa ependymoma, 218
Posterior fossa masses, 226
Posterior fossa pilocytic astrocytoma, 218
Posterior longitudinal ligament, 278
Posterior meningocele, 295
Posterior neurohypophysis, 465
Posterior reversible encephalopathy syndrome (PRES), 93, 205, 234
Posterior ring apophyseal fracture, 311
Posterior skull base anatomy, 445–446
Postoperative brain
    hemispherectomy, 143, 144
    lobectomy, 143
    stereotactic biopsy, 143
    surgical resection, 143
Post-operative cranium
    burr holes, 137, 138
    craniectomy, 139–141
    craniotomy, 137–139
    mastoidectomy, 142
    trans-labyrinthine, 142
    trans-sphenoidal, 142
Postprocessed images, 601
Postseptal cellulitis, 386
Pott's Puffy tumor, 429
    and intracranial abscess, 400
Powers ratio, 282
Practical quality applications in healthcare, 578, 579
Practical safety applications in healthcare, 579
Practice-based Learning and Improvement, 576
Preauthorization for reimbursement of elective outpatient advanced imaging, 585
Pre-ganglionic brachial plexus injury, 317
Premedication, 582
Preseptal cellulitis, 386
Prestyloid PPS, 503
Primary CNS lymphoma, 210, 224, 225
Primary laryngoceles, 568
Primary motor cortex (PMC), 44
Primary neurulation, 290
Primary progressive aphasia (PPA, 248
Prions, 170, 171

Professional competence, commitment, 575
Professional responsibilities, 575
Professionalism, 576
Progressive multifocal leukoencephalopathy, 203
Prominent central canal, 289
Protected Health Information (PHI), 585
Proton density weighting (PDw), 6
Pseudoaneurysm, 134
Pseudotumor cerebrii, 260
Psoriatic arthritis, 330
PSP (progressive supranuclear palsy), 249
Puberty to elderly, 466
Pyogenic meningitis, 357

Q

Quality assurance (QA) process, 576
Quality control (QC), 576
Quality improvement (QI) activities, 576, 578
Quality of care, 575

R

Radial (perpendicular) diffusivity, 601
Radiation necrosis, 226
Radiculomedullary arteries, 369
Radiculomeningeal/radiculoradial arteries, 369
Radiofrequency (RF) energy, 4
Radiofrequency (RF) fields, 581
Radiology information system (RIS), 586
Radionuclide cisternography, 607
Radiotracer activity, 607
Ramsay Hunt syndrome, 421
Ranula, 510, 539, 568, 569
Rathke cleft cyst, 269, 466, 467
Reactive arthritis, 330
Reactive bone marrow/soft tissue signal changes, 323
Recurrent pleomorphic adenoma, 508
Remediation, 575
Renal osteodystrophy, 340
Research integrity, 576
Resting-state fMRI (rs-fMRI), 598, 599
Retinoblastoma (RB), 391, 392
Retrogressive differentiation, 291
Retropharyngeal & danger spaces (RPS/DS), 514, 515
    edema or effusion, 515
Retropharyngeal abscesses, 535
Rheumatoid arthritis (RA), 330
Rhombencephalosynapsis (RES), 64
Right parathyroid adenoma, 608
Ringing artifact, 287
Root cause analysis (RCA), 580
Rs-fMRI, *see* Resting-state fMRI (rs-fMRI)
Rubella, 156

S

Sacral fractures, 311
Sacroiliitis, 329
Sacrum, 282
Salivary mucocele, 568
SAPHO syndrome, 339
Sarcoid, 223
Sarcoidosis, 180–182, 476
Scheuermann disease, 329
Schistosomiasis infections, 352
Schmorl's node, 339

Schwannomas, 406, 421, 439, 473
Scirrhous orbital metastasis, 390
Scottie dog sign, 273, 278
Secondary laryngoceles, 568
Secondary lymphoma, 225
Secondary neurulation, 290, 291
Sedation, 579
SEGA, see Subependymal giant cell astrocytoma (SEGA)
Segmental spinal dysgenesis (SSD), 302
Self-referral, 576
Self-regulation, 575
Sella/Parasella, imaging technique, 466
Seronegative spondyloarthropathies, 329, 330
Sialadenitis, 533–534
Sialocele (salivary mucocele), 568, 570
Sigmoid sinus dehiscence without diverticulum, 457
Sigmoid sinus diverticulum, 457
Simple, fluid-filled cysts, 263
Simple ranula, 568
Simply FTD, 248
Sinonasal adenocarcinoma, 409
Sinonasal cavity
　　aggressive/malignant lesions, 430
　　and ASB, metastatic or systemic lesions, 431
　　malignancies, 429
Sinonasal disease (infection, tumors)
　　acute rhinosinusitis, 399
　　　drainage pathways and anatomic variations, 399
　　　paranasal sinuses, 399
　　　tumor mapping, 405
Sinonasal lymphoma, 410
Sinonasal melanoma, 410–411
Sinonasal mycetoma, 402
Sinonasal polyposis, 404, 522
Sinonasal sarcoidosis, 404
Sinonasal undifferentiated carcinoma, 410
Sinusitis, and associated complications, 429
Skill-rule-knowledge (SRK) model, 577
Skull base anatomy, 423–426
Skull base osteomyelitis, 437, 525–527
Skull base/vertebral involvement, 499
Small vessel occlusion, 88
Social justice–physicians, 575
Soft tissue and ligamentous injury, 315
Solitary fibrous tumor, 223, 224, 343
Solitary SEGA, 213
Specific absorption rate (SAR), 581
SPECT perfusion imaging, 606
Speech and language system
　　fiber tracts, 47, 48
　　IFG, 46, 47
　　overview, 46
　　SMA, 47
　　supramarginal gyrus, 47
　　ventral stream, 48–50
　　vPMC, 47
Spina bifida, 289
Spina bifida occulta, 289
Spinal arthritides, 319
Spinal canal and spinal cord
　　epidural space, 283
　　spinal meninges, 283, 284
　　subarachnoid space, 284
　　subdural space, 284
Spinal canal/cord tumors, 340, 341, 347, 348
Spinal canal stenosis, 326

Spinal cavernous malformation, 374
Spinal columns, 307, 308
Spinal cord
　　abscess, 364
　　blood supply, 285
　　general anatomy, 284, 285
Spinal cord cavernous malformation, 375
Spinal cord glioblastoma, 340
Spinal cord infarction, 364, 366, 374–376
Spinal cord injury, 315
Spinal cord involvement, 363
Spinal dural arteriovenous fistula, 370–371
　　type I, 371
Spinal dysraphism, 292
　　classification and imaging role, 291
　　　CT, 291
　　　MRI, 291
　　　ultrasound, 291
Spinal epidural hematoma, 314
Spinal fractures, types, 308–312
Spinal intradural perimedullary arteriovenous fistula (Type IV), 373
Spinal intramedullary arteriovenous malformation, 371, 372
　　type II, 372, 373
Spinal juvenile (metameric) arteriovenous malformation (Type III), 372, 374
Spinal leaks, 261
Spinal ligamentous injury, 315
Spinal lipoma, 347
Spinal meninges, 283, 284
Spinal stenosis, 327
Spinal synovial cysts, 324, 325
Spinal trauma
　　diagnosis, 307
　　MRI, 307
Spinal vascular pathologies
　　arteriovenous shunting classifications, 370
　　frontal subtraction angiographic projection, 370
　　pial plexus, 369
　　superficial arterial system, 369
Spindle cell oncocytomas, 473
Spine
　　bone-forming tumors, 333–334
　　cartilage-forming tumors, 335–336
　　imaging of, 286
　　　CT, 287
　　　MRI, 287
　　　plain radiograph, 286
　　normal development, 289
　　　conus medullaris, 291
　　　gastrulation, 290
　　　primary neurulation, 290
　　　secondary neurulation, 290, 291
　　　segmentation, 291
Spin echo
　　FSE, 7
　　half-Fourier acquisitions, 7, 8
　　inversion recovery, 8
　　RF excitation, 5
　　T1 weighted (T1w), 5, 6
　　T2 weighted (T2w), 6
　　ultrafast spin echo, 7, 8
Spinocerebellar ataxias, 252
Spinous process, 273
Split cord malformation, 299
Spondylolisthesis, 325
Spondylolysis, 308, 325, 326

Spontaneous intracranial hypotension, 261, 262
Squamous cell carcinoma (SCC), 408, 409, 527
    of neck, 537
Steno-occlusive disease, 594
Stroke
    acute methotrexate toxicity, 93
    arterial vascular territories, 73, 74
    CJD, 93
    computed tomography (CT)
        Alberta Stroke Program Early CT Score (ASPECTS), 77
        ischemic infarct, 77–78
        noncontrast head CT (NCCT) imaging, 76–77
    cortical/white matter diffusion restriction, 93
    definition, 69
    extracranial cerebral arteries, 70–71
    heroin-induced leukoencephalopathy, 93
    herpes simplex encephalitis, 93
    hyperammonemia and hepatic encephalopathy, 93
    hypoglycemia, 93
    hypoxic-ischemic injury, 93
    ICA stenosis grading, 71
    intracranial cerebral arteries, 71–73
    ischemic stroke
        cardioembolism, 88–92
        classification system, 84
        large artery atherosclerosis, 84–88
        small vessel occlusion, 88
    magnetic resonance imaging (MRI)
        advantages, 78
        DWI-negative AIS, 78
        ischemic changes, 78, 80
        temporal evolution, 78, 80
        vascular signs, 80, 82
    MELAS, 93
    metronidazole toxicity, 93
    migraine, 93
    MR vessel wall imaging (VWI), 82, 84
    mTICI grading, 84
    nonketotic hyperglycemia, 94
    non-vascular distribution, 93
    pathophysiology, 69, 70
    perfusion Imaging, 82, 83
    PRES, 93
    seizures, 93
    transient global amnesia, 93
    treatment, 75–76
    tumors, 93
    venous anatomy
        intracranial venous system, 73–75
        vascular territories, 75
    Wernicke's encephalopathy, 94
Sturge Weber syndrome (SWS), 67, 68
Subacute arterial infarction, 226
Subacute combined degeneration (SACD), 236
    of cord, 364, 366
Subacute necrotizing encephalomyelopathy, 253
Subarachnoid hemorrhage (SAH), 100, 101, 129, 130
    aSAH, 109, 110
    tSAH, 109
Subarachnoid space, 284
Subarticular stenosis, 326
Subcortical arteriosclerotic encephalopathy, 204, 205
Subcutaneous mass, closed spinal dysraphism with
    lipomas with a dural defect, 295, 297
    meningocele, 295
    myelocystoceles, 295

Subcutaneous mass, closed spinal dysraphism without, 296
    dermal sinus tract, 297, 298, 300
    filar fibrolipoma, 296, 299
    intradural lipoma, 296
    intraspinal lipoma, 296, 299
    midline notochordal integration, disorder of, 298–301
    notochordal formation, disorder of, 301, 302
    persistent terminal ventricle, 297
    tight filum terminale, 297
Subdural drains and devices, 146
Subdural empyema, 400
Subdural evacuating port system (SEPS™), 146
Subdural hemorrhage (SDH), 101, 129
Subdural hygroma, 129
Subdural space, 284
Subependymal giant cell astrocytoma (SEGA), 213, 216
Subependymal nodules (SEN), 213
Subependymoma, 213, 216, 219, 341
Subglottis, 381
Sublingual gland and duct, 509
Sublingual space (SLS), 509
Submandibular space (SMS), 511
Submucosal spread and deep infiltration, 527
Subperiosteal abscess, 386, 387
Superficial cervical fascia (SCF), 499
Superficial layer of deep cervical fascia (SLDCF), 499
Superficial neck abscess, 535
Superimposition of the transverse process, 273
Superior and inferior articular processes, 273
Superior semicircular canal dehiscence, 419
Supervised ML, 586
Supplementary motor area (SMA), 43, 45, 47
Suppurative adenitis, 536
Suppurative lymphadenopathy, 572
Suppurative right retropharyngeal adenitis/abscess, 515
Suprahyoid CS, 512
Suprahyoid neck spaces, 501
    and parapharyngeal fat, 504
Supraspinous ligament, 278
Supratentorial primitive neuroectodermal tumors (PNETs), 221
Susac syndrome, 201, 202
Susceptibility related BOLD signal, 600
Susceptibility-weighted imaging (SWI), 9
swallow tail, 249
Symmetric sacroiliitis, 329
Synovial cysts, 324
Syringohydromyelia, 289, 293
Syringomyelia, 289
Systems-based practice, 576

T

Taenia solium, 351
Task-based fMRI (tb-fMRI), 598, 599
Tb-fMRI paradigms, 599
Telomerase reverse transcriptase (TERT) promoter mutation, 210
Temporal bone
    anatomy, 413–414
    incomplete partition type 2, 414, 415
    internal auditory canal, 413
    Prussak space, 413
Teratoma, 225
Teratomas, 225, 226
Tethered cord syndrome, 289
Thermal injury, 581
Thoracic spine, 282, 288

MRI, 287
Thoracolumbar fractures
 classification system, 307
Thymopharyngeal duct cyst, 564
T2 hyperintensity, 237
Thyroglossal duct cyst (TDC), 561, 562
Thyroglossal duct remnant, 539
Thyroid eye disease, 388, 389
Thyroid gland abnormalities, 517
Thyroid-associated orbitopathy, 388
Tight filum terminale, 297
Tolosa-Hunt syndrome, 478
Tonsillitis, 535
Tooth abscess, 533
Toothpaste tumors, 218
Tornwaldt cyst, 522, 565
Tortori-Donati and Rossi method, 292
Toxic and metabolic disorders of central nervous system, 231
 basal ganglia involvement
  carbon monoxide (CO) toxicity, 237, 238
  chemotherapy-associated PRES, 239
  diabetic Striatopathy, 240
  methanol, 238, 239
  parathyroid dysfunction disorder, 239
  uremic encephalopathy, 240
  Wilson's disease, 238
 brain metabolism, 231
 brainstem involvement
  osmotic myelinolysis, 236, 237
  Wernicke Encephalopathy, 237
 cerebellum involvement
  Maple Syrup Urine Disease, 240
  metronidazole toxicity, 241
 corpus callosum involvement
  Marchiafava-Bignami disease, 242
 differential diagnosis, predominant brain site involvement, 232
 imaging appearances of metabolic disorders, 231
 predominant cortical involvement
  hepatic encephalopathy, 232
  hypoglycemic encephalopathy, 232
  hypoxic-ischemic encephalopathy, 232
 predominant deep white matter involvement
  hypernatremia, 233, 234
  methotrexate toxicity, 236
  opioid-induced Leukoencephalopathy, 235
  PRES, 234
Toxic leukoencephalopathy, 235, 236
Toxic-metabolic etiologies, 231
Toxoplasmosis, 151, 172, 173
Transcallosal glioblastoma, 210
Transcallosal lesions, 227
Transitional vertebrae, 283
Transverse process, 273
Transverse process fracture, 311
Trauma, 540
Traumatic brain injury, 601
Traumatic fractures, 311
Traumatic sacral fractures, 311
Traumatic SAH (tSAH), 109
T1 relaxation, 4
T2 relaxation, 4
Truncation, 287
Tuberculoma, 164, 165
Tuberculosis, 223, 476
 meningitis, 163, 164
 parenchymal tuberculosis
  calvarial, 166
  cerebritis and abscess, 165
  miliary, 165, 166
  tuberculoma, 164, 165
  tuberculous encephalopathy, 166
Tuberculosis osteomyelitis, 351
Tuberculous abscesses, 605
Tuberculous cervical lymphadenitis, 572
Tuberculous (TB) discitis, 350, 351
Tuberculous encephalopathy, 166
Tuberculous lymphadenitis, 573
Tuberculous meningitis, 163, 164, 357
Tuberous sclerosis complex (TSC), 66, 67
Tumefactive demyelinating lesions, 226
Tumefactive perivascular spaces, 272
Tumefactive variant of demyelinating disease, 210
Tumor mimics, 226
 abscess, 226
 demyelinating process, 226
 radiation necrosis, 226
 subacute arterial infarction, 226
Tumor-induced destruction of eloquent cortex, 600
Tumors with cystic mass and enhancing mural nodule, 226

U
Ultrafast spin echo, 7, 8
Ultrasound, 291
Uncovertebral arthrosis, 323
Uncovertebral joints, 323
Undifferentiated and nonkeratinizing NPC, 527
Undue influence, 576
Unilateral facet dislocation, 313
Unique cervical vertebrae, 279
Universal Protocol, 580
Uremic encephalopathy, 240

V
Vallecular cyst, 567
Varicella, 155
Vascular devices
 aneurysm clips, 146, 147
 arterial stents, 147
 embolization coils, 147
 endosaccular flow disruption devices, 147
 liquid embolic agents, 147
 venous stents, 147
Vascular malformations, 555, 556, 559
Vascular tumors
 benign, 553
 classification, 553
 locally aggressive (borderline), 553
 malignant, 553
 true proliferative neoplasms, 553
Vasculitis/vasculopathy, 106
Vasospasm, 594
Venolymphatic malformations, 408, 559
Venous effect, 600
Venous ischemia, 364
Venous malformations, 538, 556
Venous system, 369

Venous vascular malformation in PPS, 504
Ventral premotor cortex (vPMC), 47
Ventral roots, 284
Ventricular catheters, 144–146
Ventricular vestibular folds, 381
Ventriculitis, 162
Vertebra plana, 308
Vertebral anatomy
  bones, 273
  ligament, 278
Vertebral body compression/burst fractures, 312
Vertebral body endplate degeneration, 320, 322
Vertebral defects, anal atresia, cardiac defects, tracheoesophageal fistula, renal anomalies, limb abnormalities syndrome (VACTERL), 301
Vertebral venous malformation (hemangioma), 337, 338
Very long chain fatty acids (VLCFAs), 187
Vestibular schwannoma, 451, 452
Viral myelitis by location, 357
Visceral space (VS), 502, 517, 518
Von Hippel Lindau disease (vHL), 66, 224

W
Warthin tumor, 570, 571
Wernicke encephalopathy, 237, 238
White matter, 284
Wilson disease, 238, 239, 250
World Health Organization (WHO), 527

If you have any concerns about our products,
you can contact us on
ProductSafety@springernature.com

In case Publisher is established outside the EU,
the EU authorized representative is:
**Springer Nature Customer Service Center GmbH
Europaplatz 3, 69115 Heidelberg, Germany**

Printed by Libri Plureos GmbH
in Hamburg, Germany